Pharmacognosy and Pharmacobiotechnology

PHARMACOGNOSY AND PHARMACOBIOTECHNOLOGY

Ashutosh Kar

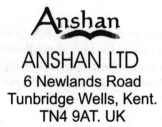

ANSHAN LTD
6 Newlands Road
Tunbridge Wells, Kent.
TN4 9AT. UK

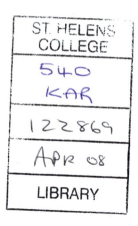
Co-published in the U. K. by

ANSHAN LTD, 6 Newlands Road, Tunbridge Wells, Kent TN4 9AT
In 2008

Tel/Fax: +44(0)1892557767
e-mail: info@anshan.co.uk
Web Site: www.anshan.co.uk

ISBN 9781905740734

British Library Cataloguing in Publication Data

A Catalogue record for this book is available from the British Library

Not for sale in India, Pakistan, Sri Lanka, Bangladesh and Nepal.

Note - every effort has been made to ensure that the drug dosage schedules in this book are accurate and in accord with the standards accepted at the time of publication. However the reader is urged to consult drug manufacturer's printed instructions, particularly regarding the recommended dose, indications and contra-indications for administration and adverse reactions, before administering any of the drugs.

Dedication

*Dedicated with humility and reverence
to the fond memory of beloved
parents who encouraged
and flared passion in
me to learn more
always.*

Thanks

*Wish to thank Leena, Ashish
and Abhijeet for their boundless
patience and eternal understanding
during completion of this text.*

Love

*Aditi, our grand-daughter, who
brought in an eternal saga of
love, and energised
our inspirations to
perform better.*

Preface to the Second Edition

Exclusively based upon the commendable comments and constructive criticisms received from various academic colleagues across the country the author has meticulously presented this entirely revised and duly expanded **Second Edition**. Moreover, the reading text material has been updated thoroughly, various biosynthetic pathways modified adequately, chemical structures and tabular contents enumerated more explicitly. Besides, the critical definitions, important statements, terminologies, names of chemical constituents have been duly highlighted so as to facilitate its readers to comprehend them accurately.

Tremendous achievement and advance in the different segments of highly sophisticated **'Research Techniques'** solely based on PC-modulated modern analytical techniques helped not only to clarify the rather complex chemical structures of unravelled chemical constituents from **Natural Products**, but also established precisely the plethora of **'Biosynthetic Pathways'** dominating the plant kingdom. The present textbook essentially comprises of nearly sixty **'biosynthetic routes'** of predominantly important natural chemical entities, such as: **alkaloids, antibiotics, glycosides, marine-derived drug substances**, and **terpenoids.**

It is, however, pertinent to add here that certain extremely preliminary aspects to the related pharmacognostical characteristic features of **'Natural Plant Products'**, namely: morphological structures, adulterants used in herbal products, habitats, method of cultivation, geographical distribution etc., have been expunged from the text, to which the students invariably obtain sufficient exposure in the early stages of their systematic curriculum follow up.

The **Second Edition** essentially comprises of **five additional chapters**, namely: (*i*) **Nutraceuticals**, (*ii*) **Enzymes and Protein Drugs**, (*iii*) **Biomedicinals from Plant Tissue Cultures**, (*iv*) **Hi-Tech Products from Plant Sources**, and (*v*) **Indian Traditional Herbal Drugs**, i.e., chapter-11 through chapter-15. The judicious and thoughtful inclusion of these five chapters would certainly expose the PG/UG students of the aforesaid disciplines to an exceptionally solid platform in the scientific pursuit of their knowledge.

It is hoped that **Pharmacognosy and Pharmacobiotechnology** will continue to enjoy its popularity amongst the august teaching fraternity, brilliant students, herbal practitioners, pharmacognosists, herbal chemists, phytochemists, biotechnologists, and above all the researchers who would like to make an illustrious career in their respective professional discipline in the New Millennium.

Finally, the author wishes to place on record his deep sense of gratitude to Shri Saumya Gupta M.D., and the entire professionals of New Age International (P) Limited Publishers and Anshan U.K., for their excellent support to bring out this edition.

Ashutosh Kar

Preface to the First Edition

Etymological evidences reveal that **'pharmacognosy'** refers to the knowledge (from the Greek *gnosis*) of drug (*Pharmacon*) substances. **Pharmacognosy** may also be referred to as— *'Study of sources, and chemical and physical properties of drugs'*. In the present context *pharmacognosy,* since Dioscorides's treatise, has spread its tentacles to investigations of a wider section of naturally occurring materials essentially comprised of plants, animals, substances originated from microorganisms and even biotechnology and genetically engineered entities. Jean Bruneton, the famous French pharmacognosist, describes pharmacognosy as— *'Study of starting materials and substances intended for therapeutics, and of biological origin, in other words obtained from plants, animals, or by fermentation from microorganisms'.*

Since the past two centuries the identification, isolation and characterization of naturally occurring substances across the world have been accomplished by the concerted efforts through a central preoccupation of innumerable research chemists and biological scientists. In the recent past, the world has witnessed an overwhelming progress towards intensification of interest more so in natural products from the herbal-based pharmaceutical industries with the epoch-making discoveries of extremely useful new drugs, namely, taxol, artemisinin ginsengoside Rg1 ginkolide A, doxorubicin and the like, from the nature's natural reserves.

The other predominant aspect is **'pharmacobiotechnology'**, an area that encompasses the intricate production of natural-product-drug substances on the basis of the copious volumes of scientific evidences amalgamated with tremendous progress and breakthroughs particularly in the fields of **'biotechnology'** and **'molecular biology'**. It is indeed an altogether newer frontier charged with innovative ideas and approaches in modern-drug-discovery scenario to modify and improve upon the quality of life of human beings on this planet. Therefore, in the present textbook, an earnest attempt has been made to deal with the newest drugs on one hand and the oldest ones on the other in a very systematic and lucid manner with a strong conviction that these all belong to the natural origins.

Interestingly, the last five decades have witnessed a quantum jump in relevant and useful publications especially with regard to books pertaining to medicinal plants, medicinal herbs, biologically active natural products, phytochemistry of medieval plants, alternative medicine; besides herbal and botanical remedies for commoners. It is, however, pertinent to mention about the legitimate exposure *vis-a-vis* the in depth knowledge of the various aspects of medicinal plants well within the broader limits of *pharmacognosy*—a professional discipline widely recognised not only amongst the pharmacy and medical herbalism academic programmes but also of utmost significance to non-medical professionals.

The present text essentially comprised of ten chapters, namely: introduction to phytochemistry, pharmacobiotechnology, carbohydrates, glycosides, terpenoids, phenylpropanoids, alkaloids, bitter principles, antibiotics, and drug molecules of marine organisms. Keeping in view the intensive and remarkable progressive advances accomplished in phytochemical and technological research, it was thought worthwhile to make adequate coverage of pharmacognosy essentially needed not only for the pharmacy degree syllabuses in general but also for the professional class in particular.

The drugs have been classified on a unique broad-based, widely accepted and literature-supported manner.

These are carefully selected and arranged in each chapter, organized on the strong footing of chemical relationships, their biosynthetic approach, thereby elaborating sufficient basic fundamentals for the better advanced knowledge and vivid understanding of the wonderful natural products as **'drugs'**.

Each individual drug belonging to various groups dealt with in the present textbook has been carefully selected based on its academic merit, status and relevance. It has been treated in a most scientific and methodical manner essentially consisting of the following highlights, namely: latest classification, authentic nomenclature, synonym(s), biological source(s), chemical structure, chemical name, molecular formula, isolation or preparation methods, characteristic features, identification test(s), derivatization, characteristics of derivatives, therapeutic uses, and biosynthetic pathways, wherever applicable. A number of important classes of compounds and their relevant features have been summarized in tabular forms selected figures in the text have been incorporated at appropriate places to make the ensuing subject matter more easily understandable to its readers biosynthetic pathways have been explicitly dealt with. The text contains more than one thousand chemical structures of drugs and their intermediates, more than fifty biosynthetic pathways and about fifteen figures.

Bearing in mind the extraordinary pace and appreciable momentum gathered by the global pharmaceutical market, followed by an encouraging number of newer drug companies joining the modern trend of market demands, there exists an enormous scope in phytochemical research and development efforts. The world-wide intensive quest for newer, safer and effective drugs from natural products is not confined only to the terrestrial plants from tropical rain forests and to animals, but also to the plants and microorganisms occurring in deep oceans surrounding this earth.

It is earnestly believed that in the present textbook modern concepts of **pharmacognosy** shall fulfil the necessary requirements of undergraduate and graduate students of various universities in India and other developing nations. Those who intend to continue their research in medicinal plants and desire to establish a strong base in the production of herbal-drug industries may also find this compilation equally informative and useful.

Addis Ababa   **Dr. Ashutosh Kar**

Contents

1 Introduction

- Pharmacognosy—A Brief History
- Importance of Natural Drug Substances
- Natural Drugs Substances: Cultivation and Production
- Phytochemistry
- Further Reading References

1.1 PHARMACOGNOSY—A BRIEF HISTORY.

'Pharmacognosy'—has been coined by the merger of two Greek words **Pharmakon** (drug) and **Gnosis** (knowledge) *i.e.*, the **knowledge of drugs.** The nomenclature—'**Pharmacognosy**' was used first and foremost by C.A. Seydler, a medical student in Halle/Saale, Germany, who emphatically employed **Analetica Pharmacognostica** as the main title of his thesis in the year 1815. Besides, further investigations have revealed that. Schmidt has made use of the terminology *'Pharmacognosis'* in the monograph entitled **Lehrbuch der Materia Medica** (*i.e.*, Lecture Notes on Medical Matter) which dates back to 1811, in Vienna. This compilation exclusively deals with the medicinal plants and their corresponding characteristics.

It is indeed quite interesting to observe that our **ancients** were duly equipped with a vast, in-depth and elaborated knowledge of plethora of drugs from the vegetable origin but unfortunately they possessed a scanty knowledge with regard to the presence of chemically pure compounds in most of them.

Camphor found its enormous use in the treatment and cure of many ailments, for instance: **internally** as—*a stimulant and carminative*; **externally** as—an **antipruritic**, *counterirritant* and *antiseptic* by the ancient Egyptians, Chinese, Indians, Greeks and Romans.

Earlier it was obtained by mere cooling of volatile oils from—ssasafras, rosemery, lavender, sage; while the Ancient Greeks and Romans derived it as a by product in the manufacture of wine. Nowadays, camphor is obtained on a large-scale synthetically (racemic mixture) from the α-pinene present in the terpentine oil (Chapter 5).

African natives used plant extracts in their ritual ceremonies whereby the subject would lose his/her complete body movements but shall remain mentally alert for 2 or 3 days. Later on, the earlier civilization also discovered a number of fermented drinks solely derived from carbohydrate—rich plant substances invariably containing **alcohols** and **vinegar**. With the passage

CAMPHOR
(A Bicyclic Ketone)

of time they also recognised certain plant products exclusively used for poisoning their spears and arrows in killing their preys and enemies as well. Interestingly, they found that some plant extracts have the unique property of keeping the new meat fresh and also to mask its unpleasant taste and flavour.

The human beings belonging to the ancient era in different parts of the globe independently discovered the inherent stimulating characteristics of a wide variety of drinks exclusively prepared from the vegetative source as stated below in Table 1.1.

Table 1.1 Stimulating Characteristics from Vegetative Sources

S. No.	Common Name	Biological origin (Family)	Part used	Active Ingredient	Distribution
1.	Guarana	*Paullinia cupana* **Kunth** (*Sapindaceae*)	Seed	Caffeine (2.5-5.0%) Tannin (Catheochutannic acid) 25%	Brazil, Uruguay
2.	Paraguay Tea or Mate	*Ilex paraguariensis* St. Hill. (*Aquifoliaceae*)	Leave	Caffeine (upto 2%)	South America
3.	Coffee Bean or Coffee Seed	*Coffee arabica* **Linne'** or *C. liberica* (*Rubiaceae*)	Seed	Caffeine (1-2%) Trigonelline (0.25%); Tannin (3-5%) Glucose & Dextrin (15%); Fatty Oil (trioleoglycerol) and palmitoglycerol (10-13%) Protein (13%)	Ethiopia, Indonasia, Sri Lanka, Brazil
4.	Coca Kola or Kolanuts	*Coca nitida* (Ventenat) Schott et Endlicher (*Sterculiaceae*)	Seed	Caffeine anhydrous (≤ 1%)	Sierra Leone, Congo, Nigeria Sri Lanka, Ghana Brazil, Indonesia Jamaica
5.	Tea or Thea	*Camellia sinensis* **Linne's O. Kuntze** (*Theaceae*)	Leave or Leaf bud	Caffeine (1-4%) Gallotannic acid (15%) Volatile oil (Yellow) 0.75%	China, Japan, India, Indonesia Sri Lanka
6.	Cacao Beans or Cacaoseeds	*Theobrome cacao* **Linne'** (*Sterculiaceae*)	Seed	Fixed Oil (35-50%) Starch (15%) Protein (15%) Theobromine (1-5%); Caffeine (0.07-0.36%)	Ecuador, Columbia Malasia, Curacao, Mexico, Trinidad Brazil, Nigeria Camerrons, Ghana Philippines, Sri Lanka

Figure 1 shows the basic nucleus of '**Xanthine**' and '**Purine**'; besides the three well-known members of the Xanthine family *viz.*, **Caffeine**, **Theophylline** and **Theobromine**.

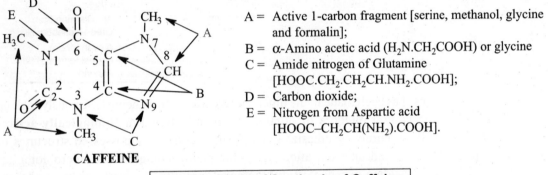

Xanthine · Purine

Caffeine:
$R_1=R_2=R_3=CH_3$;

Theophylline:
$R_1=R_2=CH_3$; $R_3=H$;

Theobromine:
$R_2=R_3=CH_3$; $R_1=H$;

Fig. 1.1   The Xanthine and Purine Structures

Figure 1.2, illustrates the mode of synthesis of caffiene essentially from the same precursors present in *Caffea arabica* as the *three* purine alkaloids (see Fig 1.1) found in order biological systems which have been studied so far at length, either from a compound which may afford an active 1-carbon fragment (*e.g.*, serine, methanol, glycine and formalin) or from formic acid.

A = Active 1-carbon fragment [serine, methanol, glycine and formalin];
B = α-Amino acetic acid ($H_2N.CH_2COOH$) or glycine
C = Amide nitrogen of Glutamine [$HOOC.CH_2.CH_2CH.NH_2.COOH$];
D = Carbon dioxide;
E = Nitrogen from Aspartic acid [$HOOC–CH_2CH(NH_2).COOH$].

CAFFEINE

Fig. 1.2   Mode of Synthesis of Caffeine

• Methionine along with the said four compounds act as active precursors of the three 'Methyl Groups' at N_1, N_3 and N_7 positions respectively.
• Glycine is responsible for the contribution of C-4, C-5 and C-7,
• Carbon dioxide contributes C-6,
• N-1 is provided from aspartate, and
• N-3 and N-9 are derived from the amide nitrogen of glutamate.

Such elaborated and intensive studies of chemical constituents present in *'Natural Products'* could only be feasible with the advent of various advancement in the field of **'Phytochemistry'**.

However, it is pertinent to mention here that the scientific reasonings for the various age-old established characteristic medicinal properties have been adequately ascertained and determined in the past two centuries. A critical survey of literatures would reveal that a few chemical entities were not only identified but also known to the therapeutic armamentarium between the said era. A few typical examples are enumerated below in a chronological order, as stated in Table 1.2.

Table 1.2   Examples of Plant Constituents in Use from 1627 to 1830

S. No.	Period	Researcher	Chemical Entity	Remarks
1.	1627-1691	R. Boyle	Alkaloid(s) (probably)	Present in Opium
2.	1645-1715	N. Lemery (French Apothecary)	Alcohol	As a solvent in extraction processes
3.	1709-1780	A.S. Marggraf (German Apothecary)	Sugar	isolated from many plant sources including Sugar-Beet
4.	1742-1786	K.W. Scheele	Organic acids oxalic, malic, citric, gallic, tartaric and prussic (HCN)	isolated from natural sources.
5.	1805	Serturner (German Chemist)	Meconic acid	Present in Opium
6.	1811	Gomeriz (Portugese Chemist)	Cinchonine	Isolated from Cinchona Barks
7.	1817	Serturner (Geman Chemist)	Morphine	An alkaloid present in Opium
8.	1817	Pelletier and Caventou (French Chemist)	Strychnine	An alkaloid from Strychnos Nux Vomica
9.	1819	- do -	Brucine	- do -
10.	1820	Meissner	Veratramine	An alkamine from Green Hellebore.
11.	1830	–	Amygdalin	A cyanophore glycoside from Bitter Almond.

Considerable progress has been made in the nineteenth century when chemists seriously took up the challenge of synthesizing a plethora of organic compounds based or **'biologically-active-prototypes'**. Some of these purely 'synthesized compounds' essentially possessed structures of ever increasing complexity; and later on, after systematic pharmacological and microbiological evaluations proved to be yielding excellent useful therapeutic results. Evidently, as most of these **'tailor-made'** compounds having marked and pronounced therapeutic indices were found to be existing beyond the realm of **'pharmacognosy'** or more specifically **'phytochemistry'**—an altogether new discipline under the banner of **'medicinal chemistry'** came into existence. However, this particular discipline almost remained dormant since the era of Parcelsus. But now, the **'medicinal chemistry'** has acclaimed deserving wide recognition across the globe due to its own legitimate merit and advantages.

In short, *three* major basic disciplines became largely prevalent with regard to the development of drugs, namely:

- **Pharmacognosy:** embracing relevant information(s) with regard to medicines exclusively derived from natural sources, for instance: plants, animals and microorganisms,
- **Medicinal Chemistry:** covering entirely the specific knowledge not only confined to the science of 'synthetic drugs' but also the basic fundamentals of **'drug-design'**, and
- **Pharmacology:** dealing particularly the actions of **'drugs'** and their respective effects on the cardiovascular system and the CNS-activities.

Over the years, with the tremendous growth of scientific knowledge and valuable informations the three aforesaid disciplines have fully-emerged as **'complete sciences'** within their own spheres.

Though copious volumes of ancient literatures in Chinese, Egyptian, Greek, Unani and Indian (Ayurvedic) systems of herbal medicines were found to contain factual and invariably exaggerated claims of their therapeutic efficacies, yet when they are evaluated intensively on a scientific basis with the advent of latest analytical techniques, such as: FT-IR, NMR, MS, GLS, HPLC, HPTLC, X-Ray Diffraction, ORD, CD and UV-spectroscopy—it has adequately and promptly provided an elaborated structure of various **complex chemical constituents**. A few select typical examples of known compounds are given in Table 1.3.

1.2 IMPORTANCE OF NATURAL DRUG SUBSTANCES

In general, natural drug substances offer *four* vital and appreciable roles in the modern system of medicine thereby adequately justifying their legitimate presence in the prevailing therapeutic arsenal, namely:

   (*i*) Serve as extremely useful natural drugs.
  (*ii*) Provide basic compounds affording less toxic and more effective drug molecules.
 (*iii*) Exploration of biologically active prototypes towards newer and better synthetic drugs.
  (*iv*) Modification of inactive natural products by suitable biological/chemical means into potent drugs.

The aforesaid aspects shall be briefly dealt with in the sections that follows:

1.2.1 Serve as Extremely Useful Natural Drugs

On a recent survey conducted by the World Health Organisation (WHO) globally, around 20,000 medicinal plants are being used profusely either in **pharmceutical industry** or in **folk medicines.** Interestingly, about 1.4% do possess well-established, widely—proven and broadly accepted un-equivocally active constituents.

De Souza *et al.*[*] in 1982 opined on a serious note that—*"the usual success rate of discovering new drugs from natural sources is solely based not only on the conception but also on the implementation of ingenious comprehensive strategies which invariably explore and exploit the untrapped potential of the natural sources"*. In fact, there are *four* ways by which the above objectives may be accomplished reasonably and legitimately, such as:

   (*a*) Isolation of novel genotypes from marine and terrestrial ecosystems,
   (*b*) Genetic engineering: creating novel and altered genotypes,
   (*c*) Biochemical manipulation of selected pathways, and
   (*d*) Supersensitive and specific selection techniques and evaluation for varied bioactivities.

---

* De Souza, NJ *et al.*, *Annu. Rep. Med. Chem*, **17**, 301, 1982.

Table 1.3   Examples of Chemical Constituents Present in Herbal Plants

S.No.	Common name(s)	Biological origin (Family)	Chemical constituents	Distribution	Uses
1.	*Artemisinin or Qinghaosu*	Artemisia annuna Linne, Linne, (Asteraceae)	ARTEMISININ	China	Treatment of cerebral malaria; Active against both chloroquine sensitive and chloroquine-resistant strains of *Plasmodium falciparum*
2.	*Doxorubicin or Adriamycin and Daunorubicin or Cerubidine*	*Streptomyces coeruleorubidus Streptomyces peucetius var caesius*	**DOXORUBICIN : R = OH;** **DAUNORUBICIN : R = H;**	—	Treatment of breast cancer, various types of carcinomas, acute Leukemia; Daunorubicin Treats acute Lymphocytic Leukmias.
3.	*Ginkgo*	*Ginkgo biloba* Linne *(Ginkgoaceae)*	**GINKGOLIDE–A**	Eastern Asia Southeastern United States.	Ginkgolides A, B, C, and M inhibit platelet-activating factor (PAF); reduces capillary fragility and blood loss from the capillary vessels that may ultimately check ischemic brain damage.

(Contd.)

4.	*Ginseng*	*Panax quinaquefolius* Linne and *Panax ginseng C.A. Mey (Araliaceae)*	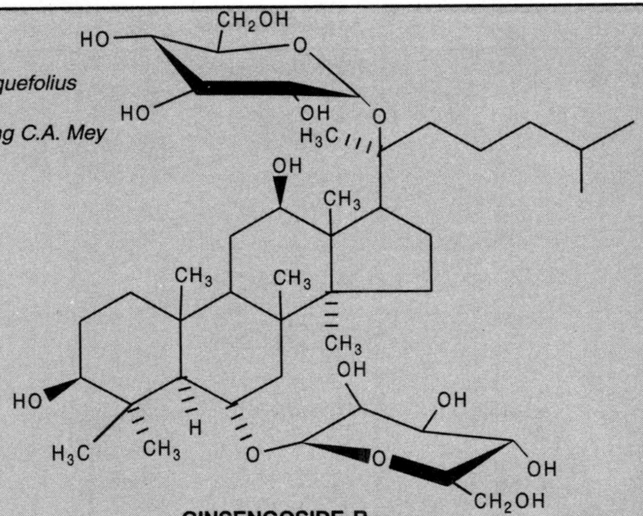 *American ginseng* (p.q.) in Eastern United States and Canada; *Asian gingseng* (P.g.) In Eastern Asia presently cultivated profusely in Korea, Japan and the former Soviet Union.	Known to possess tonic stimulant diuretic and carminative properties; reported to act significantly on metabolism, CNS 7 endocrines; Exhibits adaptogenic (antistress) activity.

GINSENGOSIDE R$_{g1}$

5.	*Gum opium or opium or Poppy Seed or Maw Seed*	*Papaver somniferum* Linne or *Papaver album* Deendolle *(Papaveraceae)*	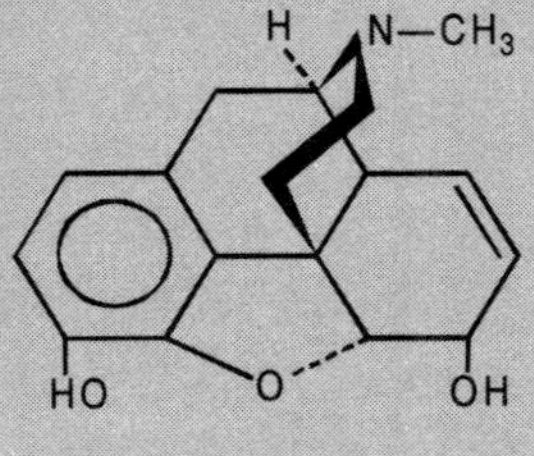 Turkish Anatolian plain extends to Northern border of Laos; India; China, Democratic peoples republic of Korea.	Strongly narcotic and hypnotic; Centrally acting analgesic.

MORPHINE

6.	*Rauwolfia sepentina*	*Rauwolfia serpentina* Linne Bentham *(Apocynaceae)*	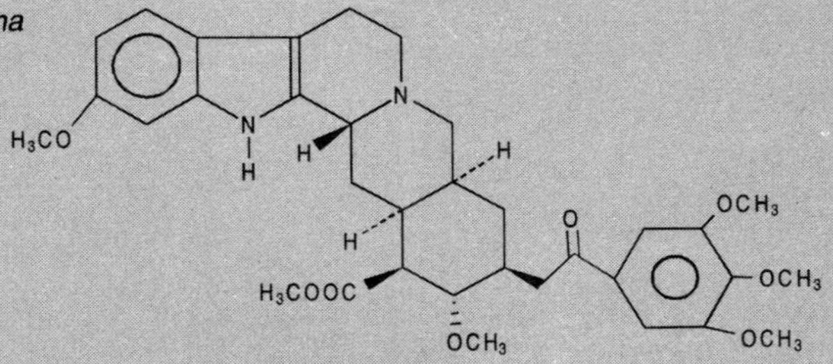 India, Myanmar, Sri Lanka; Vietnam; Malaysia; Indonesia; The Phillipines.	Treatment control of hypertension; As an antipsychotic agent.

RESERPINE

(Contd.)

7.	*Taxol or Pacitaxel or Pacific Yew*	*Taxol brevifolia* Nutt *(Taxaceae)*	**TAXOL**	Northwestern United States.	Treatment of metastatic carcinoma of the ovary after failure of first line or followup chemotherapy; Treatment of breast cancer after failure of combination chemotherapy for metastatic disease.
8.	*Curare or South American Arrow Poison*	*Strychnos castenaei* Weddell; *S. toxifera* Bentham; *S. crevauxii* G. Planchon *(Logniaceae); and Chondendron tomentosum* Ruiz et Pavon *(Menispermaceae)*	**TUBOCURARINE CHLORIDE**	Orinpoco basin; Upper Amazon regions; Eastern Ecuadorian plateau.	As a disgnostic aid in myasthenia gravis; As an adjunct to electroshock treatment in neuropsychiatry to control convulsion caused due to tetanus and strychnine poisoning.
9.	*Yohimbine*	*Pausinystalia yohimbe* (K. Schum) Pierre *(Rubiaceae)*	**YOHIMBINE**	West Africa.	Treatment of impotance in patients with vascular or diabetic problems.

(Contd.)

| 10. | **Cantharanthus or Vinca** | *Cantharanthus roseus* G. Don *(Apocynaceae)* Formerly designated as *Vinca rosea* Linne' It has a close resemblance to *Vinca minor* Linne', commonly known as Periwinkle. | | Madagascar, India, South America, Austria, South Africa, Europe, The West Indies, Southern United States. | Treatment of lymphocytic lymphoma, advanced testicular carcinoma, histocytic lymphoma, myosis fungoids, Hodgkin's disease, Kaposi's sarcoma choriocarcinoma and breast cancer Unresponsive to other diagnosis. |

A few typical examples of drugs derived from natural sources and their respective uses are given in Table 1.4.

Table 1.4   Examples of Drugs from Natural Products

S.No.	Name	Biological Origin(s)	Isolation	Synthesis	Uses
1.	Atropine	*Atropa beladona* (Linne)	1831	1883	Spastic colitis, gastro enteritis, peptic ulcer; antispasmodic.
2.	Ergotamine	*Claviceps purpurea* (Fries)	1918	1961	To prevent or abort vascular headaches, (Migraine and cluster headache)
3.	Morphine	*Papaver somniferum* (Linne)	1805	1956	As narcotic analgesics strongly hypnotic.
4.	Prostaglandins (PGE$_1$ & PGE$_2$)	C-20 Lipid Metabolites *in vitro* from essential unsaturated fatty acids of food (Linoleic acid)	1962	1969	PGE$_1$-certain congenital heart defects as a gastric antisecretory and gastroprotective agent; PGE$_2$-for termination of second trimester pregnancies.
5.	Physostigmine	*Physostigma venesonum* (Balfour)	1864	1935	In ophthalmology to treat glaucoma; decreases intraocular pressure.
6.	Quinine	*Cinchona succirubra* (Pavon et Kloyzsch)	1820	1944	For treatment of malarial fever.
7.	Scopolamine (Hyscyamine)	*Atropa belladona, Datura stramonium, Hyoscyamus nigher;* (or Egyptian henbane)	1881	1956	As CNS-depressant; in motion sickness; in preanaesthetic sedation; in obstetric amnesia along with other analgesic to calm delirium.

1.2.2   Provide Basic Compounds Affording Less Toxic and More Effective Drug Molecules

The numerous examples of naturally occurring plant products that serve as prototypes for other medicinally potent compounds either having closely related structures prepared exclusively by semisynthetic routes or possessing relatively simpler (less complex) purely synthetic structural analogues have been adequately described in various literatures. A few interesting examples of such compounds shall be described in this context as under:

1.2.3   Exploration of Biological–Active–Prototypes towards Newer and Better Synthetic Drugs

A plethora of better synthetic drug models gained considerable recognition in the therapeutic arsenal that were solely derived on the **biologically-active-prototypes.** It is, however, pertinent to mention here that these synthetic models not only possessed similar and better therapeutic index but also

S. No.	Natural	Semisynthetic	Synthetic
1.	**Morphine** (Narcotic Analgesic)	**Hydromorphone**	**Methadone**

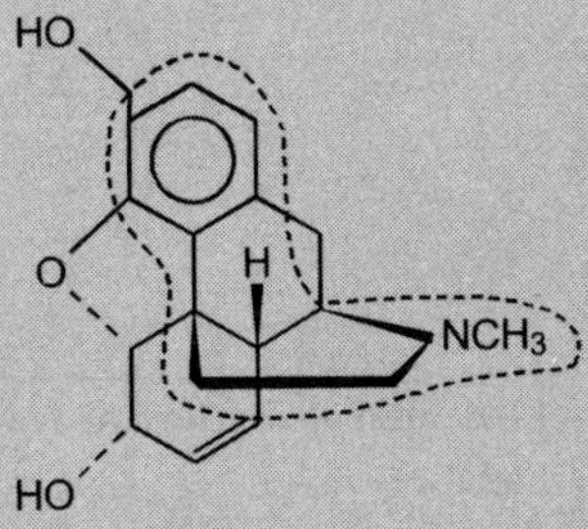

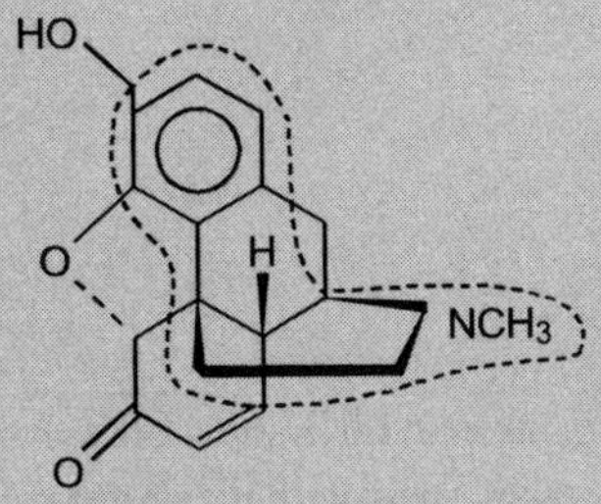

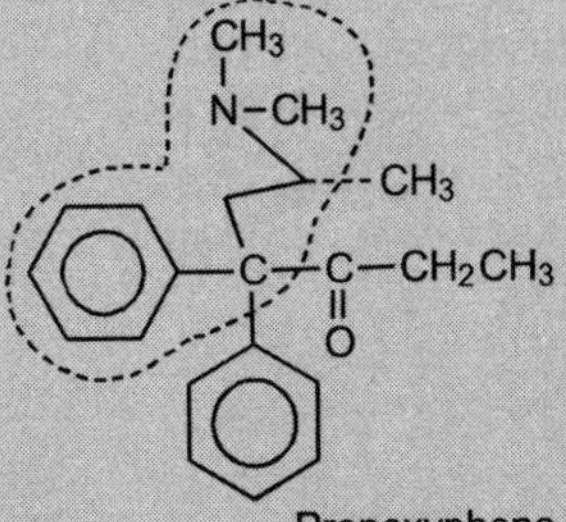

Propoxyphene

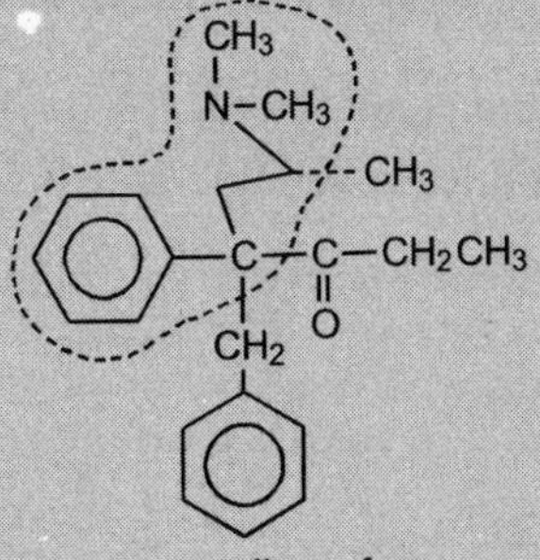

Ibuprofen

| 2. | **Salicin and salicyclic acid** (Analgesic) 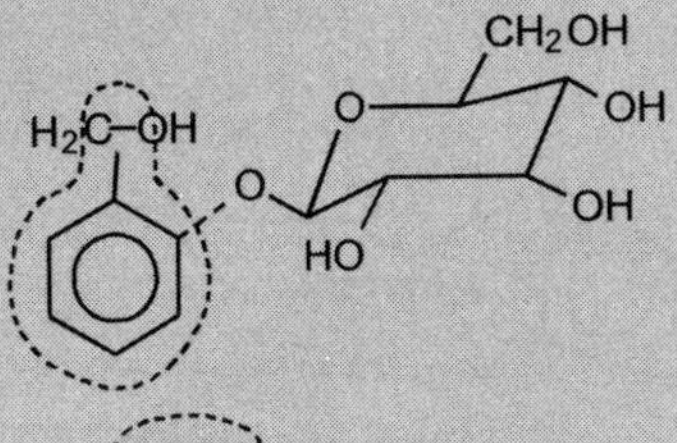 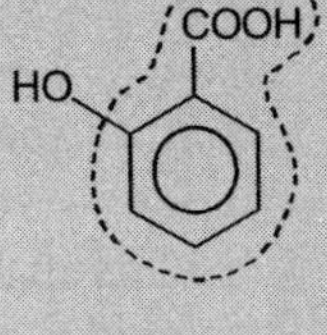 | **Acetyl salicylic acid (Asprin)** 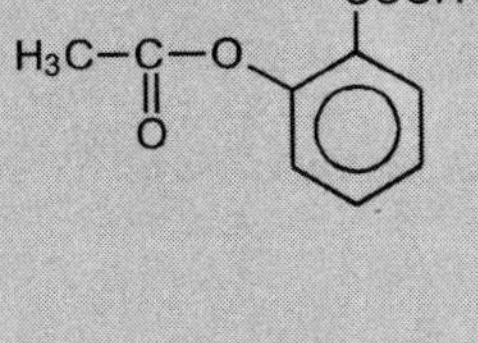 | **Ibuprofen** 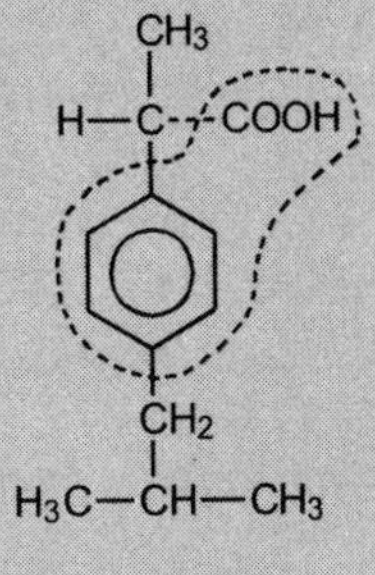 |

| 3. | **Ephedrine** (Adrenomimetic) 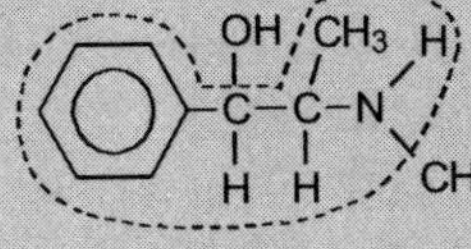 | **Phenylpropanolamine** 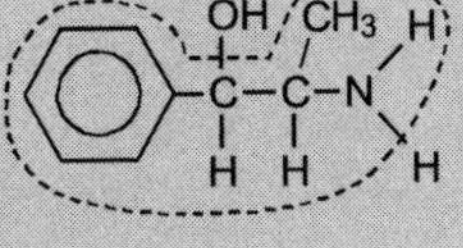 | **Tetrahydrozoline** 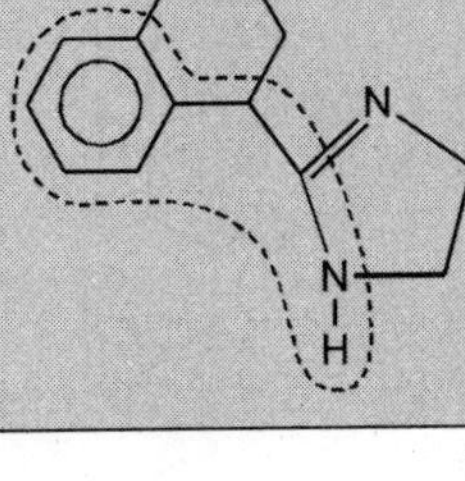 |

(Contd.)

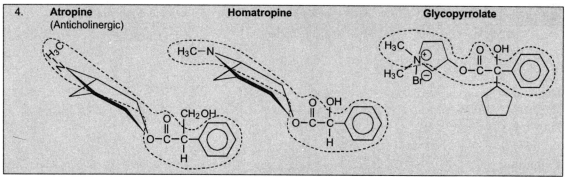

4. **Atropine** (Anticholinergic) **Homatropine** **Glycopyrrolate**

Note: The dotted areas in the above chemical structures show the presence of essential characteristic features in the natural (biological-active-prototype), semisynthetic and synthetic models.

exhibited fewer side effects than their corresponding naturally occurring constituents. A few typical examples are enumerated below:

(*a*) *Procaine from Cocaine—As Local Anaesthetic:*

Procaine Cocaine

(*b*) *trans-Diethylstillbestrol from—Estradiol—as Estrogenic Hormone:*

trans-Diethylstilibersterol α-Estradiol

(*c*) *Chloroquine from Quinine—as Antimalarial:*

Chloroquine

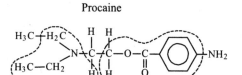

Quinine

1.2.4   **Modificaton of Inactive Natural Products by Suitable Biological/ Chemical Means into Potent Drugs**

This particular role of natural products is not only distinctly different from the rest, as discussed in section 1.2.1 through section 1.2.3, but also has its prime importance by virtue of the fact that certain constituents present in them do not exhibit any significant biological activity or chemical means surprisingly give rise to quite effective and potent drugs that are not easily obtainable by other known methods.

The following examples will expatiate the above facts squarely:

Examples:

1.   Vitamin* A from—carotene (isolation from carrots *i.e.*, *Dacus carota*)

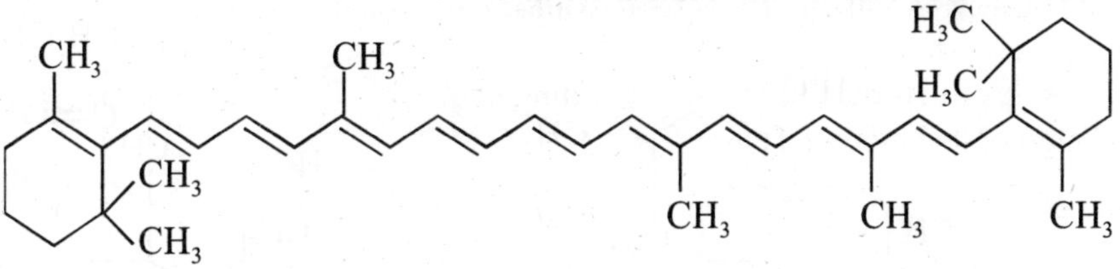

β-Carotene

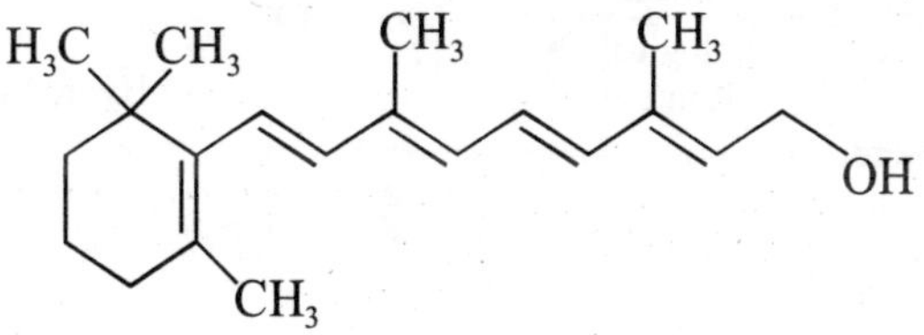

Vitamin A (Retinol)

2.   Taxol by conversation of 10–**Dasacetylbaccatin III** (Isolated from the needles of *Taxus baccata*):

10–Dasacetylbaccatin III $\xrightarrow{\text{Synthetic Route}}$ Taxol (see Table 1.3)
Taxol is an antineoplastic agent invariably used in breast cancer.

3.   Progesterone and Pregnenolone by conversion of Diosgenin (aglycone of Saponin Dioscin from *Dioscorea tokoro* Makino):

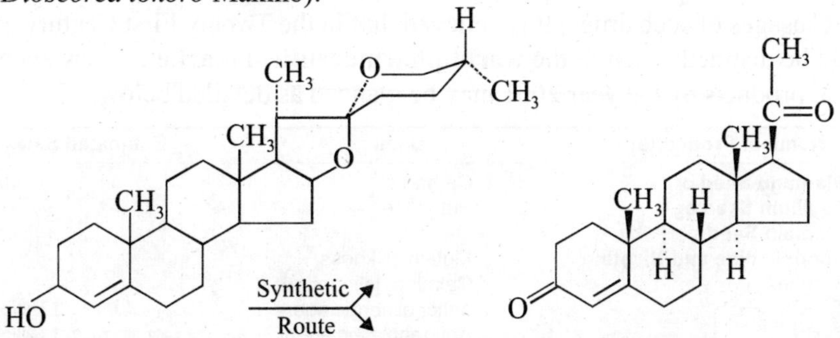

Diosgenin $\xrightarrow[\text{Route}]{\text{Synthetic}}$ Progesterone

* 2 Moles of RETINOL are produced from 1 mole of *d*-β-**Carotene** which acts as a precursor of the former.

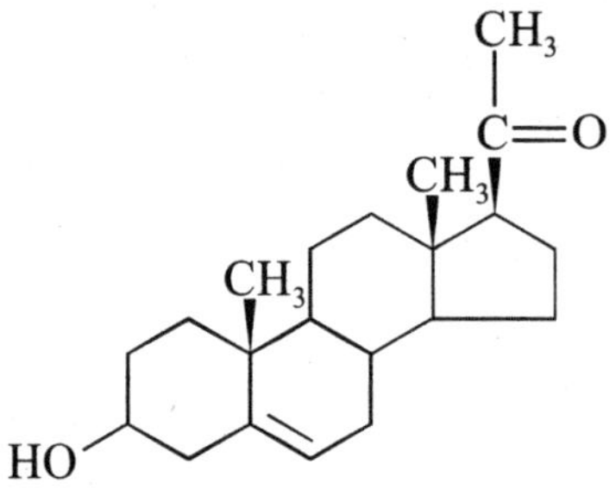

Pregnenolone

4. Hydrocortisone and Corticosterone from Stigmasteol (occurs abundantly as Phytosterol Mixture from Soyabeans and Calabar Beans)

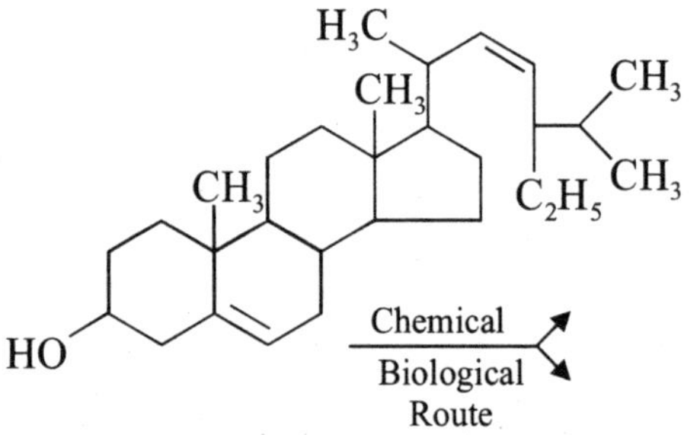

Stigmasterol

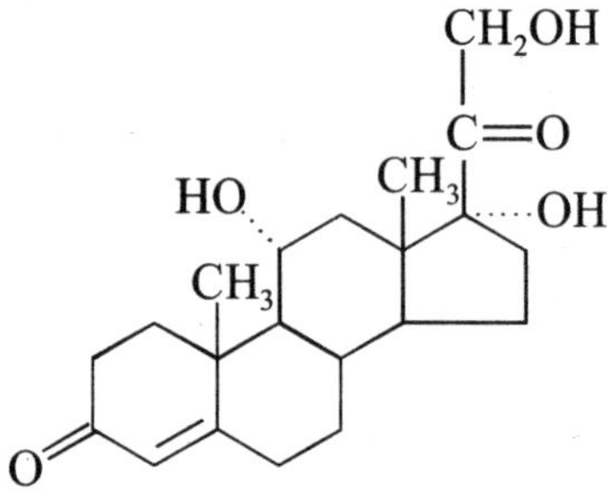

Chemical
Biological
Route

Hydrocortisone

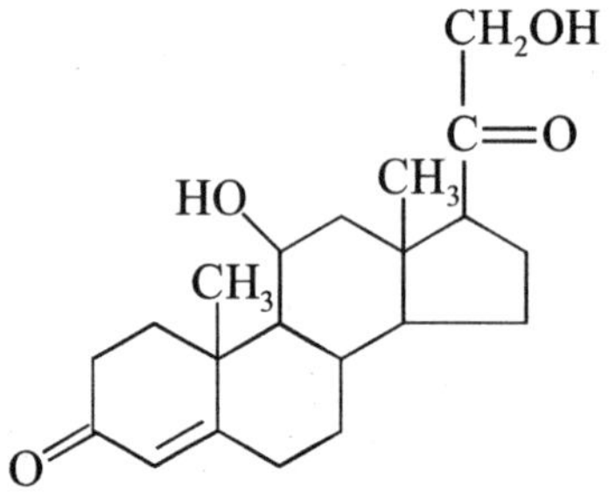

Corticosterone

In addition to the Third World nations, the technologically advanced countries like the United States have experienced a phenomenal change towards the acceptance of herbal medicines over the expanded OTC usages of such drugs. It is believed that in the Twenty First Century a quantum leap forward would be distinctly seen in the **world pharmaceutical market.** A few such projection of pharmaceutical products by the year 2001 may be glanced as detailed below:

S. No.	Name of Product(s)	Uses	Estimated Sales (USD)*/Year
1.	**Plantago Seed or Psyllium Seed or Plantain Seed**	Cathartic, Purgative	300 Million
2.	**Scopolamine and Nicotine Patches**	Motion sickness, Calming delirium, As anticholinergic agent	1 Billion
3.	**Taxol**	Antineoplastic agent	1 Billion
4.	**Vinblastine and Vincristine**	-do-	100 Billion

* **USD:** United State Dollar.

It may appear to be quite realistic and amazing that in the near future about **50% of the healthy-market-share** would be captured legitimately by **drugs belonging to the natural origin.**

It is not out of place to assert that on one hand science is advancing in a tremendous logarithmic progression towards gene-synthesis, rocket-fuels, super computers, electronic cash-transaction across the globe, fax machine, paperless offices, modern analytical computer-aided instruments, auto analysers for routine industrial analysis for on-going chemical and biological processes and final products metioulously designed and skillfully formulated life-saving drugs; while on the other hand the confidence of the people being restored at a steady pace towards the ancient herbal drugs right from the treatment of constipation to management and control of malignancies in human beings. Of course, the so-called **'Crude-Drugs'** are presently available in well refined and latest state-of-the-art packings as **over the counter (OTC) drugs** through chemists and druggists and super markets across the world. Perhaps that day is not too far when a common person will be tempted to grow medicinal plant in the kitchen garden rather than growing spring onions, lettuce, cucumber and french beans for their daily needs. It is a pity that the inhabitants of the modern society is virtually over-loaded by the usage of tonnes of chemicals used in the form of medicines for the cure of various ailments.

1.3 NATURAL DRUGS SUBSTANCES: CULTIVATION AND PRODUCTION

It is pertinent to mention here that the actual production of **'natural drug substances'** invariably adopts a number of different routes and methods based on the fact that their diversified origin as present in **plant, microbial and animal kingdom.** These *three* sources shall be discussed individually in the sections that follow:

1.3.1 Plant Products

Many countries in the world have a 'God-gifted' natural reserve of medicinal plants. Because of their judicious and cautious administration by the expertise of indigenous-systems of medicine people could survive and thus explore and conquer the world as per the historical evidence. In the past, lack of knowledge, non-availability of adequate storage facilities and proper scientific means and methods of cultivation and collection a good number of useful medicinal plants almost reached a point of not only depletion but also extinction. With the advent of scientific knowledge abundantly available these medicinal plants are now grown in an organised fashion whereby proper identification, right cultivation, due harvesting in the correct time of the year to yield maximum desired chemical constituents, and adequate prevention from spoilage and infestation due to improper storage. Nowadays, plant-extracts are available commercially across the globe so that these may be incorporated duly in several tried and tested herbal preparations. Various advanced **'analytical methods'** help a long-way in establishing the true picture of their quality, for instance: percentage of **Eugenol** present in *Clove oil* determines its quality; percentage of **Cineol** in *Eucalyptus oil* shows its purity; percentage of **Total Alkaloids** in *Datura stramonium* depicts its medicinal value.

A few countries in the world are noted for their supply of certain specialized plant extracts, namely:

India   :   Opium extracts;

China   :   Extract of *Artemisia annuna*;

United States   :   *Ginkgbo biloba* extracts (GBE)

Korea, Japan   :   *Panax ginseng* extracts;

Madagascar   :   *Catharnthus roseus* extracts;

Eastern Europe   :   Ergot produced by mechanical inoculation of rye plants with spores of a selected fungus.

1.3.2   Cell-Culture Techniques

It essentially involves the production of the **'desired secondary constituents'** that caters for a viable alternative means of **drug-plant-cultivation.** Extensive studies have revealed that under the influence of **'stress-conditions'**, for instance: reacting with a suitable pathogen-may ultimately help in simulating the yield of some specific highly desired constituents in plant-cell suspension cultures. However, the actual slow growth of the *cell-biomass* possess a serious obstacle in the wide acceptance of this innovated technique. Perhaps the day is not too far when the **plant genes** which are responsible for coding enzymes catalyzing the desired biosynthetic routes may be converted to rather **more swiftly growing bacterial or fungal cells.**

1.3.3   Microbial Metabolites

A number of **'microbial metabolites'** produced by well-defined process of fermentation give rise to certain very useful therapeutically potent drugs, especially the antibiotics and related antieoplastic agents as exemplified below:

(*a*) **As Antibiotics:** for instance:

    (*i*) **Chloromycetin** – from *Streptomyces venezualae* Bartz,

    (*ii*) **Erythromycin** – from *Streptomyces erythreus* (Walksman) Walksan & Henrici,

    (*iii*) **Gentamycin** – from *Micromonospora purpurea* MJ Weinstein *et al.*

    (*iv*) **Penicillin O** – from *Penicillium chrysogenum,*

    (*v*) **Streptomycin** – from *Streptomyces griseus* (Krainsky) Walksman et Henrici,

    (*vi*) **Tetracycline** – from *Streptomyces viridifaciens.*

(*b*) **As Antineoplastic Agents:** for examples:

    (*i*) **Dactinomycin** – from several *Streptomyces spp.*

    (*ii*) **Daunorubicin** – from *Strepomyces peucetius* G. Cassinelli; *P. orezzi.*

    (*iii*) **Mitomycin C** – from *Streptomyces caespitosus* (griseovinaceseus)

    (*iv*) **Pilcamycin** (or **Mithramycin**) – from *Streptomyces argillaceus* n. sp. and *S. tanashiensis*

Figure 1.3, illustrates the outline of the fermentation process usually accomplished in a pharmaceutical industry whereby dried drugs are produced in a large scale. However, in certain specific instances, *per se* **cephalosporins**, the end product obtained by the fermentation process is routed through semisynthetic means to yield the desired pharmaceutical substance.

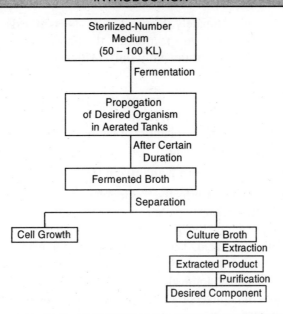

Fig. 1.3   Out-line of Fermentation Process of Drugs

It is pertinent to mention here that the production of **'genetically–engineered–drugs'**, bears fundamentally a close resemblance to the various fermentation processes normally employed for the antbiotcs. The major noteworthy difference in this specific instance lies in the fact that a gene controlling the production of the desired constituent is virtually transferred from its basic source to a fast-growing microbial cell-line whereby permitting the large-scale production in comparatively a much shorter duration.

However, it is rather a **'difficult task'** to isolate a **gene coding** for a particular antibiotic. Interestingly, in the **actinomycetin fungi,** the *'gene'* was separated conveniently from the **chromosomal genes** and cloned on naturally occurring plasmids. It has been observed that though plasmids are found in streptomycetes, only in the specific case of **methylenomycin*** *biosynthesis,* the extrachromosomal element essentially consists of several structural gene absolutely necessary for the prediction of antibiotic.

In general, a number of methods are employed to identify clones that usually harbour the plasmids carrying antibiotic-biosynthetic genes, namely:

(*a*) Mutants that are found to be blocked at different steps in the **aminoglycosidic-production-pathways** are known and also available. These 'blocked mutants' may be employed as recipients for the prediction of respective genes from **shotgun-cloning-experiments**. Shotgun cloning is the isolation of a specific DNA sequence and subsequent screening for the desired phenotype. The plasmids eventually isolated from the transformants, wherein antibiotic-biosynthesis is restored by the cloned genes, would ultimately the introduced for maximizing the final yield.

(*b*) The latest technique of **insertional mutagenesis** may be used effectively to obtain not only the mutant but also the cloned DNA in a single experiment.

---

* Member of a family of cyclopentenoid antibiotic related structurally to **sarkomycins,** and having *in vitro* activity Vs Gram positive and Gram negative organism.

(*c*) As the enzymes that are intimately involved in the **biosynthesis of aminology** essentially possess relatively wider substrate specificities, the transfer of genes between such species that cause the production of various **aminoglycosides** were invariably utilised to generate **newer antibiotics.**

If genes that code for the synthesis of chosen precursors are duly cloned interspecifically many existing aminologycosides may be produced by just a one-step-fermentation process. **Mutasynthesis*** has paved the way for the introduction of a plethora of interesting hybrids, for instance; **mutamicins, hybrimycins** and **hydroxygentamycin,** and

(*d*) Conversion of **Amikacin (I)** from **Kanamycin (II):**

Amikacin (I) is one of the most effective aminoglycosides. It may be produced chemically from **Kanamycin (II)** but this route is rather expensive and not cost-effective. However, an **aminoglycoside producing** strain of *Bacillus circulars* is capable of converting (II) into (I) by the addition of **hydroxyaminobutyric acid.** Thus, the interspecific transfer of this gene may be used to persuade successfully a kanamycin producing streptomycetes to afford (I) and this **recombinant DNA** route could prove to be an economical one.

Figure 1.4, summarizes the conversion of **Amikacin (I)** from **Kanamycin (II)** *via* **chemical and recombinant DNA routes.**

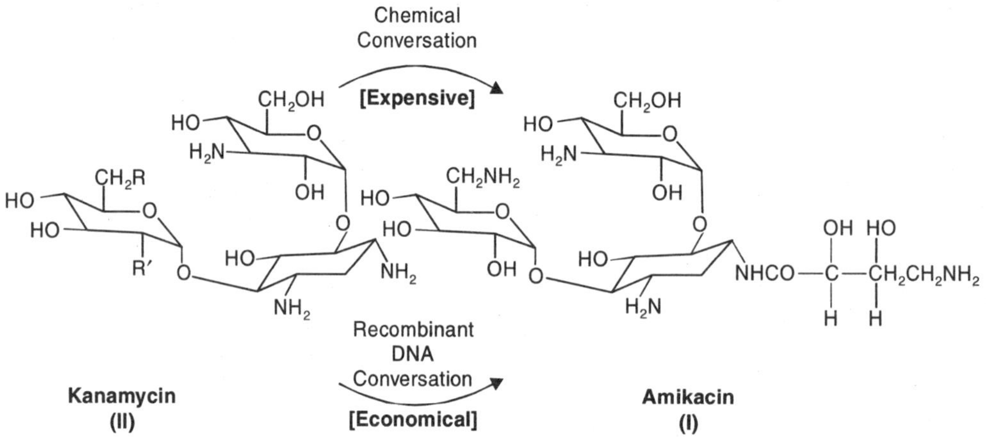

Fig. 1.4   Conversion of Amikacin(I) from Kanamycin(II)

1.3.4   Animal Derivatives

Animal Derivatives are also referred to as the **biologics** in literatures. They are invariably categorized into *two* groups, namely:

(**a**) **Prepared from the blood of animals:** Such as: *serum, antitoxins* and *globulins*. These are usually obtained by the aid of certain specific treatment particularly carved to enhance the strength of desired constituents.

---

* Here, a mutationally blocked producing organism is able to incorporate a precursor analogue to produce a modified form of antibiotic.

(*b*) **Prepared from inoculation of suitable culture medium:** For instance: *vaccines*, *toxins*, *tuberculins* collectively termed as the **'microbial products'**. These products afford protection against a host of *causative pathogenic microorganisms*. They are produced by inoculating an appropriate culture medium that may consist of living tissue along the right pathogen. The resulting product is purified suitably, and may be used as a **'drug'**.

In conclusion, it may be emphasised that even in developed countries a variety of natural products enjoy their well-deserved recognition in the therapeutic arsenal. However, their actual and precise method of production is more or less an extremely individualized aspect. Many advanced countries like United States, Germany, France. Great Britain and most parts of Europe, where medical practice is found to be oriented toward the utilisation of **preferred-single chemical entities,** a major protion of natural drugs are treated to afford either one or more active components, such as:

Ginsengoside Rg_1	from :	Ginseng;
Morphine	from :	Opium;
Reserpine	from :	Rauwolfia;
Taxol	from :	Pacific Yew;
Ergotamine	from :	Ergot;
Vincristine & Vinblastine	from :	Catharanthus;
Digoxin	from :	Digitalis;
Ginkgolide–A	from :	Ginkgo;
Artemisinin	from :	Qinghaosu, etc.

It is worthwhile to state that in **technologically-advanced nation** like China, India, Korea, Japan make use of a good number of herbal medicines having multicomponent entities with proven and advantageous therapeutic values. Mostly such preparations are available in the form of film coated tablets, capsules, syrups, powdered mixtures and dispensed under modern packing norms. Of course, there is a visible-upward tendency to adopt these preparations, from reputed manufactures in the Western World for the cure of a number of human diseases.

It is pertinent to mention here that the age-old practice of using **hydroalcoholic tinctures** and **fluid-extracts** have become more or less **obsolete nowadays.**

Various official compendia-like USP, NF, BP, Eur. P, Int. P, IP have duly incorporated the **standards of some purified natural products;** and hence, the quality in such cases may not be a significant concern at all.

1.4 PHYTOCHEMISTRY

'**Phytochemistry**' or the '**Chemistry of Natural Products**' may be strategically placed somewhere in between *natural product organic chemistry* and *plant biochemistry*. In fact, it is intimately related to the above two disciplines. However, in a broader sense phytochemistry essentially deals with the enormous different types of organic substances that are not only elaborated but also accumulated by plants. It is solely concerned with the following various aspects namely:

* Natural distribution.
* Chemical structure,
* Biosynthesis structure,
* Biosyntheses (or biogenesis),
* Metabolism, and
* Biochemical function.

Importantly, with the advent of most up-to-date analytical procedures the detailed phytochemical study of an unknown plant may be accomplished right from elucidation of chemical structure of pure constituents to the elaborated study of their biological characteristics.

Figure 1.5, illustrates the schematic development of a *'drug'* from a **'medicinal plant'** that may serve as a fruitful guide for various phytochemistry studies:

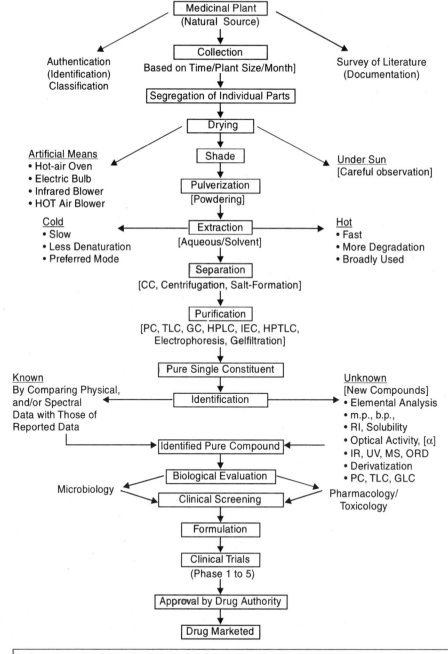

Fig. 1.5   Schematic Development of a 'Drug' from a 'Medicinal Plant'

It is, however, important to mention here that the '**living organism**' of the universe (*i.e.*; plants, microbes and animals) may be regarded as mother nature's splendid and huge BIOSYNTHETIC LABORATORY. It not only caters for the survival of the so called 'living creatures' of the earth in terms of providing a broad spectrum of **essential chemical constituents,** for instance: *proteins, fats, carbohydrates* and *vitamins* but also meticulously bring forth an enormous quantum of **physiologically active chemical entities,** such as: *alkaloids, glycosides, volatile oil* (*terpenoids*), *steroids, antibiotics, bitter principles, tannins* and the like.

The '**living organisms**' give rise to a number of interesting phytochemical aspects over the years that may be viewed closely under the following *three* heads, namely:

   (*i*) Constituents,
   (*ii*) Drug Biosynthesis (or Biogenesis) and
   (*iii*) Classification

1.4.1 Constituents

The huge number of chemical substances that are present in the plant-kingdom and animal kingdom in one form or the other are termed as '**constituents**'. These **constituents** may be further divided into **two** main categories, namely:

   (*a*) Active Constituents, and
   (*b*) Inert Constituents.

1.4.1.1 Active Constituents

The chemical entities that are solely responsible for existing pharmacological, microbial or in a broader-sense therapeutic activities are usually termed as **active constituents.** Most drugs like: *alkaloids, glycosides, steroids, terpenoids, bitter principles* are the bonafide members of this particular category.

1.4.1.2 Inert Constituents

The chemical compounds, though present in plant and animal kingdom, which do not possess any definite therapeutic values as such but are useful as an adjunct either in the formulation of a '**drug**' or in surgery are collectively known as **inert constituents.**

Examples:

   (*a*) **Plant Drugs:** The following **inert constituents** are invariably present in plants, namely:

Cellulose	: Microcrystalline forms of cellulose are used as combination binder-disintegrants in tabletting. Collodal cellulose particles aid in stabilization and emulsification of liquid;
Lignin	: To precipitate proteins, and to stablise asphalt emulsions;
Suberin	: Esters of higher monohydric alcohols and fatty acids;
Cutin	: -do-
Starch	: As pharmaceutic aid *i.e.;* tablet filler, binder and disintegrant;
Albumin	: Soyabean albumins–as emulsifiers;
Colouring Matters	: Cochineal for colouring food products and pharmaceuticals.

(*b*) **Animal Drugs:** The under mentioned **inert constituents** are mostly present in animals, namely:

Keratin	: For coating **"enteric pills"** that are unaffected in the stomach but dissolved by the alkaline into intestinal secretions;
Chitin	: **Deacylated chitin (chitosan)**–for treatment of water; sulphated chitin– as anticoagulant in laboratory animals.

It has been observed that the very presence of *'Inert Constituents'* either act towards modifying or check the absorbance and the therapeutic index of the *'active constituents'*.

Obviously, to get at the right active constituents one has to get rid of the host of 'inert constituents' by adopting various known methods of separation, purification and crystallization. Therefore, most literatures invariably refer to the former as 'secondary' plant products.

The presence of these **secondary plant products (active constituents)** are governed by **two** school of thoughts, namely:

(*a*) **Superfluous Metabolites:** *i.e.*, substances that have no value as such and perhaps their presence are due to the lack of exceretory mechanism in them and ultimately result as the **'residual lock-up'** *superfluous metabolites*, and

(*b*) **Characteristic Survival Substances:** *i.e.*, substances which exert a positive survival value on the plant wherein they are actually present. They offer more or less a **'natural defence-mechanism'** whereby these host plants are survived from destruction owing to their astringent, odorous and unpalatable features.

Examples: Poisonous alkaloidal containing plants; astringent containing shrubs; and pungent volatile oil-containing trees etc.

1. **Genetic Composition (or Heredity):** In reality, **genetic effects** exert both qualitative and quantitative alterations of the active constituents in medicinal plants.

Examples:

(*i*) **Eugenol:** It is naturally present in two different species in varying quantities as follows:
Eugenia caryophyllus (Sprengel) Bullock et Harrison: 70–95%
Syzgium aromaticm (L.) Merr et L.M. Perry: Not less then 85%.

(*ii*) **Reserpine-rescinamine group of Alkaloids:**
Rauvolfia serpentina (Linné) Bentahm: NLT* 0.15%;
Rauvolfia vomitoria Afzelius (from Africa): NLT 0.20%;
(*NLT: Not less than)

(*iii*) **Rutin:**

Fagopyrum esculatum Moznch	:	3-8%;
Sophora japonica Linné	:	20%;

(*iv*) **Menthol:**

Mentha piperita L.	:	50-60%
Mentha arvensis Linnévar	:	75-90%
(Japanese Mint Oil)		

2. Environment Factors:

The **environment factors** largely contribute to the quantitative aspect of secondary constituents *i.e.*, active constituents. It is pertinent to mention here that medicinal plants belonging to the same species which are phenotypically identical *i.e.*, they essentially bear a close resemblance with regard to their form and structure, may not, however, genotypically be the same *i.e.*, possessing the same genetic composition. This particular natural phenomenon evidently gives rise to an altogether marked and pronounced difference in their chemical composition, specially with reference to active constituents. In a more logical and scientific manner it may be said that these plants categorically belong to different chemical races.

Example:

 (*i*) **Ergotamine:** Modified strains of *Claviceps purpurea* (Fries) have been developed, exclusively for field cultivation, that are capable of producing nearly 0.35% of **ergotamine** (in comparison to the normal one producing NLT 0.15% of total **ergot alkaloids**).

 (*ii*) **Eucalyptol** (*Syn: Cineole, Cajeputol*): It is present in the fresh leaves of *Eucalyptus globus* Libillardiere to the extent of 70–85%. It has been observed that the chemical races of some species of **Eucalyptus invariably** display significant variations in the content of eucalyptus and related components present in the essential oils.

There are a number of environmental factors which may afford considerable changes in active plant constituents, for instance: *composition of soil* (mineral contents); *climate* (dry, humid, cold); *associated flora* (*Rauvolfia serpentina* and *R. vomitoria*) and lastly the methods of cultivation (using modified strains, manual and mechanical cultivation). For a specific instance it may be recalled that a soil rich-in-nitrogen content evidently gives rise to a relatively higher yield of alkaloids in the medicinal plants; whereas a soil not so abundant in nitrogen content and grown in comparatively dry zones may yield an enhanced quantum of volatile oil.

3. **Ontogeny (or Ageing of Plant):** The age of a medicinal plant has a direct impact on the concentration of the *'active constituent'*. It is, however, not always true that older the plant greater would be the active principal.

Example:

 (i) **Cannabidiol:** It is present in *Cannbis sativa* L. (*C sativa* var. Indica Auth), possessing euphoric activity; and its content attains a maximum level in the growing season and subsequently the decline commences gradually. Interestingly, the concentration of **dronabinol** (or **tetrahydrocannabinol**) starts to enhance reciprocally till the plants gets fully matured.

 (ii) **Morphine:** The well-known narcotic-anlagesic present in the air-dried milky exudate collected by incising the capsules of *Papaver somniferum* Linné or *P. album* Decandolle is found to be the highest peak just 2 to 3 week after flowering. An undue delay in harvesting from this *'critical-period'* would ultimately result into the decomposition of morphine. It is worth to be noted that a prematured harvesting of latex would certainly enhance the content of allied alkaloid like **codeine** and **thebaine.**

In short, it is a prime importance to affect the harvesting of medicinal plant at the right time so as to maximise the yield of the active principal.

1.4.1.3 *Drug Biosynthesis (or Biogenesis)*

In the recent past, a good deal of well-deserved importance and recognition have been attributed to the exclusive study of the biochemical pathways that precisely lead to the formulation of '*active constituents*' otherwise referred to as the **secondary constituents** mostly employed as *drugs*. This specific study is normally termed as **Drug Biosynthesis or Biogenesis.**

As a '**medicinal chemist**' is required to know the synthesis of **chloroquine**–an antimalarial drug from pure synthetic compounds, a '**phytochemist**' is supposed to know the biogenesis of **quinine** in the cinchona bark. With the advent of isotopically labelled organic compounds known in the early fifties it was quite possible to establish scientifically that the host of amino acids along with their corresponding derivatives more or less acted as precursors of complex alkaloids. However, these logical studies confirmed the earlier hypothesis stated above by Trier in 1912.

Figure 1.6, summarizes the various *biosynthetic pathways and their inter-relationships* that ultimately lead to the formation of different kinds of **secondary constituents** (*i.e.*, **active constituents**) belonging to the plant kingdom which are invariably employed as drugs having *potent therapeutic index*.

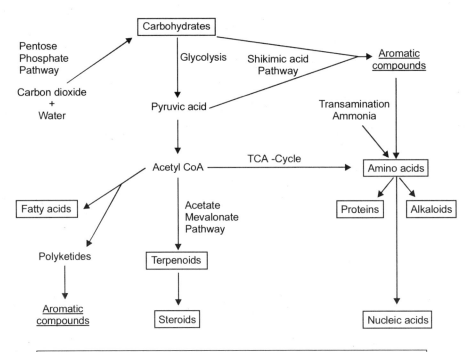

Fig. 1.6   Biosynthetic Pathways and their Interrelationships

1.4.1.4 *Classification*

A plethora of pharmacologically active naturally occurring substances derived from '**medicinal plants**' essentially comprise of rather large and complex molecules that invariably possess one or more than one of the chemical functional moieties which are responsible for attributing characteristic features for alcohol, phenols, esters, aldehydes, ketones, oxides and organic acids. In fact, the aforesaid chemical groups are often attached to the molecular skeletons (*e.g.* **aromatic, heterocyclic compounds**) of noticeable diversified nature and complexity.

In the light of the following *two* observations, the phytochemical classification is eventually done on a more rational and broader perspective:

(*a*) **Morphine** and **salicylic acid** has one phenolic—OH group in their molecule but structurally they are world-apart, and

(*b*) **Essential (or volatile) oils** mostly contain a mixture of substances, such as: *hydrocarbons, ketones*, aldehydes, and terpenes.

Therefore, ideally the phytochemical classification is solely based on the types of plant constituents present in the natural products, namely:

(*i*) Comprising of C and H only,

(*ii*) Comprising of C, H and O only,

(*iii*) Comprising 'O' into heterocyclic rings,

(*iv*) Comprising of N, S and P,

(*v*) Mostly containing Nitrogen

(*vi*) Comprising of diversified chemical entity, and

(*vii*) Mixtures.

The above phytochemical classification will be further expatiated with the help of some typical examples from the domain **'pharmacognosy'** along with their structures, wherever possible, as under:

1.4.1.4.1 Comprising of C and H only: They essentially consist of hydrocarbon present in the natural products.

Examples:

(*a*) **β-Myrcene:** It is an **unsaturated acyclic hydrocarbon** found in *oil of bay, verbena, hop* and others.

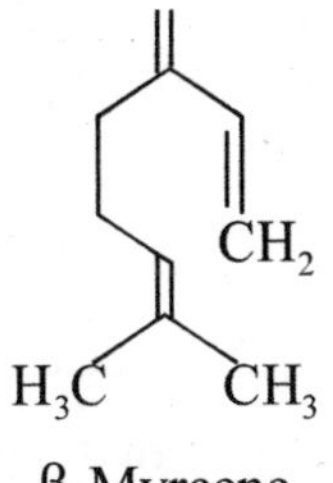

β-Myrcene

(*b*) **Ocimene:** It is also an **unsaturated acyclic hydrocarbon** found in the essential oil distilled from the fresh leaves of *Ocimum basilicum* L. and from the fruits of *Evodia rutaecarpa* (Juss.) Hook & Thoms. It exists in two modifications and forms. The *cis-* and *trans-*refers to the stereochemistry at the double-bond between C-3 and C-4.

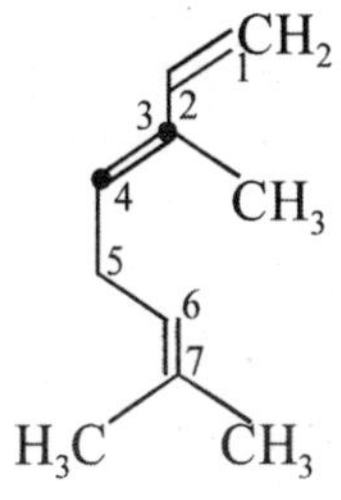

trans–β–Ocimene

(*c*) ***p*-Cymene (Dolcymene):** It is an **aromatic hydrocarbon** and occurs in a number of essential oils *e.g.*, sage, lemon, thyme, nutmeg, coriander, origanum, cinnamon.

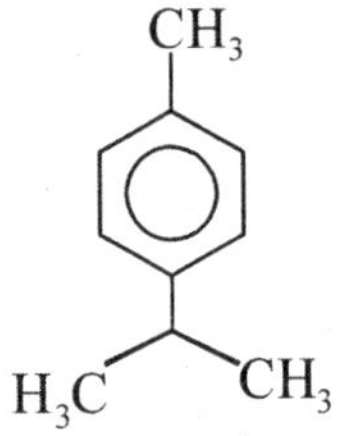

p-Cymene (Dolcymene)

(*d*) **Limonene (Syn: Cinene, Cajeputene, Kautschin):** It is an **alicyclic hydrocarbon** and further classified into *monocyclic terpene*. It occurs in various ethereal oils particularly in oils of lemon, orange, caraway, dill and bergamot.

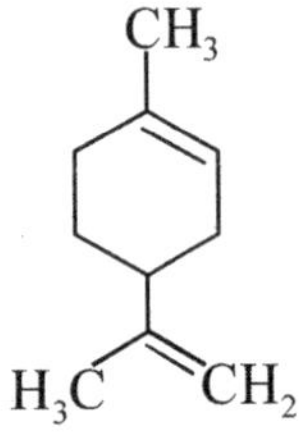

Limonene

(*e*) **α-Pinene:** It is also an **alicyclic hydrocarbon** and further classified into *bicyclic monoterpene* *d*-α-pinene obtained from Port Oxford **Cedar Wood Oil** (*Chamaecyparls lawsorliana* Parl.). *l*-α-*Pinene* obtained from **Mandarin Peel Oil** (*Citrus reticulata* Blando).

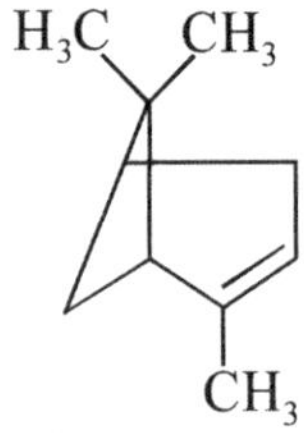

d-α-Pinene

1.4.1.4.2 Comprising of C, H, and O only: A wide spectrum of plant constituents containing C, H and O have been identified.

Examples:

(A) Alcohols:

(*a*) **Geraniol (or Lemonol):** It is an **olephenic terpene alcohol** constituting the major portion of **oil of rose** and **oil of palmarosea.** It is also found in many volatile oils, for instance: citronella, lemon grass *etc*.

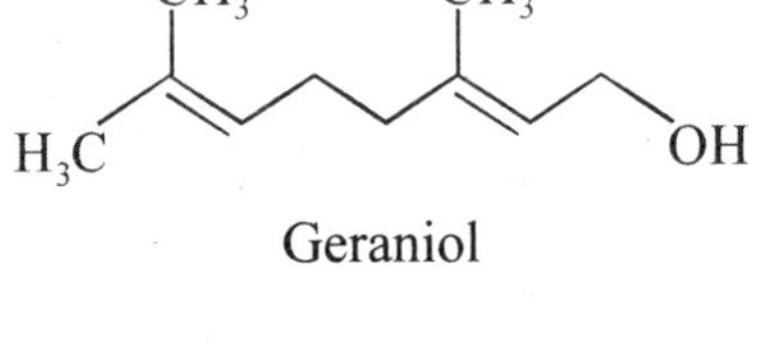

Geraniol

(b) **Menthol (or Peppermint Camphor):** It is a **monocyclic terpene** alcohol obtained from **peppermint oil** or other **mint oils** or prepared synthetically on large scale by carrying out the hydrogenation of thymol.

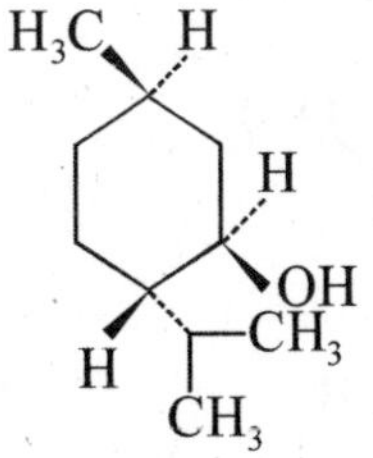

Menthol

(B) Aldehydes:

(a) **Citral**: It is an aliphatic terpene aldehyde present in oil of lemon grass, lemon, lime, ginger root and in the oils of several *Citrus species etc.* The **citral** from natural sources is a mixture of *two* isomers **geraniol** and **neral.**

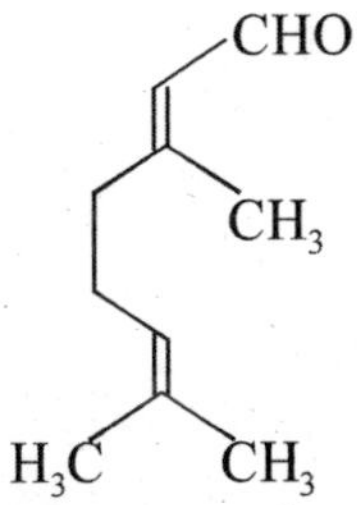

Geranial (Citral-a) 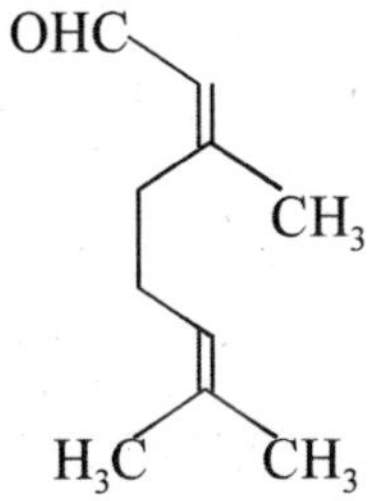 Neral (Citral-b)

(b) **Vanillin**: It is a **cyclic terpene aldehyde.** It occurs in vanilla in potato parings, in Siam benzoin, Peru balsam, clove oil etc. It is made synthetically either from **guaiacol** or **eugenol;** also from waste **(lignin)** of the wood pulp industry.

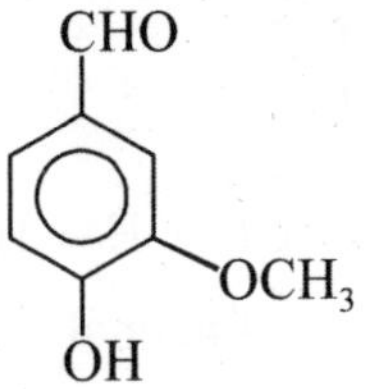

Vanillin

(C) Ketones:

(a) **Carvone**: It is a **monocyclic terpene ketone.** *dl*-**Carvone** is found in *gingergrass oil; d*-**carvone** is found in caraway seed and dill seed oils, *l*-**carvone** is found in *spearmint and kuromoji oils.*

(b) **Camphor**: It is a **bicyclic terpene ketone.** It naturally occurs in all parts of the camphor tree, *Cinnamonum camphora* T. Nees & Ebermeier; while 3/4th of the camphor consumed in USA is manufactured from **pinene** as the racemic form.

d-camphor: is found in oil of sassafras, rosemary, lavender and sage;

l-camphor: is found in lavender and artemisia;

dl-camphor: is found in oil of sage and in oil of *Chrysanthemum sinense* var. japonicum.

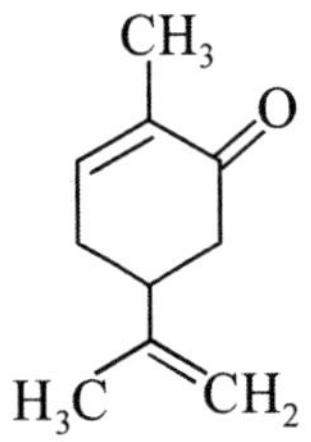

Carvone 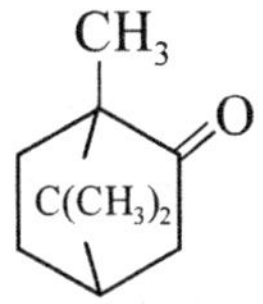   Comphor

(D) Phenols:

(*a*) **Thymol:** It is a **monocyclic phenol.** It is obtained from the volatile oil of *Thymus vulgaris* L. and *Monarda punctata* L. and several spices of *Ocimum*. Commercially it is synthesized from *p*-cymene, *m*-cresol and **piperitone.**

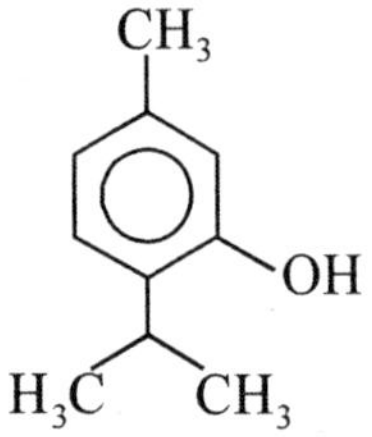

Thymol

(*b*) **Eugenol (or Allyguaicol):** It is a **dihydric phenol** and is the main constituent of several important essential oils, such as: **oil of clove, oil of cinnamon leaf, oil pimenta.**

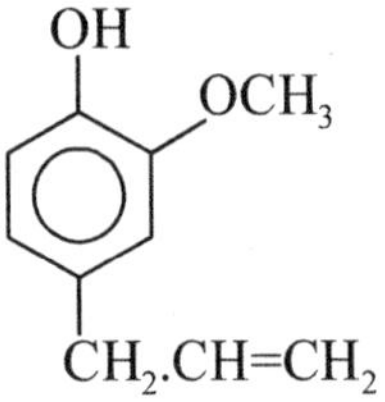

Eugenol

(*c*) **Myristicin:** It is a **trihydric phenol** occurs in **oils of nutmeg, mace, French parsley, dill oils and carrot.**

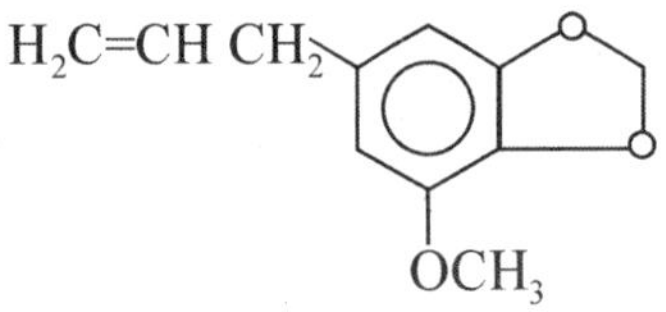

Myristicin

(*d*) **Apiole:** It is a **tetrahydric phenol** which occurs in **Dill oil** (*Anethum graveolus L.*) and known as Apiole (Dill); and also in **Parsley oil** (*Petroselinum sativum* Blanchet, Sell) and termed as Apiole (Parsley).

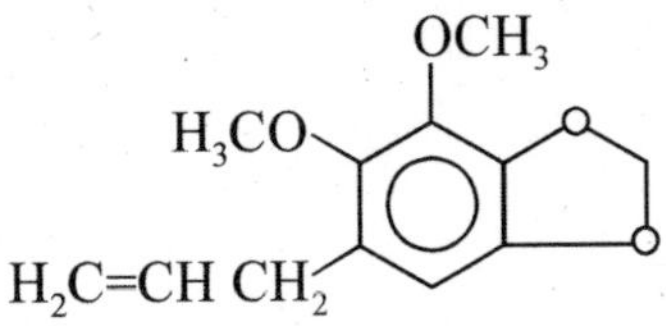

Apioile (Dill) 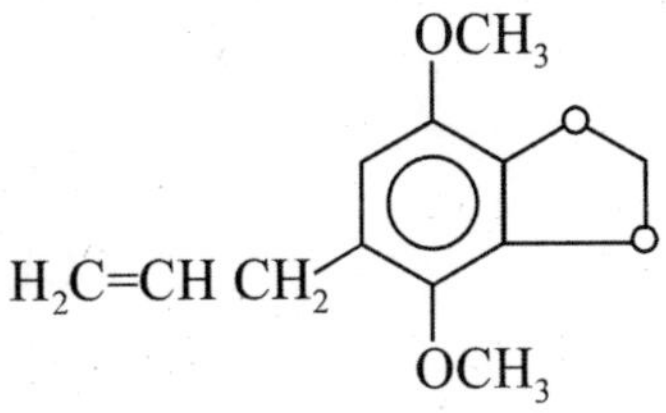   Apiole (Parsley)

(E) Quinones:

Examples:

Anthraquinone Glycosides: A plethora of glycosides having aglycone moieties related to anthracene are present in such drugs as aloe, rhubarb, senna, frangula and cascara sagrada. In general, the glycosides on hydrolysis give rise to corresponding aglycones which are di-, tri-, or tetra-hydroxyanthraquinones or invariably structural modifications of these compounds.

Examples: Frangulin-A upon hydrolysis yields **emodin** and **rhamnose** as shown below:

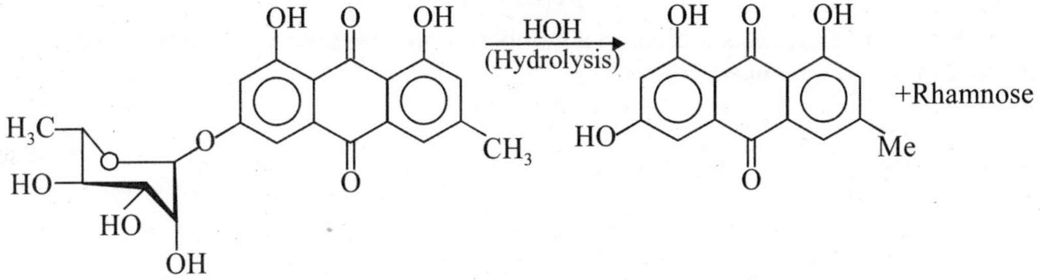

Frangulin A   Emodin (An Aglycone)

(F) Acids:

(*a*) **Caffeic acid:** It is the constituent of plant and isolated from green **coffee beans**. It probably occurs in plants only in conjugated forms *e.g.* **chlorogenic acid.**

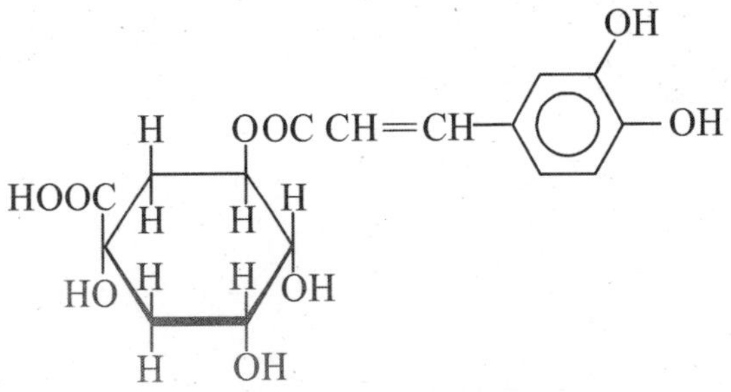

Chlorogenic acid 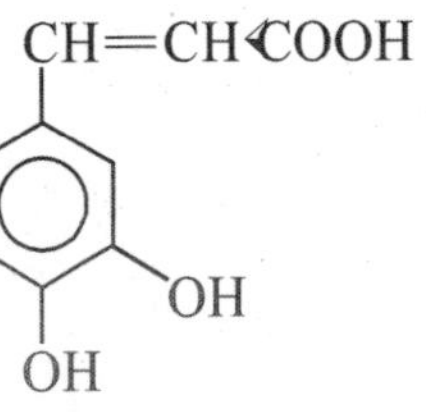   Caffeic acid (*b*) **Ferulic acid:** It is widely distributed in small amounts in various plants species. It is isolated from *Ferula foetida* Reg.

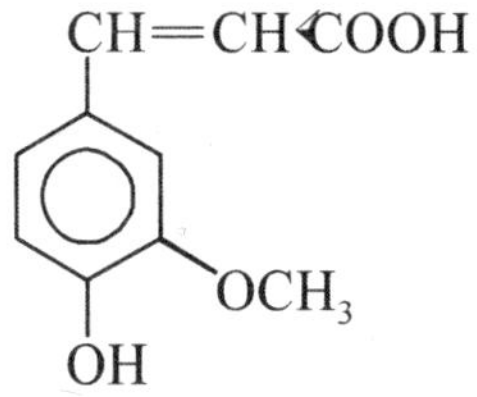

Ferulic acid

(G) Esters:

(*a*) **Pyrenthrins (Pyrethrin I & Pyrethrin II):** It is the active insecticidal constituents of **pyrethrum flowers.**

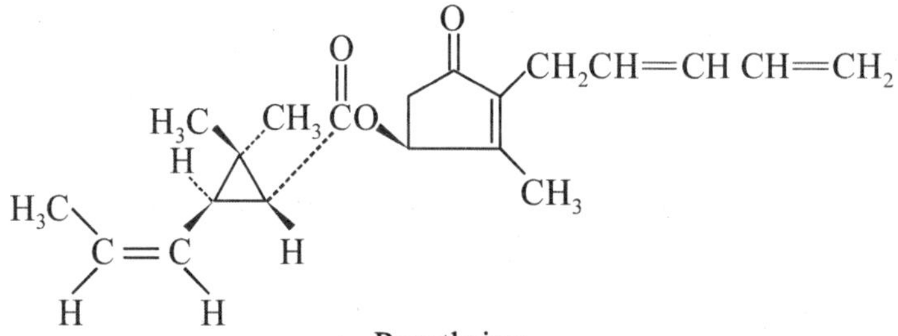

Pyrethrins

(*b*) **Methyl Salicylate:** It is present in a number of oils, namely: **wintergreen oil, betula oil, sweet birch oil, teaberry oil.**

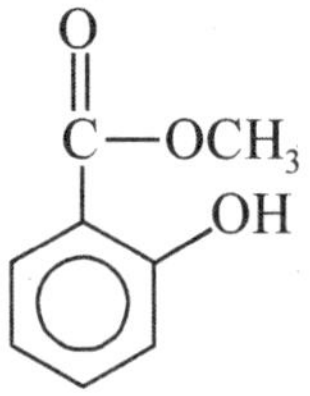

Methyl Salicylate

(H) Lactones:

(*a*) **Podophyllotoxin (Syn: Condyline, Podofilox, Martec):** It is an *antineoplastic* **glycoside** found in the rhizomes of North American *Podophyllum peltatum L.*

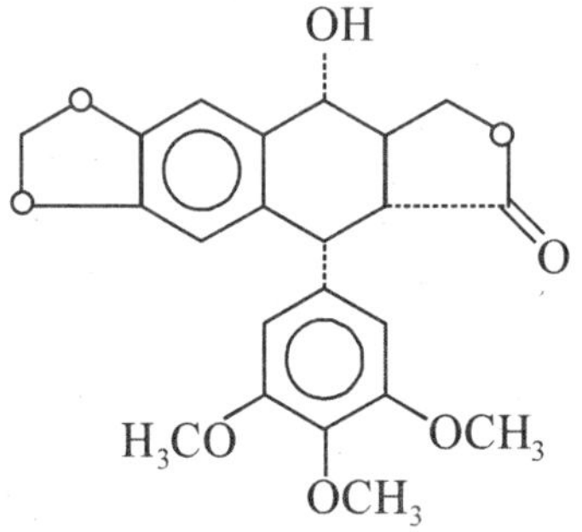

Podophyllotoxin

(b) **α-Santonin:** It is an *anthelmintic* isolated from the dried unexpanded flower heads of *Artemesia maritima* L., sens lat.

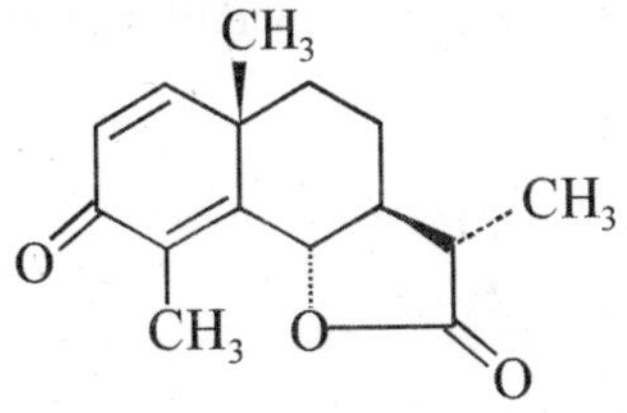

α-Santonin

(I) Terpenoids:

(a) **Gibberellins:** It represents a class of *plant growth hormones* first isolated from the cultures of *Gibberella fujikuroi* (Sawada) Wollenweber.

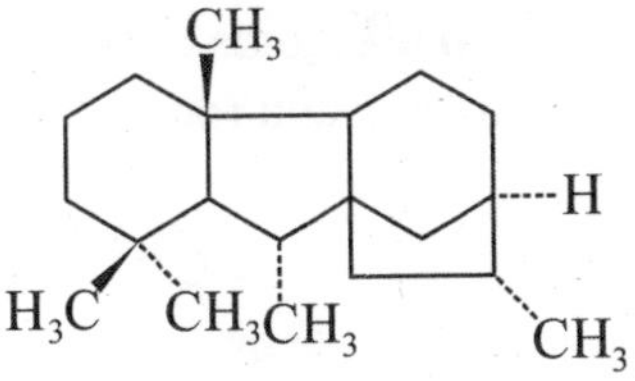

Gibberelane

(b) **Primaric Acid:** It is obtained from American rosin, French galipot and from *Pinus maritima* Mill.

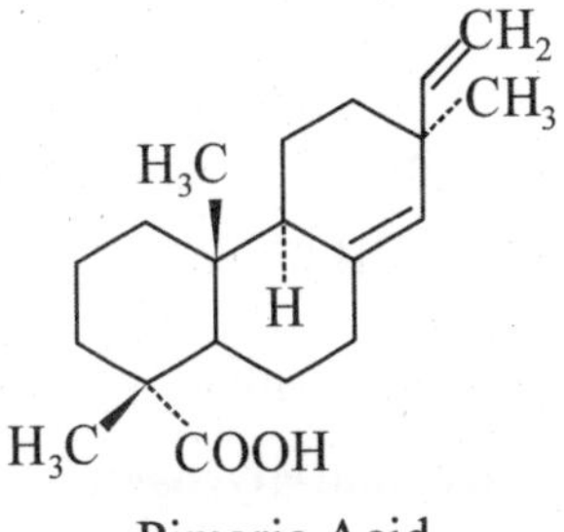

Pimaric Acid

(J) Carotenoids:

(a) **Xanthophyll (Syn: Vegetable lutein; Vegetable lutenol; Bo-Xan):** It is one of the most widerpread **carotenoid alcohol** present in nature. It occurs in egg-yolk, nettles, algae, and petals of many yellow flowers. It also occurs in the coloured feathers of birds.

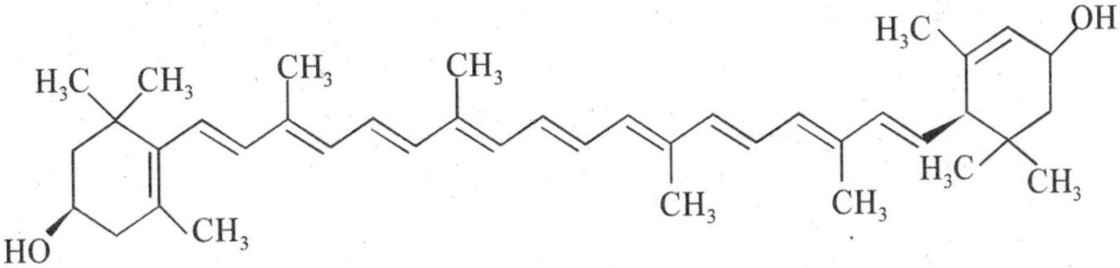

Xanthophyll

(b) **β-Carotene:** It is most abundantly distributed in the plant and animal kingdom. In plants it occurs invariably with chlorophyll. It acts as a **precursor of Vitamin A.** It was first isolated from carrots and hence bears its name. It usually represents the natures 'red' colouration in plant kingdom.

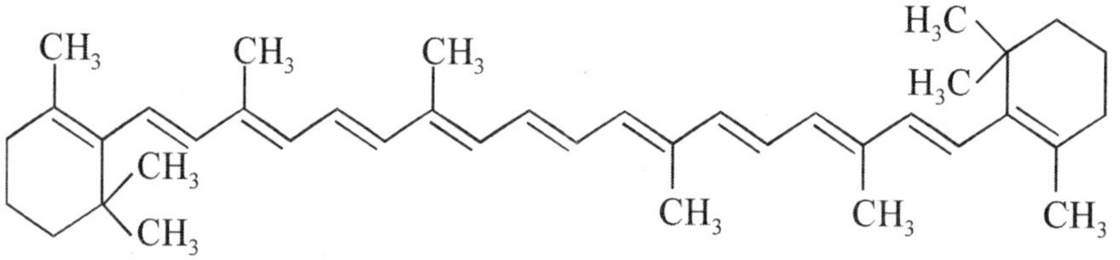

β-Carotene

(K) Steroids:

(a) **Cevadine:** It is one of the **steroidal alkaloids** obtained from *Veratrum viride. American or Green hellebore* from its dried rhizome and roots.

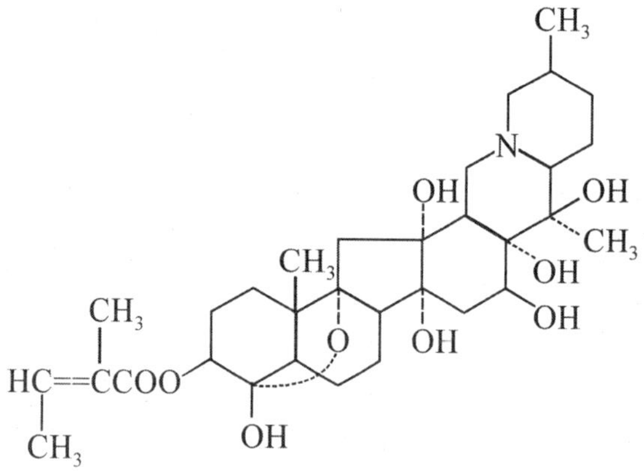

Cevadine

(b) **Digitoxin:** It is a *cardiotonic* **steroidal-glycoside** obtained from *Digitalis purpurea L;D. lanata* and other species of Digitalis. About 10 Kilo leaves yield only 6 Grams of pure **digitoxin.**

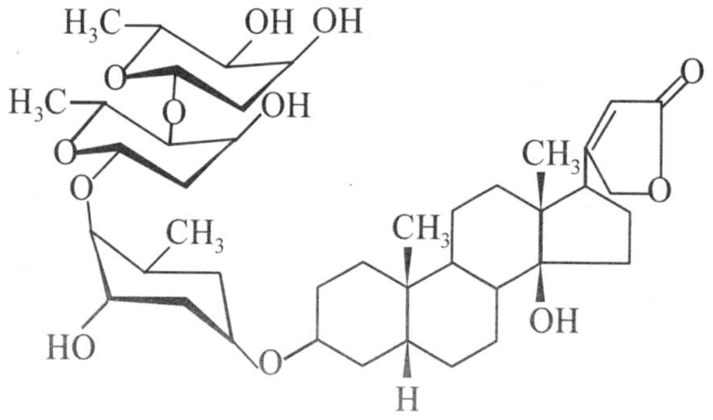

Digitoxin

(c) **Ergosterol:** It is usually obtained from yeast that synthesizes it from simple sugars such.as-glucose. The damp yeast yield about 2.5 g ergosterol; however, the particular variety of yeast is very important.

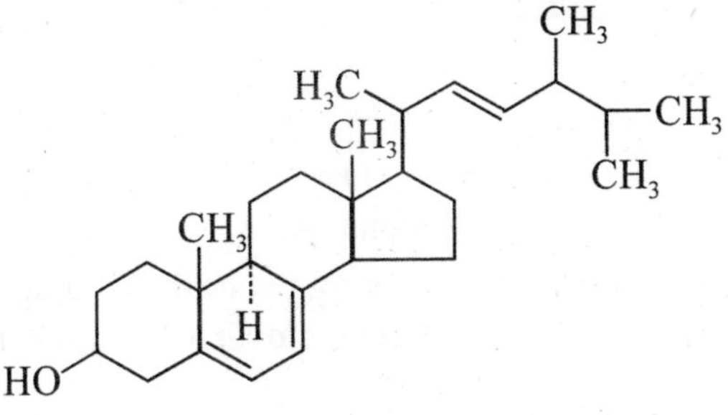

Ergosterol

1.4.1.4.3 Comprising of 'O' into Heterocyclic Rings: There are a number of natural plant constituents that essentially possess an oxygen atom into the heterocyclic ring-system. A few typical example are cited below to initiate some commendable interest in the domain of **"phytochemistry"**:

1.4.1.4.3A Furan-based Constituents: These constituents are derived from *five-membered heterocyclic ring* **'furan'**, namely:

(a) **Furfural (or 2-Furfuraldehyde):** It is a **heterocyclic aldehyde** that usually occurs in the first fraction of many essential oils, belonging to the natural order-**Pinaceae**, for instance: *Pinus palustris* **(Pine oil)** and **cade oil.** It is also present in **oil of orris rhizome, clove oil,** petit-grain, lavender and **cinnamon oils.**

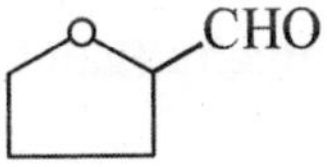

Furfural

1.4.1.4.3B Pyran-based Constituents: They are derived from *six-membered heterocylic ring* **'pyran'**, namely:

(a) **Dicoumarol (Syn: Dicoumarin: Dufalone; Melitoxin;):** It was originally isolated from **sweet clover** (Improperly cured Mililotus hay).

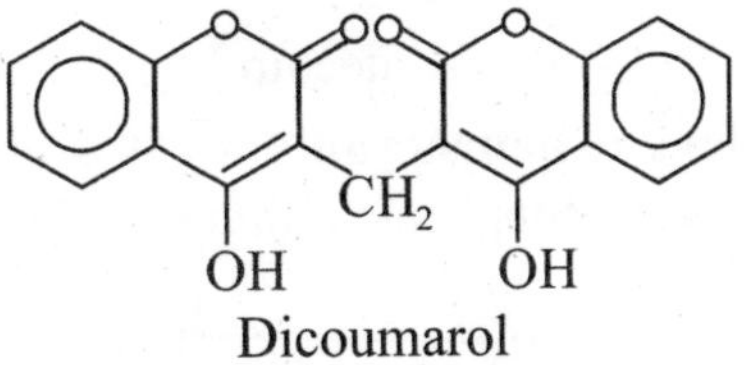

Dicoumarol

(b) **Umbelliferone (Syn: Hydrangin; Skimmetin;):** It is present in many plants and obtained by the distillation of resins belonging to the natural order **Umbelliferae**. It is the **aglucon** of *skimmin.*

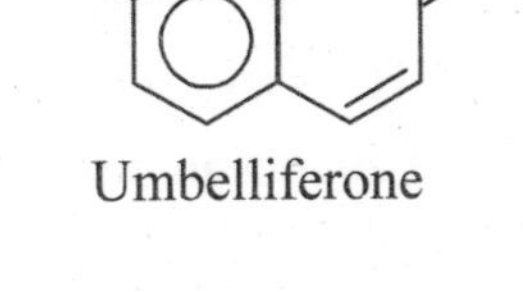

Umbelliferone

(c) **Meconic Acid (Syn: Oxychelidonic acid):** It is obtained from **opium** *i.e., Papever somniferum* which contains 4 to 6% of **meconic acid.**

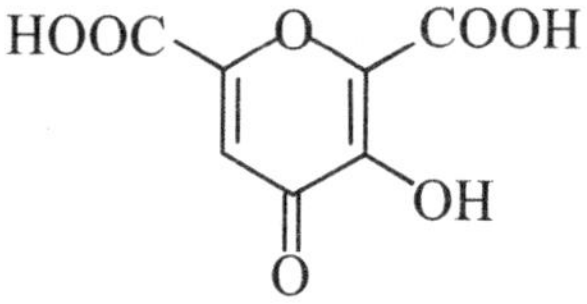

Meconic Acid

(d) **Coumestrol:** An *estrogenic factor* occuring naturally in forage crops, especially in **ladino clover** (*Trifolium repens L.*), **strawberry clover** (*T. fragiferum*) and **alfalfa** (*Medicago sativa L.*).

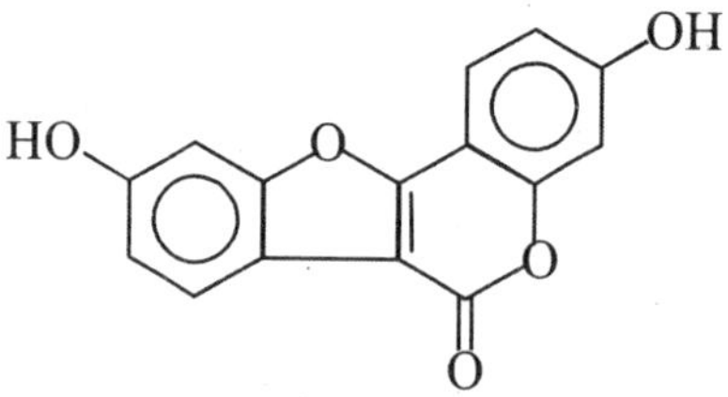

Coumestrol

1.4.1.4.3C Flavan based Constituents:

(a) **Caechin (Syn: Catechol; Cyanidol):** It is a flavonid found primarily in **higher woody plants** as **(+)–catechin** along with **(–)–epicatechin** (*cis*-form).

Source: From **mahogany wood** and **catechu** (gambir and acacia).

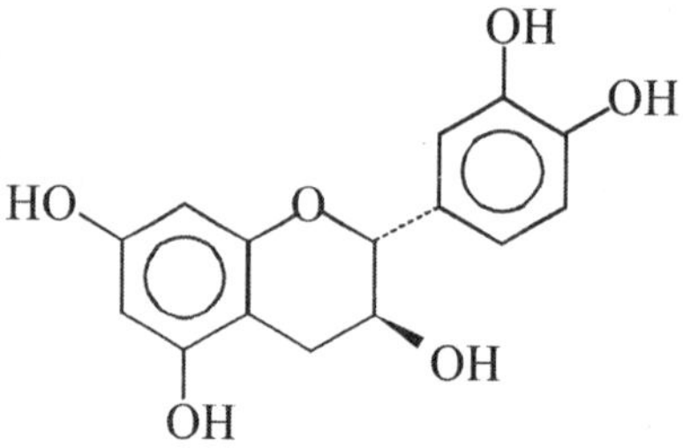

d-Catechin

(b) **Leucocyanidin (Syn: Flavan; Leucocyanidol):** It is obtained from the petals of **Asistic cotton flower** (*Gossipum spp.*) Stephens; *Butea frondosa* Koen ex Roxb. and **taxifolin.**

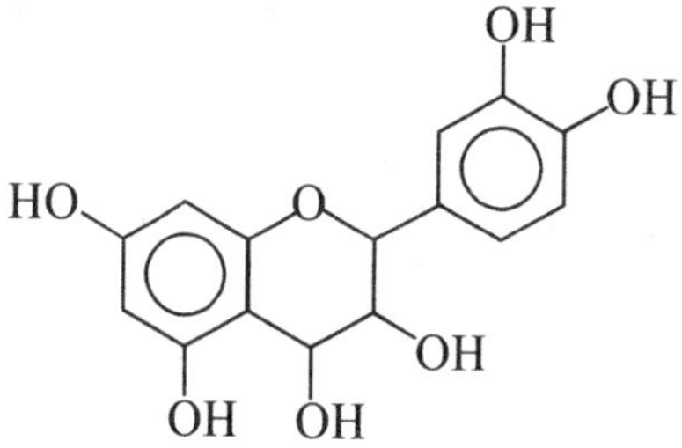

Leucocyanidin

1.4.1.4.3D Phenylbenzopyrilium based Constituents:

(*a*) **Cyanidin Choride:** It is isolated from **bananas** and prepared by the reduction of **quercitin**.

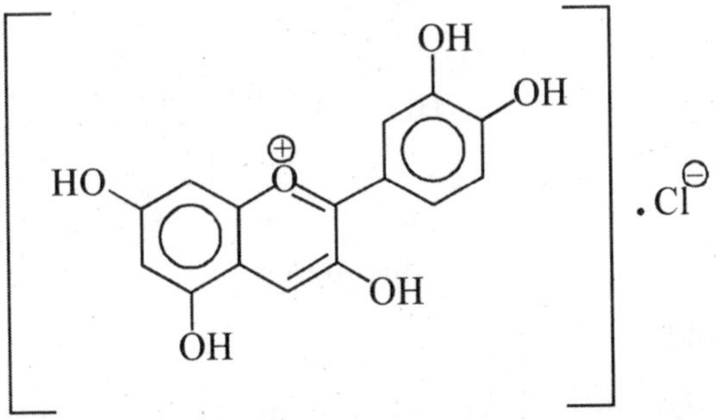

Cyanidin Chloride

1.4.1.4.3E Carbohydrates: There are several examples of well known compounds belonging to the **carbohydrates**:

(*a*) **Glucose:** It occurs naturally in the free state in fruits and other parts of plants, it is also found in the combined form in **glucosidase, in di- and oligosaccharides,** in the **polysaccharides** (cellulose and starch) and in **glycogen**.

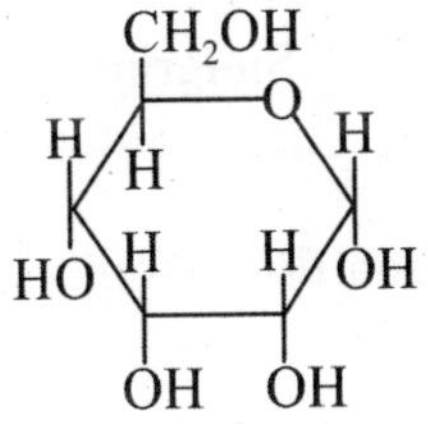

Glucose

(*b*) **Algin (Syn: Kelgin; Allose; Protanol):** It is a *gelling polysaccharide* extracted from **giant brown seaweed** [giant kelp (*Macrocystis pyrifera*) (L.) Ag]; **horsetail kelp** [*Laminaria digitata*) (L.) (Lamour)]; and **sugar kelp** [*Laminaria succharina*) (L.) (Lamour)].

(*c*) **Pectin:** It is a **polysaccharide** substance present in cell walls of all plant tissues that functions as an *intercellular cementing materials*. Orange and lemon rind serve as the richest source of pectin and contains about 30% of the same.

1.4.1.4.4 Comprising of N, S and P: It can be divided into *three* groups, namely:

(A) Comprising of N:

(*a*) **Amygdalin:** The name **amygdalin** is currently used interchangeably with **'lactrile'**. It is a *cyanogenic glycoside* that occurs in seeds of *Rosacea*, principally in bitter almonds and also in peaches and apricots.

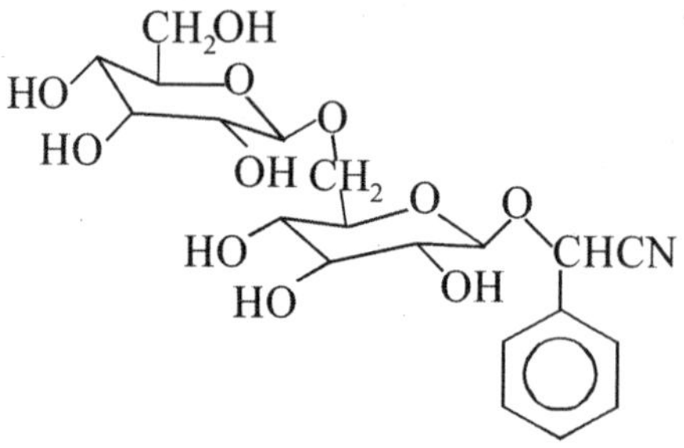

Amygdalin

(B) Comparising of N and S:

(*a*) **Sinigrin (Syn: Sinigroside: Allyl glucosinolate):** It is a **β-glucopyranoside** isolated from **black mustard seeds** *Brassica niagra* Linne, Koche., **horse raddish root** *Alliaria officinalis* Andrz.

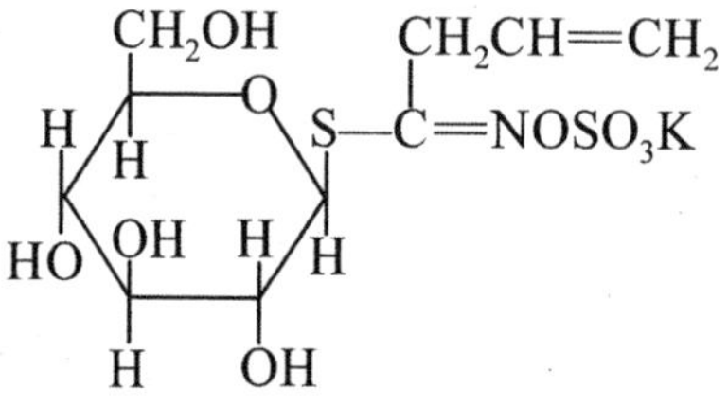

Sinigrin

(C) Comprising of P:

(*a*) **Glycerophosphoric Acid:** In fact, *three* isomers of phosphoric acid glycerol esters exist, namely:

$(HOCH_2)_2$ $CHOPO(OH)_2)$ and $HOCH_2CH(OH)CH_2O\text{—}PO(OH)_2$
β-Glycerophosphoric acid   D(+) and L(−) forms of
                                    β-Glycerophosphoric acid

The L-α-acid is the naturally occuring form; whereas the corresponding acid, found to be present in the hydrolysates of **lecithins (soyalecthin,** egg-ylk) from natural sources, arise from migration of the phosphoryl moiety from the α-carbon atom.

1.4.1.4.5 Mostly Containing Nitrogen: The various examples of naturally occurring plant substances that contain nitrogen as essential component are as follows:

(A) Amino Acids: They are mostly present in the protein hydrolysates.

(B) Proteins: These form an essential component of natural products *e.g.*, seeds, fruits, barks, leaves etc.

(C) Amines and Allied Compounds:

(*a*) **Capsaicin (*Syn:* Mioton; Zostrix):** It is the pungent principal in fruits of various species of *Capsicum, Solanaceae.* It is isolated from **aparika** and **cayenne.**

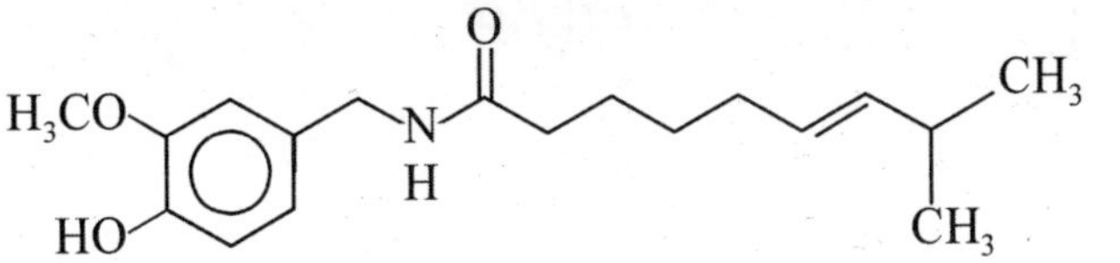

Capsaicin

(b) **Trigonelline (*Syn:* Coffearin; Gynesine; Trigenolline):** It occurs in the seeds of *Trigonella foenumgraecum* L., in coffee beans, in the seeds of *Strophanthus spp.* and the *Cannabis sativa L.,* Besides in seeds of many other plants. It is also found in **jellyfish** and in **sea urchin.**

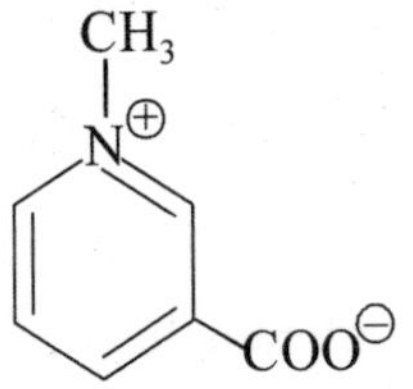

Trigonelline

(c) **Trimethylamine:** It occurs as a degradation product of nitrogenous plant and animal substances. It is widely distributed in animal tissue and especially in fish.

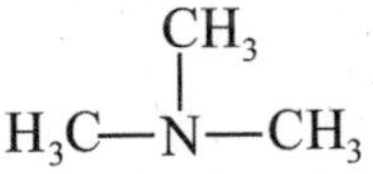

Trimethylamine

1.4.1.4.6 Comprising of Diversified Chemical Entity: The naturally occurring plant products invariably represent a class of entirely diversified chemical entity and nature. A few typical examples are cited below:

(a) **Thiamine Hydrochloride (*Syn:* Vitamin B$_1$; Aneurine Hydrochloride; Bivatin; Metabolin; Bedome; Bewon):** It occurs abuntantly in plant and animal tissues, notably in rice husk, cereal grains, eggs, milk, green leaves, yeast, liver, tubers and roots.

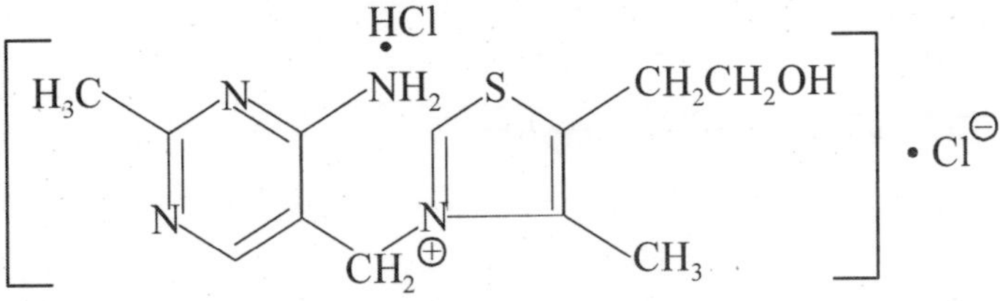

Thiamine Hydrochloride

(b) **Ascorbic Acid (*Syn:* Vitamin C; Cantaxin; Cevalin):** It is widely distributed in the plant and animal kingdom. However, the good sources are **fresh tea-leaves, citrus fruits, hip berries** and **acerola.** It was isolated from **lemons** and **paparika.**

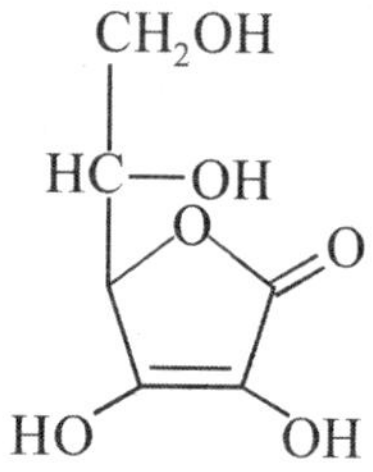

Ascorbic Acid

(*c*) **Chloramphenicol (*Syn:* Chloromycetin; Levomycetin; Klorita):** It is a broad-spetrum antibiotic obtained from cultures of the soil bacterium *Streptomyces venezualae*.

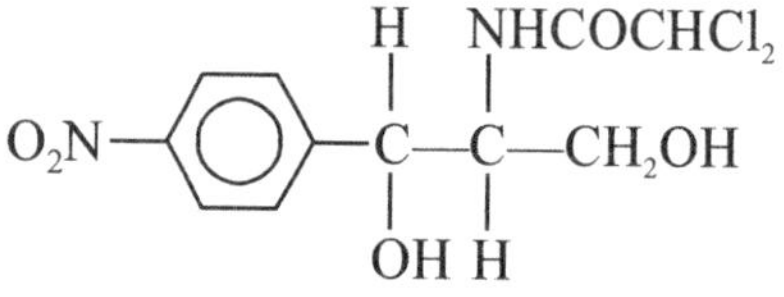

Chloramphenicol

(*d*) **Penicillium O (*Syn:* Panicillium AT):** It is an antibiotic produced by *Penicillium chrysogenum*.

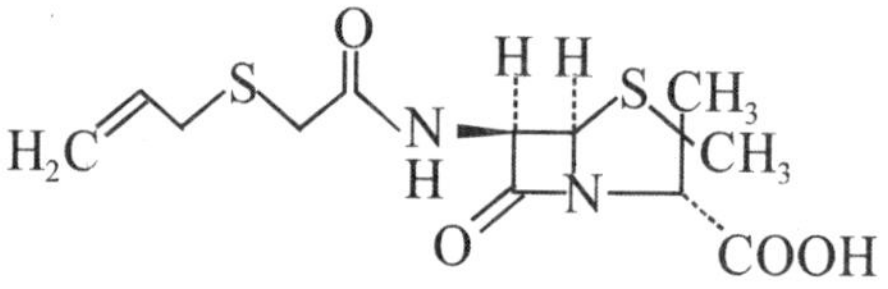

Penicillin O

1.4.1.4.7 Mixtures: A good number of naturally occurring plant substances contain a mixture of constituents, namely:

(A) Tannins:

(*a*) **Hydrolyzable Tannins**	:	**Examples:**
Chest Nut	:	Bark and wood;
Oak	:	-do-
Sumac	:	Leaves;
Turkish Tannins	:	Galls of *Cynips tinctoria*
(*b*) **Consensed Tannins**	:	**Examples:**
Eucalyptus	:	Bark;
Black catechu	:	Hearthwood;
Spruce	:	Bark;
Gambier	:	Leaves and Twigs
(*c*) **Pseudotannins**	:	**Examples of drug containing pseudotannins are as follows:**

Gallic acid	:	Rhubarb;
Catechins	:	Acacia; catechu; cocoa; guarana;
Chlorogenic acid	:	Nux-Vomica; coffee; mate;
Ipecacuanhic acid	:	Ipecacuanha

(B) Volatile Oils : **Examples**
(Syn: Essential Oils)

Oil of Chenopodium	:	p-Cymene; α-terpinene; l-limonene; methadiene;
Oil of Cinnamon	:	Cinnamaldehyde; eugenol; cinnamyl acetate;
Oil of Cloves	:	Eugenol; acetyleugenol; caryophyllene; vanillin; furfural;
Oil of Bitter Orange	:	d-Limonene; citral; decyl aldehyde; linalool; terpineol; methyl anthranilate;
Oil of Juniper	:	Pinene; cadinene, camphene; terpineol; juniper; camphor

(C) Resins:

Examples:

(a) **Rosin (Syn: Colophony: Yellow resin):** It is obtained as a residue left over after distilling off the essential oil from the oleoresin obtained from *Pinus palustris* and other species of *Pinus*.

(b) **Guaic (Syn: Guaiacum; Resin guaic)**	:	**It contains**
α-and β-Guaiaconic acid	:	$\simeq$ 70%;
Guacic acid + Guaiaretic acid + Related compounds	:	11%;
Vanillin + Guaiac Yellow + Guaiac Saponin (Guaiacin)	:	1.5%

(D) Latex:

Examples:

(a) **Opium Latex:** It is the air-dried milky exudation from incised unripe capsules of *Papaver somniferum L.,* or *P. album* Mill. It contains about 20 alkaloids, constituting about 25% of the opium, meconic acid, sulphuric acid and lactic acid, sugar, resinous and wax-like materials.

(b) **Euphorbia (Syn: Cat's hair; Snake weed; Queensland; Asthma weed; Pill bearing Spurge):** It is obtained from the dried herb of *Euphorbia hirta L.,* or *E. pilifera L.* It contains several resins and an unstable glucoside.

FURTHER READING REFERENCES

1. **'Biochemical Evolution of Plants'** in *Comprehensive Biochemistry,* Vol. 29A, M. Florkin. and E.H. Stotz (Eds.), Elsevier, Netherland, 1974.
2. **'Biochemical Systematics',** in *Plant Taxonomy,* 2nd ed., V.H. Heywood, Edward Arnold, London, 1976.

3. Grifo F *et al. in Bio-diversity and Human Health,* Grifo F and Rosenthal J (Eds) Island Press, Washington D.C., 1997.

4. Hamburger M and Hostettmann K: **Bioactivity in Plants—The Link between Phytochemistry and Medicine,** In: *Thirty Years of Phytochemistry* (1961-1991) *Phytochemistry,* **30**(12), pp. 3849-3874, 1991.

5. **'Handbook of Medicinal Herbs',** J.A. Duke, CRC-Press, London, 1st Edn., 2001.

6. Jack T: **Molecular and Genetic Mechanisms of Floral Control,** *Plant Cell,* **16,** S1-S17, 2004.

7. Jeevaratnam K *et al.*: **Biological Preservative of Foods—Bacteriocins of Lactic Acid Bacteria,** *Ind. J. of Biotech.,* **4**(4), 446-454, 2005.

8. Miller JS: *in Sampling the Green World,* Stuessy TF and Sohmer SH (Eds). Columbia University Press, New York, 1996.

9. Paul L Huang *et al.*: **Developing Drugs from Traditional Medicinal Plants: Chemistry & Industry,** pp. 290-293, 1992.

10. Radenbaugh K: **Syn Seeds: Applications of Synthetic Seeds to Crop Improvement,** CRC Press, Boca Raton (USA), 1993.

11. Topssell KBG: **Natural Product Chemistry: A Mechanistic, Biosynthetic, and Ecological Approach,** Apotekarsocieteten, Stockholm, 1997.

12. **'Toxicology and Clinical Pharmacology of Herbal Products'.** M.J. Cupp (Ed.), Humana Press, New Jersey, 1st Edn, 2000.

2 Pharmacobiotechnology

- Introduction
- Theory
- Important Means in Biotechnology
- Recombinant Proteins
- Biotechnology *Vs* Modern Pharmacy Practice

- Biotechnology Based Pharmaceuticals for the Millennium
- Biotechnology and Modern Drug Discovery
- Further Reading References

2.1 INTRODUCTION

In a broader-sense **"biotechnology"** may be defined as—'*the use of organism or enzymes for the large-scale production of useful substances ranging from not only agricultural products, food products and environmental science but also in the field of medicinal compounds, vaccines and diagnostics*'.

Interestingly, Robbers *et al*.* (1996) coined an altogether newer terminology called the **Pharmacobiotechnology** so as to specifically refer to the wide application of **"biotechnology"** to the development of *pharmaceuticals* or *pharmaceutically active substances*.

The 1980s proved to be a golden–era in the field of **biotechnology.** In this particular decade science has virtually conquered the peak of **"Everest"** when it really became absolutely possible to detect, isolate and decipher the large congregation and wide–spectrum of natural proteins that invariably play a major role in coordinating the various functions extremely critical and vital to human life and health. Thus for the first time the numerous complicated processes that were mostly responsible as the root-cause of a plethora of mysterious major and dreadful ailments have been unearthed successfully and hence, could be modulated duly.

In short, this upcoming, innovating and fool proof comparatively newer developing methodology has made an ever-lasting impact that more or less embraced the unique-top-notch blending of meaningful discoveries from various diversified fields, such as:

- Recombinant DNA–technology
- Molecular biology,
- DNA-alteration

---

* Robbers, J.E.; Speedie, M.K. and Tyler, E., '*Pharmacognosy and Pharmacobiotechnology*', Williams & Wilkins, London, 1996.

- Gene-splicing,
- Genetic engineering,
- Immunology, and
- Immunopharmacology

into an wonderful perfect scientific blend of high-tech-state–of-the-art industry.

Though, at present the viability and potential of newer range of pharmacobiotechnologically developed products is almost facing a staggering fate *vis-à-vis* the stringent US-FDA regulation and Drug Laws in the other countries of the world, it is expected earnestly with a great hope and wishful desire that in the new millenium quite a few of them , which are at present under critical phases of trials, would see the light-of-the-day with a thunderous bang to improve the quality of life of the human suffering due to the host of dreadful ailments.

It is, however, pertinent to mention here that in the recent past a number **'biotechnology-based products'** have already made a gainful entry into the Western World. A few typical examples are mentioned below:

Actimmune[(R)]	:	For chronic granulomatous disease,
Betaseron[(R)]	:	For relapsing ,remitting multiple sclerosis,
Epogen[(R)]	:	For treatment of anemia associated with chronic renal failure,
KoGENate[(R)]	:	For treatment of haemophilia A,
Leupine[(R)]	:	For autologus bone marrow transplantation,
OncoScint[(R)] **CR/OV**	:	For detection,staging and follow up of colorectal and ovarian cancer, and
Proleukin[(R)]	:	For renal cell carcinoma.

2.2 THEORY

Since 1953, the epoch making discovery of a 3D structure of DNA by the help of exclusive X-ray diffraction studies carried out by Watson and Crick* (1953) there has been a tremendous quantum growth in the development and application of **biotechnology.** These advancements shall be briefly highlighted at this juncture so as to ascertain the much–deserved-acclaim of this nescent technology not only in the field of drugs but also in various aspects of our day-to-day life, namely:

    (*i*) Mutation, Crossing-over and Recombination at Meiosis:
    (*ii*) Third revolution in modern medicine,
    (*iii*) Genetic code,
    (*iv*) Collection of specialized cells,
    (*v*) Reverse transcriptase,
    (*vi*) 3D-Proteins,
    (*vii*) From nervous systems to immune systems,
    (*viii*) Body's defence mechanism,
    (*ix*) PCR-in Forensic and Research,

---

* James Watson and Francis Crick, 1953 (Nobel Prize, 1962).

    (*x*) DNA-Metabolic Pathways,

   (*xi*) Recombinant vaccinia vector, and

  (*xii*) OKT3-Monoclonal Antibody.

2.2.1 Mutation, Crossing-over and Recombinant of Meiosis

'**Mother nature**' has been actively engaged in carrying out silently an wonderful task of 'natural' genetic experiments since the past several billion years. The outcome of these splendid and meticulous experiments are as follows:

Mutation (or Random Heredity Alteration)

It has been exploited judiciously in enhancing the yield of antibiotic and strain selection. Thus the initial yield of penicillin from **Penicillium notatum** Westling, amounting to 4 mg L^{-1} and from **Penicillium chrysogenum** Thom, amounting to 40 mg L^{-1} has been increased to a phenomenal extent of 21,000 mg L^{-1} by the **utilisation of mutation and strain selection.**

Crossing Over

It essentially refers to the simultaneous breakage and exchange of corresponding segments of the homologous chromosomes. The relentless efforts of inbreeding (hyberdization) experiments invariably give rise to a better new species, such as:

     (*i*) *Improved strains of cereals*: wheat, corn, rice producing much more yield per acre,

    (*ii*) *Improved versions of fruits*: seedless-grapes, seedless-watermelons, larger and sweeter oranges, larger and bulky tomatoes,

   (*iii*) *Improved versions of vegetables*: larger potatoes, pumpkins, tubers, cucumbers, etc.,

   (*iv*) *Improved hyberdization*: Tangelo due to crossing the tangerine with the grapefruit,

    (*v*) *Improved hyberdization in animals*: Alsetian Dogs-due to cross breeding of a German shephard dog with a wild-wolf; mule-due to crossing a donkey and a horse.

Recombination at Meiosis (or Fertilization): The innovation of such processes have brought about a revolution to the status of present diversity of life on various parts on this globe.

2.2.2 Third Revolution in Modern Medicine

According to Sadee* (1987) not only the physical characteristic features but also the gross-structures of each and every organism basically originated by virtue of the genetic code inherited and actually present within the nucleus of each cell. The major building blocks responsible for the architectural design of the cell are due to the essential components like carbohydrates, lipids, proteins and nucleic acids. Eventually the **enzymes**, which are nothing but a special class of proteins, invariably build and use such types of molecules in the course of a cell-life, *viz.*, maturation, maintenance and finally reproduction. Deoxyribonucleic acid (DNA) is the central point wherein the code for building the proteins in a cell takes place. In fact, DNA is the **genetic blueprint** of an organism. It essentially

---

  * Sadee, W. 'A Third Revolution in Modern Medicine. The World and I, Washington Times, Washington D.C., Pt I (Nov), 178; Pt II (Dec), 162 (1987).

comprises of nucleotides that are appropriately connected together in a sufficiently lengthy structure which more or less looks like a ladder.

2.2.3   Genetic Code

The human *genome** contain appropriately three billion nucleotide units of which four different nucleotides essentially comprise of the bases, namely: *adenimine, cytosine, guanine* and *thymidine* that are compactly stored into the **chromosomes.** Importantly, these possess the genetic code for about one million different type of gene. Now, each of these genes controls and regulates the synthesis of a protein that is made up of a long chain-like-sequence of amino acids ranging in number from 50 to 1000. Nirenberg *et al.* (1966) and Khorana (1966) for the first time in the world accomplished successfully the determination of the **genetic code,** In fact, they proved scientifically the manner whereby the inherent nucleotide sequence present in a gene actually regulates the particular sequence wherein the requisite number (say 20) of individual amino acids shall be combined to produce a specific protein molecule. It has been observed that one single codon is comprised of three necleotides placed in a series; and every codon represents one specific amino acid. Thus, the very sequential arrangement of a codons in the DNA, following transcription into messanger RNA (*i.e.*, mRNA), eventually establishes the particular sequence of amino acids that will ultimately give rise to a specific protein. In short, both **molecular biology** and **biotechnology** has one common goal to achieve, that is to decepher the manner by which the genes and their corresponding proteins help in the management and control of basic cellular processes.

2.2.4   Specific Sets of Genes in Each Individual Organ

It has been observed that each organ, which is nothing but a collection of specialized cells, possesses some very specific sets of genes. Since, essential organs of the body, such as: brain, heart, liver, tissue, blood etc is tantamount to carry out a certain exclusively particular set of jobs, they are supposed to be triggered of for activation and followed up by deactivation *i.e.*, turned "on" and "off" as and when required by the system.

Thus, under the supreme command of the genetic code of DNA and subsequently mediated by mRNA a broad-spectrum of proteins are duly generated by every individual cell in a continous fashion. A good number of these highly specific and specialized proteins are consumed within the cell itself, whereas the remaining are secreted directly into the extra cellular fluid. It is assumed justifiably that over a certain long duration and bearing in mind the enormous possible permutation and combination of nearly 500 amino acids, that each organism would have evolved a reasonably large excess of unique proteins having optimized characteristic functions.

2.2.5   Reverse Transcriptase (RT)

The basic underlying principle of **'modern biology'** rests on the fact stated below:

---

* **Genome:** The entire DNA capable of expressing all the genetic information in the cell.

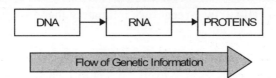

In 1970, another landmark was established with the advent **reverse trancriptase (RT)** which was responsible for the actual conversion of its own genomic RNA into a double-stranded RNA. It is, however, pertinent to mention here that the latest trends in biotechnogy profusely bank upon this particular enzyme (RT). A few typical and glaring examples of RT, sometimes also refered to as **cellular catalyst's** are enumerated as under:

- Produce the chemical building blocks of cell life, for instance: fats and carbohydrates.
- To carry out the digestion of food.
- Generate hormones which in turn regulate and monitors organism,
- Severe as fuel for energy production, and
- Production of important molecules like DNA.

2.2.6   3D-Proteins

In true sense, the proteins are responsible for the creation of the cell cytoskeleton which ultimately gives rise to an organised three-dimensional (3D) structure. Generally speaking, the proteins not only help in the transport but also regulates the movement of various molecules throughout the cellular structure. They are strategically located in the outer-cell-membrane and aids in the transportation of ions as well as nutrients across the cell-membranes Proteins play various vital roles as described below briefly:

(*a*) Regulate gene-activity by binding to DNA.
(*b*) Both proteins and peptides (smaller fragments of proteins) are usually secreted by cells as hormones like **insulin** and as **neurotransmitters.**
(*c*) Caters as carrier molecule such as hemoglobin to act as body's oxygen transport mechanism, and
(*d*) Serve as receptor sites for various hormones which in turn tunes up the cell-function as per the varying pattern of body's requirements.

2.2.7   From Nervous System to Immune System

It is virtually an open-secret that 'hormones' not only influence directly a good number of specific-cell-surface-receptors but also more or less on all functions of the body right from the **nervous system to the immune system.** By virtue of the fact that these hormones are capable of exerting highly selective, potent and above all hitting the bullseye by affording a specific action on the selective target cells have gained a wide recognition as a most promising and viable candidate for a new generation-drug in terms of the '**magic-bullet'** hypothesis laid down by Ehrlich. These hormones have the following **merits,** namely:

- When given parenterally they approach the target receptors just on the outer-periphery of the cells without even penetrating the membranes, and

- Capable of binding to **cell-surface-receptors** intimately thereby activating the cell's specific function instantly;

Example: Interleukin–2, which is still an experimental anticancer substance, may triger stimulation to certain immune cells so as to exert a direct influence on cancerous cell-growth.

2.2.8 Body's Defence Mechanism

The so called **'immune system'** of the human body actually governs its defence mechanism against all sorts of pathogenic invading organisms. The *two* vital factors that have a direct influence on the body's defence mechanism (immune system) are, namely:

    (*a*) **Memory:** the capability of recognizing and responding immediately to the previously encountered infections; and

    (*b*) **Specificity:** the capability of concentrating directly on the specific pathogens.

    The various cells which are solely responsible to the spectrum of immune responses are – **Phagocytic cells (macrophages); B-cells; Suppresor T-cells; Helper T-cells; Killer T-cells** and **Natural Killer (NK) cells;** and **Memory cells.**

2.2.9 PCR–in Forensic & Research

The DNA research on the **polymerase chain reaction (PCR)** has turned out to be a very efficacious and useful technique in the specialised field of forensic as well as research applications. Many mysteries from the scene of murder, hither to impossible to detect precisely, has now been made easy with the blood-strains collected from the victim. Likewise, the authenticity of fraternity may be established beyond any reasonable doubt with the help of DNA studies.

2.2.10 DNA–in Metabolic Pathways

The recent developments in the field of **metabolic engineering** has made a tremendous impact on the intermediary metabolism with a big bang. A few typical examples whereby DNA helps in the metabolic pathways are enumerated below:

- To facilitate and solve the branch-point-control problems,
- Introduction of identical enzymes obtained from different sources into the studied organism has brought to light not only improved and newer degree of flexibility but also introduced much better and acceptable metabolic characteristics into the older mechanism.
- To increase copies of a gene at a rate-controlling point,
- To remove a poisonous product by the addition of a single specific gene
- To accomplish an altogether new pathway into an organism that otherwise ceases short of the desired product by addition several genes.

2.2.11 Recombinant Vaccination Vector

It is now known that the **vaccinia virus** may be used as a **molecular vehicle** for transporting **foreign genes** into other organism. With the advent of both extensive and intensive research it is quite possible to exploit this **recombinant vaccinia vector** to act as a vehicle for the production of **live vaccines** for otherwise difficult ones to produce.

2.2.12 OKT3–Monoclonal Antibody

Antibodies are regarded as the body's **missile defence mechanism.** These are large protein molecules produced by WBC which seek out and destroy dreadful foreign substances. They are used gainfully in matching donors and recipients in organ transplantation, in blood typing, in the measurement and identification of hormones, toxins and various antigens in blood and fluids. The remarkable use of monoclonals as a pinpoint attack on a cancerous cell or to eradicate cells left after a conventional **chemotherapy.** They may also be utilized to transport drugs, radioactive particles and toxins to such cells. Recently, **OKT3 monoclonal antibody** has been duly cleared and approved by the US-FDA for the treatment of acute renal allograph rejection.

2.3 IMPORTANT MEANS IN BIOTECHNOLOGY

There are a number of ways and means whereby this wonderful ever-expanding field of **biotechnology** has gained enough recognition to be identified as a top-brass zone of research. A few such important tools of technology shall be discussed in the sections that follows:

2.3.1 Recombinant DNA (rDNA)

It may be defined as—**"the hybrid DNA produced by joining pieces of DNA from diferent sources".** It is usally designated as **rDNA.**

Recombinant DNA is normally formed outside the living cell with the aid of highly critical enzymes termed as **'restriction enzymes'** which will essentially cleave the DNA at particular sites. Subsequently, another type of enzymes known as **'ligases'** will help to insert the cut piece of DNA (called the **'insert'**) directly into the **Vector DNA** (*i.e.*, **viral DNA** or **plasmid**). The resulting vector DNA shall be capable of entering conveniently into a **'host'** cell or otherwise called as **microorganism.**

It is pertinent to mention here that once the **foreign DNA** (or **vector DNA**) gains an entry into the microorganism (*i.e.*, host organism), it is known as a **"recombinant organism".**

2.3.2 Restriction Enzymes

Restriction enzymes are also known as **'restriction endonucleases'.** They are found to **'digest'** DNA into corresponding short strands at very particular sites which is exclusively governed by the following *two* factors, namely:

(*a*) By a four-base-system *i.e.* four different nucleotides containing the bases – **adenine, cytosine, guanine** and **thymidine;** and

(*b*) By a relatively larger stretch of **specific DNA sequence.**

Restriction enzymes, infact just act as a pair of **"molecular scissors".** Evidently, the longer the number of bases that command a particular cleavage-site for a specific enzymes, the less frequently it will afford a cut to a long strand of DNA.

Table 2.1 illustrates the examples of a few **restriction enzymes*** and their cleavage sites respectively:

Table 2.1   Examples of Restriction Enzymes

Name of Enzymes	Generating Organism	Cleavage Site
Pvu1	Proteius vulgaris	CG ⌐ ATCG GCTA ⌐ GC
Hpa1	Haemophilus parainfluenzae	GTT | AAC CAA | TTG
Eco R1	Escherichia coli	G ⌐ AATTC CTTAA ⌐ G
Sau 3A1	Staphylococus aureus	GATCZ CTAG

Most restriction enzymes have either **'sticky ends'** or **'blunt ends'**.

2.3.3   DNA–Ligase

It has been observed that the DNA pieces cut with the same enzyme shall possess **'sticky ends'** which would anneal under the appropriate and favourable conditions when such 'pieces' are pooled together. The resulting annealed pieces usually exhibit only single strands (termed as **'nicks'**) at the specific sites where they were actually cleaved. When such mixed pieces are treated with an enzymes, termed as **DNA – ligase,** it will ultimately give rise to an **intact piece of recombinant DNA** by the combination of phosphodiester bond (at the ends of the DNA strands) with the complementary bases **(adenine, cytosine, guanine** and **thymidine).**

2.3.4   Cloning Vector

A **cloning vector** may be a **plasmid**** or a **bacterophage*****. In **genetic engineering** (*i.e.*, **gene cloning techniques)** – a gene having a close resemblance to a particular protein shall be joined together with a **cloning vector** so as to enable it get transferred into a host cell.

---

* (*a*) **Restriction enzymes** are named by using the **first letter** of the **genus name** combined with the **first two letters** of the **species name;**

   (*b*) **Strain** is designated by a capital letter (*e.g.* Eco R1) or an arabic numeral and a capital letter (eg Sau 3A1) and Roman numerals follow immediately to specify individual enzymes when a given microbe has more than one.

** These are self replicating, double-stranded, circular DNA molecules which are invariably found and maintained in the respective host-cell as an independent extrachromosomal moiety. They are normally characterised by specificity of host, size, and copy number.

*** They are viruses that infect bacteria. These are employed as cloning vectors. The foreign DNA is usually inserted into the viral genome in an analogous fashion. At times the genes could be eliminated from the bacteriophage to result a vector that might infect cells but not kill the infected cell; thus, the DNA may be expressed within the recipient bacterial cell.

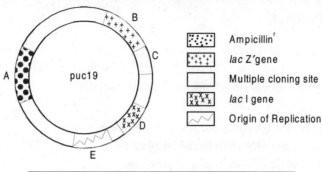

![Ampicillin pattern]	Ampicillin^r
![lac Z gene pattern]	*lac* Z'gene
![Multiple cloning site]	Multiple cloning site
![lac I gene pattern]	*lac* I gene
![Origin of Replication]	Origin of Replication

Fig. 2.1   Genetic Map of Plasmid puc19

Figure 2.1 represents the genetic map for a **plasmid puc 19** that has been used in cloning where,

        A = Ampicillin,
        B = *lac* Z gene,
        C = Multiple cloning site
        D = *lac* 1 gene, and
        E = Origin of replication.

Here, the **plasmid** contains an ampicillin resistance gene (A) that permits only the selection of plasmid – bearing organism. The multiple cloning site (C) possesses a member of restriction enzymes sites. It essentially exists very much within the *lac* **Z gene (B)** which in turn encodes β-galactosidase. In fact, **isopropylethiogalactoside (IPTG)** induces B that eventually interferes with the binding process of the repressor proteins encoded by (D) to the (B) promoter. In this manner (B) undergoes depression ultimately leading to its subsequent *transcription* and *translation*. At this juncture, any foreign genes strategically inserted into the **multiple cloning site** (C) shall positively interfere with the production of β-**galactosidase activity.** However, these would be expressed by themselves either from the promoter belonging to the gene or from the *lac* **Z gene (B)** promoter.

2.3.5   Hybridization Probes

Hybridization probes constitute another extremely important and vital technique exclusively meant for **genetic engineering.** In reality, probe is nothing but a complementary **sequence of DNA** that is specifically labelled with anyone of the **three** different means namely:

    (*a*) A radioactive substance,
    (*b*) A fluorescent material, and
    (*c*) A chromagenic material.

    Probe DNA or probes may be either **larger segments of DNA** or **synthetic oligonucleotides** or even **whole plasmids.** In usual practice, the DNA which is subjected to probe shall be conveniently bound to a solid support that could be either nitrocellulose or nylon. The product thus obtained is heated in a mixture clong with the **probe DNA.** Subsequently, the strands would separate and reanneal thereby allowing the probe to bind with its complementary sequence. Consequently, the resulting product shall determine the very presence of that segment of DNA by rendering the **hyberdized DNA** either **chromogenic or fluorescent or radioactive.**

2.3.6   Cloning Process

Literally it refers to – *'a cutting used for propagation'*. In the present context cloning means, to make identical copies. The recent advances accomplished in the field of *"Biotechnology"* the **cloning process** has been exploited in the following *six* aspects, namely:

(*i*)   DNA–cloning,
(*ii*) Cloning larger DNA fragments in specified cloning vectors,
(*iii*) Cloning Eukaryotic DNAs in bacterial plasmids,
(*iv*) Cloning Eukaryotic DNAs in phage genomes,
(*v*)   Cloning cDNAs, and
(*vi*) Expression cloning.

The above diversified **cloning processes** shall be dealt individually as under:

2.3.6.1   DNA–Cloning

The **DNA cloning** is nothing but a broad based technique whereby large quantum of a particular DNA-segment are produced. Usually, the resulting DNA segment which is to be cloned is first linked to a vector DNA, that serves as a vehicle for carrying foreign DNA into a suitable host cell, such as the bacterium *Escherichia coli*. The **vector** *(i.e., E. coli)* essentially contains sequences which in turn permits to be replicated within the host cell. In order to clone DNAs within bacterial hosts two types of vectors are commonly employed, namely:

(*a*) The DNA segment to be cloned is introduced into the bacterial cell by **first** joining it to a plasmid and **secondly**, causing the bacterial cells to take up the plasmid from the medium, and

(*b*) The DNA segment is joined to a portion of the **genome** of the bacterial virus lambda (λ) which is subsequently allowed to infect a culture of bacterial cells. Thus, a huge quantum of viral progeny are produced, each of which contains the foreign DNA segment.

It is, however, pertinent to mention here that by following either of the two methods stated above—the DNA segment once gets inside a bacterium, it will undergo the replication process with the bacterial (or viral) DNA and partitioned to the daughter cells (or progeny viral particles). In this manner, the actual number of bacterial cells which are actually formed.

Besides, **cloning** may also be employed as a versatile method to **isolate in a pure form any specific DNA fragment** amongst a relatively large heterogeneous population of DNA molecules.

2.3.6.2   Cloning Larger DNA Fragments in Specified Cloning Vectors

It has been observed that neither plasmid or **lambda phage** (λ) vectors are adequately suitable for **cloning DNAs** whose length is more than 20-25 kb*. This specific lacuna has revitalized the interest of researchers to look into the development several other vectors which might facilitate to clone much larger **segments of DNA.** However, the most important of these vectors are termed as **yeast artificial chromosomes (YACs)**

---

* **[Kilobase (kb)]:** A 1000 – base fragment of nucleic acid. A *kilo base pair* is a fragment containing 1000 base pairs.

YACs are nothing but artificial versions of a normal yeast chromosome. They normally comprise of all the elements of a yeast chromosome which are absolutely necessary for the specific structure to be replicated during **S-phase** and subsequently segregated to **daughter cells** during **mitosis,** including:

- One or more origins of replication,
- Having telomers at the ends of the chromosomes, and
- A centromere to which the spindle fibers may get attached during chromosome separation.

Invariably, the **YACs** are designed in such a fashion so as to provide essentialy:

(*a*) A gene whose encoded product permits those particular cells having the **YACs** to be selected from those that lack the element, and

(*b*) The **DNA fragment** to be cloned like other cells, subsequently the yeast cells shall pick up DNA from their respective medium that caters for the path whereby **YACs** are introduced directly into the cells.

It has been observed that **DNA fragments** cloned in **YACs** range typically from 100kb to 1, 000 kb in length. *Example:*

'The **restriction enzyme** usually recognizes the eight-nucleotide sequence GCGGCCGC, which in turn specifically cleaves mammalian DNA into fragments approximately one million base pairs long'.

Fragments of this length can now be introduced conveniently into **YACs** and subsequently cloned within host yeast cells.

2.3.6.3 *Cloning Eukaryotic* DNAs in Bacterial Plasmids***

A **foreign DNA** intended to be cloned is strategically inserted into the plasmid to give birth to a **recombinant DNA** molecule. However, the plasmid used for DNA cloning are exclusively the modified versions of those occurring in the bacterial cells. Consequently, the bacterial cells are able to take up DNA from their medium. This particular phenomenon is termed as *'transformation'* and forms the basis for **cloning plasmid in bacterial cells.**

Figure 2.2 represents the DNA cloning using bacterial plasmids. First of all the recombinant plasmids each containing a different foreign DNA insert are added to a bacterial culture (*E.coli*) which has been previously treated with Ca^{+2} ions. These bacteria are gainfully stimulated to take up DNA from their respective surrounding medium upon exposure to a brief thermal-shock treatment yielding **plasmid DNA** (purified). Secondly, **human DNA** are also obtained in the purified form. Subsequent treatment of **human DNA** and **plasmid DNA** with EcoR1*** result into the cleavage of human and bacterial DNA into various sized fragments. Now, these small fragments join together to yield recombinant DNAs with DNA ligase and thus give rise to the *plasmids*. These population of plasmids invariably contain various segments of **human DNA.** Incubation of these plasmids with

---

* **Eukaryote:** A cell or organism having a unit membrane–enclosed (true) necleus and has no extracellular form.

** **Plasmid:** An extrachromosomal genetic element that is not essential for growth and has no extracellular form.

*** **EcoR1:** Enzymes designation for *E. coli* with reocgnition sequence G AA* TTC [arrow indicate the sites of enzymatic attack; indicate the site of methylation].

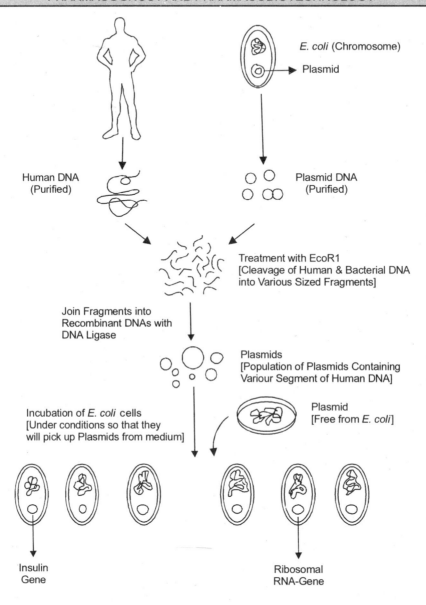

Fig. 2.2   DNA Cloning Using Bacterial Plasmids

E coli cells under controlled experimental parameters ultimately yield plasmid that are free from *E coli*. It has been observed that only a very small percentage of the cells are competent to pick up and retain one of the combinant replicate molecules. Once it is taken up the plasmid undergoes replication autonomously within the recipient and is subsequently passed on to its progeny during cell division. The isolated **recombinant plasmids** can then be treated with the same restriction enzymes used in their formation, that releases the **cloned DNA segments** from the remainder of the DNA which served as the vector. Thus, the **cloned DNA** can be separated from the **plasmid.**

2.3.6.4 Cloning Eukaryotic DNAs Phase Genomes

A *bacterophage*, or more commonly a *phage* is a virus particle which infects a bacterial cell. In fact, a phage particle normally comprises of *two* essential components: first, *a phage head* that contains the genetic material and secondly, *a tail* through which the genetic material is injected into the host cell.

Interstingly, one of the most broadly explored of these phage particles, termed ***Bacteriophage Lambda [or bacteriophage (λ)]***, has more or less turned out to be a commonly employed **cloning vector***.

The **genome**** of lambda is a linear and double-stranded DNA molecule having 50kb length.

Figure 2.3 depicts the protocol for **cloning eukaryotic DNA** fragment in lambda (λ) phase.

In usual practice, the modified strain **(mutant)***** employed in most cloning experiments contains two cleavage sites for the enzymes EcoR1 that ultimately fragments the genome into *three* large segments. However, the two outer segments essentially contain all informations required for the infectious growth, whereas the middle fragment could be rejected conveniently and replaced suitably by a piece of DNA upto 25 kb in length.

It has been observed that the genes of eukaryotes are often split, with non-coding intervening sequences–known as *introns*, thereby separating the coding regions—termed as *exons.* The two outer segments undergo *splicing*† with **eukaryotic fragment** to result into the formation of recombinant DNA. Consequently, the recombinant DNA molecules can be packaged into phage heads *in vitro* and in turn these genetically engineered phage particle may be employed to infect host bacteria. Once gaining entry into the bacteria, the **eukaryotic DNA segment** is adequately amplified along with the viral DNA and subsequently packaged into an altogether new generation of virus particle that are released when the cell undergoes *lysis*††. The released particle thus obtained infect new cells, and without any loss of time either a *plaque*††† or a clear spot in the '*bacterial lawn*' is visible distinctly at the site of infection. Each **plaque,** which is nothing but a **zone of lysis,** possesses millions of phage particle, each carrying a single copy of the same **eukaryotic DNA segment.** Interestingly, a single pertridish may accommodate more than 10, 000 different plaques.

2.3.6.5 Cloning cDNAs

It is pertinent to mention that the explanation of **cloning cDNAs** has been specifically restricted to cloning DNA fragment isolated from extracted DNA *i.e.,* genomic fragments. In other words, the isolation of a genomic DNA means the eventual isolation of a particular gene or a family of genes out of a pool of hundreds of thousands of unrelated sequences. Besides, it becomes more or less necessary to study the following different aspects during the course of isolation of **genomic fragment,** namely:

---

 * **Vector:** A genetic element able to incorporate DNA and cause it to replicate in another cell.
 ** **Genome:** The complete set of genes present in an organism.
*** **Mutant :** A strain differing from its parent because of mutation.
 † **Splicing :** The processing step whereby introns are removed and exons are joined.
 †† **Lysis:** Rupture of a cell, resulting in a loss of cell contents.
††† **Plaque:** A zone of lysis or cell inhibition caused by virus infection on a lawn of cells.

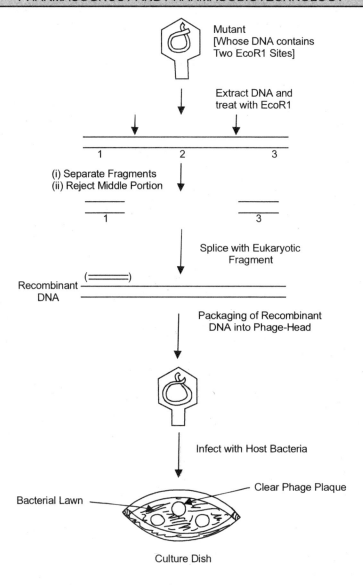

Fig. 2.3 Sequence for Cloning DNA Fragments in Lambda (λ) Phage.

- Non-coding intervening sequences,
- Regulatory sequences flanking on either sides the coding portion of a gene,
- Different members of a multigene family that invariably lie very close in the genome,
- Evolution of DNA sequences, such as: duplication and DNA of various species *vis-a-vis* their rearrangement, and
- Interspersion of transposable genetic elements'.

There are **two** aspects which are very important with **cloning cDNAs,** namely:

(*a*) Analysis of gene structure, and

(*b*) Analysis of gene expression.

Figure 2.4 illustrates the manner by which cDNAs are synthesized for cloning in a plasmid.

In order to **clone cDNAs,** *first* of all a sizable population of mRNA is isolated; *secondly*, it is employed as a template to provide a single-stranded DNA complement; *thirdly*, the resulting product (single stranded) is duly converted to a double stranded population with the help of a DNA polymerase; and *fourthly*, they are finally combined with the desired vector. It is quite evident that essentially

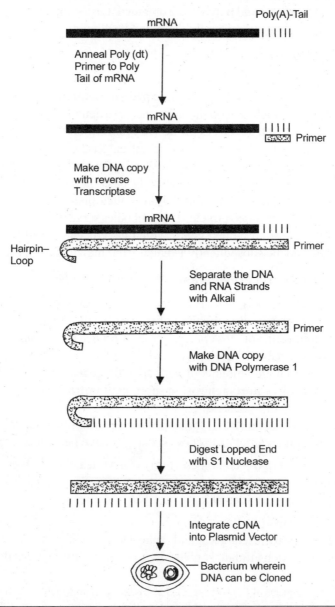

Fig. 2.4   Synthesis whereby cDNAs get Cloned in a Plasmid.

mRNA populations typically consist thousands of altogether different species, and as with experiments employing genomic DNA fragments, the clones should be invariably screened to isolate only one particular sequence from a heterogeneous population of recombinant molecule.

From Figure 2.3, it may be observed that when polypeptide (A) and mRNA are annealed, it provides a small segment of primer attached to poly(A) to the tail of mRNA. Now, with the help of **reserve transcriptase** the primer to poly(A) gets fully developed. Alkali helps in the separation of DNA and RNA strands to give rise to fully developed primer alone, which on treatment with RNA polymerase 1 yields the combined product. The resulting product when digested with S1 nuclease two separate strands of the primer and poly(A) are obtained. Lastly, integrate cDNA into the **plasmid vector** that will produce a bacterium wherein DNA can be cloned.

2.3.6.6 *Expression Cloning*

For practical applications it is quite important that such systems must be available wherein the cloned genes may be expressed. In other words, **expression cloning** is an alternative method for identifying a *phage plaque* which essentially contains a particular cDNA. In this specific method the cDNA being cloned is inserted directly in the downstream region from a strong bacterial promoter, which adequately ensures that the foreign DNA is not only transcribed but also translated in the course of the infections process. Interestingly, those phage which has originally incorporated the gene being sought must form plaques that essentially possess the protein encoded by the gene. Further identification of the plaque is performed on replica plates of employing a labeled probe which binds particularly to the encoded protein. The antibodies serve invariably as the most commonly used probe to identify the desired cloned genes which have been critically located on the replica plate whereas the genes may be subsequently isolated from the viruses on the original plate.

2.3.6.7 *Amplifying DNA: The Polymerase Chain Reaction (PCR)*

The *conventional molecular cloning techniques* may be considered *in vivo* DNA–amplifying tools. Interestingly, the latest development in the field of **synthetic DNA*** has evolved an altogether new method for the rapid amplification of DNA *in vitro*, broadly termed as the *Polymerase Chain Reaction* (PCR). In reality, PCR is capable of multiplying DNA molecules to the extent of a billion fold *in vitro*, thereby giving rise to huge amounts of very specific genes employed for various purposes, such as: **cloning, sequencing** or **mutagenesis.** In short, PCR utilizes the enzyme DNA polymerase, which eventually copies DNA molecules.

The polymerase chain reaction (PCR) for amplifying specific DNA sequences have been shown in Figure 2.5 [*Stage–A* through *Stage–F*]. These six stages have been duly explained here under:

Stage–A: The target genes (DNA–combined form) if *first* heated to affect the separation of the strands of DNA; *secondly*, a reasonably excess amount of two **oligonucleotide primers****, of which one is complementary strand, is added along with DNA-polymerase;

Stage–B: As the resulting mixture attains the ambient temperature, the excess of primers relative to the target DNA makes sure that most target strands anneal to a primer exclusively and not to each other. In this way, the primer extension ultimately gives rise to a copy of the original double-stranded DNA.

---

* **Synthetic DNA**—short fragments of DNA of specified base sequence and widely used in molecular genetics.

** **Primers:** A molecule (usually a polynucleotide) to which DNA polymerase can attach the first nucleotide during DNA replication.

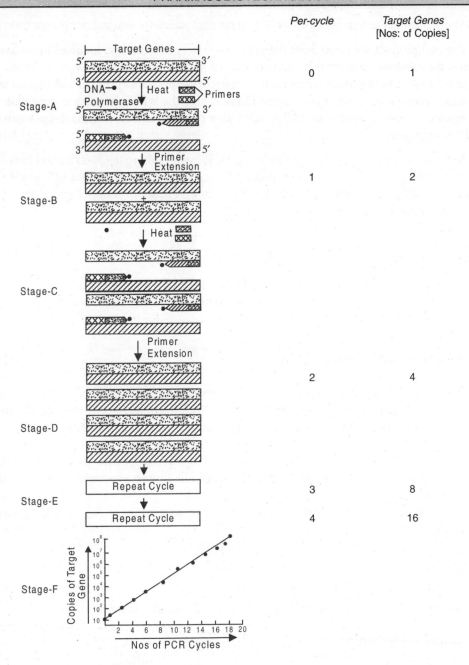

Fig. 2.5   PCR for Amplifying Specific DNA Sequences (Stage–A through Stage–F)

Stage–C: Further follow up of *three* above mentioned steps sequentially *viz*; *heating*, *primer annealing* and *primer extension* results into the formation of a copy of the original double-stranded DNA. In other words, **DNA polymerase extends the primers employing the target strands as a template.**

Stage-D: Another primer extension of the resulting product yields the second double-stranded DNA.

Stage-E: The end product obtained from the previous step is subjected to incubation for a suitable duration; and the resulting mixture is heated once again so as to separate the strands. Subsequently, the mixture is brought to the room temperature whereby the primers aptly get hybridized with the complementary regions of newly synthesized DNA. Thus, the whole process is repeated. In this particular instance, the two additional PCR-cycles give rise to 8 and 16 copies, respectively, of the original DNA sequence.

Stage-F: It represents a plot between the number of PCR cycles (along the X-axis) and the copies of the target gene (along the Y axis). The graphical illustration depicts the effect of carrying out 20 PCR cycles on a DNA preparation initially having only 10 copies of a target gene. The resulting graph is **semilogarithmic** in nature.

Advantages of PCR–Technique

PCR-technique has **two** cardinal advantages, namely:

(*a*) Each and every cycle virtually doubles the content of the original target DNA, and

(*b*) A 10^6 to 10^8 fold increase in the target sequence is actually achieved after a 20-30 PCR cycle run.

2.4   RECOMBINANT PROTEINS

After accomplishing the isolation, cloning and sequencing of a gene, it becomes absolutely necessary to express it in an appropriate *expression** system which could be either **fungal, bacterial mammalian tissue culture,** or **insect tissue culture.** The inclusion of a host organism together with the *specific vector*** gives rise to an expression system. At this juncture a *promoter**** not only augments relatively high yields of protein but also yields a secreted protein by sheer manipulation. It is, however, pertinent to mention here that the criteria of selecting an expression system are namely: economic factors and the structure of proteins.

The production of **recombinant proteins** and peptides can be accomplished to a fairly reasonable extent by the following *three* techniques, namely:

(*a*) Bacterial systems,

(*b*) Gylcosylation, and

(*c*) Mammalian tissue culture expression systems.

These techniques shall be discussed briefly in the sections that follows:

2.4.1   Bacterial Systems

It essentially makes use of the microorganism *E. coli* which being considerably inexpensive, but unfortunately they fail to yield an active protein invariably. Ideally, a constant endeavour is always

---

* ***Expression:*** The ability of a gene to function within a cell in such a way that the gene product is formed.

** ***Vector:*** An agent normally an insect or other animal, able to carry pathogens from one host to another. OR A genetic element able to incorporate DNA and cause it to be replicated in another cell.

*** ***Promoter:*** The site on DNA where the RNA polymerase begins transcription.

made to look for cheaper, dependable and reproducible methods whereby newer active protein is produced first on a smaller scale and then scaled up to a pilot and finally to the commercial scale without any compromise on the quality of protein.

It has been observed that the proteins produced by bacterial systems essentially have an **N-formylmethionine** (designated as '**f-Met**') at the N terminus because that is considered to be a critical signal for the exact initiation of *translation,** to a stage whether either a cleavage site is introduced or the resulting protein is cleaved and secreted in the process.

It has been observed that when proteins are overexpressed in a bacterial system of *E.coli*, they exhibit a tendency to aggregate in intracellular bodies usually termed as ***inclusion bodies.*** They may prove to be either beneficial or harmful for the subsequent protein recovery that could be accomplished by anyone of the following *two* methods usually adopted.

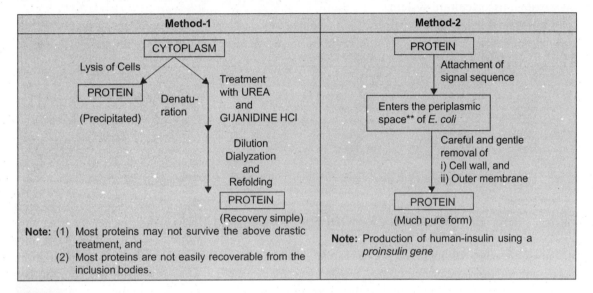

2.4.2 Glycosylation

Glycosylation mainly contributes in enhancing the molecular weight of several mammalian glycoproteins. It also helps in modifying activity of the protein of choice. It has been observed that the eukaryotic proteins which are usually either secreted or inserted in membranes enter through the golgi apparatus and endoplasmic reticulum right into the eukaryotic cell and are duly glycosylated during this particular phenomenon. *O-glycosylation* takes place upon threonines or serines in the protein sequence, whereas *N-glycosylation* occurs exclusively at the aspargine residues which are essentially part of the sequence.

Precisely, a recombinant protein which has duly undergone the process of glycosylation for improving its activity should be produced only in the eukaryotic cells. Thus, **glycosylation** may be accomplished by using specific yeast cells, such as:

---

* ***Translation:*** The synthesis of protein using the genetic information in a messenger RNA as a template.
** ***Periplasmic space:*** The area between the cytoplasmic membrane and the cell wall in gram negative bacteria (*e.g. E. coli*).

Yeast		Characteristics
Saccharomyces cereviseae	:	Attached oligosaccharides having more than 100 mannose residues.
Pichia pastoris	:	Transfection* with a baculovirus expression system.

2.4.3 Mammalian Tissue Culture Expression Systems

The **mammalian tissue culture expression systems,** for instance: *Chinese hamster ovary cells*, are invaribaly transfected with a *viral vector*. In reality, they require a very complex media for the production of protein, besides the entire process shows slower growth and very poor yields thereby making it an expression system. Of course, there exists an ample genuine scope whereby the exhorbitant cost may be brought down considerably by the advent of more stable and more efficient mammalian tissue culture systems.

Once a protein has been developed by the help of biotehnology it is essential that its identification and determination of its purity is established by known modern–analytical techniques, such as:

Characteristics		Techniques used
Molecular Weight of Protein	:	Polyacrylamide electrophoresis to assess any proteolytic, cleavages
Bioactivity	:	Bioassay;
Charge	:	Isoelectric focussing electrophoresis to assess any amino acid substitution;
Hydrophobicity or charges	:	High performance liquid chromatography
In charge		to assess folding errors;
Purity	:	Capillary electrophoresis and pyrogenicity;
Confirmation of identity	:	X-ray crystallography with respect to initially identified protein.

2.5   BIOTECHNOLOGY *VS* MODERN PHARMACY PRACTICE

In the recent past, **'biotechnology'** has already gained a tremendous magnitude of commendable success in the most upcoming field of modern pharmacy practice. These multifold plus points may be further expatiated with the help of the following *four* cardinal aspects, namely:

(*a*) A host of *modern drug substances* available in the therapeutic armamentarium belong to the class of **protein** and **peptides.** Therefore, they essentially require prime consideration towards their stability, dosage forms, storage, administration and lastly the probable side-effects as compared to the relatively much smaller synthetic drug molecules;

(*b*) The proper selection of the recombinant products would heavily depend upon not only the correct choice of the expression system but also the small differences existing in the structure which may result from the use of various known expvression systems;

(*c*) A plethora of new drug class have evolved as a result of the advent of more in-depth knowledge of pathophysiology besides newer modes of therapies for such diseases that could not be successfully treated earlier; and

(*d*) A good number of **'diagnostic products',** available in the form of **'kits',** are solely based on *monoclonal antibody technology.* They have been exclusively developed for the proper

---

* **Transfection:** The transformation of a prokaryotic cell by DNA or RNA from a virus.

diagnosis of *thyroid disorders, anaemia, fertility for pregnancy, allergies, cancer,* and finally the *management of several hormone-related imbalances* (*i.e.,* disorders). In short, *diagnostic products* represent one of the **largest biotech startups.**

It is worth while to mention here that since the world-wide recognition of **biotechnology** an enormous progress has already been accomplished in modern pharmacy practice. A few typical and classical instances shall be cited as under, namely:

(*i*) Human proteins as drugs,

(*ii*) New Drug Classes,

(*iii*) Vaccines,

(*iv*) New Diagnostic Agents, and

(*v*) DNA probes and RELP analysis.

The aboresaid various aspects shall now be treated individually in the sections that follows:

2.5.1   Human Proteins as Drugs

It has been established beyond any reasonable doubt that DNA, the genetic material, not only directs the production of the proteins which essentially comprise the structure of, but also regulate the processes in the living system.

Genetic engineering fundamentally comprises of picking up a particular gene from a chromosome of one brand of organism and then inserting the same into the chromosome of another. In other words, **genetic engineering** is nothing but a sheer manipulation of DNA in a deliberate and controlled manner. It really allows the wisdom and skill of biotechnologists to lay hand on specific individual components of complex living systems and subsequently produce them on a large-scale either in comparatively much simple micro-organisms or mammalian cells inside fermentation tanks.

However, the production of human proteins exclusively by the aid of **genetic engineering** exclusively guided by the following *three* factors, namely:

(*a*) Ability to isolate the DNA of interest,

(*b*) Selection of an appropriate organism (*e.g. E. coli; B. subtilis*) wherein the selected DNA is first inserted and then produced and

(*c*) Ability to extract and purify the resulting product after fermentation.

Various categories of human proteins are invariably used as drugs, such as: **hormones, blood products** and **lymphokines.** These specialized proteins shall be discussed briefly as under:

2.5.1.1   Hormones

Interestingly, hormones are relatively simple protein molecules that usually serve as a medium organ-to-organ communication in the body. Examples:

1. **Human Insulin: Insulin** is a protein essential for correct sugar metabolism and is produced in the body by the pancreas. *Humulin*[R] (Eli Lily) was the first approved and marketed clinical product produced by recombinant DNA technology in *E. coli* (1983). Soonafter in 1987, NOVO–

a Danish company evolved a continuous process for the production of genetically engineered human insulin from *yeast cells.*

2. **Calcitonin gene-related peptide(CGRP): Calcitonin** being a thyroid hormone which helps in the regulation of calcium retention in bones. It has been observed that patients either suffering from **Paget's disease*** or post menopausal condition thereby rendering the bones structurally weakened. **Cloned CGRP** was developed by Sandoz (Basel, Switerland) with a view that the peptide could be useful in the treatment of cardiovacular diseases.

2.5.1.2 Blood Products

Interestingly, more than fifty proteils naturally occurring in human blood have been successfully cloned either in mammalian cells or in *E.coli*, but only a handful of these have gained access for detailed clinical studies. A few typical examples will be cited below:

(*a*) **Tissue Plasminogen Activator (tPA)**: It is a protein generated by the body cells that is exclusively involved in the dissolution of unnecessary and unwanted blood clots. However, tPA is formed by natural cells of the body exactly in a similar manner as the interferons, but the former is produced in such a small quantity that its isolation in sizable quantities poses a difficult problem for its ultimate utility either in research or medicinal purposes. With the advent of biotechnology it is now possible to *clone* the **human tPA gene** into bacterial cells and thus produce any amount required. When tPA is administered intravenously to a patient suffered from heart attack, it reaches directly to the culprit blood clot that blocks the cardiac vessel thereby acting as a *'Cardiac-drano' i.e.* it helps in clearing off the blocked passage quickly and swifty.

(b) **Factor VIII**: The **genetically engineered Factor–VIII** is used exclusively for the treatment of haemophillia.

2.5.1.3 Lymphokines

Lymphokines represent a class of small proteins, which essentially include substance like: **interleukins, interferons** and **tumour-necroses factor,** and are usually secreted most naturally by cells of the immune system. They exert a *hormone-like action* through cell-to-cell interactions rather than spread out over the entire body. Perhaps this aspect offers a clear line of demarcation with regard to their usage as pharmaceutical substances as most drugs need to be administered systemically.

Examples: A few typical examples of **lymphokines** are enumerated below along with their applications in therapeutic domain:

(*i*) **α-Interferon:** for rare cancer *hairy cell leukemia;*

(*ii*) **Interleukin–2:** for cancer

(*iii*) **Tumour Necrosis Factor (TNF)**–for killing tumour cells and causing a generalized wasting syndrome.

---

* **Paget's disease:** A chronic form of osteilis with thickening and hypertrophy of the long bones and deforming of the flat bones.

2.5.2 New Drug Classes

The **recombinant DNA technology** has paved the way in the management and control of a number of diseases related to body's immune system. In the past two decades the US-FDA approved quite a few recombinant DNA products that are being used as drugs across the world. Recently, the exact role of **cytokines** has been revealed in order to understand the intricacies of the relatively complex immune system.

The most recent and epoch-making developments with regard to the new drug classes are the *novel vaccines, proteins, hormones, glycoprotein, blood-clotting proteins* and *immunoactive drugs*. A few typical examples have been enumerated in Table 2.1, to stress upon the versatility of newer **recombinant DNA products.**

Table 2.1   Approved Biotechnology Medicines

S. No.	Name of the Product	Brand Name (Mfg. Co.)	Indication
Vaccines:			
1.	Hepatitis B vaccine	Engerix B(R) (Smith Kilne Beecham)	Hepatitis B prevention. Comprise of highly specific antibodies that more or less act as *'magic bullets'*.
2.	Human Insulin	Humulin(R) (Eli-Lilly); Novalin(R) (Nova Nordisk)	To combat insulin dependant diabetes; it is the first human health product used in medicine.
Proteins			
3.	Interleukin- 2 Recombinant	Proleukin(R) (Chiron/ Cetus)	For metastatic renal cancer. A protein drug through which immune cells communicate with each other.
4.	Interferon Alfa-2a, Recombinant	Roferon-A (Hoffman-LaRoche)	For hairy cell leukemia; AIDS related Kaposi's sarcoma; Antiviral activity, especially against RNA Viruses; Enhances the targetting of monoclonal antibody-tethered cytotoxic drugs to cancer cells.
5.	Interferon alfa – 2b, Recombinant	Intron-A (Schering Alferon) (Interferon Sciences)	For hairly cell leukemia; AIDS related Kaposi's sarcoma, chronic hepatitis types B & C; *Condylomata acuminata*.
Hormones:			
6.	Somatropin	Humatrope(R) (Eli-Lilly); Protropin(R) (Genentach)	Identical to human pituitary derived somatropin; for human growth hormone deficiency in childern.
7.	Calcitonin	Cibacalcin(R) (Ciba); Miacalcin(R) (Sandoz) Calcimar(R) (Rhone-Poulenc Porer)	To decrease osteoelastic activity thereby inhibiting the movement of bone salts from bone to the blood; also decreases renal tubular secretion of calcium.
Glycoprotein (Purified)			
8.	Alteplase Recombinant	Actirase(R) (Genentech)	For acute mycocardial infarction; Pulmonary embolism.

(Contd.)

(Table 2.1 contd.)

S. No.	Name of the Product	Brand Name (Mfg. Co.)	Indication
Blood Clotting Proteins:			
9.	Antihemophilic Factor	Profilate[R] (Alpha) Hemofil T[R] (Hyland); KoGENate[R] (Miles); Recombinant[R] (Baxter)	For the management and control of severe hemorrhage in the patient with hemophilia A.
Immunoactive Drugs:			
10.	Muromonab CD3	Orthcloue OKT3 (Ortho)	For acute alograft rejection in renal transplant patients; and cardiac transplant patients.

2.5.3   Vaccines

Vaccine is a suspension of infectious agents, or some part of them given for the purpose of establishing resistance to an infectious disease. Traditionally, vaccines comprise of *four* general classes, namely:

(*a*) Those containing living attenuated infectious organisms, for example, **vaccine for poliomyelitis;**

(*b*) Those containing infectious agents either by chemical or physical means, for instance: *vaccines used to protect human beings against typhoid fever, rabies and whooping cough.*

(*c*) Those containing soluble toxins of microorganisms sometimes used as such, but usually forming toxoids such as : *vaccine used in the prevention of diphtheria and tetanus*, and

(*d*) Those containing substances extracted from infectious agents, for examples: *capsular polysaccharides extracted from pneumococci.*

At this juncture, it is worthwhile to draw a line between the **traditional vaccines** as stated above and the **recombinant vaccines** (or **subunit vaccines**) obtained exclusively by the aid of genetic engineering techniques known so far are described below:

S. No.	Traditional Vaccines	S. No.	Recombinant Vacines (or Subunit Vaccines)
1.	Prepared either by attenuating or killing the pathogens with a view to disabling the disease causing function of the pathogens.	1.	By the help of genetic engineering techniques it is quite possible to eliminate the potential vaccine induced illness by separating effectively the *immune activation function of pathogens* from the disease producing functions.
2.	Immune activating molecules remained unharmed.		
3.	Modified pathogens on being injected into a subject induce immunity to the modified pathogen thereby preventing the disease.	2.	First , all the gene(s) solely dedicated for encoding the cell surface molecules that eventually trigger the immune activation function is isolated.
Disadvantages:		3.	Secondly, these genes are removed from the pathogens genome by endonuclease action and subsequently inserted into a cloning vehicle that later on employed to transform either a bacteria (*E. coli*) or yeast (*Saccharomyces cereviseae*) host cell.
(*a*) In certain instances, the *whole virus vaccine (i.e., the attenuated pathogens)* invariably revert back to their virulant state in the produced disease in the vaccinated subject rather than preventing it,			

(Contd.)

(*Table contd.*)

S. No.	Traditional Vaccines	S. No.	Recombinant Vacines (or Subunit Vaccines)
	(*b*) Possibility of certain pathogens being escaped from attenuation (or being killed). (*c*) Impurities may be incorporated through the method of production based on different *animal species. They may be removed by very tedious and exensive procedures.* **Advantages:** Inspite of various serious adverse reactions they have been used successfully in combating diseases like; Polio, Small pox, Yello fever, Measles, Mumps, Tetanus and Diphtheria.	4. 5. 6. 7.	A series of antigenic molecule are synthesized by the host cells that may be suitably isolated, purified and made into a vaccine. When this recombinant vaccine is injected into a subject, the individual affords an immune response against the antigen. The synthesis of suitable memory B cells is the net result of the immune response. The immunized subject on being exposed to a pathogen that essentially bears that specific antigen on its cell surface, the resulting immune response swifty erradicates the pathogen totally. **Advantage:** As it contains only the immune-activating subunit* of the pathogen, it is incapable of inducing the disease state in the subject.

* **Recombinant vaccines** only contain a subunit of the original pathogen, hence they are also termed as **'Subunit Vaccines'**.

2.5.3.1 Specificity of Vaccines

Whether it is a *whole virus vaccine* or a *subunit vaccine* both exert their action by including an immune response against a specific subset of molecules that could be the reason why a vaccine specifically prepared against one influenza strain fails to response against an altogether different strain. Based on this observation the health authorities in hospitals and OPDs always advise the youngsters, the elderly ones and above all the chronic ones to receive the shot against influenza every year periodically. It has been duly observed that each outbreak of flu is invariably caused by a different and newer influenza virus which means logically to produce new vaccines with each outbreak of the disease. The same logical explanation holds good for polio whereby three different strains give rise to three types of vaccines to control and prevent the same disease.

2.5.3.2 Search for AIDS Vaccines

Human Immunodeficiency Virus (HIV) belongs to the class of viruses termed as *retroviruses* which differ from most of the cell types. Here they usually comprise of RNA as their only major genetic material in comparison to the more common DNA. It has been observed that whenever a HIV virus infects a cell it not only injects its RNA but also the specific genetic material usually an enzyme termed as *reverse transcriptase.* Now, the reverse transcriptase affords the synthesis of a DNA molecule complementary to the viral RNA inside the host cell. Thus the virally derived DNA exert the *'infective assault'* upon the host cell and ultimately leads to a condition commonly known as **Acquired Immunodeficiency Syndrome (AIDS).**

It is pertinent to mention here that HIV is not adequately suitable for production of vaccine by virtue of the following *four* aspects, namely:

(*a*) Being an extremely complex virus it may conveniently get lost in the inner portion of the infected cells thereby leaving absolutely no trace of viral antigens on the cell surface. At the end, the overall immune system may appear to behave as if no outside viral were ever present, (*b*) Unfortunately, till date no appropriate animal model has been established for human HIV infection, which has slowed down the active research and subsequent screening through an elaborated experimental laid-down procedure.

(*c*) Consideration of ethical aspects with regard to human screening of any probable and potential AIDS vaccines, and

(*d*) HIV possesses its unique ability to insert pieces of its self-genome right in the genome of the infected host, thereby rendering the genetic material invisible to the respective host human-system.

Keeping in view the above serious limitations encountered a good number of **AIDS vaccines** have been prepared meticulously and tested adequately. A few such examples are illustrated below:

(*i*)	**Thymosin Alpha 1** (Immunomodulator) Manufactured by Alpha 1 Biomedicals (Bethesda, MD)	: For AIDS in combination with PEF-II-2 and Retrovir[R] (under Phase I/II Clinical Trial)
(*ii*)	**Soluble CD4** (Product of Recombinant DNA technology)	: This protein interacts with HIV and thereby blocks its attachment to intact CD4 T cells.

2.5.4   New Immunodiagnostic Agents

Immunodiagnostic agents are regarded as stranded tools in the physicians diagnostic regimens. They afford an improved testing technology whereby diagnosis could be faster, cheaper and easier.

2.5.4.1 *Monoclonal Antibodies (MABs)*

Antigen recognition by antibodies, that more or less acts like an anchor in body's defence mechanism system to combat dreadful diseases, has been judiciously explored for quite sometime towards the logical development of newer diagnostic tests for various ailments making use of antibodies from animal sources.

Hybridoma Technology The **hybridoma technology** is the process whereby the fusion of an immortal cell with a lymphocyte to produce an immortal lymphocyte. In other words, the antibody producing cells are duly fused with the respective tumour cells which results into the production of a hybrid that could be grown in an appropriate laboratory culture and which reproduces antibodies of a single specificity **(monoclonal antibodies).**

The tremendous growth in the field of **pharmacbiotechnology** in the recent past has broadened the scope of monoclonal antibodies (MABs) in *two* vital aspects of immunodiagnostics, namely:

    (*i*) MABs in diagnostics, and

    (*ii*) MABs in Imaging and Therapy.

2.5.4.2 *MABs in Diagnostics*

More recently MABs have gained rapid and wide recognition into the ever-expanding field of health-care diagnostics. There are usually *four* important techniques that find their utility in diagnostics, for instance:

(a) **Immunoassays:** Most immunoassays make use of radioactive antibodies [*i.e.* **radio-immunoassays (RIA)**] whereby the sample showing positive test which allow the antibody to get bound to it and thus the radioactivity will be retained onto the sample. However, the stringency and authenticity of RIA tests mostly restrict it to centralized specialist disgnostic facilities exclusively;

(b) **Enzyme Immunoassays (EAI):** In this particular instance a specific colour-producing enzyme is coupled to the antibody. Thus, the outcome of the results may be read either directly by a naked eye or spectrophotometerically;

(c) **Enzymes- Cascade Technique*:** Here, several enzyme reactions taking place are coupled to generate an appreciable amplification of the original binding signal which is either read by a naked eye or spectrophotometerically; and

(d) **Fluorescence Immunoassays (FIA) and Luminescence Immunoassays (LIA):** Precisely, these are nothing but related techniques wherein the *'lable'* either exhibits fluorescence or light respectively.

Examples:

1. **Pregnancy Dipstick Test:** Based on MABs the pregnancy dipstick test determines the pregnancy either at home or in a clinical laboratory.

2. **Ovulation Dipstick Test:** Another dispstick test based on MABs ascertains the positive or negative ovulation in a subject , and

3. **AIDS Test:** MABs based AIDS test kit is available to identity its presence in donated blood sample(s).

2.5.4.3 MABs in Imaging and Therapy

Ironically, the most acute and severe hinderances ever encountered in the treatment of cancer virtually lies in the fact that *malignant cells* have a very close resemblance to the *normal cells*. It is, therefore, quite possible that the therapeutic agents that are actually intended to destroy (kill) malignant cells also destroy normal cells perhaps due to their close similarity. However, it has been established beyond any reasonable doubt that the surfaces of malignant cells do differ in certain respects from those of normal cells. As we have seen earlier that MABs only recognise specific antigens on cells, they are being fully exploited to image cancerous tumours particularly in an intense on-going clinical research programme and in therapy against a variety of malignancies, such as: lymphomas, melanomas, colon and breast cancer.

A few typical examples have been duly expatiated below, namely:

(a) **Glastrointestinal Cancer**:** MABs is employed singly to combat gastrointestinal cancer. The underlying principle being that when the antibodies opt to bind to the turnover, they invariably exhibit a tendency to attract the cells of the immune system to act against the prevailing cancerous tissue.

(b) **Lung, Breast, Prostate and Pancreas Cancer:** It is however, pertinent to mention here that enough research activities have triggered off in the recent past towards the development of monoclonal conjugates of *two* important class of drugs namely:

---

* Developed by I Q (BIO) in Great Britain.

** A collaborative research by Centocor (USA) & Hoffman – LaRoche (Switzerland).

(*i*) **Anthracycline Drugs*:** Such as antibodies having quinones and related structures, eg. Adriamycin[R] (Adrio); Bufex[R] (Bristol);

(*ii*) **Desacetyl Vinblastine**:** When desacetyl vinbiastin *ie.* a chemical enity obtained either from the plant source or produced by plant cell culture, is conjugated to a monoclonal which consequently acts specifically on lung, prostate, breast and pancreas malignant cells.

(*c*) **Drug Targetting and Tumour Imaging:** Another theory of **drug targetting** *vis-s-vis* **tumour imaging** is based on the use of highly specific and relatively *small molecular size toxins* [*e.g.*, castor seed) and toxin from bacteria (microorganism source)] conjugated with monoclonals. It has been observed that the same monoclonals that are being employed to target may also be used to image tumours via conjugation to radioactive elements. Once the conjugate has been injected, whole-body-scanning methods may be carried out to localize and quantify the malignant thereby helping the physicians either to intiate a preliminary diagnosis or to ascertain if the patient is giving due response to the conventional therapy.

2.5.5   DNA Probes and RFLP Analysis

Probe that are specific to different *genes* as well as *DNA fragments* have paved the way for the diagnosis of a number of prenatal problems. Besides, the genetic probes makes it possible to establish future outset of some ailments for instance: emphysema (*i.e.*, pathological distention of interstitial tissues by gas or air) and Huntington's disease (*i.e.*, an inherited disease of the CNS which usually has its outset between ages 25 and 55).

The cross section of **recombinant DNA** and medicine invariably occurs when genetically engineered probes help in the cure and management of human ailments. DNA probe is a radioactive labeled DNA fragment that acts as a complementary to a particular gene or gene segment. Thus, suitable probes may be employed to analyse not only the abnormal genes but also the human genome, Interestingly, prenatal medicine makes use of probes to ascertain the presence of the genes in some ailments, namely: *Cystic fibrosis**** and *Tay-Sachs disease*****.

In addition, **DNA probe** is considered to be the most versatile and powerful technique for the identification of individuals.

The application of **DNA probe** as diagnostics has been extended to test for AIDS, understand the course and causes of cancer, genetic disease (*e.g.*, *muscular dystropy, sickle cell anaemia*) and bacterial infections (*e.g.*, *walking pneumonia, Legionnaire's disease*).

Restriction Length Fragment Polymorphism (RELP) Analysis   Each and every human being born on this earth essentially inherits one set of genes from its father and another one from its

---

* A collaborative research of Carbo-Erba (Italy) and Cytogen (New Jersey, (USA).

** Eli – Lilly (USA).

*** A single gene defect manifesting in multiple body systems as chronic obstructive pulmonary disease, pancreatic exocrine deficiences, urogenital dysfunction and abnormally high electrolyte concentration in the sweat.

**** An inherited disease transmitted as an autosomal recessive trait. Because of the lack of the enzymes hexosaminidase A, which is important in sphingolipd metabolism, sphingolipids accumulate in the cells, especially those of the nerves and the brain. Death normaly occurs before the age of 4. There is no specific therapy.

mother which in most cases have been found to be identical. Invariably, mutation of genes that one inherits from one or other of one's parents ultimately leads to diseases like muscular dystropy and haemophilia. Besides, these distinct differences occurring between the two sets of DNA there exists many thousands of relatively *'Silent'* differences usually termed as **restriction length fragment polymorphisms (or RELP).**

The enormous progress made in the field of *biotechnology* has made it possible to afford the diagnosis of genetic defects prenatally. The following steps are performed sequentially:

(*a*) Cells from the growing foetus are first drawn by sophisticated methods, namely: **Chorionic vili sampling and aminocentesis,**

(*b*) DNA preparations are subsequently made by standard methods,

(*c*) Specific enzymes that chop DNA in strategic positions are usually employed so as to trace **'silent'** genetic markers and also the **RELPs,** associated with the prevailing ailments,

(*d*) Carrying out a close comparison between the *'pattern of silent genetic markers'* on the foetal DNA and those on the paternal and maternal DNA, it is now relatively possible to ascertain with a high degree of probability, whether the foetus under investigation is either normal or diseased.

In addition to the above mentioned diseases **RELP analysis** has also been judiciously and effectively extended to some more gruesome diseases such as: *schizophrenia, Alzheimer's disease* and *complications of heart.*

2.5.6 Enzyme Linked Immunosorbant Assay (ELISA)

The unique covalent attachment of enzymes to antibody molecules provided an immunological method that not only affords high specificity but also high sensitivity. **ELISA** utilizes antibodies to which enzymes (*eg: peroxidase, alkaline phosphatase* and *3-galactosidase* have been covalently bound in such a fashion that neither the enzyme's catalytic characteristics nor the antibody's specificity are changed.

It is however, pertinent to state that **ELISA** may prove to play a major role in pin-pointing the early diagnosis of plethora of human ailments or medical conditions that are of major public health significance, for instance:

Diseased Condition	Primary(P)/Confirmatory (C)
• Pregnancy	P
• Leprosy (*Mycobacterium leprae*)	P
• Syphillis (*Treponema pallidum*)	P
• Tuberculosis (*Mycobacterium tuberculosis*)	C
• Leishmaniasis	C
• Hepatitis	P
• AIDS	P
• T3-T4, TSH (Thyroid hormones)	P

In fact *two* fundamental **ELISA methodologies** are prevalent, namely:

(*a*) **Direct ELISA:** It is meant for detecting *antigen* exclusively, for instance:

   (*i*) Virus particles from faecal sample, and

   (*ii*) Virus particles from a blood sample.

Method of Testing:

   (*i*) Specimen is first added to the wells of a microtitre plate that has been duly precoated with antibodies specific for the antigen to be detected. If the antigen (*i.e.* **virus particulates**) is present in the sample, it would be trapped by the available antigen binding sites present on the antibodies.

   (*ii*) The unbound material is washed out and a second antibody (containing a **conjugated\ enzyme**) is added,

   (*iii*) As the second antibody is also specific for the antigen it gets bound to any available remaining exposed determinants,

   (*iv*) After giving a proper wash, the enzymes activity of the bound material present in every microtiter well is estimated by adding the substrate of the enzymes, and

   (*v*) The characteristic colour thus produced is found to be directly proportional to the amount of antigen present.

(*b*) **Indirect ELISA:** It is meant for detecting *antibodies* present in human serum. It is invariably employed to specifically detect antibodies to **human immunodeficiency virus (HIV).**

Method of Testing (HIV- ELISA):

   (*i*) The microtiter plates are first and foremost coated with a disrupted preparation of HIV particles (approximately 200ng of disrupted HIV particle is needed in each and every well)

   (*ii*) The resulting plates are subjected to a brief incubation period so as to ensure plates of the antigens to the surface of the microtiter wells.

   (*iii*) Now, a diluted serum sample is added and the mixture thus obtained is again incubated so as to permit **HIV–antibodies** to bind to **HIV antigens.**

   (*iv*) In order to detect the presence of antigen–antibody complexes, a *second antibody* is now introduced, which is essentially an enzyme conjugated anti-human IgG preparation,

   (*v*) Again after a short incubation (with the second antibody) followed by a washing step to ensure complete removal of any unbound second antibody, and

   (*vi*) The enzyme activity is now determined with the production of a colour which is directly proportional to the quantum of anti-human TgG antibody bound.

Note:

1. **It is a positive indication by virtue of the fact that the binding of the second antibody and the antibodies from the patients serum ultimately recognised the HIV antigens *i.e.*, the patient possesses antibodies HIV, and the same has been exposed to HIV.**

2. **Always the control sera* are also assayed simultaneously along with any sample(s) so as to measure the extent of background absorbance in the particular assay.**

---

* **Control sera:** which is known to be HIV–negative

However, the **'Indirect ELISA-Test'** for the detection of antibodies to HIV, the casual agent of AIDS, has been depicted in Figure 2.5 along with the various sequential procedural details for both positive and negative test *vis-à-vis* the graphic representation between the quantum of antibody and the intensity of the colour produced.

2.6 BIOTECHNOLOGY BASED PHARMACEUTICALS FOR THE MILLENNIUM

From a recent survey (1993)* it has been broadly accepted that *biotechnology* based pharmaceuticals (or **Biotechnology Drugs**) will enhance tremendously to combat today's complex ailments. In the last two decades American Pharmaceutical concerns have grossly shifted their interest towards life-saving medicinals based solely on biotechnology that is shown by the quantum jump of their on-going research projects from a meager 2% (in 1980) through 33% (in 1993) to a maximum of upto 70% (in 1993) for larger pharmaceuticals**.

S. No.	Methodology	Positive Test	Negative Test
1.	Miceotitre wells are coated with antigen preparation from disrupted HIV particles(*)		
2.	Patient serum sample is added. HIV specific antibodies bind to HIV antigen		
3.	Washing is done with buffer		
4.	Human anti-IgG antibodies conjugate to enzymes (E⊥E) is added		
5.	Washing is done with buffer		
6.	Substrate for enzyme is added and quantity of colored product(.) is measured, which is directly proportional to the antibody concentration.		
	Colour Intensity	+ + + +	−

* Mossionghoff G: Biotehcnology medicines in Development (1993).
** Study by the Boston Consulting Group (BCG); April, 1993.

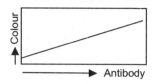

Fig. 2.6 Indirect ELISA Test for Detecting Antibodies to HIV, the Casual Agent of AIDS.

Interestingly, the **biotechnology based pharmaceuticals** for the millenium may be broadly categorised under the following *five* heads; namely:

(*i*) Genetically engineered vaccine,

(*ii*) Gene-splicing and DNA recombinant procedures,

(*iii*) Antibodies in biotechnology,

(*iv*) Gene Therapy

(*v*) 3-D Picture of the 'Lock' and 'Keys'

These different categories shall be discussed briefly in the sections that follows:

2.6.1 Genetically Engineered Vaccine

In general, **vaccines** preparations made of either *dead organisms or living attenuated microorganisms* which may be administered to man or animal to specifically stimulate their immunity to infection by the same or closely related organisms. It has been observed that once an individual's immune system has positively responded to a particular antigen, it gives rise to a state of resistance that will remain for a reasonably long period of time. Thus, *vaccines* are regarded as important **immunizing agents.**

Interestingly, many viruses invariably possess an outer-coat made of protein. When human subjects or animals become immune to virus diseases, it is achieved by virtue of the fact that their immune systems to recognize the particular *virus protein-coat* and subsequently make corresponding antibodies to it. Now, mostly the pharmaceutical concerns actively engaged in **gene-cloning** maintains a keen interest in *'yeast'* as possible host for the expression of cloned gene.

Following are the examples of some **genetically engineered vaccines,** namely:

(*a*) **Hepatitis B Surface Antigen (HBSAG):** It is prepared by cloning a coated protein gene in yeast, extracting the protein formed by the genetically altered yeast, and obtaining from it the desired vaccine. It confers immunity to **Hepatitis B** without exposure to the virus itself.

(*b*) **Viral Vaccines:** In reality, **viral vaccines** are of *two* types, namely:

(*i*) those consisting of inactivated viruses that are incapable of mutiplication in the body, for instance, *Salk Poliovaccine*; and

(*ii*) those consisting of viruses that multiply at low rates in the body, but do not exhibit the symptoms of the disease, such as: *Sabin Oral Polio Vaccine*

(*c*) **Whooping Cough Vaccine:** It is essentially a **bacterial vaccine** that consists of dead cells and provides a long-term immunity.

(*d*) **Vaccines from Live Attenuated Viruses:** Both *Small Pox Vaccine and Measles Vaccine* obtained from live attenuated viruses induce a high degree of immunity in the vaccinated subjects, effective for a long duration and thus prove to be highly effective in the control and management of the respective diseases.

(*e*) **Influenza Vaccine:** The vaccine of influenza viruses that have been grown in chick embryos and subsequently rendered non-infectious either by UV irradiation or by formalin. It prevents influenza by its parentral injection and the duration of immunity rarely exceeds a year because of the fact that the causative agent (virus) of influenza is capable of undergoing mutation rather frequently.

It is pertinent to mention here that by the turn of the century the development of **synthetic vaccines** *via* **genetic combination** and **gene cloning** would likely to promote legitimately their medicinal utility and availability.

Figure 2.7 illustrates the various steps involved for the preparation of **vaccine** from hepatitis virus by the method of **genetic engineering.**

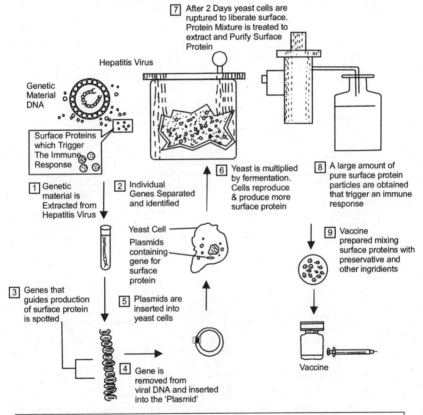

Fig. 2.7   Preparation of Vaccine from Hepatitis Virus by the Technique of Genetic Engineering

2.6.2   Gene Splicing and DNA Recombinant Procedures

The techniques invariably referred to as **'gene-splicing'** are well defined means of judiciously and constructively rearranging the genetic code to give rise to an organism with an altogether new, altered and most desirable features. It essentially comprise of the following *five* cardinal aspects namely:

(*i*) A simple microbe may be empowered to generate a specific chemical, (*ii*) This desired characteristic informative feature or product is strategically located on the DNA molecule,

(*iii*) **'Engineering'** aspect is mainly concerned with **cutting out** only that particular section of the string and subsequently grafting this into another organism.

(*iv*) **'Splicing'** is generally carried out with a specific set of enzymes termed as *'litigation enzymes',* that would help in sticking the fragments once again, and

(*v*) In fact, **'cutting'** and **'splicing'** involves more or less a very delicate surgery and these functions are actually accomplished *chemically* in solution only.

A brief description of **recombinant DNA (rDNA)** has already been made in section 3.1 in this chapter.

Figure 2.8 vividly depicts the basic **gene-splicing** and **recombinant DNA** procedures in an elaborated sequential manner.

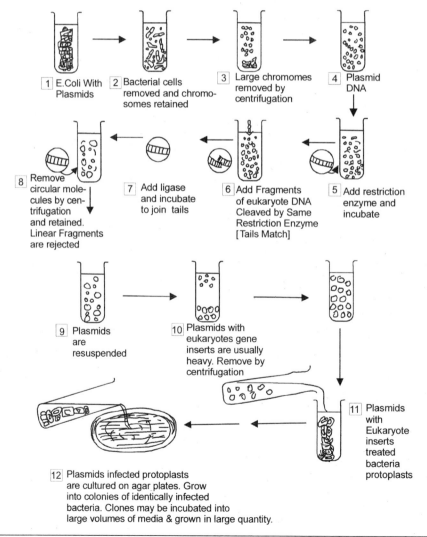

Fig. 2.8   Basic Gene Spilcing and Recombinant DNA Procedure in Sequential Order.

First of all the bacterial cells are removed from the mixture of *E.coli* with plasmids and the resulting chromosomes are retained. Secondly, the large chromosomes are removed by centrifugation and the resulting plasmid. DNA is treated with restriction enzymes and incubated accordingly. Thirdly, add to it fragments of **eukaryote DNA** cleaved by the same restriction enzymes and add ligase; incubate to join tails. Fourthly, the circular molecules are removed by centrifugation and retained, whereas the linear fragments are rejected. Fifthly, the plasmids are resuspended and the ones with eukaryotes gene-inserts being heavier are removed by centrifugation. Sixthly, these segregated heavier plasmids are treated with bacterial protoplasts, Seventhly, the plasmids infected protoplasts are duly cultures on agar plates, grown into colonies of identically infected bacteria. Finally, the resulting clones may be incubated into large volumes of media and produced in large quantity.

2.6.3 Antibodies in Biotechnology

An extremely important and versatile aspect of **recombinant DNA technology** is the application of **antibodies** in biotechnology. In fact, **antibodies** are produced by the **B-cells** (or **plasma cells**) exclusively. They are virtually composed of four protein chains that one are interconnected by *'disulphide bonds'*. It has been observed that the surface of the antibody essentially bears a highly *specific marking (or 'lock')* that would promptly recognize the particular foreign particle (or 'key') with which it readily undergoes complexation or binding. It has now been well established that different antibodies are actually generated in each individual person for their characteristic and highly specific interaction with antigens. In other words, antibodies play the role of the *immune surveillance* in the living system. Certain antibodies have the job of surveying foreign cells or molecules and mark the invading antigenic entity distinctly for destruction by other immune system cells. Consequently, the marked **antigens** are actually removed from the living system thereby leaving the unmarked ones *in situ*.

It is understood that there exists approximately 4000 strategic locations in the human genome which are responsible for various genetic disorders (diseases). Interestingly, out of this lot only 30 (*i.e.* 1200) have been studied in sufficient details. It has been observed that certain abnormalities found on the genes are usually termed as 'point mutations'. In all these instance, a single nucleic acid base present in a gene is normally replaced by a different one. Therefore, in the encoded protein the net result would be visualised by the exchange of a single amino acid.

Example: The genes encoding the *hemoglobin protein sequences* invariably possess a minimum of forty 'point mutations'.

It is pertinent to state here that the **molecular probing,** with regard to the characteristic alteration in the shape of blood cells in *sickle-cell anemia*,* would go a long way in revealing these types of abnormalities parentally, or in the early stage of life so as to make it possible to institute a suitable remedial measure or a preventive action adequately *(i.e.; 'gene therapy')*.

Figure 2.9 clearly illustrates that the manner by which genetic defects could be detected in a logical way in *foetal cells.*

It has been noticed that quite often variance do take place in the genetic code on account of error into the *chemical sequence.* The defects of this sort are invariably caused by chemical change or by inheritance and ultimately results into specific disease condition. At this particular juncture the

---

* *Sickle Cell Anemia:* The gene for sickle cell anemia is hemoglobin S. Thus each RBC has both normal hemoglobin A and abnormal hemoglobin S. These will not become sickled until extremely low concentration of oxygen occur.

prenatal examination of the *foetal cells* would help in locating the **faculty genes** and thus, identify particular subjects who may develop certain disease. The DNA is carefully removed from the *foetal cells* and with the help of an appropriate enzyme the DNA is cleaved whereby the same is unwound into respective single strands. In this particular instance, one nucleotide base (say, 'A') is defective giving rise to a situation termed as *'point mutation'*. Now, a purely synthetic DNA is manufactured in the laboratory whose genetic sequence will allow it to bind to the *'point mutation'* i.e; its 'T' with a defective 'A'. A radioactive tag (-) is then attached to the probe which is subsequently mixed with the **foetal DNA.** This specific radioactive tag makes it possible for investigators to know whether the bases get bound or not. In this particular instance (Figure 2.9), they do, thereby suggest that the foetus under investigation may develop the blood disease.

Occaissionaly variance do occur in the genetic code due to error into the chemical sequence. Defects of this by chemical change or by inheritence and results into disease condition. Timely prenatal screening may locate faulty genes & thus, identify particular subjects who may contract certain diseases.

The DNA is carefully removed from the foetal cell.

An enzyme is employed to cleave the DNA. It is unwound into respective single strands. In this instance, one nucleotide base is defective giving rise to a situation termed as a "*Point mutation*".

(a) A purely synthetic DNA is prepared in the lab. Its genetic sequence will allow it to bind to the '*Point mutation*'. (*i.e.* its 'T' with a defective 'A').

(b) This probe is mixed with the foetal DNA. The radioactive tag makes it possible for researchers to know whether the bases get bound. In this instance, they do, thereby indicating that the foetus may develop the blood disease.

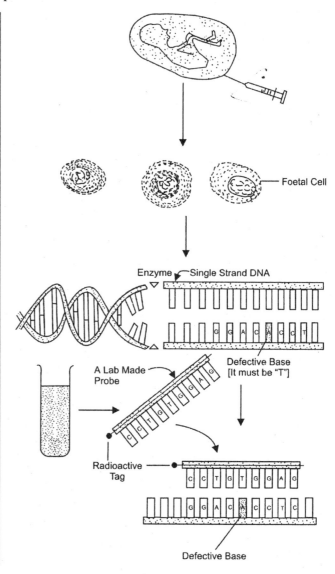

Fig. 2.9 Searching for Genetic Defects in Foetal Cell.

2.6.4 Gene Therapy

It has been adequately proved that there exists two probable cellular targets essentially required for carrying out the process of *'gene replacement therapy'* namely: the **Somatic Cell*** and the **Germ Cell****.

In the light of the ethical issues inherent in **'gene therapy'**, *five* narrowly cardinal objectives have been put forward by the scientific review committees, namely:

  (*i*) Research should be limited to somatic cells only, so that a treated individual cannot pass genetic alterations to offspring,

 (*ii*) Risk to the patient must be outweighed by the potential therapentic benefit,

(*iii*) Target diseases must be limited to those that involve a known defect in a single gene, and the normal gene must be cloned and available,

(*iv*) Disease must involve cells that can be isolated from a patient, altered in tissue culture and subsequently reimplanted in the patient, and

 (*v*) Planned well-defined procedures must meet strict safety standards in animal trials, before attempts are made with human beings.

Targets of human **gene therapy** essentially include several serious ailments such as:

(*a*) **Lesch-Nyhan Syndrome: [M. Lesch, b: 1939, William Leo Nyhan, b: 1926, U.S. Pediatricians]** A functional lack of a single enzymes *i.e. hypoxanitin – guanine phosphoridbosyl transferase,* produced by a single gene, which is essential for purine metabolism, gives rise to an inherited metabolic disease that affects only males, in whom mental retardation, aggressive behaviour, self-mutation, and renal failure are exhibited, and

(*b*) **Tumour Necrosis Factor (TNF)**: Another effort is exclusively focussed on new approaches in the treatment of cancer, whereby immune system cells known to be associated with tumours are suitably modified to produce a protein with appreciable anti-tumour activity termed as TNF. Alternatively, TNF is a protein mediator or cytokine released primarily by **macrophages** and **T lymphocytes** that helps regulate the immune response and some **hematopoietic functions.**

There are *two* factors, namely:

  (*i*) **Alpha (TNF-a)** : [*Syn*: Cachectin – produced by macrophages, and

 (*ii*) **Beta (TNF- b)** : [*Syn*: Lymphotoxin]- produced by activated CD4*** + T cells.

Interestingly, **gene therapy** is a process by which a patient is cured by altering his or her *genotype*****. **Severe Combined Immunodeficiency *(SCID)******** is treated by **gene therapy** for a variety of valid reasons, such as:

---

  * *Somatic Cell:* [Gr. Soma = body] Petaining to nonproductive cells or tissues;

 ** *Germ Cell:* A cell whose function is to reproduce the organism. It usually has a single set of chromosomes. Germ cells are called 'ova' in females and 'spematozoa' in males.

 *** *CD4:* A protein on the surface of cells that normally helps the body's immune system combat disease. HIV attaches itself to the protein to attack WBC, causing a failure of host defence.

**** *Genotype:* The precise genetic constitution of an organism (Phenotype the observable characteristics of an organism).

***** *SCID:* A syndrome marked by gross functional impairment of both humoral and cell-mediated immunity and by susceptibility to fungal, bacterial and viral infections.

(*i*) There is no possible cure for the disease and is fatal at an early age,

(*ii*) **SCID,** results from an alteration in a specific gene that has been isolated and cloned and thus is available for use in treatment.

(*iii*) **SCID,** results from the hereditary absence of a single enzymes **adenosine deaminase (ADA), and**

(*iv*) The cells that usually express a gene are a type of WBC that can be easily removed from a patient, cultured *in vitro*, genetically modified and then reintroduced into the patient by transfusion.

In the recent past, the somatic cells have been regarded as **'targets'** for **gene therapy.** It has been observed that **adenosine deaminase defficiency (ADD),** a very serious type of disorder of the immune system, takes place once in each 200, 000 newly born babies. **Adenosine deaminase (ADA)** plays a vital role for the production as well as maintenance of *two* of the most important cell types that are found to be active in the immune response, namely: **B-lymphocytes** and **T-lymphocytes.** In the absence of these aforesaid cell types the childern are susceptible to every possible infection to which they are exposed.

Examples:

(*i*) The case of David, the ***'Bubble Boy'*** from Texas (USA) in 1971, represents a typical example wherein he suffered from ADA deficiency causing severe immune dysfunction. Eventually, David had SCID and died at the age of 13 years probably due to a series of infections spread out through his entire body as a result of the *total collapse of prevailing immune systems*.

(*ii*) Blaese and Anderson (1990) isolated **T-cells** from the blood of a 4-year old girl suffering with ADD. They were successful in the transformation of these isolated T-cells with a tailor made, ***genetically nonmutant ADA gene.*** The resulting **engineered T-cells,** having the inserted **ADA gene,** were subsequently inducted to the same child through blood transfusion. The investigators had a strong prediction that the newly administered gene will not only function properly but also help in the synthesis of enough ADA to restore normal immune function required by the affected child.

2.6.5   3D Picture of the 'Lock' and 'Keys'

The explanation of **'lock'** and **'keys'** has been made in Section 2.6.3 of this chapter. With the advent of latest developments in the fields of science and technology and the unique combination of X-ray crystallographic studies, molecular mechanic calculations and supercomputers have tremendously helped in revealing the three-dimensional (3D) arrangement vividly. Based on this 3D picture of the **'lock'** scientists are in a position to design specifically shaped drug molecules **('keys')** that would conveniently fit into the active sites of the 3D protein (or the folded protein). In this way, it has really paved the way towards a quantum jump for a realistic and rational approach to drug design. It is earnestly expected that in the near future this 3D-picture of the **'lock'** and **'keys'** would certainly prove to be a great asset.

2.7 BIOTECHNOLOGY AND MODERN DRUG DISCOVERY

In the past two decades, an exponential growth has emerged in the field of modern drug discovery exclusively based on '*biotechnology*'. An unique blend of wisdom, skill, knowledge and an enormous strength of perseverance with regard to the most advanced and sophisticated techniques of **recombinant DNA technology, gene splicing, cloning of genes, genetically engineered vaccines** and the like have given birth to the discovery of a plethora of drug substances. Interestingly, these newer types of drugs would certainly prove to be beneficial in treating some of the most dreadful human ailments besides improving the quality of life.

These '*biotechnology medicines*' may be broadly categorised into *two* heads, namely:

(*a*) Approved medicines, and

(*b*) Medicines under development.

The two different categories of biotechnology medicines shall be exemplified in the sections that follow.

2.7.1 Approved Medicines

A number of medicines that have been approved by several drug authorities are enumerated below:

S.No	Name of the Product	Company	Indication (s)
1.	Activase(R) (Alteplase)	Genentech (S. San Francisco CA)	Acute myocardial infarction Pulmonary embolism;
2.	Actimmune(R) (Interferon gamme –1b)	Genentech (S. San Francisco CA)	Chronic granulomatous disease
3.	Beta seron(R) (Interferon beta – 1b)	Berlex Laboratories (Wayne, NJ)	Multiple sckerosis
4.	Cerezyme(R) (Imiglucerase)	G-enzyme	Type-1 caucher's disease
5.	Epogen(R) (Epoctin alfa)	Amgen (Thousand Oaks, CA)	Anemias of chronic renal disease; AIDS, cancer; chemotherapy
6.	Engerix-B(R) (Hepatitis B vaccine)	Smith Kline Beecham (Philadelphia, PA)	Hepatitis –B prevention
7.	Humatrope(R) (Somatropin)	Eli-Lilly (Indianapolis, IN)	Human growth hormones deficiency in childern
8.	Humulin(R) (Human insulin)	Eli-Lilly (Indianapolis, IN)	Diabetes;
9.	Intron-A(R) (Interferon alfa-2b)	Schering Plough (Madison, NJ	Hairy-cell leukemia; genital warts; AIDS-related Kaposi's sarcoma; hepatitis – C; hepatitis B
10.	Leukine(R) (Sargramostim)	Immunex (Seattle, WA)	Myeloid recognition after bone marrow trans-plantation
11.	Neopogen(R) (Filgrastim)	Amgen (Thousand Oaks, CA)	Neutropenias due to myclosuppressive chemotherapy; myeloid reconstitution after bone marrow transplantation
12.	Orthoclone OKT3 (Muromonab CD-3)	Ortho Biotech (Raritan, NJ)	Reversal of acute kidney transplant rejection; reversal of heart and liver transplant rejection
13.	Proleukin(R) (Aldesleukin)	Chiron (Emeryville, CA)	Renal cell carcinoma;
14.	Recombivax HB(R) (Hepatitis B vaccine)	Merck (Rahway, NJ)	Hepatitis B prevention
15.	Recombinate(R) (Antihmophilac factor	Baxter Healthcare/ Hyland Division	Hemophilli A

2.7.2   Medicines Under Development

A good number of medicines are in the last phase of clinical trial *i.e.*, Phase-III with regard to their development status in USA. A few typical examples of drugs under this class are mentioned below:

S. No.	Name of Product	Company	Indication(s)	(Class)
1.	P1XY 321	Immunex (Seatle, WA)	Chemotherapy-induced neutropenia and thronbocytopenia	Colony-stimulating factors
2.	Procrit(R) (Epoetin alfa)	Ortho Biotech (Raritan, NJ)	Prevention of anemi associated with surgical blood loss; autologous blood donation adjuvant	Erythropoetin
3.	Epidermal growth factor	Intraptics (Inrvine, CA)	Corneal and cataract surgeries	Growth factor
4.	Recombinant human platelet derived growth factor–BB(PDGF)	Chiron (Emeryville, CA)	Wound healing	Growth factor
5.	Nutropin(R) (Somatropin for injection)	Genentech (S. San Francisco, CA)	Turner's Syndrome*	Human Growth Hormones
6.	Beta Interferon	Biogen (Cambridge, MA)	Multiple sclerosis	Interferon
7.	Immuneron (Interferon gamma)	Biogen (CambridgeMA)	Rheumatoid arthritis	Interferon
8.	Roferon-A(R) (Interferon alfa 2a)	Hoffman Roche (Nutley, NJ)	Chronic myclogenous leukemia; Hepatitis C	Interferon
9.	Recombinant human interleukin-3	Sandoz Pharmaceutcials (East Hanover, NJ)	Adjuvant to chemotherapy autologous bone marrow transplants	Interferon
10.	Anti-LPS Mab	Chiron (Emeryville, CA)	Sepsis	Monoclonal Antibodies
11.	CentoRX (Mab)	Centocor (Malvern, PA)	Anti-platelet prevention of blood clots	Monoclonal Antibodies
12.	ES™ (Mab)	Pfizer (New York, NY)	Gram-negative sepsis	Monoclonal Antibodies
13.	Myoscint (Mifarmonab)	Centocor (Malvern, PA)	Cardiac imaging agents	Monoclonal Antibodies
14.	Antitumor necrosis factor	Miles Ine; (West Haven, CT)	Sepsis syndrome	Tumor necrosis factors
15.	Melacine (Therapeutic vaccine)	Ribi Immunothem (Hamilton, MT)	Stage III-IV Melanoma	Vaccines
16.	VaxSyn® HIV-1 (gp 160)	MicroGene Sys (Menden, CT)	AIDS	Vaccines
17.	Antril (Interleukin I receptor antagonist)	Synergen (Boulder, CO)	Severe sepsis	Others

* A congenital endocrine disorder caused by failure of the ovaries to respond to pituitary hormone simulation;

2.7.3   Human Clone

Severino Antinori and **Robert Edwards** jointly produced the first test-tube baby and created a history in the world. Now, Antinori, a 53 year old Italian embryologist wants to repeat the history by creating the world's first **human clone**. Inspite of severe glaring ethical challenges, Antinori with the help of first human *in vitro fertilization* (**IVF**) technique enabled a 62 year old woman in 1994 to become the oldest to have a baby. He advocates and argues strongly that the technology of cloning is nothing but a logical and legitimate extension of IVF that may help in fertile couple to bear childern.

After decades of constant dedicated efforts the scientists have developed the key techniques to "reset" the DNA of living cells that essentially possessed specialist functions so they behaved as though they were a *newly fertilized embryo* which grew into a **clone of the adult.** In early 1998, the experts at the University of Hawaii succeeded the **cloning of mice.**

Thus, the prospect of *'human cloning'* is now perceived as an absolute reality in the near future. In view of the above rapid development in biotechnology the US government and the European parliament have made strict legislations to outlaw its practice on human beings. Although, it has been entirely left upto individual American and European states to accept or reject it outright. In Britain, the strict control of the **Human Fertilization and Embryology Authority (HFEA)** which has strongly pronounced its obvious intension to block and reject any requests to do work related to human cloning.

Antinori argues and seeks support from the world body for him to go ahead with human clone—

"What about the man who does not produce any sperm at all? What should he do? If he cannot reproduce himself why should he not reproduce his 'genes' in this way—this is one of the few cases where it is acceptable to clone".

our medicines and how we keep healthy.

'Functional-food' was first developed by the US Institute of Medicine as food wherein the concentration of one or more ingredients have been duly manipulated to enhance their all-out contribution towards a healthy and complete diet.

Since 1969, when the very idea of healthy foods was first conceived , a host of such products slowly gained entry for the human consumption, for instance:

- Bran and soy; low-fat, low-salt and no-sugar products
- Ginseng—based products
- Fish oil supplement products,
- Extra-strong cabbage,
- Specially designed pasta, and
- Genetically altered porridge

Besides, some specially produced vegetables and other eatables also took due cognizance of their added therapeutic value such as:

Name of Product	Indication
Special broccoli	For cancer
Tomatoes	To prevent prostate malignancies
Spagetti	For arthritis
Egg sandwich	To prevent heart disease
Cornflakes	To minimise the risk of breast cancer

Likewise, the genetically altered rapessed oil plant to result hybrids that produce a substantial amount of β-**carotene,** the well known precursor of Vitamin-A, commonly found in rather very small concentrations in carrots, palm oil etc. It has also been proved logically* that if one consumes

---

* According to Dr. G. Kishore, the St. Louis based Chief Biotehcnologist at Monsanto (USA).

a tablespoon of this oil daily, one would have an adequate amount of Vitamin-A required by the body. Perhaps, it would help a long way in providing between 250m to 1 billion people around the world, having various stages of Vitamin-A deficiency, and saving 10m childern dying each year globally as a result of this deficiency, as an alternative *'functional food'*.

2.8 BIOTECHNOLOGY: SOME THOUGHT PROVOKING NEWER IDEAS

Since, the intensive and extensive research has gained a surmountable momentum in '**biotechnology**' a number of newer thought provoking ideas have been put forward by the scientists, such as: *potato vaccine, functional food revolution* and *human clone*. These different aspects shall be discussed briefly in the sections that follows:

2.8.1 Potato Vaccine

A researcher in US has recently developed a **genetically engineered potato** that could afford protection against food poisoning and diarrhoea. Charles Arntzen* has successfully transferred the antibiotic gene of *E.coli* into the genetic material of potato. As the potato could not be tricked into producing enough *E.coli* proteins to elicit an immune response, an *'artificial gene'* identical to the bacterium was duly synthesized. It has been observed that small chunks of raw potato incorporated with the **synthetic gene** were administered orally by 14 volunteers, antibodies against *E.coli* appeared in the gut. According to the researcher this *'vegetable vaccine'* is going to be a very effective strategy for delivering oral vaccines as it goes straight into the gut. It is earnestly believed that this **engineered potato** may prove to be the forerunner of many edible vaccines against a wide range of diseases, including *cholera* and *hepatitis B*.

2.8.2 Functional Food Revolution

The time is not far when it is all set to convert our kitchens into culinary pharmacies;. Interestingly, it is termed as **functional food revolution.** This new concept of 'functional food' bears an attitude which is poised to revolutionise the manner we normally take.

FURTHER READING REFERENCES

1. Cleveland J *et al.* Bacteriocins: Safe, natural antimicrobials for Food Preservation, *Int. J. Food Microbiol.*, **71,** 1-20, 2001.
2. De Souza NJ, *Coleus Forskohlii* Briq.: **The Indian Plant Source for Froskolin,** In SP Chaudhuri (Ed) *Recent Advances in Medicinal, Aromatic, and Spice Crops,* Today and Tomorrow's Printers and Publlishers, New Delhi, Vol. I, pp. 83-91, 1991.
3. Ellaiash *et al.*: Optimization of process Parameters for Alkaline Protease Production under solid state fermentation by alkalophilic *Bacillus* sp., *Asian J. Microbiol Biotechnol Environ Sci.*, **5,** 49-54, 2003.
4. Gennaro, A.R., **'Remington : The Science and Practice of Pharmacy',** Mac Publishing Company, Easton, Pennsylvania Vol. I & II 19th edn. 1995.

---

* A plant biologist from the Boyce Tompson Institute for Plant Research in New York.

5. Karp, G., **'Cell and Molecular Biology : Concept and Experiments'**, John Wiley and Sons Inc., New York, 1996.

6. Madian, M.T., J.M., Martinko and J.Parker, **'Brock's: Biology of Microorganism'**, Prentice Hall, International, Inc., New Jersey, 8th ed., 1997.

7. Misawa M and Nakemishi TM, **Antitumour Compounds Production by Plaut Cell Cultures:** In Bajaj VPS (Ed) *Medicinal anad Aromatic Plants* II, Springer Verlag, New York, pp. 192-207, 1988.

8. Otta SK and Kurmasagar I, *Detection of monodon baculovirus and white spot syndrome virus in apparently healthy **Penaceous monodon** postlarvae from India by polymerase chain reaction, Aquaculture,* 220, 59-67, 2003.

9. Peters, P. **'Biotechnology'**, Wm C. Brown Publishers, Dubuque, 1993.

10. Sandmann G: Genetic *Manipulation of Carotenoid Biosynthesis: Strategies, Problems and Achievements, Travels Plant Sci.,* **6,** 14-17, 2001.

11. **'The International Biotechnology Handbook'**, Euromonitor Publishers Limited, London, 1988.

12. Wilson, M., and S.S. Lindow : ***'Release of Recombinant Microorganisms, Ann. Rev. of Microbiol.* 47,** 913-944, 1993.

3   Carbohydrates

• Introduction	• Carbohydrate Biogenesis
• Classification	• Further Reading References

3.1   INTRODUCTION

The Germans first and foremost introduced the word **'kohlenhydrates'** which was later on coined to **carbohydrates.** The name obviously suggests that these compounds are essentially the hydrates of carbon. In reality, all carbohydrates comprise of carbon, hydrogen and oxygen; whereas, the last two elements are found to exist in the same proportions as in water (*i.e.*, H_2O – 2:1). However, it has been observed that there are certain compounds that do conform to the said **'hydrate rule'** *i.e.*, maintain the ratio of H and O (2:1) but do not belong to the category of carbohydrates, for instance:

    (*i*)   Formaldehyde   [HCHO]   2:1
    (*ii*)   Acetic Acid   [CH_3COOH]   2:1
    (*iii*)   Lactic Acid   [$C_3H_6O_3$]   2:1

    Besides, there exist such compounds that evidently show the chemical properties of carbohydrates but do not necessarily abide by the above mentioned **'hydrate rule',** for example:

S.No.	Name	Emperical Formula	Structure	Remarks
1.	**Cymarose**	$C_7H_{14}O_4$	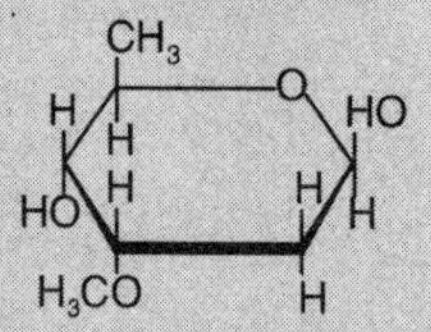	*Apocynum cannabinum* L. *A. androsaemifolium* L., *A. venetum* L.
2.	**Digitoxose**	$C_6H_{12}O_4$	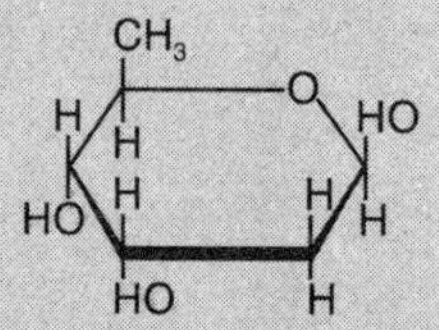	Obtained by mild hydrolysis of the glycosides eg; digitoxin, gitoxin and digoxin

(Table contd.)

3.	**Rhamrose**	$C_6H_{12}O_5$	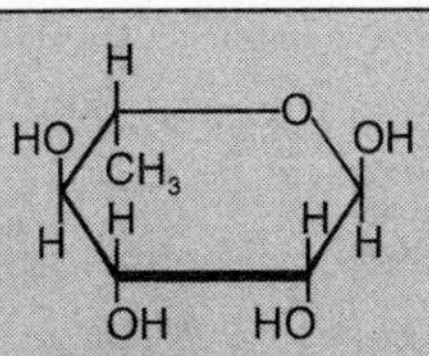	*Rhus toxicoden*dron L.
4.	**Sarmentose**	$C_7H_{14}O_4$	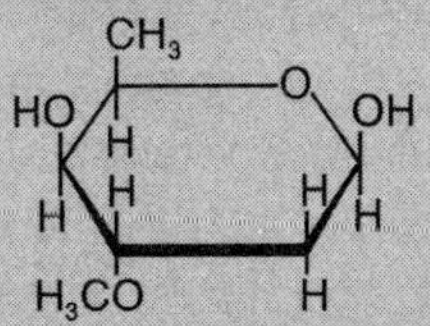	Hydrolysis of sarmentocymarin, a glycoside isolated from seeds of *Strophanthus sarmentosus* DC by the enzymatic method.
5.	**Oleandrose**	$C_7H_{14}O_4$	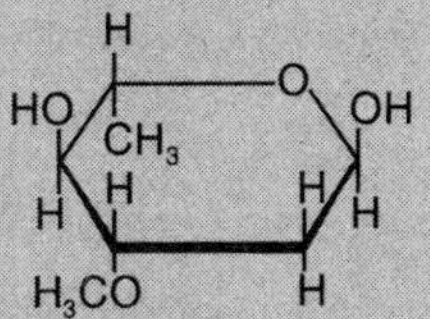	*Nerium oleander* L. (Laurier Rose)
6.	**Digitalose**	$C_7H_{14}O_5$	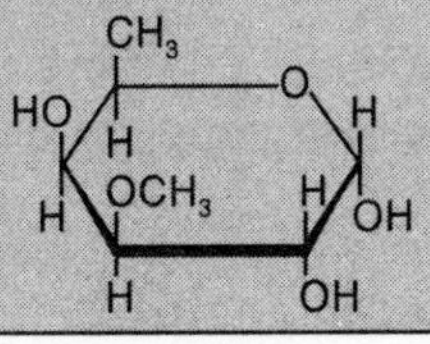	Obtained by hydrolysis of the glycoside from the seeds of *Strophanthus eminii* Aschers & Pax.

In view of the above cited glaring examples with regard to various anomalies the terminology **'Carbohydrates'** has still been retained to represent not only the sugars but also those substances that are related to them basically in structure and other characteristic features.

Invariably, the carbohydrates belong to the chemical class of the aldehydes, ketone alcohols, and also the condensation polymers of these partially oxidized polyalcohols collectively known as **'Polysaccharides'** or **'Oligosaccharides'**.

Glycan is the generic term for polysaccharide and in the systematic nomenclature the latter is assigned a suffix "-an". Generally, the polysaccharide may be classified into *two* broad heads, namely:

(*a*) **Homoglycan:** The polysaccharide is termed as homoglycan when it contains only one type of monosaccharide unit, and

(*b*) **Heteroglycan:** The polysaccharide is known as heteroglycan when it involves more than one kind of monosaccharide unit.

However, a more accurate and precise demarkation of polysaccharides essentially makes use of nomenclature that includes, *first* the type of monosaccharide building unit, and *secondly,* the exact position and configuration of the glycosidic linkage involved.

Examples:

(*i*) **Homoglycan:** *e.g., Cellulose.* It may also be expressed as β-1, 4 –D-glycan by virtue of the following reasons, namely:

• Prevailing attached unit is D-glucose,

- D-glucose bears the β-configuration at the anomeric C-atom (*i.e.*, C-1),
- C-1 is linked to C-4 of the next identical unit of D-glucose.

(*ii*) **Heteroglycan:** *e.g., D-gluco-D-mannose.* It is made up of D-glucose and D-mannose. The two altogether different monosaccharides usually show up in an orderly manner. In this particular instance, the diheteroglycan is composed of two different types of monosaccharides that has been arranged in an alternating and regular fashion.

It is worhwhile to mention at this juncture that plant kingdom provides a variety of complex polysaccharrides, such as: **cellulose, starch, dextran, inulin** and the like. These complex polysaccharides yield the respective sugar residues upon hydrolysis, for example:

Pentosans $\xrightarrow{\text{Hydrolysis}}$ Pentoses, Arabinose, Xylose, Ribose;

Hexosans $\xrightarrow{\text{Hydrolysis}}$ Hexoses, Glucose, Fructose;

Fructan $\xrightarrow{\text{Hydrolysis}}$ Inulin that results Fructose;

Glucan $\xrightarrow{\text{Hydrolysis}}$ Strach that gives Glucose.

Nevertheless, the starch and sugars find their abundant applications not only as food or food supplements, but also as indispensable adjuvants in the formulation of a wide range of pharmaceutical products all over the globe.

3.2 CLASSIFICATION

In broader sense the **polysaccharides** or **glycan** may be classified into *two* major groups, namely:

(*a*) Homoglycans, and

(*b*) Heteroglycans

These two major groups would be described in details with the help of important representative members in the sections that follows:

3.2.1 Homoglycans

A large number of plant products belonging to this particular category are namely: *honey, starch, hetastarch, inulin, lichenin, dextran, cyclodextrins, cellulose, cotton, and dextrin.*

3.2.1.1 Honey

Synonyms   Madhu, Madh, Mel, Honey (English);

Biological Source   Honey is a viscid and sweet secretion stored in the honey comb by various species of bees, such as: *Apis dorsata, Apis florea, Apis indica, Apis mellifica,* belonging the natural order *Hymenotera* (Family: *Apideae*).

Geographical Source   Honey is available in abudance in Africa, India, Jamaica, Australia, California, Chili, Great Britain and New Zealand.

Preparation   Generally, honey bees are matched with social insects that reside in colonies and produce honey and beeswax. Every colony esentially has one *'queen'* or *'mother bee'*, under whose command a huge number of *'employees'* exist which could be mostly sterile females and in certain seasons male bees. The *'employees'* are entrusted to collect nector from sweet smelling flowers from far and near that mostly contains aqueous solution of sucrose (ie; approximately 25% sucrose and 75% water) and pollens. Invertase, an enzyme present in the saliva of bees converts the nector into the invert sugar, which is partly consumed by the bee for its survival and the balance is carefully stored into the honey comb. With the passage of time the water gets evaporated thereby producing honey(ie; approximately 80% invert sugar and 20% water). As soon as the cell is filled up completely, the bees seal it with wax to preserve it for off-season utility.

The honey is collected by removing the wax-seal by the help of a sterilized sharp knife. The pure honey is obtained by centrifugation and filtering through a moistened cheese-cloth. Invariably, the professional honey collectors smoke away the bees at night, drain-out honey, and warm the separated combs to recover the beeswax.

Description

Appearances	:	Pale yellow to reddish brown viscid fluid,
Odour	:	Pleasant and characteristic,
Taste:	:	Sweet, Slightly acrid,
Specific gravity	:	1.35-1.36
Specific rotation	:	+3° to –15°
Total Ash	:	0.1-0.8%

However, the taste and odour of honey solely depends upon the availability of surrounding flowers from which nector is collected. On prolonged storage it usually turns opaque and granular due to the crystallisation of dextrose and is termed as **'granular honey'**.

Chemical Constituents   The average composition of honey rangles as follows: Moisture 14-24%, Dextrose 23-36%, Levulose (Fructose) 30-47%, Sucrose 0.4-6%, Dextrin and Gums 0-7% and Ash 0.1-0.8%. Besides, it is found to contain small amounts of essential oil, beeswax, pollen grains, formic acid, acetic acid, succinic acid, maltose, dextrin, colouring pigments, vitamins and an admixture of enzymes eg; diastase, invertase and inulase. Interestingly, the sugar contents in honey varies widely from one country to another as it is exclusively governed by the source of the nector (availability of fragment flowers in the region) and also the enzymatic activity solely controlling the conversion of nector into honey.

Substituents/Adulterants   Due to the relatively high price of pure honey, it is invariably adulterated either with artificial invert sugar or simply with cane-sugar syrup. These adulterants or cheaper substituents not only alter the optical property of honey but also its natural aroma and fragrance.

Uses

1. It is used as a sweetening agent in confectionaries.
2. Being a demulsent, it helps to relieve dryness and is, therefore, recommended for coughs, colds, sore-throats and constipation.
3. Because of its natural content of easily assimilable simple sugars, it is globaly employed as a good source of nutrient for infants, elderly persons and convalescing patients.

3.2.1.2 Starch

(Corn starch, Potato Starch, Rice Starch, Wheat Starch)

Synonym   Amylum

Biological Source   Starch comprises of mostly polysaccharide granules usually separated from the fully grown grains of Corn [*Zea mays* Linn.]; Rice [*Oryza sativa* Linn.] ; and Wheat [*Triticum aestivum* Linn.] belonging to the family *Gramineae* and also from the tubers of Potato [*Solanum tuberosum* Linn.] family *Solanaceae*.

Geographical Source   USA, Canada, Australia, China, India, CIS – countries (Russia), Thailand, Indonesia, Vietnam, Pakistan and many other tropical and sub-tropical countries are the major producers of starch in the world.

Preparation   In general, cereal grains *e.g.,* corn, rice and wheat mostly comprise of starch bundles, oil, soluble protein and the insoluble protein termed as *'gluten'*; whereas the potato contains starch, mineral salts (inorganic), soluble proteins and vegetable tissues. Obviously, various specific methods are normally employed to separate starch either from cereal grains or from potato. These methods are briefly enumerated below, namely:

(*a*) Methods for Maize (Corn) Starch

Maize grains are first washed with running water to get rid of dust particles and adhered organic matters. They are now softened by soaking in warm water (40-60°C) for 48 to 72 hrs charged with a 0.2-0.3% solution of SO_2 to check the fermentation. The swollen grains are passed through '**Attrition Mill'** to split and partly crush them to separate the embryo and the epicarp. It is extremely important to isolate the germ (embryo) which may be accomplished by addition of water, whereby the germs float and are segregated by skimming off promptly. The corn oil, a rich source of Vitamin E, is recovered from the germ by the process of expression. After removal of the germ the resultant liquid mass is subsequently freed from the accompanying **cell debris** and **gluten** (insoluble protein) by passing through a number of fine sieves. The milky slurry thus obtained is a mixture of starch and gluten particles which is then subjected to centrifugation by custom-designed **starch purification centrifuges.** Thus, the starch which being relatively heavier settles at the bottom and the gluten being lighter floats on the surface and removed quickly by a jet of water. Consequently, the starch is washed thoroughly with successive treatment of fresh water, centrifuged or filter pressed and ultimately dried either on a *moving belt dryer* or *flash dryer.*

(*b*) Method for Rice Starch

The rice* is adequately soaked in a solution of NaOH (0.5% w/v) till such time when the gluten is softened and dissolved partially. The resulting grains are wet-milled and taken up with water. The suspension is purified by repeatedly passing through sieves and the starch is recovered by centrifugation. Finally, the starch is duly washed, dried, powdered and stored in HDPE** bags.

(*c*) Method for Wheat Starch

Wheat being an extensively used common staple food, therefore, its utility for making starch is restricted by many government authorities. First of all the wheat flour is made into a stiff ball of

---

* Broken pieces of rice obtained during the polishing are mostly used for preparation of rice starch.
** **HDPE :** High density polyethylene.

dough which are kept for a short duration. The gluten present in the dough swells up and are shifted to grooved-rollers that move forward and backward slowly. Constant sprinkling of water is done which carries off the starch along with it whereas gluten remains as a soft elastic mass. The shurry of starch is purified by centrifugation, washed, dried, powdered and packed in HDPE bags.

(*d*) Method for Potato Starch

The tubers of potato are thoroughly washed to get rid of the sticking soil. These are subsequently chopped into small pieces and made into a fine pulp by crushing in a **Rasping Machine.** The resulting slurry is passed through metallic sieves to remove the cellular matter as completely as possible. The starch suspension (slurry) is purified by centrifugation, washed, dried and the stocked in HDPE bags.

Description

Starch occurs in nature as irregular, angular, white masses that may be easily reduced to power.

Appearance	: White – rice and maize starch,
	Creamy white – Wheat starch,
	Pale yellow – potato starch,
Odour	: Odourless
Taste	: Bland and mucilaginous.

Nevertheless, all the four types of starch mentioned above do possess a definite shape and characteristic features as illustrated in Fig. 3.1

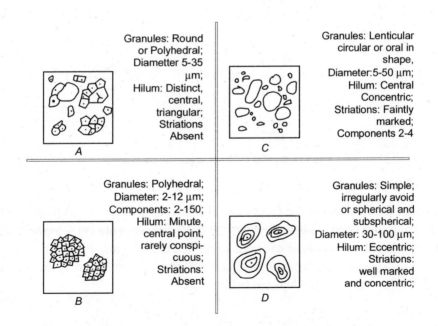

Granules: Round or Polyhedral; Diametter 5-35 µm; Hilum: Distinct, central, triangular; Striations Absent

A

Granules: Lenticular circular or oral in shape, Diameter:5-50 µm; Hilum: Central Concentric; Striations: Faintly marked; Components 2-4

C

Granules: Polyhedral; Diameter: 2-12 µm; Components: 2-150; Hilum: Minute, central point, rarely conspicuous; Striations: Absent

B

Granules: Simple; irregularly avoid or spherical and subspherical; Diameter: 30-100 µm; Hilum: Eccentric; Striations: well marked and concentric;

D

Fig. 3.1 Characteristic Features of (*A*) Maize Starch, (*B*) Rice Starch, (*C*) Wheat Starch, (*D*) Potato Starch.

Chemical Constituents

In general, under ideal experimental parameters hydrolysis of starch in acidic medium yields glucose in theoretical proportion that essentially represent the main building block of the starch molecule. It has been established that starch molecule is essentially made up of *two* **complex polysaccharides,** namely:

(*a*) Amylopectin: (α-Amylose)

Amylopectin is insoluble in water and swells in it thereby giving rise to a thick paste upon boiling with water. It produce a distinct violet or bluish red colouration with iodine* solution (0.1 N). It has a highly branched structure that is composed of several hundred short chains of about 20-25 **D-Glucose units** each. Interestingly, one terminal of each of these chains is joined through C-1 to a C-6 with the next chain and so on and so forth as shown below:

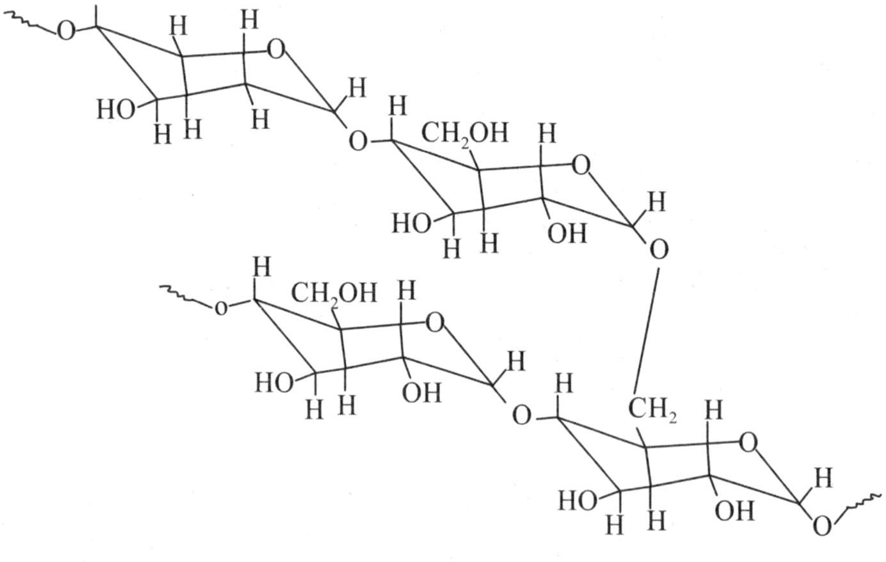

Amylopectin (Chair – Conformations Anticipated)

(*b*) Amylose: (β-Amylose)

Amylose is water soluble and gives an instant bright blue colour with iodine solution (0.1 N). Based on the fact that amylose upon hydrolysis yields the only **disaccharide (+) – Maltose** and the only **monosaccharide D-(+) – Glucose,** it has been suggested that amylose is comprised of chains of a number of D-(+) – glucose units, whereby each unit is strategically linked by an **alpha–glycoside bondage** to C-4 of the next unit as depicted below:

---

* Iodine colour reaction is influenced by the starch-chain ie; longer the branching the colour varies from Blue→Blue violet→Red→Brown.

Amylose (Chair Conformations Anticipated)

Amylose invariably constitutes upto 25% of the total starch content; however, the proportion varies with the particular species under consideration. Amylose is found to be either absent or present to a very small extent ($\leq$ 6%) in some glutinous or waxy starches available in the plant kingdom.

Substituents and Adulterants

A number of biological species containing starch is generally employed to substitute (adulterate) the conventional commercially available starch used as **food** and as **pharmaceutical adjuvants,** namely:

S.No.	Name	Biological Source	
1.	Topioca Starch or Cassava Starch	*Manihot esculenta* Pohl., *Manihot aipi* Pohl., *Manihot utilissima* Pohl.	Family: Euphorbiaceae
2.	Sago Starch	*Metroxylon sagu*	Family: *Palmae*
3.	Brazilian Arrowroot Starch or Sweet-Potato Starch	*Ipomoea batas Lam.*	Family: *Convolvulaceae*
4.	Nuts Starch	*Tapa bispinosa* Roxb.	Family: *Onagraceae*

Uses

 1. It possesses both absorbent and demulcent properties.
 2. It is employed in dusting powder because of its unique protective and absorbent property.
 3. It is used in the formulation of tablets and pills as a vital disintegrating agent and a binder.
 4. It is utilized as a diagnostic aid for the proper identification of crude drugs.
 5. It is employed as a diluent (or filler) and lubricant in the preparation of capsules and tablets.
 6. It is used as an indicator in iodimetric analyses.
 7. It is an antidote of choice for iodine poisoning.
 8. Dietetic grades of corn starch are marked as **'Maizena'** and **'Mondamin'.**
 9. **'Glycerine of starch'** is used not only as an emollient but also as a base for the suppositories.
10. It is the starting material for the large scale production of liquid glucose, glucose syrup, dextrose and dextrin.
11. It finds its extensive industrial application for the sizing of paper and textile.
12. It possesses nutrient properties as a food and in cereal based weaning foods for babies *e.g.*, **Farex**[R] (Glaxo) and **Cerelac**[R] (Nestle).

13. It is used topically and externally to allay itching.
14. It is used profusely in laundry starching.

3.2.1.3 Hetastarch

Hetastarch is a semisynthetic material that essentially comprises of more than 90% amylopectin, which has been treated with *pyridine* and *ethylene chlorohydrin,* so as to give rise to 7 to 8 hydroxyethyl substituents present for every **10 D-glucopyranose units** of the starch polymer. The molecular weight is approximately 450, 000 daltons.

Amylose Derivative

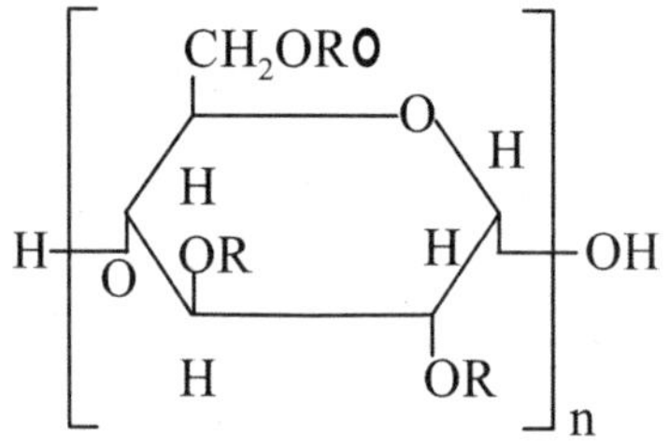

Where R or R′ = H or CH_2 CH_2 OH

Amylopectine Derivative   It specifically differs from the amylose derivative in that the sequence is frequently interrupted by a unit in which R is the residue of an additional *o*-**hydroxyethylated α-D-glucopyranosyl** moiety that essentially constitutes the first unit in a branch or sub-branch of the polymer.

Uses
1. It serves as a **'Plasma Volume Expander'.** A 6% solution is osmotically equivalent to a 5% albumin solution. But in the blood, it draws up certain quantum of water either from the intestinal or intracellular fluids, thus expanding the blood volume slightly in excess of the volume infused. This acquired expansion lasts for 24 to 36 hours.
2. It is employed in the management and treatment of **hypovolemic shock*.**
3. It is also used as a suspension medium for **leukapheresis**.**
4. It is employed as a **cryoprotective*** agent for erythrocytes.

3.2.1.4 Inulin

It is found to bear a close resemblance to starch except that it is a *levulan* rather than a **dextran.** The following characteristic features make it altogether different from starch, namely:

- Gives yellow colouration by iodine.
- Does not gelatinize with water.

---

* Shock caused due to diminished blood volume.
** The separation of leukocytes from blood, which are then transfused back into the patient.
*** A chemical that protects cells from the effect of cold.

- Not commonly found in plants in the form of granules having concentric layers, and
- Upon hydrolysis in acidic medium yields fructoses.

Synonyms   Dahlin; Alantin; Alant starch.

Biological Source   It occurs in certain plants of the *Compositae* family, such as:

Inula helenium Linn.	: Roots contain inulin;
Eupatorium cannabinum Linn.	: Plant contains inulin;
Cynara scolymus Linn.	: Flower heads contain inulin;
Carpesium cernuum Linn.	: Roots contain inulin;
Calendula officinalis Linn.	: Roots contain inulin;
Aretium lappa Linn.	: Roots contain 45% inulin.

Geographical Source

A. lappa – Western Himalayas from Kashmir to Simla;

C. officinalis – India, Pakistan;

C. cernuum – Temperate Himalayas and Nilgiri Hills (India);

S. scolymus – Throughout India; *E. canabinum*—Temperate Himalayas;

I. helenium – Europe and Asia.

Preparation   Isolated from *dahlia tubers* and from other members of the family *Compositae*.

Description   The crystals are spherical in shape when prepared from water.

Chemical Constituents

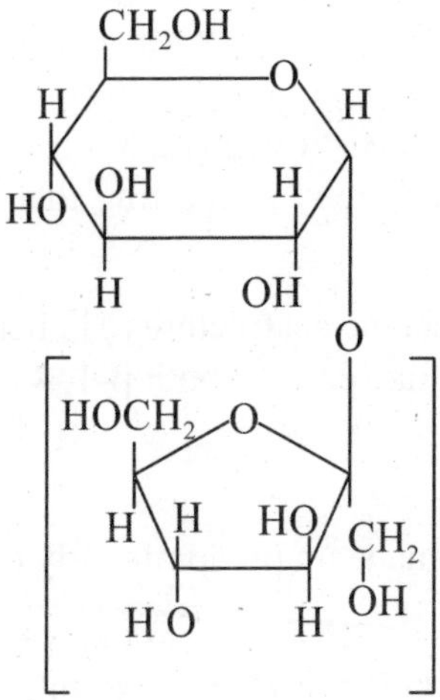

Inulin

[Structure of INULIN showing arrangement of *Fructofuranose* residues in chain]

Inulin is quickly hydrolyzed by acids to D-fructose by the enzymes inulase but does not undergo hydrolysis by the amylases. However, methylated inulin upon hydrolysis gives rise to 3,4,6-trimethylfructose as a major product and 1,3,4,6- tertamethylfructose as a minor product, thereby suggesting that the fructose residues are present in the furanose form and the adjacent units are joined through C-1 and C-2 (*i.e.*, the glycosidic hydroxyl moiety).

3,4,6-Trimethyl Fructose
(Furanose-Form)
(Major Product)

1,3,4,6 – Tetramethyl Fructose
(Furanose-Form)
(Minor Product)

Uses

1. It is used in **culture media** as a fermentative identifying agent for certain bacterial species.
2. It is filtered exclusively by the glomeruli and is neither secreted nor reabsorbed by the tubules. Hence, it is employed as a **diagnostic agent** for evaluation of glomerular filteration *i.e.*, renal–function test (or kidney function test).
3. It is considered to be valuable in the diet of the diabetic patients.

3.2.1.5 Lichenin

Synonym Moss starch; Lichen starch;

Biological Source *Cetraria islandica (L.) Ach., Family: Parmeliaceae.* It is known as Iceland Moss.

Description It is a cellulose like polysaccharide which occurs as a cell wall component in lichens. It is readily soluble in hot water to give rise to a colloidal solution. It is more rapidly hydrolyzed than cellulose. It produces cellobiose upon acetylation with acetic anhydride and sulphuric acid. It is a white powder.

On methylation followed by hydrolysis it yields 2,3,6-trimethylglucose as a major component and tetramethylglucose as minor one thereby suggesting that the chain present in lichenin is not branched at all as in cellulose.

Chemical Constituents The exact chemical structure of lichenin molecule is yet to be established; however, it has been indicated that it may contain both β-1, 4 and β-1, 6 linkages.

3.2.1.6 Dextran

Dextran is a carbohydrate substance made up predominantly of D-glucose units *i.e.* $(C_6H_{10}O_5)_n$. It is α–1, 6 linked polyglucan.

Synonyms Dextraven; Expandex; Gentran;Hemodex; Intradex; Macrose; Onkotin; Plavolex; Polyglucin.

Biological Source A number of organisms produce dextrans; however, only *two* of them, namely; *Leuconostoc mesenteroides* and *L. dextranicum,* belonging to the family *Lactobacteriaceae*, have been used commercially.

Preparation Commercially, dextrans are manufactured by the process of fermentation of sucrose (a disaccharide) either by cell-free enzymatic fermentation technique or by whole culture technique.

The enzymes that are responsible for producing dextrans from sucrose as a substrate are collectively known as 'dextran-sucrases'.

   Native dextran possesses a very high moleculer weight, whereas the clinical dextrans have lower moleculer weights, for instane; Dextran 40 [Gentran 40[R] (Baxter); Rheomacrodex[R] (Pharmacia)]; Dextran 70 [Hyskon[R] & Macrodex[R] (Kabi Pharmacia)]; Dextran 75 [Gentran 75[R] (Baxter)]; These may be accomplished by controlled depolymerization e.g., ultrasonic vibration, fungal dextranase and acid hydrolysis.

Description   Dextrans obtained by the precipitation from methanol vary considerably with regard to their characteristic physical and chemical properties which solely depends upon the individual method of preparation.

Chemical Constituents   The interaction between 'n' molecules of sucrose and 'x' number of glucose moieties yields dextran together with 'n' molecules of fructose as shown in the following equation:

$$n\text{Sucrose} + (\text{Glucose})_x \longrightarrow (\text{Glucose})_{x+n} + n\text{Fructose}$$
$$\qquad\qquad\quad \text{Primer} \qquad\qquad \text{Dextran}$$

Uses

1. Dextran 40 is employed as an isotonic solution either to prime pumps or to improve flow in surgery concerned with *cardiopulmonary bypass*. Thus, it exerts its effect by lowering the viscosity of blood and improving flow; and the latter is caused due to hemodilution.
2. Dextrans as a whole helps in minimising platelet adhesiveness, which property is gainfully exploited in their usage for *prophylaxis of thrombosis and thromoembolism both during and after surgery.*
3. Both Dextran 70 and Dextran 75 find their extensive use as plasma extender for the control and management of *hypovolemic shock*. Hypertonic solutions usually afford the dehydration of tissues, whereby the abstracted water being added to the plasma causing increase in its volume. For this reason they are quite useful in the prevention and treatment of *toxemia of pregnancy* and *nephrosis*.
4. Dextran 70 and Dextran 75 are used in 6% solutions to prevent pending shock caused by hemorrhage, trauma, and severe burns.
5. Dextran 40 (10% solution) is not only used to lower blood viscosity but also to improve microcirculation at low flow rates.
6. Dextrans are employed in the formulation of fat-soluble vitamins (viz. Vitamin A, D, E, K).
7. It is also used in preparing sustained released tablets.
8. Dextrans find their abundant applications in various types of confectionaries, for instance: ice-creams, candies, jellies, syrups and cake–topings.
9. It is employed as an adjunct in cosmetic preparation exclusively meant for soothening wrinkles.

3.2.1.7 Cyclodextrins

Cyclodextrins invariably consist of 6, 7 or 8 molecules (viz. α, β and γ cyclodextrin) in a 1, 4-configuration to result into the formation of rings having various diameters. In fact, based on the geometry of the chiral isomer, only one would possibly gain entry into the cavity in the ring while the other is excluded evidently.

Synonyms   Cyloamyloses; Cycloglycans; Schardinger dextrins.

Biological Source   Starch on being treated with the amylase of *Bacillus macerans,* a specific enzyme, gives rise to a mixture of cyclodextrins. They are naturally occuring carbohydrates.

Preparation   It is obtained from the action of *B. macerans* amylase on starch to yield homogeneous cyclic $\alpha - (1{\rightarrow}4)$ linked D-gluco-pyranose units.

Description   The various rings constituting the cyclodextrins appear to be as doughnut shaped. However, **α-cyclodextrin** *i.e.*, the smallest of the lot, has a diameter about two times that of 18-crown–6 (viz., as crown ethers) and its hole (4.5°A across) is approximately two times as broad.

Chemical Constituents   **Cyclodextrins** mainly are comprised of *three* different types, as detailed below:

S.No.	Name/Mol. Formula	Chemical Name	Shape
1.	α-Cyclodextrin ($C_{36}H_{60}O_{30}$)	Cyclohexamylose	Hexagonal plates, or blood–shaped needles
2.	β-Cyclodextrin ($C_{42}H_{70}O_{35}$)	Cycloheptaamylose	Parallelogram shaped crystals
3.	γ–Cyclodextrin ($C_{48}H_{80}O_{40}$)	Cyclooctamylose	Square plates or rectangular rods.

The structure of α-cyclodextrin may be represented in Figure 3.2, in *two* different manners, namely:

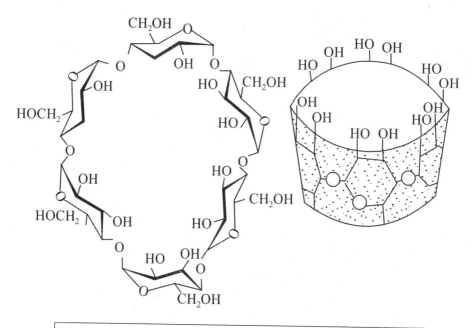

**Fig. 3.2   A Schematic Representation of α-Cyclodextrin:
(a) Chair-conformation Based (b) Doughnut Shaped.**

(*a*) Chair-conformation based cyclic structure, and
(*b*) Doughnut shaped or like a tiny-pail with the bottom knocked out.

Uses

1. As enzyme models based on the fact that , like enzymes, they first and foremost *bind* the substrate and then, through substituent groups, *act on it.*
2. As a complexing agent to explore the various types of enzyme action.
3. It may be employed as an additive to the mobile phase (in HPLC*), but it invariably gets bound to an innert support material.

3.2.1.8 Cellulose

Cellulose represents one of the most widely distributed and abundantly available organic matter on this planet. It is, in-fact, the most important structural element of *higher-plant-cell walls*. In nature, wood (40-50% cellulose) caters as the major source of cellulose for industrial utilities, whereas cotton (98% cellulose) provides the balance requirement globally.

Geographical Source   It has been observed that nearly thirty billion MT of carbon is transformed annually into organic compounds by higher plants and out of this approximately 1/3rd is converted into cellulose. As cellulose is profusely utilized in the form of wood to build houses, paper industry and textile industry, a considerable amount of research has been duly conducted on this well-known polysaccharide.

Preparation   The scientific and large-scale methods for preparing cellulose essentially involves the removal of excess of the non-cellulose substances *e.g.* **Lignin.** In fact, there are *three* well defined and established procedures whereby the undesired *'lignin content'* present in wood shavings are removed exhaustively, namely:

(*a*) *Treatment with Sodium Bisulphite [Sulphonate Process]:* The small wood chips are boiled with a solution of sodium bisulphite whereupon the lignin is removed as *lignosulphonate,*
(*b*) *Treatment with Sodium Hydroxide [Soda Process]:* The wood chips on being boiled with sodium hydroxide solution removes the lignin content as soluble products, and
(*c*) *Treatment with NaOH and Na₂SO₄ [Sulphate Process]:* The sodium sulphide (Na_2S) obtained by the interaction of NaOH and Na_2SO_4 will remove most of the lignin component from the wood shavings.

However, the traces of lignin may be removed by bleaching with chlorine. The remaining mixture of hemicellulose and cellulose are subsequently extracted by subjecting it to alkaline treatment. The readily soluble hemicellulose are removed by treatment with higher concentration of NaOH solution, whereas the cellusans (Xylans) may be removed by treatment with a 5% solution of NaOH.

Description   **Cellulose** has molecular weights ranging from 250,000 to 1,000,000 or even more. It is assumed that at least 1500 glucose units may be present in each molecule. Based on the findings by X-ray analysis and electron microscopy it is revealed that these long chains lie side by-side in bundles, held together by H-bonds available between the huge number of adjoining –OH moieties. Further, these bundles are twisted together to give rise to rope-like structures, that ultimately are clubbed together to yield the normal apparently visible fibers. Interestingly, in the case of wood

---

* **HPLC:** High performance liquid chromatography.

these cellulose **"ropes"** are meticulously embedded in lignin to afford a structure that resembles to concrete reinforced structures used for making buildings.

Chemical Constituents   **Cellulose** is comprised of chains of D-glucose units, whereby each unit is joined by a glycosidic linkage to C-4 of the next unit.

Cellulose

Cellulose   **Cellulose** derived from various sources and also from different modes of preparations usually display great differences not only in their mean chain length but also in their degree of homogenity. Generally, the cellulose that are distinctly more homogenous are the most suitable for industrial utilities.

Uses

1. The viscose when forced through a spinnerette into an acid-bath, it gives rise to the generation of **cellulose** as fine filaments that yield threads of a substance termed as RAYON.
2. **Cellulose** undergoes an analogous reaction to produce *cellulose xanthate*, that is made to dissolve in alkali to yield a viscous colloidal dispersion known as **VISCOSE.**
3. Methyl, ethyl and benzyl ethers of cellulose are proved to be important in the commercial production of films, textiles and various types plastic materials.

3.2.1.9 Absorbent Cotton

Synonyms   Purified cotton; Cotton wool; Surgical cotton.

Biological Source   Cotton comprises of the *epidermal trichomes* (or hairs) from the seeds of different species of *Gossypium,* such as : *G. herbaccum; G. hirsutum; G. barbedense*; belonging to the family *Malvaceae.* In fact, absorbent cotton or purified cotton consists exclusively of the trichomes that are completely freed from adhering impurities, fat, properly bleached and finally sterilized.

Geographical Source   Cotton is produced on large scale in USA, Egypt, China, India, South America and certain parts of Africa. Egyptian cotton–yarn enjoys a world-wide reputation. Both India and China are not only self-sufficient in the production of absorbent cotton but also exports a substantial quantity to various countries.

Preparation   The **cotton** plant after flowering bears fruits which are also called **'capsules'** or **'balls'.** These are usually 3-5 celled. Once the fruit ripens they open-up widely that contains a number of seeds per loculus. The brown coloured seeds are normally surrounded with a thick mass of white hairs. The *long-lint hairs* are known as **'staple'** or **'floss';** whereas the *short-fuzz hairs* are called *'linters'.* The cotton fibres (*i.e.,* mass of white hairs) along with their seeds are collected manually by hand picking. The raw cotton is subjected to a mechanical process called **'ginning'** whereby only the hairy substance is collected separately and the undesired substances, such as: dirt, leaf-fragments and other foreign materials are removed separately. **'Delintering'** is the mechanical process which discards the short hairs that eventually passed along with the cotton fibres obtained from the *'ginning'* process. The raw segregated long-sized cotton hairs are subsequently freed from colouring matters and traces of wax and oil coating the hairs which render them non-absorbent. The treated absorbent cotton obtained above is processed through the *'carding machine'* so as to arrange the fibres in parallel direction and also to get rid of immature fibres completely. Short fibres are once again removed by *'combing'* mechanically. Finally, the processed cotton fibres are defatted (with alkali) washed, bleached (with chlorinated soda) and then washed (with diluted mineral acid). It is again washed, dried, recarded and sterilized.

Description White, soft, fine, filament like hairs appearing under the microscope as hollow, flattened and twisted bands, striate and slightly thickened at the edges, practically odorless and tasteless. Cotton fibres are usually 2.5 to 4.5 cm in length and 25 to 35 μ in diameter.

Chemical Constituents Absorbent cotton is mostly cellulose 93-94% and moisture 6-7% (for structure see under section 3.2.1.8)

Uses

1. It is employed as surgical dressings.
2. It is mostly used in the textile industry to prepare a wide range of fibres.
3. It is invariably employed as its derivatives to be recognized as the most versatile adjunct in pharmaceutical formulations, for instance:

Microcrystalline cellulose – as Tablet Disitegrant
Carboxymethyl Cellulose (CMC) – as Binder and thickening agent;
Cellulose acetate phthalate – as an Enteric coating material;
Ethyl Cellulose ⎫ – as Binder and Film
Methyl Cellulose ⎬ coating substance;
Hydroxypropyl methyl Cellulose ⎭
Oxidised Cellulose – as local Haemostatic;
Purified *'Rayon'* – as Surgical aid;
Pyroxylin – as an ingredient in the preparation of Collodian and nail polishes.

4. It is used as a filtering medium and also as an insulating material.
5. Pharmaceutical grade cotton seed oil is used as an emolient and in the preparation of *Steroidal Hormone Injections*.
6. It is used for making explosives.

3.2.1.10 Dextrin

Synonyms British Gum; Starch Gum; Leiocom; Pyrodextrin; Torrefaction dextrin; Canary dextrin; Yellow dextrin; White dextrin.

Preparation Dextrin is prepared by carrying out the incomplete hydrolysis of starch with dilute acid or by heating dry starch.

Various types of dextrin are prepared as detailed below namely:

(*a*) **British Gum, Starch Gum:** It is produced at high temperature in the absence of acid.

Characteristic features:

(*i*) Dark brown colour, odourous,

(*ii*) High viscosity, very soluble in cold water,

(*iii*) Does not reduce Fehling's Solution, and

(*iv*) Gives reddish-brown colour with iodine.

(*b*) **Canary Dextrin, Yellow Dextrin:** It is prepared by hydrolyzing starch at high temperature for a longer duration but in the presence of small quantum of acid.

Characteristic features:

(*i*) Light brown to yellow colour, slight odour, and

(*ii*) Low viscosity, very soluble in cold water.

(*c*) **White Dextrin:** It is prepard by hydrolysis at low temperature for a shorter duration but in the presence of large quantum of acid.

Characteristic features:

(*i*) White colour, odourless,

(*ii*) Slightly soluble in cold water, and gives a red colour with iodine, and

(*iii*) Very soluble in hot water and gives a blue colour with iodine.

Uses

1. As an excipient for dry extracts and pills.
2. It is used for preparing emulsions and dry bandages.
3. It is employed for thickening of dye-pastes and mordants used in printing fabrics in fast colours.
4. It is used for sizing paper and fabrics.
5. It is employed for preparing felt and printing tapestries.
6. It is used for preparing printer's inks, glues and mucilage.
7. It is employed for polishing cereals.
8. It is extensively used in making matches, fireworks and explosives.

3.2.2 **Heteroglycans**

In general, **Gums** represent a heterogenous group of acidic substances, that essentially possess in common the characteristic property of swelling in water to form either gels or viscous, sticky, solutions. It has also been advocated that gums are the resulting products obtained from normal plant metabolism. In addition, it is also believed that gums may have been produced from starch or cellulose through hydrolysis, followed by oxidation to uronic acids and finally undergoing the process of esterfication or formation of salt accordingly.

In actual practice, the **natural gums** may be classified into *four* different groups, namely:

(*a*) Exudate Gums

(*b*) Seed Gums

(*c*) Marine Gums, and

(*d*) Microbial Gums

These different types of gums would be discussed along with some typical examples in the sections that follows:

3.2.2.1 Exudate Gums

It has been observed that a large number of plants which grow in a semiarid environment generate **exudate gums** in sufficient amount when either an incision is made on their bark or they get damaged that invariably helps to seal off the cracked wound thereby preventing dehyration of the plant.

A plethora of exudate gums find their abundant applications as a pharmaceutical aid, namely: **Acacia, Tragacanth** and **Karaya Gum.**

3.2.2.1.1 Acacia

Synonyms Indian Gum; Gum Acacia; Gum Arabic.

Biological Source According to the USP, **acacia** is the dried gummy exudation from the stems and branches of *Acacia senegal* (L.) Willd; family; *Leguminoseae,* or other African species of Acacia. It is also found in the stems and branches of *Acacia arabica,* Willd.

Geographial Source The plant is extensively found in India, Arabia, Sudan and Kordofan (North-East Africa), Sri Lanka, Morocco, and Senegal (West Africa). Sudan is the major producer of this gum and caters for about 85% of the world supply.

Cultivation and Collection Acacia is recovered from wild as well as duly cultivated plants in the following manner, such as:

(*a*) **From Wild Plants:** The Gum after collection is freed from small bits of bark and other foreign organic matter, dried in the sun directly that helps in the bleaching of the natural gum to a certain extent, and

(*b*) **From Cultivated Plants:** Usually, transverse incisions are inflicted on the bark which is subsequently peeled both above and below the incision to a distance 2-3 feet in length and 2-3 inches in breadth. Upon oxidation, the gum gets solidified in the form small translucent beads, sometimes referred to as *'tears'.* Tears of gum normally become apparent in 2-3 weeks, which is subsequently hand picked , bleached in the sun, garbled, graded and packed.

Description

Colour: Tears are usually white, pale-yellow and sometimes creamish-brown to red in colour. The power has an off-white, pale-yellow or light-brown in appearance.

Odour: Odourless (There is a close relationship between colour and flavour due to the presence of tannins).

Taste: Bland and mucillagenous.

Shape & Size: Tears are mostly spheroidal or ovoid in shape and having a diameter of about 2.5-3.0 cm.

Appearance: Tears are invariably opaque either due to the presence of cracks or fissures produced on the outer surface during the process or ripening. The fracture is usually very brittle in nature and the exposed surface appears to be glossy.

Chemical Constituents Acacia was originally thought to be composed only of *four* chemical constituents, namely : **(–) arabinose; (+) – galactose; (–)–rhamnose** and **(+) glucuronic acid.**

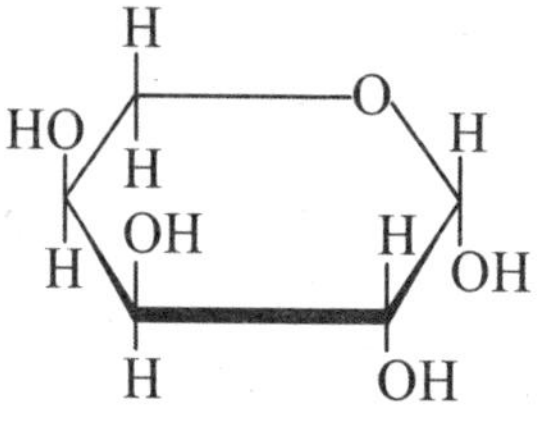

(−)–Arabinose 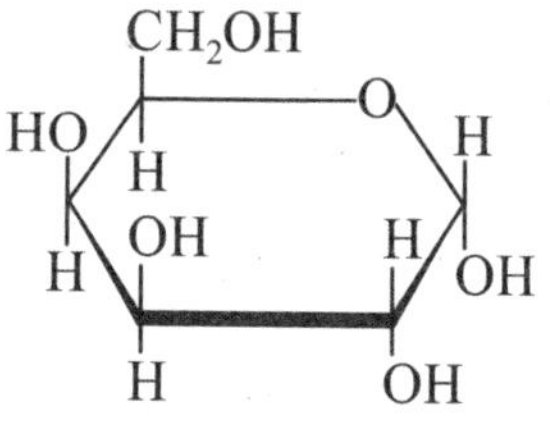   (+)–Galactose

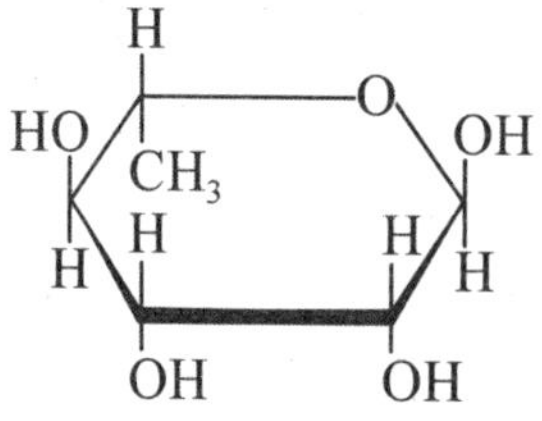

(−)–Rhamnose 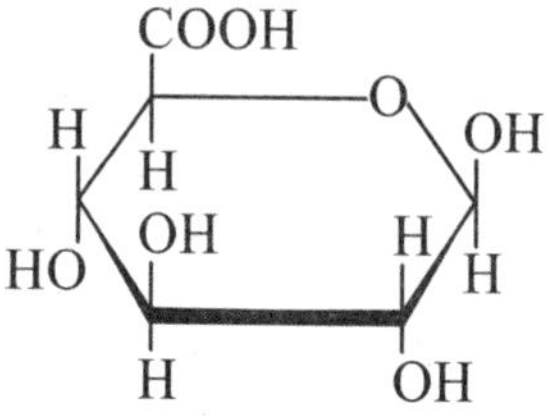   (+)–Glucuronic Acid

On subjecting the gum acacia to hydrolysis with 0.01 N H_2SO_4 helps in removing the combined product of (−) – arabinose and (+) – galactose, whereas the residue consists of the product (+) – galactose and (+) – glucuronic acid. These two products are formed in the ratio of 3:1.

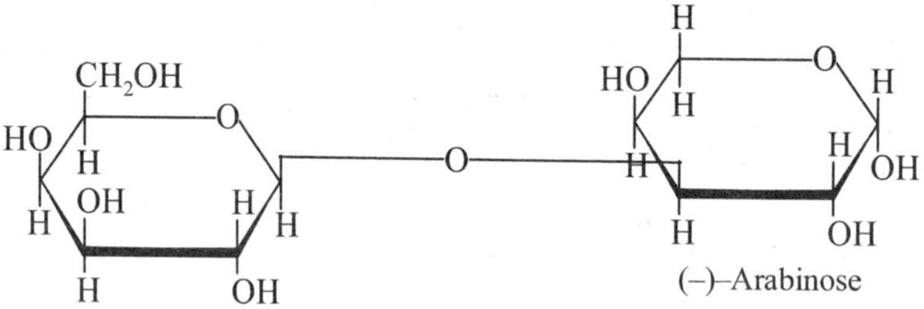

(+)–Galactose   [3 Parts]   (−)–Arabinose

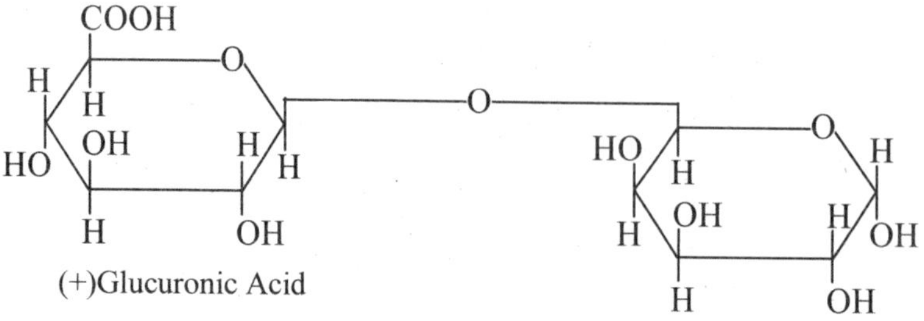

(+)Glucuronic Acid

[1 Part]   (+)–Galactose

It also contains a **peroxidase enzyme.**

Chemical Tests

1. **Lead Acetate Test:** An aqueous solution of acacia when treated with lead-acetate solution it yields a heavy white precipitate.

2. **Borax Test:** An aqueous solution of acacia affords a stiff translucent mass on treatment with borax.

3. **Blue Colouration due to Enzyme:** When the aqueous solution of acacia is treated with benzidine in alcohol together with a few drops of hydrogen peroxide (H_2O_2), it gives rise to a distinct–blue colour indicating the presence of enzyme.

4. **Reducing Sugars Test:** Hydrolysis of an aqueous solution of acacia with dilute HCl yields reducing sugars whose presence are ascertained by boiling with Fehling's solution to give a brick-red precipitate of cuprous oxide.

5. **Specific Test:** A 10% aqueous solution of acacia fails to produce any precipitate with dilute solution of lead acetate (a clear distinction from Agar and Tragacanth); it does not give any colour change with Iodine solution (a marked distinction from starch and dextrin); and it never produces a bluish-black colour with $FeCl_3$ solution (an apparent distinction from tannins).

Uses

1. The mucilage of acacia is employed as a demulscent.
2. It is used extensively as a vital pharmaceutical aid for emulsification and to serve as a thickening agent.
3. It finds its enormous application as a binding agent for tablets *e.g.*, cough lozenges.
4. It is used in the process of *'granulation'* for the manufacture of tablets. It is considered to be the gum of choice by virtue of the fact that it is quite compatible with other plant hydrocolloids as well as starches, carbohydrates and proteins.
5. It is used in conjuction with gelatin to form conservates for microencapsulation of drugs.
6. It is employed as colloidal stabilizer.
7. It is used extensively in making of candy and other food products.
8. It is skillfully used in the manufacture of spray – dried *'fixed'* flavours – stable, powdered flavours employed in packaged dry-mix products (puddings, desserts, cake mixes) where flavour stability and long shelf-life are important.

3.2.2.1.2 Tragacanth

Synonym   Gum Tragacanth

Biological Source   The dried gummy exudation from *Astragalus gummifer* Labill. (white gavan) or other Asiatic species of *Astragalus* belonging to the family of *Leguminoseae*.

Geographical Source   It is naturally found in various countries, *viz.*, Iran, Iraq, Armenia, Syria, Greece and Turkey. A few species of *Astragalous* are located in India, *viz.*, Kumaon, Garhwal and Punjab.*Persian tragacanth* are exported from Iran and North Syria, whereas the *Smyrna tragacanth* from the Smyrna port in Asiatic Turkey.

Collection   The thorny shrubs of **tragacanth** normally grow at an altitude of 1000-3000 meters. As an usual practice transverse incisions are inflicted just at the base of the stem, whereby the gum is given out both in the pith and medullary rays. Thus, the absorption of water helps the gum to swell-up and subsequently exude through the incisions. The gummy exudates are duly collected and dried rapidly to yield the best quality white product. It usually takes about a week to collect the gum exudates right from the day the incisions are made; and this process continues thereafter periodically.

Description
   Colour: White or pale-yellowish white
   Odour: Odourless

Taste: Tasteless

Shape: Curved or twisted ribbon –like flakes marked with concentric ridges that is indicative of successive exudation and solidification. Fracture is normally short and horny.

Size: Flakes are usually 25 × 12 × 12 mm.

Appearance: Translucent

Chemical Constituents   Interestingly, tragacanth comprises of two vital fractions: *first*, being water-soluble and is termed as **'tragacanthin'** and the *second*, being water-insoluble and is known as **'bassorin'**. Both are not soluble in alcohol. The said two components may be separated by carrying out the simple filtration of a very dilute mucilage of tragacanth and are found to be present in concentrations ranging from 60-70% for bassorin and 30-40% for tragacanthin. Bassorin actually gets swelled up in water to form a gel, whereas tragacanthin forms an instant colloidal solution. It has been established that no methoxyl groups are present in the tragacanthin fraction, whereas the bassorin fraction comprised of approximately 5.38% methoxyl moieties. Rowson (1937) suggested that the gums having higher methoxyl content *i.e.*, possessing higher bassorin contents, yielded the most viscous mucilages.

Chemical Test

1. An aqueous solution of tragacanth on boiling with conc. HCl does not develop a red colour.
2. Ruthenim Red* solution (0.1% in H_2O) on being added to powdered gum tragacanth whereby the particles will not either acquire a pink colour or are merely stained lightly.
3. When a solution of tragacanth is boiled with few drops of $FeCl_3$ [aqueous 10% (w/v)] it produces a deep-yellow precipitate.
4. It gives a heavy precipitate with lead acetate.
5. When tragacanth and precipitated copper oxide are made to dissolve in conc. NH_4OH it yields a meagre precipitate.

Substituents/Adulterants   **Karaya gum** which is sometimes known as **sterculia gum** or **Indian tragacanth** and is invariably used as a substitute for gum tragacanth.

Uses

1. It is used as a demulcent in throat preparations.
2. It is employed as an emolient in cosmetics (*e.g.*, hand lotions).
3. It is used as a pharmaceutical aid as a suspending agent for insoluble and heavy powders in mixtures.
4. It is effectively employed as a binding agent for the preparation of tablets and pills.
5. It is also used as an emulsifying agent for oils and waxes.
6. A substantial amount find its application in calico printing and in confectionary.
7. It is used in making medicinal jellies *e.g.*, spermicidal jelly.
8. A 0.2-0.3% concentration is frequently used as a stabilizer for making ice-creams and various types of sauces *e.g.*, tomato sauce, mustard sauce.
9. It is used to impart consistence to troches.
10. The mucilages and pastes find their usage as adhesives.

---

* Ruthenium oxychloride ammoniated, $C_{16}H_{42}N_{14}O_2R_{u3}$, soluble in water and used in microscopy as reagent for pectin and gum.

3.2.2.1.3 Karaya Gum

Synonyms   Gum Karaya; Kadaya; Katilo; Kullo; Kuteera; Sterculia; Indian Tragacanth; Mucara.

Biological Source   **Karaya Gum** is the dried exudate of the tree *Sterculia urens* Roxb; *Sterculia villosa* Roxb; *Sterculia tragacantha* Lindley and other species of *Sterculia, belonging to the family: Sterculeaceae.* It is obtained from *Cochlospermum Geographical Source: gossypium, De Candolle or other species of cochlospermum Kunth –family: Bixaceae.*

Geographical Source   The *S. urens* is found in India especially in the *Gujarat* region and in the central provinces.

Preparation   The gum is obtained from the *Sterculia* species by making incisions and, thereafter, collecting the plant excudates usually after a gap of 24 hours. The large irregular mass of gums (tears) which weigh between 250 g to 1 kg approximately are hand picked and despatched to the various collecting centres. The gum is usually tapped during the dry season spreading over from March to June. Each healthy fully grown tree yields from 1 to 5 kg of gum per year; and such operations may be performed about five times during its lifetime. In short, the large bulky lumps (tears) are broken to small pieces to cause effective drying. The foreign particles *e.g.*, pieces of bark, sand particles, leaves are removed. Thus, purified gum is available in *two* varieties, namely:

(*a*) **Granular or Crystal Gum:** Having a particle size ranging between 6 to 30 mesh, and

(*b*) **Powdered Gum:** Having particle size of 150 mesh

Description

Colour : White, pink or brown in colour

Odour : Slight odour resembling acetic acid

Taste : Bland and mucilageous taste

Shape : Irregular tears or vermiform pieces.

It is water insoluble but yields a translucent colloidal solution.

Chemical Constituents   **Karaya gum** is partially acetylated polysaccharide containing about 8% acetyl groups and about 37% uronic acid residues. It undergoes hydrolysis in an acidic medium to produce (+)–galactose, (–)–rhamnose, (+)–galacturonic acid and a trisaccharide acidic substance. It contains a branched heteropolysaccharide moiety having a major chain of 1, 4-linked α–(+)–galacturonic acid along with 1, 2-linked (–)–rhamnopyranose units with a short (+)– glucopyranosyluronic acid containing the side chains attached 1→3 to the main chain *i.e.*, (+)–galactouronic acid moieties.

Chemical Test   It readily produces a pink colour with a solution of Ruthenium Red.

Substituent/Adulterant   It is used as a substitute for **gum tragacanth.**

Uses

1. It is employed as a denture adhesive.
2. It is used as a 'binder' in the paper industry.
3. It is also employed as a thickening agent for dyes in the textile industry.
4. It is widely used as a stabilizer, thickner, texturizer and emulsifier in foods.

5. It is used as a bulk laxalive.
6. It finds its usage in lozenges.
7. It is employed extensively in wave set solution and in skin lotions.
8. It is used in preparations concerned with composite building materials.

3.2.2.2 Seed Gums

Seed Gums are hydrocolloids contained in some seed embryos where they actually play the role as polysaccharide food reserves.

A few typical examples of seed gums are described below, such as: Plantago seed; Pectin; Locust bean gum; and Guar gum.

3.2.2.2.1 Plantago Seed
The origin of the word '**Plantago**' is from the Latin and means sole of the foot, referring to the shape of the leaf. Likewise, *'Psyllium'* is from the Greek and means *flea-*describing the seed.

Synonyms   Psyllium seed; Plantain seed; Flea seed; Ispaghula; Isapgol; Isabgul.

Biological Source   It is the dried ripe seeds of *Plantago psyllium L.,* or *Plantago arenaria* Waldst & Kit *(P. ramosa* Asch.) (Spanish or French psyllium seed) or of *Plantago ovata* (blond or Indian plantago seed) or of *Plantago amplexicaulis* belonging to the family: *Plantaginaceae.*

Geographical Source   *P. amplexicaulis* is grown on the Panjab plains, Malwa and Sind and extending to Southern Europe.

P. psyllium is an annual pubescent herb practically native to the Mediterranean countries. It is grown in France and constitutes the main bulk of the American imported psyllium seed.

P. ovata is extensively grown in Pakistan; besides it is found to be native to Mediterranean countries and Asia.

Preparation   The crops are grown usually on light, well drained sandy loamy soils; and during their entire growth peroid the climate must be cool and dry. The ripe and matured fruits are normally collected after a span of about three months. The seeds are separated by thrashing lightly on a solid support. The dust and foreign particles are removed by sieving and against a current of mederate air-blast.

Description
  Colour : Pinkish grey to brown
  Odour : No characteristic odour
  Taste   : Bland and mucilageous
  Weight : 100 seeds weigh between 0.15-0.19 g

Figure 3.3 gives an account of the dorsal surface as well as the ventral surface of *Ispaghula seed* and *Psyllium seed* along with their overall shape, size and outersurface.

Chemical Constituents   **Plantago** seeds generally comprise of approximately 10% of mucilage invariably located in the epidermis of the testa together with proteins and fixed oil. The mucilage essentially consists of **pentosan** and **aldobionic acid.**

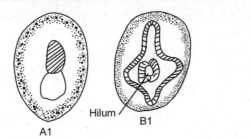 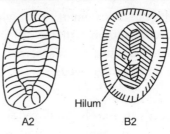

ISPAGHULA SEED
A1–Dorsal Surface
B1–Ventral Surface

PSYLLIUM SEED
A2–Dorsal Surface
B2–Ventral Surface

Shape : Ovate or boat shaped
Size　: Length = 1.8-3.5 mm, Width = 1.0-1.7 mm.

Outersurface: The *Convex surface* has a central brown oval spot, whereas the *Concave surface* bears a deep furrow having its hilum covered with a thin whitish membrane.

Fig. 3.3　Dorsal and Ventral Surfaces of *Ispaghula Seed* and *Psyllium Seed*.

$$(C_5H_8O_4)_n$$

Pentosan

The various products of hydrolysis are, namely: **xylose, arabinose, rhamnose** and **galacturonic acid.**

Chemical Tests

1. Its mucilage gives a distinct red colouration on treatment with Ruthenium Red solution.
2. **Swelling Factor*:** It establishes the purity of the drug and ranges between 10 to 14. It is easily determined by transferring accurately 1.0g of the drug in a 25 ml measuring cylinder duly filled with 20 ml of water with intermittent shaking. The exact volume occupied by the seeds after a duration of 24 hours of wetting is noted carefully which represents the *swelling factor* of the seeds under investigation.

Substituents/Adulterants A number of species of **Plantago** have been studied extensively for their mucilage contents. Interestingly, *Plantago rhodosperma* which is particularly habitated in Missouri and Lousiana (USA) and *Plantago wrightiana* are worth mentioning. The former species

---

* **Swelling Factor:** It represents the quantitative swelling due to the presence of mucilage present in the drug substance.

contains mucilage to the extent of 17.5% whereas the latter contains about 23%. However, these two species compare favourably with the official drug.

In addition to the above, a few species like *P. purshii, P. aristata* and *P. asiatica* are also employed as a substitute for **plantago seeds.**

Uses

1. Plantago seeds are mostly employed as demulscent and in the treatment of chronic constipation.
2. It is also used in amoebic and bacillary dysentary.
3. Mucilage of the isapgol is invariably employed in the preparation of tablets (*e.g.*, granulation)
4. It is used as a stabilizer in the ice-cream industry
5. The crushed seeds are employed as a poultice for rheumatic pain
6. The *acid form of polysaccharide* is obtained by carefully removing the cations from the mucilage by treatment with cation-exchange resins and spray drying the resultant products. This *'specialized product'* finds its enormous applications as a tablet disintegrator, as enteric coating substance and finally employed in the sustained release drug formulations.

3.2.2.2.2 Pectin **Pectin,** in general, is a group of polysaccharides found in nature in the primary cell walls of all seed bearing plants and are invariably located in the middle lamella. It has been observed that these specific polysaccharides actually function in combination with both cellulose and hamicellulose as an intercellular cementing substance. One of the richest sources of pectin is lemon or orange rind which contains about 30% of this polysaccharide.

Pectin is naturally found in a number of plants namely: lemon peel, orange peel, apple pomace, carrots, sunflower-heads, guava, mangoes and papaya. The European countries, Switzerland and USA largely produce pectin either from apple pomace or peels of citrus fruits. Evaluation and standardization of pectin is based on its '*Gelly-Grade*' that is, its setting capacity by the addition of sugar. Usually, pectin having 'gelly grade' of 100, 150 and 200 are recommended for medicinal and food usuages.

Biological Sources **Pectin** is the purified admixture of polysaccharides, obtained by carrying out the hydrolysis in an acidic medium of the inner part of the rind of citrus peels, for instance: *Citrus limon* (or Lemon) and *Citrus aurantium* belonging to the family *Rutaceae*, or from apple pomace *Malus sylvestris* Mill (*Syn: Pyrus malus* Linn, family: *Rosaceae*).

Geographical Source Lemon and oranges are mostly grown in India, Africa and other tropical countries. Apple is grown in the Himalayas, California, many European countries and the countries located in the Mediterranean climatic zone.

Preparation The specific method of preparation of **pectin** is solely guided by the source of raw material *i.e.*, lemon/orange rind or apple pomace; besides the attempt to prepare either low methoxy group or high methoxy group *pectins*.

In general, the preserved or freshly obtained lemon peels are gently boiled with approximately 20 times its weight of fresh water maintained duly at 90°C for a duration of 30 minutes. The effective pH (3.5 to 4.0) must be maintained with food grade lactic acid/citric acid/tartaric acid to achieve maximum extraction. Once the boiling is completed the peels are mildly squeezed to obtain the liquid portion which is then subjected to centrifugation to result into a clear solution. From this resulting solution both proteins and starch contents are suitably removed by enzymatic hydrolysis. The remaining solution is warmed to deactivate the added enzymes. The slightly coloured solution is effectively decolourized with activated carbon or bone charcoal. Finally, the pectin in its purest form is obtained by precipitation with water-miscible organic solvents (*e.g.*, methanol, ethanol, acetone), washed with small quantities of solvent and dried in a vaccum oven and stored in air-tight containers or polybags.

Note: As Pectin is fairly incompatible with Ca^{2+}, hence due precautions must be taken to avoid the contact of any metallic salts in the course of its preparation.

Description

Appearance	:	Coarse or fine- powder
Colour	:	Yellowish white
Odour	:	Practically odourless
Taste	:	Mucilaginous taste
Solubility	:	1. Completely soluble in 20 parts of water forming a solution containing negatively charged and very much hydrated particles.
		2. Dissolves more swiftly in water, if previously moistened with sugar syrup, alcohol, glycerol or if first mixed with 3 or more parts of sucrose.

Chemical Constituents Pectin occurs naturally as the partial methyl ester of α (1→4) linked (+) – polygalacturonate sequences interrupted with (1–2) – (–) – rhamnose residues. The neutral sugars that essentially form the side chains on the pectin molecules are namely: (+) – galactose, (–) – arabinose, (+) – xylose, and (–) – fructose.

Schneider and Bock (1938) put forward the following probable structure for **pectin galacturonan:**

Pectin Galacturonan

Chemical Tests

1. A 10% (w/v) solution gives rise to a solid gel on cooling.
2. A *transparent gel* or *semigel* results by the interaction of 5 ml of 1% solution of pectin with 1 ml of 2% solution of KOH and subsequently setting aside the mixture at an ambient temperature for 15 minutes. The resulting gel on acidification with dilute HCl and brisk shaking yields a voluminous and gelatinous colourless precipitate which on warming turns into white and flocculent.

Uses

1. It is employed mostly as an intestinal demulscent. It is believed that the unchanged molecules of polygalacturonic acids may exert an adsorbent action in the internal layers of the intestine, thereby producing a protective action along with *Kaolin* to prevent and control diarrhoea.

2. As a pharmaceutical aid pectin is used frequently as an emulsifying agent and also as a gelling agent preferably in an acidic medium.

3. It is employed extensively in the preparation of jellies and similar food products *e.g.*, jams, sauces, ketchups.

4. Poectin in the form of pastes exerts a bacteriostatic activity and hence, is used frequently in the treatment of indolent ulcers and deep wounds.

5. A combination of *pectin* and *gelatin* find its application as an encapsulating agent in various pharmaceutical formulations to afford sustained-release characteristics.

3.2.2.2.3 Locust Bean Gum

Synonym   Carob Flour; Arobon; Carob Gum; Ceratonia; Johannisbrotmehl;

Biological Source   The Gum essentially consists of the hydrocolloid from the powdered endosperm of tree pods of *Ceretonia siliqua* Linn, belonging to the family *Leguminoseae* **(St. John's bread).** It normally takes about 15 long years for a full-grown tree to yield seeds which , therefore, restricts the provision of a regular production of the gum to cater for the ever-expanding needs for the hydrocolloids.

Geographical Source   The tree is found in abundance in Egypt, Cyperus and Sicily. It is very sensitive to low temperature. It is also commercially grown in countries like: Algeria, Greece, Israel, Italy, Morocco, Portugal and Spain.

Preparation   The locust bean pods comprise of about 90% pulp and 8% kernnels. The kernnels are separated from the pods mechanically by means of **Kibbling Machine.** The kernnels comprise of mainly the endosperm (42-46%), husk (30-33%) and germ to the extent of 25%. First of all the seeds are duly dehusked and splitted lengthwise the seeds are duly dehusked and splitted lengthwise to facilitate the separation of the endosperm from the **embryo*** (*i.e.*, the yellow germ). The dried gum is pulverised and graded as per the mesh-size *e.g.*, 150, 175 and 200 mesh sizes available in the European market.

Description

Colour	:	Translucent white, yellow green
Odour	:	Odourless
Taste	:	Tasteless and mucilaginous. Acquires a leguminous taste when boiled with water
Solubility	:	Insoluble in alcohol. Dispersable in concentration upto 5%
Viscosity	:	As it is a neutral polysaccharide, hence pH has no effect on viscosity between 3-11.

Chemical Constituents   Locust bean gum comprises of *proteins*, for instance: albumins, globulins and glutelins; *carbohydrates,* such as: reducing sugar, sucrose, dextrins, and pentosans; besides ash, fat, crude fiber and moisture.

---

* Embryo enhances the rate of fermentation of gum solutions and hence it must be removed as completely as possible.

Chemical Tests The mucilage of this gum when gently boiled with 5% KOH solution it yields a clear solution; but agar and tragacanth gives rise to a yellow colour, whereas karaya gum produces a brown colour.

Substituent Adulterant In food industry it is employed as a substitute for strach.

Uses
1. It is used as a stabilizer, thickner and binder in foods and cosmetics.
2. It is widely employed as a sizing and finishing agent in textiles.
3. It finds its abundant use as fiber - bonding in paper manufacture.
4. It is used as an adsorbent - demulcent therapeutically.
5. It is employed as drilling mud additive.

3.2.2.2.4 Guar Gum

Synonyms Guar flour; Decorpa; Jaguar; Gum cyamopsis; Cyamopsis gum; Burtonite V-7-E.

Biological Source **Guar gum** is the ground endosperms of *Cyamopsis tetragonolobus* (L.) Taub; belonging to family *Leguminoseae*.

Geographical Source It grows abundantly in tropical countries like: Indonesia, India, Pakistan and Africa. In USA, southern western regions it was introduced in the year 1900 and its large-scale production commenced in early 1950's.

Preparation First of all the fully developed white seeds of Guar gum are collected and freed from any foreign substances.

The sorted seeds are fed to a mechanical **'splitter'** to obtain the *bifurcated guar seeds* which are then separated into husk and the respective cotyledons having the *'embryo'*. The gum is found into the endosperm. Generally, the guar seeds comprise of the following:

Endosperm	:	35 to 40%
Germ (or Embryo)	:	45 to 50%, and
Husk	:	14 to 17%

The **cotyledons,** having a distinct bitter taste are separated from the endosperm by the process called **'winnowing'**. The crude guar gum *i.e.*, the endosperms is subsequently pulverised by means of a *'micro-pulveriser'* followed by grinding. The relatively softer cotyledons sticking to the endosperms are separated by mechanical *'sifting'* process. Thus, the crude guar-gum is converted to a purified form (*i.e.*, devoid of cotyledons), which is then repeatedly pulverized and shifted for several hours till a final white powder or gramular product is obtained.

Description
Colour	:	Colourless; Pale-yellowish white powder
Odour	:	Characteristic smell
Taste	:	Mucilagenous
Solubility	:	Insoluble in alcohol with water it gives a thick transparent suspension

Chemical Constituents It has been found that the water soluble fraction constitutes 85% of Guar gum and is commonly known as **Guaran.** It essentially consists of linear chains of $(1 \rightarrow 4)$ –β-Dmannopyranosyl units with α–D-galactopyranosyl units attached by $(1 \rightarrow 6)$ linkages. However, the ratio of D-galactose to D-mannose is 1:2.

Guaran

Chemical Tests
1. On being treated with iodine solution (0.1 N) it fails to give olive-green colouration.
2. It does not produce pink colour when treated with Ruthenium Red solution (distinction from sterculia gum and agar)
3. A 2% solution of lead acetate gives an instant white precipitate with guar gum (distinction from sterculia gum and acacia)
4. A solution of guar gum (0.25 g in 10 ml of water) when mixed with 0.5 ml of benzidine (1% in ethanol) and 0.5 ml of hydrogen peroxide produces no blue colouration (distinction from gum acacia).

Uses
1. It is used therapeutically as a bulk laxative.
2. It is employed as a protective colloid.
3. It is also used as a thickner and its thickening property is 5 to 8 times more than starch.
4. It finds its use in peptice ulcer therapy.
5. It is used as an anorectic substance *i.e.*, it acts as an appetite depressant.
6. It is employed both as a binding and a disintegrating agent in tablet formulations.
7. It is used in paper sizing.
8. It is abundantly employed as film forming agent for cheese, salad dressing, ice-cream and soups.
9. It is used in pharmaceutical jelly formulations.
10. It is widely used in suspensions, emulsions, lotions, creams and toothpastes.
11. It is largely used in mining industry as a flocculant and also as a filtering agent.
12. It is also employed in water treatment plants as a coagulant aid.

3.2.2.3 Marine Gums

A variety of algae and seaweeds comprise of **marine gums** as components of cell walls and membranes or present in the intracellular regions where they actually serve as reserve food material.

A few typical examples of marine gums would be discussed in the sections that follow.

3.2.2.3.1 Algin

Synonyms Sodium alginate; Alginic acid sodium; Sodium polymannuronate; Kelgin; Minus; Protanal;

Biological Source **Algin** is a gelling polysaccharide extracted from the giant brown seaweed (*giant kelp. Macrocystis pyrifera* (L.) Ag., *Lessoniaceae*) or from *horsetail kelp (Laminaria digitata* (L.) *Lamour, Laminariaceae)* or from *sugar kelp (Laminaria saccharina* (L.) *Lamour)*. Some other common species are *Laminaria hyperborea* and *Ascophyllum nodosum*

Geographical Source The different varieties of seaweeds are invariably found in the Pacific and Atlantic Oceans, more specifically along the coastal lines of USA, Canada, Scotland, Japan and Australia. In India the Western coast of Saurashtra is also a potential source of algin. However, USA, and UK are the largest producers of algin in the world.

Preparation The **algin** (or sodium alginate) is the sodium salt of alginic acid which is a purified carbohydrate extracted from brown seaweed (algae) by the careful treatment with dilute sodium hydroxide. The brown colour of the crude algin is due to the presence of a carotenoid pigment associated with it which may be eliminated by treating the aqueous solution with activated carbon and spray drying the powder.

Description
- **Colour** : Yellowish-white, cream coloured, buff coloured
- **Odour** : Odourless
- **Taste** : Tasteless
- **Solubility** : Insoluble in alcohol, ether, chloroform and strong acids, freely soluble in water
- **Viscosity** : A 1% (w/v) aqueous solution at 20°C may show a viscosity ranging between 20-400 *centipoises*.

Chemical Constituents Alginic acid is mainly comprised of D-mannuronic acid residues which on methylation and hydrolysis gives rise to the formation of 2,3 dimethyl-D- mannuronide. Therefore, the ring as well as bridge oxygen atoms involve C-4 and C-5 and the carboxyl groups are absolutely free to react (to form sodium salts), whereas the aldehydic moieties are duly utilized by the respective glycosidic linkages. It has been observed that these mannuronic acid entities are joined by β-1, 4-glycosidic linkages. The resulting structure could be either linear or very slightly branched.

Alginic Acid

Chemical Tests
1. The aqueous solution of algin gives an instant white copious precipitate with calcium chloride solution.

2. A 1% (w/v) aqueous solution of algin yields a heavy gelatinous precipitate with diluted sulphuric acid.
3. It is not precipitated by saturated ammonium sulphate solution (distinction from agar and tragacanth)
4. It gives effervescence (liberates CO_2) with carbonates.
5. It readily reacts with compounds having ions of alkali metals (*e.g.*, Na^+, K^+, Li^+) or ammonium (NH_4^+) or magnesium (Mg^{2+}) to produce their respective alginates (salts) that are *water soluble* and forms thick and viscous solutions characteristic of *hydrophillic colloids.*

Uses
1. It is extensively used in the manufacture of ice-creams where it serves as a stabilizing colloid, ensuring creamy texture thereby checking the growth of ice-flakes (or crystals).
2. It is also used in the flocculation of suspended solids in most water treatment plants.
3. It is employed as a stabilizing and thickening agent in food and pharmaceutical industry.
4. It is used as a film and film-forming agent in the rubber and paint industry.
5. It is widely used in the textile industry as absorbable haemostatic dressings.
6. It is employed as a binding and distintegrating agent for tablets and lozenges.

3.2.2.3.2 Agar

Synonyms   Agar-agar; Gelose; Japan-agar; Chinese-isinglass; Bengal isinglass; Ceylon isinglass; Layor carang; Vegetable gelatin.

Biological Source   **Agar** is the dried hydrophilic colloidal polysaccharide complex extracted from the agarocytes of algae belonging to the class *Rhodophyceae*. It is also obtained as the dried gelatinous substance from *Gelidium amansii* belonging to the family *Gelidaceae* and several other species of red algae, such as *Gracilaria* (family: *Gracilariaceae)* and *Pterocladia (Gelidaceae)*. The predominant agar-producing genera are, namely; *Gelidium; Gracilaria; Acanthopeltis; Ceramium and Pterocladia.*

Geographical Source   **Agar** is largely produced in Japan, Australia, India, New Zealand, and USA. It is also found in Korea, Spain, South Africa and in the Coastal regions of Bay of Bengal (India) together with Atlantic and Specific Coast of USA.

Preparation   It is an usual practice in Japan where the **red-algae** is cultivated by placing poles or bamboos spread in the ocean which will serve as a support and shall augment the growth of algae on them. During the months of May and October the poles are removed and the algae are carefully stripped off from them. The fresh seaweed thus collected is washed thoroughly in water and subsequently extracted in digestors containing hot solution of dilute acid (1 portion of algae to 60 portions of diluted acid). The mucilagenous extract is filtered through linen while hot and collected in large wooden troughs to cool down to ambient temperature so as to form solid gel. The gel is mechanically cut into bars and passed through a wire netting to form strips. The moisture from the strips is removed by successive **freezing and thawing*** and finally sun dried and stored as thin agar strips.

 Alternatively, the mass of gel if frozen and subsequently thawed and the dried agar is obtained by vaccum filtration. The crude agar is usually formed as flakes which can be powdered and stored accordingly.

---

* To bring down to room temperature from –20 to –30ºC.

Description

   Colour : Yellowish white or Yellowish grey
   Odour : Odourless
   Taste : Bland and mucilaginous
   Shape : It is available in different shapes, such as: bands, strips, flakes, sheets and coarse powder
   Size : Bands: width = 4cm; Length = 40 to 50 cms
            Sheets: Width = 10-15cm; Length = 45 to 60 cms
            Strips: Width = 4mm; Length = 12 to 15 cms

India produces about 250 MT of good quality agar using *Galidiella accrosa* as the raw material. It is insoluble in cold water in organic solvents. It readily dissolves in hot solutions and it forms a translucent solid mass which characteristic is very useful in microbiology for carrying out the *Standard Plate Count.*

Chemical Constituents   **Agar** can be separated into two major fractions, namely: (*a*) *Agarose*-a neutral gelling fraction; and (*b*) *Agaropectin*—a sulphated non-gelling fraction. The former is solely responsible for the *gel-strength of agar* and consists of (+) –galactose and 3,6-anhydro-(–)-galactose moieties; whereas the latter is responsible for the *viscosity of agar solutions* and comprises of sulphonated polysaccharide wherein both uronic acid and galactose moieties are partially esterified with sulphuric acid. In short, it is believed to be a complex range of polysaccharide chains having alternating α–(1→3) and β–(1-4) linkages and varying *total charge content.*

Chemical Tests

1. It gives a pink colouration with Ruthenium Red solution.
2. A 1.5-2.0% (w/v) solution of agar when boiled and cooled produces a *stiff-jelly.*
3. Prepare a 0.5%(w/v) solution of agar and add to 5 ml of it 0.5 ml of HCl, boil gently for 30 minutes and divide into two equal portions:
   (*a*) To one portion add $BaCl_2$ solution and observe a slight whitish precipitate due to the formation of $BaSO_4$ (distinction from Tragacanth), and
   (*b*) To the other portion add dilute KOH solution for neutralization, add 2 ml of Fehling's solution and heat on a water bath. The appearance of a brick red precipitate confirms the presence of galactose.

Substituents/Adulterants   **Gelatin** and **isinglass** are usually used as substituents for **agar.**

Uses

1. It is used in making photographic emulsions.
2. It is also employed as a bulk laxative.
3. It is extensively used in preparing gels in cosmetics.
4. It is widely used as thickening agent in confectionaries and dairy products.
5. It is used in the production of ointments and medicinal encapsulations.
6. In microbiology, it is employed in the preparation of bacteriological culture media.
7. It is used for sizing silks and paper.
8. It finds its enormous usage in the dyeing and printing of fabrics and textiles.
9. It is also used as dental impression mould base.
10. It is employed as corrosion inhibitor.

3.2.2.3.3 Carrageenan

Synonyms   Irish moss; Chondrus.

Biological Source   **Carrageenan** refers to closely associated hydrocolloids which are obtained from different red algae or seaweeds. The most important sources of carrageenan are namely: *Chondrus crispus* (Linn.) stockhouse and *Gigartina mamillosa* (Goodnough and Woodward) J. Agardh belonging to the family *Gigartinaceae*).

Geographical Source   The plants are abundantly found along the north-western coast of France, the coast of Nova Scotia, and the British Isles.

Preparation   In general, the plants are collected mostly during June and July, and spread out on the bench for natural drying. They are then exposed to the sun rays directly whereby bleaching takes place. Now, they are treated with a brine solution, and ultimately dried and stored.

Description   The *Chondrus* is more or less an allusion to the cartilage-like characteristic features of the dry thallus; whereas *Gigartina* is an absolute allusion specifically to the fruit bodies which appear as raised tubercles on the thallus.

Chemical Constituents   The **carrageenan** bears a close physical resemblance to agar. However, its hydrocolloids are mostly galactans having sulphate esters, which are present in excess amount in comparison to agar. Carrageenan polysaccharides essentially comprise of chains of 1, 3 linked β – (+) – galactose and 1,4-linked α- (+) – galactose moieties that are invariably substituted and later on modified to the 3, 6- anhydro derivative. In fact, carrageenans may be further separated into *three* major components, namely: **k-carrageenan; i-carrageenan;** and **λ-carrageenan.**

Uses
1. Both **k-and i-carrageenans** proved to be good gelating agents because of the fact that they tend to orient in stable helics when in solution.
2. The λ-carrageenan does not form stable helics and hence represent the nongelling portion of the carrageenans which serves as a more useful thickner.
3. The fairly stable texture and supported by excellent rinsability of the hydrocolloids these are immensely useful in the formulations of toothpastes.
4. They are used as bulk laxative.
5. They are employed as a demulscent.
6. They constitute as an important ingredient in a large number of food preparations.

3.2.2.4 Microbial Gums

Microbial Gums are produced by certain selected miroorganisms in the course of fermentation. The resulting exopolysacharides are usually isolated from the fermentation broth by appropriate procedures.

A few typical examples are described below, for instance: Xanthan Gum; Chitin.

3.2.2.4.1 Xanthan Gum

Synonyms   Polysaccharide B-1459; Keltrol F; Kelzan.

Biological Source   The Polysaccharide Gum is produced by the bacterium *Xanthomonas campestris* on certain suitable carbohydrates.

Preparation   One of the latest techniques of **'biotechnology'** *i.e.,* **'recombinant DNA technology'** has been duly exploited for the commercial production of xanthan gum.

Methodology: First of all the genomic banks of *Xanthomonas campestris* are meticulously made in *Escherichia coli* by strategically mobilizing the broad-host-range cosmids being used as the vectors. Subsequently, the conjugal transfer of the genes take place from *E. coli* into the nonmucoid *X. campestris*. Consequently, the wild type genes are duly separated by virtue of their unique ability to restore mucoid phenotype. As a result, a few of the cloned plasmids incorporated in the wild type strains of *X. campestris* shall afford an increased production xanthan gum.

Interestingly, the commercial xanthan gums are available with different genetically controlled composition, molecular weights and as their respective sodium, potassium or calcium salts.

Description   It is a cream coloured, odourless and free flowing powder. It dissolves swiftly in water on shaking and yields a highly viscous solution at relatively low concentrations. The aqueous solutions are extremely pseudoplastic in character. It gives rise to a strong film on evaporation of its aqueous solutions. It is fairly stable and resistent to thermal degradation. The viscosity is independent of temperature between 10 to 70°C. It is fairly compatible with a variety of salts.

Chemical Constituents   **Xanthan gum** is composed of chiefly D-glucosyl, D-mannosyl and D-glucosyluronic acid residues along with variant quantum of O-acetyl and pyruvic acid acetal. The primary structure essentially comprises of a cellulose backbone with trisaccharide side chains and the repeating moiety being a pentasaccharide.

Uses
1. Its potential in chemically enhanced oil recovery is well known.
2. The inherent pseudoplastic property of its aqueous solutions rendered both toothpastes and ointments in enabling them to hold their shape and also to spread readily.
3. It is extensively employed in pharmaceuticals due to its superb suspending and emulsifying characteristic features.

3.2.2.4.2 Chitin   **Chitin,** is the nitrogen containing polysaccharide which invariably occurs in certain fungi *e.g.,* ergot. It is also commonly found in some invertebrate animals eg, crab, shrimp, lobster-specifically located in the exoskeleton of the body. Besides, it is located in the appendages of insects and crustaceans.

Biological Source   The mycelia of *Penicillium* species contain approximately 20% of chitin. The relatively hard crustacean shells of crab and lobster are reported to contain 15 to 20% chitin, whereas the rather soft crustacean shells of shrimp contain between 15 to 30% chitin. It is found in the spores of many fungi and yeasts.

Preparation   The hard or soft **crustacean shells** are first ground to fine powder and then treated with dilute HCl (5%) for a duration of about 24 hours whereby most of the calcium* and other impurities are eliminated completely as soluble $CaCl_2$. The above extract containing the proteins derived from the shells are eliminated by treating it with proteolytic enzymes like *pepsin* or *trypsin*.

---

* Crustacean shell contain approx. 60-75% of calcium carbonate.

The resulting pink coloured liquid extract is bleached by H_2O_2 in an acidic medium for 5-6 hours at room temperature. The bleached product is subjected to deacetylation at 120°C with a mixture of 3 parts of KOH, 1 part EtOH and 1 part ethylene glycol. The deacetylation process is repeated several times till the *'acetyl content'* reaches a minimum level. **Chitin** is obtained as an amorphous solid substance.

Description   It is an amorphous solid. It is practically insoluble in water, dilute acids, dilute and concentrated alkalies, alcohol and other organic solvents. It is soluble in concentrated HCl, H_2SO_4, anhydrous HCOOH and H_3PO_4 (78-97%). There exists a wide difference with regard to the solubility, molecular weight, acetyl value and specific rotation amongst chitins of different origin and obtained from different methods.

Chemical Constituents   **Chitin** may be regarded as a derivative of cellulose, wherein the C-2 hydroxyl groups have been duly replaced by acetamido residues. In fact, it is more or less a cellulose like biopolymer mainly consisting of unbranched chains of β-(1→4) -2- acetamido -2-deoxy-D-glucose. It is also termed as N-acetyl-D-glucosamine. It contains about 6.5% of nitrogen.

Chitin

Chemical Tests
1. **Chitin** affords a brown colour with Iodine solution which turns into red violet on acidification with sulphuric acid.
2. **Chitin sulphate** gives rise to a characteristic strain with acidic dyes, such as: picric acid and fuchsin.
3. When chitin is heated with strong KOH solution under pressure it fails to dissolve, but undergoes deacetylation to form acetic acid and other products collectively termed as *chitosans*.
4. Hydrolysis of **chitin** in the presence of strong mineral acids forms acetic acid and glucosamine.
5. When **chitin** is dissolved in dilute nitric acid (50%) and allowd to crystallise overnight it forms beautiful spherocrystals of chitosan. These crystals on being examined under polarised light, by making use of crossed nicols, a distinct cross is observed.

Uses
1. **Chitosan** *i.e.*, **deacetylated chitin,** finds its application in water treatment operations.
2. It is used in pholographic emulsions.
3. It is used in improving the dyeability of synthetic fibers and fabrics.
4. Therapeutically it is used in wound healing preparations.
5. It shows considerable adhesivity to plastics and glass.
6. It is used as a sizing agent for cotton, wool, rayon and for synthetic fibers.

3.3   CARBOHYDRATE BIOGENESIS

One of the most vital aspects of pharmacognosy which has gained paramunt importance and legitimate recognition in the recent past is the intensive and extensive studies involving the various biochemical pathways that has ultimately led to the production of **'secondary constituents'** invariably employed as **'drugs'.** This type of specific and elaborated study is frequently termed as **biogenesis** or **drug biosynthesis.** It is quite pertinent to mention here that as it is absolutely necessary for a medicinal chemist to understand the intricacies of chemical synthesis of a potent drug substance, such as: naproxen, chloramphenicol etc., exactly in the same vein a pharmacognosist must possess a thorough knowledge of the biogenesis of drugs of natural origin.

A Swiss chemist G. Trier, as far back in 1912, not only predicted but also postulated that amino acids and their corresponding derivatives invariably act as the precursors of relatively complex naturally occurring alkaloids mostly used as potent therapeutic agents. Interestingly, soonafter the second half of the twentieth century, there had been a tremendous progress in the era of **isotopically labelled organic compounds** that facilitated the affirmation as well as confirmation of the earlier speculated theories.

With the advent of most advanced knowledge in sciences it has been established that the carbohydrate biogenesis usually takes place due to the *Photosynthesis* from carbon dioxide (CO_2) as the starting material occurring abundantly both in all plants and in certain purple bacteria as depicted below:

$$nCO_2 + n\ H_2O + \underset{\text{(energy)}}{\text{Light}} \longrightarrow \underset{\text{(carbohydrate)}}{(CH_2O)n} + nO_2 \qquad\qquad (a)$$

However, the general pattern of **'Carbohydrate Biogenesis'** may be shown explicitly in the following Fig. 3.4.

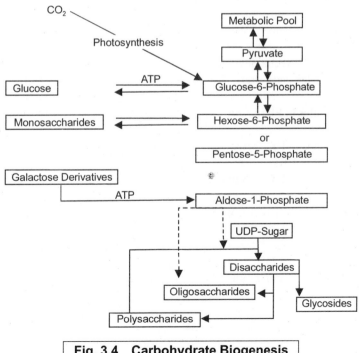

Fig. 3.4   Carbohydrate Biogenesis

Calvin and coworkers established the various steps involved in the chemical reactions ultimately leading to the overall Eq. (*a*). They have also shown that D-ribose-1, 5-diphosphate is the primary acceptor of CO_2. However, the exact mechanism of this particular step whereby CO_2 gets assimilated has been studied at length with radio labelled $^{14}CO_2$ and *Chiorella* (a fresh water algae).

Besides, the following Eq. (*b*) evidently illustrates the distribution of radiocarbon originating from $^{14}CO_2$ after completion of one full photosynthetic cycle:

$$
\begin{array}{c}
\overset{*}{}\qquad\qquad\qquad\qquad \overset{*}{}\quad\overset{*}{} \\
\overset{*}{}\qquad\qquad\qquad\qquad \overset{*}{}\quad\overset{*}{} \\
2\overset{*}{C}HO.\overset{*}{C}HOH.\overset{*}{C}H_2OP \longrightarrow \overset{*}{C}H_2OP{-}\overset{*}{C}O{-}\overset{*}{C}HOH{-}\overset{*}{C}HOH{-}\overset{*}{C}HOH{-}\overset{*}{C}H_2OH
\end{array}
\qquad (b)
$$

From Eq. (*b*) it may be inferred that a triose phosphate having the identified radiocarbon distribution shall ultimately result after completing a single full cycle. It would most logically lead to hexose phosphate which should invariably contain relatively higher amounts of $^{14}CO_2$ (*i.e.*, radio labelled carbon), till such time after a series of recycling slots, give rise to an even distribution of radio active carbon spread over the entire hexose molecule.

FURTHER READING REFERENCES

1. Baird JK: **Gums: Kirk-Othmer Encyclopedia of Chemical Technology,** 4th ed., Vol. 12, Wiley, New York, pp. 842–862, 1994.
2. BeMiller JN: **Carbohydrates: Kirk-Othmer Encyclopedia of Chemical Technology,** 4th ed., Vol. 4. Wiley, New York, pp. 911–948, 1992.
3. Bugg TDH: **Bacterial Peptidoglycan Biosynthesis and its Inhibition,** *Comprehensive Natural Products Chemistry,* Vol. 3, Elsevier, Amsterdam, pp. 241–294, 1999.
4. Davidson, R. L; (Ed); **Handbook of Water Soluble Gums and Resins,** McGraw Hill Book Co., London, 1980.
5. Dea ICM: **Industrial Polysaccharides,** *Pure appl. Chem.* **61,** 1315–1322, 1989.
6. Dewies, D.D., J. Giovenelli, and T. Ress, '**Plant Biochemistry'.** Blackwell Scientific Publications, Oxford (UK), 1964.
7. Franz G: **Polysaccharides in Pharmacy-Current Applications and Future Concepts,** *Planta Medica,* **55,** 493–497, 1989.
8. Hoppe, H.A., T. Levring, and Y. Tanaka: (Eds), **Marine Algae in Pharmaceutical Science.,** Vols. 1-2, Walter de Gruyter, Berlin, 1979, 1982.
9. Livington JN and Schoen WR: **Glucagon and Glucagon-Like Peptide-I,** In Ann. Reports. *Med. Chem.,* **34,** 189-198, 1999.
10. Phillips, G.O., P.A. Williams, and D.J. Wedlock: (Eds), '**Gums and Stabilizers for the Food Industry',** Oxford University Press, Oxford (UK) 1992.
11. Pigman, W.W, M.L. Wolfram and R.S. Tipson; (Eds), '**Advances in Carbohydrate Chemistry',** Vol. 1, Academic Press, New York, 1945, 1984.
12. Walter, R.H., (Ed), '**The Chemistry and Technology of Pectin',** Academic Press Inc., Sar Diego (USA), 1991.

---

* Radio labelled carbon.

13. Whistler, R.L., and J.N. Bemiller: (Eds), **'Industrial Gums, Polysaccharides and their Derivatives'**, Academic Press, New York, 1959.

14. Weymouth-Wilson AC: **The Role of Carbohydrates in Biologically Active Natural Products,** *Nat. Prod. Rep.* **14,** 99–110, 1997.

15. Yalpani, M,: (Ed), **'Progress in Biotechnology,** Vol. 3, **Industrial Polysaccharides,** Elsevier Science Publishers, B.V. Amsterdam, 1987.

4 Glycosides

- Introduction
- Classification
- Biosynthesis of Glycosides
- Profile of Glycosides in Natural Plant Sources
- Further Reading References

4.1 INTRODUCTION

Glycosides, in general, are defined as the condensation products of sugars with a host of different varieties of **organic hydroxy** (occasionally *thiol*) **compounds** (invariably monohydrate in character), in such a manner that the hemiacetal entity of the carbohydrate must essentially take part in the condensation. It is, however, pertinent to state here that the *polysaccharides* are also encompassed in this broad-based overall definition of **glycosides**. The noncarbohydrate moiety is usually termed as **aglycone** (or **aglycon**), or a **genin**.

The rather older or trivial names of glycosides usually has a suffix 'in' and the names essentially included the source of the glycoside, for instance: **strophanthidin** from *Strophanthus*, **digitoxin** from *Digitalis*, **barbaloin** from *Aloes*, **salicin** from *Salix*, **cantharidin** from *Cantharides*, and **prunasin** from *Prunus.* However, the systematic names are invariably coined by replacing the "ose" suffix of the parent sugar with "oside". The *stereochemical anomeric prefix* α *or* β and the *configurational prefix (D- or L-)* immediately precede the sugar nomenclature, and lastly the *chemical name of the aglycone* precedes the name of the sugar. It may be expatiated with the help of the following examples:

(*a*) **Aloin (or Barbaloin):** 10-Glucopyranosyl-1, 8-dihydroxy-3-(hydroxymethyl)-9 (10H)-anthracenone;
(*b*) **Salicin:** 2-(Hydroxymethyl) phenyl- -D-glucopyranoside;
(*c*) **Amygdalin:** D-Mandelonitrile–β-D-glycosido-6-β-D-glucoside;
(*d*) **Digitoxin:** 3-[0-2, 6-Dideoxy-β-D-ribo-hexopyranosyl -(1 $\rightarrow$ 4)-O-2, 6-dideoxy-β-D-ribo-hexopyranosyl (1 $\rightarrow$ 4), 2, 6-dideoxy-β-D-ribo hexopyranosyl) oxy]-14-hydroxycard- 20(22)-enolide.

Interestingly, the **glycosides** may be regarded as internal acetate. The two series of stereoisomeric glycosides are usually termed as **α and β glycosides**. Thus, taking into consideration the simple example of **methyl D-glucosides**, these α and β structures may be represented as shown below:

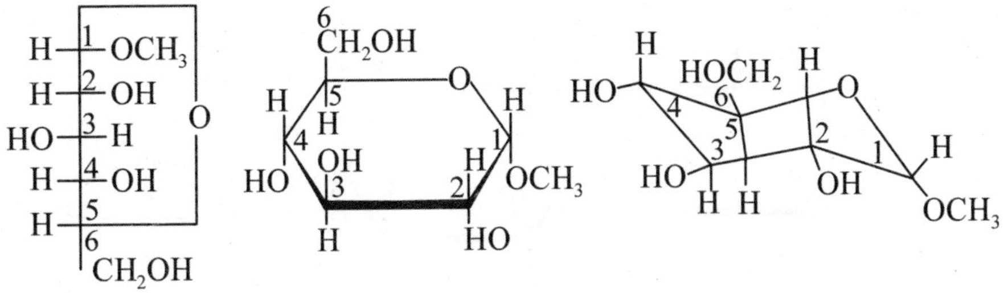

Fig. 4.1   Methyl-α-D-Glucoside

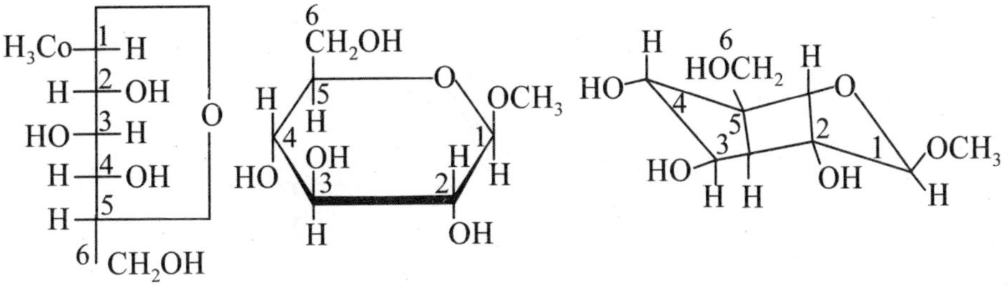

Fig. 4.2   Methyl-β-D-Glucoside

Figures 4.1 and 4.2 represent the **open-chain structure, cyclic structure and boat configuration of methyl–α-D-glucoside and methyl–β-D-glucoside** respectively. In this particular instance the glycosidic likage is established by dehydration involving a *hydroxy group* of the *aglycone portion* (*i.e.*, methyl alcohol) and the *hydroxyl group* on the *hemiacetal carbon of the carbohydrate* (in question), thereby ultimately resulting into the formation of an *acetal type of structure.*

α-Configuration   If the —OCH$_3$ moiety (generalized as OR′) is in opposite steric sense as the —CH$_2$OH moiety on C-5 (for D-family sugars), the glycosidic structure is designated as **α-configuration.**

β-Configuration   If the -OCH$_3$ moiety is in the same steric sense as the CH$_2$OH group on C-5, the glycosidic structure is designated as **β-configuration.**

It has been observed that the substantial quantum of naturally occurring glycosides essentially possess the **stereo-configuration.** However, this observation may be further expatiated with the help of the following typical examples of **β-amygdalin** and **β-salicin**:

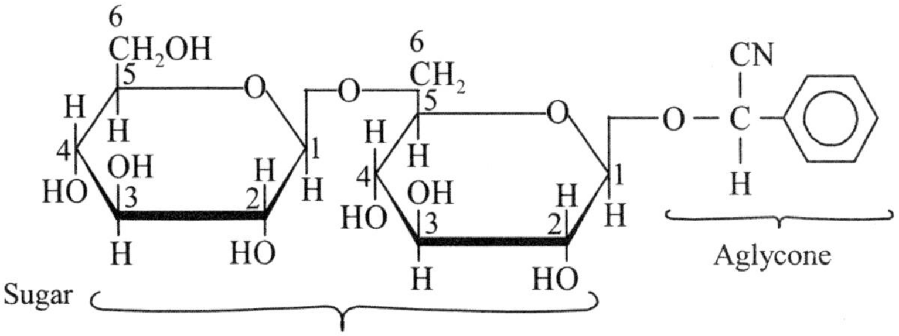

β-Amygdalin

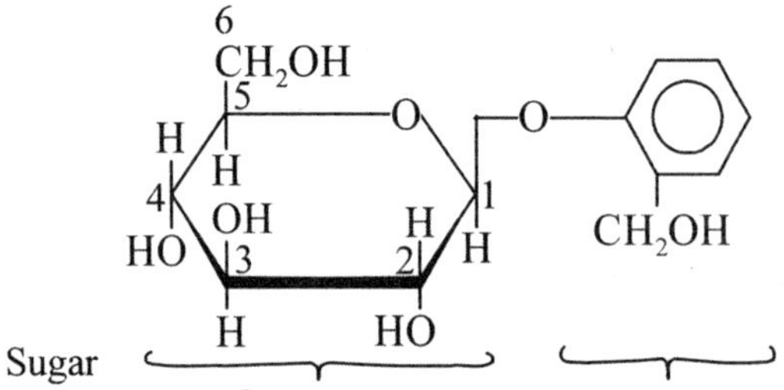

β-Salicin

Sailent Features (β-Amygdalin):

(*i*) Glycosidic linkage is β-because it is hydrolysed by **emulsin** (an enzyme),

(*ii*) The linking oxygen is on the same side of the plane of the ring as the CH_2OH moiety on C-5.

(*iii*) It contains several asymmetric C atoms *i.e.,* **chiral centres,** and

(*iv*) It is **optically active**.

Salient Features (β-Salicin):

1. Hydrolysed by emulsin, hence it has **β-configuration,**
2. The linking oxygen is on the same side of the plane of the ring as the CH_2OH moiety on C-5,
3. It has several **chiral centres,** and
4. It is **optically active.**

Glycosides, are found to exert a wide spectrum of therapeutic actions, both in modern medicines and in traditional medicaments, ranging from *cardiotonic, analgesic, purgative,* and *anti-rheumatic, demulcent* and host of other useful actions.

The Glycosidic Linkages   The exact point of linkage between the carbohydrate (sugar) and non carbohydrate (aglycone) moieties is an '**oxygen bridge**' that essentially connects the reducing group present in carbohydrate to either an alcoholic or a phenolic group present in the non carbohydrate. Such glycosides are collectively termed as **O-glycosides.** However, if the 'O' is replaced by 'S' it is called **S-glycosides;** if replaced by 'N' is known as **N-glycosides;** and if replaced by 'C' is termed as **C-glycosides.**

These **four** types of glycosides shall be described briefly at this juncture with appropriate examples from the domain of medicinal plants.

4.1.1 O-Glycosides

The **O-glycosides** are usually represented as follows:

$$—OH \quad HO—C_6H_{11}O_5 \longrightarrow —O—C_6H_{11}O_5 \quad \textit{O-Glycoside}$$

These are most abundantly found in nature in the higher plants, such as: senna, rhubarb and frangula.

Examples: Rhein-8-glucoside obtained from rhubarb.

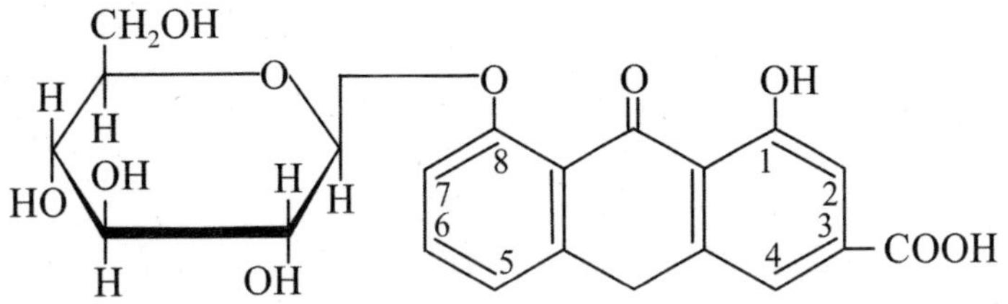

Rhein-8-Glycoside

4.1.2 S-Glycosides

The **S-glycosides** are normally designated as below:

$$—SH \quad HO—C_6H_{11}O_5 \longrightarrow S—C_6H_{11}O_5 \quad \textit{S-Glycoside}$$

The presence of S-glycosides is more or less restricted to isothiocyanate glycosides, such as: **Sinigrin,** obtained from black mustard seeds. (*i.e.*, **Brassica campestris** Family: *Cruciferae*)

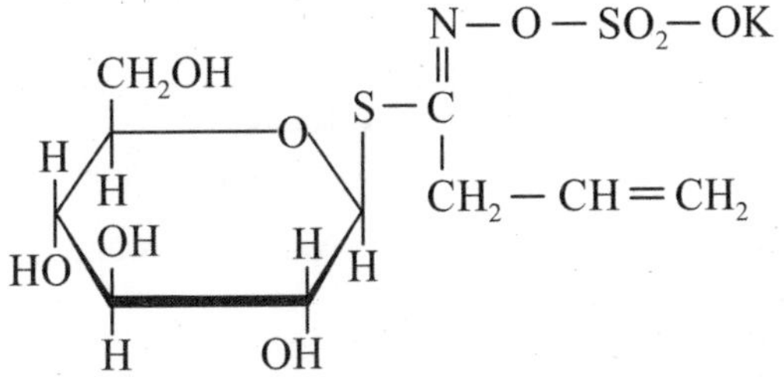

Sinigrin

4.1.3 N-Glycosides

The **N-glycosides** may be represented as shown below:

$$=N—H \quad HO—C_6H_{11}O_5 \longrightarrow \quad =N—C_6H_{11}O_5 \; \textit{N-Glycoside}$$

The most typical example of N-glycosides is the nucleosides, wherein the respective amino group of the base ultimately reacts with —OH group ribose/deoxyribose.

Examples: Adenosine: It is widely distributed in nature *e.g.*; from yeast nucleic acid.

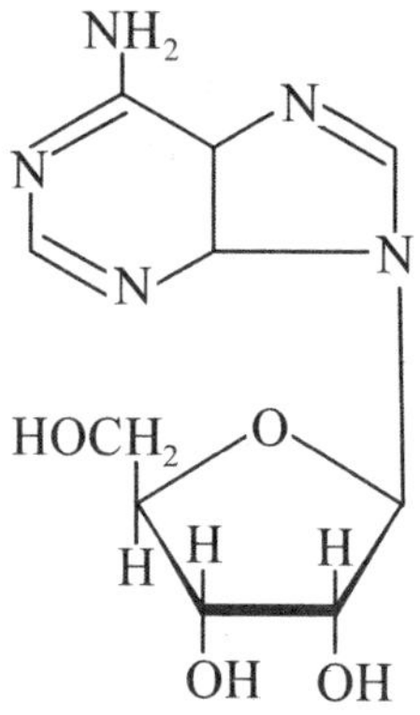

Adenosine

4.1.4 C-Glycosides

The **C-glycosides** may be designated as shown under:

$$\geqslant CH \quad HO—C_6H_{11}O_5 \longrightarrow \geqslant C—C_6H_{11}O_5 \quad \textit{C-Glycoside}$$

C-Glycosides are present in a variety of plant substances, such as: **aloin** in Aloe; **cascaroside** in Cascara.

(*i*) **Aloin or Barbaloin:**

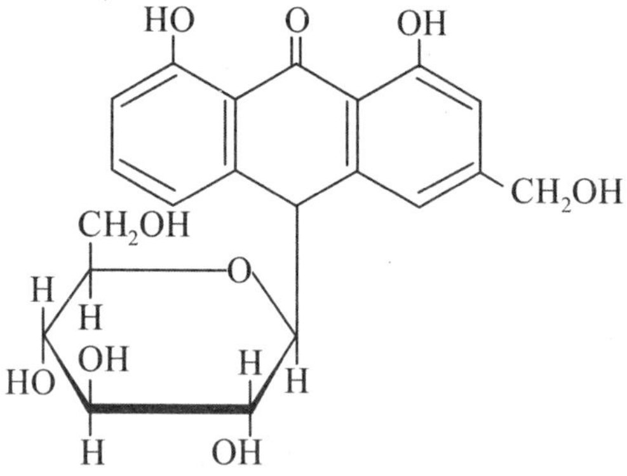

Aloin (or Barbaloin)

(*ii*) **Cascarosides (A, B, C and D):**

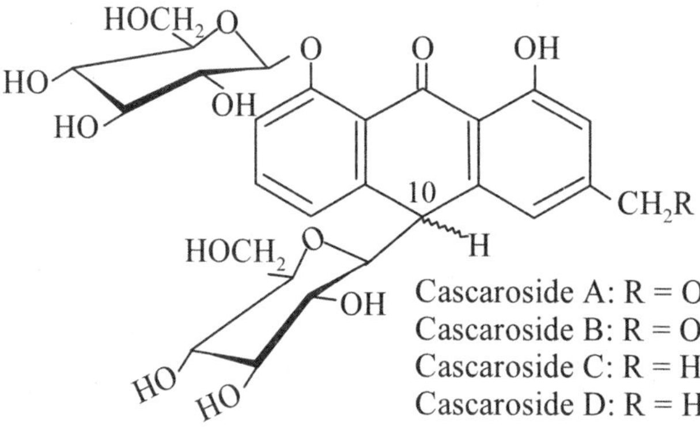

Cascaroside A: R = OH, (12S)
Cascaroside B: R = OH, (10R)
Cascaroside C: R = H, (10S)
Cascaroside D: R = H, (10R)

Cascarosides

4.2 CLASSIFICATION

In reality, the most befitting classification of glycosides is rather a hard-nut-to-crack. In case, the classification is to be governed by the presence of sugar moiety, a good number of rare sugars are involved, if the aglycone function forms the basis of classification, one may come across groups from probably all major categories of plant constituents identified and reported. Of course, a therapeutic classification offers not only a positive edge over the stated classification but also affords an excellent means from a pharmaceutic viewpoint, but it grossly lacks a host of glycosides which are of great pharmacognostic interest.

The most acceptable **classification of glycosides** is based on the chemical nature of the **aglycone moiety** present in them, namely:

- (*i*) Anthracene glycosides
- (*ii*) Phenol glycosides
- (*iii*) Steroid glycosides
- (*iv*) Flavonoid glycosides
- (*v*) Coumarin and Furanocoumarin glycosides
- (*vi*) Cyonogenetic glycosides
- (*vii*) Thioglycosides
- (*viii*) Saponin glycosides
- (*ix*) Aldehyde glycosides
- (*x*) Bitter glycosides
- (*xi*) Miscellaneous glycosides

All these **different categories of glycosides** would be discussed individually with appropriate examples in the sections that follows:

4.2.1 Anthracene Glycosides (or Anthraquinone Glycosides)

Anthracene glycosides represent a major class of glycosides. They are abundantly found in various dicot plant families, such as: *Ericaceae, Euphorbiaceae, Leguminoseae, Lythreaceae, Polygonaceae, Rhamnaceae, Rubiaceae* and *Verbenaceae* to name a few. Interestingly, some monocots belonging to the family *Liliaceae* also exhibits the presence of anthracene glycosides. Besides, they are also present in certain varieties of **fungi** and **lichens**.

A plethora of glycosides having their aglycone moieties closely related to anthracene are present in noticeable amounts in a variety of drug substances, for instance: *aloe, cascara, frangula, sagrada* and *senna.* These drugs are invariably employed as **cathartics**.

4.2.1.1 Aloes

Synonym: Aloe

Biological Source: Aloe is the dried latex of leaves of various species of Aloes, namely:
Aloe barbadensis Miller (or **Curacao Aloe**);
Aloe ferox Miller (or **Cape Aloe**);

Aloe perryi Baker (or **Socotrine Aloe**);
Aloe africana Miller and *Aloe spicata* Baker (or **Cape Aloe**).

All these species belong to the family *Liliaceae.*

Geographical Source

Curacao, Barbados, Aruba and Bonaire (West Indian Islands)	: Curacao Aloes or Barbados Aloes
Cape Town (South Africa)	: Cape Aloes
Socotra and Zanzibar Islands	: Socotrine or Zanzibar Aloes

It is also cultivated in Europe and the North West Himmalayan region in India.

Preparation

General Method   The leaves are transversely cut at the base and the incised ends placed downwards in a 'V' shaped trough having a hole at its bottom. The latex drains down the trough and is collected in individual receptacles placed beneath. The latex is evaporated in a kettle made of copper till it attains such a consistency that it may be poured into metallic ingots where it gets solidified. When the latex is concentrated gradually and then cooled slowely, it gives rise to an opaque product. The aloe thus obtained is termed as *'hepatic'* or *'livery'* aloe. If the latex is concentrated rapidly, followed by sudden cooling the resulting product appears to be transparent and relatively brittle in nature. The broken surface has a vitreous or glassy surface. Such a product is commonly known as *'vitreous'*, *'lucid' or 'glassy'* aloe.

Description

S. No.	Properties	Curacao Aloes	Cape Aloes	Socotrine Aloes	Zanzibar Aloes
1.	Colour	Brownish black opaque mass	Dark brown or greenish brown to olive brown mass	Brownish yellow opaque mass	Liver brown colour
2.	Odour	Strong odour resembles with *Iodoform*	Sour and distinct odour	Unpleasant odour	Characteristic but agreeable odour
3.	Taste	Intense bitter taste	Nauseating and bitter taste	Extremely bitter and nauseous taste	Bitter taste
4.	Texture	Waxy and somewhat resinous	Breaks with a glassy fraction	Fractured surface looks conchoidal	A dull, waxy, smooth and even fracture

Chemical Constituents   **Aloe-emodin** occurs in the free state and as a glycosides in various species of Aloe and also in *Rheum* (Rhubrb). **Curaeao aloes** contains about two and half times the amount of aloe emodin when compared to **cape-aloes.**

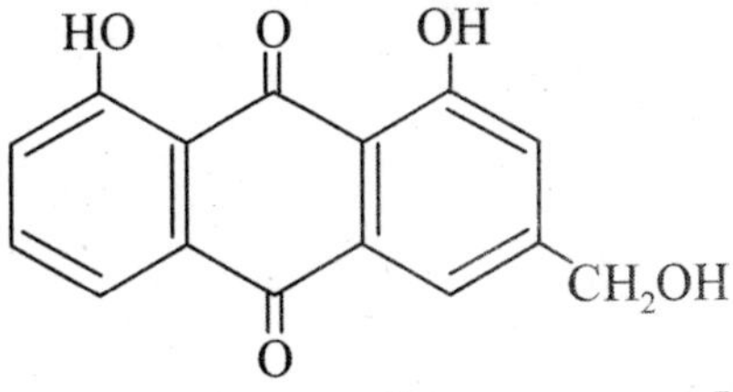

Aloe-Emodin
(Free State)

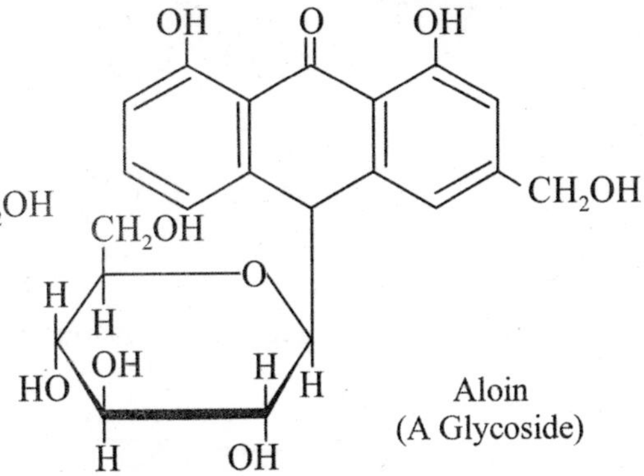

Aloin
(A Glycoside)

Interestingly, the glycosides of anthranols, dianthrones, and oxanthrones *i.e.*, the reduced derivatives of anthraquinones, invariably found in various plant substances. These plant products do make an appreciable contribution to the inherent therapeutic values of the naturally occurring substances. The structural relationships of emodin are represented as shown in Figure 4.3.

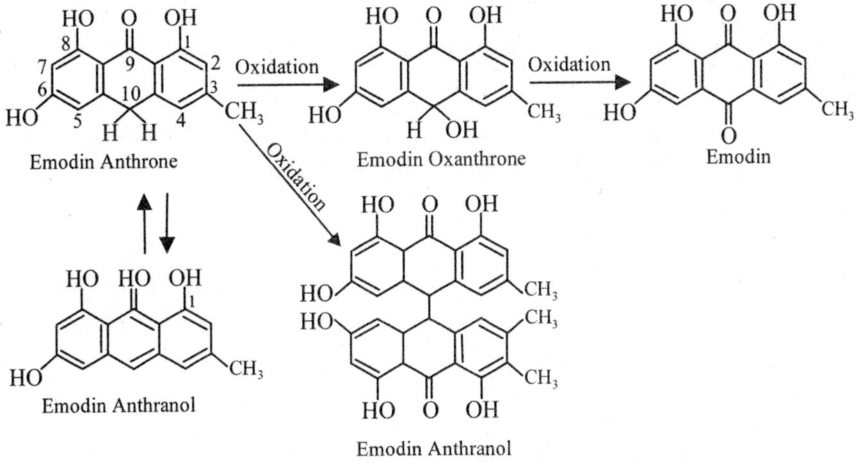

Fig. 4.3 Emodin: Structural Relationships of its Derivatives.

Both **anthrones** and **anthranols** mostly occur either as free or combined as glycosides. From a close look at their respective structures it may be observed that they are reduced anthraquinone derivatives. Both anthrone and anthranol are isomeric in nature; however, the latter may be partially converted to the former, which is essentially a non-fluorecent substance and is not soluble in alkaline solutions. Generally, the anthrones are converted on oxidation into their corresponding anthraquinones, namely: oxanthrone and dianthrone. Hence, it has been observed that prompt oxidation usually takes place in the powdered crude drug rather than the rhizomes itself.

Besides, **aloin** (or **barbaloin**) the aloes also contain **isobarbaloin** (Curacao aloes), β-**barbaloin**) = (Cape aloes), aloe emodin and resins. The principal resin present in the aloes is known as **aloesin**.

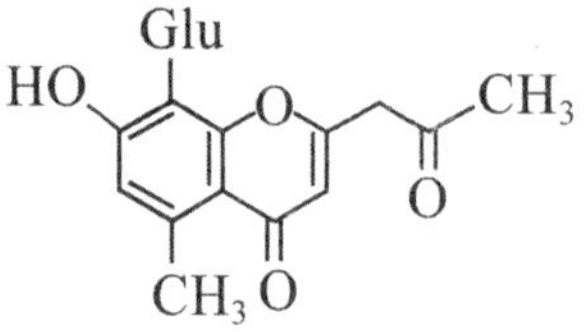

Aloesin

γ-Coniceine, which is a piperidine alkaloid is found in *Aloe gililandii, A. ballyi*, and *A. ruspoliana (Liliaceae)*

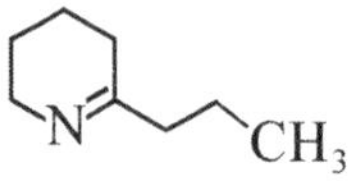

γ-Conieceine

Aloe yields not less than 50% of water soluble extractives. It also contains volatile oil to some extent that imparts a characteristic odour to it.

Chemical Tests   The overall chemical tests for *aloes* may be divided into *two* separate heads, namely: (*a*) General Tests, and (*b*) Special Tests

(*a*) **General Tests:** For this prepare a 0.1% (w/v) aqueous solution of aloes by gentle heating, add to it 0.5g of Kiesulgur and filter through. Whatman Filter Paper No. 42 and preserve the filtrate for the following tests:

1. *Borax Test (or Schoenteten's Reaction):* To 5 ml of the above test solution add 0.2 g of pure borax and heat gently till it gets dissolved. Transfer a few drops of the resulting solution into a test tube filled with distilled water, the appearance of a green coloured fluoroscence due to the formation of *aloe emodin anthranol* shows its presence.

2. *Bromine Test:* When equal volumes of the test solution and bromine solution are mixed together, it yields a pale-yellow precipitate due to the production of tetrabromaloin.

3. *Modified Borntrager's Test:* It is known that aloin (or barbaloin) belongs to the class of **C-glycoside** which does not undergo hydrolysis either by heating with dilute acid or alkali, but it may be decomposed with ferric chloride due to oxidative hydrolysis. Hence, the **Modified Borntrager's test** employing $FeCl_3$ and HCl is used as stated below:

First of all heat together 0.1 g of powdered aloe with about 2 ml of $FeCl_3$ solution(5% w/v) and 2 ml of dilute HCl (6N) in a test tube over a pre-heated water bath for 5 minutes. Cool the contents and extract the liberated anthraquinone with carbon tetrachloride. Now carefully separate the lower layer of CCl_4 and add to it ammonia solution. The appearance of a rose-pink to cherry red colour confirms its presence.

(*b*) **Special Tests**

1. **Nitrous Acid Test:** Crystals of sodium nitrite together with small quantity of acetic acid when added to 5 ml of the above test solution of aloe, the following observations are noted:
   (*a*) *Curacao Aloes:* A sharp pink to caramine colour due to the presence of isobarbaloin.

(*b*) **Cape Aloes:** A faint pink colour due to isobarbaloin.

(*c*) **Socotrine and Zanzibar aloes:** *Colour* comparatively lesser change in colour.

2. **Nitric Acid Test:** The Test solution of aloes when made to react with nitric acid, it gives rise to various shades of colour due to different types of aloes available commercially as shown below:

Caracao Aloe	:	Deep brownish red
Cape Aloes	:	Initial brownish colour changing to green
Socotrine Aloes	:	Pale brownish yellow
Zanzibar Aloes	:	Yellowish brown

3. **Cupraloin Test (or Klunge's Isobarbaloin Test):** To 10 ml of a 0.4% (w/v) aqueous solution of aloe add a drop of the saturated solution of copper sulphate, immediately followed by 1 g of NaCl and 20 drops of ethanol (90% v/v). It produces different shades of colours depending on the variety of aloes used:

Carocao Aloes	:	A wine red colour lasting for few hours,
Caoe Aloes	:	A faint colouration changing to yellow quickly,
Socotrine Aloes	:	No colouration
Zanzibar Aloes	:	No colouration

Uses

1. Though, both aloes and aloin are official drugs, the former is mostly used as a purgative by exerting its action mainly on colon, whereas the latter is generally prepared over the former now-a-days.
2. Aloes find its usefulness as an external aid to painful inflammatory manifestations.
3. It constitutes an important ingredient in the **'Compound Tincture of Benzoin'** (or **Friar's Balsam**).
4. Aloe gel made from the mucilaginous latex of *A. vera* is frequently employed in the treatment and cure of radiation burns to get immediate relief from itchings and pains.
5. Aloe usually causes gripping and is, therefore, administered along with carminatives.

4.2.1.2 Rhubarb

Synonyms: Rheum; Radix rhei; Rhubarb rhizome.

Biological Source: Rhubarb is the rhizome and roots of *Rheum officinale* Bail., *R. palmatum* L., *Rheum emodi* Wall ; *R. webbianum* Royle, belonging to the family *Polygonaceae*. The rhizome and roots are mostly collected from 6-7 year old plants just prior to the following season. They are commercially available either with intact cortex or partially decorticated.

Geographical Source   It is obtained largely from cultivated as well as wild species of *Rhubarb* grown in regions extending from Tibet to South East China. It is also found in Germany and several European countries. In India it is grown extensively in Kashmir, Kullu, Sikkim, Uttar Pradesh, Panjab. It is also found in Nepal. It is cultivated in Southern Siberia and North America.

Preparation   The rhizomes are collected either in spring or in autumn from 6 to 10 year old plants., grown at an altitude of more tha 3, 000 meters. These are duly cleaned, decordicated and dried. The relatively larger rhizomes are cut into small pieces either longitudinally or transversely. The cut fragments are threaded and dried in the shade. They are also dried artifically in an atmosphere of hot wooden boxes and exported for commercial consumption.

Description   **Rhubarb** is usually found to be compact, rigid, cylindrical conical or barrel shaped with 8-10 cm length and 3-4 cm thickness. They appear to be mostly longitudinally wrinkled, ridged or furrowed; whereas a few of them do exhibit transverse annulations or wrinkles. Interestingly, the flat pieces are prepared from large rhizomes that are normally cut longitudinally and, therefore, they appear to be largely as plano-convex with tapering at both ends. These two varieties of pieces possess a sharp characteristic odour and a bitter astringent taste. The surface is often smeared with a bitter yellowish powdery substance, which on being removed gives rise to a rather smooth surface that appears to be pale brown to red in colour.

Chemical Constituents   **Rhubarb** essentially contains mainly the anthraquinone glycosides and the astringent components. The former range between 2 to 4.5% and are broadly classified into *four* categories as stated below:

(*a*) **Anthraquinones with —COOH moiety**—*e.g.*, Rhein; Glucorhein;

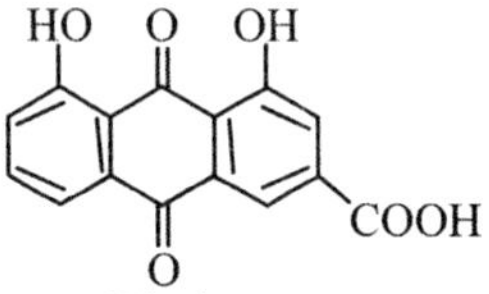

Rhein

(*b*) **Anthraquinones without —COOH moiety**—*e.g.*, Emodin; Aloe-Emodin; Chrysophanol; Physcion;

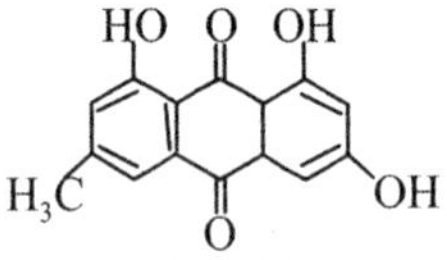

Emodin 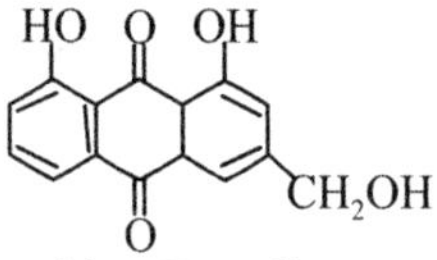   Aloe-Emodin 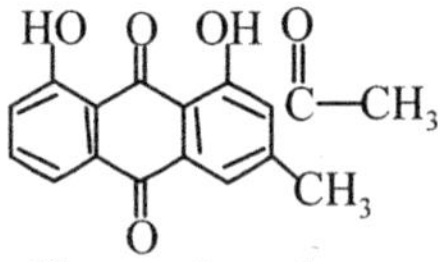   Chrysophanol 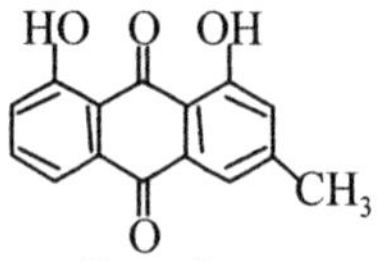   Physcion

(*c*) **Anthrones and Dianthrones of Emodin**—as shown below:

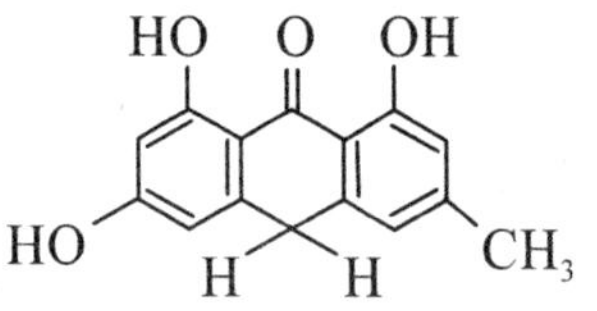

Emodine Anthrone 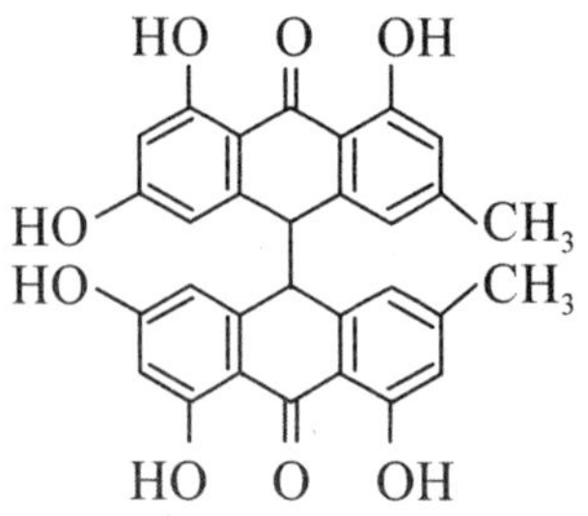   Emodin Dianthrone

(*d*) **Heterodianthrones**—*e.g.* Palmidin A, B, and C, which are produced from two different anthrone molecules, as stated under:

Palmidin A : Aloe-emodin anthrone + Emodin anthrone
Palmidin B : Aloe-emodin anthrone + Chrysophanol anthrone
Palmidin C : Emodin anthrone + Chrysophanol anthrone

However, the astringet portion of rhubarb chiefly comprises with the following components, namely: **gallic acid** as *α- and β-glucogallin*; **tannin** as *d-catechin* and *epicatechin*.

α-Glucogallin   β-Glucogallin

d-Catechin   Epicatechin

Rhubarb in addition to the above constituents, consists of **rheinolic acid, pectin, starch, fat** and **calcium oxalate**. The calcium oxalate content ranges between 3-40% in various species of rhubarb which reflects directly on the corresponding **ash values** (*i.e.*, total inorganic contents).

Chemical Tests
1. The Rhubarb powder on being treated with ammonia gives rise to a pink colouration.
2. Rhubarb gives a blood-red colouration with 5% potassium hydroxide.
3. It gives a positive indication with modified Borntrager's test (see under Aloes).

Uses
1. It is used mainly in the form of an ointment in the treatment and cure of chronic eczema, psoriasis and trichophytosis—as a potent *keratolytic agent*.
2. It is employed as a bitter stomachic in the treatment of diarrhoea.
3. It is also used as a purgative.

4.2.1.3 Cascara Sagrada

Interestingly, the very name 'cascara sagrada' is *Spanish* for the sacred bark; *Rhamnus* is the ancient classical name for buckthorn, and *Purshianus* was attributed as a mark of honour and respect to the great German botanist Friedrich Pursch.

Synonyms Sacred bark; Chitten bark; Chittin bark; Purshiana bark; Persian bark; Bearberry bark; Bearwood; Cascara bark; Cortex *Rhamni purshianae*.

Biological Source   **Cascara sagrada** is the dried bark of *Rhamanus purshiana* DC., belonging to family *Rhamnaceae*, from which a naturally occurring cathartic is extracted. It is usually collected at least one year prior to its use.

Geograhical Source   It is invariably obtained from cultivated as well as wild shrubs and small trees grown in Northern Idaho, West to Northern California, North Carolina, Oregon, in Kenya and Western Canada.

Preparation   The bark is collected, during the dry season (April to August) from the 8 to 9 years old trees that have gained a height of 16-18 meters with their stems having a diameter of 8 to 10 cm, by inflicting longitudinal incisions on the fully developed stems. In usual practice, the *coppicing technique* is employed for the collection of bark. The bark is carefully stripped off from the branches and the stems. They are subsequently allowed to dry in shade by putting their inner-surface facing the ground so as to permit the completion in the enzymatic conversion of the anthranol derivative *i.e.*, glycosides (an emetic principle) to its anthraquinone derivative usually present in the fresh drug, thereby exerting a milder cathartic activity. During this span of one year the drug must be duly protected from rain or humid environment so as to check the growth of mould.

Description

Colour	:	Outside-purplish brown; Inside reddish brown.
Odour	:	A typically nauseatic odour.
Taste	:	Persistently bitter.
Size	:	Occurs in varying sizes of thickness between 1 to 4 mm.
Shape	:	Mostly occurs in quills or channels. Also available in small, flat and broken segments.

However, internally the bark exhibits longitudinal striations; whereas externally the bark appears to be quite smooth and usually displays the presence of seattered lenticles, lichens and cork. Besides, mostly insects and liveworts are found on the exterior surface of the bark.

Chemical Constituents   The **cascara sagrada** bark is found to contain **two** major types of anthracene compounds, namely:

  (*a*) *Normal O-Glycosides*   These are based on emodin like structures and constitute about 10 to 20% of the total glycosides, and

  (*b*) *Aloin-like C-Glycosides*   These comprise of about 80 to 90% of the total glycosides.

The two **C-glycosides** are known as **barbaloin** and **deoxybarbaloin** (or **chrysaloin**) as given below:

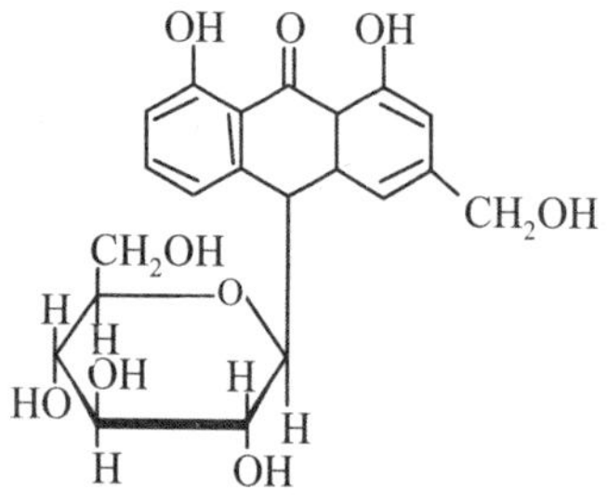

Barbaloin (Aloin) 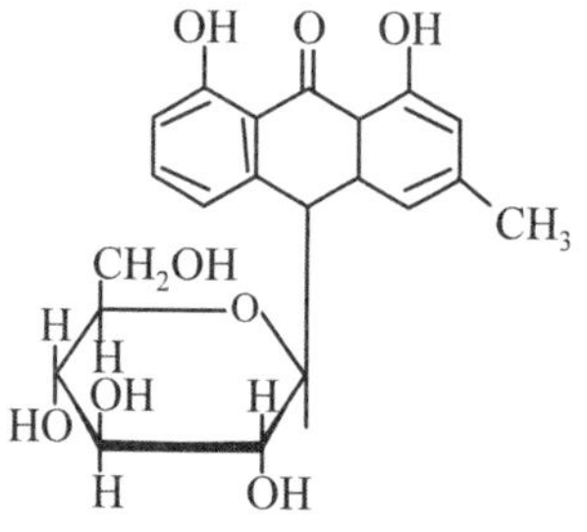   Deoxybarbaloin (Chrysaloin)

The main active constituents are *four* glycosides usually designed as Cascarosides A, B, C and D. From extensive and intensive studies of these cascarosides by *optical rotary dispersion* (ORD) technique it has been established that the *cascarosides A and B* are solely based on optical isomers of **barbaloin** ; whereas *cascarosides C and D* on optical isomers of **deoxybarbaloin.** However, from a close inspection of all the four basically primary glycosides of **barbaloin** and **deoxybarbaloin** it may be revealed that they possess the characteristic features of **O-glycosides** as well as **C-glycosides**.

Glycosides	Type	R	Configuration
CASCAROSIDE	A	OH	(10 S)
CASCAROSIDE	B	OH	(10 R)
CASCAROSIDE	C	H	(10 S)
CASCAROSIDE	D	H	(10 R)

Salient Features   The **sailent features** of the various **glycosides** are as follows:

(*i*) About six anthracene derivatives isolated and identified in the drug belong to the category of **O-glycosides** which are solely based on **emodin,**

(*ii*) Dried cascara bark normally produces not less than 7% of the total hydroxyanthracene derivatives, calculated as **cascaroside A,** and

(*iii*) The remaining cascarosides must make up at least 60% of this total quantum.

Perhaps the presence of a *'lactone'* in the drug attributes a bitter taste to it.

Casanthranol is the purified version of a mixture of **anthranol glycosides** highly water-soluble and duly extracted from **cascara sagrada**. It has been reported that each gramme of casanthanol contains not less than 200 mg of the entire hydroxyanthracene derivative, calculated as cascaroside A, out of which not less than 80% of the respective derivatives mainly consists of cascarosides.

Chemical Test   It gives a positive indication with **Modified Borntrager's test** because of the presence of **C-glycosides**.

Substituents/Adulterants   The barks of *Rhamanus californica* and *R. fallax* are generally used as a substitute for **cascara sagrada** bark. Sometimes the *frangula bark* is also used as a substitute for this drug. However, the former types of barks (*Rhamnus species)* exhibit a more uniform coat of lichens along with broader medullary rays when compared to the original drug species.

4.2.1.4 Frangula

Synonyms   Buckthorn bark; Alder buckthorn; Black dogwood; Berry alder; Arrow wood; Persian berries;

Biological Source   **Frangula bark** is the dried bark of *Rhamnus frangula* Linne belonging to the family *Rhamnaceae.*

Geographical Source   The plant is a shrub which grows abundantly in Europe, the Mediterranean coast of Africa and Western Asia.

Preparation   The preparation of **frangula bark** resembles to that of cascara bark (see section 4.2.1.3). Just like the cascara bark, the frangula bark must be aged for at least a period of one year before it is used therapeutically so as to permit the reduced forms of the glycosides with harsh action to be oxidised to comparatively milder forms.

Chemical Constituents   The seed, bark and rootbark of *Rhamnus species*, specifically in *Alder Buckthorn (Rhamnus alnifolia L' Her.); in Rhamnus carthartica* L., in *Rhamnus purshiana* DC (*Cascara sagrada)* consists of the *two* important glycosides *Frangulins A and B*, which were initially thought to be isomeric compounds. Later on *two* more glycosides known as **glucofranguIns A and B** have also been reported . However, the structures of **Frangulins A* and B**** along with **Glucofrangulins A and B** are given below:

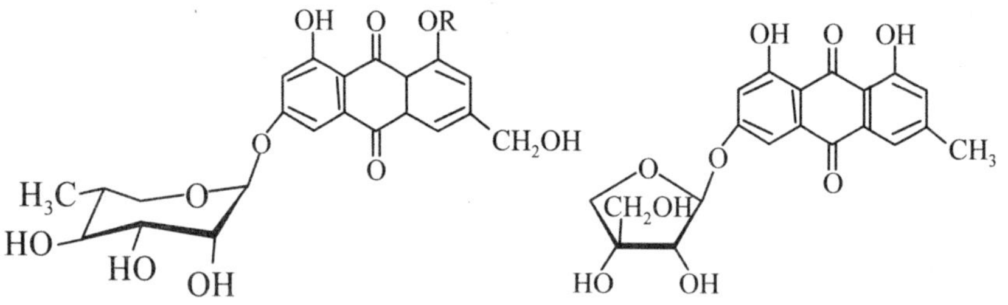

Frangulin A : R=H;
Glucofrangulin A : R = β-D-Glucopyranose

Frangulin B : R = H;
Glucofrangulin B : R = β-D-Glucopyranose

Besides, *frangulin* the **frangula bark** contains emodin (see Section 4.2.1.2) and chrysophanic acid as shown below:

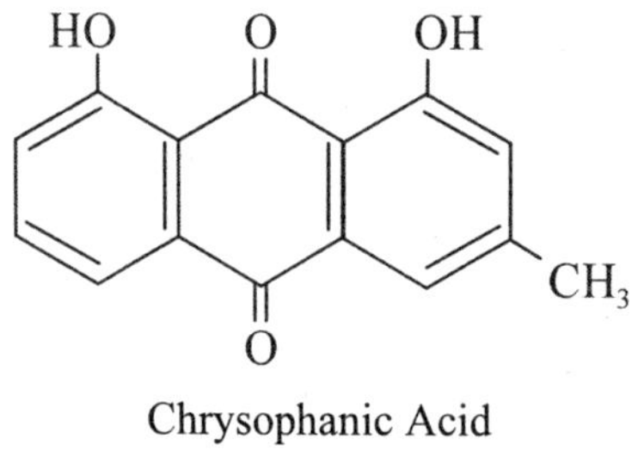

Chrysophanic Acid

---

* Horhammer, Wagner, Z. *Naturforsch*, 27B, 959, 1972.
** Wagner, Demuth, *Tetrahedron Letters*, 5013, 1972.

Substituents/Adulterants As the activity of **Frangula Bark** corresponds to that of *cascara sagrada,* it finds a good substitute and comparable usage in Europe and the Near East. Interestingly, the drug substances obtained from the ripe and duly dried fruits of *Rhamnus catharticus* Linn., are invariably employed in Europe and the Near East for their recognised cathartic therapeutic activity.

Uses It is mostly used as a cathartic.

4.2.1.5 Senna

Senna was first used in the European medicine as early as the 9th or 10th century by the Arabs. An Egyptian native Issae Judaeus (850 to 900 A.D.) was reported to be the pioneer in bringing and introducing the drug to Egypt from Mecca,

Synonyms Senna leaf; Sennae folium; Tinnevelley Senna; Indian Senna;

Biological Sources Senna is the dried leaflets of *Cassia senna* L. (*Cassia acutifolia* Delile, (Alexandria senna), or of *Cassia angustifolia* Vahl (Indian or Tinnevelley Senna) belonging to the family *Leguminoseae*. However, the modern taxonomists recommend to club together both the commonly available species of senna, namely: *Alexandria senna and Thinnevelley senna*—under one name as *Senna alexandria Mill.*

Geographical Source *C. acutifolia* grows wild in the vicinity of Nile River (Egypt) extending from Aswan to Kordofan; whereas, *C. angustifolia* grows wild in the Arabian Peninsula, Somalia, India, and Northwest Pakistan. In India the drug is cultivated in Southern part- Tinnevelly, Mysore and Madurai; Northern part- Jammu, Western part Pune and Kutch region of Gujrat.

Preparation After a duration of 2-3 months of sowing the Alexandra senna is harvested both in April and in September by cutting off the tops of the plants approximately 15 cm from the ground level and subsequently allowing them to dry in the sun. Later on, the unwanted stems and pods are segregated from the leaflets with the help of sieves using mechanical vibrators. The portion that passes through the sieves, is now *'tossed'* carefully, whereby the leaves are colleted on the surface and the relatively heavier stalk fragments at the bottom. The dried leaves are now graded, packed in bags and stored in dry place. The commercial drug at present is distributed through Port Sudan located on the Red Sea, and from the Port of Tuticorin, in India.

Description

Features		Alexandria senna	Tinnevelley senna
Colour	:	Pale greyish green	Yellowish green
Odour	:	Slight	Slight
Taste	:	Mucilagenous slightly bitter and characteristic	Mucilagenous, bitter and characteristic
Size	:	Length = 2-4 cm, Width = 7-12 mm;	Length = 2.5-5cm Width = 3-8 mm
Shape	:	Ovate -lanceolate;	Lanceolate
Texture	:	Thin and brittle	Thin and flexible

Chemical Constituents The principle active constituents of senna are *four* sennosides A, B, C and D, which are the dimeric glycosides having their aglycones composed of either *rhein* and/or aloe-emodin moieties *i.e.*; 10, 10′ -*bis* (9, 10-dihydro-1, 8-dihydroxy-9-oxoanthracene-3-carboxylic acid).

The structure of the above *four* glycosides are as given below:

Glycosides	R	C-10 & C-10'	Characteristics
Sennoside-A	—COOH	*trans-*	Optically active, a levoratory isomer present in large concs; water insoluble
Sennoside-B	—COOH	*meso-*	Intramolecularly compensated present in large concs; more water soluble
Sennoside-C	—CH$_2$OH	*trans-*	Aglycone (–) isomer; present in small concs;
Sennoside-D	—CH$_2$OH	*meso-*	Aglycone (+) isomer; present in small concs.

Besides, relatively small quantities of monomeric glycosides and free anthraquinones are also present in senna pods, such as: **rhein–8-glucosides, rhein-8-diglucoside, aloe emodin-8-glucoside, aloe-emodin anthrone diglycoside, rhein, aloe-emodin and isorhamnetin.**

It also contains **kaempterol** (a phytosterol), mucilage, resins, myricyl alcohol, chrysophanic acid, calcium oxalate and salicylic acid.

Specific method of extraction for the sennosides: Exclusively for commercial purposes, the sennosides are extracted as their corresponding calcium sennosides in varying strengths because of its enhanced stability.

Methodology: The drug powder (about 80-100 mesh size) is duly macerated with either 80% acetone or 90% methanol for a period of 6 hours, followed by 2 hours with cold water. This process helps to achieve an extract that contains between 17-18% sennosides and enables to extract about 65% of sennosides from the crude drug.

The sennosides and other anthracene derivatives may be extracted by the help of a mixture of polyethylene glycols (in 70% v/v ethanol) and solutions of non-ionic surfactants.

However, the isolation of individual sennosides may be achieved by employing non-polar synthetic resins having porous structural features.

Alternatively, the drug powder is macerated with citric acid in methanol which is followed by a repeated extraction with a mixture of methanol, toluene and ammonia. The resulting extract is treated with a concerntrated solution of calcium chloride to salt out the sennosides as their respective calcium salts.

Chemical Tests

1. **Modified Borntrager's Test:** It gives a pink to red colouration for the presence of anthraquinone glycosides (see under section 4.2.1.1).
2. The mucilage of senna gives a distinct red colouration with Ruthenium Red solution.

Substituents and Adulterants   Tinnevelley senna is invariably found to be adulterated with the following *three* cheaper varities of senna namely:

(*a*) Dog senna ie; *Cassia abovata,*
(*b*) Palthe senna ie; *Cassia auriculatad,* and
(*c*) Arabian Senna or Mecea senna or Bombay senna *i.e.*; wild variety of *Cassia angustifolia* Vahl. from Southern Arabia.

    Dog senna   : It contains approximately 1% of anthraquinone derivatives.
    Palthe senna   : It contains no anthraquinone glycosides
    Arabian senna : It is brownish-green in appearance.

Uses

1. Senna and its branded preparations, for instance: Glaxenna[R] (Glaxo); Pursennid[(R)] (Sandoz); Helmacid with senna[(R)] (Allenburrys); are usually employed as purgative in habitual constipation. The glycosides are first absorbed in the small intestinal canal after which the aglycone portion gets separated and ultimately excreted in the large intentine (colon). The released anthraquinones irritate and stimulate the colon thereby enhancing its peristaltic movements causing bulky and soft excretion of faces.
2. The inherent action of senna is associated with appreciable griping , and therefore, it is generally dispensed along with carminatives so as to counteract the undesired effect.

4.2.2   Phenol Glycosides

A variety of **phenol glycosides** are widely distributed in nature. It has been found that quite a few simple phenol glycosides have their aglycone portion loaded with either phenolic moieties or more often with alcoholic moieties or carboxylic acid functions. Invariably, the natural vegetative plant products, such as: Willow bark (containing *Salicin*) and Bearberry leaves (containing *arbutin*) have been employed therapeutically since ages, the former as antipyretic and the latter both as urinary antiseptic and as diuretic.

A few frequently used **phenol glycosides** commonly found in natural plant products are described below; such as: **Arbutin; Gaultherin; Salicin; Populin; Glucovanillin.**

4.2.2.1 *Arbutin*

Synonyms   Ursin; Arbutoside; Uvasol; Uvaursi; Bearberry leaves; Busserole.

Biological source   It occurs in the dried leaves of *Bergenia crassifolia* (L.) Fritsch, belonging to the family *Saxifragaceae.*

It is also obtained from the dried leaves Uva-Ursi or Bearberry *Arctostaphylos uva-ursi* (Linne') Sprengel, belonging to family *(Ericaceae)* and other related plants *e.g.*, **coactylis** or adenotricha Fernald and McBride (family *Ericaceae*). Besides, it is extracted from the leaves of blueberry, cranberry and pear trees (*Pyrus communis* L., family; *Rosaceae*).

Geographical Source   Bearberry is mostly grown in various parts of North and Central Europe, North America, Canada and Scotland.

Description   **Arbutin** occurs in white needles that are promptly soluble in water and ethanol. It is very hygroscopic in nature.

Chemical Constituents   The structure of **arbutin** is given below:

Arbutin

It has a β-D-glucopyranoside function attached to the *para* position of a phenol.

It yields upon hydrolysis, either by dilute acids or by emulsin, one mole each of D-glucose and hydroquinone.

Arbutin   Hydroquinone D-Glucose

Besides, the leaves also contain **methyl arbutin, quercetin, gallic acid, ursolic acid** and **tannin.** However, **arbutin** forms a complex with hexamethylenetetramine that may be used as a means to separate it from **methylarbutin.**

Methyl   Quercetin   Gallic Acid   Ursolic Acid
Arbutin

Chemical Tests

1. **Arbutin** yields a blue colouration with ferric chloride solution.
2. Its presence in crude drug may be detected by frist moistening the powdered tissues with dilute HCl, warming cautiously over a watch glass on a low flame and carefully collecting the sublimate as crystals of hydroquinone that forms on another watch glass.

Important Features   The presence of **gallotannin** usually helps in preventing certain specific enzyme, for instance: **β-glucosidase** from splitting **arbutin** that justifiably explains why the crude plant extracts are more effective therapentically, as compared to **pure arbutin.**

Uses

1. It is used as a diuretic.
2. It finds its application as an antiseptic agent on the urinary tract.
3. It also exerts astringent actions.

4.2.2.2 Gaultherin

Synonyms   Monotropitoside; Monotropitin; Methyl salicylate 2-glucoxyloside.

Biological Source   It occurs in the leaves of the Canadian Wintergreen plant *Gaultheria procumbens* L., in *Monotropa hypopitys* L., belonging to family *Ericaceae* It is also found in the bark of *Betula lenta* L., family *Betulaceae*; in *Spiraea ulmaria* L., and *S. filipendula* L., family *Rosaceae*.

Geographical Source   It grows in the hills of India, Burma and Ceylon.

Description   It has a needle-shaped star formation look when crystallised from acetone (99%). It is soluble in water and alcohol.

Chemical Constituents   When **gaultherin** is hydrolysed with 3% H_2SO_4, it forms one mole each of **methyl salicylate, D-glucose** and **D-xylose** as shown below:

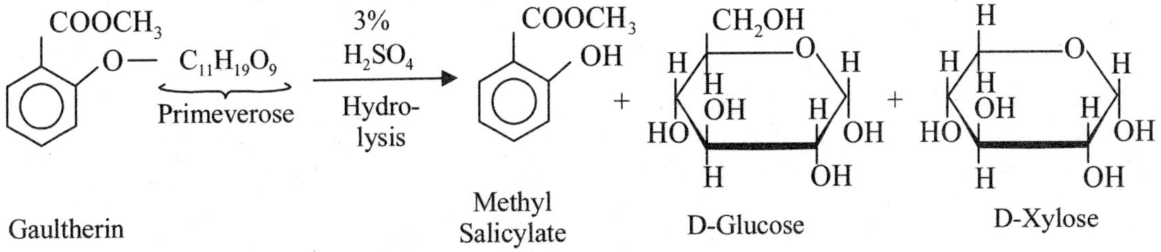

Gaultherin — Methyl Salicylate + D-Glucose + D-Xylose

However, **gaultherin** (or **monotropitin**) on being subjected to hydrolysis by the enzyme *gaultherase* gives rise to the production of one mole each of **primeverose** [*i.e.*; **6- (β-D-xyloside)-D glucose**] a disaccharide and methyl salicylate.

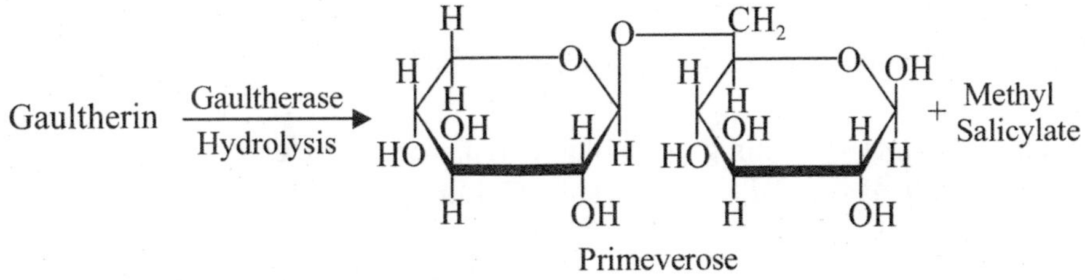

Gaultherin $\xrightarrow[\text{Hydrolysis}]{\text{Gaultherase}}$ Primeverose + Methyl Salicylate

4.2.2.3 Salicin

Synonyms   Salicoside; Salicyl alcohol glucoside; Saligenin β-D-glucopyranoside.

Biological Source   It is obtained from the bark of poplar (*Populus*) and willow (*Salix*) and also found in the leaves and female flowers of the willow. It is specifically found in *two* species of *Salix*, namely: *Salix fragilis* and *Salix purpurea* , belonging to the family *Salicaceae*. It is also found in the root bark of *Viburnum prunifolium* L., family : *Caprifoliacea* and in *Spiraea ulmaria,* family: *Rosaceae.*

Geographical Source   It grows in China, Europe and in India.

Preparation   The powdered bark is macerated with hot water for several hours whereby the **glucoside (salicin)** and tannin are extracted collectively. The resulting liquid extract is filtered, concentrated under vacuum and treated with lead acetate to remove the tannins as a precipitate. It is subsequently treated with hydrogen sulphite to remove the excess of lead. The clear filtrate is neutralized with ammonia, allowed to concentrate, chilled to obtain the crystals of salicin. The crude **salicin** may be further purified by treating its solution with animal charcoal and concentrating followed by cooling.

Description   It occurs as colourless crystals or prisms or scales. It has a very bitter taste. It is highly soluble in hot water and practically insoluble in ether. It is a levoratatory substance [$(\alpha)_D$: –63°].

Chemical Constituents   It is hydrolysed in the presence of the enzyme **emulsin** by yielding one mole each of **saligenin** (aglycone) and **D-glucose** as stated below:

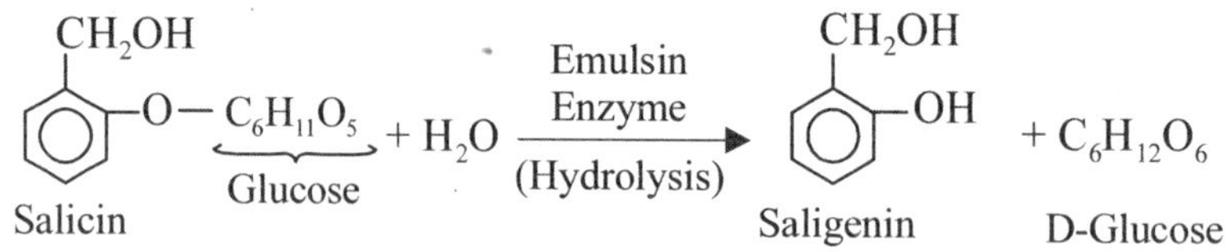

When hydrolysis is done in an acidic medium by boiling for a prolonged duration, two moles of **saligenin** combine together to provide **saliretin** (water insoluble) with the loss of a mole of water, which may be summarised as shown under:

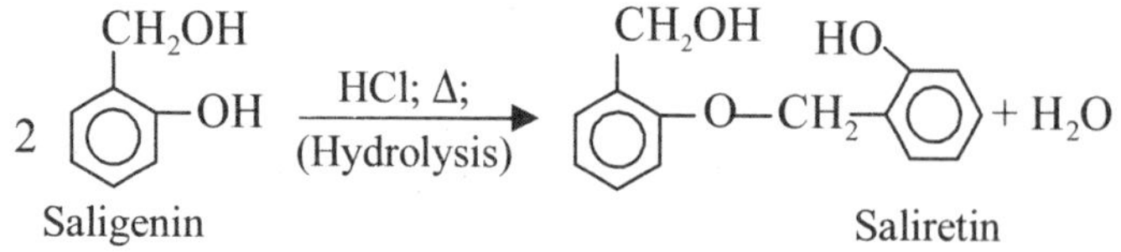

Chemical Tests
1. It gives an instant bright red colour with concentrated sulphuric acid that fades out on the addition of water.
2. Its hydrolysed product saligenin gives a blue colour with ferric chloride.
3. On oxidation with potassium dichromate and sulphuric acid and heating yields salicylaldehyde having a characteristic odour.

4. It gives specific colours with the following reagents:

Frachde's Reagent : Violet colour
Mandelin's Reagent* : Purple red colour
Erdmann's Reagent** : Bright red colour

Uses

1. It is used as an analgesic
2. It has been employed as a bitter stomachic.
3. It is also used as an antirheumatic agent.
4. It is used as a standard substrate in evaluating enzymes preparations containing β-glycosidase.

4.2.2.4 Populin

Synonyms Populoside; Salicin benzoate.

Biological Source It occurs in the bark leaves of *Populus tremula* L., *P. nigra* L., *P. nigral*. L. var *italica* Duroi, *P. canadensis* Moench., *P. grandidentate* Michx., and *P. tremuloides* Miehx., belonging to the family *Salicaceae*. It is perhaps also found in *Salix helix, Salix purpureae* L. var helix (L.) Koch.

Preparation It may be prepared either from *salicin* by melting with benzoic anhydride, or from *salicin* and benzoyl chloride in the presence of KOH as shown below:

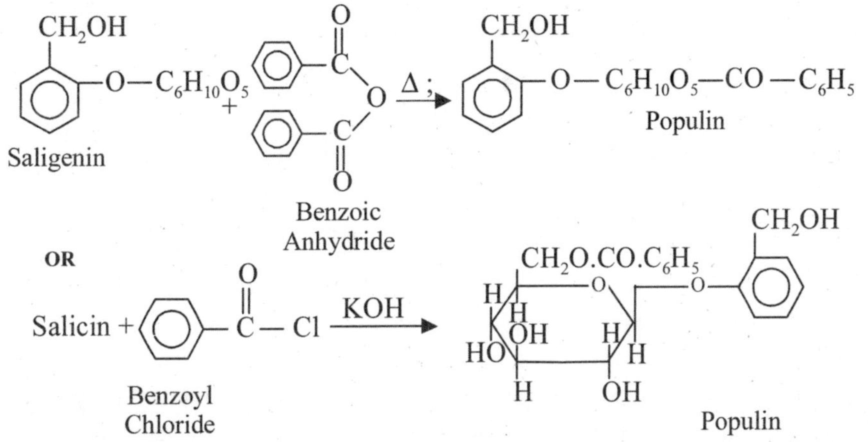

Description It occurs as white needles having a sweet taste like licorice. It is readily soluble in alcohol and hot water, but sparingly soluble in cold water and almost insoluble in solvent ether.

Chemical Constituents **Populin** on hydrolysis with alkalies [eg., $Ba(OH)_2$] yields salicin and benzoic acid, whereas, its hydrolysis in an acidic medium gives benzoic acid, saligenin and glucose. However, its enzymatic hydrolysis with **taka-diastase** provides **salicin** and **monobenzoyl glucose**.

Chemical Tests It gives exactly identical reactions with conc. H_2SO_4 and Frachde's Reagent as those with salicin.

---

* *Mandelin's Reagent:* Dissolve 0.5 g of ammonium vanadate in 15 ml of water and dilute to 100 ml with sulphuric acid. Filter the solution through glass wool.
** *Erdmann's Reagent:* A 1% (w/v) aqueous solution of ammonium diamminetetrakis–(nitrito–N) cobaltate (1–).

4.2.2.5 *Glucovanillin*

Synonyms   Vanilloside; Avenein; Vanillin -D-glucoside. It is obtained from the green fruit of vanilla.

Preparation   It is prepared from **coniferin** by oxidation with chromium-6-oxide (CrO_3) as follows:

Glucose
Coniferin

Glucovanillin

Description   It has a needle-like appearance having a bitter taste. It is readily soluble in hot water and alcohol; but almost insoluble in ether.

Chemical Constituents   **Glucovanillin** is the chemical constituent present in the green fruit of vanilla.

Uses
It is mostly used in pharmaceutical preparations as a flavoring agent.

4.2.3 Steroid Glycosides

Steroid glycosides are also referred to as **'Cardiac glycosides'** in many available books on phytochemistry. In fact, there exists enough evidence in literatures to reveal that a host of medicinal plants comprise of cardiac or cardiotonic glycosides, collectively known as **'steriod glycosides'**, and they have since been employed as *arrow poisons* or *cardiac drugs*. Interestingly, from a therapeutic perspective this particular group of compounds may be regarded as one of the most important of all naturally occurring plant products.

    The **cardiac glycosides** are basically steroids with an inherent ability to afford a very specific and poweful action mainly on the cardiac muscle when administered through injection into man or animal. As a word of caution, a small amount would exhibit a much needed stimulation on a diseased heart, whereas an excessive dose may cause even death.

    Generally, the **steroid glycosides** are invariably employed in the therapeutic domain primarily for *two* vital reasons, namely: (*a*) to enhance the tone, excitability and above all the contractibility of the cardiac muscle; and (*b*) to increase the diuretic action, due principally to the enhanced renal circulation (an inherent secondary action).

    A few important plant products belonging to this category are discussed in the sections that follows, namely:

4.2.3.1 Digitalis

Synonyms   Foxglove; Purple foxglove; Fairy gloves; Digifortis; Digitora; Pil-Digis; Neodigitalis.

Biological Source   **Digitalis** comprises of the dried leaves of *Digitalis purpurea* L., belonging to the family *Scrophulariaceae*. [The word *purpurea* has been derived from the purple colour of flowers]. It is pertinent to mention here that the fresh leaves must be dried immediately in the dark at a temperature not exceeding 60°C so that the final dried leaves should not contain more than 5% of inherent moisture. This is, however, extremely important to retain the glycosides in a good undecomposed condition.

Geographical Source   It is grown in Southern and Central Europe, England, Holland, Germany, United States and India. In India, it is grown in Kashmir and Nilgiri Hills.

Preparation   Good quality **digitalis** is grown specifically from the seeds of selected strains that will invariably yield only leafy plants enriched with glycoside contents. Even the soil is usually sterilized by steam before commencement of sowing. Mostly it grows both appreciably and luxuriantly at an altitude ranging between 1600-300 meters preferably in a shady environment. In actual practice, the sowing of seeds is performed in autumn (October/November) , and the seedlings are virtually transplanted in the fields in the following springs (March/ April). The leaves are normally hand picked in the *afternoon* during August / September in the *first* and *second* year, when almost 2/3rd of the flowers have fully bloomed. The leaves collected in the first year are found to contain the highest percentage of glycosides. The basal leaves and the ones located at the top are collected at the end. The discoloured leaves are sorted out and rejected outright. The selected leaves are duly spread on perforated trays (usually a thin bed), the trays are stacked one above the other in a well-closed dark drying shed heated by a stream of hot air maintained strictly at a temperature not more than 60°C. The dried leaves having a misture content not more than 5% are carefully packed in suitable air-tight containers, charged with appropriate dehydrating agents and shipped for export.

Note   The therapeutic potency *vis-à-vis* the activity of the leaves is solely due to the glycoside content. Surely, the presence of moisture and certain enzymes, namely; *oxidase* and *digipurpuridase,* are chiefly responsible for the ultimate deterioration of the glycosides of the leaves. In case, the leaves are made to dry at a temperature beyond 60°C, it has been observed that there is a drastic loss in potency on account of *chemical degradation* (irreversible).

Description

Colour	:	Dark greyish green
Odour	:	Slight
Taste	:	Bitter
Size	:	Length: 10-14 cm; width: 4-15 cm
Shape	:	Orate-lanceolate to broadly ovate

Special Features   The digitalis leaves are more or less pubescent venation together with pronounced and marked veinlets on the under surface. The leaves are invariably crumpled and broken.

Chemical Constituents   Nativelle (1868), Kiliani (1891), and Stoll (1938) were the pioneers who contributed valuable informations with regard to the chemical constituents present in *digitalis* through their extensive and intensive studies.

It has been reported that **digitalis** essentially contains *three* important *primary glycosides* namely: *Purpurea glycoside A*, *Purpurea glycoside B*, and *Purpurea glycoside C*, which upon hydrolysis give rise to *digitoxin, gitoxin* and *gitalin* respectively. These **secondary glcosides** on further hydrolysis yields noncarbohydrate moieties (called *aglycones or genins*) *digitoxigenin, gitoxigenin* and *gitaligenin* or *gitaloxigenin* respectively. The series of all these hydrolysed products and their structures are summarised below.

Besides, the crude drug also contains a good number of other *glycosides* (*e.g.*; **digitalin, diginin**); *saponins* (*e.g.*; **digitonin, gitin** and **digitosaponin**); tannins, gallic, formic, acetic, succinic and benzoic acids; fatty acids and enzyme *digipuridase* solely responsible for hydrolysis of purpurea glycosides.

Chemical Tests A plethora of chemical colour reactions have been evolved to be used as the qualitative tests either for the various glycosides or their corresponding aglycones in the chemical laboratory. However, the exact positions of the respective **glycosides** or their **aglycones** may be detected either on the paper charomatograms or on the thin layer chromatographic plates by virtue of the production of specific colours or by exposing the chromatograms under UV light so that the components would be detcted by their fluorescence. All these specific tests are summarised in Table 4.1.

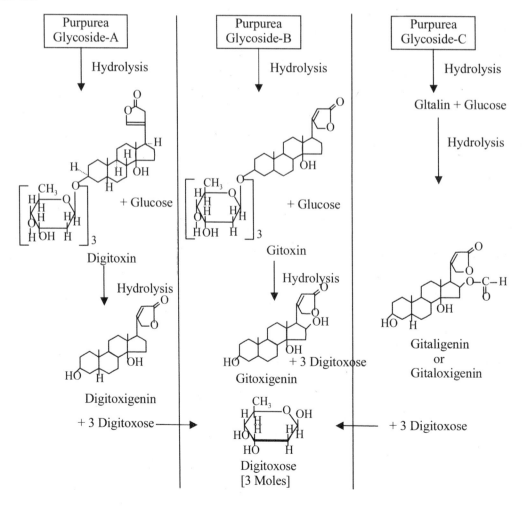

Table 4.1 Colour Tests of Glycosides

S.No	Specific Tests	Experimental Procedures	Inferences
1.	Kellar-Kiliani Test	The glycoside is dissolved in glacial acetic acid containing a trace of $FeCl_3$, add the same amount of $FeCl_3$ dissolved in conc. H_2SO_4 along the side of the test tube to settle at the bottom (for α-deoxy sugars eg; digitoxose)	A reddish brown colour changing to bluish green colour appears at the junction of two reagents within 2-5 minutes spreading slowly into the acetic acid layer.
2.	Legal Test	A few mg of the glycoside (except scillaren) is dissolved in a few drops of pyridine. To this is added a drop of sodium nitroprusside soln. (2% w/v), add a drop of NaOH soln. (20% w/v)	Appearance of a pink or deep red colour indicates its presence.
3.	Baljet Test	The aglycone portion of the glycoside is mixed with Baljet reagent*	Appearance of an orange or red colour shows its presence.
4.	Raymond Test	Dissolve a small quantity of the glycoside in 1 ml of ethanol (50%) Add to it 0.1 ml of Raymonds Reagent** and 2/3 drops of NaOH solution (20% w/v) (for activated methyene group at C-21 in the lactone ring)	Appearance of a violet colour slowly changing to blue gives an affirmative test.
5.	Tollen's Test	Dissolve a small amount of the glycosde in a few drops of pyridine. To this is added a few ml of Tollen's Reagent*** & heated gently (if required).	Appearance of a silver mirror shows a positive test.
6.	Xanthydrol Test	Add to the glycoside solution 0.5 ml of xanthydrol solution**** (for 2-desoxy sugars only)	Development of red colour shows its presence.
7.	Antimony Trichloride Test	To a solution of glycoside add a solution of antimony trichloride and trichloroacetic acid, and then heat the mixture (for *Cardenolides* & *Bufadienolides*)	Appearance of a blue or violter colour shows its presence.
8.	Kedde Test	A solution of glycosides is treated with a small amount of Kedde's Reagent***** (for *Cardenolides* & *Cardinolide aglycones*)	Development of a blue or violet colour that fades out in 1 to 2 hours shows its presence.

* **Baljet Reagent:** Aqueous solution of picric acid (1% w/v) and NaOH soln. (10% w/v). Both solutions mixed immediately before use and filtered.
** **Raymond's Reagent:** A 1% (w/v) solution of m-dinitrobenzene in ethanol (or methanol)
*** **Tollen's Reagent:** To a 0.1 N soln. of $AgNO_3$ is added dilute NH_4OH till the white precipitate intially formed gets dissolved after further addition of NH_4OH.
**** **Xanthydrol Reagent:** A solution of 0.125% (w/v) xanthydrol in glacial acetic acid containing 1% HCl.
***** **Kedde's Reagent:** Mix equal volumes of a 2% (w/v) soln. of 3, 5 dinitrobenzoic acid in methanol and a 7.5% (w/v) aqueous soln. of KOH

Substituents/Adulterants   The **digitalis** leaves have been frequently adulterated with the following varieties of leaves, namely:

1. *Great mullein leaves:* The leaves of *Verbascum thapsus* belonging to the family *Scrophularineae* are usually mixed with the genuine drug leaves which may be identified and distinguished microscopically by the abundant presence of huge woolly and branched candelabra trichomes.

2. *Primose leaves:* The leaves of *Primula vulgaris* belonging to the family *Primulaceae* are invariably mixed to **digitalis**, that may be identified microscopically as follows:

(a) *P. vulgaris* has uniseriate covering trichomes , that are normally 8-9 celled long, and

(b) *P. vulgaris* leaves have straight lateral veins.

3. *Comfrey leaves:* The leaves of *Symphytum officinale* belonging to the family *Boraginaceae* are mixed with **digitalis**, which may be distinguished by the presence of multicellular trichomes seen at the top in the shape of a hook.

Uses

1. **Digitalis** enhances the force of contradiction of heart muscle which ultimately affords an increased carrdiac output, decreased size of heart, decreased venous pressure and above all the decreased blood volume. Hence, digitalis together with its various marketed preparations are employed profusely as vital cardiotonics in the management and control of different kinds of congestive heart failure, atrial flutter, atrial fibrillation, supraventricular tachycardia and premature extra systoles.

2. **Digitalis** has a tendency to exert an overall cumulative effect in the body, and hence it gets eliminated rather gradually. Therefore, it is extremely important to monitor the dosage regimen by a physician whether he relies on branded products or natural drug preparations eg., Digitoxin injection, Lanoxin, Prepared digitalis and Digitalis tinture.

4.2.3.2 *Allied Drugs of Digitalis*

Three important allied drugs of **digitalis** which shall be discussed in this section are, namely:

(*a*) *Digitalis lanata,*

(*b*) *Digitalis lutea, and*

(*c*) *Digitalis thapsi.*

4.2.3.2.1   Digitalis Lanata   The drug is almost three times more potent in comparison to *Digitalis purpurea* discussed earlier.

Synonyms   Wooly Foxglove leaf, Grecian Foxglove; Austrial Digitalis.

Biological Source   The dried leaves of *Digitalis lanata* Ehrhart, belonging to family *Scrophularineae.*

Geographical Source   It is a biennial or perennial herb which being indigenous to Southern and Central Europe. It is also cultivated abundantly in India, Holland, United States and Ecuador.

Preparation   The preparation of *D. lanata* leaves is quite similar to the one described under section 4.2.3.1 earlier.

Description   The leaves are usually 5-15 cm in length, sessile, linear lanceolate to oblong lanceolate; margin- entire apex-acute; veins leave the mid-rib at an acute angle.

Chemical Constituents   Stoll and Jucker* (1955) first isolated from its leaves *three* chemically pure *primary glycosides* usually termed as *Lanatoside A, Lanatoside B, and Lanatoside C.* These primary glycosides are also known as **Digilanid A, Digilanid B,** and **Digilanid C** respectively.

However, the inter-relationship of digitalis glycosides found in *Digitalis lanata* may be represented in the following flowchart.

---

* Stoll, A.; and E. Jucker, **'Modern Methods in Plant Analysis',** Springer Verlag, Berlin, 1955

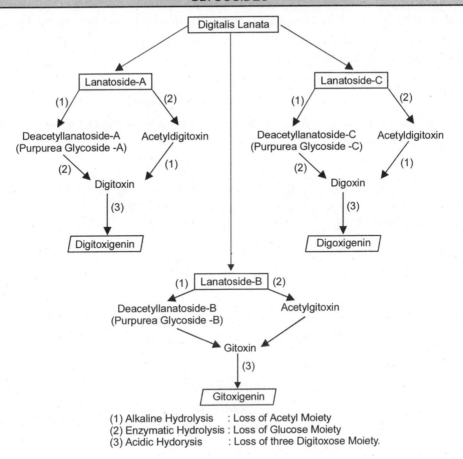

(1) Alkaline Hydrolysis : Loss of Acetyl Moiety
(2) Enzymatic Hydrolysis : Loss of Glucose Moiety
(3) Acidic Hydorysis : Loss of three Digitoxose Moiety.

4.2.3.2.2 Digitalis lutea

Synonym Straw Foxglove.

Biological Source The dried leaves of *Digitalis lutea* Linn. belonging to family *Scrophulariacea*.

Geographical Source It is found in Europe and USA.

Description The leaves have a length of 28 cm and width of 6 cm, but they usually attain only half of their size.

Chemical Constituents The chemical constituents of *D. lutea* have not been fully reported, but it does not contain calcium oxalate.

Uses
1. It is used as a common substitute for the *official drug*.
2. It is potent as *D. purpurea*.
3. It is mostly used for the same purpose as that of *D. purpurea* , but it is found to exert much lesser irritation.

4.2.3.2.3 Digitalis Thapsi

Synonyms Spanish Foxglove; Spanish digitalis.

Biological Source   The dried leaves of *Digitalis thapsi* Linn. belonging to the family *Scrophulariacea*.

Geograhical Source   It is grown in Italy and Spain.

Description   The leaves are mostly yellowish green in colour; and have lanceolate with decurrent lamina and crenate margin. It also contains calcium oxalate crystals.

Uses   Its therapeutic efficacy is almost 1.25 to 3 times more potent than *D. purpurea* and its actions are similar to those of the latter.

4.2.3.3 *Squill*

A survey of literature reveals that the *Squill bulbs* was thoroughly and repeatedly investigated since 1879. However, Stoll in 1933 was first able to separate and isolate two glycosides in their purest form, namely: **Scillaren A** and **Scillaren B**. These *two* naturally occurring glyosides are usually present in the crude drug in the ratio 2:1 (*i.e.*, 2 parts of Scillaren A and 1 part of Scillaren B).

Generally, the squill is available in *three* varieties, namely:

(*a*) European Squill
(*b*) Indian Squill, and
(*c*) Red Squill.

These *three* varieties would be described in the sections that follows:

4.2.3.3.1   European Squill

Synonyms   Sea, onion, Bulbus Scillae; Meerzweibel, White Squill, Squill bulb; Scila.

Biological Source   **European squill** is the fleshy inner bulb scales of the white variety of *Urginea maritima* (L.) Baker (*Scilla maritima* L.) belonging to family *Liliaceae*.

Geographical Source   It is found to be indigenous to those countries located near the Mediterranean region, such as: France, Malta, Italy, Greece, Spain, Algeria and Morocco.

Preparation   Normally the white squill yields fully grown and healthy bulbs that have a height ranging between 18-20 cm and a diameter varying between 12-15 cm. These bulbs are grown in partially submerged condition in sandy soil in the mediterranean coastal region. The bulbs are usually collected in late August soonafter the flowering season. The roots and the thin external scaly layers are removed and discarded. While the central fleshly bulbs are collected separately. These bulbs are then cut into transverse slices and subsequently dried either in sun rays or by artificial heating devices.

Description
    Colour : White; Whitish yellow;
    Taste : Bitter and gummy;
    Size   : Length = 3.5-5 cm; Width = 5-8 mm; Thickness = 2-5 mm;
    Shape : Available as strips with tapering both ends.

Chemical Constituents   Squill has the following glycosides, namely:

        Glucoscillaren A = Scillarenin + Rhamnose + Glucose + Glucose;
             Scillaren A = Scillarenin + Rhamnose + Glucose;
      Proscillaridin A = Scillarenin + Rhamnose.

Scillaridin A; Scilliglaucoside; Scillipheoside; Glucoscillipheoside; Scillicyanoside.

The structures of these glycosides are as shown below:

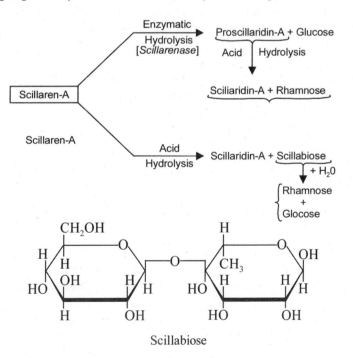

Glucoscillaren A : R $= C_{18}H_{32}O_{14}$;
Scillaren A : R $= C_{12}H_{21}O_9$;
Proscillaridin A : R $= C_6H_{11}O_4$;
Scillarenin : R $=$ H

In addition to the above cardiac glycosides, the drug also comprises of **flavonoids, calcium oxalate, xanthoscillide, sinistrin** (an *inulin* like carbohydrate) and an irritation causing volatile component.

The following flowchart evidemtly illustrates the various steps involved in the *acidic* and *enzymatic hydrolysis* of *Scillaren A* as shown below.

Stoll was first to separate the *two* glycosides from **squil bulbs** and named them as **Scillaren A** and **Scillaren B**. They have the following characteristic features.

Chemical Test   Scillaren A on interaction with acetic anhydride and H_2SO_4, it gives rise to a red colour which changes gradually first to blue and finally to bluish green colour.

Scillabiose

Characteristics of Scillaren A and Scillaren B

S.No.	Properties	Scillaren A	Scillaren B
1.	Nature	Crystalline	Amorphous
2.	Colour	Colourless	White/ Yellowish white
3.	Taste	Bitter	Very bitter
4.	Odour	Odourless	Odourless
5.	Solubility	Comparatively less water soluble	More soluble in water ethanol and methanol
6.	Activity (in Frog assay)	Less active (3 times to reference drug)	More active (5 times to reference drug)
7.	Stability	Less stable	More stable

Uses

1. It is a potent cardiotonic without having any cumulative effect (unlike *Digitalis*).
2. It is mostly employed in small doses as an effective expectorant specially in chronic bronchitis.
3. It causes emesis in relatively higher doses.
4. The **squill glycosides** usually produce copious diuresis.
5. By virtue of the fact that the **squill glycosides** possess high therapeutic index and rapid elimination they invariably maintain compensation in such patients where a prolonged treatment is required.

4.2.3.3.2   Indian Squill

Synonyms   Scilla; Sea onion; Jangli Pyaj; Urginae.

Biological Source   **Indian squill** comprises of the dried slices of the bulbs of *Urginbea indica* Kunth; belonging to the family *Liliaceae*.

Geographical Source   It is grown in India along the sea coasts of Konkan and Saurashtra; and also on the dry hills of the lower Himalayan range located at an altitude of 1500 meters.

Preparation   The method of preparation of dried slices of **Indian squill** is very much alike the **European squill.** It loses approximately 80% of its weight after sun drying.

Description

     Colour   :   Yellowish to White
     Odour   :   Slight and characteristic
     Taste   :   Acrid, bitter and mucilaginous
     Size   :   Length = 30-60 cm; Breadth = 3-8 mm
     Shape   :   Usually 4 to 8 slices are placed one on the top of other and gives it a curved shape.

Characteristic Features

1. It has an overall diameter of 15 cm
2. The dried slices are translucent in appearance which become flexible and rather tough soon after gaining moisture.

Chemical Constituents   **Indian Squill** essentially comprises of cardiac glycosides (0.3%), alcohol soluble extractives (20-40%), mucilages (40%) and calcium oxalate.

     The two major **cardiac glycosides** present in the drug are **Scillaren A** and **Scillaren B** (see Section 4.2.3.3.1).

Substituents/Adulterants The bulbs of different species of Ledebouria (*Scilla*, Linn) are sold in the Indian bazars, under vernacular names which are equivalent to *'small squill'*.

Ledebouria hyacinthoides, is used as a substitute for squill. It has a scaly bulb, about the size and shape of a small pear, composed of very amooth and fleshyscales, which are so *imbricated* that they might be mistaken for entire coats if not carefully examined.

Uses

1. It is largely employed as a cardiotonic , stimulant and also an expectorant.
2. It is used as a very effective expectorant both in asthma and chronic bronchitis.
3. It possesses anticancer activity against human epidermoid carcinoma of the masopharynx in tissue culture.
4. It is in no way a perfect replacement for *Digitalis* since it possesses not only irritant effect but also is very poorly absorbed systemically.

4.2.3.3.3 Red Squill It is the red variety of **European squill** *Urginea maritima* (L.) Baker belonging to family *Liliaceae*. In fact, the red colour is attributed due to the presence of anthrocyanin pigments present in the mesophyll cells of scales.

The glycoside present in the **red squill** is known as **scilliroside** having the following structure.

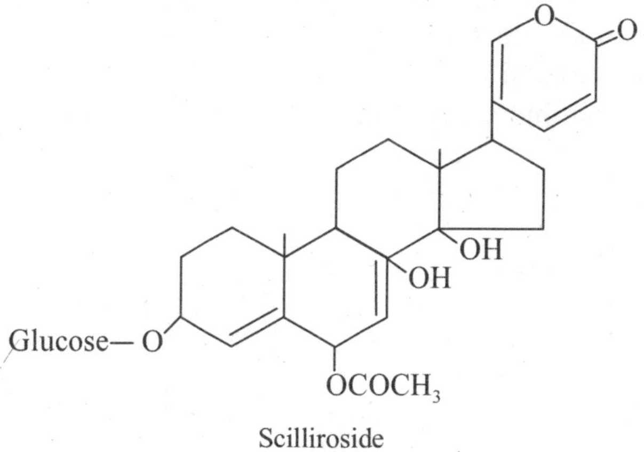

Scilliroside

It is slightly soluble in water, but is soluble freely in lower alcohol, ethylene glycol, dioxane and glacal acetic acid. It is mostly used as a rat poison.

4.2.3.4 Strophanthus

Synonyms Semino stropanthi.

Biological Source These are the dried and ripe seeds of *Strophanthus hispidus* De*, or of *Strophanthus kombe* Oliver, belonging to the family *Apocynaceae*, deprived of the awns.

---

* De = De Candolle

Geographical Source   Strophanthus plants are elimbers, which being perennial large & woody, found to be indigenous in the vicinity of Shire river, Nyanza and Tanganyika lakes of Eastern tropical Africa.

Preparation   The ripe **strophanthus** fruit comprises of two fully developed follicles each about 30cm broad with tapering at both ends and consisting of a number of seeds. The ripe fruits are collected from the wild plants, the seeds are subsequently separated and freed from their awns.

Description

Colour	:	Greyish green to light yellowish brown
Odour	:	Slight unpleasant
Taste	:	Bitter
Size	:	Length 1- 2 cm; Breadth = 3-5 mm; Thickness = 2 mm
Shape	:	Lanceolate to linear-lanceolate, acute at the apex, rounded or blunt at the base
Weight	:	For 100 seeds 3-4 g
Specific feature	:	On treating with 80% H_2SO_4 the endosperm exhibits a deep Emerald green colour.

Chemical Constituents   The seeds of **strophanthus** usually contain *three* vital glycosides, namely: **K-strophanthoside, K-strophanthride β** and **cymarin**. Interestingly, all these glycosides undergo hydrolysis to yield **strophanthidin**.

The structure of **strophanthidin** and its allied glycosides are given below:

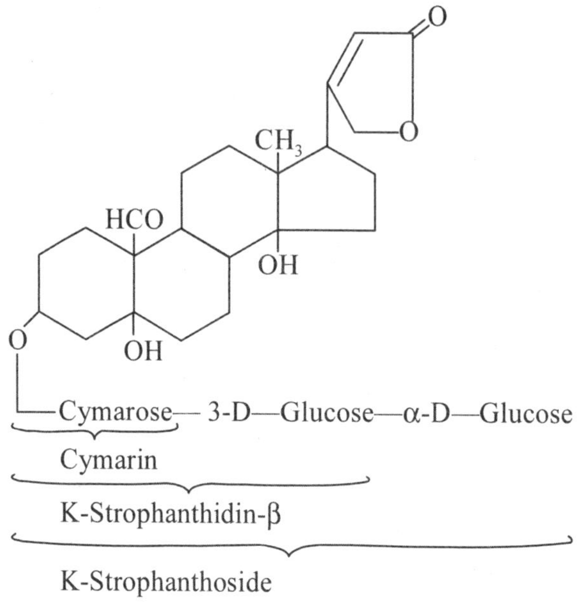

K-Strophanthoside   It is the main constituent of *S.kombe*, the aglycone is known as **strophanthidin** that has the following characteristic features, namely:

(a) Three—OH moieties at positions C-3, C-5 and C-14.

(b) An aldehydic (—CHO) function is present at C-10 which being an essential requirement.

(c) At C-17 an unsaturated 5-membered lactone ring, and

(d) At C-3 an 'O' atom forms a bridge to the sugar compotent(s) essentially comprising of cymarose, β-D-glucose and α-D-glucose.

Acidic hydrolysis of K-strophanthoside gives rise to the aglycone strophanthidin along with a triose sugar known as **strophanthotriose** that comprise of one mole of **cymarose** and two moles of **glucose**.

Enzymatic hydrolysis of **K-strophanthoside** using the enzymes-*glucosidase*, usually present in yeast, helps in cleaving off the terminal α-D glucose thereby yielding the secondary glycoside known as **K-strophanthidin β**. Further hydrolysis of the resulting product with *strophanthobiase,* the former yields the glycosides **cymarin** which comprises of the aglycone **strophanthidin** along with one mole each of **cymarin** and **β-D-glucose**.

Strophanthobiase

However, it is worth noting that the acidic hydrolysis of **K-strophanthoside** gives rise to the aglycone **strophanthidin** and **strophanthobiase** which being a disaccharide (or **biose**) It may be observed that the terminal *glucose* possesses an *alpha linkage*, while the one attached to *cymarose* bears a *beta linkage.*

Chemical Tests

1. Generally, the **strophanthus glycosides** exhibit an emerald green colouration on the addition of sulphuric acid.

2. Dissolve about 0.1g of **strophanthin** in 5 ml of water and add to it a few drops of ferric chloride solution followed by a 1-2 ml of concentrated sulphuric acid; the appearance of an initial red precipitate that finally turns green within a period of 1-2 hours.

3. To 50 mg of **strophanthin** add 5 ml of water, shake and add 2 ml of 2% tannic acid solution, the appearance of a distinct precipitate affirms its presence.

4. It shows positive **Baljet Test, Legal Test** and **Keller Killiani Test** (see Section 4.2.3.1).

Uses

1. It is used intravenously for treating emergency cardiac conditions. However, orally strophanthin is not so active.

2. These glycosides have been found to exert less cumulative effect unlike the digitalis glycosides.

3. Overall their therapeutic actions are very much similar to those of *Digitalis.*

4.2.3.4.1 Allied Drugs

G-Strophanthin

Synonyms Ouabain; Gratus strophanthin; Acocantherin; Gratibain; Astrobain; Purostrophan; Strophoperim; Strodiral.

Biological Source G-Strophanthin is obtained from the seeds of *Strophanthus gratus* (Wall & Hock)Baill. It also occurs in the wood of *Acokanthera ouabio* Cathel and *A. schumperi* belonging to the family *Apocynaceae.*

Geographical Source The wood is grown in Ethiopia and Somaliland.

Chemical Constitutents The seeds contain the glycoside **G-strophanthin** (or **Ouabain**) as given below:

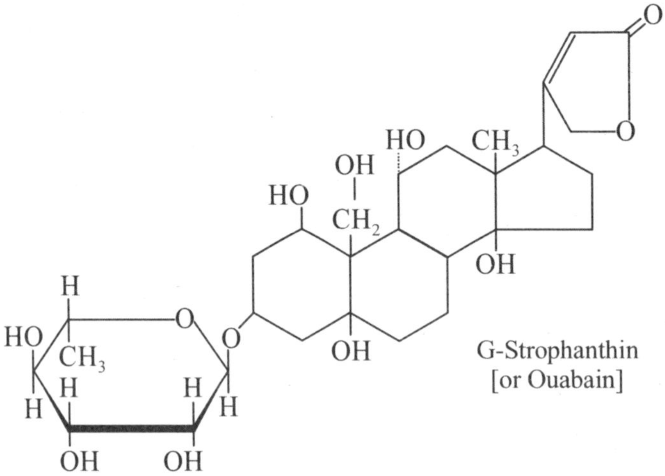

G-Strophanthin
[or Ouabain]

   Ouabain on hydrolysis gives rise to an aglycone termed as G-strophanthidin (or Ouabagenin) and L-rhamnose as the residual sugar moiety.

Description G-Strophanthin mostly occurs as colourless small shining crystals, which are odourless and have an extremely bitter taste. It is readily affected by light, but is quite stable in air. It is practically insoluble in ether, chloroform and ethyl acetate, whereas it is sparingly soluble in cold water (1:75); freely soluble in hot water and alcohol (1:100).

Chemical Tests

1. Mix a few crystals of oubain with a mixture of conc. H_2SO_4 and water (4:1), the appearance of a brownish red colour, which deepens slowly and ultimately shows a green fluorescence.

2. **Froehde's Test:** Mix a few crystals with a drop of Froehde's reagent, evaporate to dryness, cool and add a drop of H_2SO_4—the development of a blue colour takes place.

3. **Mandalin's Test:** Moisten a few crystals with Mandalin's reagent, evaporate to dryness, cool and then add one drop of conc. H_2SO_4—the appearance of a green colour ocurs.

Uses

1. It is an important cardiotonic, which is usually administered intravenously in acute cardiac failure, due to its inherent rapid onset of action.
2. It is invariably employed as a *'reference standard'* for comparison of **cardiac glycosides**.
3. It also exerts diuretic action.

4.2.4 Flavonoid Glycosides

Flavonoid constitute one of the largest class of naturally occuring plant products mostly phenols either in the free state or as their respective glycosides. As the very name suggests they are usually yellow-coloured compounds (*flavous* is a *latin* word yellow colour). Interestingly, more than 2000 different chemical compounds have been isolated, identified and reported from plant sources. In fact, their chemical structures are solely based upon a C_6—C_3—C_6 carbon skeleton having a **pyran** or **chroman** ring bearing a second benzene (aromatic) ring strategically positioned at C—2, C—3 or C—4 as shown below:

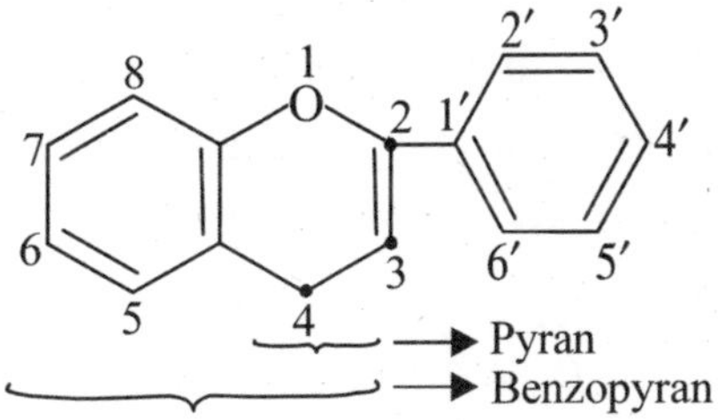

In nature they are invariably available as: **flavones, flavanones, flavonols, isoflavones,** and **anthocyanidins***. In certain specific instances either the 6-membered heterocyclic ring **(pyrones)** is replaced by a 5 membered heterocyclic ring **(aurones)** or exists in an open-chain isomeric form **(chalcones)**. Besides, the normally existing glycosylated derivatives found in nature, other types of derivatives, such as methylated, acetylated, prenylated, or sulphated ones also exist. Nevertheless, it has been established that a large variety of **flavonoids** exert a wide range of activities in nature, namely: antimicrobial agents, signaling molecules, or stress metabolites.

The structures of a few typical **flavonoids** are represented here as follows:

---

* **Anthocyanidins** are the colored aglycones found as a large number of pigments from flowerd and fruits (**Gr. Antho** flower + **Gr. Kyanos**, blue). Investigations of these pigments were initiated by Willstatter in 1914 and later on extended by Karner R Robinson, GM Robinson and others.

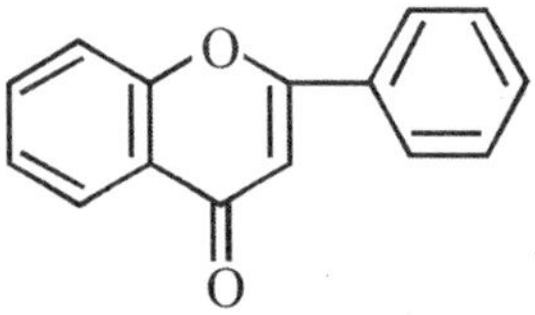

Flavones

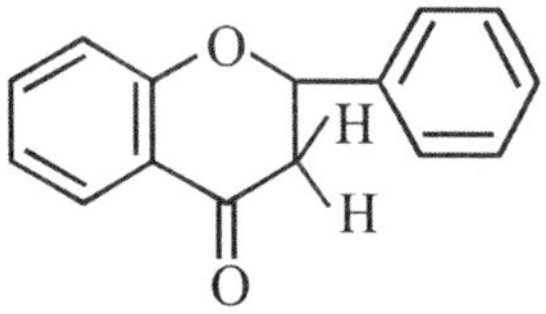

Flavanones

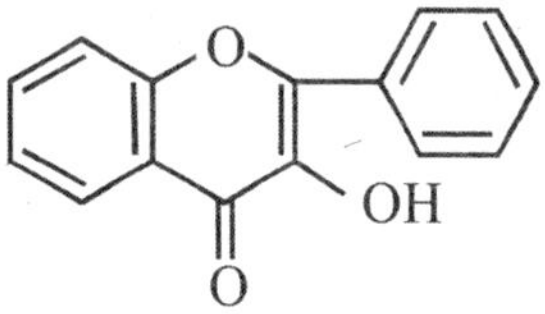

Flavonols

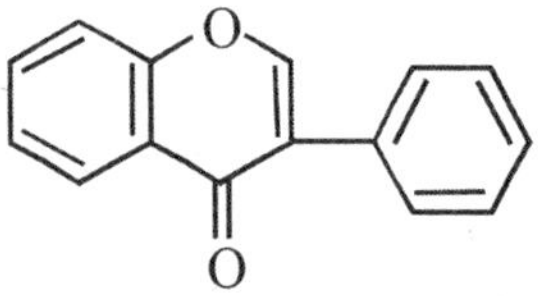

Isoflavones

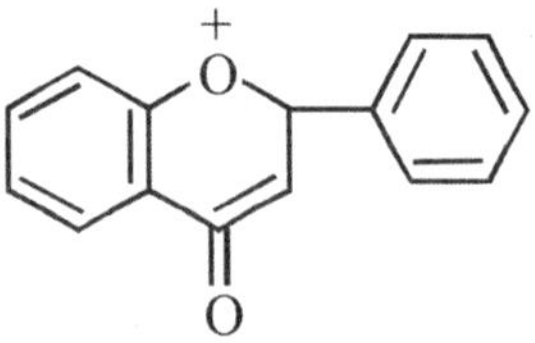

(a)
Anthocyanidins
[Oxonium Form]

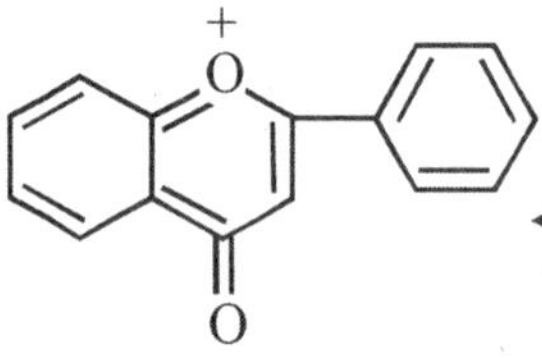

(b)
Anthocyanidins
[Oxonium Form]

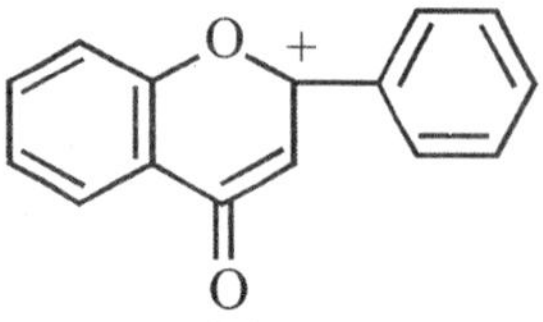

(c)
Anthocyanidins
[Carbonium Form]

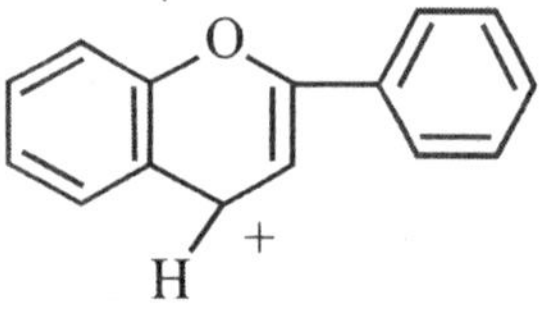

(d)
Anthocyanidins
[Carbonium Form]

The structure (*a*) is more stable, because it has a **naphthalenoid system** of linkages, whereas (*b*) contains a **quinonoid system.**

The structures of only the key portions of **pyrones, aurones** and **chalones** are as follows:

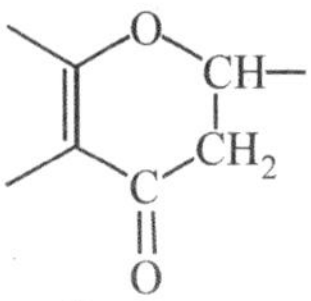

Pyrones
(6-membered)

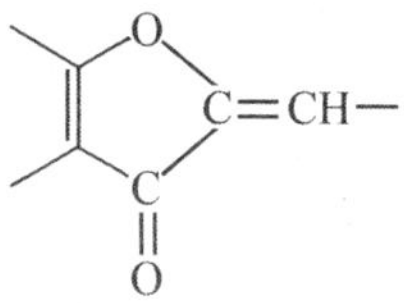

Aurones
(5-membered)

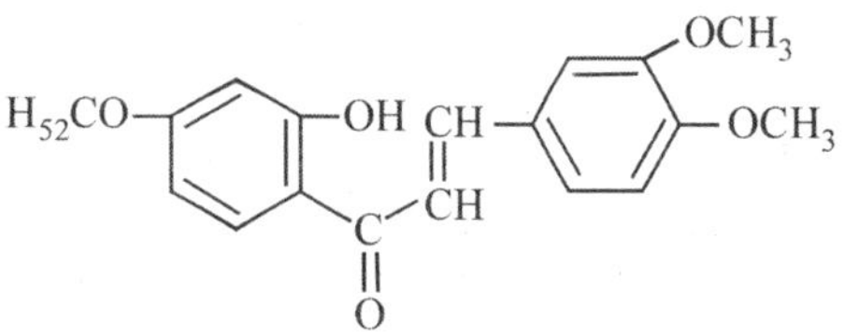

Chalones
(Open-Chain isomeric form)

The **flavonoid glycosides** mostly occur as **O-glycosides** or **C-glycosides** contained in the cell sap of relatively younger tissues of higher plants belonging to several families, such as: *Compositae, Leguminosae, Polygonaceae, Rutaceae* and *Umbelliferae* . It has been observed that a host of natural plant products containing **flavonoid glycosides** exert a variety of therapeutic effects, namely: antiasthmatic, antispasmodic, diuretic, fungicidal and oestrogenic activities.

A few typical **flavonoid glycosides** shall be discussed in the sections that follows, namely:

(*a*) Flavone Glycosides,

(*b*) Flavonol Glycosides,

(*c*) Flavanone Glycosides,

(*d*) Chalcone Glycosides,

(*e*) Isoflavonoid Glycosides, and

(*f*) Anthocyanidin Glycosides.

4.2.4.1 *Flavone Glycosides*

The two important members of this class of glycosides are **Apiin** and **Diosmin** which are described here under:

4.2.4.1.1 **Apiin**

Synonyms   Apioside, Apigenin 7-apiosyglucoside.

Biological Source   **Apiin** usually occurs in the seeds and leaves of *Petroselinum sativum* Hoffm, and *Apium petroselinum* Linn., known as **parsley,** and also in *Apium graveolens* L., and *Anthemis nobilis*. L, called as **celery,** family *Umbelliferae.* It has also been found to be present in the ray florets of *Marticaria chamomilla* Linn., and some other ray florets belonging to the family *Compositae.*

Geographical Source   The fruits are grown in Persia, Greece, Northwest Himalaya and Europe.

Description   It is a very small fruit, almost globular in shape. The taste is at first like anise, but afterwards bitter. The colour is like anise, but generally faint. It occurs as colourless needles.

Chemical Constituents   The structure of **apiin** is given below:

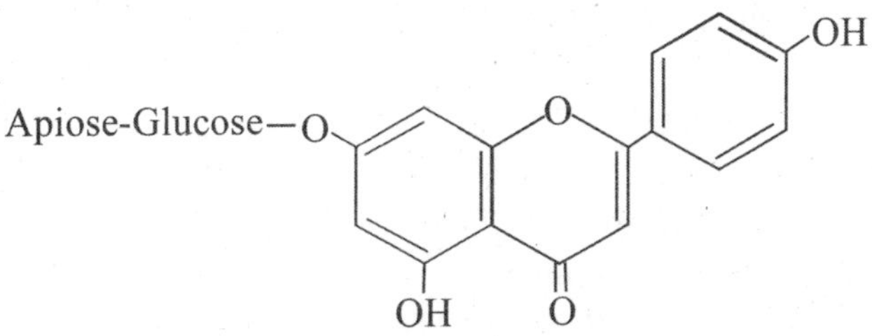

Apiin

Apiin is neither hydrolysed by the enzyme emulsin, nor by yeast or yeast extract. However, it undergoes hydrolysis in an acidic medium to yield *glucose, apiose* (pentose sugar) and *apigenin* (aglycone) which is 4, 5, 7-trihydroxyflavone.

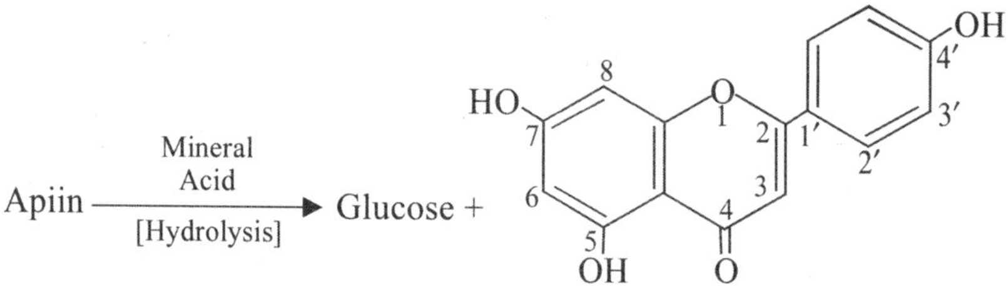

Apigenin
[4',5,7-trihydroxyflavone]

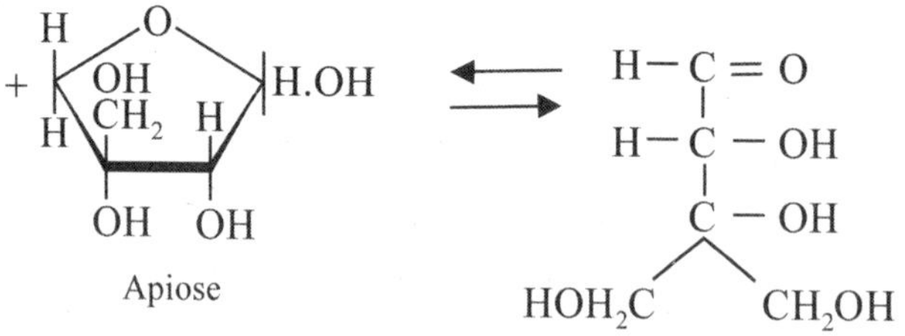

Apiose

Apiose

Apiin when treated with dilute sulphuric acid (0.5 to 1%) undegoes cleavage only at *apiose moiety* thereby giving rise to **7- glucoapigenin** as shown below:

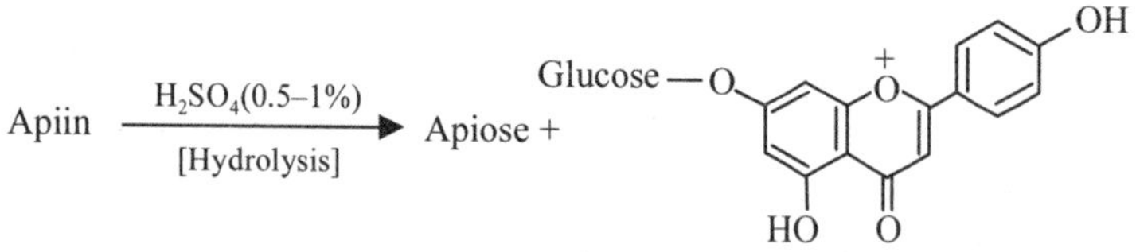

7-Glucoapigenin

Chemical Tests

1. It gives a yellow precipitate with basic lead acetate.
2. It produces a reddish brown colour with $FeCl_3$.
3. It gives an intense yellow colour with NH_4OH solution
4. It yields a pale yellow colour with NaOH solution.

4.2.4.1.2 Diosmin

Synonym   Barosmin.

Biological Source   It occurs in the dried *Buchu* leaves *i.e.*; various species of *Barosma crenulata*, *Barosma serratifolia* and *Barosma betulina* belonging to family *Rutaceae*. It has also been isolated from *Serophularia nodosa, Hyssopus officinalis, Mentha crispa, Mentha pulegium* and from species of *Conium, Dahlia* etc.

Description   It occurs as pale yellow needles.

Chemical Structure   The chemical structure of **diosmin** (5, 7, 3'-trihydroxy-4'-methoxyflavone-7-rhamnoglucoside) is given below:

Diosmetin (Aglycone)

Disomin upon hydrolysis yields rhamnose, glucose and the aglycone diosmetin.

Chemical Test   A solution of **diosmin** in concentrated sulphuric acid exhibits a slight fluorescence.

4.2.4.2 Flavonol Glycosides

The two well known glycosides belonging to this class are namely: **Rutin** and **Quercetin,** whereas the less important ones are—**galangin, gossypin, hibiscitrin, kaempferin** and **avecularin.**

4.2.4.2.1   Rutin

Synonyms   Melin; Phytomelin; Eldrin; Ilixanthin; Sophorin; Globularicitrin; Paliuroside; Osyritrin; Osyritin; Myrticolorin; Violaquercitrin; Birutan; Rutabion; Rutozyd; Tanrutin.

Biological Source   **Rutin** is found in many plants, especially the **buckwheat plant** (*Fagopyrum esculentum* Moench; family: *Polygonaceae*); in **forsythia** [*Forsythia suspensa (Thunb).)* Vahl ver. *Fortunei* (Lindl). Rehd., family *Oleaceae]*; in **hydrangea** (*Hydrangea paniculata* Sieb., family: *Saxifragaceae); in **pansies** (Viola sp. *Violaceae); from leaves of *Eucalyptus macroryncha* F.v. Muell., family : *Myrtacea);* in *Fagopyrum tartaricum* Gaertn: family: *Polygonaceae);* in *Ruta graveolens* L., (family: *Rutaceae); in buds of *Sophora japonica* L., (family: *Leguminoseae);* in fresh leaves of **tobacco plants,** *Nicotiana tabacum* L., (family : *Solanaceae);* in **cotton seed** *Gossypium hirsutum;*(family *Malvaceae*); in *Viola tricolor,* (family : *Violaceae).*

Geographical Source   The various plants like eucalyptus, tobacco, and cotton grow abundantly in tropical countries like India, Africa, Ceylon and United Stated, Australia and China.

Preparation   Based on experimental evidences it has been observed that the glycoside content in plants declines sharply as they mature; however, the highest yields are usually obtained from the **buckwheat leaves and flowers** as soon as the plants attain the blossom-stage.

The dried and ground plant material (say 150 g) is extracted with two successive quantities (2 × 200 ml) of ethanol (80% v/v). The resulting filtered hydro-alcoholic extract is carefully evaporated under vaccum in a rotary evaporator till it reaches upto 50-60 ml. The content of the flask is mixed with an equal volume of ether and the ethereal layer is separated. The aqueous layer is once again extracted with the same volume of ether and the ethereal layer separated. Both the ethereal layers are discarded and the aqueous layer is evaporated under reduced pressure to 10 ml. Keep the concentrated residual liquid in a refrigerator (0-5°C) overnight when a solid crystalline substance appears. Separate it from the mother liquor. The crude rutin, thus obtained may be further purified by *Column Chromatography*, using magnesium silicate as an adsorbent and ethanol as an eluant.

Description   It has a pale yellow crystalline needle like apprearance. It is practically insoluble in water, ether, petroleum ether and chloroform. It is fairly soluble in ethanol and acetone.

Chemical Structure   The structure of **rutin** (or 5, 7, 3′, 4′ tetrahydroxy flavonol -3-rhamnoglucoside) is given below:

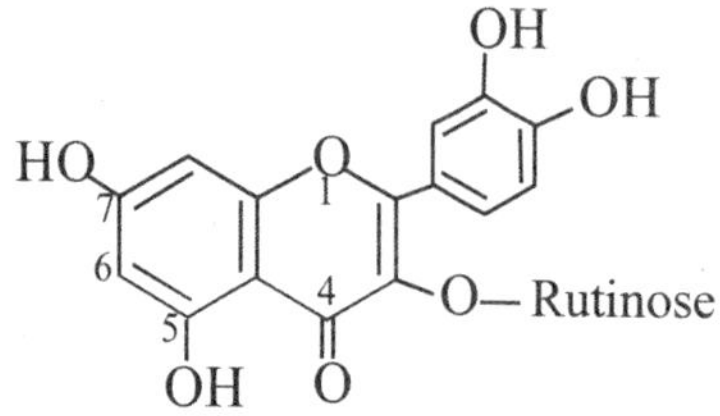

Rutin 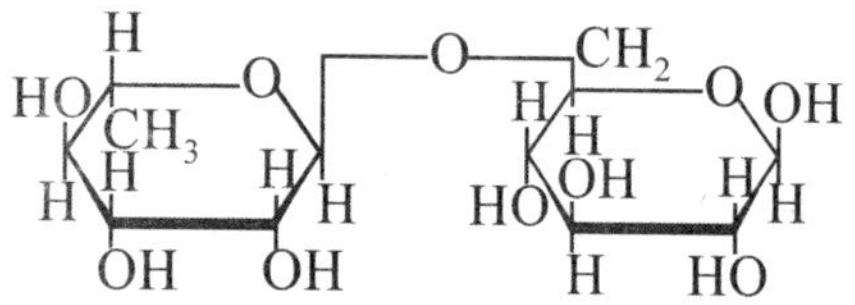   Rutinose

Rutin on refluxing with dilute mineral acid (200 ml of 0.1N H_2SO_4 + 1 g rutin) for 90 minutes gives rise to the aglycone known as **quercetin** plus the corresponding sugars.

Chemical Tests

1. It gives a distinct yellow precipitate with basic lead acetate.
2. It yields a greenish brown colour with ferric chloride.
3. It produces a silver mirror with ammonical silver nitrate solution (Tollen's Reagent)

Uses

1. **Rutin** is used to decrease the capillary fragility (*i.e.,* to enhance the tensile strength of capillary walls), reduce capillary permeability by tissue injury, and minimise the destruction of epinephrine in body tissues.
2. It has been mostly used in certain disease condition to reduce capillary bleeding promptly.
3. It is found to be useful in the treatment of retinal harmorrhages.

4.2.4.2.2   Quercetin

Synonyms   Quercitroside; Quercimelin; Quercitin – 3-L-rhamnoside; Thujin; Quercitin; Quercetin.

Biological Sources   Quercetin occurs in the bark of *Quercus tinctoria* and some other species of *Quercus*. It is also obtained from *Alsculus hippocastarum* L., **horse chest nut,** belonging to family *Hippocastanaceae*. Besides, it is also found in *Thuja occidentalis* L., *Morus alba* L., *Humulus lupulus* L., *Fraxinus excelsior* L., *Vitis vinifera* and a host of other plants.

Geographical Source   *A. hippocastanum* is found in India and the African continent.

Description   The crystals are yellow in colour when obtained from ethanol or methanol. It is practically insoluble in cold water and ether. *Flavine yellow shade* obtained from the **quercitron bark** by extraction under high pressure steam which is used exclusively in dyeing fabrics.

Chemical Structure   The structure of **quercetin** is as shown below:

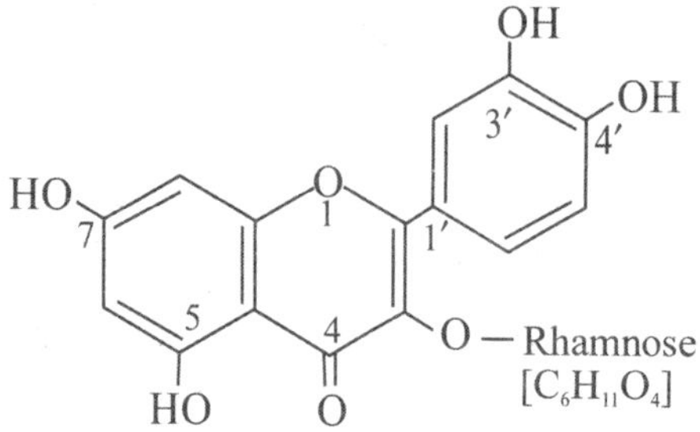

Quercitin

Quercitin on hydrolysis in an acidic medium gives rise to **rhamnose** and **quercetin** (*i.e.*, 5, 7, 3′, 4′-tetrahyroxy flavonol).

It has been observed that the fully methylated *quercetin* upon hydrolysis yields 5, 7, 3′, 4′-tetramethyl flavonol which amply suggests that the residue is duly attached at C-3 of the aglycone moiety and also **quercitin** is nothing but quercetin-3-rhamnoside.

Chemical Tests

1. It exhibits a brown fluorescence under the UV-light.
2. It gives a distinct yellow precipitate initially with a solution of basic lead acetate, but it gets dissolved on further addition of the reagent in excess.
3. It reduces Tollen's reagent to give a silver mirror.
4. It gives a negative test with Fehling's solution *i.e.*, not yielding brick red precipitate.

Uses   It has been used as textile dye.

4.2.4.3 *Flavanone Glycosides*

Flavanone glycosides are most abundantly distributed amongst the citrus fruits. **Hesperidin** is the glycoside most commonly found in this particular class. However, the comparatively less important glycosides belonging to this category are, namely: **naringin, citronin** and **liquiritin. Hesperidin** shall be discussed in details here.

4.2.4.3.1 Hesperidin

Synonyms   Cirantin; Hesperitin 7-rhamnoglucoside; Hesperetin-7-rutinoside.

Biological Source   **Hesperidin** is the most predominant flavonoid in lemons and sweet orange *Citrus sinensis* (Linn.) Osbeck. It is also found in the rind or peel or unripe, green citrus fruits, for instance: **Bitter Orange** (*Citrus aurantium* Linn.); Lemons *(Citrus limon* Linn); **Citron** (*Citrus medica* Linn.).

Geographical Source   Citrus fruits are abundantly grown in the tropical African countries *e.g.*; Togo, Nigeria, Ghana, besides the Mediterranean regoins.

Preparation   The glucoside may be isolated by adopting the laid down detailed procedures as in Section 4.2.4.2.1. It is also present in the dried orange peel upto 8% and it occurs in the highest concentration in the white portion of the peel usually termed as *albedo*.

Description   **Hesperidin** is a colourless needle like crystals. It seems to be closely related to Vitamin P (*Citrin*). It is readily soluble in hot water, sparingly soluble in alcohol and cold water, and practically insoluble in ether, benzene and chloroform.

Chemical Structure   The Structure of **hesperidin** is given as under:

The hesperidin chalone, comprising of an embedded phloroglucinol ring is promptly converted to flavones (*e.g.*, **hesperidin**) in an acidic medium, when heated or allowing it to stand in the dry state for a long duration. However, **methylation of the hesperidin chalone** helps in the ultimate methylation of one of the phenolic moieties present in the phloroglucinol portion of the chalone not only stablizies the corresponding **methyl chalone** but also prevents closure of the ring to produce the **flavones** [see structure on next page].

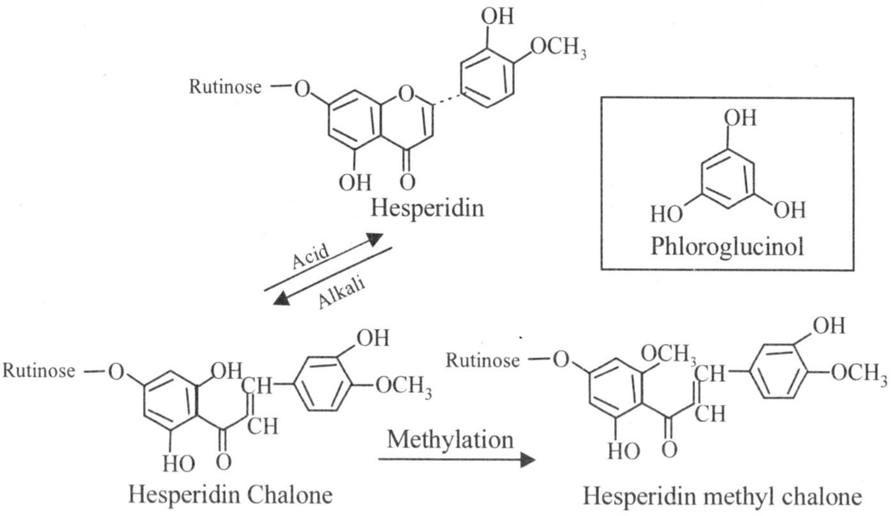

Hesperidin

Phloroglucinol

Hesperidin Chalone

Hesperidin methyl chalone

Uses

1. It is normally used in conjunction with ascorbic acid to minimise capillary fragility.
2. It is also indicated in the prevention and management of capillary fragility or permeability in hypertension, cardiovascular and cerebrovascular disease, and also in habitual and threatened abortion.

4.2.4.4 Chalcone Glycosides

Chalcones are characterised usually by the presence of the following essential structure:

$$Ar(A) — CO — CH = CH — Ar(B)$$

Evidently, the two aromatic rings (A and B) are linked by the *three carbon -aliphatic chain* which does not actively take part in the formation of a *hetero-ring* as is normally found in other types of flavonoid compounds. Likewise, the **dihyrochalones** shall have the following general structure:

$$Ar(A) — CO — CH_2 — CH_2 — Ar(B)$$

Also, the **chalone** yields a flavanone on treating with 10% H_2SO_4. These *two* reactions may be represented as follows:

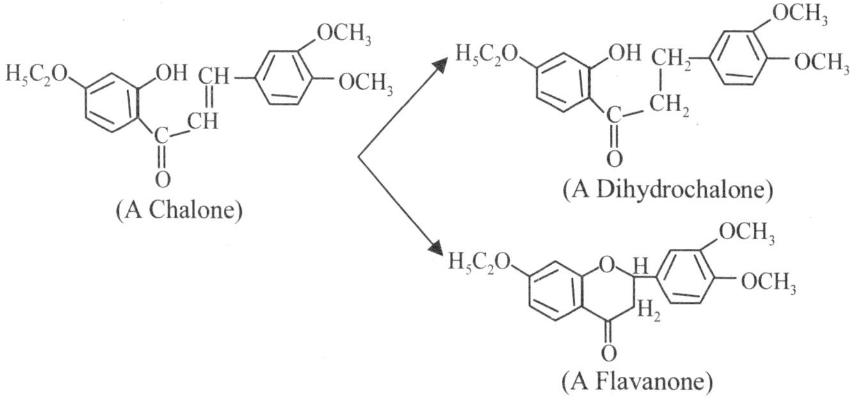

(A Chalone)

(A Dihydrochalone)

(A Flavanone)

Interestingly, the **chalones** and **flavanones** are closely related to each other and they are also fully *intercovertible*.

Examples:

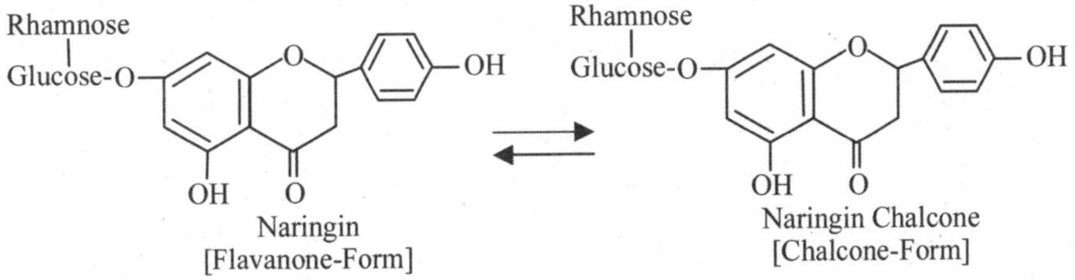

Naringin
[Flavanone-Form]

Naringin Chalcone
[Chalcone-Form]

(a)

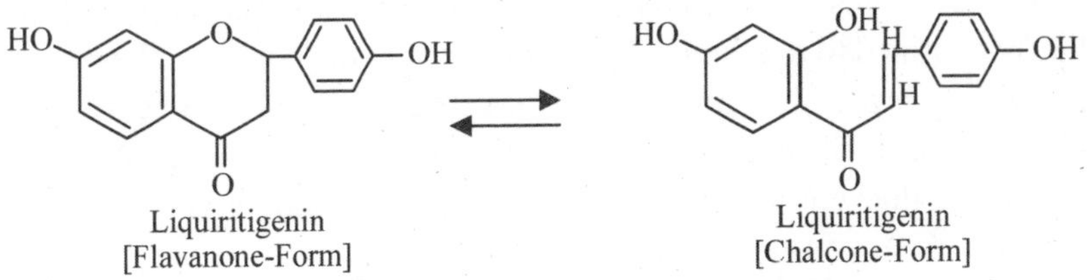

Liquiritigenin
[Flavanone-Form]

Liquiritigenin
[Chalcone-Form]

(b)

A few typical examples are described below:

4.2.4.4.1 Carthamin

Synonyms Safflor carmine; Safflor red; Carthamic acid.

Biological Source Carthamin is the coloring principle obtained from *Carthamus tinctorius* L., belonging to family *Compositae* (Safflower).

Geographical Source It is grown throughout a large portion of Inida. It is one of the most ancient crops cultivated in Egypt as a dye-yielding herb. It is also grown in Russia, Mexico, United States, Ethiopia and Australia.

Description It is a dark red granular powder having a green luster. It is slightly soluble in water and practically insoluble in ether. It is found to be soluble in alcohol and in dilute alkali carbonates.

Chemical Structure The structure of **carthamin** is as given below:

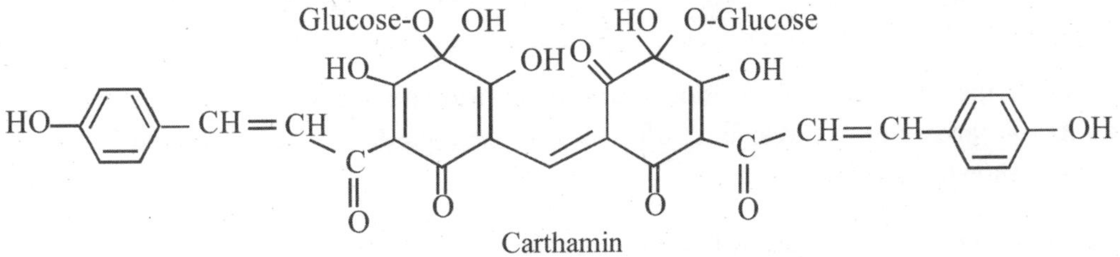

Carthamin

Carthamin on being treated with diilute hydrochloric acid gets converted to ite isomeric yellow compound known as **isocarthamin.**

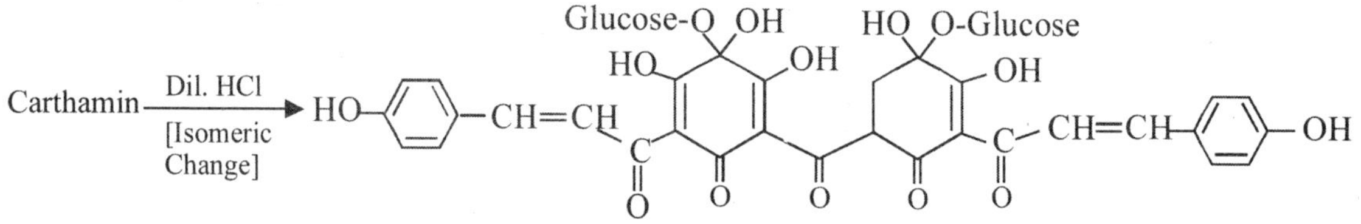

Isocarthamin

Uses

1. It is used as a dye.

4.2.4.5 Isoflavonoid Glycosides

Unlike most other flavonoids, the isoflavonoid glycosides possess a rather limited taxonomic distribution, chiefly confined to the family *Leguminosae*. On the contrary, their chemical structures display an exceptionally broad spectrum of modifications. Wong (1975)* carried out an extensive review of the chemistry as well as taxonomic distribution of isoflavonoids. A few major classes of isoflavonoids along with their enormous prevailing structural variations are exemplified in Table 4.1.

Table 4.1   Major Classes of Isoflavonoids

S.No	Name	Biological Source	Chemical Structure	Uses
1	**Tephrosin** (Toxicarol; Hydroxydequelin)	From leaves of *Tephrosia vogelli* Hook.f., (*Legumonoseae*) In derris root, cube root;	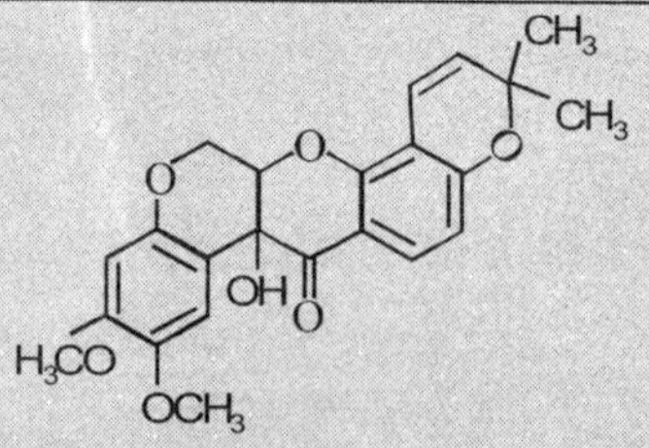	Toxic to fish, insects and crustaceae. Not toxic to human
2.	**Sophoricoside** (Genistein-4'-glucoside)	From the green pods of *Sophora japonica* L., (*Leguminosae*)	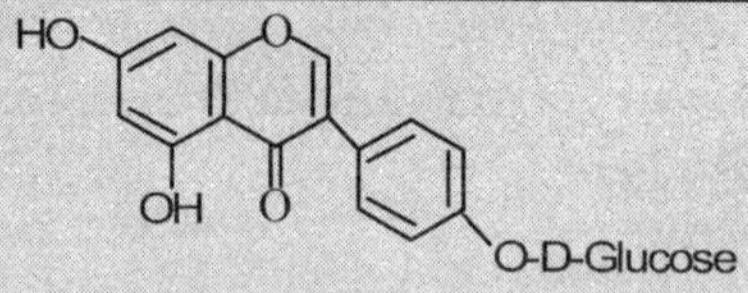	Not reported
3.	**Prunetrin** (Glucoside prunetin)	From the bark of *Prunus avium* L., var Bigarreau Napolean (*Rodaceae*)	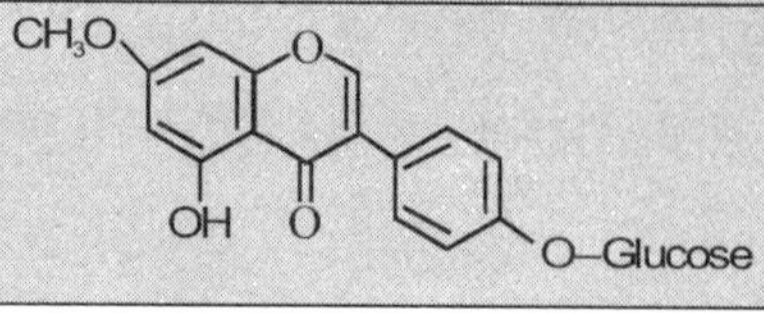	Not reported

However, there exists a close relationship with the structure of **isoflavones** to the skeleton of the **rotenoids** (or **rotenone**), whereas both of them may be regarded as being derived from *3-phenyl chroman* as shown below:

---

* Wong, E *'The Flavonoids'* Chapman & Hall, London, p. 743-800, 1975.

Isoflavone
[Genistein]

Rotenoid
[Rotenone]

3—Phenyl Chroman

4.2.4.6 Anthocyanidin Glycosides

In addition to chlorophyll, **anthocyanins** represent the most important class of natural plant pigments visible to the naked eye. **Anthrocyanidine** (aglyconoes) are structurally closely related to each other. It has been established that there exist *six* prominent **anthrocyanidines** whose chemical structres are entirely based on the structure of **pelargonidin**. These six aglyconoes differ from **pelargonidin** by having one or two additional hydroxyl or methoxyl moieties strategically positioned at C-3′ and C-5′ in the latter, as shown in Table 4.2.

Pelargonidin (R = R′ = H)

Table 4.2 Six Major Anthocyanidins and Biological Source

S.No.	Anthocyanidins	R	R′	Biological Source(s)
1.	Pelargonidin	H	H	Flowers of *Pelargonium graveolens* L'Herit., and *P. roseum* (R. Br.in) Ait. Family: *Geraniaceae*.
2.	Cyanidin	OH	H	Flowers of *Althaea roaea* cav., Family: *Malvaceae*.
3.	Peonidin	H_3CO	H	Tubers from *Peony officinalis* Linn., Family: *Ranunculaceae*.
4.	Delphinidin	OH	OH	From the whortleberry *Vaccinium myrtillus* Linn., family: *Ericaceae*.
5.	Petunidin	OH	OCH_3	Flowers of *Petunia hybrida*, family: *Solanaceae*.
6.	Malvidin	H_3CO	OCH_3	Flowers of *Malva sylvestris* Linn., family: *Malvaceae*.

It is, however, pertinent to mention here that the sugar components are invariably attached to C-3′ position, and more rarely to C-5′ position. It is worth mentioning here that in the flavone glycosides the attachement is normally at C-7 position. These sugar moieties may be:

Monosaccharides : *e.g.*: arabinose, galactose, glucose and rhamnose

Disaccharides : *e.g.*: rhamnoglucosides (present in *Antirhinum sp.*)

Trisaccharides : *e.g.*: 5-glucosides-3-rutinoside (present in some *Solanaceae* species such as: *Atropa* and *Solanum*.)

Leucoanthocyanidins (or Proanthocyanidins) **Procanthocyanidins** represent a group of highly water soluble naturally occuring plant pigments that are closely related to anthocyanidins. However, they may be easily differentiated from other flavonoids by virtue of the fact that the **procanthocyndins** are easily converted into their corresponding anthocyanidins on being boiled either with alcoholic or aqueous hydrochloric acid.

In general, they are considered equivalent to *flavan 3, 4-diols* chemically, which may be present either in their monomeric/ polymeric forms or as their corresponding derivatives. Examples: **(-)-Melacacidin** obtained from *Acacia melanoxylan* and other related species.

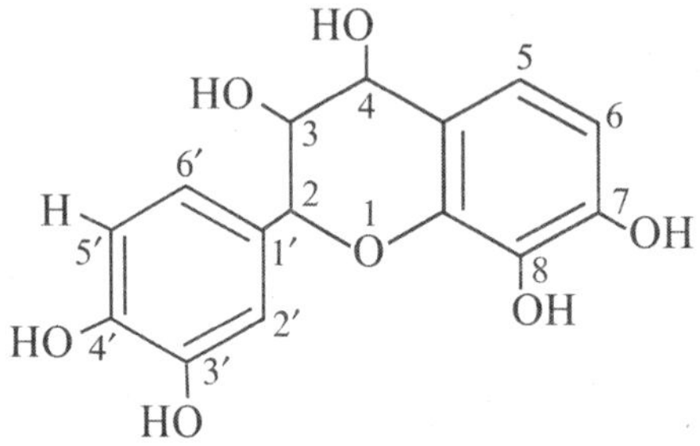

(-) – Melacacidin (2,3 – *cis* & 3, 4 – *cis*)

The **isomelacidin** has the 2,3-*cis* and 3,4 –*trans*. configuration

4.2.5 Coumarin and Furanocoumarin Glycosides

Generally, **couramin** and its derivativces **furanocoumarin** are found to be present in a plethora of naturally occuring plants. Nevertheless, the coumarin is presnet either in the free state or its corresponding glycosides form in nature, but it has been observed that the former being most common.

The *two* different types of glycosides of this group shall be discussed separately under the following heads:

4.2.5.1 Coumarin Glycosides

These are reported to be present in about 150 different species spreading over to nearly 30 different families, of which a few important ones are, namely: *Caprifoliaceae, Leguminosae, Oleaceae, Rubiaeeae, Solaneceae,* and *Umbelliferae.*

This basic nucleus of coumarin is considered to be derived from o-hydroxy cinnamic acid (or o-coumarin acid) by its dehydration to yield the fused lactone ring as shown below:

It has been observed that invariably most naturally occurring **coumarins** essentially bear an oxygen atom either as hydroxyl (OH) or alkoxyl (—OCH_3 or —OC_2H_5) at C-7 position.

A few important naturally occurring **coumarin glycosides** along with their respective biological sources have been summarised in Table 4.3.

2.5.1.1 Coumarin **Coumarin** is abundantly found in a variety of natural products which are used profusely as a flavouring agent in pharmaceutical preparations.

Synonyms Tonka bean camphor; Cumarin; Coumarimic anhydride.

Table 4.3 Coumarin Glycosides and Biological Sources

S.No	Name	Biological Source	Chemical Structure	Uses
1.	Acsulin	Horse chest nut tree; Fruit and bark of *Aesculus hippocastanum* Linn., family *Hippocastanaceae*	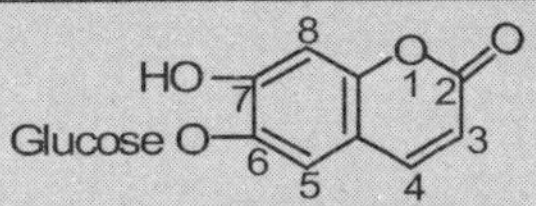	Fruit and bark in diarrhoea
2.	Cichorin	Flowers of the chicory plant: *Cichorium intybus* Linn., family: *Compositae*	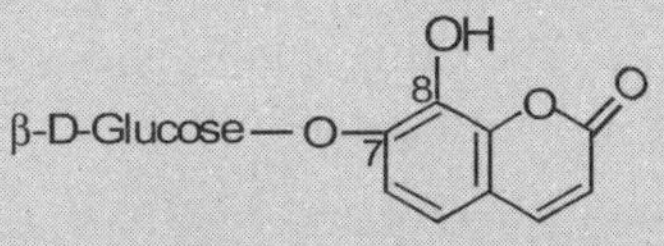	Used as tonic, febrifuge, and in diarrhoea
3.	Daphnin	Bark of various species of *Daphne* eg: *Daphne* mezerium family: *Thymelaceae*	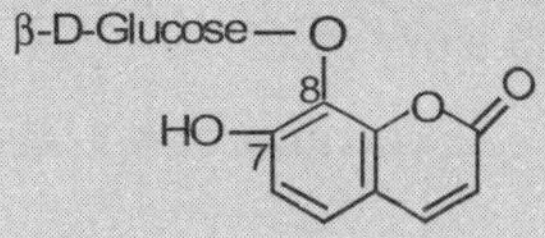	As a febrifuge
4.	Fraxin	From bark of the common European ash: *Fraxinus excelsir* Linn., family: *Oleaceae.*	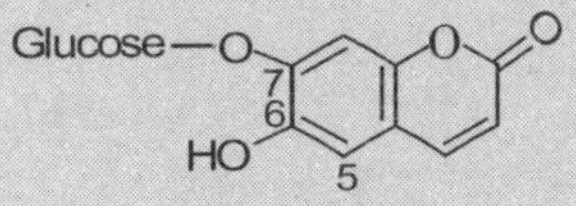	Bark used as a bitter astringent, tonic and febrifuge.

Biological Source It is found in the *tonka seed*, also known as **tonquin beans** or **tonco seed** *i.e.*, *Dipteryx odorata* Wild, and *Dipteryx oppositifolia* L., belonging to family *Leguminosae*. It is also obtained from *Woodruff (Asperula species)* and in **sweet clover** *i.e.*; *Melilotus alba* Dess., family : *Leguminosae.*

Geographical Source These plants are found in Europe, India and in the African continent.

Description

> **Colour** : Colourless
> **Odour** : Pleasant and fragrant odour resembling that of vanilla beans.
> **Taste** : Burning Taste
> **Shape** : Orthorhombic, rectangular plates.

Chemical Structures **Coumarin** has the following structure:

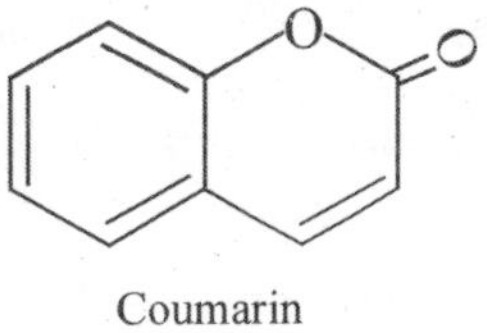

Coumarin

Uses It is mostly employed as a pharmaceutical aid.

4.2.5.2 *Furanocoumarin Glycosides*

In general, the **furanocoumarins** are obtained by the fusion of the **'furan ring'** to the coumarin nucleus either at C-6 and C-7 positons or at C-7 and C-8 positions. A few typical examples belonging to this class of glycosides are discussed in the sections that follows, namely: **Khellol glucoside; Psoralea;** and **Cantharides.**

4.2.5.2.1   Khellol Glucoside

Synonyms   Khellinin; 2-Hydroxy-methyl-5-methoxyfuranochrome glucoside.

Biological Source   It is obtained from the seeds of *Eranthis hyemalis* Linn., family *Ranunculaceae, Ammi visnaga* Lam family *Umbelliferae.*

Geographical Source   The drug is indigenous to Egypt specially the Nile Delta and also to the Mediterranean region. It is cultivated in India.

Preparation   The annual herb plant usually bears flowers from March to April. The harvesting is carried out when the ripening of first fertilized flowers takes place. The plants are cut and preserved in stacks, preferably in a dry place, whereby all the fruits are ripened.

Chemical Structure   The **furanocoumarin** derivative **khellol glucoside** has the following strutcure.

Khellol Glucoside: $R_1 = H$;

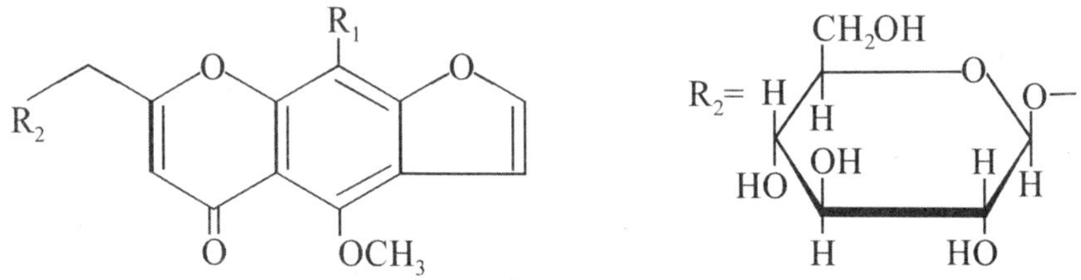

$R_2 = $ [structure]

Khellin: $R_1 = OCH_3$; $R_2 = H$;
Visnagin: $R_1 = R_2 = H$;

The drug also contains *two* well known aglycones **khellin** and **visnagin** as shown above.

Description   The characteristic features of **khellol glucoside, khellin** and **visnagin** are summarised in Table 4.4.

Table 4.4   Characteristic Features of Khellol Glucoside, Khelin and Visnagin

S.No	Characteristic Features	Khellol Glucoside	Khellin	Visnagin
1.	Colour	Colourless crystals	Colourless crystals	Colourless thread like needles.
2.	Odour	No specific odour	Odourless	Odourless
3.	Taste	—	Bitter	—
4.	Solubility	Soluble in acetic acid, hot ethanol; slightly soluble in hot methanol; practically insoluble in acetone, ethyl acetate, ether, chloroform, cold alkali	Sol. In water 0.025 g/ 100 ml at 25°C, in acetone 3.0 g; in methanol 2.6 g; in isopropanol 1.25 g; in ether 0.5 g; in skelly solve B 0.15 g; More soluble in hot water and methanol	Very slightly soluble in water, sparingly soluble in alcohol; and freely soluble in chloroform.

Uses

1. It is mostly used as a coronary vasodilator
2. Khellin has proved to be a potent smooth muscle relaxant
3. Khellin is employed as coraonary vasodilator, in angina pectoris, renal and uterine colic pains, bronchial asthma and whooping cough.

Note **Khellin is found to be fairly stable when mixed with the usual tabletting excipients.**

4.2.5.2.2 Psoralen

Synonyms *Lata-kasturi* (Bengali); *Bahuchi* (Sanskrit).

Biological Sources They are the dried ripe fruits of *Psoralea corylifolia* Linn., belonging to the family *Leguminosae*. **Psoralen** is also found naturally in more than two dozen plant sources, namely: Bergernot, Limes, Cloves: family *Rutaceae;* Figs.: family *Moraceae*.

Geographical Sources It is grown almost throughout India as a weed in abandoned locations. It is also found in Ceylon. Several species of *Psoralea* have been used medicinally in America.

Description

Colour	:	Dark chocholate to black
Odour	:	Pungent and characteristic after crushing the fruits
Taste	:	Unpleasant, bitter and acrid
Size	:	3 to 5 × 2 to 3 mm
Shape	:	Pods are ovoid, oblong beam shaped

Chemical Constituents The fruits of *P. corylifolia* invariably contain **fluorocoumarin** compounds known as **psoralen** and **isopsoralen** as shown below:

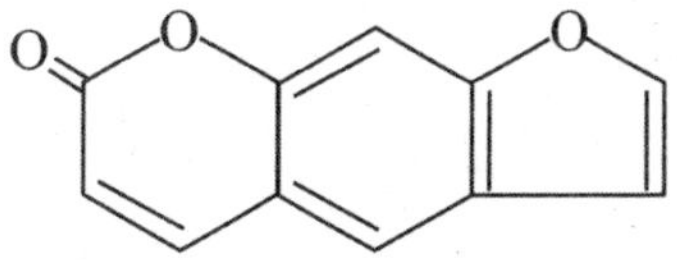

Psoralen 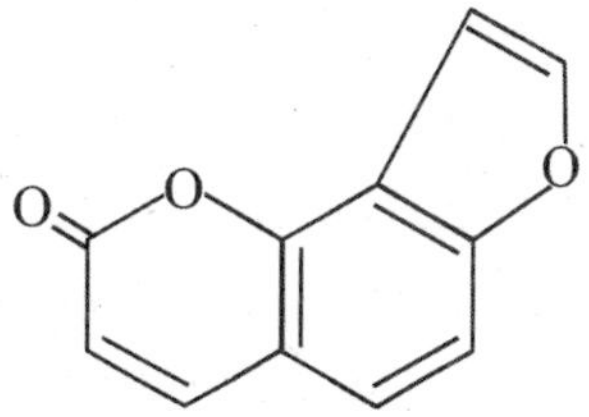   Isopsoralen

The seed kernel of *P. corylifolia* is found to conatin **psolaridin** as given below:

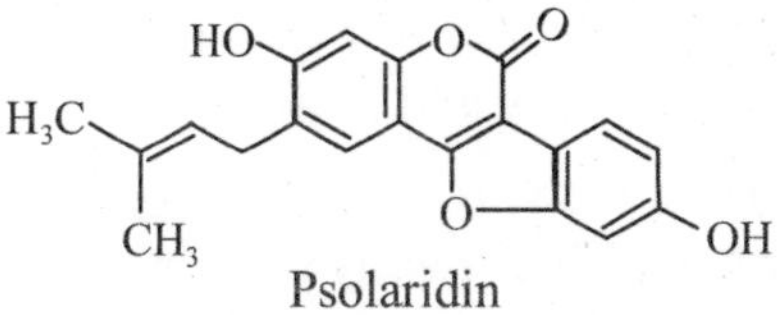

Psolaridin

The plant also contains substituent components of the *linear* molecule, such as: **8-methoxypsoralen** and **5-methoxypsoralen** (or **bergapten**); besides *angular* molecules, such as: **anglicin** and **isobergapten**.*

---

* It has been observed that the naturally occurring **psolarens** lower the phototoxic potential whereas the **anglicins** may enhance it.

8-Methoxypsoralen   5-Methoxypsoralen   Angelicin   Isobergapten
                 or
                 Bergapten

However, in the recent past *two* more compounds, namely: **psoralenol** and **bavachromanol** have been reported.

Besides the fruit contains a variety of other chemical constituents, for instance: fixed oil (10%); resin (8.9%); essential oil (0.05%) and small amounts of raffinose and a pigment.

Chemical Tests (For Psoralen)

1. To a small amount of drug add a minimum quantity of alcohol for complete dissolution. Add to this 3 volumes of propylene glycol, 5 volumes of acetic acid and 43 volumes of water and shake well. The appearance of a blue fluorescence under UV-light indicates its presence.
2. The drug is dissolved in minimum amount of alcohol and on addition of a little sodium hydroxide solution exhibits a yellow fluorescence in UV-light.

Uses

1. The seeds are recommended in leprosy, leucoderma and other skin manifestations. They are also used for snake bite and scorpion sting.
2. The oleroesin extracts of seeds are employed to cure leucoderma patches.
3. The seeds also find their use as stomachic, anthelmintic, diuretic and diaphoretic.
4. It is used orally as a laxative.

4.2.5.2.3 Cantharides Beetles

Synonyms   Spanish fly; Blistering fly; Blistering beetles.

Biological Sources   *Cantharides* comprises of the dead and dried insects of *Cantharis vesicatoria* Linn., (*Lyatta vesicatoria*) belonging to the family *Meloidae*. **Cantharides** contains the **furanocoumarin** derivatives **cantharidin** ranging from 0.6 to 1%.

Geographical Sources   These beetles are invaribaly found in the Southern and Central Europe residing on the plants belonging to the family *Oleaceae* and *Caprifoliaceae*. The various countries that are commercially engaged in the collection of **cantharides** are namely: Russia (now known as CIS countries), Rumania, Italy, Spain, Sicily and India.

Preparation   The fully developed insects, that are brilliant green in apprearance with a distinct metallic lusture, are invariably collected in the early morning on a large spread cloth by vigorously shaking the branches of the shrubs. The beetles are sacrificed either by exposing them to the vapours of chloroform, sulphur dioxide and ammonia in a closed chamber or dipping them into vinegar. The dead beetles are dried artificially at a controlled temperature not exceeding 40°C.

Description

    Colour : Brilliant green or Bronze green
    Odour : Characteristic odour

Size : Length = 10-20 mm: Width = 3-6 mm.

Chemical Constituents **Cantharides** essentially contains an important **vesicating*** principle termed as **canthraridin,** which is nothing but the anhydride of cantharidic acid, located in the soft portions of beetles.

Besides, **cantharides** also contains resin, formic, acetic, uric acids and fat (12-15%)

Cantharidin

Substituents/Adulterants **Cantharides** beetles are mostly substituted by *Mylabris species,* the well known Chinese cantharis having a close resemblance to the former ones. Mylabris essentially comprises of the dried beetles of *Mylabris cichorii* or *Mylabris pustulata* abundantly found in China and India, and contains **cantharidin** ranging between 1 to 1.2%.

Uses

1. **Cantharidin** has proved to a hair growth stimulant and hence used in hair oil.
2. **Cantharides beetles**, in general, is a vesicant, rubefacient and counter irritant.

4.2.6 Cyanogenetic Glycosides

The **cyanogenetic glycosides** are named so because they yield either hydrocyanic acid upon hydrolysis or they essesntially possess a hydrocyanic acid in the aglycone moiety. They are also designated as **'cyanophore glycosides'**. Interestingly, about 110 families belonging to the plant kingdom have been reported to contain the **cyanogenetic glycosides**; however, *Rosaceae* being the most prominent one amongst them.

It is pertinent to mention here that **cyanogenetic glycoside** containing drug substances, as such do not exert any specific therapeutic activity, but they are invariably employed as viable pharmaceutical aids, such as: flavouring agents.

A large number of **cyanogenetic glycosides** were isolated and identified from various plant sources, namely: Linamarin, Linustatin, Lotaustralin and Lucumin as shown in Table 4.5.

A few important examples of naturally occurring drug substances containing **cyanogenetic glycosides** shall be discussed here, namely; Bitter almond, Wild cherry bark and Linseed. These drugs shall be discussed in the pages that follows:

4.2.6.1 Bitter Almond

Synonym Amygdala amara.

---

* **Vesicating** = Causing blisters.

Table 4.5   Cyanogenetic Glycosides and Biological Source

S.No	Name	Biological Sources	Chemical Structure
1.	**Linamarin** (Manihotoxine; Phaseolunatin)	Clover (*Trifolium repens;* Birds foot trefoil (*Lotus corniculatus*); and other legume pasture plant. *Acacia* spp. (*Leguminosae*); seedlings of flax (*Linum usitatissimum,* fam *Linaceae*);cassava (*Mahihot esculentum*) fam: *Euphorbiaceae*); *Passiflora* spp. (*Passifloraceae*) and several other families	
2.	**Linustatin**	Seed meal of flax (Linum *usitassimum,* fam: *Linaceae*); also present in certain *Passiflora* spp. (fam: *Passifloraceae*)	
3.	**Lotaustralin**	*Lotus corniculatus* Linn., *australis, Trifolium repens* and other legume herbs; *Haloragis ereta* (*Haloragidaceae*); *Linum usitatissimum*(*Linaceae*); Passiflora spp. (*Passifloraceae*) and certain *Trictum* spp. Including *T. monococcum* (*Graminaceae*)	
4.	**Locumin** (Lucuminoside; Prunasin xyloside)	Seeds of *Calocarpum sapota* (*Sapotaceae; (S)* – Epilucumin *i.e.*; the epimer is present in *Anthemis altisssima* (*Compositae*), alongwith two cyanogenic glycoside, *Anthemis* glycosides A and B	

Biological Source   **Bitter almond** comprises of the dried ripe kernels of *Prunus amygdalus* Batsch. *Var amara* (DC) Focke; *Prunus communis* Arcang., *P. amygdalus* Bail; and *Amygdalus communis* Linn., belonging to family *Rosaceae.*

Geographical Source   **Bitter almond** trees are mostly native of Persia and Asia Minor. They are also cultivated in the cooler parts of Panjab and Kashmir, Italy, Sicily, Portugal, Spain, Southern France and Morocco.

Description

   Colour : Brown

   Odour : No specific odour

   Taste : Bitter

Size	: Length = 1.5 to 2 cm; Breadth = 12.5 mm; Thickness = 8 mm
Shape	: Oblong, ellipsoidal, rounded at one end and pointed at the other.
Solubility	: Insoluble in ether, but soluble in water and boiling alcohol.

Preparation   The cyanogenetic glycoside **amygdalin** is usually obtained from either the cake of bitter almond or other prunaceous seeds after the expression of the fixed oil. The cake is subjected to extraction with ethanol (95%, v/v), and the resulting alcoholic extract is concentrated to a small volume preferably under vacuum and mixed with a large volume of ether, when the desired glycoside will separate out as a crystalline product.

Chemcial Constituent   **Bitter almond** contains a colourless crystalline cyanogenetic bitter glycoside commonly termed as **amygdalin** present to the extent of 1-3% as given below:

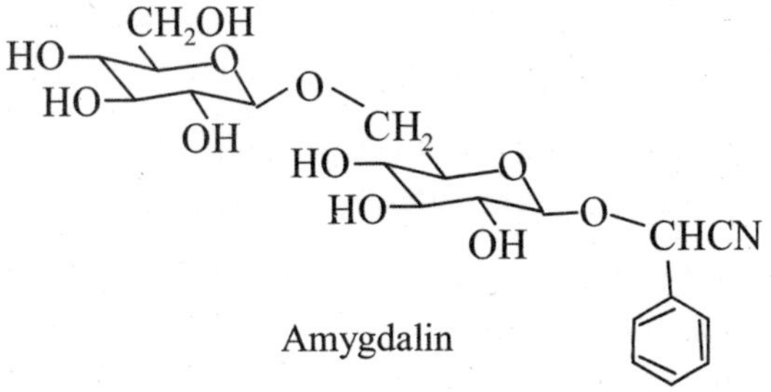

Amygdalin

   Amygdalin upon enzymatic hydrrolysis with **emulsin** gives rise to one mole each of benzaldehyde and hydrocyanic acid plus two moles of glucose as follows:

$$\underset{\text{Amygdalin}}{C_{20}H_{27}NO_{11}} + 2H_2O \xrightarrow[\text{(Hydrolysis)}]{\text{Emulsin}} \underset{\text{Benzaldehyde}}{C_6C_5\text{—CHO}} + \underset{\substack{\text{Hydro–}\\\text{Cyanic acid}}}{HCN} + \underset{\text{Glucose}}{2C_6H_{12}O_6}$$

   Besides, **bitter almond** contains fixed oil (40-50%), proteins (20%), volatile oil (0.5%) and an enzyme emulsin.

   The enzymatic hydrolysis of **amygdalin** takes place in the following *three* steps, namely:

(*a*) The enzyme **amygdalase** helps to cleave the glycoside amygdalin first into one mole each of glucose and **prunasin** (or mandelonitrile glucoside),

(*b*) The enzyme **prunase** helps to liberate the second molecule of glucose with the formation of the aglycone *mandelonitrile* (or benzaldehyde cyanohydrin), and

(*c*) The enzyme **hydroxynitrilase** helps to break down the mandelonitrile into one mole each of benzaldehyde and hydrocyanic acid.

All these *three* steps may be summarised as given below:

It is, however, assumed that the enzyme **emulsin,** isolated from the kernels of bitter almonds, comprises of several enzymes, such as: **amygdalase, prumase, hydroxynitrilase** etc.

Chemical Tests The general tests of the **cyanogenetic glycosides** by means of microchemical reactions in naturally occurring crude drugs are based on their hydrolysis to yield hydrocyanic acid. In fact, there are *four* speciifc and characteristic reactions to detect the presence of liberated HCN, namely:

1. **Ferriferrocyanide Test:** Macerate 1 g of the powdered drug with 5 ml of alcoholic KOH (5% w/v) for five minutes. Transfer it to an aqueous solution containing $FeSO_4$ (2.5 %w/v) and $FeCl_3$ (1% w/v), and maintain at 60-70°C for 10 minutes. Now, transfer the contents to HCl (20%) when the appearance of a distinct prussian blue colour confirms the presence of HCN.

2. **Precipitation of Hg from $HgNO_3$:** The reduction of aqueous mercurous nitrate solution (3% w/v) to metallic Hg by HCN being observed by an instant formation of black metallic Hg in the cells.

3. **Grignard Reaction Test:** First of all, dip a strip of white filter paper into a solution of picric acid (1 % w/v in water) drain and then dip into a solution of sodium carbonate (10% w/v in water) and drain. Now, place the crushed and moistened drug material in a small Erlenmeyer flask, and subsequently suspend the strip of the prepared sodium picrate paper above the material and stopper the flask with an air tight cork. Maintain the flask in a warm place for 1 hour when the liberated HCN would turn the sodium picrate paper from its original yellow colour to brick red colour due to the formation of sodium isopurpurate **(Grignard's Reaction).**

4. **Cuprocyanate Test:** First of all, saturate pieces of filter paper in a freshly prepared solution of guaic resin dissolved in absolute ethanol and allow them to dry completely in air. Now, carefully moisten a piece of the above paper with a very dilute solution of $CuSO_4$ and place it into contact with a freshly exposed surface of the drug. In case, HCN is generated, it will give rise to a distinct stain on the paper.

Uses

1. Bitter almonds are employed as sedative due to HCN content.
2. The fixed oil of bitter almond finds its use as demulscent in skin-lotion.
3. It is also employed in the preparation of amygdalin and bitter almond water.

Note

1. The misleading term *Vitamin B$_{17}$*, has sometimes been applied to **amygdalin**.
2. Bitter almond oil must not be used for flavouring of foods and confectionaries.

4.2.6.2 Wild Cherry Bark

Synonyms   Viginian Prune Bark; Wild Black Cherry Cortex; Pruni.

Biological Source   It is the dried bark of *Prunus serotina* , Ehrk, and *Prunus macrophylla* Sieb et Zucc, belonging to family *Rosaceae.*

Geographical Source   **Wild Cherry bark** is found to be indigenous to the Eastern States of USA and certain parts of Canada. However, in the United States it is found abudantly in Dakota, Florida, Missisipi, North Carolina and Virginia.

Preparation   It has been established that the **wild cherry bark** possesses the highest potency only during the autumn. Therefore, the bark is mostly collected during this period. As the inner layer of the bark contains a substantial amount of HCN, hence soonafter collection it is necessary to get rid of the inner layer of cork. Consequently, after the removal of cork as well as a portion of the cortex, the exposed surface of the bark exhibiting phloem more or less give rise to an uniform dark brown coloured product, which is commercially known as **Rossed Bark**. The resulting rossed bark is dried in the shade and stored carefully in a dry place for onward trasmission to several countries as a valued export material.

Description

Colour	:	Dark-brown colour
Odour	:	Mostly very faint; but when slightly moisten it has an odour resembling to that of benzaldehyde (bitter almond like)
Taste	:	Bitter and astringent
Size	:	Length = 10 cm; Width = 4 cm; Thickness = 3-4 mm
Shap	:	Mostly curved or chanelled
Fracture	:	Short and granular
Inner Surface	:	Reddish brown and longitudinally striated
Outer Surface	:	*'Rossed Bark'* - Rough with pale buff coloured lenticel scars; *'Unrossed Bark'*—Reddish brown to brownish black, smooth, glassy and exfoliating cork having prominent whitish lenticels.

Chemical Constituents   **Wild cherry bark** essentially contains a **cyanogenetic glycoside** termed as **prunasin** (or **mandelonitrile glucoside**) as shown below:

d-Prunasin

d-Prunasin undergoes hydrolysis in the presence of the enzyme *prunase*, usually present in the bark itself, to yield one mole each of bnzaldehyde, glucose and hydrocyanic acid.

Besides, the drug also contains *p*-coumaric acid, scopoletin *i.e.*, β-methylesculetin, benzoic acid and trimethyl gallic acid.

p-Coumaric Acid   Scopoletin   Benzoic Acid   Trimethyl Gallic Acid

Chemical Tests   The chemical tests are same as described under Section 4.2.6.1.

Uses
 1. The syrup of wild cherry is mostly employed as a flavoured vehicle in cough syrup.
 2. It is also used as a sedative expectorant.

4.2.6.3 Linseed

Synonym   Flax seed.

Biological Source   It consists of the dried fully ripe seeds of *Linum usitatissimum* Linn. belonging to family *Liliaceae.*

Geographical Sources   It is cultivated extensively as a source of fibres in Algeria, Egypt, Greece, Italy and Spain; as a source of oil in Afghanistan, India and Turkey; and in Russia (now CIS – countries) for both oil and fibre. It is also found in several temperate and tropical zones.

Preparation   **The cyanogenetic glycoside** *linamarin* is prepared from the defatted oil meal, seed-skins or embryos of flax by standard methods available for glycosides.

Description
    Colour : Reddish brown
    Odour : Characteristic odour
    Shape : Oval and strongly flattened
    Size : Length = 4-6 mm; Width = 2-3 mm.

Chemical Constituents The ripe seeds of linseed contain small quantitites of a **cyanogenetic glycosides** known as *linamarin* (or *phaseolunatin*) as given below:

Interestingly, **linamarin** evolved HCN with linseed meal only but not with emulsin. However, pure linamarin is a bitter needle like crystalline substance. It is freely soluble in water, cold alcohol, hot acetone, slightly in hot ethyl acetate, ether, benzene, chloroform and practically insoluble in petroleum ether.

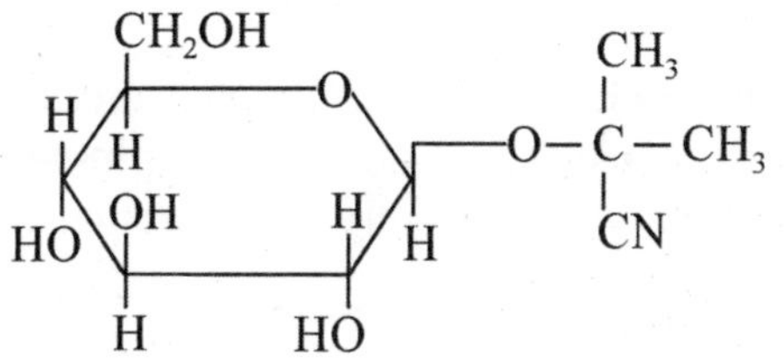

Linamarin

Besides, linseed seeds comprise of fixed oil (33-43%) mucilage present in testa (6%), proteins (25%) and an enzyme called *linase*.

Linamarin upon enzytmatic hydrolysis yields HCN which actualy renders the seeds highly poisonous.

Chemical Test The mucilage of linseed seed gives a distinct red colour on being treated with Ruthenium Red Solution.

Uses

1. Therapeutically, the linseed oil is mostly recommended for the external applications only; liiments and lotions.
2. It is employed in the treatment of scabies and other skin disease in combination with pure flowers of sulphur.
3. As the linseed oil has an inherent very high **'iodine value'** it is used mostly in the preparation of non staining **'Iodine Ointment'** and several other products such as: **'Cresol with Soap'.**
4. Commercially, it is one of the most important **'drying oil';** and, therefore, substantially huge amounts are exclusively used for varnishes and paints.
5. Linseed oil finds its extensive application in the manufacturer of soap, grease, polymer, plasticizer, polish and linoleum.

4.2.7 Thioglycosides

This speicific group of glycosides is also referred to as **'Thiocynate Glycosides'** or **'Sulphurated Glycosides'** or **'Glucosinolate Compounds'** or **Isothiocyanate Glycosides'** in various literatures. The aglycone portion of such glycoside essentially contains isothiocynate residue having sulphur plus nitrogen atoms. The general structure originally assigned to these aglycones (Formula A) has now been replaced by a more favourable one (Formula B).

In general, the **thioglycosides** are specifically abundant in several families, such as: *Cruciferae, Capparidaceae* and *Rosaceae*. More tham forty **thiocyanate glycosides**, having a variety of

$$R-N=C \begin{smallmatrix} \diagup O.SO_2.OX \\ \diagdown O.C_6H_{11}O_5 \end{smallmatrix}$$

(Formula-A)

$$R-C \begin{smallmatrix} \diagup N-O.SO_2.OX \\ \diagdown S.C_6H_{11}O_5 \end{smallmatrix}$$

(Formula-B)

configurations in the side chain, have been isolated and identified. In fact, most glycosides belonging to this category invariably comprise of a sulphuric acid residue which on hydrolysis gives rise to a potassium salt resepctively.

The *three* principal **thioglycosides** commonly known are as follows: **Sinigrin**—in **Black Mustards; Sinalbin**—in **White Mustards;** and **Gluconapin**—in rape seeds. These naturally occurring plant drugs shall be discused individually in the sections that follows.

4.2.7.1 *Black Mustard*

Synonym   Brown Mustard.

Biological Sources   These are dried ripe seeds of *Brassica nigra* Linn., Koch or *Brassica juncea* Linn, Czern & Coss, belonging to family *Cruciferae.*

Geographical Sources   *B. nigra* is extensively cultivated in various parts of Europe and United States. *B. juncea* is widely grown in different parts of India and the CIS-countries (*i.e.,* Russia).

Preparation   The **thioglycoside** *sinigrin* is obtained from the defatted black- mustard seed by employing standard methods. It is usually present in the seeds to the extent of 4%.

Black mustard seeds are powdered and defatted with petroleum ether. The defatted meal is boiled with ethanol to destroy the enzyme. The resulting marc is squeezed while hot, dried at 100°C and maceraed in cold water for 3-4 hours with constant stirring, since **sinigrin** is fairly soluble in cold water. The liquid content is decanted and maceration is repeated a number of times to ensure complete extraction of the **thioglycoside**. The combined aqueous extract is collected and treated with mild alkalies, such as : $BaCO_3$, so as to neutralize any free acidity. The liquid is now concentrated under vaccum to a syrupy consistency. The resulting syrup is boiled with ethanol (95% w/v) for about 2-3 hours to allow sinigrin to dissolve and at the same time to precipitate the mucilageous components. The alcholoic extracts are filtered and allowed to cool slowly when **sinigrin** crystallizes out (approximately 4%).

Description

Colour   : Black, dark brown or reddish brown
Odour   : Whole seed-none; Crushed seed-pungent characteristic odour.
Taste   : Bitter
Size   : Approx. 0.9-1.0 mm in diameter
Shape   : Mostly spherical in shape

Special Features   Seeds are normally covered with a brittle testa and the kernel is oily and greenish yellow in colour. The approx. weight of 100 seeds ranges between 150 to 170 mg.

Chemical Constituents   The **black mustard** seed contains a thioglycoside *i.e.,* a **β-glucopyranoside** termed as **sinigrin**. It is also known as myronate potassium or allyl glucosinolate as shown under:

Sinigrin

However, **sinigrin** undergoes complete hydrolysis in the presence of an enzyme *myrosin* to yield one mole each of allyl iso-thiocyanate, glucose and potassium hydrogen sulphate as given below:

$$C_{10}H_{16}KNO_9S_2 + H_2O \xrightarrow[\text{(Hydrolysis)}]{\text{Myrosin}} S=C=N-CH_2-CH=CH_2 + \quad C_6H_{12}O_6 + KHSO_4$$

| Sinigrin | Allyl iso-thiocyanate | Glucose | Pot.hydrogen Sulphate |

The **allyl iso-thiocyanate** *i.e.*, the volatile oil component of mustard is solely responsible for the characteristic pungent dour of musturd oils.

Besides, it contains fixed oil (30%), proteins (20%), and volatile oil (0.7-1.3%).

Chemical Tests

1. The powdered **black mustard** seeds on being treated with sodium hydroxide solution yields bright yellow colouration
2. Chromatographic Evaluation
   (*a*) Paper chromatography of the mustard oil in a solvent system consisting of butanol-acetic acid water; and subsequently spraying the chromatogram with 0.02 N silver nitrate solution, drying at 100°C and finally spraying with 0.02 N potassium dichromate produces yellow spots against a red background of silver chromate thereby confirming the presence of *sinigrin*.
   (*b*) The thiourea derivatives are used as reference compounds along with the mustard oil spots in paper chromatography using the solvent system consisting of water saturated chloroform or butanol-ethanol-water. The chromatogram is sparyed with *Grote's Reagent* (*i.e.*, a mixture of sodium nitroprusside, hydroxylamine and bromine) which distinctly yields blue spots with thiourea derivatives as well as *sinigrin*.

Uses

1. A paste of **black mustard** seed is mostly employed in the form of plaster or poultice as a rubefacient and counter irritant.
2. In higher doses, when administered internally, it acts as an emetic.
3. **Black mustard** seeds are invariably used as a widely accepted condiment in the preapration of pickles, curries and vegetables.
4. The fixed oil is widely employed as a popular edible oil.

4.2.7.2 White Mustard

Synonyms *Brassia alba* Hook f. & Th., *Sinapis alba* Linn.

Biological Source   These are the dried ripe seeds of *Brassia alba* H.f. & T., belonging to family *Cruciferae*.

Geographical Source   The plant is grown in India as a garden crop. It is a weed usually arising from cultivation in Panjab.

Preparation   The powdered **white mustard** seeds are defatted with a suitable solvent (*e.g.*, petroleum ether, n-hexane) and the dried marc is extracted with boiling ethanol (95% v/v). The thioglycoside is purified by dissolving in warm water, decolourised with activated charcoal, filtered and the resulting filtrate is crystallied out.

Chemical Constituents   The main constituent of **white mustard** is the **thioglycoside** known as **sinalbin** (or *sinapine glucosinalbate*) having the following structure:

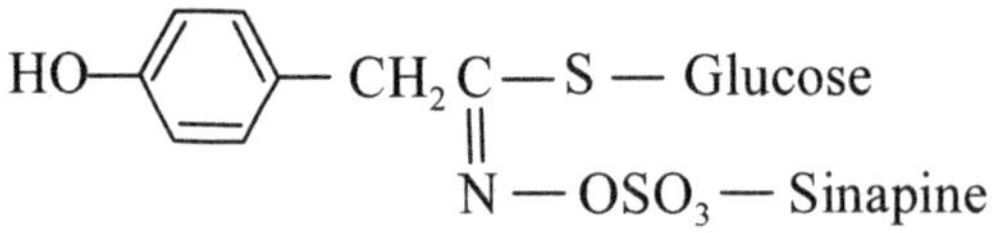

$$HO-\langle\bigcirc\rangle-CH_2\underset{\underset{N-OSO_3-\text{Sinapine}}{\parallel}}{C}-S-\text{Glucose}$$

Sinapine

The enzymatic hydrolysis of **sinalbin** by the enzyme *myrosin* gives rise to one mole each of glucose, acrinyl isothiocynate and sinapine acid sulphate as shown (see page 214).

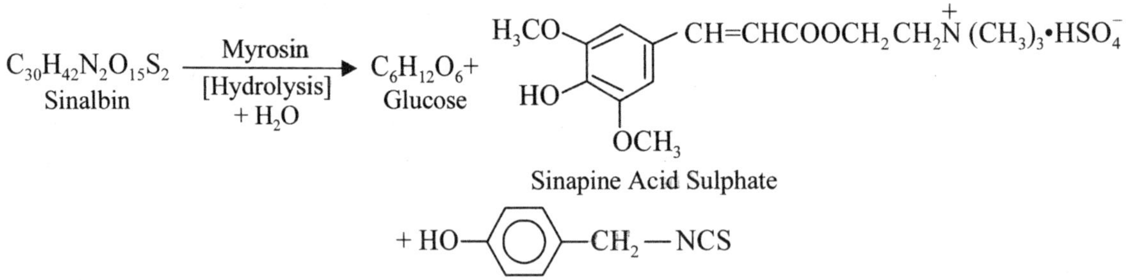

$$C_{30}H_{42}N_2O_{15}S_2 \xrightarrow[\substack{\text{[Hydrolysis]} \\ + H_2O}]{\text{Myrosin}} C_6H_{12}O_6 +$$

Sinalbin   Glucose

$$H_3CO-\langle\bigcirc\rangle-CH=CHCOOCH_2CH_2\overset{+}{N}(CH_3)_3\bullet HSO_4^-$$
$$HO-$$
$$\overset{|}{O}CH_3$$

Sinapine Acid Sulphate

$$+ HO-\langle\bigcirc\rangle-CH_2-NCS$$

Acrinyl Isothiocyanate
(*p*-Hydroxy Benzyl Isothiocyanate)

Chemical Tests
1. The hydrolysed product of sinalbin *e.g.*; sinapine acid sulphate and other salts are crystalline and give rise to a distinct bright yellow colouration in an alkaline medium .

Uses
The paste of **white mustard** seed is frequently employed in the form of a plaster or poultice as counter irritants and rubefacients.

4.2.8 Saponin Glycosides

In general a group of plant glycosides commonly referred to as **saponin glycosides**, usually share in different extents, the following *two* specific characteristics namely:

   (*a*) They produce foam in aqueous solution, and
   (*b*) They cause haemolysis of Red Blood Corpuscles (RBC).

The **saponin glycosides** are broadly regarded as haemotoxic in nature by virtue of the fact that they afford the haemolysis of erythrocytes, which render most of them as *'fish poisons'*. Invaribaly, they possess a bitter and acrid taste, besides causing irritation to mucous membranes. They are mostly amorphous in nature, soluble in alcohol and water, but insoluble in non-polar organic solvents like benzene, n-hexane etc.

Interestingly, the naturally occurring plant materials consisting of **saponin glycosides** have been extensively employed in various parts of the globe for their *exclusive detergent characteristics*, for instance: In South Africa the bark of *Quillaia saponaria* belonging to family *Rosaceae* and in Europe the root of *Saponaria officinalis* belonging to family *Caryophyllaceae*.

Sapogenins—The *aglycone* of the **saponin glycosides** are collectively known as *sapogenins*. *Sapotoxins*—the harmful and poisonous sapogenine/ saponins are aften referred to as *sapotoxins*.

Based on the nature of the **'aglycone'** residue present in the **saponin glycosides**, they are broadly classified into the following *two* categories, namely:

(*i*) Tetracyclic triterpenoid saponins (or Steroidal saponins), and

(*ii*) Pentacyclic triterpenoid saponins.

These *two* categories of **saponin glycosides** will be discussed with suitable examples from plant sources in the sections that follows:

4.2.8.1   Tetracyclic Triterpenoid Saponins (or Steroidal Saponins)

Due to the enormous pharmaceutical importance a plethora of plants have been screened thoroughly for the detection of **steroidal saponins**. They are not only confined to *monocot plants* but also extended to *dicot plants*, such as:

Monocot Plants : Family—*Amaryllidaceae, Dioscoreaceae* and *Liliaceae*

Dicot Plant   : Family—*Apocynaceae, Leguminosae and Solanceae*

However, from a commercial angle the steroidal saponins occupy a very important position in the therapeutic armamentarium which is evidenced by the following glaring examples, such as: used as raw material for the synthesis of a number of medicinally potent **steroids** *e.g.*, vitamin D, **sex hormones**—like testosterone, progesterone, oestradiol etc., **cardiac glycosides** *e.g.*, digoxin, digitoxin; **corticosteroids** *e.g.*, cortisone acetate, cortceosterone, aldosterone; **oral contraceptives** *e.g.*, mestranol, norethisterone; and **diuretic steroid** *e.g.*, spironolactone.

A few typical examples of naturally occurring medicinal plants containing **tetracyclic triterpenoid saponins** shall be described in the sections that follow, namely: dioscorea, solanum khasianum and shatvari.

4.2.8.1.1   Dioscorea

Synonyms   Rheumatism root; Yam.

Biological Source   It essentially comprises of the dried tubers of *Dioscorea delitoidea* Wall., *Dioscorea tokora* Makino, and *Dioscorea composita* and other species of *Dioscorea* belonging to the family *Dioscoreaceae*.

Geographiacal Source   *D. delitoidea* is grown in United States and Mexico. It is cultivated from Nepal to China at an altitude ranging from 3,000 to 10,000 feet. It is also found growing abundantly in North Western Himalayas from Kashmir to Panjab in India.

Preparation   Generally, the saponins do have high molecular weight and hence their isolation in the purest form poses some practical difficulties.

The tubers are washed, sliced and extracted with hot water or ethanol (95% v/v) for several hours. The resulting extract is filtered, concentrated under vacuo and the desired glycosides is precipitated with ether.

However, there are various ways and means to obtain the respective steroidal saponins from the aqueous/ alcoholic extracts as stated below:

For Acid Saponins   : Lead Acetate is employed to precipitate the steroidal saponins from aqueous extract.

For Neutral Saponin : Basic lead acetate is used to precipitate the neutral steroidal saponins from aqueus extract.

Nevertheless, a few saponins are also precipitated from their aqueous solutions either by the addition of $Ba(OH)_2$ solution or by the addition of $(NH_4)_2SO_4$ solution.

Note   The Barayata-Saponin Complex is sometimes employed for the estimation of Saponins.

Description

    Colour : Slightly brown

    Odour : Odourless

    Taste   : Bitter and acrid

    Size   : Varies dependig on the actual age of the rhizomes (tubers)

Chemical Constituents   The major active constituent of **dioscorea** is *diosgenin* usually present in the range of 4-6%. **Diosgenin** is the *aglycone* of saponoin **dioscin**

Diosgenin

Besides, the rhizomes contain starch to the extent of 75% but it has no edible utility because of its bitter taste. They also contain phenolic compounds and an enzyme *sapogenase*.

Uses

1. **Dioscorea** is mostly employed in the treatment of rheumatic arthritis.
2. **Dioscorea** has a tremendous potential as a commercial product because of its high content of diosgenin, which in turn is invariably employed as a starting material for the synthesis of a host of important therapeutic drugs, for instance: *sex-hormones, oral contraceptives* and several *corticosteroids*.

4.2.8.1.2   Solanum Khasianum

Biological Source   It consist of the dried and full grown berries of *Solanum khasianum* CR belonging to the family *Solanaceae*.

Geographical Source   The plant grows indigenously on the *Khasia Mountains* in Assam (India).

Preparation   The plant usually grows in various climatic and agricultural conditions. Almost after a duration of six months the plants are normally harvested for the collection of berries. They are dried immediately either in an artificial environment at low temperature (50-60°C) or dried preferably in shade so as to bring down the initial large moisture content to enable its prolonged storage life.

The dried berries are powdered by mechanical grinders and the oil is removed by solvent extraction. The defatted material (marc) is then extracted in a soxhlet assembly with ethanol (95% v/v) The resulting alcoholic extract is filtered, concentrated under vacuo, treated with HCl (12N) and refluxed for at least six hours. The alcoholic extract thus obtained is made alkaline by the addition of ammonia and the eontents are again refluxed for a duration of 1 hour. The contents of the flask is filtered and the residue is washed, dried and taken up in chloroform. The resulting mixture is fltered and the steroidal alkaloid solasodine is obtained as a solid residue soonafter evaporating the solvent.

Description   The berries have a yellowish to greenish colouration with flattened smooth brown seeds.

Chemcial Constituents   The berries mostly comprise of the steroidal saponin **Salosanine** as shown below:

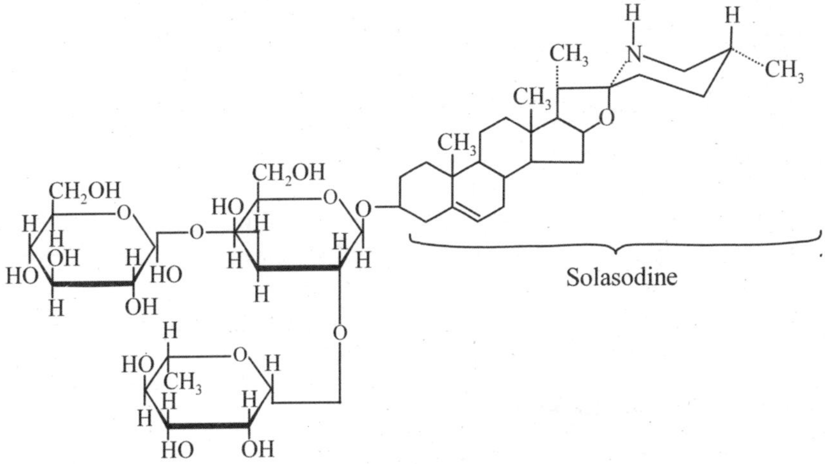

Solasonine

Solasonine also occurs in various *Solanum species* namely : *Solanum aviculare* Forst F., *Solanum sodomeum* L., *Solanum xanthocarpum* Schrad & Wendl, m *Solanum nigrum* Linn., *Solanum torvum* Sw.,￼ and *Solanum verbascifolium* Linn.

Besides, the berries contain a **steroidal glycoalkaloid** known as **solasodine** (Approx. 3%) and a greenish yellow fixed oil (8-10%).

Uses   **Solasodine** is the hydrolysed product of **solasonine** which is mostly used as a starting material for the synthesis of steroidal drugs, such as: **19-NOR steroids, pregnane** etc.

4.2.8.1.3   Shatavari

Synonyms   Shatamuli.

Biological Source   The **shatavari** mostly comprises of the dried roots and the leaves of the naturally occurring plant known as *Asparagus racemosus* Will, belonging to the family Liliaceae.

Geographical Source   It is widely distributed throughout the tropical regions of Africa, Australia, Asia and India. It is also found in the Himalayan range up to an altitude of 4000-4500 feet. It occurs as a wildely grown plant in the dry and deciduous forests of Maharshtra State in India.

Preparation   The roots usually occur in the form of a cluster or fascicle at the base of the stem. The leaves are mostly linear green and needlelike. The **steriodal spanonin** is extracted by the standard methods.

Chemical Constitutents   The **shatavari** contains *four* **steriodal saponins** usually designated as **shatavarin I-IV** present collectively to the extent of 0.2%; however, **shatavarin I** is the major glycoside present.

R=H:Sarsasapogenin
R=—GLU—GLU—GLU: Shatavarin-I
                      |
                   Rhamn
R=—GLU—GLU: Shatavarin-IV
              |
           Rhamn

Uses
1. The roots are employed mostly as galactogogue to promote the flow of milk.
2. The roots are used invariably as tonic and diuretic.
3. The **steroidal saponin Shatavari-I** is reported to exert antioxytocic activity.
4. The roots are extensively employed as a medicinal oil for the control and management of nervine disorders and rheumatism.
5. In the Ayurvedic System of Medicine it is widely used both in threatened abortion and safe delivery because of its distinct uterine blocking activity.

4.2.8.2   *Pentacyclic Triterpenoid Saponins*

This particular class of saponin essentially contains the sapogenin component with **pentacyclic triterpenoid** nueleus, that is eventually linked with either sugars or uronic acids. It is pertinent to mention here that the sapogenin may be further classified into *three* major categories namely: **α-Amyrin, β-Amyrin** and **Lupeol**.

α-Amyrin   β-Amyrin   Lupeol

Interestingly, the most important derivative of this specific class of saponins is the *triterpenoid acids* that are present in different drugs. The general structure of the tritenpenoid acid is given below and a few commonly found such acids are summarized herewith:

[
A Triterpenoid Acid
The–COOH moiety present
at C-4, C-17 and C-20
]

The typical examples of some naturally occurring plants containing the **pentacyclic triterpenoid saponins** shall be described in the sections that follow.

Triterpenoid Acids in Plants

S.No	Name (Source)	R'	R''
1.	**Gypsogenin; Githagenin; Albasapogenin;** (*Agrostemma, Githago* L., Scop.)	—CHO	—H
2.	**Hederagenin; Caulosapogenin;** Melanthigenin; (*Hedera helix* L.)	—CH$_2$OH	—H
3.	**Oleanolic acid; Oleanol;** Caryophyllene; (*Olea europaea*)	—CH$_3$	—H
4.	**Quillaic acid; Quillaja sapogenin;** (*Quillaia sapogenin Molina*)	—CHO	—OH

4.2.8.2.1 Ginseng

Synonyms   Panax; Energofit; Pannag; Ninjin.

Biological Source   **Ginseng** is the dried root of different naturally occurring species of Panax, namely: *Panax ginseng* C.A. Mey or *Aralia quinquefolia* Deene & Planch **(Korean Ginseng);** *Panax japonica* **(Japanese Ginseng);** *Panax notoginseng* **(Indian Ginseng)** belonging to family *Araliacea*e.

Geographical Source   The plant is found extensively in Korea, Russia and China, but off late it has been cultivated on a large commercial scale in Japan, Canada and United States.

Preparation   The plants are usually harvested 3 to 5 years after transplantation. It is usual practice to affect the actual harvesting between July to October.

White Ginseng   It is obtained by removing the outer layers of the roots. However, it has been established that the removal of outer layers may tantamount to serious loss of the active components.

Red Ginseng   It is obtained by first subjecting the roots to stearning and after that they are dried in an artificial environment between 50-60°C. The *two* types of roots sare subsequently graded and packed.

Description
   Colour   : Yellowish- brown,, white or red

Odour   : None
Shape   : Tuberous and corpulent
Appearance   : Translucent and bears the stem scars.

Chemicals Constitutents   **Ginseng** chiefly comprises of a complex mixture of **triterpenoid saponins** which may be either a **steroidal triterpene** or a pentacyclic related to oleonic acid. However, these glyscosides have been classified into *three* major heads, namely:

(*a*) Ginsenosides,

(*b*) Panaxosides, and

(*c*) Chikusetsu Saponins.

Ginsenoside Rg$_1$, is one of the major saponins that has been isolated and identified in ginseng, with a **steroidal triterpene aglycone** known as (20S)-**protopanaxatriol** as shown below:

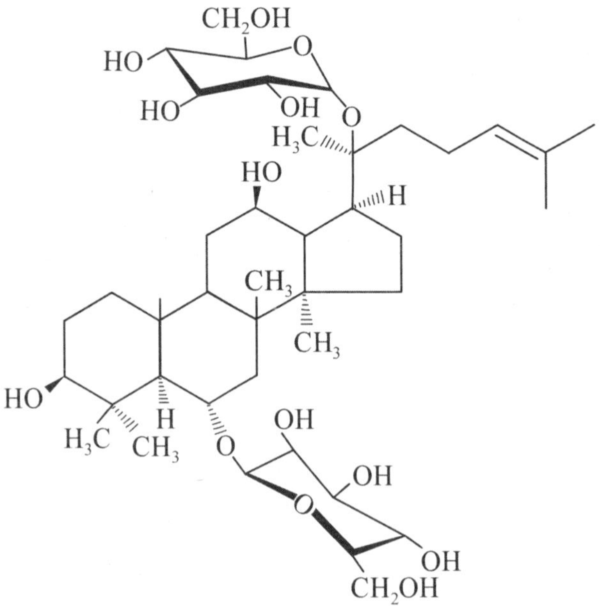

Ginsenoside Rg$_1$

In all, about 13 **ginsenosides** have been isolated and identified. Interestingly, **panaxasides** undergo decomposition yielding *oleanolic acid, panaxadipol* and *panaxatriol* as given below:

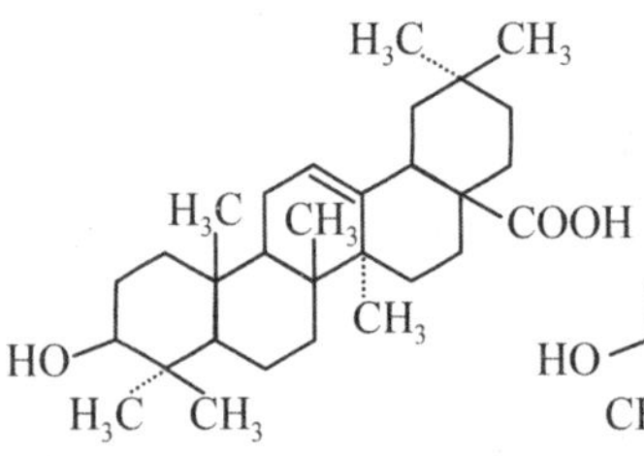

Oleanolic Acid 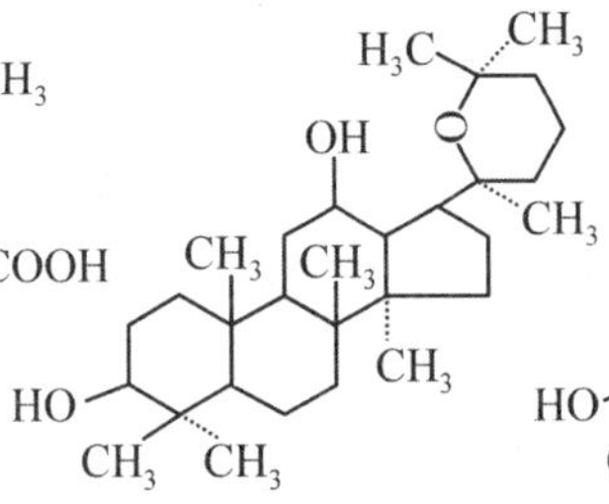   Panaxadiol 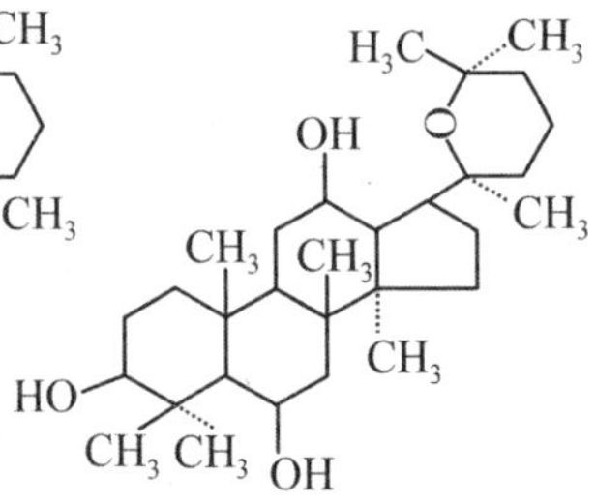   Panaxatriol

Uses

1. In the Chinese system of medicine ginseng is the most favourite remedy for a variety of ailments *e.g.*, as a general tonic, stimulant, carminative and diuretic activities.
2. It also possesses adaptogenic (antistress) properties and is found to exert positive action on the metabolism, the endocrine system and the central nervous system.
3. In the **orient ginseng** is used abundantly in the treatment of anaemia, diabetes, insomnia, gastritis, neurasthenia and specifically to cure sexual impotence.
4. It is found to enhance the natural resistance (*i.e.*, non-specific resistance) and increases the ability to overcome both exhaustion or illness to a great extent.
5. It prolongs the life of elderly persons and cures giddiness.

4.2.8.2.2   Liquorice

Synonyms   Glycyrrhiza; Liquorice root; Glycyrrhizae radix.

Biological Sources   Liquorice is the dried, peeled or unpeeled, roots, rhizome or stolon of *Glycyrrhiza glabra* Linn., invariably known in commerce as Spanish liquorice, or of *Glycyrrhiza glabra* Linne. var *Glandulifera* Waldstein et Kitaibel, mostly known in commerce as Russian liquorice, or of other varieties of *Glycyrrhiza glabra* Linne., which produce a sweet and yellow wood, belonging to family *Leguminosae.*

The word **Glycyrrhiza** has been derived from the Greek origin that means *sweet root*; and **glabra** means *smooth* and usually refers to the smooth, pod-like fruit of this particular species. Nevertheless, the fruits of the *glandulifera* variety has a distinct gland like swellings.

Geographical Sources   Liquorice is grown in the sub-Himalayan tracts and Baluchistan. It is cultivated on a large scale in Spain, Sicily and Yorkshire (England) *G. glabra* var *violaceae* is found in Iran; whereas *G. glabra* var *glandulifera* exclusively grows in Russia (the '*Russian Liquorice*').

The following are the *three* commonly grown varieties of *Glycyrrhiza glabra*, namely:

(*a*) *G. glabra* var. *violaceae* (or *Persian Liquorice*): This specific species bears violet flowers,

(*b*) *G. glabra* var *gladulifera* (or *Russian Liquorice*): It has a distinct big stock together with a number of elongated roots, but it has not got any stolon, and

(*c*) *G. glabra* var. *typica* (or *Spanish Liquorice*): This specific plant bears only purplish-blue coloured papilionaceous flowers. It possesses a large number of stolons.

Preparation   The roots are usually harvested after 3 to 4 years from its plantation when they mostly display enough growth. The rhizomes and roots are normally harvested in the month of October, particularly from all such plants that have not yet borne the fruits. thereby ascertaining maximum sweetness of the sap. The rootlets and buds are removed manually and the drug is washed with running water. The drug is first dried under the sun and subsequently under the shade till it loses almost 50% of its initial weight. The large thick roots of the Russian Liquorice are usually peeled before drying. It is an usual practice in Turkey, Spain and Israel to extract a substantial quantity of the drug with water, the resulting liquid is filtered and evaporated under vacuo and the concentrated extract is molded either into sticks or other suitable forms.

4.2.8.2.3 Senega

Synonyms   Senega snakeroot; Seneca snakeroot; Rattlesnake root; Radix senegae; Senega root.

Biological Source   **Senega** is the dried root and root stock of Polygala *senega* L., or *Polygala senega* var *latifolia* Torret Gray or *Polygala alba* Nutt. belonging to family *Polygalaceae.*

Geographical Source   The plant is grown in North America and Eastern Canada. Presently, the drug is chiefly sourced from the cultivated species in Japan. However, the species grown in North West United States is known as *Northern Senega*, whereas the one found in Canada, Minnesota and Mannitoba is called as *Western Senega*.

Preparation   The root is collected from the wild plants normally in summer. The stems are promptly cut off and the roots are sorted out, washed thoroughly and dried either in the shade or artificial environment between 50-60°C.

Description

Colour	:	Brownish grey
Odour	:	Characteristic odour of methyl salicylate
Taste	:	First sweet and then acrid taste
Size	:	Length = 5 to 20 cm; Diameter = 3 to 10 cm
Appearance	:	A large knotty crown with a long tapering root normally curved, twisted having two or more large branches
Fracture	:	Short in the bark and splintery in the wood.

Chemical Constituents   **Senega** essentially contains two **saponin glycosides** that are *triterpenoid in character*, namely: **senegin** (4%) and **polygallic acid** (5.5%).

Hydrolysis of **senegin** gives rise to one mole each of **senegenin, senegenic acid** and **presenegenin.** It has been established that **senega** contains certain other derived forms of **presenegenin** known as **Senegin II** as shown below:

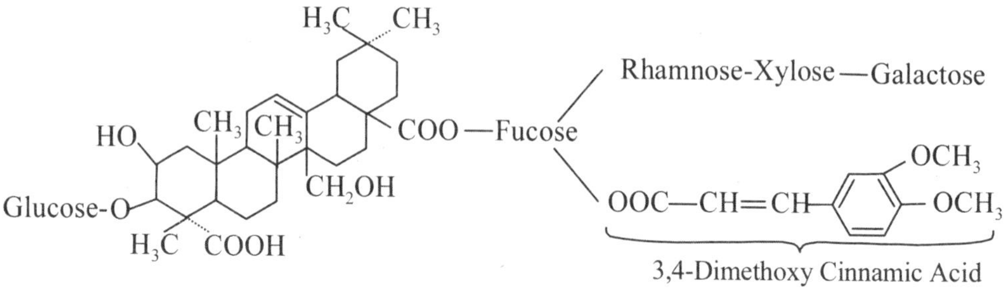

Senegenin-II

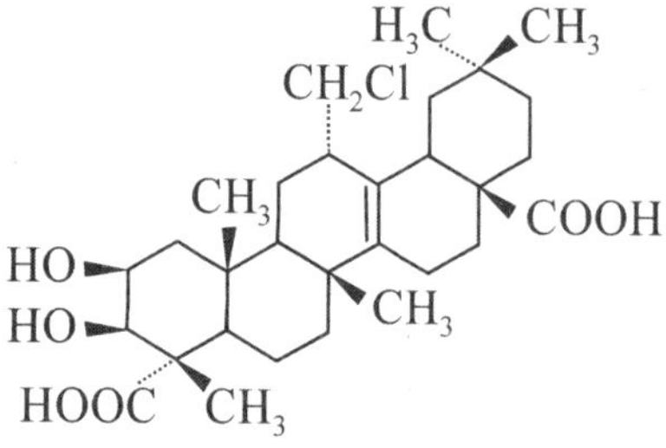

3,4-Dimethoxy Cinnamic Acid

Senegenin

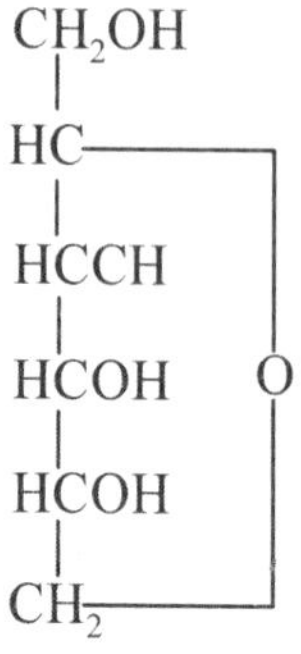

Polygalitol
[1,5-Anhydrosorbitol]

The sweet taste of the drug is owing to the presence of **1, 5-anhydrosorbitol** (or **polygalitol**). Besides, the **senega root** contains fixed oil, resin, sucrose, proteins, sterol and methyl salicylate (which is formed by the enzymatic hydrolysis of the glycosides called as **primveroside**).

Substituents and Adulterants   The roots obtained from *Polygala chinensis* Linn., grown almost throughout India at an altitude of 5000 feet is mostly used as an adulterant in **Senega root.**

Uses
1. The **senega root** is used extensively as an expectorant and in chronic bronchitis to relieve the spasms.
2. It is also employed as an emetic.

4.2.8.2.4   Bacopa

Synonyms   Herpestis; Brahmi.

Biological Sources   It comprises of the fresh stems and the fresh leaves of *Bacopa monnieri* Linn., Pennell or *Bacopa monnniera* Wettst., or *Herpestis monniera* Linn., H.B. & L., belonging to family *Serophulariaceae.*

Geographical Sources   The plant is grown extensively throughout the marshy places in India, Ceylon and Singapore. The plant is glabrous, succulent and creeping herb.

Preparation   The leaves along with stems are collected from the fully grown plant and are dried preferably in shade. The leaves are separated from the stems and packed separately in polybags.

Description
    Colour : Green
    Odour : None
    Taste : Bitter
    Size : Length = 1.2-1.8 cm; Breadth = 2.5-10 mm
    Shape : Leaves sessile, broad, entire, ovate-oblong or spathulate with black spots.

Chemical Constituents   The leaves contain **saponin glycosides** known as **bacoside A** and **bacoside B** which on acid hydrolysis give rise to **triterpenoid aglycone** termed as **bacogenin A** and **bacogenin B** respectively. It also contains **asiatic acid** and **brahmic acid** as depicted below:

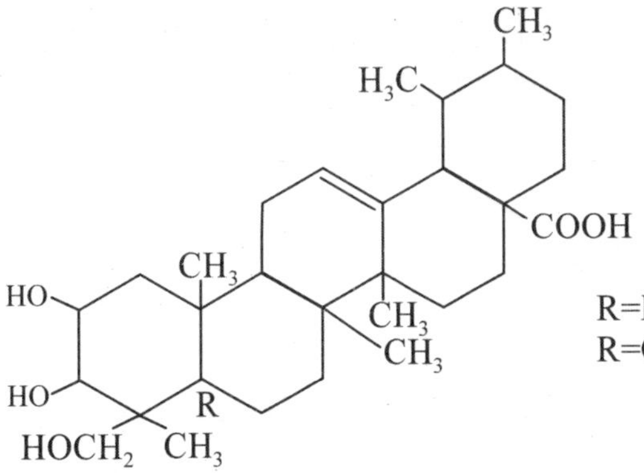

R=H; Asiatic Acid
R=OH; Brahmic Acid

Uses
1. It is used in the treatment of insanity and epilepsy

It also contains another glycoside known as **glucovanilline alcohol**, which upon hydrolysis yields **vanillic alcohol** and glucose. The vanillic alcohol on oxidation gives **vanillin.**

Uses

1. It is mostly used as a pharmaceutical aid for flavouring various liquid preparations.
2. Interestingly, the pleasant odour and flavour of **vanilla** are not only confined to **vanillin,** but more or less collectively on account of **vanillin** along with other fragrant chemical constituents.
3. **Vanillin** enhances the chocholate flcvour of cocoa based malted milk foods.

4.2.10   Bitter Glycosides

In general, bitters are the edible natural products mostly consumed before any normal meals to stimulate as well as enhance the appetite. However, the **bitter glycosides** as a class do possess almost similar activities like the bitters such as: digestive, stomachic and febrifuge.

Therapeutically, the bitters have been found to exert their stimulant effects on the gustatory (*i.e.*; related to the sense of taste) nerves located in the mouth and ultimately give rise to an improved gastric juice secretion in the stomach.

The **bitter glycosides** have been found not confined to the same chemical class, but the most important ones amongst them essentially possess the *pyran cyclopentane ring*.

A number of **bitter glycosides** isolated from natural plants have been put into actual therapeutic practice, namely: **Picrorhiza, Gentian,** and **Chirata,** which shall be discussed in the sections that follow.

4.2.10.1   Picrorhiza

Synonyms   Indian Gentian; Katki.

Biological Source   It is the dried rhizome of *Picrorhiza kurroa* Royle ex Benth., belonging to family *Serophulariaceae.*

Geographical Sources   It is a perennial herb grown abundantly and distributed on the Alpine Himalayas extended from Kashmir to Sikkim at an altitude between 3000 to 5000 meters. It is also found in China.

Preparation   The plant is either propogated by seeds or by rhizomes. The rhizomes are collected from the cultivated and naturally growing plants washed dried and packed.

Description

Colour	:	*Externally*—Dark Greyish brown
		Internally—White blackish
Odour	:	Slight and unpleasant
Taste	:	Bitter
Size	:	Length = 3-5 cm; Diameter = 0.5-1 cm
Shape	:	Mostly cylindrical small fragments having longitudinal wrinkled and annulations at the tip.
Special Features	:	The stems and conical buds along with the drugs usually form a part of the drug itself. The roots are invaribaly wrinkled in the longitudinal fashion having transverse cracks. They are greyish to brown in appearance, while the fracture is tough.

Chemical Constituents The therapeutically potent constituents of the drug essentially comprises of *three* vital **bitter glycosides,** namely: **Picroside I, Picroside II** *and* **Kutkoside** as given below:

S.No	Glycoside	R_1	R_2	R_3
1.	Picroside I	H	H	*Trans*-Cinnamoyl
2.	Picroside II	Vanilloyl	H	H
3.	Kutkoside	H	Vanilloyl	H

In fact, chemically both **Picroside** and **Kutkoside** are **C-9 monoterpene iridoid glycosides** having an epoxy moiety present in the cyclopentane ring.

Besides, it also contains organic acids, resin, sugar and tannins.

Uses
1. It is mostly employed as a vital bitter tonic
2. It is also used as a stomachic and febrifuge.
3. In large doses it exerts its action as a laxative
4. It also finds its usefulness in the treatment of jaundice.
5. Its alcohlic extract exhibits remarkable antibacterial effect.

4.2.10.2 Gentian

Synonyms Yellow Gentian; Pale Genetian; Bitter Root; Gentian Root; Radix; Radix Gentianae; Gentiana.

Biological Source Gentian is the dried rhizomes and roots of *Gentiana lutea* L., belonging to family *Gentianaceae.*

Geographical Source It is perennial herbaceous tree which is found to be native to the hilly zones in Central and Southern Europe. It is also grown on Vosges mountains, Yugoslavia (now known as Serbia and Crotia) and Jura.

Preparation The long rhizomes and fully grown fleshly roots of 2 to 5 year aged plants are dug up carefully and collected preferably in autumn. The roots and rhizomes are washed thoroughly to get rid of the adhered soil and then sliced into a longitudianal fashion. The freshly sliced pieces of roots and rhizomes generally appear white in colour and do not have any odour. However, during the process of gradual drying in small heaps at a controlled temperature of 50-60°C fermentation commences which eventually turns them into dark or yellow coloured product that have a characteristc odour.

4.2.11 **Miscellaneous Glycosides**

There are a number of glycosides which do not fall into the various classifications discussed under Sections 4.2.1 to 4.2.10 ; therefore, they have been grouped together under the present head *i.e.*, **'Miscellaneous Glycosides'** A few imortant members of this group shall be described here briefly.

4.2.11.1 *Steroidal Alkaloidal Glycosides*

They are sepecifically abundant in *two* families, namely: *Liliaceae* and *Solanaceae*. Just like saponins, the **steroidal alkaloidal glycosides** do possess significant haemolytic activities, such as:

S.No.	Name	Biological Source (Family)	Steroidal Alkaloidal Glycosides	Uses
1.	**Bitter Sweet**	*Solanum dulcamara* Linn., (Solanaceae)	Solanidine	Skin disease, psoriasis
2.	**Tomato**	*Solanum lycopersicum* Linn., (Solanaceae)	Rubijervine	Antifungal
3.	**Potato or White Flower Potato**	*Solanum tuberosum* Linn., (Solanaceae)	Solanine	—

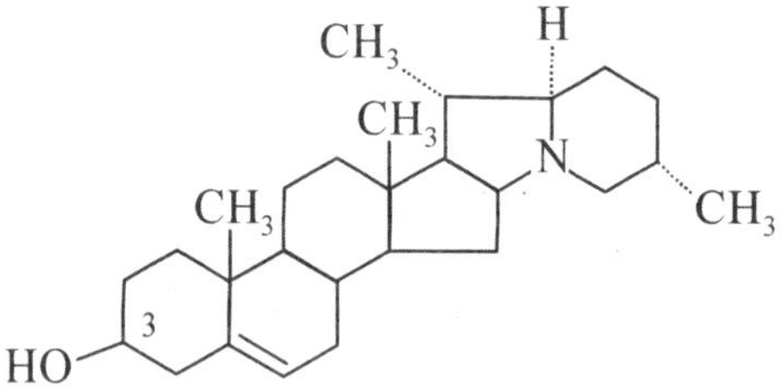

Solanidine

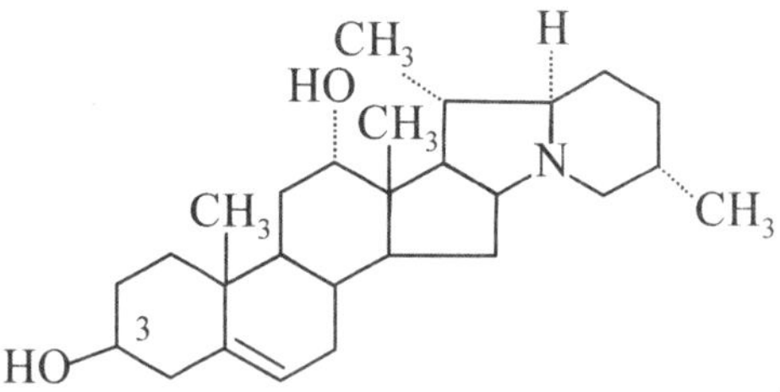

Rubijervine

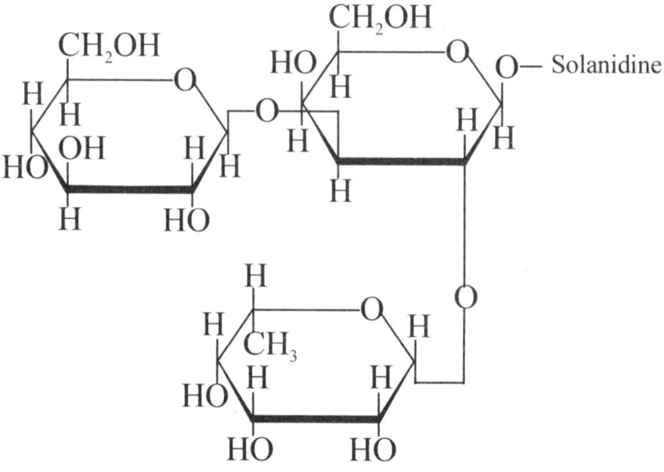

Solanine

The sugar components are usually attached at C-3 in **solanidine** and **rubijervine** which may be galactose, glucose, rhamnose or xylose and their quantity may vary from one to four.

4.2.11.2 Antibiotic Glycosides

Streptomycin is the glaring example of an **antibiotic glycosides** produced by the soil Actinomycete, *Streptomyces griseus* (Krainsky) Waksman et Henrici belonging to family *Actinomycetaceae*. It is usually formed by the combination of the genin **Streptidine** a nitrogen containing cyclohexane derivative and **Stretobiosamine** a disaccharide representing two-thirds of the streptomycin molecule, through a glycosidic linkage as shown below:

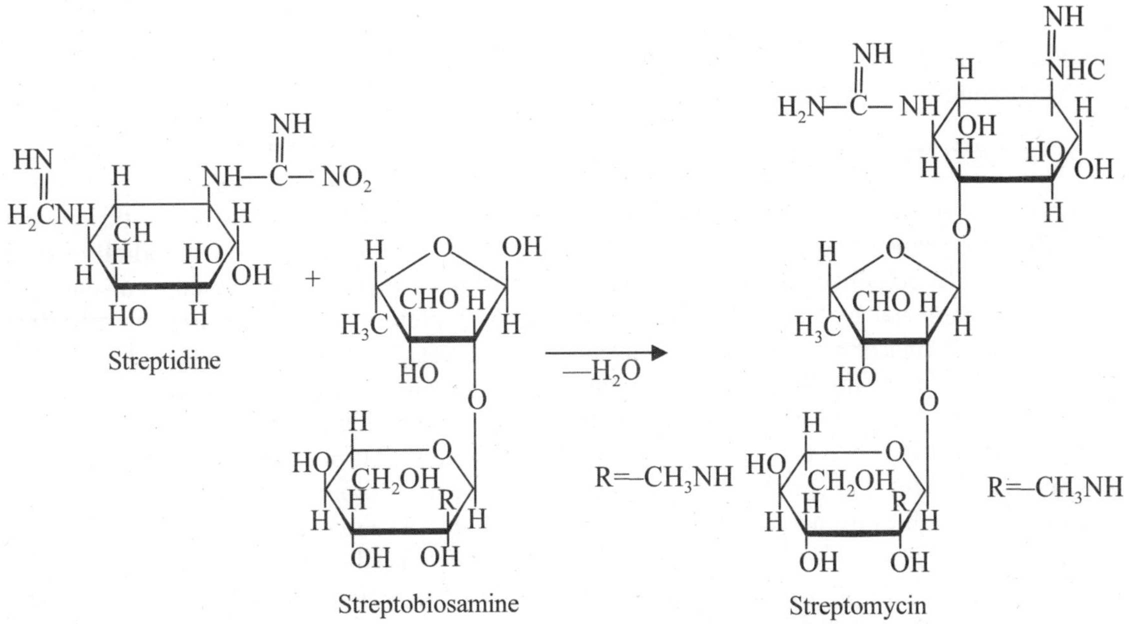

Streptidine + Streptobiosamine → Streptomycin

4.2.11.3 Glycosidal Resins

The *Jalap* and *Scammony* are the two well known examples of the **glycosidal resins** occurring in the natural products, namely: *Jalap*—from the dried tuberous root of *Exogonium purga* (Hayne) Lindl. (*E. jalap* Baill., *Ipomea purga* Hayne), belonging to family *Convolvulaceae; Scammony*—from the dried roots of *Convulvulus scammonia* L., belonging to family *Convolvulaceae*. The glycosidal nature of these resins are evidenced by the presence of sugars, such as glucose, rhamnose and fucose on hydrolysis.

4.2.11.4 Nucleosides (Nucleic Acids)

These naturally occurring substances are of prime biological importance and essentially possess *three* vital components namely: *first,* a **sugar moiety** *e.g.; ribose or 2-desoxyribose; secondly,* a **purine or pyrimidine base** *e.g.; adenine, guanine* and *cytosine; and thirdly, a phosphoric acid.*

A **base-sugar unit** is known as a **nucleoside**, whereas a **base-sugar phosphoric acid unit** is known as **nucleotide**.

An example of a **nucleotide** and a **nucleoside** is given here under:

Nucleotide

Nucleotide : An odenylic acid unit of RNA
Nucleoside : Adenosine with the adenine as the heterocyclic base.

4.3 BIOSYNTHESIS OF GLYCOSIDES

Generally, the naturally occurring living plant could be regarded as the most sophisticated and meticulously designed biosynthetic laboratory not only confined to the **primary metabolites** such as: Amino acids, carbohydrates, terpenes, fatty acids which are mostly consumed as a source of edible food material by human beings, but also for a plethora of **secondary metabolites** of enormous pharmaceutical significance, for instance: glycosides, flavonoids, alkaloids, essential oils and the like. Interestingly, such naturally found chemical substances which specifically attribute plant drugs their marked and pronounced therapeutic activities are collectively termed as 'phytopharmaceuticals'. Therefore, a higher plant is nothing but an intricate **solar energised biochemical reactor** that is exclusively responsible for the mass production of primary as well as secondary metabolites from air, water, minerals and sunlight - a source of UV radiations.

However, the *primary metabolites* are more or less widely distributed in nature practically in all organisms that are essentially required for the overall growth as well as physiological development by virtue of their basic cell metabolism. Nevertheless, the **secondary metabolites** are biosynthetically engineered products solely derived from the primary ones and are confined in their distribution strategically ie; being restricted to a particular taxononic group. These products may be regarded either as various chemical adaptations to environmental stresses or they may be considered as nature's protective, defensive or offensive chemical entities against the host of microorganism, fungi, insects and higher herbivorous predators.

Thus, with regard to cellular economic cognizance the secondary products are mostly tedious to form and subsequently accumulate, and hence, invariably show up in the plant kingdom in relatively much lesser amounts in comparison to the **primary metabolites**. The **secondary metabolites** are also regarded to be as the waste products of the plant metabolic processes.

The different biosynthetic reactions taking place in the plant cells are based on certain enzymes. In fact, it is the control of enzymatic activity on the plant metabolism which ultimately governs a specific biosynthetic pathway. In general, the enzymatic reactionbs in plants ae reversible. Under the influence of specific enzymes the **secondary metabolites** are either synthesized or hydrolysed in plants.

The biosynthetic pathways in plants may be duly elucidated and extensively studied by the aid of isotopically labelled precursors. Nowadays, with the advent of 'tracer technology', it is a lot easier to introduce isotopes into the anticipated precursors of plant metabolites and employed as specific **'markers'** in the elaborated biogenetic experiments. It is now quite possible to unfold the mysteries of biosynthetic pathways with the use of radioactive carbon (^{14}C), hydrogen (^{3}H), sulphur (^{35}S) and phosphorus (^{32}P).

The biosynthesis of different categories of glycosides shall be discussed briefly in the sections that follow.

<h3>4.3.1   Biosynthesis of Anthracene Glycosides</h3>

The **biosynthesis of anthracene glycosides** may be considered under the following *two* heads, namely:

(*a*) *Emodin and Other Related Derivatives:*The indepth knowledge with regard to the biosynthesis of **anthracene aglycones** has been duly established from an elaborated study with microorganisms, specifically *Penicillium islandicum* as shown below:

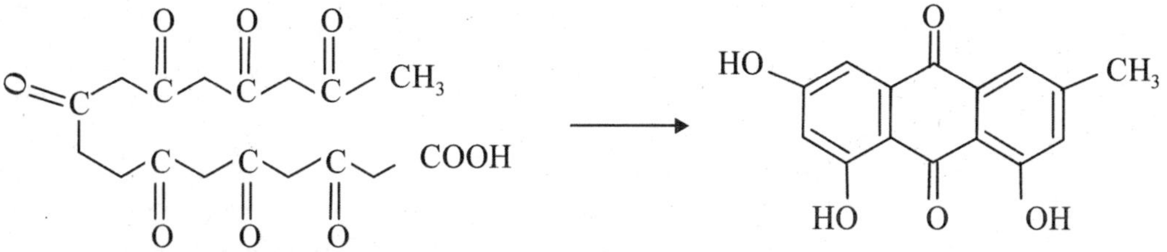

Poly—β-Ketomethylene Acid
[An intemediate with
8-Acetate Units]

Emodin & other Related
Derivatives

In this particular instance, an intermediate **poly β-ketomethylene acid** is assumed to have formed from 8 acetate units which on being subjected to intramolecular condensation gives rise to **anthraquinones** *i.e.*; **emodin** and other related derivatives.

(*b*) *Alizarin:* Another metabolic pathway for the formation of **anthraquinone** is established and recognised through the **shikimic acid—mevalonic acid mediators** as could be seen functional in certain plants belonging to the family *Rubiaceae* as given below:

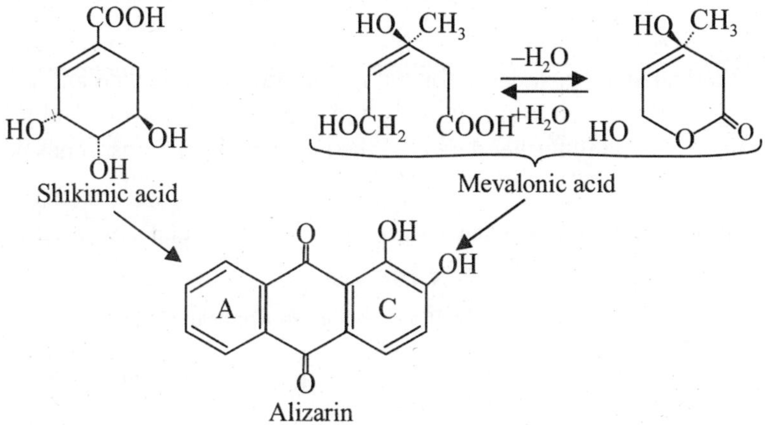

Shikimic acid

Mevalonic acid

Alizarin

The **biosynthesis of alizarin** reveals that the *ring A* in alizarin molecule has been derived from the **shikimic acid**, whereas the *ring C* in alizarin has been incorporated by the **mevalonic acid** component.

4.3.2   Biosynthesis of Phenol Glycosides

The **biosynthesis of Phenol Glycosides** *arbutin* takes place from the shikimic acid *via* phenylalanine (an amino acid)—cinnamic acid—hydroquinone and finally to the desired glycoside as indicated below:

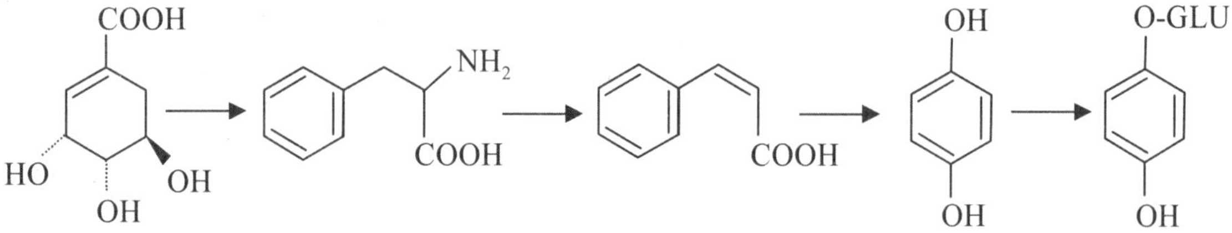

| Shikimic Acid | Phenylalanine | Cinnamic Acid | Hydroquinone | Arbutin |

4.3.3   Biosynthesis of Steroid Glycosides

Biotransformation of **steroids and cardiac glycosides** (*e.g.*, **gitoxin, digitoxin**) by plant cell cultures have been studied extensively and have been reviewed by Reinhard* (1974), Stohs and Rosenberg** (1975), Stohs*** (1977), and Furuya**** (1978).

However, in general the **steroidal aglycones** of **cardioactive glycosides** may be assumed to have formed as a broad based overall mechanism of **steroid biogenesis** as shown below:

Acetate $\longrightarrow$ Mevalonate $\longrightarrow$ Isopentenyl $\longrightarrow$ Squalene $\longrightarrow$ Steroid
                                             Pyrophosphate

The steroidal molecule is considered to have generated with the head to tail linkage of several acetate units.

4.3.4   Biosynthesis of Flavonoid Glycosides

Recently, both extensive and intensive research at the enzymatic level has more or less confirmed the original hypothetical steps postulated for the incorporation of acetate and phenylalanine into flavonoids. In fact, studies related to enzymology and regulation of flavone and flavonol glycoside biosynthesis has unfolded many further details of the individual reactions. It has been reported that

---

    * Reinhard, E., **In Tissue Culture and Plant Science**—1974, (H.E. Street Ed.), Academic Press, New York, pp. 433-459, 1974.

   ** Stohs S.J., and H. Rosenburg., *Lloydia*, 38, 181-194, 1975.

  *** Stohs, S.J., 'In plant **Tissue Culture and its Biotechnological Applications**', (W. Barz, E. Reinhard and M.H. Zenk, eds), Springer-Verlag, New York, pp. 142-150, 1977.

**** Fuarya, T., In **'Frontiers of Plant Tissue Culture'**, (T.a. Thorpe-ed.) The Boostore, University of Calgary, Alberta, Canada, pp. 191-200, 1978.

more than 20 different **flavonoid glycosides** occurrig in irradiated parsley cells are based on only three **flavone** and three **flavonol** aglycones all of which have essentially very similar substitution modes (Kreuzaler and Hahlbrock*, 1973). The chemcial structures of the aglycones and their probable reactions are as shown here under.

It may be observed that except for the characteristic C-3 hydroxyl moiety of **flavonols** the six aglycones essentially differ only with respect to substitution at C-3' position.

Another school of thought suggests that the flavonoid glycoside aglycones may be obtained from the major pathways ultimately leading to the synthesis of aromatic compounds in the biological systems, namely:

(*a*) Acetate Pathway, and

(*b*) Shikimic Acid Pathway

It has been observed that one 6-carbon fragment of the C_6-C_3-C_6 compounds derived from the **acetate pathways** gets combined with the remaining 9 carbon fragment ontained from the **shikimic (phenyl propanoid) pathway** as stated below:

Explanation

1. The C_6–C_3 segment, perhaps in the oxidation form of a cinnamic acid molecule, gets combined with three molecules of acetate to yield first a C_{15} **chalcone** moiety an intermediate and subsequently the **flavanone** residue.

2. The simultaneous introduction of removal of OH moieties from the aromatic rings B and A gives rise to the production of a good number of derivatives,

3. Flavonoids are first formaed by the introduction of the hydroxy group at position 3, whereas dehydrogenation at positions 2 and 3 results in the formation of flavonols, and

4. Evidently, the simultaneous occurance of a variety of glycosides having the same aglycone in a specific plant species strongly supports the well established hypothesis that **glycosylation** usually takes place at a late stage of **flavonoid biosynthesis**.

4.3.5   Biosynthesis of Coumarin and Furanocoumarin Glycosides

It has been established experimentally that by using grafts of *Melilotus alba* on *Trigonella foenum graecum*, practically no **coumarin** is formed in the shoots of *M. alba*; therefore, it may be inferred that the roots are absolutely essential for coumarin synthesis, perhaps since they provided an important precursor (Reppel and Wagenbreth, 1958)**. However, more recently it has been shown with the aid of reciprocal grafting experiments involving parsnip (*Pastinacia sativa*) that **furanocoumarins** in this species are usually generated in the fruits where they accumulate, and of course, no evidence for translocation could be observed (Beyrish, 1967)***.

There are two experimentally demonstrated pathways whereby natural products incorporating the bezopyran nucleus are usually formed, namely:

---

* Kreuzaler, F., and K., Hahlbrock, *Phytochemistry,* **12,** 1149-1152, 1973.
** Reppel L., and D. Wagenbreth, *Flora* (Jena), **146,** 212-227, 1958.
*** Beyrish, T., *Planta Med.* **15,** 306-310, 1967.

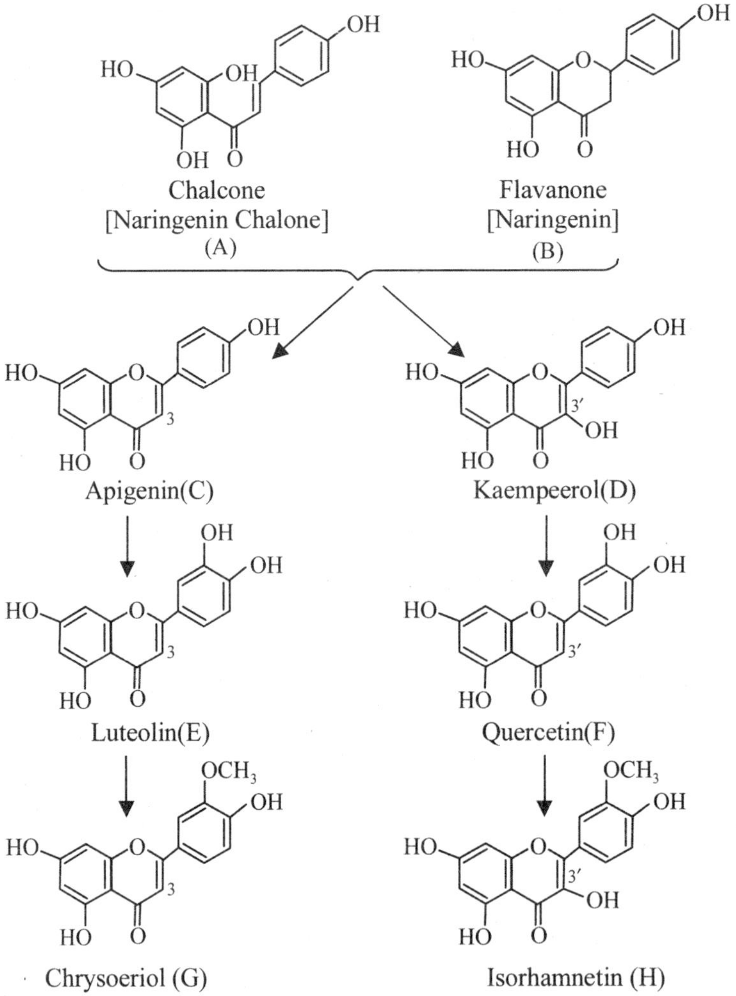

Chalcone
[Naringenin Chalone]
(A)

Flavanone
[Naringenin]
(B)

Apigenin(C)

Kaempeerol(D)

Luteolin(E)

Quercetin(F)

Chrysoeriol (G)

Isorhamnetin (H)

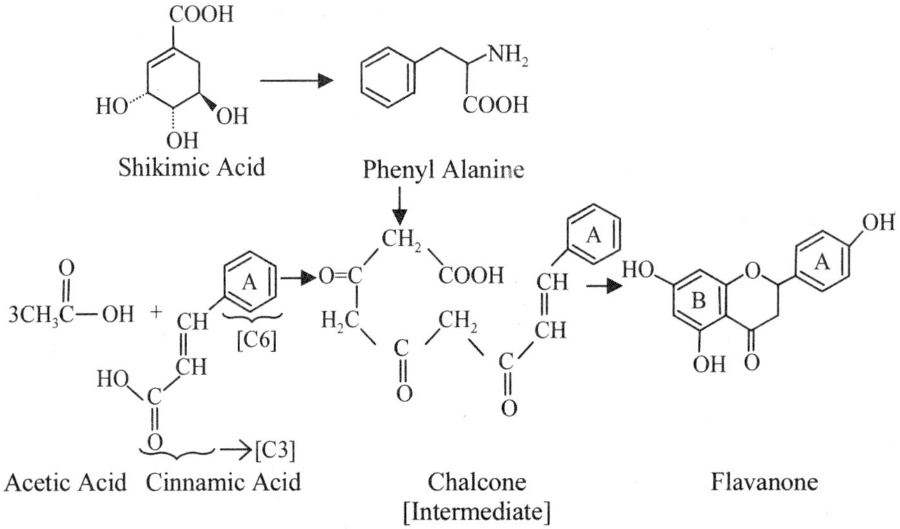

Shikimic Acid

Phenyl Alanine

$3CH_3C-OH$ + Acetic Acid   Cinnamic Acid

[C6]

[C3]

Chalcone
[Intermediate]

Flavanone

(a) In 3- and 4-phenylcoumarins, the aromatic components of this nucleus is derived from polyketide, wherein the 3 aliphatic carbon atoms and the phenyl substitute is found to originate from shikimic acid *via* a **phenylpropanoid** intermediate, and

(b) The coumarin originates *via* the shikimate-chorismate pathway leading to **phenylpyruvic acid**, from which arise L-phenylalanine by transmination and *trans*-cinnamic acid in turn by the action of phenylalanine ammonia lyase. Generally, two types of **furanocoumarins** are recognised, namely: *Linear furanocoumarin* and *Angular furanocoumarin* as shown below:

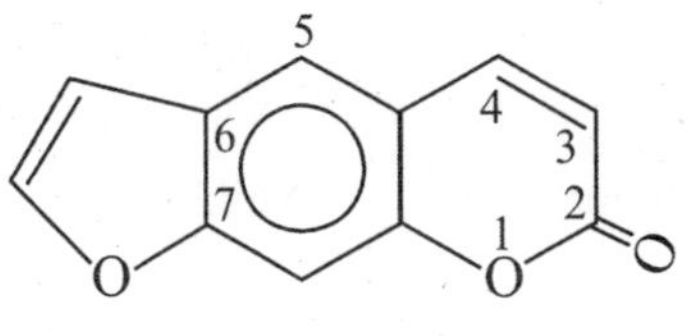

Linear
Furanocoumarin
(A)

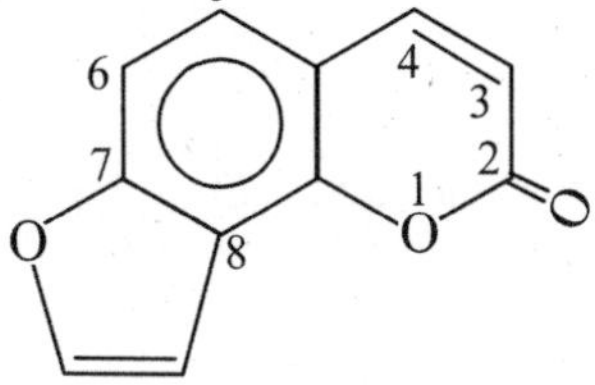

Angular
Furanocoumarin
(B)

In (A), the furan ring is fused at C-6 & C-7 positions of the benzopyran nucleus (eg., *psoralens)*, whereas in (B) the fusion is between C-7 and C-8. However, the latter is less widely distributed than the former.

4.3.6 Biosynthesis of Cyanogenetic Glycosides

Cyanogenesis is the ability of living organisms that exist freely in the higher plants but instead it is released from the **cyanogenetic precursors** as a result of the enzymatic action. Now, it has been well established that these precursors are normally glycosides of **hydroxynitriles** (or **cyanohydrins**). Once the cellular integrity of a cyanophoric plant tissue is disrupted, the **cyanogenetic glycosides** in turn are brought in contact with the respective catabolic enzymes that helps to hydrolyze the glycosides and ultimately give rise to the formation of hydroxynitriles.

There are two important **cyanogenetic glycosides**, namely: **dhurrin** nad **prunasin** which are present in a variety of plant families and genera as stated below*:

S.No.	Glycoside	Family	Genera
1.	**Dhurrin**	*Gramineae*	Sorghum spp.
		Proteaceae	Macadamia, Stenocarpus
		Trochodendraceae	Trochodendron
2.	**Prunasin**	*Caprifoliaceae*	Sambucus
		Compositae	Achillea,Centaurea, Chaptalia
		Leguminosae	Acacia Spp. (Australia), Holocalys
		Myoporaceae	Eremoophila
		Myrtaceae	Eucalyptus
		Oliniaceae	Olinia
		Polypodiaceae	Cystopteris, Pteridium
		Rosaceae	Cotoneaster Spp. Cydonia
		Saxifragaceae	Jamesia
		Scrophulariaceae	Linarria Spp.

* Seigler, D.S., *Prog, Phytochem.,* **4**, 83-120, 1977.
Seigler, D.S., *Rev Latinoam Quim*, **12**, 39-48, 1981.

The two amino acids *Tyrosine* and *Phenylalanine* are considered to have derived from the **Shikimic Acid Pathway** and **Phenylalanine Pathway** as depicted below:

(*a*) **Shikimic acid Pathway:** It is based on studies carried out with *E. coli* as follows:

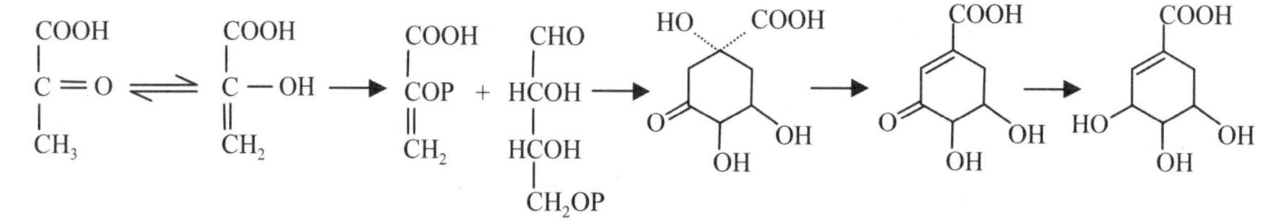

| Pyruvic Acid (*Keto*-form) | Pyruvic Acid (*enol*-form) | Phospho-enolpyruvic acid | Erythrose-4-P., | 5-Dehydro-quinic Acid | 5-Dehydro-Shikimic Acid | Shikimic Acid |

(*b*) **Phenylalamine Pathway:** It starts with **Shikimic acid** as the starting material as shown under:

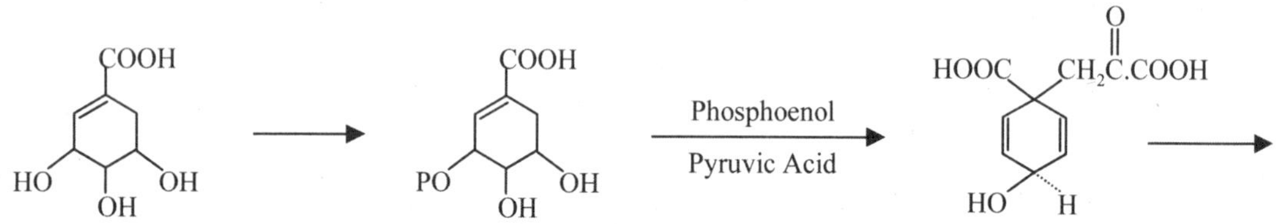

Shikimic Acid   5-Phospho-shikimic Acid   Prephenic Acid

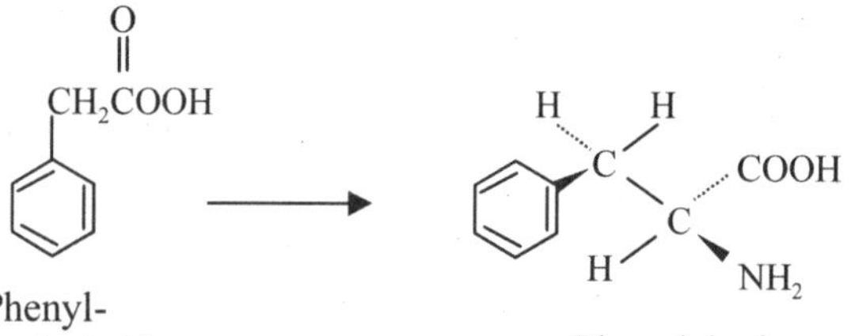

Phenyl-Pyruvic Acid   Phenylalanine

(*c*) **Tyrosine from Phenylalanine:** It is obtained by the oxidation of phenylalanine.

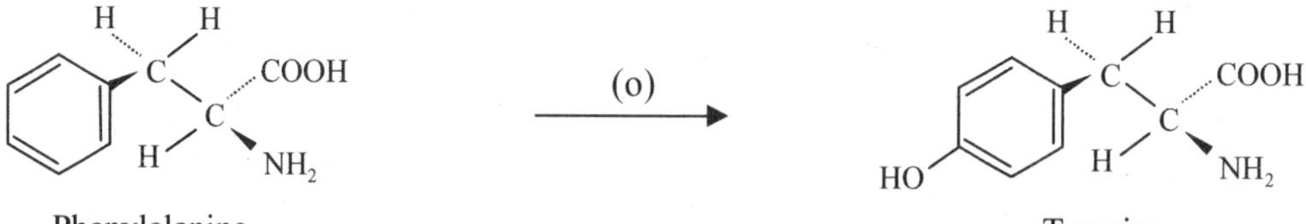

Phenylalanine   Tyrosine

(*d*) **Dhurrin from Tyrosine:** It is obtained from tyrosine as shown below:

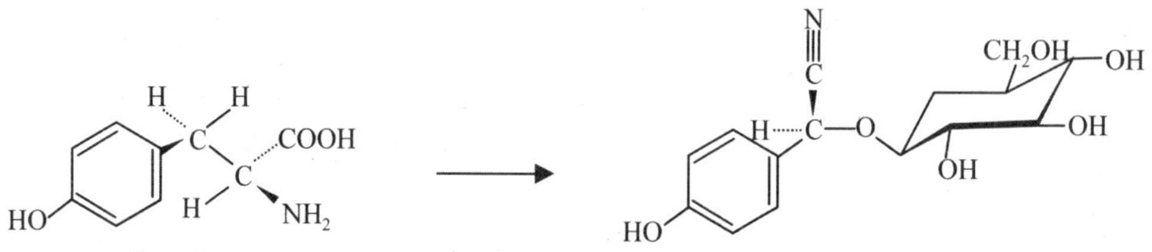

Tyrosine   Dhurrin

(*e*) **Prunasin (or Prulaurasin) from Phenylalanine:** It is obtained from phenylalanine as given below:

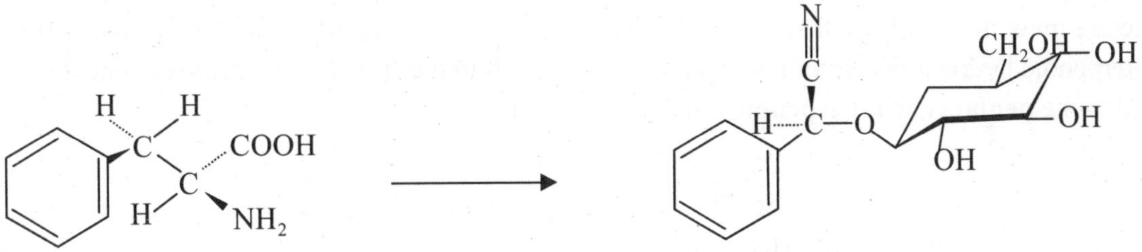

Phenylalanine

Prunasin
(Prulaurasin)

It has been established that labelled **shikimic acid** and labelled **tyrosine** were equally effective precursors of the hydroxylated aglycone of *Dhurrin*, a **cyanogenetic glycoside** produced by *Sorghum vulgare* Linn. belonging to family *Gramineae*.

Likewise, introducing labelled phenylalanine to young cherry laurel plants ie; *Prunus laurocerasus*, has proved that the amino acid acts as a precursor of *Prunasin* in young peach seedlings.

4.3.7 Biosynthesis of Thioglycosides

The seeds of a number of plants belonging to the mustard family comprise of glycosides, the aglycones of which are invariably isothiocyanates. Hence, these glycosides are also known either as **thioglycosides** or as **glucosinolates** and mostly form a group of bound toxins.

It has been observed that the aglycone portions of **thioglycosides** may largely consist of either aliphatic or aromatic derivatives. It is established experimentally that the carboxy-labelled acetate is being inorporated in the allyl moiety of *Sinigrin* usually present in *Brassica juncea*.

$$2 \ CH_3.\overset{*}{C}OONa \longrightarrow$$

Sodium Acetate

Sinigrin

4.3.8 Biosynthesis of Saponin Glycosides

Saponins are usually of *two* types, namely: *first*, the **steroidal saponins** which essentially have a spiroketal side chain, and *secondaly,* the **triterpenoid saponins**. It has been proved that labelled acetate and mevalonate are duly incorporated into **spiroketal steroids** as well as **pentacyclic triterpenoids**. It is, however, pertinent to mention here that the major pathway adopted by both types of sapogenins is more or less identical and that it involves head to tail coupling of various acetate units. It is asumed that a branching takes place most probably after the formation of the triterpenoid hydrocarbon **squalene**, that ultimately leads to the **spiroketal steroids** in one direction and to the **pentacyclic triterpenoids** in the other as shown below:

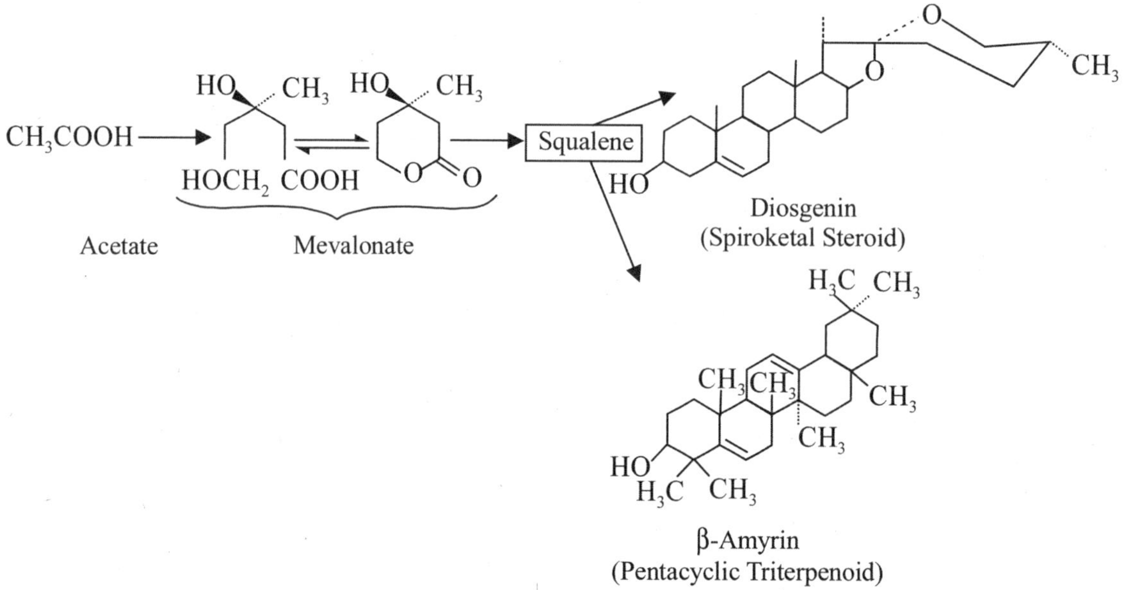

Acetate   Mevalonate

Diosgenin
(Spiroketal Steroid)

β-Amyrin
(Pentacyclic Triterpenoid)

4.3.9   Biosynthesis of Aldehyde Glycosides

It has been established that the aromatic nuclei of **aldehyde glycosides** are usually from the C_6-C_3 precursors formed *via* the *Shikimic Acid Pathway*. However, the conversion of **cinnamic acid** to **vanillin** is considered to be the most propable route as shown under:

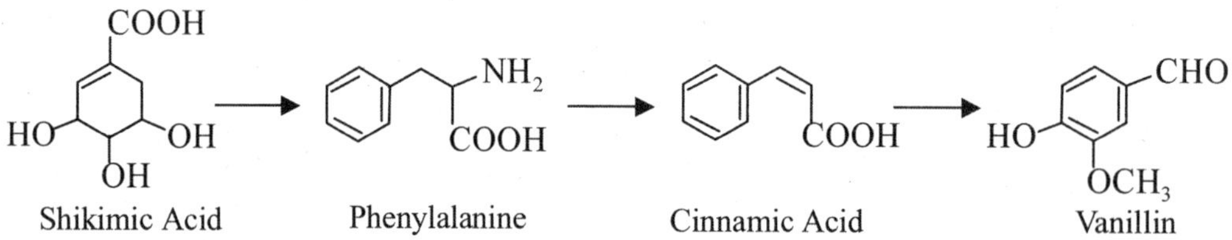

Shikimic Acid   Phenylalanine   Cinnamic Acid   Vanillin

4.4   PROFILE OF GLYCOSIDES IN NATURAL PLANT SOURCES

The variety of glycosides occurring in natural plant sources are so numerous that it is not quite possible to include all of them in one chapter in the present context. Hence, it is thought worthwhile to summarize them in the following Table 4.6:

Table 4.6   Summary of Glycosides in Natural Plant Sources

S. No.	Class	Name	Biological Source (Family)	Major Glycosides	Uses
I	Anthracene Grycosides	Aloe	*Aloe barbadensis;* A. Ferox; A. perryi; A. africana; A. spicata (Liliaceae)	Aloin, Aloe-emodin,	Purgative
		Rhubarb	Rheum officinale; R. palmatum; R. emodi; R. webbianum; (Polygonaceae)	Rhein; Aloe emodin;	Bitter Stomachic; Purgative
		Cascara sagrada	Rhamrnus purshiana (Rhamnaceae)	Barbaloin; Deoxybarbaloin Carcaroside-A, B, C & D	Cathartic, Tonic and Stomachic
		Frangula	Rhamnus frangula (Rhamnaceae)	Frangulin A & B; Glucofrangulin-A & B	Cathartic
		Senna	Cassia senna; C., angustifolia; (Leguminosea)	Sennoside A, B, C & D	Purgative
		Chrysarobin	*Andira araroba (Leguminoseae)*	Chrysophano anthranol	Ringworm
II	Phenol Glycosides	Bearberry (Uvs ursi)	*Bergenia crassifolia (Saxifragaceae)*	Arbutin	Diuretic
		Canadian Wintergreen Plant	Gaultheria procumbens and Monotropa hypopitys (Ericaceae)	Gaultherin	—
		Poplar and Willow	Salix fragilis and Salix purpurea (Salicaceae)	Salicin Populin	Analgesic Bitter Stomachic
		Khatta	Citrus aurantium (Rutaceae)	Hesperidin	—
		Irridis rhizoma (Orris root)	Iris kumaonensis (Iridaceae)	Iridin	Cathartic, stimulant, Diuretic
		Apple	*Malus sylvestris (or Pyrus malus) (Rosaceae)*	Phlorizin	—
III	Steroid Glycosides	Digitalis (Fox Glove)	*Digitalis purpurea* (Serophulariaceae)	Purpurea Glycosides A, B, & C; Digitoxin	Cardiotonic
		Digitalis	Digitalis lanata (Scrophulariaceae)	Lantosides A, B & C; Digoxin	Cardiotonic
		European Squill (Sea Onion)	Urginea maritima (Scilla maritima) (Liliaceae)	Glucoscillaren Scillaren –A; Scillarenin; Proscillaridin	Cardiotonic
		Indian Squill (Scilla)	Urginea indica (Liliaceae)	Scillaren-A; Scillaren-B	Rat poison
		Red Squill (Red variety of European Squill)	Urginea maritima (Liliaceae);	Scilliroside	Cardiotonic
		Strophanthus	Strophanthus hispidus (or S. kombe) (Apocyneceae)	Cymarin; K-Strophanthidin-β; K-Strophanthosi de	Cardiotonic
		Ouabain	Strophanthms gratus (Apocyneceae)	G-Strophanthin (Ouapain)	Cardiotonic
		Oleander	Nerium oleander (Apocynaceae)	Oleandrin	Cardiac Stimulant
		Black Hellebore	Helleborus niger (Ranunculaceae)	Hellebrin	Cardiotonic

(Contd.)

(*Table 4.6 contd.*)

		Adonis	Adonis vernalis (Renunculaceae)	K-Strophanthin; Adoniotoxin	Cardiotonic
		Thevetia	Thevetia nerifolia (Apocynaceae)	Thevetin- A	Cardiotonic
IV	**Flavonoid Glycosides**				
A	Flavone Glycosides	Parsley	Petroselinum sativum and Apium petroselinum (Umbelliferae)	Apin	Stimulant; Diuretic;
		Buchu	Barsoma crenulata B. serratifolia; B. betulina; (Rutaceae)	Diosmin	—
B	Flavonol Glycosides	Buck Wheat	Fagopyrum esculatum (Polygonaceae)	Rutin	Decrease capillary fragility
		Ring	Crategus oxycantha (Rosaceae)	Quereitrin	Textile dye
C	Flacanone Glycosides	Lemons, Sweet Oranges; Bitter Oranges;	Citrus sinensis; Citrus limon; C. aurantium, C. medica, (Rutaceae)	Hesperidin	Minimise capillary fragility
D	Chalone Glycosides	Safflor Red	Carthamus tinctorius	Carthamin	Dye
E	Isoflavonoid Glycoside	Sharapunkha	Tephrosia purpurea (Leguminosae)	Tephrosin	Fish poison
		Gilas	Prunus avium (Rosaceae)	Prunetrin	—
		Green Pods	Sopora japonica (Leguminosae)	Sophoricoside	—
F	Anthocyani-din Glycosides	Pelargonium Flower	Pelargonium gravecolens and P. roseum (Geraniaceae)	Plargonidin	Diuretic
		Althaea Flower	Althaea rosea (Malvaceae)	Cyanidin	—
		Peony Tuber	Peony officinalis (Ranunculaceae)	Peonidin	—
		Whortle Berry	Vacinium myrtillus (Ericaceae)	Delphinidin	—
		Petunia Flower	Petunia hybrida (Solanaceae)	Petunidin	—
		Malva Flower	Malva sylvestris (Malvaceae)	Malvidin	—
V	**Coumarin and Furanocou marin Glycosides**				
A	Coumarin Glycosides	Horse-chestnut Tree;	Alsculus hippoeastanm (Hippocastanacea)	Aesculin	Fruit and bark in diarrhoea Tonic
		Chicory Flower	Chicorium intybus (Compositae)	Chicorin	Febrifuge Diarrhoea
		Daphne Bark	Daphne mezerium (Thymelaceae)	Daphnin	Febrifuge
		European Ash	Fracinus exclsior (Oleaceae)	Fraxin	Tonic; Febrifuge; Bitter Astringent;
		Tonka Seed	Dipteryx odorata D. oppositifolia (Leguminoseae)	Coumarin	Pharmaceut ical aid
B	Furanocour-marin	Honey Plant (Visnaga)	Ammi Visnaga (Umbelliferae)	Khellin; Khellol; Glucoside;	Coronary vasodiltor
		Psoralea Fruit	Psoralea Corylifolia (Leguminosae)	Psoralen, Isopsoralen Psolaridin	In leprosy and leucoderma
		Cantharides	Cantharis	Cantharidin	Vesicant

(Contd.)

(*Table 4.6 contd.*)

		Beetles (Spanish Fly)	vesicatoria (Mesloidae)		rubefacient and hair growth stimulant
		Mylabris (Chinese cantharides)	Mylabris sidae (Coloeoptera)	Cantharidin	Rubefacient, Counter irritant
VI	**Cyanogenetic Glycosides**	White Clover	*Trifolium repens* (Leguminsoae)	Linamarin	—
		Flax	Linum usitassimum (Linaceae)	Linustatin	Demulscent as poultices
		Lotus Legumes	Lotus corniculatus (Leguminosae)	Lotaustralin	—
		Calcocarpum seeds	Calcocarpum sapota (Sapotaceae)	Lucumin	—
		Anthemis Seeds	Anthemis altissima (Compositae)	Anthemis Glycosides A and B	—
		Bitter Almond	Prunus amygdalus P. communis; Amygdalus communis; (Roseceae)	Amygdalin	Sedative; Demulscent in skin lotion
		Wild cherry Bark	Prunus serotina P. macrophylla (*Rosaceae*)	d-Prunasin	Sedative expectorant
VII	**Thioglyco- sides**	Black Mustard	*Brassica nigra Brassica juncea* (Cruciferae)	Sinigrin	Rubefacient Counter irritation
		White Mustard	Brassica alba (*Cruciferae*)	Sinalbin	Rubefacients, Counter Irritation;
VIII	**Saponin Glycosides**				
A	Tetracyclic Triterpenoid Saponins	Rheumatism Root	Dioscorea delitoidea; C. tokora; D. composita	Diosgenin	As a starting material for some potent steroidal drugs
		Solanum Berries	Solanum khasianum (Solanaceae)	Solasonine	Starting material for synthesis of steroidal drugs
		Asparagus Roots	Asparagus recemosus	Sarsapogenn; Shatavarin-I, Shatavarin-IV	Tonic Diuretic
B	Pentacyclic Triterpenoid Saponins	Ginseng	Panax ginseng, P. japonica; P. notoginseng; P. quinquefolium; P. pseudo ginseng; (Araliaceae)	Ginsenoside-Rg_1 Panaxosides	General tonic; Stimulant; Carminative, Diuretic
		Liqorice	Glycyrrhiza glabra; (Leguminosae)	Glycyrrhizin	Demulscent Expectorant
		Senega	Polygala senega Polygala alba; (Polygalaceae)	Senegin-II	Expectorant; Emetic
		Bacopa	Bacopa monnieri (Scrophulariaceae)	Bacogenin A, Bacogenin B	Insanity; Epilepsy
		Soap Bark	Quillaja saponaria (Rosaceae)	Quillaia Sapotoxin	Foam producer
		Sarsaparilla	Smilax aristolochiaefolia; S. regelii (Liliaceae)	Sarsapogenin; Smilagenin	Rheumatism, Skin ailments, Syphilis

(Contd.)

(*Table 4.6 contd.*)

IX	**Aldehyde Glycosides**	Vanilla Beans (Vanilla Pods)	*Vanilla planifolia* Vanilla tahitenis *(Orchidaceae)*	Glucovanillin	Pharmaceut-ical aid;
X	**Bitter Glycosides**	Indian Gentian	*Picrorhiza kurroa* (Scrophulariaceae)	Picroside I, Picroside II, Kutposide	Tonic, Stomachic, Febrifuge, Laxative
		Bitter Root	Gentiana lutea (Gentianaceae)	Gentiopeirin, Amarogentin	Bitter tonic in dyspepsia and anorexja
		Bitter stick (East Indian Balmony)	Swertia (Ophelia) Chirata *(Gentianaceae)*	Chiratin, Amarogenin	Bitter tonic Febrifuge Diuretic Epilepsy
XI	**Miscellaneous Glycosides**				
A	Steroidal Alkaloidal Glycosides	Bitter Sweet	Solanum dulcamara (Solanaceae)	Solanidine	Psoriasis skin diseases
		Tomato	Solanum lycopersicum (Solanaceae)	Rubijervine	Antifungal
B	Antibiotic Glycosides	Streptomycin	Streptomyces griseus (Streptomyce-taceae)	Streptomycin	Antibiotic
C	Nucleosides (Nucleic Acids)	Adenosine	Base-sugar unit as a nucleoside	Adenosine	RNA, DNA formation

FURTHER READING REFERENCES

1. Baker, W., and W.D., Ollis., In: **Recent Developments in the Chemistry of Natural Phenolic Compounds,** Ed by W.D. Ollis, Pergamon Press, Oxford, 152, 1961.
2. Bonner, J., and J.E. Varner., **'Plant Biochemistry',** Academic Press, London, 1965.
3. Britton, G., **'The Biochemistry of Natural Pigments',** Cambridge University Press, Cambridge, 1983.
4. Conn, E.E., **'The Biochemistry of Plants',** Vol. 7, *Secondary Plant Products*, Academic Press, London, 1981.
5. Ciba Foundation Symposium: 140, **Cyanide Compounds in Biology,** John Wiley & Sons Ltd., Chichester (U.K.), 1988
6. Griffith, J.Q., Krewson, C.S. amnd J. Naghski, Eds., **'Rutin and Related Flavonoids',** Mack Publishing Company, Easton Pennsylavania, 1959.
7. Glasby, J.S. **'Encyclopedia of the Terpenoids',** Vols I & II, Jphn Wiley & Sons Ltd. Chichester (U.K.), 1982.
8. Harborne, J.B., Ed. **'Biochemistry of Phenolic Compounds',** Academic Press Inc., New York, 1964.
9. Mann J., Davidson R.S., Hobbs J.B., Banthrope D.V., and Hardborne J.B.: **Natural Products: Their Chemistry and Biological Significance,** Longman, Harlow, 1994.
10. Poulton, J.E., **Cyanogenic Compounds in Plants and Their Toxic Effects. In Handbook of Natural Toxins** Vol I., Keeler, R.F., Tu A . T. Eds., Marcel Dekker Inc., New York, 1983.
11. Shibata, S., Tanaka, O., Shoji, J., and H. Saito., **Chemistry and Pharmacology of Panax, In Economic and Medicianl Plant Research,** Vol I., Wagner, H., Hikino, H., Farnsworth, N.R., Eds., Academic Press, Inc., Orlando, 1985.
12. Thompson, R.H., **'Naturally Occurring Quinones',** Butterworth, London, 1957.
13. Torsell K.B.G.: **Natural Product Chemistry. A Mechanistic, Biosynthetic and Ecological Approach,** Apotekarsocieteten, Stockholm, 1997.
14. Wright, S.E., **'The Metabolism of Cardiac Glycosides',** Springer Verlay, Berlin, 1960.

5

Terpenoids

5.1 INTRODUCTION

A plethora of naturally occurring plant products have been found to be related wherein they are comprised of one or more units of **isoprene** (C_5H_8)-a hydrocarbon:

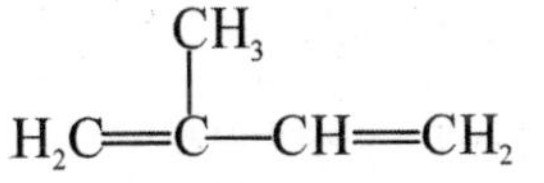

$$H_2C\!\!=\!\!\overset{\overset{\displaystyle CH_3}{|}}{C}\!\!-\!\!CH\!\!=\!\!CH_2$$

Isoprene

In general, **terpenoids**, may be defined as natural products whose structures are considered to be divided into several isoprene units; therefore, these compounds are invariably termed as **isoprenoids**. Besides, this particular group of compounds is sometimes collectively referred to as the **terpenes** in relatively older texts. Logically, the *–oid* suffix seems to be more acceptable and convincing, as it is in the same vein for steroids, alkaloids, flavonoids, etc., However, the-*ene* suffix must be solely confined to the unsaturated hydrocarbon belonging to this specific class of compounds.

It has now been established experimentally that the **isoprene units** come into being through the biogenetic means starting from acetate *via* mevalonic acid. Each such unit essentially consists of five-carbons having two unsaturated bonds and possesses a branched chain. The **terpenoids** usually have a number of such **isoprene units** joined together *in a head to tail manner*, as exemplified below:

Terpenoids are broadly classified on the basis of the number of **isoprene units** incorporated into a **specific unsaturated hydrocarbon terpenoid molecule,** such as:

(*a*) **Monoterpenoids:**	These are built up of *two* isoprene units and have the **molecular formula** $C_{10}H_{16}$;	
(*b*) **Sesquiterpenoids:**	These are composed of *three* isoprene units and have the **molecular formula** $C_{15}H_{24}$;	
(*c*) **Diterpenoids:**	These are comprised of *four* isoprene units and have the **molecular formula** $C_{20}H_{32}$;	

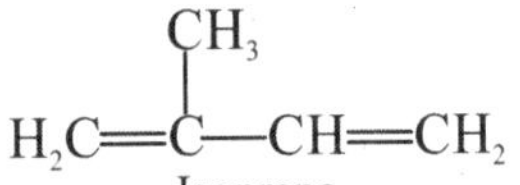

$H_2C=\overset{\overset{\displaystyle CH_3}{|}}{C}-CH=CH_2$

Isoprene
(2-Methyl buta 1,3 Diene)

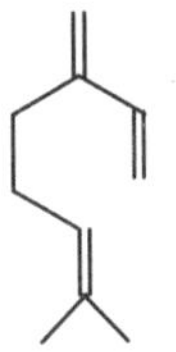

Myrcene

$\begin{bmatrix} \text{Acyclic} \\ \text{Monoterpenoid} \end{bmatrix}$

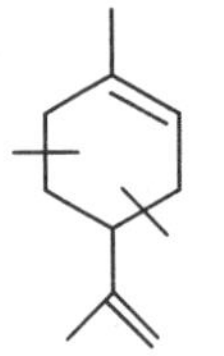

Limonene

$\begin{bmatrix} \text{Monocyclic} \\ \text{Monoterpenoid} \end{bmatrix}$

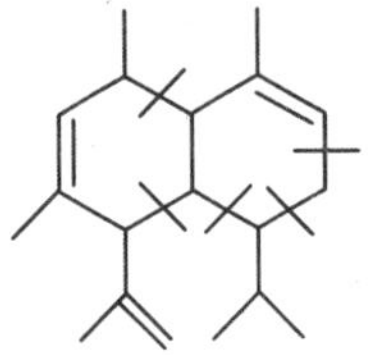

Cadinene

$\begin{bmatrix} \text{Bicyclic} \\ \text{Sesquiterpenoid} \end{bmatrix}$

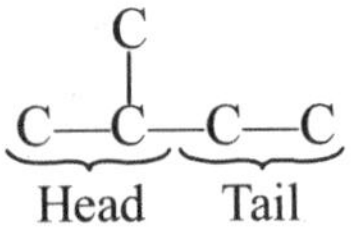

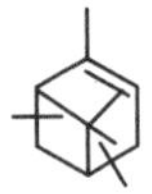

$\underset{\text{Head}}{C-\overset{\overset{\displaystyle C}{|}}{C}}-\underset{\text{Tail}}{C-C}$

α-Pinene

$\begin{bmatrix} \text{Bicyclic} \\ \text{Monoterpenoid} \end{bmatrix}$

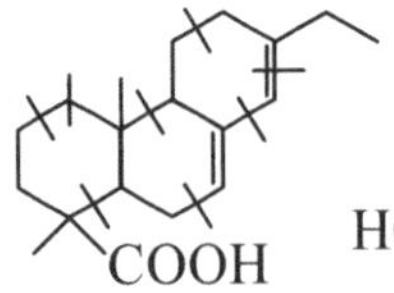

Abietic Acid

$\begin{bmatrix} \text{Tricyclic} \\ \text{Diterpenoid} \end{bmatrix}$

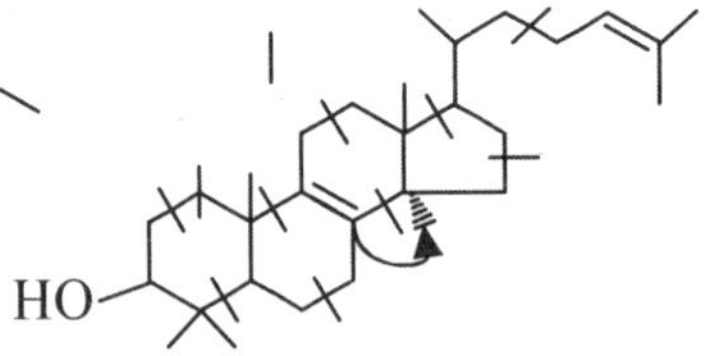

Lanosterol

$\begin{bmatrix} \text{Tetracyclic} \\ \text{Triterpenoid} \end{bmatrix}$

(d) **Triterpenoids:**   These contain *six* isoprene units and have the **molecular formula** $C_{30}H_{48}$; and

(e) **Tetraterpenoids**   These are made up of *eight* isoprene units and have the **molecular**
    (or Carotenoids):   **formula** $C_{40}H_{64}$.

Biogenetic Isoprene Rule   The very idea and basic concept that **terpenoids** are essentially built up of several **isoprene units** is commonly termed as the **biogenetic isoprene rule** as could be observed from the various typical examples cited earlier.

Meroterpenoids   It has been observed that a good number of other natural products do exist which essentially belong to mixed biosynthetic origin and are mostly made up from **isoprene** as well as **nonisoprenoid** entities.

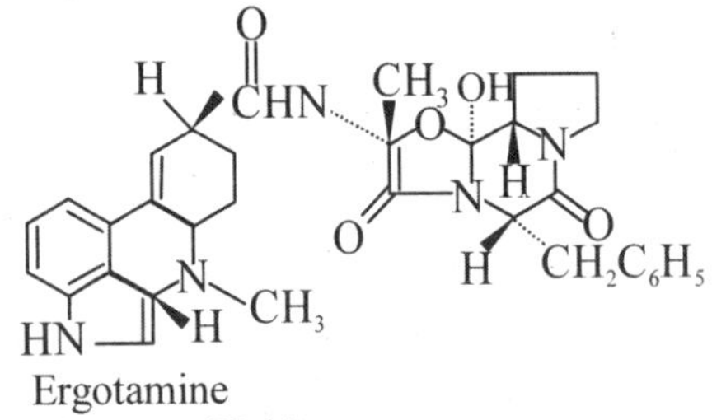

Ergotamine
[One Isoprene Unit]

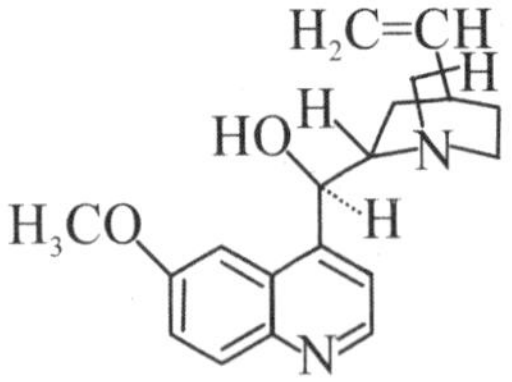

Quinine
[One Monoterpenoid Unit]

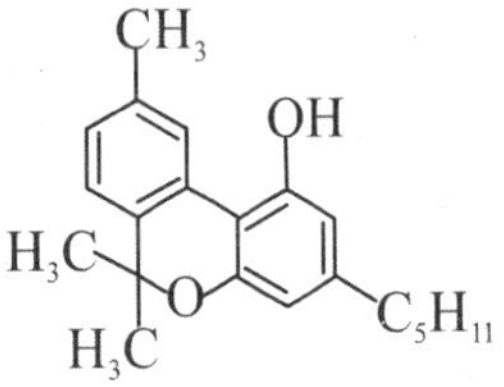

Cannabinol
[Two Isoprene Unit]

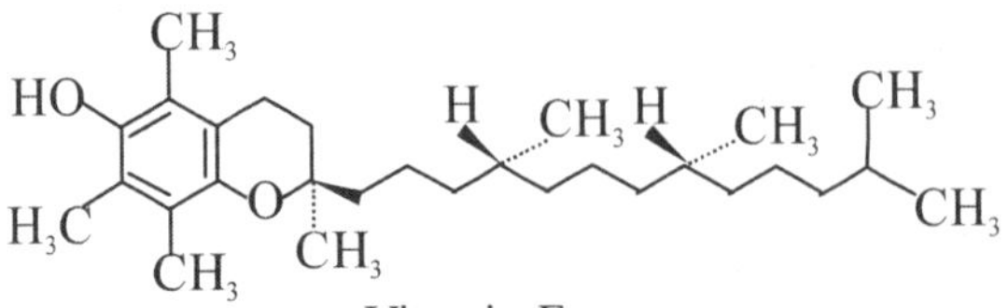

Vitamin-E
[One Isoprene Unit]

Examples   A few typical examples are: *ergotamine, quinine, cannabinol* and *vitamin-E.*

More than 20, 000 naturally occurring large variety of **terpenoids** have been duly isolated and characterized, and thus constitute a major congregation of such products when compared to any other individual class of natural products. In fact, the **chemical ecology** rests heavily and predominantly on the occurrence of profusely distributed **plant terpenoids**, and hence, the latter play a broad-spectrum of highly specific and characteristic roles in the plant kingdom, such as: **insect propellents** and **antifeedants, phytoalexins, attractants for pollingranes, pheromones, defensive substances against herbivorous animals, allelochemicals, signal molecules** and above all the **plant growth hormones.** Terpenoids usually engage in a variety of probable interactions, for instance: plant and plant, plant and microorganism, and plant and animal.

The International Union of Pure and Applied Chemistry (IUPAC) recommends a systematic mode of nomenclature of **terpenoids**; however, the names suggested by it are not only lengthy but also quite cumbersome. Therefore, the old and the trivial names of most **terpenoids** are used most frequently even today for naming the relatively common substances: examples:

Trivial Name	IUPAC Name
Geraniol	3, 7- Dimethyl-2, 6-octadien-1-ol;
Limonene	1-Methyl-4-(1-methylethynyl)- cyclohexene;
β-Myrecene	7-Methyl-3-methylene-1, 6-octadiene;

Carbon-Skeleton in Terpenoids   A comparative study of carbon-skeleton in terpenoids has revealed that a great majority of monocyclic terpenes essentially possess a *para menthane* carbon skeleton; besides, derivatives of **cyclopentane** and **methylated cyclohexanes** also exists invariably.

Generally, *two* different methods of tackling the structural problems normally encountered in **terpenoids** are adopted, namely:

(*i*) **Dehydrogenation:** Mostly the terpene hydrocarbon, *dienes,* upon dehydrogenation give rise to *p*-cymene. Having identified the prevailing carbon-skeleton in it, the exact location of the double bonds in the existing framework may be established by oxidative degradation to the corresponding simple aliphatic acids, and

(*ii*) **Oxidation:** Tilden was pioneer for the strategic incorporation of nitrosyl chloride (O=N–Cl) function by the help of a specific reagent (**Tilden Reagent**) so as to characterize and ensure the purity of the starting material *via* formation of definite crystalline derivatives of the corresponding terpenes under investigation. It has been established by Tilden's study that the olefenic linkage reacted specifically with this reagent to yield the respective **nitrosochloride adduct,** as shown below:

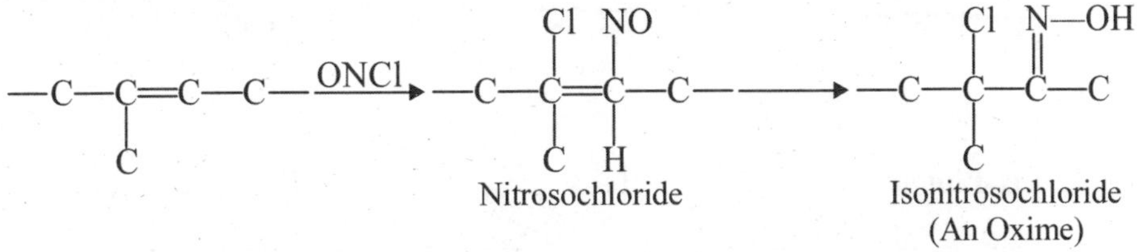

Nitrosochloride   Isonitrosochloride
                                        (An Oxime)

In a situation, where the C-atom possesses both nitrosomoiety and a H-atom, the former undergoes **isomerization** readily to yield isonitrochloride an oxime. However, in the absence of this specific characteristic feature the nitrosochloride is fairly stable.

It has been observed that when the substance is **monomeric*** the corresponding nitrosochloride provides a distinct blue colouration, which also ascertains the presence of tetrasubstituted ethylenes.

5.2 CLASSIFICATION

Based on the extensive distribution of **terpenoids** in the vast plant kingdom they are classified broadly as follows, namely:

  (*i*) Monoterpenoids
 (*ii*) Sesquiterpenoids
(*iii*) Diterpenoids
 (*iv*) Triterpenoids
  (*v*) Tetraterpenoids and Carotenoids
 (*vi*) Volatile Oils (or Essential Oils)
(*vii*) Resins and Resin Combinations
(*viii*) Oleoresins
 (*ix*) Oleo-Gum-Resins
  (*x*) Balsams

These different classes of naturally occurring substances shall be discussed individually in the sections that follows:

5.2.1 Monoterpenoids

In general, **monoterpenoids** represent a structurally diverse class of compounds may be categorised into nearly 35 varying structural analogues. However, the most commonly occurring structural variations are of the following types, namely:

Name	Chemical Structure	Type
Myrcene	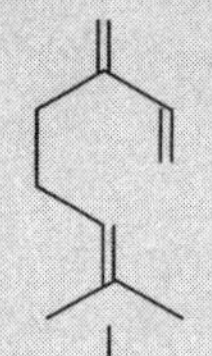	Acyclic
***p*-Menthane**	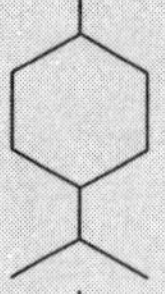	Monocyclic
α-Pinene	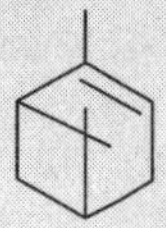	Bicyclic

---

* **Monomeric:** An entity or a unit from which polymer is formed.

It has been found that a large number of **monoterpenoid** derivatives belonging to these categories invariably occur naturally in the purest optically active form; however, certain plant species do have both enantiomers, such as: *Pinus* species contain both (+)- and (–)-α – pinene.

A few typical examples of monopenoids found in naturally occurring plant species are described under: *camphor, eucalyptol, menthol* and *thymol*.

5.2.1.1 Camphor

Synonyms   Gum camphor; Japan camphor; Formosa camphor. Laurel camphor.

Biological Source   It occurs in all parts of the camphor tree, *Cinnamonum camphora*. T. Nees & Ebermeier, belonging to family *Lauraceae*.

Geographical Source   The word *camphora* is derived from the Arabic *Kafur*, meaning chalk. The **camphor** tree, which is a huge evergreen plant, is found to be indigenous to Japan, China and Taiwan. It has also been naturalized specifically in the Mediterranean region eg; Algeria, Tunsia, Libya, Egypt, Italy and Greece. Besides it is grown in South Africa, Ceylon, Brazil, Jamaica, Florida and California. History reveals that Borneo camphor (from Borneol) arrived in Arabia in the sixth century and in Europe in the twelth century. Earlier, the worlds 80% supply of natural camphor was provided by Taiwan (Formosa) alone and the rest 20% by Japan and Southern China. Soonafter the second World War (1945) the commercial production of **synthetic camphor** has more or less catered for the ever increasing demand of **camphor** in the world market.

Preparation   It is prepared from the chipped wood by subjecting it to steam distillation and subsequently collecting the distillate in specifically designed chambers where camphor will solidify on its miner walls upon colling and may be collected later on from the bottom of the chamber. The crude solidified camphor is purified by mixing it with a suitable proportion of soda lime, sand and charcoal; and subjecting the mass to sublimation at controlled temperature when pure crystals of camphor would be collected as a sublimate. It is finally compressed into either small cubes or thin plates, wrapped and exported.

Camphor from Volatile Oils   It may be prepared from volatile oils by *two* simple methods, namely:

Methods-I   In case, the oil contains a substantially large proportion of **camphor**, it may be separated by deep freezing or sudden chilling; and if the camphor content in oil is not so much it is mostly fractionated and the camphor containing fraction is chilled to recover camphor.

Method-II   **Camphor** may be recovered from volatile oils by the instant production of insoluble complexes with strong mineral acids eg; sulphuric acid 80% (30N).

Synthetic Camphor (or Borneol Camphor)   The **camphor** is obtained commercially from α-pinene present in the turpentine oil through several steps sequentially *e.g.*, treatment with HCl, isomerization, treatment with KOH and finally oxidation with HNO_3 as given below:

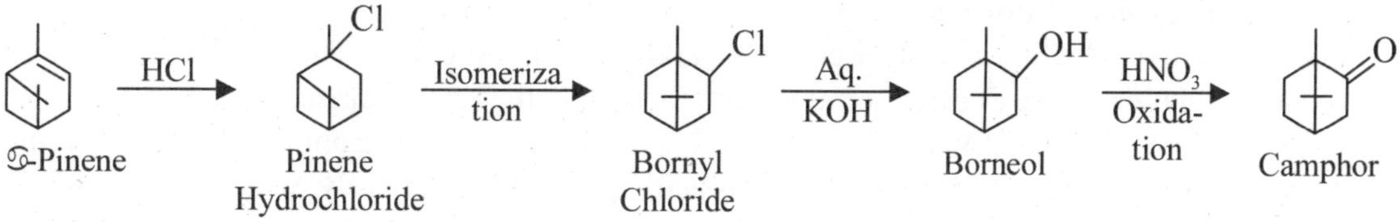

α-Pinene $\xrightarrow{\text{HCl}}$ Pinene Hydrochloride $\xrightarrow[\text{tion}]{\text{Isomeriza}}$ Bornyl Chloride $\xrightarrow[\text{KOH}]{\text{Aq.}}$ Borneol $\xrightarrow[\text{Oxida-tion}]{HNO_3}$ Camphor

Description

Colour	: Translucent mass with crystalline fraction
Odour	: Characteristic odour
Optical Activity	: Natural camphor = Dextro rotatory (+ 41° to 43°) Synthetic camphor = Racemic mixture;
Solubility	: Soluble in water (1:600)

Chemical Structure   **Camphor** is a **bycyclic terpenoid ketone** as given below:

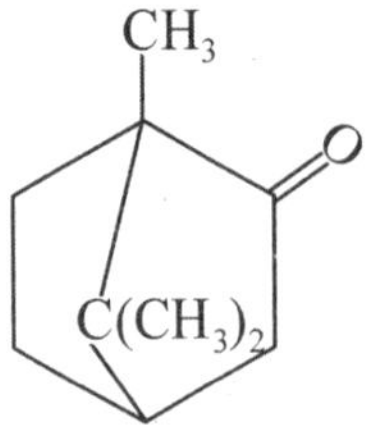

Camphor

In the presence of platinum black it undergoes hydrogen at ambient temperature giving rise to **isoborneol** as the major product and traces of **borneol**.

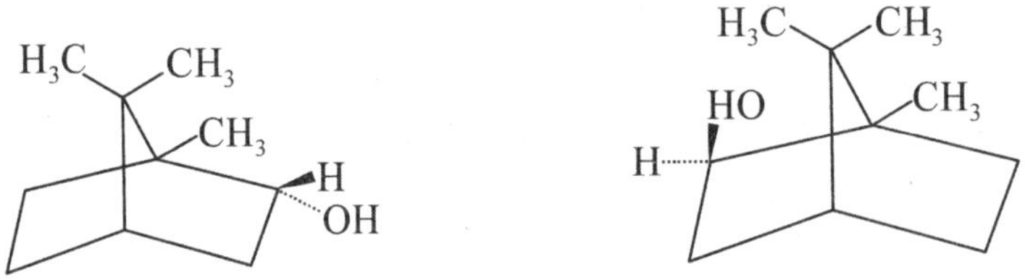

S-Borneol

1-Isoborneol

Its prolonged hydrogenation often yields **camphene**.

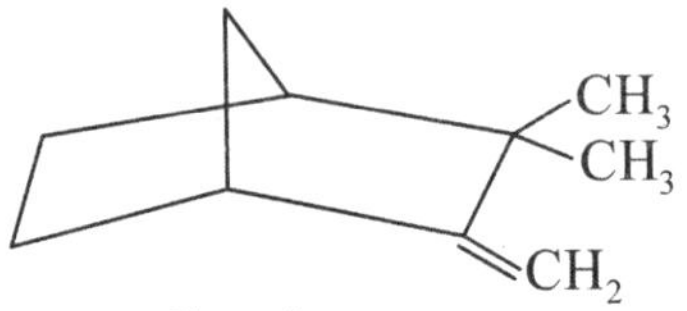

Camphene

Chemical Tests

1. Its semicarbazone derivative using semicarbazine hydrochloride has a m.p. 247-248°C for d-camphor.
2. Its 4-dinitrophenyhydrazone derivative has different mp *e.g.*, *d*- and *l*- = 175°C and *dl* = 164°C.

Camphor in presence of Borneol

1. **Borneol** is first esterified with stearic acid to yield a high-boiling ester. The resulting mixture on steam distillation removes camphor as the product while the ester remains in the flask.
2. **Borneol** forms an adduct with either succinic anhydride or phthalic anhydride upon heating to yield borneol acid auccinate and borneol acid phthalate respectively, which are soluble in

NaOH solution. Camphor (unreacted) is subsequently extracted with ether from the alkaline medium.

3. **Camphor** forms an oxime ($>C=N-OH$) with hydroxylamine which is then dissolved in sulphuric acid; the unreacted borneol is removed by extraction with ether.

Distinction between Natural Camphor and Synthetic Camphor   A drop of freshly prepared vanillin solution (1: 100 in dilute HCl) and sulphuric acid when added to powdered natural camphor, it gives rise to an instant yellow colouration changing to red, violet and finaly blue. The **synthetic camphor** fails to respond to this test and gives a distinct bright smoky flame.

Uses
1. It is used as a topical antipruritic in concentrations ranging between 0.1 to 0.3%
2. It is mostly used as a counterirritant (11%) particularly for fibrositis and neuralgia associated with inflamed joints, sprains and other inflammatory manifestations.
3. It is also employed as antipyretic, antiseptic, antifungal and carminative agent.
4. It is employed as a safe and effective measure for reducing cough when applied externally, in the form of an ointment, on the chest and throat of children.
5. It exerts its stimulant, rubefacient, antispasmodic and analgesic activities.
6. It stimulates the nerve endings in the skin and causes substantial relief of pain due to the masking of deeper visceral pain with a milder pain arising from the skin at the same level of innervation.

5.2.1.2 Eucalyptol

Synonyms   Cineole; Cajeputol.

Biological Source   It is obtained from the leaves of *Eucalyptyus globulus* Labill, belonging to family *Myrtaceae.*

Geographical Source   The eucalyptus tree is a native of Australia and Tasmania. It is largely cultivated in Calfornia, Spain, Portugal and India. In India it is abundantly found in the Himalayan region, Nilgiri district, Kumaon Hills and Assam.

Preparation   A number of volatile oils from certain *Eucalyptus species* invariably contain eucalyptol as high as 30 to 70%. It also occurs in **cajuput oil** (40%) and in **laurel leaf oil** (50%). However, **eucalyptol** may be isolated from these oils by adopting one of the following methods:

Method 1   By subjecting the volatile oil to fractional distillation and collecting the fractions between 170-180°C to obatin crystals of **cineole** at −10°C (m.p. + 1.5°C)

Method-2   **Cineole** forms addition compounds with halogen acids, *e.g.,* $C_{10}H_{18}O$ HCl and $C_{10}H_{18}O$. HBr; with phosphoric acid as $C_{10}H_{18}O \cdot H_3PO_4$ which also serve as a means of its purification, and

Method 3   **Eucalyptol** yields an addition product with a 50% (w/v) alcoholic solution eg; $C_{10}H_{18}O$. $C_6H_6O_2$ (mp 82-85°C), from which the former may be generated.

Note: This method is mostly applicable to such volatile oils that have a higher cineole content.

Synthetic Method   **Eucalyptol** may be prepared synthetically by the dehydration of **terpin hydrate** as given below:

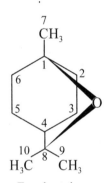

Terpin Hydrate   Eucalyptol

Description

Colour   : Colurless or pale yellow liquid.
Odour   : Camphoraceous and aromatic.
Taste   : Pungent and leaves a cold sensation.
Solubility : Water insoluble; soluble in paraffin, fixed oils and ethanol 90%.

Chemical Structure

Eucalyptol

Eucalyptol is an epoxy or oxido derivative of p-menthane. and is also known as 1,8-epoxy-p-methane or 1,8-oxido-p-menthane. It is found to be quite stable and hence may be distilled over metallic sodium safely without undergoing any change whatsoever. It is not affected by the action of reducing agents.

Chemical Tests

1. When a drop of **eucalyptol** is carefully treated with a drop of 5% (w/v) solution of hydroquinone in alcohol on a slide, it forms either colourless prisms or rhomboids; but with a 50% (w/v) solution of resorcinol in alcohol leaf-like crystals are obtained.
2. It forms characteristic addition compounds with HCl, HBr and H_3PO_4 with well defined melting points.

Uses

1. It is used internally as a stimulating expectorant to relieve severe cough and in bronchitis in the form of inhalatious.
2. It is abundantly employed externally as a mild anaesthetic and antiseptic for the treatment of various inflammatory conditions.

3. It also finds its use as a decongestant nasal drops.
4. It is profusely used in room sprays, lotions and all types of cosmetic preparations.
5. It is also used as a flavouring agent in pharmaceutical preparations *e.g.*; mouth washes, and gargles.

5.2.1.3 *Menthol*

Synonyms   1-Menthol; 3-Menthanol; Menthan-3-ol; Peppermint camphor, Hexahydrothymol.

Biological Sources   It is found in the **peppermint oil** obtained from the fresh flowering tops of the plants commonly known as *Mentha piperita* Linn., or other allied species of *Mentha,* belonging to family *Labiatae.*

Geographical Source   Various mentha species are duly cultivated in various parts of the world. It grows both abundantly and widely in Europe, while it is cultivated in Japan , Great Britain, Italy, France, United States, CIS countries, Bulgaria and India.

Preparation   It is normally prepared from *Japanese Peppermint Oil,* from the flowering tops of *Mentha avensis* Linne' var *piperascens,* by subjecting it to refrigeration below –22°C whereby the menthol crystallizes out distinctly. The crystals of **menthol** are separated by filteration and squeezes between layers of filter papers to remove the adhering oil and finally purified by recrystallization.

   Synthetic racemic menthol is prepared by the hydrogenation of either **pulegone** or **thymol** as shown below:

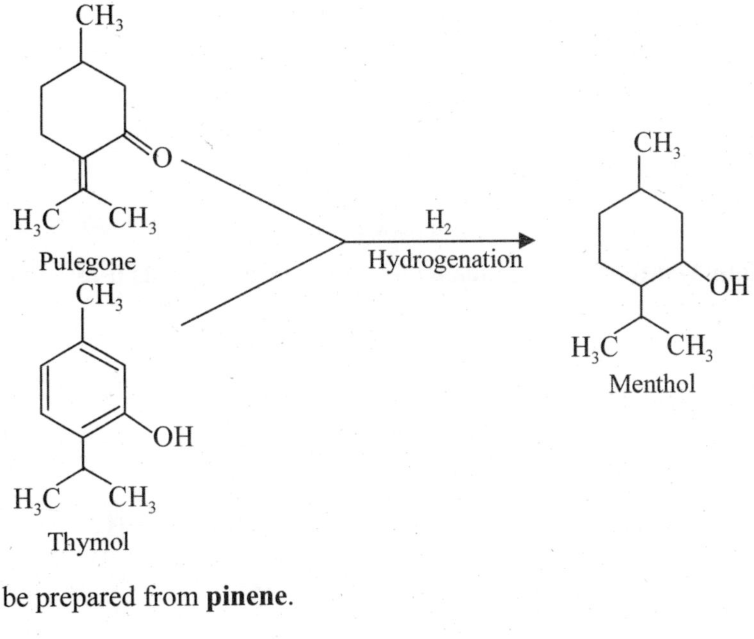

It may also be prepared from **pinene.**

Description

Colour : Colourless
Odour : Pleasant peppermint like odour

Taste   : Characteristic, aromatic and cooling taste

Shape   : Hexagonal cyrstals usually needle like, prisms; crystalline powder; fused masses.

Chemical Structure   **Menthol** has three chiral centres (*), hence it would give rise to eight (2^3) optically active isomers and four racemic forms. **Menthol** on oxidation gives menthone (a ketone), by the sacrifice of one chiral centre; therefore, the resulting menthone must exist in four (2^2) optically active isomers and two recemic forms and all, these have been actually prepared.

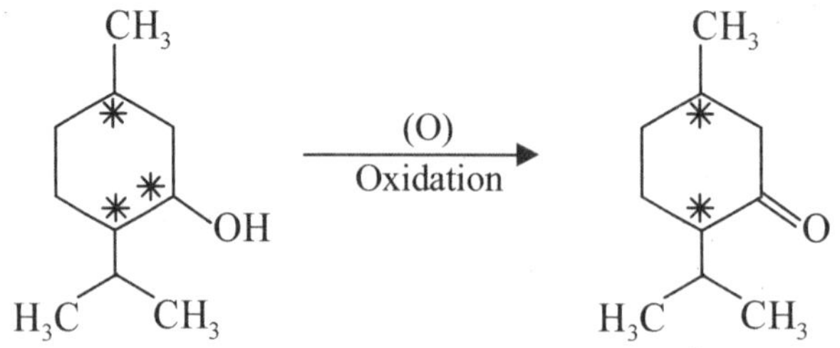

Menthol   Menthone

Special Features   following are the special features of **menthol**, namely:

   (*a*) **Dehydrogenation: Menthol** first on dehydration yields two isomeric forms of p-menthane, which on subsequent dehydration gives rise to **p-cymene** as follows:

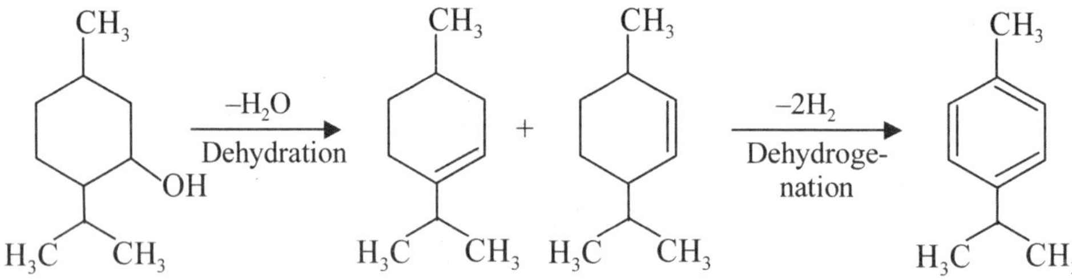

Menthol   *p*-Menthone   *p*-Cymene
                   (Isomeric Forms)

   (*b*) **Reduction: Menthol** on reduction with hydroiodic acid yields **p-menthane** as under:

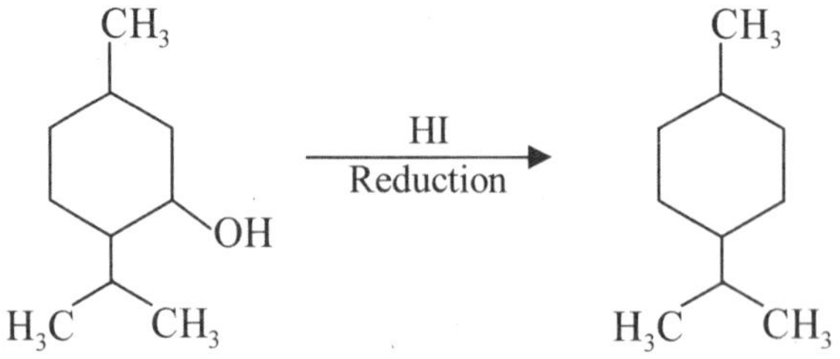

Menthol   *p*-Menthane

Chemical Tests

1. When 10 mg crystals menthol are first dissolved in 4 drops of concentrated sulphuric acid and then a few drops of vanillin sulphuric acid reagent are added it shows an orange yellow colouration that ultimately changes to violet on the addition of a few drops of water.

2. A few crystals of **menthol** are dissolved in glacial acetic acid and to this solution a mixture of 3 drops of H_2SO_4 and 1 drop of HNO_3 are added. It fails to produce either green or bluish green colouration (**Thymol** gives a green colouration).

3. **Menthol** provides a plethora of compounds of diagnostic value for differential identification, for instance: **menthoxy acetate; p-nitrobenzoate; d-camphor sulphonate; acid phthalate; phosphoric acid-complex;** and **3,5-dinitrobenzoate.**

Uses

1. It is used profusely in various types of mouth washes, toothpastes and similar oral formulations.

2. It finds its enormous use as a flavouring agent for chewing gums, candies, throat lozenges and also certain mentholated cigarettes.

3. It is mostly used on the mucous membranes or on the skin to serve as a counterirritant, antiseptic and as a mild stimulant at a concentration ranging between 1 to 16%.

4. It is employed in conjunction with other allied substances *e.g.*, **camphor, eucalyptus oil (eucalyptol)** in various pharmaceutical preparations, such as: expectorants, nasal sprays, and inhalants to cause immediate relief from symptoms of nasal congestion, sinusitis and above all bronchitis.

5. **Menthol** at a lower concentration ranging from 0.1 to 1%, when applied to the skin helps in the dilatation of blood vessels affording a cold feeling followed usually by a depression of the sensory cutaneous receptors thereby exhibiting an antipruritic action. Perhaps this could be the reason for its logical inclusion in formulations meant for treating sunburns, minor burns, douche powders, athelete's foot and poison ivy rash.

5.2.1.4 Thymol

Synonyms Thyme camphor; m-Thymol; 3-*p*-Cymenol; 3-Hydroxy-*p*-cymene;

Biological Sources It is obtained from the essential oil of *Thymus vulgaris* L., (Thyme oil); *Monarda punctata* L., **(Horsemint oil),** and *Monarda didyma* L., **(Oswego tea oil),** belonging to family *Lbiatae*. It may also be derived from *Carum capticum* Bentham er Hooker, **(Ajowan oil),** belonging to family *Umbelliferae*, and several species of *Ocimum,* for instance: *Ocimum gratissimum* L. **(Tulsi oil),** belonging to family *Labiatae*.

Geographical Source *T. vulgaris* is grown and cultivated abundantly in many parts of Europe, Australia and North Asia.

Preparation **Thymol** may be extracted from **thyme oil** by agitation with dilute aqueous alkali solution (= 5% w/v in water). The aqueous layer is first separated and subsequently made acidic with dilute acid, when **thymol** gets separated as an oily layer floating on the surface that may be recovered either by extraction with ether or by steam distillation.

Another means of obtaining **thymol from thyme oil** is to subject the latter to very low temperature ($-25°C$) when thymol separates as crystals.

Synthetic Thymol The **thymol** of commerce may be prepared synthetically by anyone of the following routes, namely:

(a) **From Menthone: Menthone** is first treated with bromine. and then quinoline to produce **thymol:**

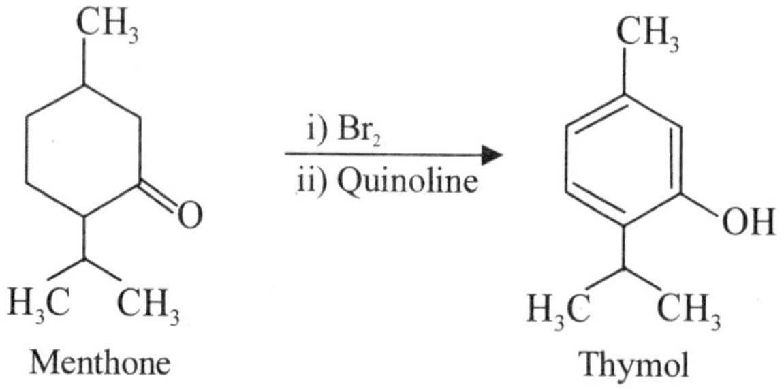

CH₃

i) Br₂
ii) Quinoline

CH₃

OH

H₃C   CH₃
Menthone

H₃C   CH₃
Thymol

(b) **From m-Cresol:** *m***-Cresol** on being treated with isopropanol in the presence of a suitable catalyst yields **thymol.**

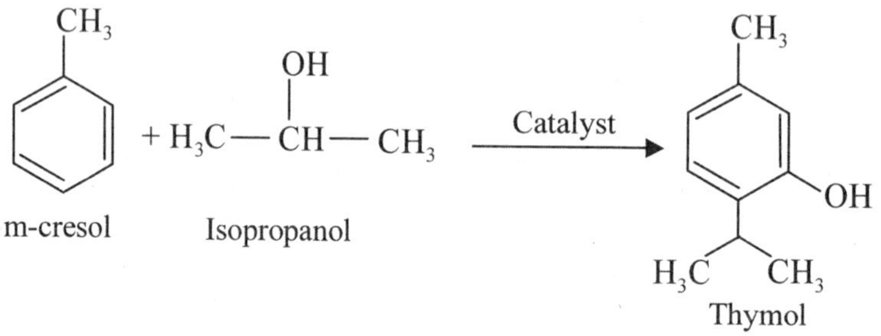

CH₃

OH
+ H₃C — CH — CH₃

Catalyst

m-cresol   Isopropanol

CH₃

OH

H₃C   CH₃
Thymol

(c) **From Piperitone:** When pipertone, usually obtained from the Australian Eucalyptus oils, is treated with ferric chloride it gives rise to **thymol.**

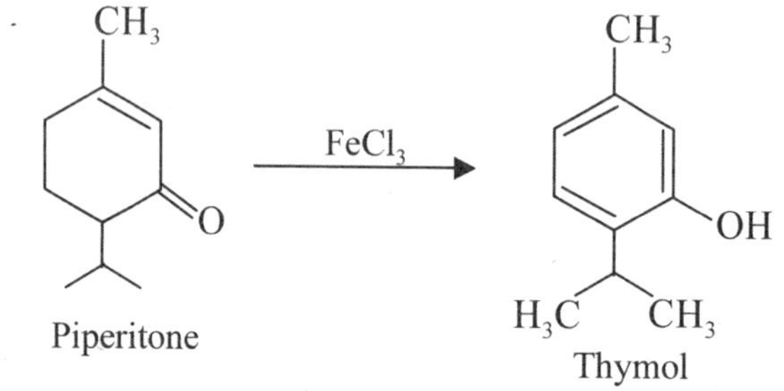

CH₃

FeCl₃

CH₃

OH

H₃C   CH₃
Thymol

Piperitone

Description

Colour : Transparent, colourless

Odour   : Aromatic thyme—like odour

Taste   : Pungent taste

Solubility : In water (1: 1200); in alcohol (1:1), in glycerol (1: 1000); Freely soluble in ether, chloroform, carbon disulphide, benzene and glacial acetic acid; soluble in fixed oil and volatile oil.

Chemical Structure   The phenolic OH moiety present in **thymol** enables it to form salts of acetate and carbonate easily which are used as antiseptic and anthelmintic respectively.

Thymol

Thymol when disolved in NaOH solution and treated with an I_2-KI solution it forms thymol iodide that finds its use as an anti-infective and antifungal agent.

Thymol   Thymol Iodide

Chemical Tests

1. **Thymol** when fused with phthalic anhydride develops bright violet red to intense red colouration, and on adding dilute alkali it gives an intense blue coluration due to the formation of thymolphthalein.

2. **Thymol** on being dissolved in concentrated sulphuric acid yields the corresponding thyme-sulphuric acid $[C_6H_2(SO_3H) (CH_3). (C_3H_7).OH]$, which produces a distinct violet colour with ferric chloride solution.

3. An alcoholic solution of **thymol** on being treated with $FeCl_3$ solution does not produce any colouration.

   Note: Carvacrol on identical treatment gives a green colouration.

4. A small crystal of **thymol** is dissolved in 1 ml of glacial acetic acid and to this is added one drop of HNO_3 and six drops of sulphuric acid, when it exhibits a deep bluish green colour.

5. Dissolve 0.1 g of **thymol** in 2 ml of NaOH solution (10% w/v) and heat in a water bath to produce either a clear colourless solution or a pale red solution, that ultimately turns darker in shade on keeping without the separation of oily drops. If the resulting solution is shaken with a few drops of chloroform it gives a violet colouration.

6. **Thymol** forms definite derivatives with various reagents *e.g.*, napthylurethane derivative (m.p. 160°C); phenylurethane derivative (106-107°C).

Uses

1. It is invariably employed as an antifungal and antibacterial agent.

2. It is a vital component in several analgesic and topical antiseptic formulatios in low concentrations ranging between 0.1 to 1% in personal health care products.
3. It is widely employed in preparation exclusively intended for mouthwashes, gargles, oral preparations and as a local anaesthetic in toothache.

5.2.2 Sesquiterpenoids

The **sesquiterpenoids** are found to be extensively distributed in nature and by all means represent the most abundantly prevailing class of **terpenoids.** A few typical examples are cited below:

S. No.	Name	Biological Source (Family)	Geographical Source	Uses
1.	β-Cadinene	*Juniperus communis* Linn., (*Cupressaceae*); Oil of Cade	United States, Europe, Canada, India in Western Himalayas (12,500-14,000 ft)	For scenting soaps
2.	β-Caryophyllene	*Syzygium aromaticum* (l.) Merrill & Perry (*Jambrosa caryophyllus* Niedenzu; *Eugenia caryophylata* Thumb) (*Myrtaceae*) Clove oil	Moluccas Islands (volcanic island in Eastern Indonesia), Zanzibar, Tanzania (Pemba Islands), Madagascar, Ceylon, Malaysia, Haiti and Southern India	Antitoothache; Antiseptic in tooth-pastes, mouth wshes; As a spice; stimulant aromatic carminative; Perfumery; preparing vanilline (from Eugenol)
3.	Abscisic Acid	*Found in sycamore, birch, rose leaves, cabbage, potato, lemon, avocado*	Mostly in tropical countries	An essential plant growth and development hormone

$$\begin{pmatrix} \text{β-Cadinene} \\ \text{Bicyclic} \\ \text{Sesquiterpenoid} \end{pmatrix} \qquad \begin{pmatrix} \text{β-Caryophyllene} \\ \text{Bicyclic} \\ \text{Sesquiterpenoid} \end{pmatrix} \qquad \begin{pmatrix} \text{Abscisic Acid} \\ \text{Monocyclic} \\ \text{Sesquiterpenoid} \end{pmatrix}$$

Sesquiterpenoids may be classified into *four* major categories namely: **acyclic, monocyclic, bicyclic** and **tricyclic sesquiterpenoids,** as summarized in Table 5.1.

Sesquiterpenoid Lactones Interestingly, another class of compounds essentially bearing such characteristic features as an **∝-methylene ⲩ-lactone system; ∝, β-unsaturated carbonyls,** and **epoxides** and obviously chemically distinct from the **sesquiterpenoids** are collectively termed as **sesquiterpenoid lactones.** The specific and vital **biological nucleophilies** *e.g.*; thiol and amino moieties present in the enzymes, help in the augmentation of faster and reactive approach to receptor sites by these **sesquiterpenoid lactones.** Thus, the overall effect is evidenced by a marked and pronounced biological activities, for instance: modified antimicrobial activity, enhanced antitumour properties.

Table 5.1 Classification of Sesquiterpenoids with Summarized Details

S. No.	Type of Sesquiter-penoids	Name	Biological Source (Family)	Geographical Source	Nos of Double Bonds	Specific Gravity	Structure	Characteristic Features	Uses
I	**Acyclic**	α-Farnesene, β-Farnesene,	Citronella oil from leaves of *Cymbopogon winterianus* and *C. flexuosus* (Steud.) Melabar Lemongrass Wats (*Graminaceae*)	Ceylon, India (Malabar Coast)	4	0.84	β-Farnesene α-Farnesene	Ozonolysis cleaves-β farnesene into acetone, formalin, succinic and levulinic acid components	Perfume in toiletaries;
II	**Monocyclic**	Zingiberene	From rhizomes of *Zingiber offocinale* Roseoe, (*Zingiberaceae*); Jamaica Ginger	South East Asia, West Indies, Australia, Africa, Jamaica, Taiwan, Mauritius, India	3	0.87-0.98	Zingiberene	Has 3 double bonds and 2 of which are conjugated Dehydragenation on with S yields cadalene-a napthalene hydrocarbon	Stomachic Carminative
III A	**Bicyclic** *Napthalene Derivatives*	β-Cadinene	From essential oils of juniper species and cadars (oil of cade) *Juniperus communis* Linn., (*Cuperessaceae*)	Canada, USA, Europe, India	2	0.90-0.92	β-Cadinene	Heating with S it gets transformed into cadalene-a napthalene hydrocarbon	Scenting soaps
B	*Azulene Derivatives*	Guaiazulene	From chamomile oil, *Achillea millefolium* Linn., (*Compositae*) [Syn: *A lanulosa* Nutt]	Europe, Africa	2	0.90-0.92	Guaiazulene	Unsaturated hydrocarbons Catalytic hydrogenation yields deahydroazulenes	Anti inflammatory
IV	**Tricyclic**	α-Santalene	Sandalwood oil from the wood of *Santalum album* Linn., (*Santalaceae*)	India, Malaysia	1	0.91-0.935	α-Santalene	A tricyclic saturated hydocarbon with a 6-carbon side chain	Scenting soaps

In general, the **sesquiterpenoid lactones** are classified into *three* major group as summarized below:

S. No.	Class	Name	Biological Source	Geographical Source	Special Features	Uses
1.	**Germacra-nolides**	Germacranolide	Leaf of Labrador Tea *Geranium macrorrhizum (Geraniaceae)*	Europe,	Has a ten membered carbon skeleton ring	—
2.	**Eudesma-nolides**	Eudesmanolide	*Magnolia obovata (Magnoliaceae)*	Europe North America	Has two fused six membered carbon skeleton ring	Neurotrophic activity
3.	**Guaian-olides**	Guaianolide	*Guaiacum officinale*Linn., *(Zygophyllaceae) Packwood Tree; Brazil Wood*	Tropical America	Has a five membered ring fused to a seven membered ring	Antioxidant

Germacranolide   Eudesmanolide   Guaianolide

It would be worthwhile to mention some typical examples of natural products that have the **sesquiterpenoid lactone** functions, namely: **artemisinin**.

5.2.2.1 Artemisinin

Biological Source   It is obtained from the leaves and the closed, unexpanded flower heads of *Artemisia annua* Linn., belonging to family *Asteraceae.*This particular herb has been used in the Chinese system of medicine exclusively for the treatment of malaria since more than one thousand years.

Geographical Source   The plant grows abundantly in China.

Chemical Structure   Though the herb was used for its wonderful proven therapeutic efficacy for more than a decade centuries, but its active principal **artemisinin** was isolated and identified in 1972.

Artemisinin

It has been established experimentally that the presence of an internal peroxide linkage strategically located in the seven membered ring is an absolute necessity for it to exert the unique antimalarial property.

Modifications in Structure   On account of the poor water solubility of **artemisinin** an attempt was made to improve either its water solubility ir its lipid solubility. In the former instance, *Sodium artesunate i.e.*, the sodium salt of its hemisuccinate ester was developed; while in the latter instance, *Artemether i.e.*, its corresponding methyl ether analogue was produced. Evidently, **sodium artesunate** is employed for intraveneous injections and artemether is used as a potent long acting drug.

Uses
1. The drug and its derivatives are used as fast acting blood schizontocides in the control and management of malarial fever caused by *plasmodium vivax* strain.
2. These drugs are found to be active against both chloroquine resistant and chloroquine sensitive strains of *Plasmodium falciparum.*
3. These drugs are found to show extremely encouraging therapeutic effects specifically in the treatment of *Cerebral malaria* by virtue of their significant rapid clearance of the prevailing parasites when compared to either chloroquine or quinine (synthetic antimalarials)

Note: **The chances of recurrence is quite substantial by the treatment of artemisinin and its derivatives; therefore, it is always necessary to adopt the course of a combination therapy employing other antimalarials.**

5.2.2.2 Parthenolide

Biological Source   It is obtained from the leaves of *Tanacetum parthenium* (L.) Schultz-Bip, belonging to family *Asteraceae*. It is commonly known as *feverfew* and has been employed for centuries as an effective *febrifuge* (antipyretic) which perhaps suggested the original nomenclature.

It is also obtained from *Chrysanthemum parthenium* (L.) Bernh. Family *Compositae;* and *Magnolia grandiflora* (L.) family *Magnoliaceae.*

Geographical Source   The plant *M. grandiflora* is a native of North America and also cultivated in Indian gardens.

Chemical Structure   Parthenolide is a **sesquiterpenoid lactone** having the following structure with the chemical name 4, 5$\propto$-epoxy-6 β-hydroxy germacra-1 (10), 11(13)-dien-12-oic acid γ-lactone.

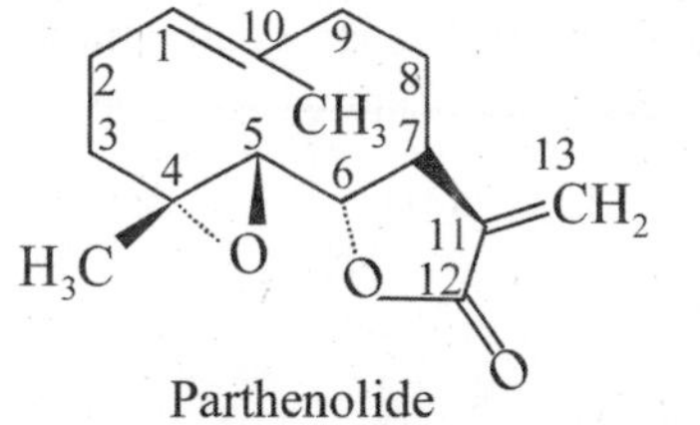

Parthenolide

It has an additional epoxide bridge between 4-and 5α-positions.

Uses
1. It is found to act as a **serotonin antagonist** thereby causing an inhibition of the release of serotonin from blood platelets.

2. Based on the findings conducted by an elaborated double blind placebo-controlled clinical trials have established that the drug is significantly effective in the prophylaxis of migraine by reducing considerably the severity as well as the frequency of the pain due to headache.

3. A normal dose of 125 mg per day of good quality dried leaves either in the form of tablets or capsules are used in the therapeutic practice as an antipyretic or febrifuge.

5.2.2.3 *Matricarin*

Biological Source It is obtained from the dried flower heads of *Matricaria chamomilla* L., and *Artemnisia tilesii* Ledeb, belonging to family *Compositae*. It is also found in *Matricaria recutita* Linne., family *Asteraceae* which represent the drug usually termed as **German Chamomile**. Besides, an allied plant source *Chamaemelum nobilc* Linne, normally known as **Roman Chamomile** also comprises of identical components and used alike.

Geographical Source In general, the above two **chamomiles** are cultivated abundantly in various parts of Europe.

Chemical Structure Its chemical name is 8α-acetoxy-4α-hydroxyguaia-1(10), 2-dien-12, 6α-olide.

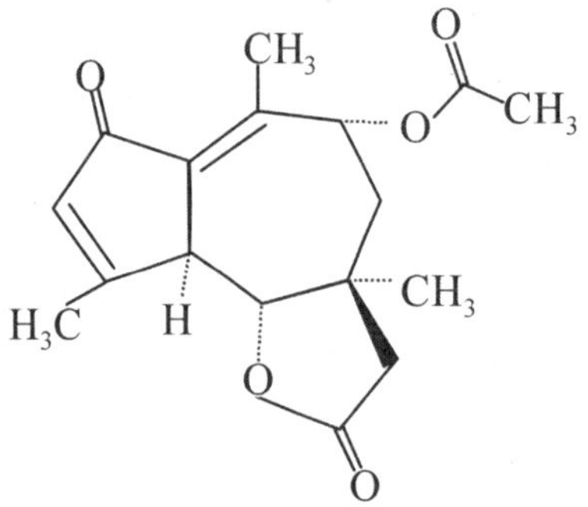

Matricarin

Uses

1. **Chamomile** has acclaimed to be the most popular *'herbal tea'* in the United States because of its definite anti-inflammatory and antipasmodic therapeutic properties.

2. The volatile oil of *M. chamomilla* contains the *sesquiterpenoid* **(-)-α-Bisabolol (Bisabolane)** which exerts anti-inflammatory activity.

3. An infusin (tea) when consumed over a long span results into a cumulative overall positive effect which certainly justifies its age-old usage as an unique home-remedy and healthy beverage not only in Europe but also in the United States.

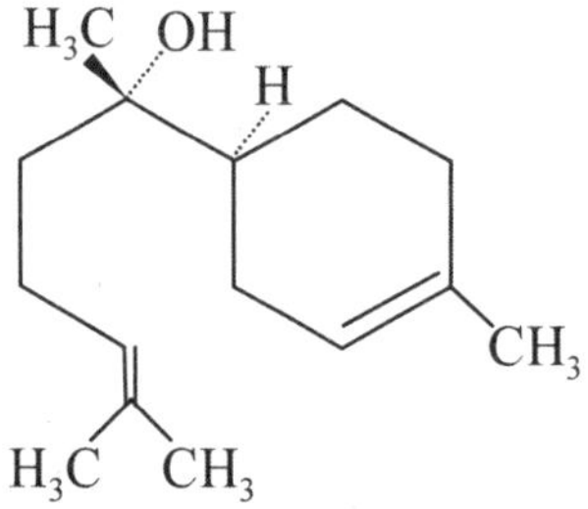

(–)-α-Bisabolol (Bisabolane)

5.2.3 Diterpenoids

Generally, **diterpenoid** represent a broad class of non-volatile C_{20} compounds that have been essentially obtained from **geranyl pyrophosphate**.

Geranyl Pyrophosphate

It has been observed that they mostly originate from the plant or fungal sources, but they are invariably formed by certain insects as well as **marine organisms.**

Characteristic Features Following are some of the characteristic features of **diterpenoids**, namely:

(*a*) Most of them are carboxylic compounds having upto five aromatic rings.

(*b*) Certain members of this class are acyclic compounds,

(*c*) Mostly occur as hydrocarbons or highly oxygenated compounds based on their degree of oxidation,

(*d*) Invariably isolated as optically active solids which may occur as the antipodal stereochemical cofigurations and the normal configurations; the former ones are called the *ent* series, while the latter ones possess and A/B ring fusion and are related to the steroid stereochemically.

A few typical examples of **diterpenoids** shall be discussed in the sections that follow.

5.2.3.1 *Colforsin*

Synonyms Forskolin; Beforsin (obsolete)

Biological Source It is obtained from the root of *Coleus forskohlii,* Briq., belonging to family *Labiatae.* The word *coleus* has been derived from the Greek *coleus* equivalent to sheath *i.e.*; the natural formation of the fused filaments of the flower which form a staminal sheath around the style; and the word **forskohlii** is due to the honour bestowed upon the Finnish botanist Forskal.

Geographical Source The plant is extensively distributed within the subtropical to temperate climatic zones on the hilly regions of Burma, Africa, Nepal, Ceylon and Thailand. It is also found on the dry, sunny slopes of hills at an attitude ranging between 300 to 1800 meters. It is cultivated in India.

Chemical Structure It was first discovered in India during a general sereening studies of **potential medicinal plants***. Its chemical name is 7β-acetoxy-8, 13-1α, 6β, 9α-trihydroxylate-14 en-11-one.

---

* Bhat, S.C. *et al., Tetrahedron Letters,* 1669, 1977

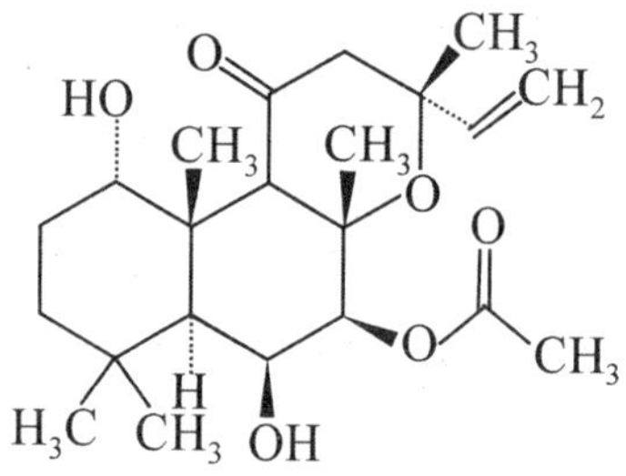

Forskolin

Uses

1. It is used in the purification of adenylate cyclase; and as a result it serves as a vital research tool in cyclic AMP-related investigations.
2. It also finds enormous use in glaucoma and hypertension.
3. It possesses significant therapeutic potential in diseases like: congestive cardiomyopathy and bronchial asthma wherein the excessive long term usage of β-adrenergic agonist drugs (*e.g.*; **propranolol, labetalol**) ultimately results into the desensitization of the receptors and a loss of drug efficacy.

5.2.3.2   *Ginkgolide–B*

Biological Source   It is obtained from the root bark and leaves of *Ginkgo biloba* L., belonging to family *Ginkgoaceae.*

Geographical Source   It is cultivated in the south eastern United States. The priests in China and Japan have confined this specimen to their temple grounds. It is a dioecious tree attaining a maximum height of 30 meters and has been cited in literatures as a living fossil that still survived unchanged in the region of eastern Asia since 200 million years.

Chemical Structure   **Ginkgolide-B** is the most active member of the family significant therapeutic efficacy in the treatment of severe sepsis, whereas the corresponding A and C analogues are devoid of such activities.

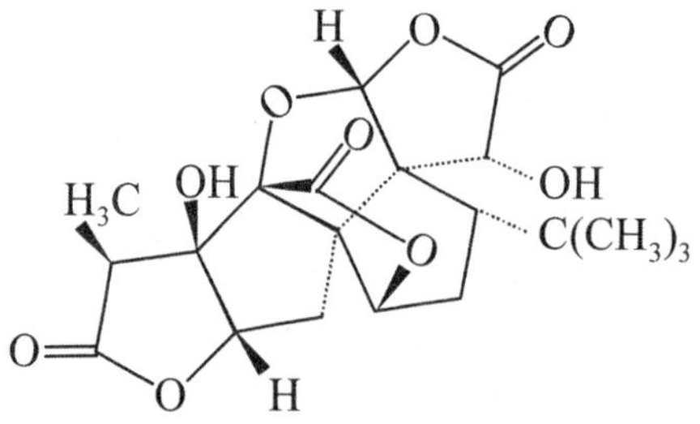

Ginkgolide-B

Uses

1. The standardized dehydrated acetone–water extract of the dried leaves equivalent to 6% **terpenoids** and 24% **flavone glycosides** is sold commercially in Europe as an approved drug to enhance blood fluidity and circulation.

2. In the United States only the tablets containing 40mg of the Ginkgo is allowed to be sold as a ditary suppliment.

3. **Ginkgolides A,B, C and M** have been shown to check the platelet activating factor (PAF) thereby preventing the bronchoconstriction, hypotension, cutaneous vasodilatation and finally the release of inflammatory compounds.

5.2.3.3 *Taxol*

Synonym   Paclitaxel; Taxol A; NSC – 125973.

Biological Source   It is obtained from the bark of the **Pacific Yew tree,** *Taxus brevifolia Nutt* belonging to the family *Taxaceae.*

Geographical Source   The plant is a native to the northwest United States. It is a small, not so growing evergreen tree.

Preparation   Keeping in view the paucity of the drug it look quite sometime to isolate **taxol** and establish its chemical structure. The very complexity of its chemistry has more or less turned its total synthesis into a not so viable and feasible economic exercise. However, an attempt is being made to enhance its availability through the semisynthetic route whereby the **taxol precursors** are usually obtained by extraction from the needles of largely available species of *Taxus.*

Example   The chemical component, 10-descetylbaccatin III, isolated from the needles of *Taxus baccata* Linn., may be conveniently converted to **taxol** *via* simple synthetic route.

Note: **The needles, in comparison to the bark, may be harvested without causing any injury to the plant whatsoever, and thus provides a rather more easily renewable plant source for the drug.**

Chemical Structure   The chemical structure is provided in Chapter 1 (Table 1.1).

Characteristic Features   **Taxol** has the following characteristic features, namely:

(*a*) It has a taxane ring system,

(*b*) It has a four membered octane ring

(*c*) An ester side chain at C-13 of the taxane ring is a prime requirement for taxol's cytotoxic activity, and

(*d*) The presence of an accessible hydroxyl moiety at C-2 of the ester side chain renders an appreciable enhancement of the cytotoxic activity.

Uses

1. **Taxol** is primarily employed in the treatment and management of *metastatic carcinoma of the ovarian glands* after the failure of follow-up chemotherapy.

2. It is also used in the treatment of breast cancer usually after the observed failure of combination chemotherapy for metastatic disease.

3. Because of its hydrophobic nature the injectable concentrate of taxol formulation meant for intravenous infusion is normally solubilized duly in polyoxyethylated caster oil. However, before injection it should be appropriately diluted in normal saline or dextrose solution or combination thereof.

5.2.4   Triterpenoids

Triperpenoids, generally are obtained by biogenesis from six isoprene units, They are found to share commonly the acyclic precursor **squalene** (C_{30}). Based on the various possible modes, whereby ring closure in squalene takes place may ultimately give rise to a large number of triterpenoids having a variety of skeleton structures. In actual practice, more than 4000 naturally occurring triterpenoids have been isolated and identified, and over 40 varying skeleton types have been established.

The **triperpenoids** may be categorized into two major groups, namely: the tetracyclic and the pentacyclic compounds: the former ones of the steriodal types with C-27 carbon atoms present in the skeleton while the latter are of the triterpenoid types with C-30 carbon atoms as shown below:

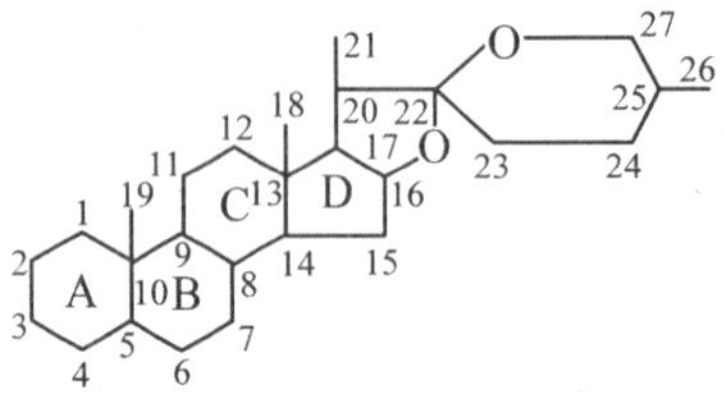

(Steroidal Triterpenoid)
[C-27]

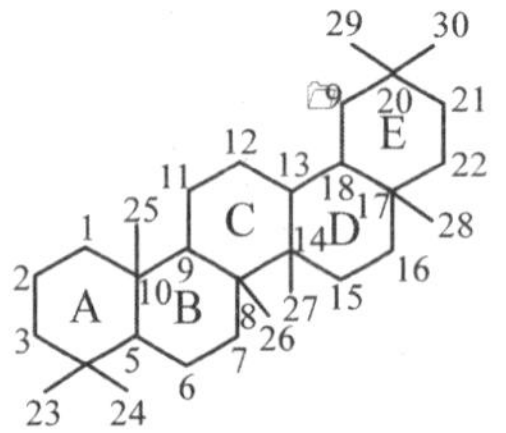

(Pentacyclic Triterpenoid)
[C-30]

However, the steroidal types (C-27) and the triterpenoid types(C-30) may be distinguished by virtue of the fact that the former yields Diel's hydrocarbon on dehydrogenation with Se at 360°C, while the latter gives either naphthalene or pinene end products.

Interestingly, both these types of compounds may easily combine with sugar moieties at C-3 position to yield the corresponding **glycosides**. Nevertheless, the **free triterpenoids** are invariably associated with natural latex, resins, or cuticle of plants.

A few typical examples shall be discussed in the sections that follows:

5.2.4.1   Cucurbitacin-B

A group of **tetracyclic triterpenoids**, usually termed as **"bitter principles of cucurbits"** that essentially possess distinct antineoplastic and anti-gibberellin activity.

Biological Sources   **Cucurbitacins** are obtained from a number of species belonging to cucurbitaceous plants known since antiquity due to their useful as well as toxic properties.

It is obtained primarily from most plants belonging to the *Cucurbitaceae* family, namely: *Luffa acutangula* (Linn.) Roxb. **(Ridged or Ribbed gourd);** *Luffa cylindricaa* (Linn.) M. Roem (*Luffa aegyptiaca* Mill ex Hook f. **(Dish-cloth gourd, Vegetables sponge, Spongegourd)**], *Luffa echinata* var *longystyla* Clarke (supposed to be a hybrid of *L. graveolens* Roxb. And *L. aegyptica* Mill); and *Luffa graveolens* Roxb. It is also found in various species belonging to family viz., *Begoniaceae, Cruciferae, Datisceae, Euphorbiaceae,* and *Scrophulariaceae.*

Geographical Source   It is found in Eastern Himalayas, Sikkim, Bihar and Bengal abundantly.

Chemical Structure   It has been observed that **cucurbitacin B** and E are the most commonly identified principles of these plant sources.

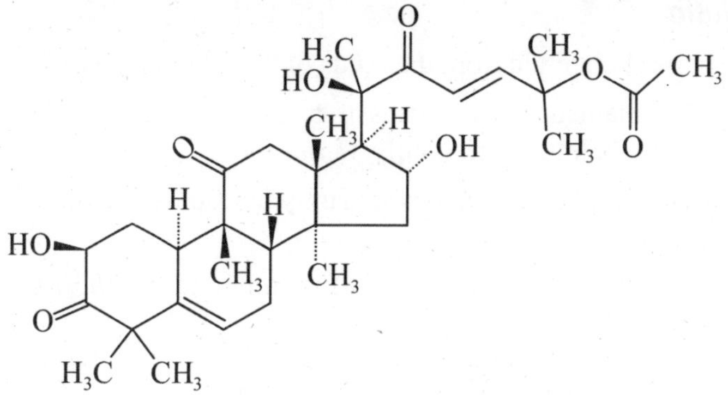

Cucurbitacin-B

Uses

1. It has antineoplastic and anti-gibberellin activity.
2. The plants have been employed as vermifuges, narcotics, emetics and antimalarials.
3. They have also been implicated in sporadic livestock poisoning in South Africa.

5.2.4.2 Quassin

Synonyms   Nigakilactone D; Nortriterpenoid, Quassane.

Biological Source   It is one of the bitter constituents of the wood of *Quassia amara* L., belonging to family *Simaroubaceae,* usually known in commerce as *Surinam quassia.* It is also obtained from the dried wood of *Pierasma quassioldes* Benn., *Picrasma excelsa (Picroena excelsa* or *Aeschrion excelsa)* belonging to family *Simaroubaceae.*

Geographical Source   It is found abundantly in Surinam and Jamaica.

Chemical Structure   It has a **triterpenoid** structure as given below:

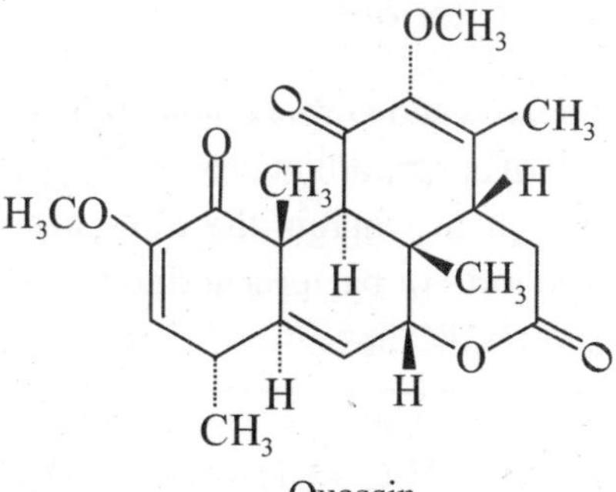

Quassin

Uses

1. Its bitterness threshold is found to be 1: 60,000; and hence used as bitter tonic.
2. It also finds its application as an insecticides and an anthelmintic for the expulsion of threadworms.
3. It is also used as a febrifuge.
4. **Quassin** possesses antifertility activity, thereby inhibiting testosterone secretion of rat Leydig cells.

5.2.4.3 Azadirachitin

It is a **tetranontriterpenoid** obtained from the seeds of the **Neem tree** and the **Chinaberry tree.**

Biological Sources   It is obtained from the seeds of *Azadirachta indica* A. Juss., (*Melia ozadirachta* L.) and *Melia azedarach* L., belonging to family *Meliaceae.*

Geographical Sources   The plant is found abundantly in tropical countries like India, Africa and Burma.

Chemical Structure   Its chemical structure was first reported by *Thornton** in 1993, as shown below:

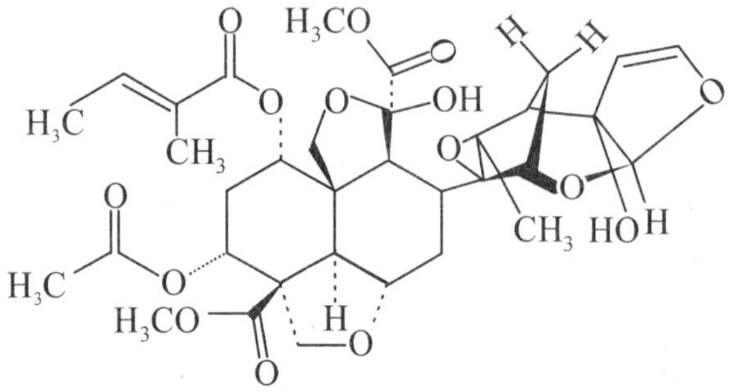

Azadirachtin

Uses

1. It is a highly active feeding deterrent and growth regulator.
2. It is used experimentally as insect control agent.
3. It helps in insect ecdysis and growth inhibition**.

It is, however, pertinent to mention here that the **triterpenoids** which are exclusively used as drugs are described in the chapter on **'Glycosides'**.

5.2.5 Tetraterpenoids and Carotenoids

A plethora of natures yellow, orange, red and purple colours are mostly by virtue of the presence of **carotenoids**. The essentially consist of an important group of C_{40} **tetraterpenoids**. Invariably, there are two specific regions in a living plant wherein the **biogenesis of carotenoids** usually occur, namely: chloroplasts and chromatophores of bacteria and fungi.

There are two characteristic features that have been observed in such types of naturally occurring compounds, namely:

(a) Additional isopentenyl moieties (H_3C—CH=CH—CH_2CH_3) could be embedded onto the tetraterpenoid backbone to result into the formation of either C_{45} or C_{50} carotenoids, as seen in certain microbes.
    Example   **Homocarotenoids**, and

---

* Thornton, M.D., '*Phytochemistry*', **12**, 391, 1973.
** Reimhoed, H, and K.P. Sieber, '*Z. Naturfoesch.*', 36C, 466, 1981.

(b) Oxidation of C_{40} carotenoids aften yields such carotenoids that do possess less than 40 carbon atoms,

Example **Apocarotenoids**

So far nearly 600 **carotenoids** have been duly isolated and identified from naturally occurring sources, such as: plants, bacteria, fungi and marine organisms. The ones obtained from the marine sources are found most abundantly and usually contain acetylenic moieties ($HC\equiv CH$).

Characteristic Features of Carotenoids Some characteristic features of **carotenoids** are enumerated below:

(*i*) Most widely known carotenoids are either simple unsaturated hydrocarbons having the basic lycopene structure or their corresponding oxygenated analogues, usually termed as **Xanthophylls,**

(*ii*) Eight isoprene units are found to be joined head to tail in **lycopene** to give it a conjugated system that eventually is responsible for attributing the chromophoric character to the molecule *i.e.*; producing colour, and

(*iii*) Cyclization of **lycopene** at both terminals of the molecule yields a bicyclic hydrocarbon commonly known as **β-carotenes**, which occur most abundantly in the higher plants.

Interestingly, both in plants and micro-organisms the **carotenoids** have been observed to serve *three* major roles, namely: *first*, as **photosynthetic pigments**; *secondly*, as **photoprotective agents**; and *thirdly*, as **membrane stabilization substances**. In contrast, **carotenoids** in animals serve as a precursor of vitamin A and other retenoids. Besides, they also act not only as cancer preventive agents but also as **photoprotective agents**. Perhaps the protective characteristic features of carotenoids, in general, may be due to the easy accessibility to various singly oxygen atoms and ample free radicals, collectively checking the oxidation damage to cells and catering as **antioxidants.**

With the advent of various innovative aspects of biotechnology a quantum jump in the availability of carotenoid production is very much on the cards.

5.2.5.1 *Vitamin A*

Synonyms Retinol, All-trans-retinol; Oleovitamin A; Biosterol; Lard factor; Vitamin A alcohol; Acon; Afaxin; Agiolan; Atav; Avibon; Avitol; Axerol; Epiteliol; Testanol; Vaflol; Vogan;

It mostly occurs in animals (not in plants) such as: milk fat, fish liver oil. However, the naturally occurring carotenoids are duly converted into **Vitamin A** by the liver. It is mainly extracted from fish liver oils where it invariably occurs in the esterified form.

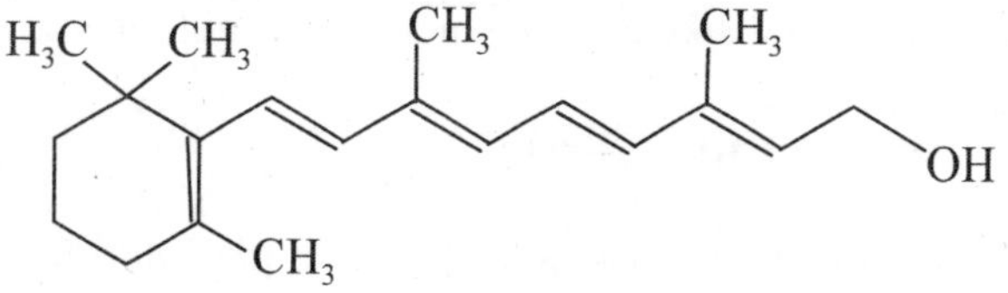

Vitamin-A

However, **total synthesis of Vitamin A** has been accomplished from **β-ionone** and a propargyl halide.

It gets easily absorbed from the normal intestinal tract to the extent of 80-90% and is subsequently stored in body tissues, mostly in the liver. It has been observed that approximately one third of the Vitamin A consumed is usually stored in the body.

The most abundntly found dietary sources of Vitamin A are namely: fish- liver oils (*e.g.*, cod-liver oil); dairy products (*e.g.*, butter, cream, whole milk powder, cheese)., animal organs (*e.g.*, liver, kidney, heart).

Biochemcially, **carotene** and **provitamin A** substances *i.e.*, allied **β-carotenoids** undergo cessation by the presence of **β-carotene oxygenase** in the mucosal cells of the intestine to give rise to **retinal;** and a substantial portion of which is readily gets reduced by NADH to **retinol.**

Uses
1. It is particularly useful in the proper maintenance of vision, growth and tissue differentiation.
2. The vitamin is employed mainly as a prophylactic when there exists an insufficient normal dietary intake
3. It helps in the synthesis of specific **glycoproteins.**

Vitamin A Derivatives   There are *two* important derivatives of **vitamin A** which find there usage in therapeutic domain, namely:

     (*a*) **13-*cis* Retinoic Acid (Synonym**   Isotretinoin; Isotrex; Accutane; Roaccutane).

Uses
1. It is used in acute recalcitrant cystic acne.
2. It is invariably employed in keratinization disorders of the skin, that are mostly preneoplastic.

     (*b*) **All–*trans* Retinoic Acid (Synonyms**   Tretinoin; Vitamin A acid)

All-*trans*-Retinoic Acid

Uses
1. It is generally used for the treatment of acne vulgaris by virtue of the fact that it enhances epidermal cell mitosis and epidermal cell turnover.
2. It is used in several formulations like cream, solution and gel meant for tropical applications.

5.2.6   Volatile Oils (or Essential Oils)

Volatile oils are the odorous and volatile products of various plant and animal species. As they have a tendency to undergo evaporation on being exposed to the air even at an ambient temperature, they are invariably termed as **volatile oils, essential oil** or **ethereal oils.** They mostly contribute to the odorferous constituents or *'essences'* of the aromatic plants that are used abundantly in enhancing the aroma by seasoning of eatables.

The nature has so meticulously provided specialized secretary structures within the plants which are primarily responsible for the generation of volatile constitutents, as shown in the following Table 5.2.

Table 5.2   Specialized Secretary Structures *Vs* Plant Sources

S.No	Specialized Secretary Structures	Biological Source	Family
1.	Glansular hairs	*Lavandula angustifolia* (Lavender oil)	*Lamiaceae*
2.	Oil tubes (or vittae)	*Foeniculum vulgare* (Fennel) *Pimpinella anisum* (Aniseed)	*Apiaceae*
3.	Modified parenchymal cells	*Piper nigrum* (Black pepper)	*Piperaceae*
4.	Schizogenous (or lysigenum) passages	*Pinus palustris* (Pine oil) *Citrus limon* (Lemon oil)	*Rutaceae*

These volatile oils are usually formed by two modes namely; *first*, by hydrolysis of some glycosides; and *secondly*, by the protoplasm directly. It has been observed that the volatile oils are present in different parts of a plant as given in Table 5.3.

Table 5.3   Plant Organs Containing Volatile Oils

S.No	Plant Organs	Biological Source (S)	Family
1.	Petals (Rose oil)	*Rosa gallica; R. alba; R. damascena* and *R. centifolia*	*Rosaceae*
2.	Flowering Tops (Lavender oil)	*Lavandula angustifolia*	*Lamiaceae*
3.	Leaves (Citronella oil)	*Cymbopogon winterianus* and *C. nardus;*	*Poaceae*
4.	Bark (Cinnamon oil)	*Cinnamomum camphora*	*Lauraceae*
5.	Fruit (Caraway oil)	*Carum carvi*	*Apiaceae*
6.	Wood (Pine oil)	*Pinus palustris*	*Pinaceae*
7.	Buds (Clove oil & Chamomile oil)	*Syzygium aromaticum* and *Matricaria chamomilla*	*Compositae*
8.	Rhizomes (Ginger oil & Calamus oil)	*Zingiber officinale, Acorus calamus;*	*Zingiberaceae* *Araceae*
9.	Seeds (Gramis of Paradise & Cardamom)	*Aframonum melegueta* *Elletaria cardamomum*	*Zingiberaceae*

Volatile oils differ from the fixed oils in many respects which may be enumerated below:

S.No	Characteristic Features	Volatile oil	Fixed oil
1.	Chemical Constituents	Mostly consist of terpenoids;	Mostly consist of glyceryl esters of fatty acids;
2.	Spot Test	Does not leave any spot on filter paper	Leaves a permanent grease spot on paper
3.	Saponification Test	Not applicable	Saponifies with alkalies.
4.	Rancidity	Not applicable	Becomes rancid on storage
5.	Exposure to air and light	Easily oxidised and undergo resinification	Not applicable
6.	Fragrance	Distinctly marked and specific	Not applicable

In general, it has been observed that a single volatile oil invariably comprises even more than 200 different chemical components, and mostly the trace constituents are solely responsible for attributing its characteristic flavour and odour.

5.2.6.1 Preparation of Volatile Oils

There are in all *four* established methods whereby the preparation of **volatile oils** from various plant sources may be accomplished, namely:

   (*i*) Direct Steam Distillation,
   (*ii*) Expression,
   (*iii*) Extraction and
   (*iv*) Enzymatic Hydrolysis.

These methods are described in the sections that follows:

5.2.6.1.1   Direct Steam Distillation   In case of direct steam distillation, the freshly cut drug is introduced into the distillation flask. The generated steam is made to pass through the drug material as shown in Fig. 5.1, and the volatile oil content along with the steam on being passed through the water condenser is collected in **Florentine Flasks** of the type FLW or FHW depending on whether the resulting oil is lighter than water or heavier than water.

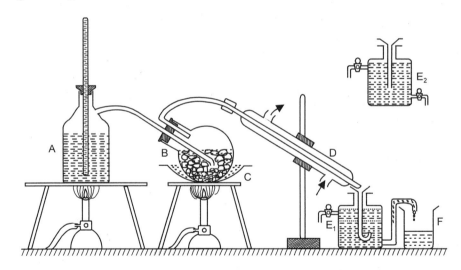

Fig. 5.1   Assembly for Preparation of Volatile Oils by Steam Distillation

The various parts of the assembly for the preparation of **volatile** oils by steam distillation are as follows:

        A = Steam generator (Copper),
        B = Distillation Flask,
        C = Sand bath,
        D = Water condenser,
        E1 = Florentine Flask for **oils lighter than water** (OLW),

E2 = Florentine Flask for **oils heavier than water** (OHW), and

F = Beaker.

Caution   The distillation flask is heated initially to start the process of steam distillation. Once the distillation commences the heat of the steam entering the flask not only maintains the high-temperature required but also in removing the volatile components to the water condenser for ultimate collection in the respective Florentine Flask.

In actual practice, however, there are *three* **different modes of distillation** depending exclusively on the condition of the plant substance, namely:

(*a*) **Water Distillation:** It is mostly applicable to such plant material which is dried initially in air and the constituents are not degraded by boiling upto 100°C.
Example: **Turpentine Oil**—In this instance, the crude turpentine oleoresin is added directly into the distillation flsk and subsequently subjected to distillation.

(*b*) **Water and Steam Distillation:** It is often suitable for such plant material, whether fresh or dried, the constituents of which undergo degradation by direct boiling.
Example: **Clove Oil, Cinnamon Oil**—In this case, the crude drug is first macerated with water for several hours, prior to steam distillation.

(*c*) **Direct Steam Distillation:** It is invariably applicable to fresh drugs that is loaded with sufficient natural moisture and hence no maceration is required.
Example: **Pippermint Oil, Spearmint Oil**—In this instance the freshly cut drug is added directly into the distillation flask prior to steam distillation.

5.2.6.1.2   Expression   A number of volatile oils mostly undergo decomposition on being subjected to distillation. Likewise, volatile oils found in the rind of the fruit, such as: **orange, lemon** and **bergamot peel,** are best obtained by extrusion *i.e.,* by the application of pressure. Even on a commercial scale these oils are produced by extrusion so as to preserve the natural fragrance that otherwise get deteriorated by distillation process.

In actual practice, however, the expression may be accomplished by any one of the *four* following processes, namely:

(*a*) **Sponge Method:** The citrous fruit (*e.g.,* **orange, lemon, grape fruit, bergamot**) is first washed to remove the dirt, and then cut into halves to remove the juice completely. The rind is turned inside out by hand and squeezed when the secretary glands rupture. The oozed volatile oil is collected by means of the sponge and subsequently squeezed in a vessel. The oil floating on the surface is separated.

(*b*) **Scarification Process (Ecuelle a Piquer): Ecuelle a piquer** is a specially designed apparatus (Fig. 5.2) first introduced on the Revieras in France, which is nothing but a large bowl meant for pricking the outer surface of citrous fruits. It is more or less a large funnel made of copper having its inner layer tinned properly. The inner layer has numerous pointed metal needles just long enough to penetrate the epidermis. The lower stem of the apparatus serve two purposes; *first,* as a receiver for the oil; and *secondly,* as a handle. Now, the freshly washed lemons are placed in the bowl and rotated repeatedly when the oil glands are punctured (scarified) thereby discharging the oil right into the handle. The liquid, thus collected, is transferred to another vessel, where on keeping the clear oil may be decanted and filtered.

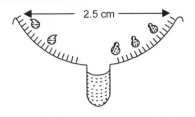

Fig. 5.2   Ecuelle a Piquer

(c) **Raspings Process:** In this process the outer surface of the peel of citrous fruits containing the oil gland is skillfully removed by a grater. The **'raspings'** are now placed in horsehair bags and pressed strongly so as to ooze out the oil stored in the oil glands. Initially, the liquid has a turbid appearance but on allowing it to stand the oil separates out which may be decanted and filtered subsequently.

(d) **Mechanical Process:** A substantial quantum of volatile oil across the globe is now prepared by various mechanical means solely based on the above principles. However, the use of heavy duty centrifugal devices may also be incorporated so as to ease the separation of oil/ water emulsions invariably formed. It is pertinent to mention here that with the advent of modern mechanical devices the oil out put has increased appreciably and the older methods have only remained for the sake of history.

5.2.6.1.3   Extraction   The extraction process is particularly useful for such plant sources which either contain very small amount of volatile oils or the oil contents are extremely succeptible to decomposition by the exposure to steam. In such cases the recovery of volatile oils is not commercially feasible.

Examples: Volatile oils obtained from various flowers like **Jasmine** *(Jasminum officinale* Linn. Ver *grandiflorum* Bailey: family – *Oleaceae);* **Sweat violet** *(Violaodorata* Linn, family – *Violaceae);* **Gardenia** *(Gardenia lucida* Roxb., family – *Rubiaceae);* **Acacia** *(Acacia farnesiana* Willd., family– *Leguminosae);* **Narcissus** *(Narcissus tazetta* Linn., family –*Amaryllidaceae)*; and **Mimosa** *(Mimosa pudia* Linn., family – *Leguminosae).*

In general, the **extraction of volatile oil** from natural sources is carried out by *two* different methods, namely:

(i) Extraction with volatile solvents *e.g.,* Hexane, Benzene and

(ii) Extraction with non-volatile solvents *e.g.,* Tallow, Lard, Olive oil

These two extraction processes shall be discussed briefly in the sections that follows:

5.2.6.1.3.1   Extraction with Volatile Solvents   The plant material containing the volatile oil is usually extracted with a low boiling volatile solvent, such as n-hexane, benzene, petroleum ether etc., either by adopting the method of hot continuous extraction (Soxhlet extraction) or by percolation. The resulting volatile oil containing solvent is removed under reduced pressure when the volatile oil will remain in the flask.

Advantages   There are several advantages of this process, namely:

1. It is possible to maintain an uniform temperature (usually 50°C) during most of these extractions which ultimately ensures the retention of a more intense and natural fragrance which otherwise cannot be achieved by distillation (perhaps due to chemical degradation of constitutents).

2. **Floral Concretes:** The ultimate concentrated and purified volatile oils are collectively designated as **'floral concretes'**. In actual practice, these floral concretes represent an admixture of natural odoriferous components of flowers, plant waxes, colour pigments and certain albuminous material. Hence, most of them are solid in consistency and partly soluble in 95% alcohol.

5.2.6.1.3.2 Extraction with Non-Volatile Solvents This process is usually employed for the preparation of the finest brands of perfume oil *i.e.*, the natural flower oils. In this instance, the volatile oil content usually present in the fresh plant sources eg., flower petals, is so scanty that oil removal is not commercially viable by any other methods. *Grassein* Southern France, is the well-known centre for the extraction of **flower volatile oil** in the world.

There are *three* methods that are used for the **extraction of volatile oils** from flowers with non-volatile solvents, namely:

(*i*) Enfleurage Method,
(*ii*) Pneumatic Method, and
(*iii*) Meceration Method.

These methods would be described briefly as under.

(*a*) **Enfleurage Method:** A thick layer of molten lard and tallow (beef fat) is applied on either surfaces of pre-cleaned glass plates that are securely placed in a covered wooden frame (or the chasis) Each glass plate is liberally sprinkled with fresh flower petals to cover its top surface only. These plates are now stacked one over the other and enclosed in the wooden frame, whereby each layer of the flower shall be enclosed between two layers of the fat. Such batteries of loaded plates are allowed to remain for 24hours, after which the flowers are removed and recharged with fresh lots. This very process is repeated religiously for several weeks till the fatty layers appear to be fully saturated with the essential oils of the flowers or until a certain desired concentration of it is accomplished.
Example: Jasmine *flowers*—The whole process lasts nearly seventy days.

The flowers are subsequently removed (**defleurage**) and the fat is separated carefully and stirred with absolute alcohol. The latter will dissolve the volatile oil portion thereby leaving the former undissolved in alcohol. The alcoholic extract is reasonably chilled and filtered to get rid off any traces of residual fat. Three successive extraction procedures are repeated so as to affect the complete recovery of volatile oil and the resulting solution is employed as such in the *perfume industry* and is commonly termed as the **'Tripple Extract'**.

The volatile oil may be recovered from the **'Triple Extract'** by anyone of the following methods, namely: *first*, fractional distillation under vacuum at 0°C; *secondly*, evaporation under vacuum at 0°C; *thirdly*, the alcoholic extract is diluted with water and saturated with NaCl, when the oil will seaparate with the retention of fresh natural ordour.

(*b*) **Pneumatic Method:** The basic principle of this method is very much like the **'enfleurage method'**. In this particular instance, the current of warm-air is made to pass through the flowers , and the subsequent air loaded with suspended volatile oil particles is then routed through a fine spray of molten fat in a closed chamber wherein the volatile oil gets absorbed promptly, and

(c) **Maceration Method:** The fresh flower petals are gently and carefully heated in molten fat (lard, tallow, or fixed oil), stirred frequently until complete exhaustion takes place. The flowers are then strained, squeezed and the exuded fat is returned to the main bulk of the fat, unless and until a desired concentration is achieved. The volatile oil containing fat is allowed to cool and is recovered by three successive extractions with absolute alcohol.

5.2.6.1.4   Enzymatic Hydrolysis   It has been observed that the volatile oil is normally found in plant substances in the form of odourless glycosidal combinations. However, the odoriferous components are liberated free only by hydrolysis of such aforesaid **glycosides**. A few typical examples of such volatile components are given below:

5.2.6.1.4.1   Volatile Oil of Bitter Almond (Benzaldehyde)   It is found to be present in the kernels of bitter almond in the form of the glyoside **amygdalin:**

Amygdalin   Benzaldehyde

5.2.6.1.4.2   Volatile Oil of Black Mustard   The volatile oil component is present is *allyl isothiocyanate* in the form of the naturally occurring glycosides **sinigrin:**

Sinigrin   Allyl Isothio-   Glucose
                        cyanate

5.2.6.1.4.3   Eugenol   It occurs invariably in the form of glycosides combination as **gein** present in the roots of *Geum urbanum* Linn. belonging to family *Rosaceae.*

Gein   Eugenol   Glucose

5.2.6.1.4.4 Methyl Salicyalate It is found to occur in the form of glycosidal combination as **gaultherin** (*Synonym:* monotropin or monotropitiside) in the leaves of *Gaultheria procumbens* Linn. belonging to family *Ericaceae*. The glycosides **gaultherin** undergoes hydrolysis in the presence of the enzyme *gautherase* to yield the aglycone methyl salicylate and the corresponding sugars glucose and xylose.

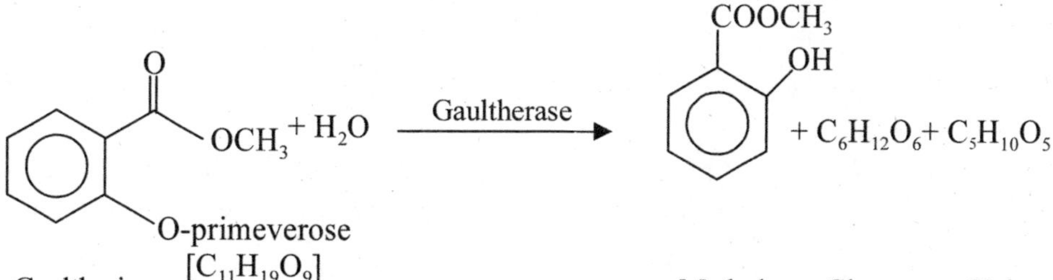

Gaultherin $[C_{11}H_{19}O_9]$ O-primeverose

Gaultherase

Methyl Salicylate   Glucose   Xylose

$+ C_6H_{12}O_6 + C_5H_{10}O_5$

5.2.6.2 Quantitative Determination of Volatile Oil in a Plant Material

The necessity to determine the volatile oil quantitatively from a plant material is mostly accomplished by a specially designed apparatus , which helps in ascertaining the raw material to be employed for commercial production. Such a determination is also extremely helpful in establishing and appraising the quality of spices and **oleoresins**.

Clavenger devised an apparatus to determine the volatile oils which essentially has several advantages, namely: (*a*) **Compactness in size,** (*b*) **Cohobation of distillation waters,** and (*c*) **Reasonably accurate estimation of volatile oil content by employing relatively smaller quantum of the raw material.** However, the apparatus also possesses an additional merit for *steam-rectification* of small quantities of essential oils.

Apparatus It consists of a round bottomed flask of varying capacity from 1 L to 2 L which is provided with a hanging type heating mantle and regulator. The mouth of the round bottomed flask is connected with a specifically designed trap to collect the volatile oil which could be either heavier than water or lighter than water as shown in Figure 5.3.

The various vital components of the apparatus for the **quantitative estimation of volatile oils** are as follows:

A = RB–flask,
B = Heating Mantle (Hanging type),
C = Drug and water
D = Bend insulted with asbestos/ cotton pad
E = Water condenser
F = Inlet – for water
G = Outlet – for water
H = Volatile oil collected in a graduated stem
 I = Excess water reintroduced in round bottomed flask

Methodology A known weight of the drug either as such powdered or cut into small pieces is introduced into the round bottomed corning flask (1 L or 2 L capacity) along with a distillation

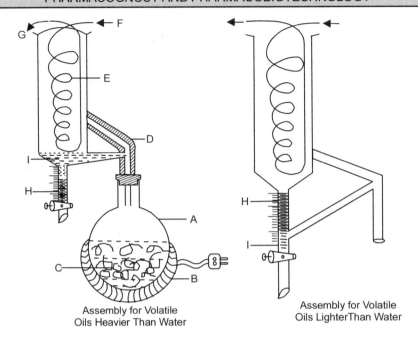

Assembly for Volatile
Oils Heavier Than Water

Assembly for Volatile
Oils LighterThan Water

Fig. 5.3   Apparatus for Quantitative Estimation of Volatile Oils

medium which often is fresh water or a mixture of water and glycerin. The quantity of this medium is usually 3 to 6 times the weight of the drug substance. The distillation is done for about 5-6 hours. The distillate is collected in a specially designed trap (or receiver). The stem of which is graduated upto 5 ml with each ml mark is subdivided into 1/10 the ml. In case, the volatile oil is heavier than water the trap on the left hand side of Fig. 5.3 is used; and when the volatile oil is lighter than water the trap on the right hand side is employed.

5.2.6.3   Physical Characteristics of Voltaile Oils

It is a well known fact that the volatile oils usually differ from each other with regard to their chemical constitutions. However, they invariably possess a number of physical characteristics as stated below, namely:

(a) **Odour:** Most volatile oils do possess very pleasant and characteristic odour which vary considerably from one specimen to another.

Detection   When a drop of the volatile oil is soaked on a filter paper, an expert may judge its quality and genuinity and may also differentiate between the authentic pure sample from the adulterated one by their individual odours.

(b) **Nature:** In general, the volatile oils are mobile liquids at ordinary temperatures. However, there are a few exceptions, for instance:
(i) **Anise Oil:** It solidifies at 15°C and melts at 17°C,
(ii) **Rose Oil:** It solidifies at 17°C and melts at 19°C, and

(*iii*) **Oil of Mentha and Oil of Thyme:** They distinctly deposit a solid substance upon chilling *i.e.*, menthol and thymol respectively, and leaving behind a liquid portion as a 'mother liquor'. The former is termed as **"Stearoptene"** and the latter is known as **"Oleoptene".**

(*c*) **Volatility:** The essential oils are mostly volatile completely, with the exception of a few of them *e.g.*, **'oil of lemon', 'oil of orange',** that contain also an additional non-volatile substance of gummy nature. Both the volatile and their pure components do possess high vapour pressures, and hence evaporate completely and rapidly when exposed to atmosphere.

Detection Volatile oils do not leave a stain when soaked on a piece of filter paper, whereas a fixed oil does. Thus, it also checks its adulteration.

(*d*) **Colour:** Invariably, the colour of freshly obtained volatile oils are more or less colourless, but on prolonged storage they usually undergo both oxidation and resinification thereby rendering it dark in colour. The darkened volatile oil can be redistilled to obtain once again the colourless sample.

Prevention The volatile oils must be stored in a cool, dry place and preferably filled upto the brim in amber glass bottle having an airlight stopper.

(*e*) **Refractive Index:** The refractive index of volatile oils vary from 1.42 to 1.61. They are mostly characterized by high refractive indices.

Detection The pure authentic volatile oils have definite refractive index as specified in official compendia, whereas the adulterated oils will show different values.

(*f*) **Optical Rotation:** A large number of volatile oils exhibit optical activity by virtue of the chemical constitution of the oil(s) or its constitution. It gives some vital informations with regard to the source and anthenticity of the oil sample, namely:

(*i*) Both optical rotation and specific rotation offer a fairly dependable and reliable clue whether the volatile oil is either genuine or adulterated,

(*ii*) It also establishes the source and variety of the volatile oil, for instance: **American oil of Turpentine is dextro-,** whereas the French oil of **Turpentine is levo-,** and

(*iii*) It ascertains whether the chemical constituent is either isolated from the volatile oil or obtained synthetically, for example: **Menthol** isolated from **pippermint oil** is exclusively *levo*-rotatory, whereas the **synthetic menthol** could be either *racemic or levo*. Likewise, the natural camphor is *dextro,* whereas the synthetic one could be either *racemic* or *levo.*

(*g*) **Specific Gravity:** The specific gravity of volatile oils ranges between 0.8 to 1.17. Interestingly, the volatile oil listed in various official compendia are lighter than water (*i.e.*, specific gravity less than 1), such as: **Oil of Anise** d_{25}^{25} 0.978-0.988; **Oil of Balm** d_{15}^{15} 0.89-0.925; **Oil of Basil** d_{20}^{20} 0.905-0.930; **Oil of Bergamot** d_{25}^{25} 0.875-0.880 etc. In contrast, there are certain volatile oils whose specific gravity is more than 1 *i.e.*, these are heavier than water, for instance: **Oil of Cherry Laurel** d_{20}^{20} 1.054-1.066; **Oil of Cinnamon** d_{25}^{25} 1.045-1.063; **Oil of Clove** d_{25}^{25} 1.038-1.060; **Oil of Garlic** d_{15}^{15} 1.055-1.098; **Oil of Parsley** d_{15}^{15} 1.040-1.100; **Oil of Sasaafras** d_{25}^{25} 1.065-1.077 etc.

(*h*) **Solubility:** The majority of volatile oils are immiscible with water, but are soluble in absolute alcohol and several other organic solvents *e.g.*, ether, chloroform, carbon disulphide, acetone, hexane, ethyl acetate etc.

Exceptions

(*i*) **Oil of Rose** gives a turbid solution due to the very presence of paraffin hydrocarbons that are very sparingly soluble in alcohol, and

(*ii*) Many a times certain volatile oils on being dissolved in organic solvents render them turbid due to the presence of traces of moisture which may be eliminated by treating the volatile oil with a small amount of powdered anhydrous sodium sulphate crystals.

In addition to the above stated physical parameters there are certain other equally valuable and important characteristic data for the identification as well as detection of adulteration in a sample of volatile oil, namely: **boiling range, flash point, evaporation residue, molecular refraction** and the like.

5.2.6.4 *Chemical Characteristics of Volatile Oils*

It has been observed that plethora of volatile oils are found to be more or less *'complex mixtures'* essentially comprising of different class of chemical constituents. Therefore, they are found to vary widely in the chemical composition and *vis-à-vis* their therapeutic applications.

However, there are a few exceptions to the above observation wherein only one chemical entity is solely present in the naturally occurring volatile oil namely:

(*a*) **Oil of Bitter Almond**—contains *benzaldehyde* exclusively, and

(*b*) **Oil of Winter Green**—contains *methyl salicylate* exclusively

In fact, there are more than 500 different chemical compounds that have been duly isolated, purified and identified in volatile oils over the years with the advent of most sophisticated physico-chemical methods of analysis, such as: **UV-visible spectroscopy, IR-Spectroscopy, NMR – spectrometry, GC – analysis, HPLC–analysis, Mass spectrometry, X-ray diffraction analysis, optical rotary dispersion (ORD) analysis, HPTLC** and the like.

The chemical constituents of volatile oils are recognized as **'terpenes'** that may contain one or several **isoprene units** as shown below:

Myrcene	Limonene	۞-Pinene
Acyclic Monoterpene	Monocyclic Terpene	Bicyclic Monoterpene
(2-Isoprene Units)	(2-Isoprene Units)	(2-Isoprene Units)

A few examples of some **terpene hydrocarbons** are summarized below:

Group	Emperical Formula	Isoprene Units	Example
Hemiterpene	C_5H_8	01	Isoprene
Monoterpene			
Acyclic	$C_{10}H_{16}$	02	Myrcene
Monocyclic	$C_{10}H_{16}$	02	Limonene
Bicyclic	$C_{10}H_{16}$	02	α-Pinene
Sesquiterpene	$C_{15}H_{44}$	03	Santalene
Diterpene	$C_{20}H_{32}$	04	Resin of Turpentine
Triterpene	$C_{30}H_{48}$	06	Saponins
Polyterpene	$(C_5H_8)_n$	∞..............	Rubber

Phenylpropanoids   There is another major class of volatile oil constituents that invariably contains a C_6 phenyl ring and an attached C_3-propane side chain.

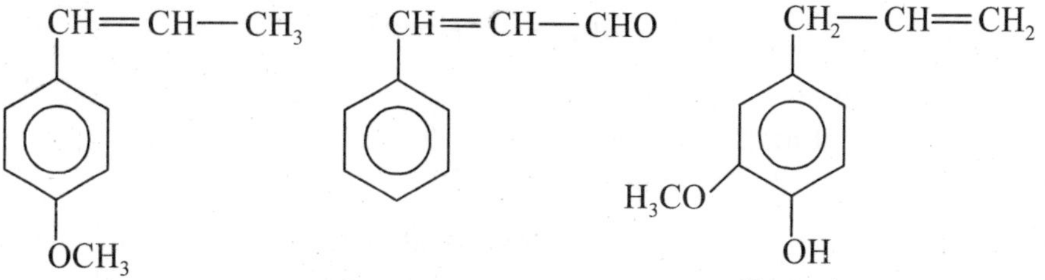

Anethole	Cinnamaldehyde	Eugenol
(Anise Oil)	(Cinnamon Oil)	(Clove Oil)

5.2.6.5   Classification of Volatile Oils

The most acceptable classification whereby volatile oils and volatile-oil containing drugs may be grouped together are as follows, namely:

 (*i*) Hydrocarbon volatile oils,
 (*ii*) Alcohol volatile oils,
 (*iii*) Aldehyde volatile oils,
 (*iv*) Ketone volatile oils,
 (*v*) Phenol volatile oils,
 (*vi*) Phenolic ether volatile oils,
 (*vii*) Oxide volatile oils, and
 (*viii*) Ester volatile oils.

These volatile oils shall be discussed in the sections that follows.

5.2.6.5.1   Hydrocarbon Volatile Oils   It has been observed that **terpene hydrocarbons** usually occur in most of the volatile oils obtained from natural sources. They may be further classified into *three* categories, namely:

 (*a*) Unsaturated acyclic hydrocarbons,
 (*b*) Aromatic hydrocarbons, and
 (*c*) Alicyclic hydrocarbons.

5.2.6.5.1A   Unsaturated Acyclic Hydrocarbons   Two typical examples of chemical constituents belonging to the category of **unsaturated acyclic hydrocarbons** are given below:

(*i*) β-Myrcene

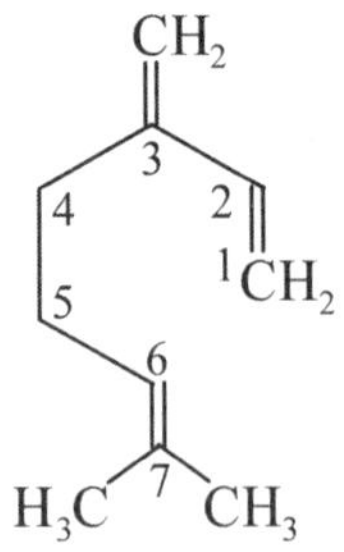

β-Myrcene

Chemical Structure   It is 7-methyl-3-methylene-1, 6-octadiene.

Occurance   It is found in several essential oils, such as: **Oil of Bay** (or Myrcia oil) – *Myrcia acris* (Family : *Myricaceae);* **Oil of Hops** – *Humulus lupulus* Linn., (family: *Moraceae);* and **Oil of Turpentine** – *Pinus logifolia* Roxb., (family: *Pinaceae*).

Isolation   The **oil of bay** is treated with sodium hydroxide solution and the remaining undissolved portion which mostly contains myrcene, is repeatedly subjected to fractional distillation under vacuo (it is also obtained by pyrolysis of **β-pinene**).

Characteristic Features   It has a pleasant odour. It is lighter than water d_4^{20} 0.794, n_D^{20} 1.4709 and UV_{max} (ethanol): 226 nm (ε16, 100). It is practically insoluble in water, but soluble in alcohol, chloroform, ether and glacial acetic acid.

Identification

   (*a*) **β-Myrcene** on reduction with sodium and alcohol (absolute) gives rise to **dihydromyrcene** ($C_{10}H_{18}$) which on subsequent bromination yields **tetrabromodihydromyrcene** (mp 88°C), and

   (*b*) It readily forms addition compounds with α-naphthoquinone (mp 80-81.5°C) and with maleic anhydride (mp 34-35°C).

Use   It is used as an intermediate in the manufacture of perfumery chemicals.

(*ii*) Ocimene (or *trans*-β-Ocimene)

Chemical Structure   It is 2,6 dimethyl 2,5,7 octatriene.

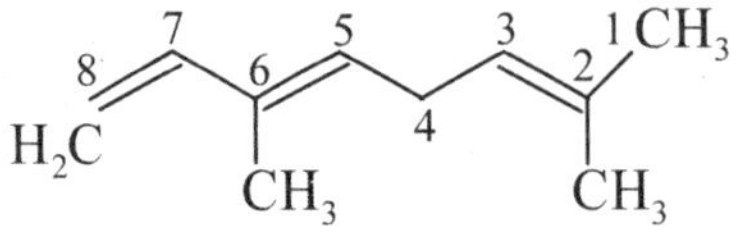

trans-β-Ocimene

Occurrence   *trans*-β Ocimene is found in the volatile oil obtained from the leaves of *Ocimum basilium L.,* (*Labiatae*); *Baronia dentigeroides* Cheel (*Rutaceae*); *Litsea zeylanica* C & T Nees (*Lauraceae*) and *Homoranthus flavescens* A. Cunn., (*Myrtaceae*).

Isolation The volatile oil obtained from the fresh leaves of *O. basilicum* is treated first with NaOH solution to get rid of the phenolic constituents i.e; *eugenol* present in the range of 30-40% of the oil. The undissolved fraction of the oil is taken up in an appropriate solvent, solvent removed under vacuum and the resulting volatile oil is subjected to fractionation under vacuum so as to obtain the desired main constituent.

Characteristic Features

trans-β-Ocimene : d_4^{20} 0.799; n_D^{20} 1.4893; UV_{max} (ethanol) 232 nm (ε 27, 600)

cis-β-Ocimene : d_4^{20} 0.799; n_D^{20} 1.4877; UV_{max} (ethanol) 237.5nm (ε 21, 000)

The **Ocimene** (*trans-* or *cis-*) undergo oxidation most readily and with relatively shorter exposure to air to form a yellow resin. However, in an atmosphere free from oxygen ocimene may be preserved unaltered. Its bp ranges between 176-178°C (decomposes).

Identification

(*a*) Reduction with sodium and absolute alcohol yields **dihydromyrcene** which on bromination yields **tetrabromodihydromyrcene** (mp 88°C),

(*b*) It yields ocimenol – an alcohol on hydration with sulphuric acid (50%) in glacial acetic acid solution,

(*c*) Its phenylurethane derivative has mp 72 °C, and

(*d*) Ocimene upon oxidation with $KMnO_4$ in alkaline solution affects complete degradation to form acids, the lead salts of which has a rhombic crystalline form, whereas the corresponding lead salts of myrcene treated in a similar fashion has a needle form thereby differentiating between **ocimene** and **myrcene** distinctly.

Uses It is used in perfumery.

5.2.6.5.1B Aromatic Hydrocarbons A typical example of aromatic hydrocarbon is that of **para-cymene** as detailed below:

(*i*) *para*-Cymene

Chemical Structure It is 1-methyl-4 (1-methyl ethyl) benzene (*Syn:* Dolcymene)

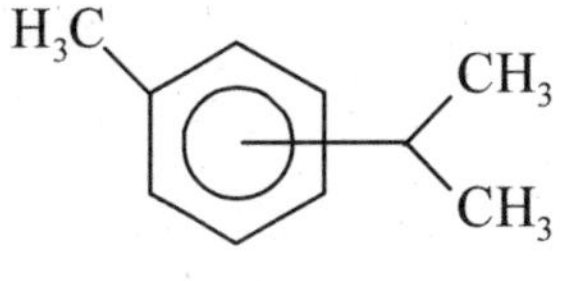

para-Cymeme

Occurrence It occurs in a number of essential oils, such as: oils of lemon, nutmeg, corriander, cinnamon, sage and thyme. *p*-**Cymene** has been reported in a number of volatile oils either due to conversion from cyclic terpenes *e.g.*, **pinene** or **terpinene** or from various terpene analogues *e.g.*, citral, carvone, sabinol etc.

Isolation The *p*-cymene fraction obtained by the fractional distillation of volatile oils may be freed from terpenes having identical boiling points by subjecting it to oxidation with cold $KMnO_4$

solution, whereby the former being resistant to the oxidising agent is recovered in its pure form. However, pure *p*-cymene may be prepared from **thymol**.

Characteristic Features *para*-**Cymene** is a colourless liquid and is found to be inactive optically. Its fragrance resembles to that of the aromatic hydrocarbons closely.

Identification

(*a*) Its boiling point is 177.10°C.

(*b*) It melts at –67.94°C.

(*c*) Its specific density d_4^{20} 0.8573 and d_4^{25} 0.8533.

(*d*) Its specific rotation n_D^{20} 1.4909 and n_D^{25} 1.4885.

(*e*) *p*-**Cymene** on oxidation with hot concentrated potassium permanganate solution gives rise to *p*-hydroxy- isopropylbenzoic acid having a melting point 155-156°C.

Uses

(*i*) It is employed in the formulation of certain imitation (artificial) essential oils.

(*ii*) It is used profusely for the preparation of scented soaps and toileteries.

(*iii*) It also finds its application in the masking of undesirable odours.

5.2.6.5.1 Alicyclic Hydrocarbon The alicyclic hydrocarbons are also termed as **'monoterpenes'** *or* **'true terpenes'** having the emperical formula $C_{10}H_{16}$. Generally, they may be classified into *two* categories, namely:

(*i*) Monocyclic Terpenes, and

(*ii*) Bicyclic Monoterpenes

These two types of alicyclic hydrocarbons shall be discussed individually with some typical examples as under:

A. Monocyclic Terpenes

Basically, the cyclic terpenes are the extended structural homologues of *cyclohexane* usually derived by varying extent of dehydrogenation. The parent molecule is **methyl-isopropyl cyclohexane** (or *para*-**Menthane**)

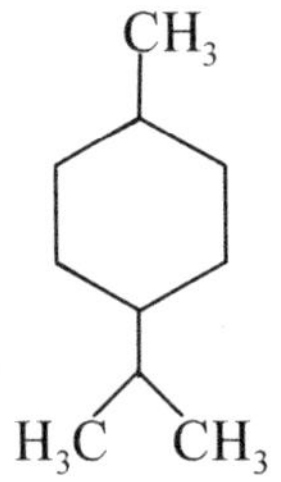

para-Menthane

The structure of the monocyclic terpenes is expressed with reference to the saturated parent substance **'menthane'** *i.e.*; **hexahydrocymene**. Consequently, the three **isomeric menthanes** viz; *ortho-, meta- and para-*, theoretically yield the **monocyclic terpenes** respectively.

A number of isomere that have been derived form various degree of dehydrogenation of *p*-menthane resulting into the formation of a series of *p*-menthenes are given on page 255:

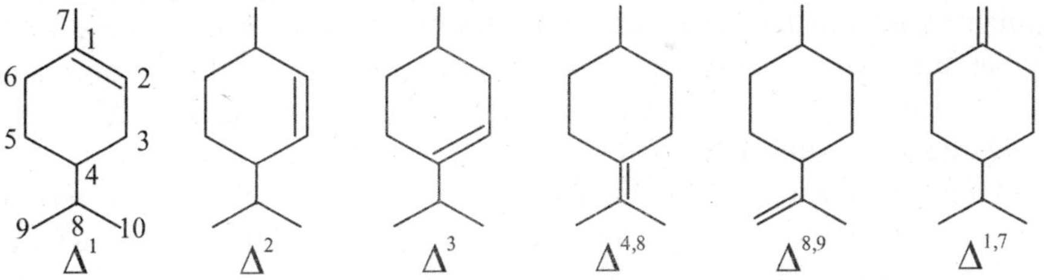

para-Menthenes

Interestingly, all the six different species of menthenes have been systematically characterized and identified. However, the most important and abundantly found in various essential oils is Δ^3 menthene, which is observed as a natural constituent of thymol oil and is very closely related to menthol, the main constituent of **pippermint oil.**

Furthermore, the subsequent dehydrogenation of ***para*-menthane** yields correspondingly the **dihydro-*p*-cymenes,** also termed as ***para*-menthadienes.**

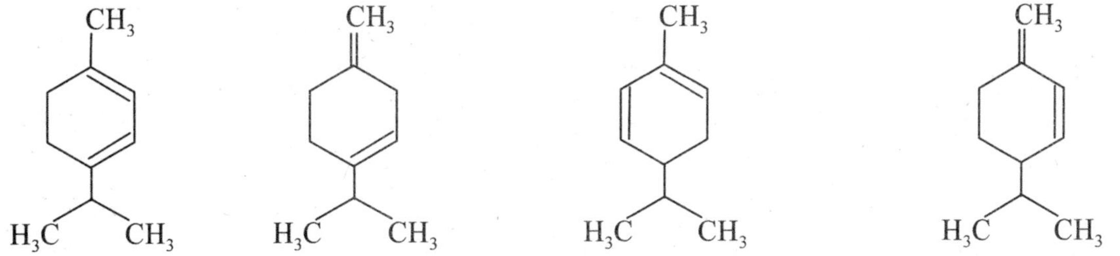

		∝-Phellandrene ($\Delta^{1,5}$)		β-Phellandrene ($\Delta^{1(7),2}$)	
∝-Terpenene ($\Delta^{1,3}$)	β-Terpenene ($\Delta^{1,7}$)	*l-Form*	*d-Form*	*l-Form*	*d-Form*
bp173.5–174.8°;	bp173.–174.°;	bp$_{16}$ 58–59°	bp$_{16}$ 66–68°	bp$_{12}$ 53°	bp$_{11}$57°
$d_4^{19.6}$ 0.8375	d_4^{22} 0.838	d_4^{20}0.8410	d_4^{25}0.8463	d_{15}^{15} 0.8497	d_4^{20} .8520
n_D^{20} 1.4784	n_D^{22} 1.4754	n_D^{20} 1.4709	n_D^{25} 1.4777	n_D^{20} 1.4800	n_D^{20} 1.4788

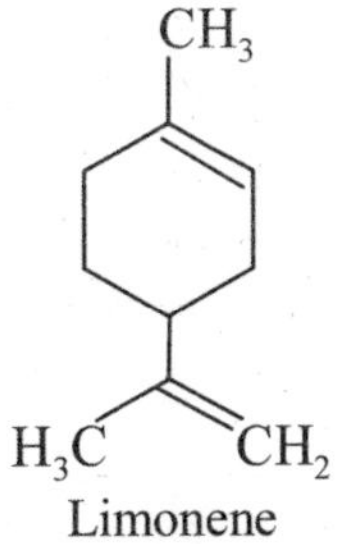

Limonene
($\Delta^{1,8(9)}$)

l-Form	*d-Form*
bp$_{763}$ 175.5–176.5°	bp$_{763}$ 175.5–176°
$d_4^{20.5}$ 0.8407	d_4^{21} 0.8402
n_D^{21} 1.4740	n_D^{21} 0.14743

There are *five* important members belonging to this particualr group, namely: **α-terpene, β-terpene, α-phellandrene, β-phellandrene** and **limonene** that are very frequently found in a variety of essential oils.

It is pertinent to mention here that the alicyclic (cyclic) hydrocarbons are invariably found to be more stable than the corresponding acyclic hydrocarbons. Nevertheless, the **monocylic terpenes** usually undergo isomerization, oxidation and polymerisation very rapidly especially when these are subjected to distillation at atmospheric pressure.

Bearing in mind the diagnostic and therapeutic efficacies of the **monocyclic terpernes** one has to consider the possibility that certain structural configurations like: **geometrical isomerism, stereoisomerism, boat and chair form of isomers** do exist amongst them as depicted below:

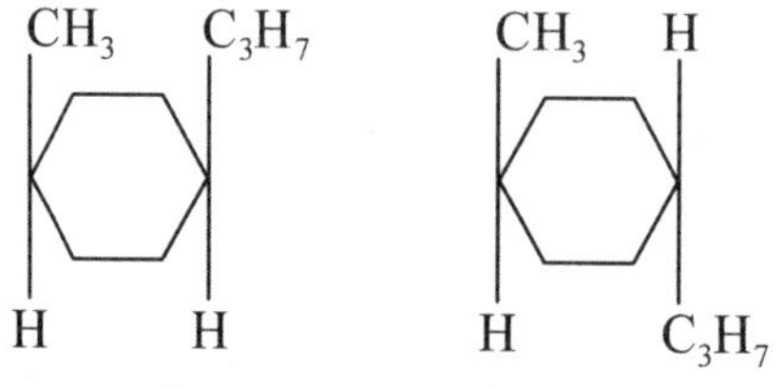

cis-Isomer   *trans*-Isomer

[Geometrical isomers]

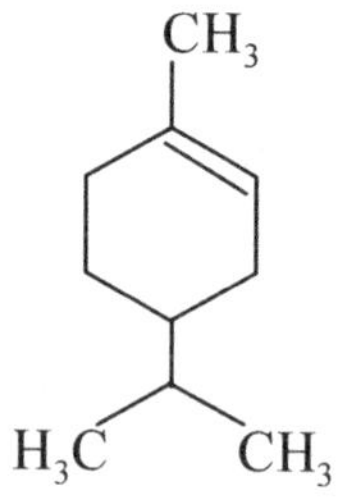

para-Menthene(Δ^1)
–a mixture of *d*-, *l*-and *dl*-forms
[Steroisomers]

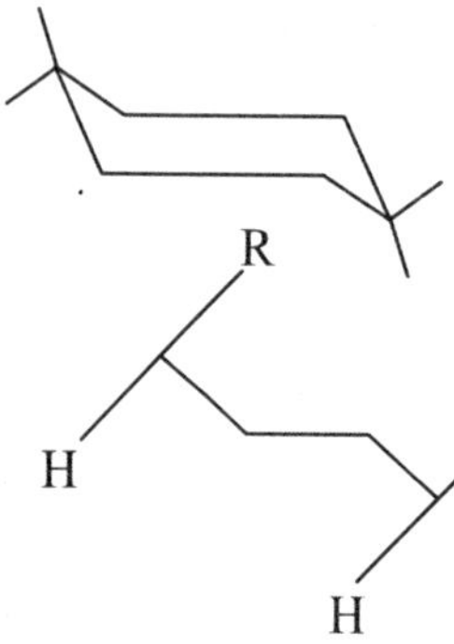

'Chair'-Form 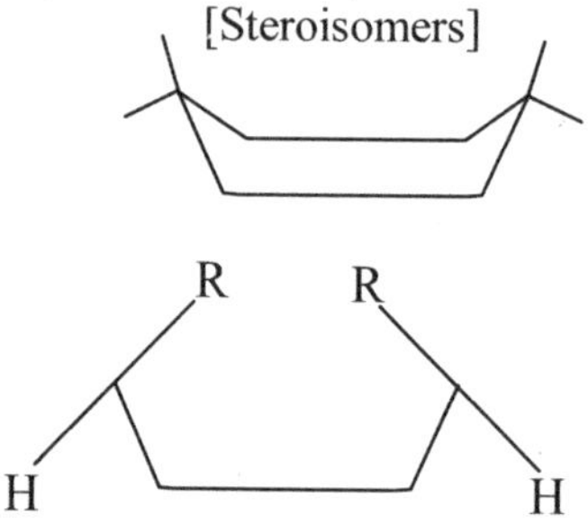   'Boat'-Form

A few typical examples of the **'monocyclic terpenes'** are described here under:

(*i*) Limonene

Chemical Structure   It is 1-methyl-4-(1-methyl ethynyl) cyclohexane (Synonym: Cinene, Cajeputene, Kautschin)

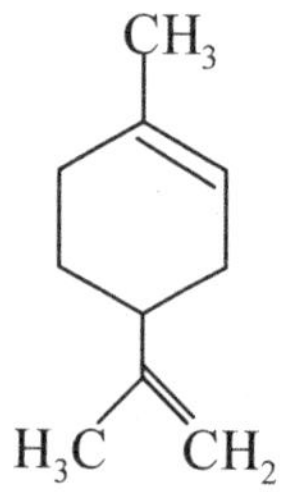

Limonene

Occurrence   It occurs in various ethereal oil, specially oils of lemon, orange, caraway, dill and bergamot. It is also found in grapefruit, bitter orange, mandarin, fennel, neroli and celery.

Isolation **d-Limonene** is isolated from the **mandarin peel oil*** (*Citrus reticulata Blanco, Rutaceae*). It may also be isolated from the ethereal oils of lemon, orange, caraway and bergamot either by careful *fractional* distillation under reduced pressure (vauum) or *via* the preparation of adducts, such as: tetrabromides (mp 104-105°C) and the desired hydrocarbon may be regenerated with the help of pure zinc powder and acetic acid.

Characteristic Features It is colourless liquid having a pleasant lemon-like odour. It is practically insoluble in water but miscible with alcohol. **Limonene** when protected from light and air is reasonably stable, otherwise it undergoes oxidation rapidly. When it is heated with mineral acids, the former gets converted to **terpentine** and to some extent *p*-cymene. On the contrary , the action of mineral acids on limonene in cold yields **terpin hydrate** and **terpineol** (alcohols) due to hydration. However, limonene could be regenerated from these alcohols upon heating. The racemic mixture *i.e.* *dl*–**limonene** is also termed as **dipentene (inactive limonene)**, which on being treated with HCl in the presence of moisture yields **dipentene dihydrochloride** (mp 50-51°C) from methanol. Dehydrogenation of dipentene or limonene with sulphur rapidly yields *p*-cymene. Autoxidation of limonene gives rise to **carveol** and **carvone** which may be observed in poorly stored orange oils by a distinct and marked caraway like odour.

Carveol   Carvone

Identification

(*a*) **Limonene** on bromination yields tetrabromide derivative which is crystallized from ethyl acetate (mp 104-105°C).

(*b*) It forms monohalides with dry HCl or HBr, and the corresponding dihalides with aqueous HCl or HBr.

(*c*) Its nitrosochloride derivative** serves as an useful means of identification having mp ranging between 103-104°C.

Uses

(*i*) It is used in the manufacture of resins.

(*ii*) It is employed as a wetting and dispersing agent.

(*iii*) It is widely employed for scenting cosmetics, soaps as well as for flavouring pharmaceutical preparations.

---

* Kugler Kovate, *Helv Chim Acta,* **46,** 1480, 1963
** Prepared by the action of amyl nitrite and hydrochloric acid

(*ii*) Sylvestrene

Chemical Structure

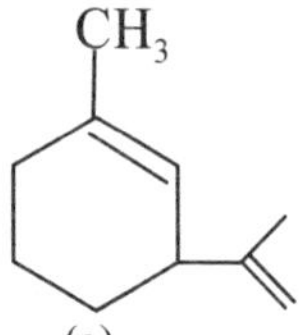

(a)	(b)
$\Delta^{1,8(9)}$ *meta*-Menthadiene	Δ *meta*-Menthadiene

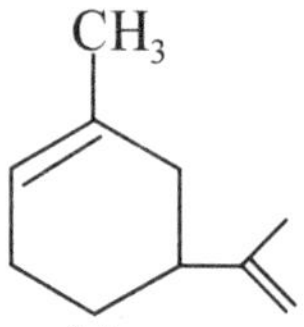

Sylvestrene is generally found to be a mixture of two hydrocarbons (*a*) and (*b*) as shown above, wherein one of these forms predominates over the other. It is mostly available as its *d*-and *l*-isomers; whereas the racemic mixture is known as **carvestrene.**

Occurrence   It is observed that **sylvestrene** does not occur as a *natural product*, but it is obtained from either of the two **bicyclic monoterpene hydrocarbons,** namely: **3-Carene** and **4-Carene,** during the course of its isolation from the respective dihyrochloride.

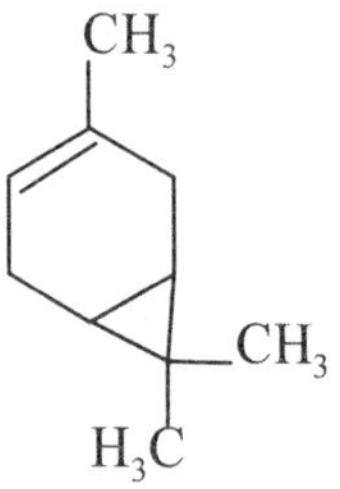

4,7,7-Trimethyl-3-norcarene;
Δ^3-Carene;
3-Carene

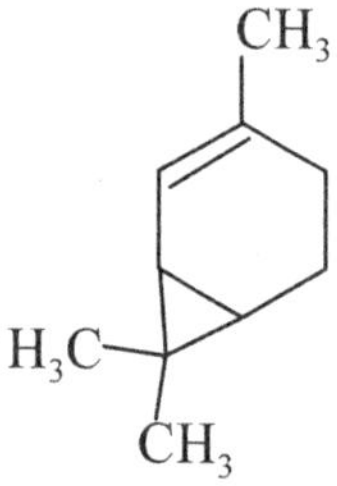

4,7,7-Trimethyl-4-norcarene;
Δ-Carene;
4-Carene

Isolation   The **turpentine** obtained from *Pinus sylveris* L., may contain as much as **42% of 3-carene,** whereas turpentine from *Pinus longifolia* Roxb. (*Pinaceae*) about **30% of 3-carene.** **Sylvestrene** is isolated in a relatively pure form by preparing the corresponding dihydrochloride.

Characteristic Features   It is a colourless oil with an agreeable **limolene** – like odour. It is considered to be one of the most stable **terpenes.** It is neither isomerized by heating nor by the interaction of alcoholic sulphuric acid. On being heated to 250°C it undergoes polymerization.

Identification

   (*a*) **Sylvestrene** yields the following *'dihalides'* by interaction with solutions of glacial acetic acid-hydrogen halides, for instance: dihydrochloride (mp 72°C); dihydrobromide (mp 72°C); and dihydroiodide (mp 66-67°C).

   (*b*) The nitrosochloride derivative prepared by the action of amyl nitrite and hydrochloric acid has a mp 107°C.

   (*c*) It is dextrorotatory.

Uses   It does not find any substantial usage either in the perfume or flavour industries.

B. Bicyclic Monoterpenes

The **bicyclic monoterpenes,** as the name suggests essentially possess two cyclic rings which are condensd together. This class of compound is relatively more complex in nature in comparison to the monocyclic species. The second ring system usually conatin 2, 3 or 4 C-atoms in common and the rings may be having 3, 4, 5 or 6 membered rings.

The **bicyclic monoterpenes** may be regarded as chemical entities derived from:

(*a*) *para-Menthane* – by direct fusion of 2–C atoms and the formation of a simple bridge, and
(*b*) *Methylated Cyclohexanes*– by having a bridge with either –CH_2– or $C(CH_3)_2$ – moieties.

In general, the **'bicyclic monoterpenes'** are classified into *five* categories, namely:

(*i*) Thujane;   (*ii*) Pinane;   (*iii*) Carane
(*iv*) Camphane; and   (*v*) Fenchane.

These *five* distinct categories shall be discussed briefly with typical examples as given below:

I. Thujane

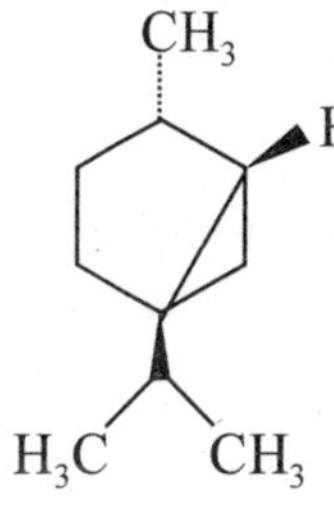

Thujane 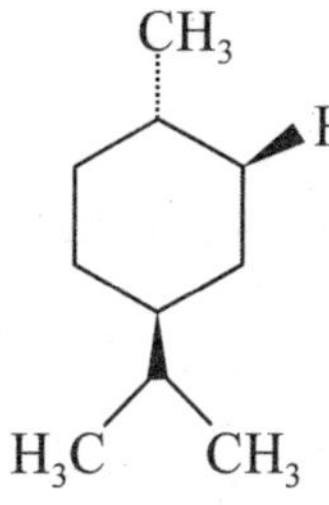   *para*-Menthane

4-Methyl-1-(1-methyl ethyl) bicyclo[3.1.0] hexane.

Eventually, **thujane** is derived from **p-menthane** with direct union between C-2 and C-4. It comprises of a 3-memberd and a 6-membered ring. The *'bridge'* in this particular instance does not have the isopropyl group in it.

Example: *Sabinene*

A Sabinene

Chemical Structure

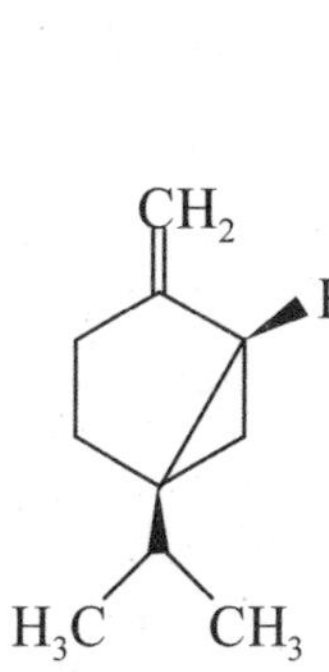

Sabinene   ⑤-Thujane

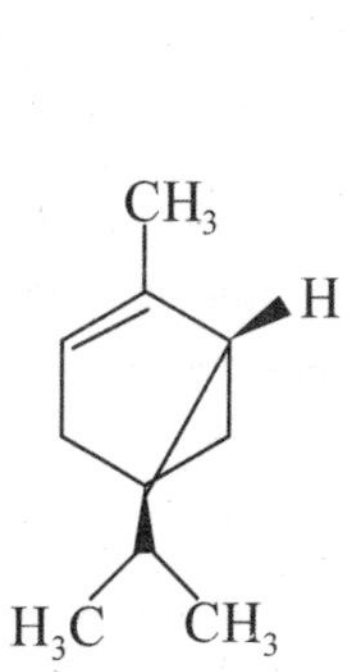

4-Isopropyl-p-methylene bicyclo-2, 4-hexane.

Occurrence   It is the major constituent (≈30%) in **oil of savin** obtained from young shoots of *Juniperus sabina* L., *Cupressaceae.* It is also present in oils of cardamom and majoram.

Isolation   It is obtained by the fractional distillation of **oil of savin** under reduced pressure.

Characteristic Features   It is a liquid, lighter than water. It is found to be isomeric with **α-thujane.**

Identification   **Sabinene** either on boiling with dilute sulphuric acid or on shakig with cold dilute sulphuric acid yields:

(*i*)   different forms of terpinene, and
(*ii*) 1, 4-terpin.

| α-Terpinene | β-Terpinene | Γ-Terpinene | 1,4-Terpin |

II. Pinane   It is formed from *p*-menthane by forming a bridge between C-3 and C-6 positions, thereby resulting into the formation of a 4-membered ring system and a parent 6-membered ring system.

p-Menthane   α-Pinene

Example   α-Pinene.

Chemical Structure   2,6,6-Trimethyl bicyclo[3,1,1] hept-2-ene;

Occurrence   It is obtained from oil of turpentine which contains 58-65% **α-pinene** along with 30% **β-pinene**. It is also widely distributed in essential oils belonging to the family *Coniferae*. It has been reported to be present in oils of American pippermint, corriander, cumin and lemon.

Isolation

(*i*)   It is isolated from the essential oils stated above by the help of chromatographic techniques.
(*ii*) Mostly isolated by the fractional distillation from essential oils, preferable under reduced pressure followed by further purification. The fraction collected between 155-165°C is converted to crystalline form of nitrosochloride (treated with amyl nitrite and hydrochloric acid) from which the desired product is liberted by treatment with aniline.

Characteristic Features It is a colourless oil which has a tendency to resinification on exposure to air. The various physical parameters of its isomers are given below:

dl-form : bp_{760} 155-156°C; d_4^{20} 0.8592; n_D^{20} 1.4664

d-form : bp_{760} 155-156°C; d_4^{20} 0.8591; n_D^{20} 1.4661;

l-form : bp_{760} 155-156°C; d_4^{20} 0.8590; n_D^{20} 1.4662.

The *l*-form is usually found in the *French Turpentine Oil*, whereas the *d*-form is found in the *American, German* and *Swedish Turpentines*.

Identification It may be characteristized by–

(*a*) Preparation of its nitrosochloride derivative mp115°C, which is devoid of optical activity,

(*b*) Preparation of its hydrochloride derivative mp 132°C, and $[\alpha]_D^{20}$ – 33.24 °C (in alcohol), and

(*c*) Preparation of its adduct with malic anhydride (crystalline) mp 169°C.

Uses

1. It is abundantly used as a starting material for the large-scale preparation of **synthetic camphor** as given below:

2. **Turpentine oil** is cooled to –10°C first and then hydrogen chloride gas is passed through it to obtain the pinene hydrochloride. The latter undergoes isomerization to yield bornyl chloride which on treatment with alkali gives rise to borneol. This on oxidation with nitric acid yields pure synthetic camphor.

3. It also finds its application in the production of insecticides, solvents, plasticizers, perfume bases and synthetic pine oil.

III. Carane *para*-**Menthane** with a bridge between C-3 and C-8 results into the formation of **carane,** which comprises of a 3-membered ring imbeded into the 6-membered parent ring as given below:

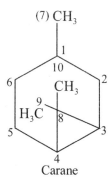

Carane

Example

A 3-Carene

Chemical Structure 3,7,7 Trimethylbicyclo [4,1,0] hept-3-ene (*a*); 4,7,7–Trimethyl-3 norcarene (*b*).

(a)   (b)

Occurrence It is a constituent of **turpentine.** The **turpentine** obtained from *Pinus sylvestris* L., contains upto 42%; turpentine from *Pinus longifolia* Roxb; *Pinaceae* about 30%.

Isolation It is isolated from the **turpentine oil** by the usage of chromatographic techniques.

Characteristic Features It is a sweet and pungent odour essential oil having a more agreeable odour than that of **turpentine.** It is practically insoluble in water but miscible with most fat solvents and oils. The *d*-form possess physical characteristics, *e.g.*; d_{15}^{15} 0.8668; d_{30}^{30} 0.8586; bp_{705} 168-169°C; $[\alpha]_D^{20}$ + 17.69; n_D^{30} 1.468.

Identification The *d*-form gives rise to the nitrosoate derivative ($C_{10}H_{16}N_2O_4$), which may be prepared by treating **d-Carene** with amyl nitrile, acetic acid and nitric acid. Its prism decomposes at 147.5°C.

Uses It is used as an antiseptic, carminative, stimulant, stomachic and diuretic.

IV. Camphane It is formed with a direct bondage between C-1 and C-8 in the structure of *p*-menthane. It essentially comprise of *two* five-membered rings besides a six-membered ring.

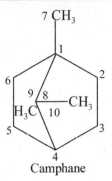

Camphane

Example

A Camphene

Chemical Structure   2,2, Dimethyl-3-methylenebicyclo-[2,2,1] heptane;

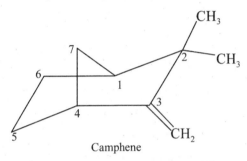

Camphene

Occurrence   It mostly occurs in a large variety of essential oils, for instance:

  (*i*) Turpentine oil (*levo and dextro* forms),
 (*ii*) Cypress oil (dextro form),
(*iii*) Camphor oil (dextro form in species of *Lauraceae*),
(*iv*) Bergamot oil, and
  (*v*) Oils of Citronella, Neroli, Ginger, and Valerian).

Camphene occurs in a number of species, namely: *Achillea, Milefolium, Acorus calamus, Anethum graveolens, Artemisia, Cinnamonum, Foeniculum vulgare, Juniperus, Kaempferia galanga, Myristica fragans, Peumus boldus, Pinus ellottii, Piper nigrum, Pistacia lentiscus, Rosamarins officinalis, Satureja, Schinus molle, Thymus, a* and *Valeriana officinalis.*

Isolation   **Camphene** is isolated by the chromatographic techniques from rectified turpentine oil.

Characteristic Features   **Camphene** obtained from alcohol found in cubic crystals (*dl*-form) having an insipid odour.

dl-form: mp 51 to 52°C; bp$_{760}$- 158.5 to 159.5°C; d$_4^{54}$ 0.8422; n$_D^{54}$ 1.45514.

Solubility   Soluble in ether, dioxane, cyclohexane, cyclohexene and chloroform. Practically insoluble in water and moderately soluble in alcohol.

***d*-form** :   mp 52°C; $[\alpha]_D^{17}$ + 103.5°; (C=9.67 in ether); d_4^{50} 0.8486; n_D^{50} 1.4605;

***l*-form** :   mp 52°C; $[\alpha]_D^{21}$ – 119.11°; (C=2.33 in benzene); d_4^{54} 0.8422; n_D^{40} 1.4620.

Identification   It forms large dodecahedra on being subjected to slow sublimation

Uses

1. As an important constituent of **eucalyptus oil** which is used as a counter-irritant, antiseptic and expectorant.

V. Fenchane   It is a trimethyl cyclohexane with a methylene (—CH_2—) bridge. It consists of *two* five-membered and a six-membered ring.

Example   *d*-Fenchone

Chemical Structure

Fenchane   *d*-Fenchone

    (1S) – 1,3,3,-Trimethylbicyclo [2,2,1]-heptan-2-one.

Occurrence   It occurs in fennel oil and in the essential oil of *Lavondula stochas* L., *Libitatae*.

Isolation   It is isolated from the **fennel oil** by column chromatography which mostly contains this ketone to the extent of 20%.

Characteristic Features   It is a colourless oily liquid having a camphor like odour. It attributes the bitter taste to the drug. It is very soluble in absolute alcohol and ether; but practically insoluble in water.

D_4^{18} 0.948; mp 6.1°C; bp_{760} 193.5°C; $[\alpha]_D^{20}$ + 66.9°; n_D^{18} 1.4636.

Identification   The pH of its saturated solution is 6.82.

Uses

1. It is employed extensively in foods and in perfumes.
2. It also finds its application as counterirritant.

5.2.6.5.1   Biosynthesis of Monoterpenoids   The hypothetic mechanism for the biosynthetic formation of monoterpenoids *viz*., **myrcane, carane, thuzane, bornane, menthane, pinane** and **fenchane** as individual class has been shown in Fig. 5.4.

5.2.6.5.2   Alcohol Volatile Oils   A good number of alcohols occur abundantly in a plethora of volatile oils, which may be judiciously classified into the following heads, namely:

(*a*) Acyclic (aliphatic) alcohols,

(*b*) Monocyclic (aromatic) alcohols,

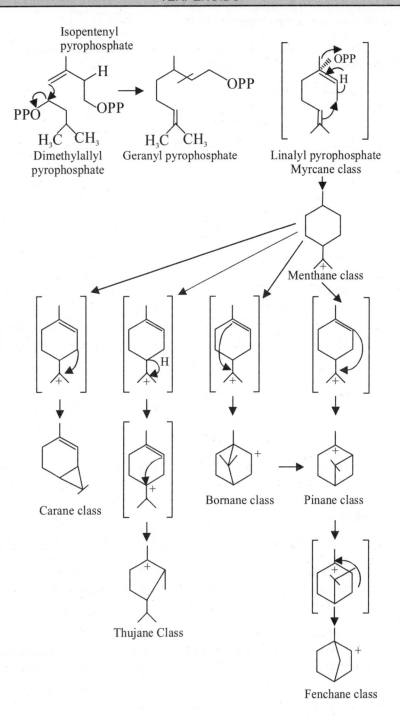

Fig. 5.4   Probable Mechanism for Biosynthesis of Various Monoterpenoids.

(Adapted from 'Pharmacognosy and Pharmacobiotechnology' by Robbers J.E. *et al.*, 1996)

(*c*) Alicyclic (terpene and sesquiterpene) alcohols.

These *three* distinct categories of 'alcohol volatile oils' shall be discussed briefly along with certain typical examples from the plant kingdom.

5.2.6.5.2.1 Acyclic (Aliphatic) Alcohols In general, a number of acyclic alcohols, such as: methyl, ethyl, isobutyl, isoamyl, hexyl and other higher alcohols occur widely in volatile oils, but being water soluble they are usually eliminated during steam distillation.

They may be further sub divided into *two* important categories, namely:

(*a*) Saturated aliphatic alcohols, and
(*b*) Unsaturated aliphatic alcohols.

which shall be discussed along with suitable examples.

5.2.6.5.2.1A Saturated Aliphatic Alcohols Volatile oils normally contain a few saturated monohydroxy alcohols belonging to the paraffin series, most of which are found to be esterified with fatty acids. In the course of steam distillation these esters undergo hydrolysis to yield the lower members of saturated aliphatic alcohols together with the lower fatty acids rarely.

A variety of substances are duly formed on account of the degradation of complex plant constituents *e.g.*, methanol, ethanol (a by product of fermentation due to plant starches), furfural and butanedione (diacetyl), which ultimately are located in the **distillation waters of volatile oils.**

Furfural

Butanedione (Diacetyl)

Isolation of aliphatic alcohols may be accomplished from the volatile oils by fractional distillation, by forming their respective derivatives *e.g.*, *para*-hydroxybenzoates, acid phthalates and calcium chlorides.

The saturated aliphatic alcohols may be identified by the preparation of their respective cyrstalline derivatives, such as: *para*-nitrobenzoates, 3,5 dinitrobenzoates, phenylurethanes, and napthylurethanes.

The presence of ethanol as an 'adultrant' in volatile oil may be carried out by treating it with iodine, potassium iodide, sodium hydroxide solution (0.5N) and heating the resulting mixture to give rise to the yellow crystals of iodoform (mp 119°C).

5.2.6.5.2.1B Unsaturated Aliphatic Alcohols The unsaturated aliphatic alcohols frequently occurring in volatile oils are nothing but **terpene-derivatives** wherein the six membered carbon ring is found to be broken at one point only. A few important typical members of this category are as follows:

Examples

1. Geraniol

Chemical Structure 3,7-Dimetyl-2,6-octadien-8-ol; Lemonol.

Geraniol

Occurrence   It is an **olefinic terpine alcohol** which constitute the major part of **oil of rose, oil of palmarose** (95%), **oil of geranium** (40-50%), **oil of citonella** (30-40%) and also in the essential **oil of lemon grass** etc.

Isolation

Method 1: **Geraniol** may be readily isolated in its pure form from volatile oil fractions by virtue of the fact that it readily forms a distinct crystalline derivative with anhydrous calcium chloride [$2C_{10}H_{18}O \, CaCl_2$]. The resulting compound is practically insoluble in organic solvents, such as: chloroform, ether, petroleum ether or benzene and hence can be readily decomposed with pure distilled water into geraniol and calcium chloride. The separated oil thus obtained is rapidly washed with luke-warm water and subjected to steam distillation finally.

Method 2: It may also be isolated and purified, of course, much less conveniently, by forming its solid acid phthalate (mp 47°C) which yields a crystalline silver salt.

Characteristic Features   It is an oily liquid having a marked and pronounced agreable rose-like odour. However, the odour of its **geometrical isomeride 'Nerol'** is definitely found to be more refreshing than that of geraniol.

Its physical characteristics are as under:

bp_{757} 229-230°C; d_4^{20} 0.8894; n_D^{20} 1.4766; UV max: 190-195 nm (ε 18000).

It is practically insoluble in water, but soluble in ether, ethanol. The characteristic features of its corresponding acetate, butyrate and formate analogues are stated below:

Derivative	Mol. Formula	Odour	bp (°C)	d	Solubility
Aceatate	$C_{12}H_{20}O_2$	Sweet, fragrant,	242 (decomposes)	~ D_{15}^{15} 0.9174	Insoluble in water. Very soluble in ethanol; miscible with ether
Butyrate	$C_{14}H_{24}O_2$	Fragrant odour	bp_{18} 152	D_4^{17} 0.901	Insoluble in water; soluble in ethanol and ether
Formate	$C_{11}H_{18}O_2$	Odour of roses and of green rose leaves	bp_{15} 113-114°	D_4^{20} 0.927	Insoluble in ether and ethanol

Identification

1. It is characterized conveniently by preparing its specific derivatives, for instance: 3-nitrophthalate (mp 109°C) diphenyl urethane (mp 82.2°C), and α-naphthylurehane (mp 47-48°C).
2. When treated with 5% sulphuric acid **geraniol** gives rise to mainly **terpin hydrate** as given below:

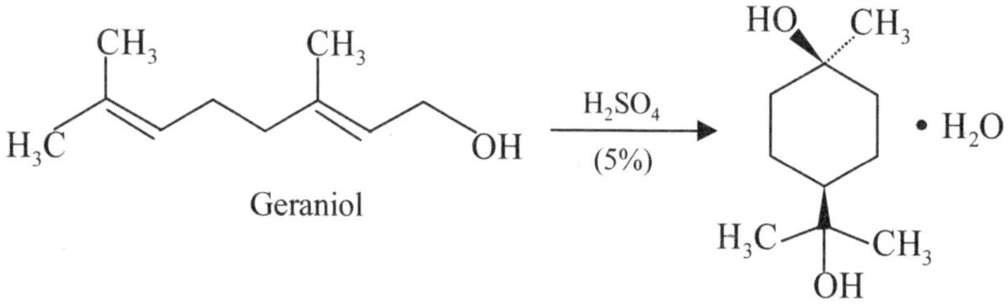

cis-Terpin hydrate

3. The interaction of **geraniol** with phosphoric acid and gaseous hydrogen chloride yields diterpene together with other terpenes as depicted below:

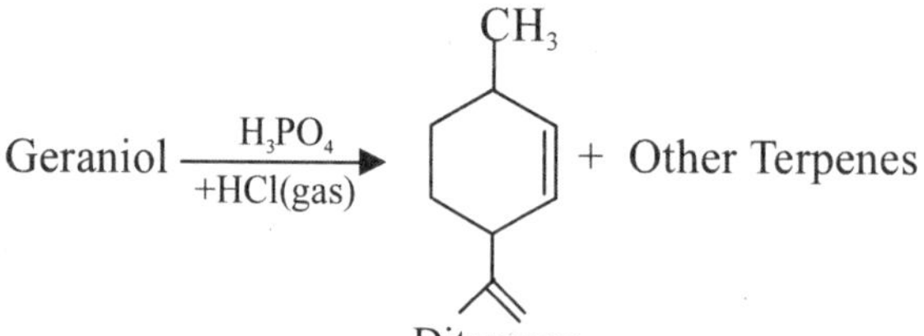

4. In the presence of mineral acids **geraniol** undergoes *cyclization* to give rise to **α-terpineol** as given under:

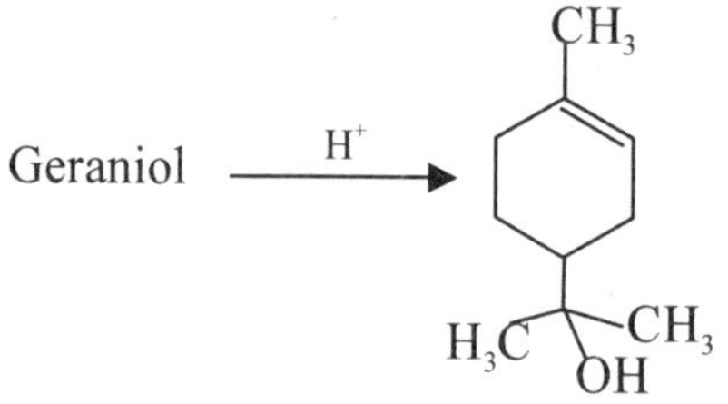

Uses
1. It finds its wide application in a plethora of formulations used as rose scents.
2. It is also employed as insect attractant.
3. It is employed extensively in perfumery *e.g.*; **butyrate** for compounding artificial attar of rose; **formate** as an important constituent of *artificial neroli oil* and of *artificial orange blossom oil*.
4. It is used in soap, cosmetic and flavour industries.

3. Nerol

Chemical Structure   *cis*-2,6-Dimethyl-2,6-actadien-8-ol; It is the *cis*-isomer of **geraniol**

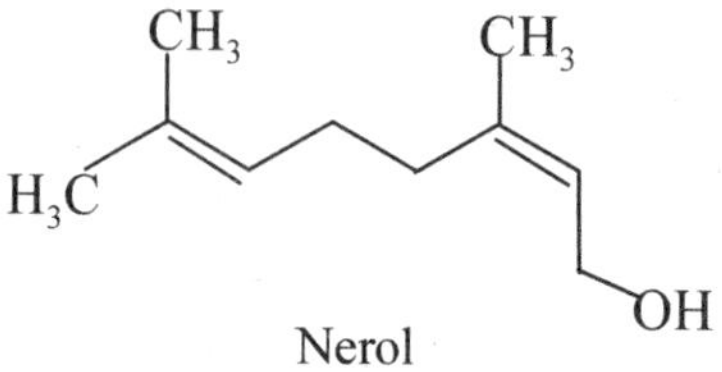

Nerol

Occurrence   Nerol is found in a number of essential oils, specifically **oil of Neroli** (usually obtained from the fresh and tender flower of orange), **oil petit grain** (normally prepared from not fully matured fruits of bitter orange) and also in **oil of bergamot** (conventionally prepared from *Citrus auranti var. bergamia).*

Isolation **Nerol** may be isolated from admixture with geraniol in volatile oils by treatment with anhydrous calcium chloride, when the former that does not form any complex with $CaCl_2$ is separated conveniently by either centrifugation or filtration techniques.

Characteristic Features It is an oily liquid having the odour of sweet rose. It is optically inactive. It has the physical parameters as : bp_{745} 224-225°C; d^{15} 0.8813; UV max: 189-194 nm (ε 18000). It is soluble in absolute alcohol.

Identification
1. It is characterized by the preparation of its tetrabromide derivative $C_{10}H_{18}Br_4O$ (mp 116-118°C).
2. It also gives rise to the diphenylurethane analogue (mp 52-53°C).
3. It forms needles of allophanate ($C_{12}H_{20}N_2O_3$) (mp 84-86°C) from petroleum ether (40-60°C).

Uses It is used extensively as a base for the manufacture of perfumes.

2. Linalool

Chemical Structure 3,7-Dimethyl-1,6-octadien –3-ol;
$(CH_3)_2C=CHCH_3CH_2C-(CH_3)(OH)CH=CH_2$ **or**

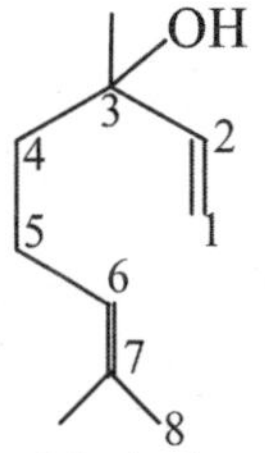

Linalool

Occurrence It is the major constituent of **linaloe oil.** It also occurs in a variety of essential oils, namely: Ceylon Cinnamon (*Cinnamonum verum), Artemisia balchanorum, Acorus calamus, Aloysia triphylla, Artemisia dracunculus, Camellia sinensis, Cananga odorta, Glechoma hederaceae, Humulus lupulus, Lantana camara, Laurus nobilis, Lavanchula angustifolia, Myrica, Myristica fragrans, Narcissus tazetta, O. imum basilicum, Peunus boldus, Piper nigrum, Prunus armeniaca, Robinia pseudoacacia, Rosmarinus officinalis, Salvia, Satureja, Syzygium aromaticum, Thymus and Tilla europaea.*

Isolation It is conveniently isolated from the saponified volatile oil by subjecting it to careful fractional distillation.

Characteristic Features The various typical examples whereby **linalool** reacts with organic acids, anhydrides and inorganic acids are given below:

(*a*) **Organic Acids:** It is very sensitive to organic acids and gets rapidly isomerized to **geraniol.** Hence, its esters cannot be obtained in the purest form by ordinary methods.

Linalool → Geraniol (Organic acids)

(b) **Inorganic Acids**

(i) **With Chromic Acid:** It undergloes oxidation to yield **Citral.**

Linalool → Citral (Chromic acid (O))

(ii) **With Formic Acid or Conc. Sulphuric Acid:** It undergoes dehydration to yield **α-terpinene** and **dipentene.**

Linalool → α-Terpinene + Dipentene (Formic Acid, Cone.H_2SO_4)

(iii) **With 5% (w/w) Sulphuric Acid Solution**

Linalool → Terpin Hydrate (H_2SO_4 (5%w/w))

(iv) **With Glacial Acetic Acid and Acetic Anhydride: Linalool** on being heated with glacial acidic acid and acetic anhydride gives rise to a mixture of esters of **geraniol, α-terpineol** and **nerol** as follows:

Linalool   Geraniol   ᵟ-Terpineol   Nerol

It has the following physical characteristic features, namely:

dl-form: bp_{720} 194-197°C; d^{15} 0.865;

d-form: (*Coriandrol*): bp_{760} 198-200°C; d_4^{20} 0.8733; n_D^{20} 1.4673; $[\alpha]_D^{20}$ + 19.3°;

l-form: (*Licareol*): colourless liquid; bp_{760} 198°C; d^{20} 0.8622; n_D^{22} 1.4604; $[\alpha]_D^{20}$ -20.1°.

Identification

1. Phenylurethane derivative: mp 65-66°C
2. α-Naphthylurethane derivative: mp 53°C
3. On oxidation with chromic acid mixture it gives rise to **citral** that may be further ascertained by forming its semicarbazone derivative mp 171°C.

Uses

1. It is used extensively in perfumery instead of bergamot or **French lavender oil** because it has an odour quite similar to these essential oils.
2. Its esters, specially the **linalyl acetate** finds its abundant usage in perfume, cosmetic, soap and flavour industries.

5.2.6.5.3   Aldehyde Volatile Oils   In general, the aldehydes occurring in a large number of volatile oils are mostly either of aliphatic or aromatic nature.

The former type (aliphatic aldehyde), with the exception of **citral** and **citronellal,** obviously do not exert any significant role in volatile oils. Interestingly, the lower members of this series, such as: formaldehyde and acetaldehyde do occur most frequently in the **'distillation water'** of volatile oils. Probably the presence of these lower aliphatic aldehydes are attributed due to degradation and decomposition of relatively more complex chemical constituents in plant products. Owing to their solubility in water, these aldehydes invariably get dissolved in the **'distillation water'** but may generally occumulate in the *'oil of cohobation',* in case the distillation waters are redistilled (cohobated).

On the contrary, the latter type (aromatic aldehyde) plays a vital role in the essential oils, for instance: volatile oil of bitter almond almost entirely comprise of *benzaldehyde,* whereas that of cassia contains *cinnamic aldehyde* chiefly.

In a broader perspective the **'terpene aldehyde'** may be classified into *four* major categories, namely:

(*a*) Aliphatic terpene aldehydes,
(*b*) Cyclic terpene aldehydes,

(*c*) Aromatic terpene aldehydes, and

(*d*) Heterocyclic terpene aldehydes.

These *four* types of **terpene aldehydes** shall be discussed briefly with the help of some typical examples in the sections that follows:

5.2.6.5.3.1 Aliphatic Terpene Aldehydes   The two important members of this particular class are namely, **citral** and **citronellal.**

A. Citral

Chemical Structure   3,7-Dimetyl-2,6-octadienal; ($C_{10}H_{16}O$); **Citral** from natural sources is a mixture of two geometric isomers **Geranial** and **Neral.**

Geranial (Citral-a)   Neral (Citral-b)

Occurrence   It occurs abundantly in the **oil of lemon grass** (75 to 85%) [*Cymbopogan flexuosus* (Ness) stapf. And *Cymbopogon citratus* (DC) stapf. Family : *Graminae*]. It is also present to a limited extent in **oils of verbena, lemon, lime, orange and ginger root.** It is reported to be present in various other species, namely: *Ocimum pilosum (*35%), *Liptospermum citratum, Eucalyptus staigeriana* and in the leaf oils of several *Citrus species* etc.

Isolation   The rich **citral** containing volatile oils *e.g.*, **lemon grass oil** is thoroughly shaken with 5%(w/v) sodium bisulphite solution for about 25-30 minutes. The resulting crystalline adduct is first separated on a Büchner funnel, and subsequently washed with solvent ether or ethanol to remove the impurities. The crude citral is usually regenerated by decomposing the sodium bisulphite adduct with dilute sodium hydroxide solution carefully. Finally, the pure citral is obtained by distilling the crude citral cautiously under reduced presure (bp_{26} 92–93°C).

Separation of Geranial (Citral-a) and Neral (Citral-b)   Tiemann* observed that **geranial** may be obtained free from **neral** during the process of regeneration from the bisulphate adduct, by taking the strategic advantage of the fact that the crystalline sodium bisulphite adduct of **geranial** is sparingly soluble, whereas the corresponding adduct of **neral** is readily soluble in water.

Tiemann** further observed that neral may be isolated from the regular citral (mixture) by shaking it for a short time with alkaline cyanoacetic acid solution (NC.CH$_2$.COOH), when **geranial** reacts with this acid much faster than **neral.** Thus, we may have:

---

* Tiemann, Semuler, *Ber.* **26**, 2708 (1893).

** Tiemann, Semular, *Ber.* **31**, 3310, 3317 (1898).

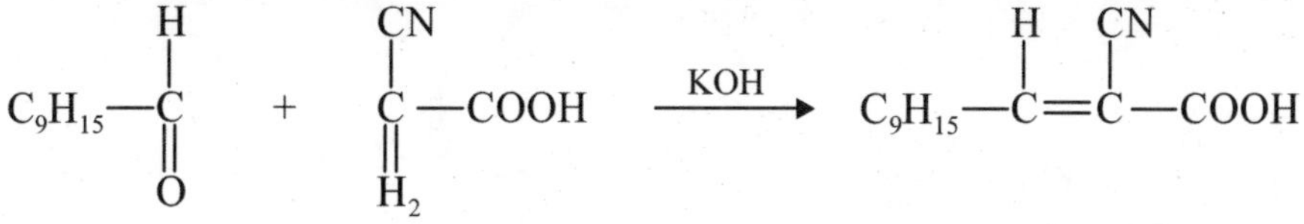

Geraniol + Cyanoacetic Acid → Geranial-Cyanoacetic Anhydride

Identification

1. By virtue of the presence of two ethylenic and one aldehydic linkage **citral** is very sensitive to oxidizing agents (even exposure to air) to yield **linalool** having an intensified yellow colour.
2. Geranial on treatment with ammoniacal silver nitrate (**Tollen's Reagent**) gives rise to **geranic acid** ($C_{19}H_{15}COOH$).
3. Hydrogenation of **geranial** with sodium amalgam in faintly acidic solution yields **citronellal** and **citronellol.**
4. Treatment with potassium bisulphate or diluted sulphuric acid **geranial** gets converted to *para-cymene* with the loss of a molecule of water.
5. Citral when digested with acetic anhydride and sodium acetate gives rise to its *enolic* form as given below:

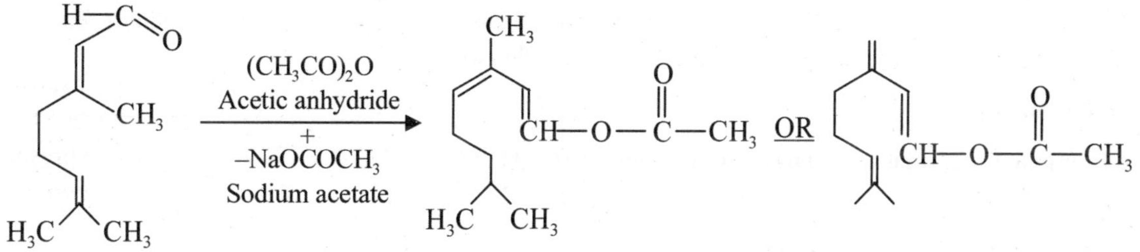

Geranial (Citral-a)   Citral-enol-acetate

6. **Syntheses of Pseudo- and α and β-Ionones:** Citral undergoes condensation with substances containing a *reactive methylene group* as depicted below in sections (a) and (b) respectively:

(*a*)

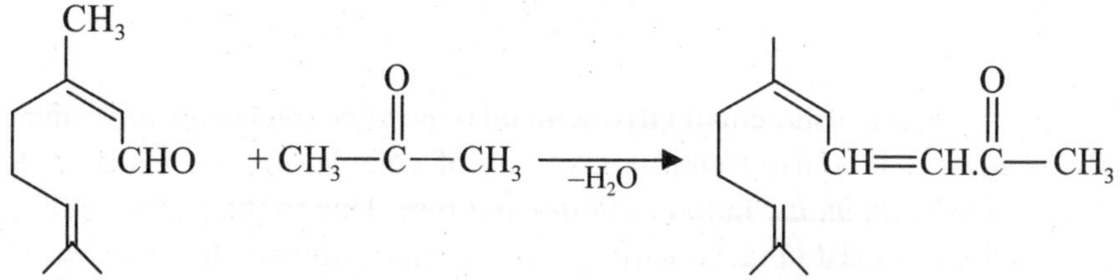

Citral   Acetone   Pseudo-ionone (△-Ionone)

Interaction of acetone and **citral** gives rise to the formation of **pseudo-ionone** (or **ψ-ionone**) with the loss of water molecule.

(*b*)

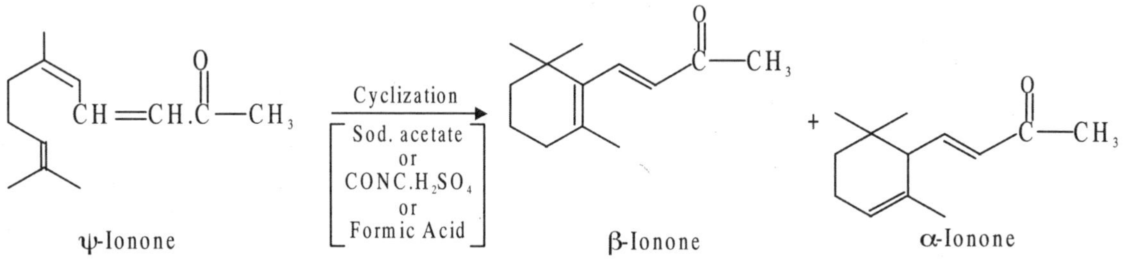

ψ-Ionone   Cyclization [Sod. acetate or CONC.H₂SO₄ or Formic Acid]   β-Ionone   +   α-Ionone

In general, the aliphatic ketone **pseudo ionone** undergoes cyclization with the aid of a variety of reagents, namely: sodium acetate, conc. sulphuric acid, formic acid, dilute mineral acids, sodium bidulphate etc., as stated above.

7. Citral may also be identified by the preparation of derivatives such as:

    (*i*) the 2,4-dinitrophenyl hydrazones: Citral-a mp 108-110°C; and Citral-b mp 96°C;

    (*ii*) the semicarbazones: Citral –a mp 164°C and Citral-b mp 171°C.

Uses

1. It is used extensively in the synthesis of **vitamin A, ionone** and **methylionone.**
2. It is employed as a flavour for fortifying **lemon oil.**
3. It is used widely in perfumery for its distinct citrus effect in lemon and verbena scents , in cologne odours and in perfumes for coloured toilet soaps.

B. Citronellal

Chemical Structure   3,7-Dimethyl-6-octenal; ($C_{10}H_{18}O$);

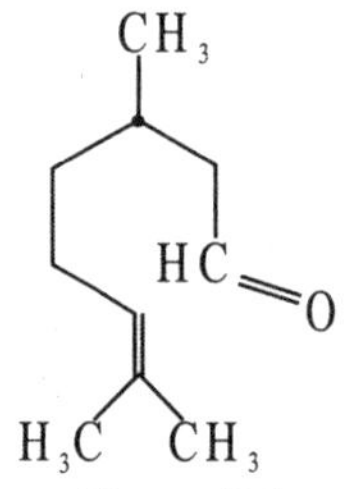

Citronellal

Occurrence   It is the chief constituent of **citronella oil** (*Cymbopogon winterianus* and *Cymbopogon nardus,* family: *Poaceae*). It is also found in a variety of volatile oils, for instacne: lemon, lemon grass, melissa* (*Melissa officinalis,* fam: *Lapiatae*) and rose. Due to the presence of one asymetric C-atom in citronellal it can exist in racemic (*dl*-) form , *d*- and *l*-forms. However, the *d*-form occurs as the chief constituent in the **oil of citronella** obtained from *Eucalyptus citriodora* and other species of *Eucalyptus* (fam: *Myrtaceae*) whereas the l-form occurs exclusively in **Java Lemon Oil.**

---

* Spoon, *Chem. Weekbl.,* **54,** 236 (1958).

Isolation   It may be conveniently isolated from essential oils by the formation of its crystalline bisulphite adduct. Interestingly, **citronellal** esentially possesses an ethylenic and an aldehyde moiety by virtue of which three different bisulphite adducts are possible theoretically as given below:

| Dihydrodisulphonic derivative | Hydrosulphonic derivative | Normal bisulphite derivative |

Note   **These three structural analogues have been prepared actually under various experimental parameters. However, the complete decomposition and subsequent regeneration of the desired aldehyde (i.e. Citronellal) may be accomplished easily by treating the 'normal bisulphite adduct' either with dilute mineral acids or with alkali carbonates. Strong alkalies eg., NaOH and KOH must be avoided so as to cause resinification of the aldehyde.**

Separation of Citronellal from Citral   There are two separate procedures adopted for the separation of **citronellal** from **citral** as discussed here under:

(a) **Tiemann's Method*:** It is based on the fact that citronellal reacts exclusively with a concentrated solution of sodium sulphite and sodium bicarbonate, whereas citral reacts even with a dilute solution.

(b) **Gildemeister Hoffmann's Method**:** It is solely guided by the fact that with *neutral sodium sulphite*, citronellal yields hydrosulphonic derivatives from which the latter cannot be recovered. However, the reaction shall commence only if:

(i) right from the beginning a strong current of pure CO_2 is made to pass through the reaction mixture, or

(ii) another acid is added gradually to the reaction mixture in sufficient quantities.

The said reaction of **citronellal** with neutral sulphite may afford its separation from citral, which also reacts rapidly with neutral sodium sulphite.

Characteristic Features   It is a colourless liquid having a pleasant melissa like odour. It has the following physical characteristic features. bp_1 47°C; bp_{760} 203-204°C; n_D^{20} 1.4460; $[\alpha]_D^{25}$ + 11.50°; d = 0.848-0.856; It is very slightly soluble in water but readily soluble in alcohols.

Under improper storage conditions it slowly undergoes decomposition, polymerization and resinification.

Under direct sun-light it yields a complex mixture which consists of acetone, **β-methyl adipic acid, isopulegol** and **menthone.**

---

* Tiemann, *Ber,* **32,** 834 (1899).

** Gildemeister Hoffmann *die Aetherischen Oele vol IV,* 307-356 (4th ed. 1956)

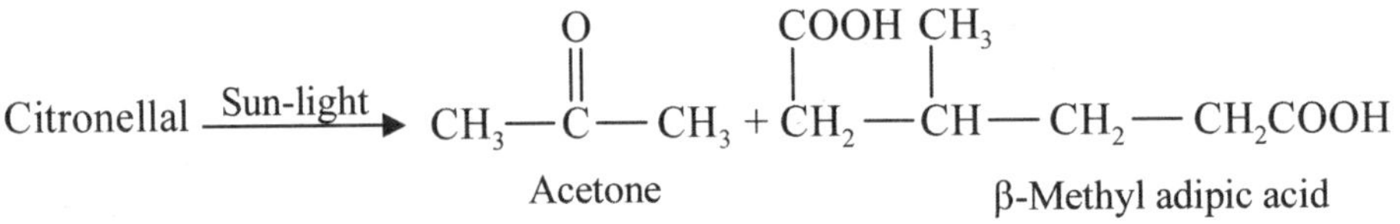
Citronellal
Sun-light
$CH_3-C(=O)-CH_3 + CH_2(COOH)-CH(CH_3)-CH_2-CH_2COOH$
Acetone
β-Methyl adipic acid

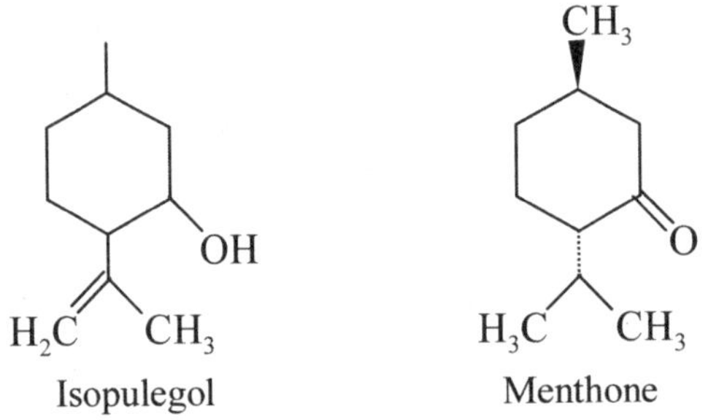
OH
H_2C
CH_3
Isopulegol
CH_3
O
H_3C
CH_3
Menthone

Strong alkalies, such as: NaOH and KOH, usually resinifies citronellal. Therefore, it is always preferred to make use of relatively weaker alkalies, for instance: Na_2CO_3, K_2CO_3, for its regeneration from its corresponding bisulphite adduct.

Reduction of citronellal with sodium amalgam yields **citronellol** *i.e.*, a terpene alcohol, due to catalytic hydrogenation as shown below:

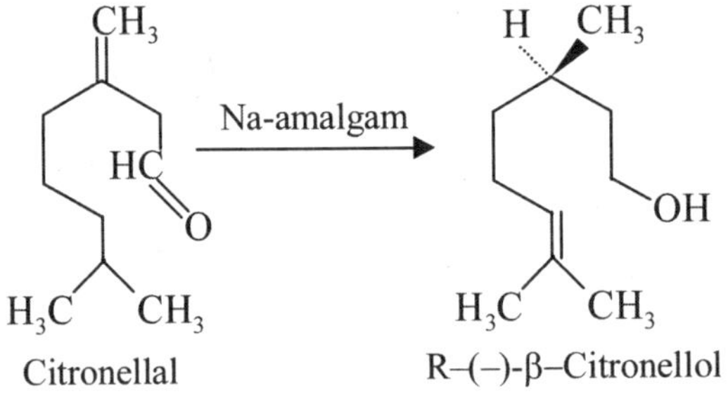
CH_3
HC
O
H_3C
CH_3
Citronellal
Na-amalgam
H
CH_3
OH
H_3C
CH_3
R-(–)-β–Citronellol

Identification

1. Its semicarbazone derivative has mp 91-92°C.
2. Its dinitrophenyl hydrazone derivative has mp 76.5°C.

Uses

1. For the manufacture of **citronellal** used in perfumery.
2. It is used largely in soap perfumes and as insect repllant.
3. It is employed as artificial citrus flavour.

*5.2.6.5.3.2 **Cyclic Terpene Aldehydes*** The **cyclic terpene aldehyde** are of two types *viz.*, monocyclic and bicyclic. A few typical examples from each category shall be discussed in the sections to follow:

A. Monocyclic Terpene Aldehydes

Examples: Perillaldehyde, Safranal and Phellandral

1. Perillaldehyde

Chemical Structure 4-(1-Methylethenyl)-1-cyclohexene-1- carboxaldehyde; ($C_{10}H_{14}O$).

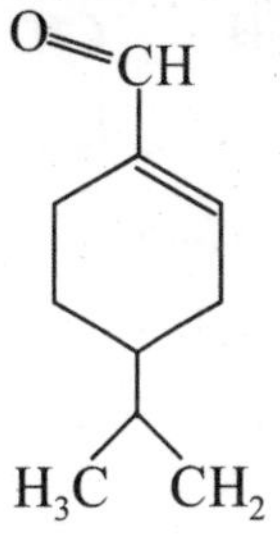

Perillaldehyde

Occurrence   It is found in essential oils of *Perilla arguta* Benth; *Labiatae*; *Sium latifolium L., Umbelliferae*; Mandarin peel oil *Citrus reticulata* Blanco; *Rutaceae* etc.

Isolation   It may be isolated from the respective essential oil, *first* by forming its crystalline sodium bisulphite adduct; and *secondly*, regenerating the desired product with alkali very carefully.

Characteristic Features   The physical characteristic of the *d-* and *l-*isomers are as follows:

d-form :   Liquid, bp_{745} 273°C; bp_7 98-100°C; d_4^{20} 0.953; n_D^{20} 1.5058; $[\alpha]_D^{20}$ + 127° (C = 13.1 in CCl4).

l-form :   Liquid, bp_{10} 104-105°C; d_4^{20} 0.9645; n_D^{20} 1.5069; $[\alpha]_D^{20}$ – 146°.

Identification   It forms oxime ($C_{10}H_{15}NO$) known as: **1-perillaldehyde-α-syn-oxime; perillartine; "perilla sugar"**. Previously, it was commonly referred to as **1-perillaldehyde-α-anti-oxime.** The needles have mp 102°C, UV max (alcohol). 232 nm (ε 21800). It is about 2000 times as sweet as sucrose.

Uses
1. The oxime is used as a sweetening agent in Japan.

2. Safranal

Chemical Structure   2,6,6-Trimethyl-1,3-cyclohexadiene-1-carboxaldehyde; ($C_{10}H_{14}O$).

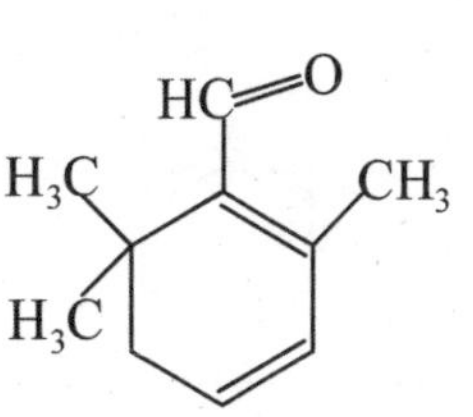

Safrnal

Occurrence   It is the chemical constituent obtained from the dried stigmas and tops of the styles of *Crocus sativus* (Fam; *Iridaceae*); The fresh drug comprises of **protocrocin** which upon drying undergoes decomposition to yield one mole of **crocin** (a coloured glycoside) and two moles of **picrocrocin** (a colourless **bitter glycoside**). It is the latter that on hydrolysis gives rise to safranal which is solely responsible for attributing the characteristic odour of the drug (saffron). These transformations are as given below:

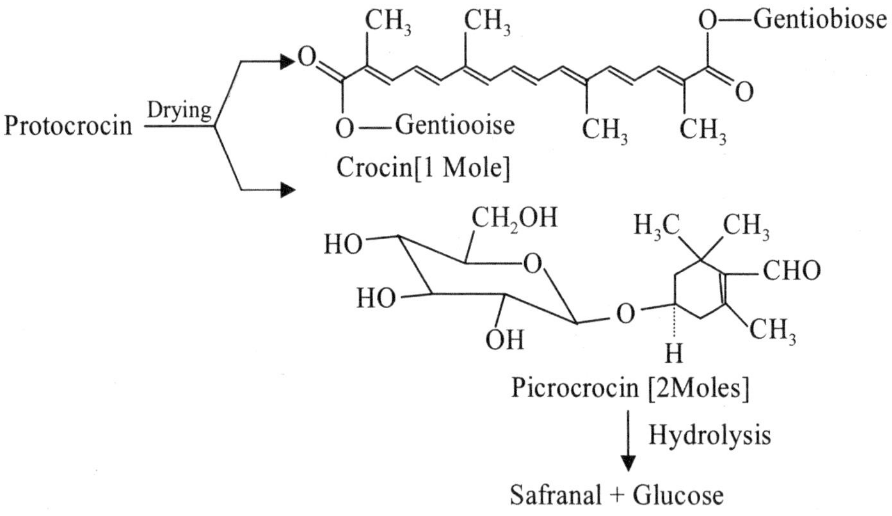

Crocin[1 Mole]

Picrocrocin [2Moles]

Safranal + Glucose

Isolation   The stigmas and tops of the styles of *C. sativus* are first dried under shade and then subjected to hydrolysis in controlled conditions to yield safranal. The resulting product is treated with pure sodium bisulphite to obtain the safranal sodium bisulphite adduct from which the desired product is regenerated by treatment with dilute alkaline solution.

Characteristic Features   It is a liquid having a pleasant characteristic odour. It has the following physical properties namely:

$bp_{1.0}$ 70°C (bath temparature); d^{19}_4 0.9734; n^{19}_D 1.5281. It is freely soluble in organic solvents like: methanol, ethanol, petroleum ether and glacial acetic acid.

Uses   It is employed as a flavouring agent in confectionery products.

3. Phellandral

Chemical Structure   4-Isopropyl-1-cyclohexen aldehyde; ($C_{10}H_{15}O$).

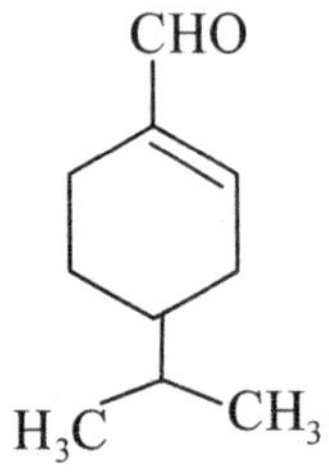

Phellandral

Occurrence   It was first and foremost found in the essential oil of *Phellandrium aquaticum*. It also occurs in the essential oil obtained from the flowers of lavender (*Santolina chamaecyparissus* L., family: *Asteraceae*) and several *Eucalyptus species*.

Isolation   It is usually isolated through its sparingly soluble crystalline sodium bisulphite compound, from which **phellandral** is generated by treatment with dilute alkaline solution carefully.

Characteristic Features It is an oil having an odour very much reminiscent of cuminaldehyde. It undergoes rapid oxidation either on exposure to air or with silver oxide to give rise to **phellandric acid** (mp 144-145°C)

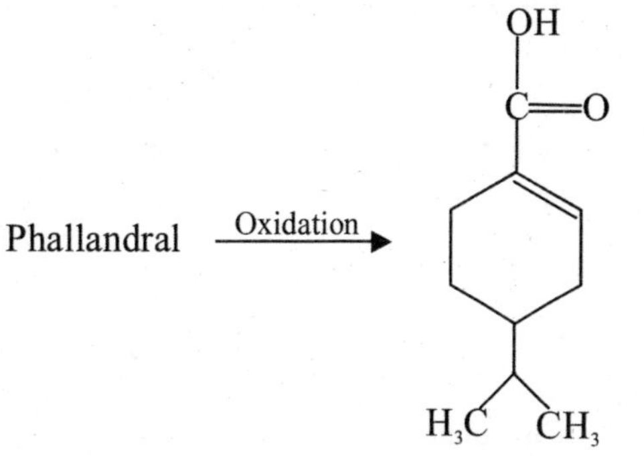

Phallandral →(Oxidation)

Phellandric Acid

Identification It may be identified by preparing its corresponding derivative, such as: oxime, semicarbazone and phenyl hydrazine etc.

Uses Due to its resemblance of odour of cuminaldehyde it finds application in perfumery.

B. Bicyclic Terpene Aldehydes

Example: Myrtenal.

Chemical Structure

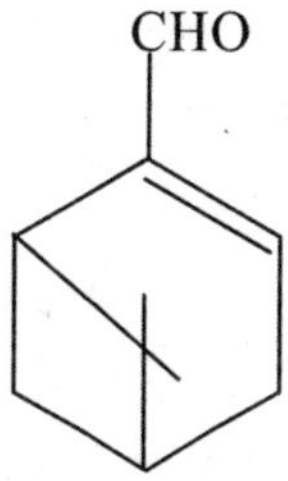

CHO

Myrtenal

It is a naturally occurring **oxygenated pinane derivative.**

Occurrence The leaves of boldo contains essential oil to the extent of 2%* (*Peumus boldus* Molina, family: *Monimiaceae*).

Isolation The aldehyde is successfully isolated by preparing its sodium bisulphite adduct first and then regenerating it by treatment with mild alkaline solution cautiously.

Uses
1. The aromatic leaves are frequently used as mild diuretic, especially in liver ailments like jaundice.
2. It is also recommended for urogenital inflammations *e.g.*; gonorrhea in Latin America

---

* Bruns, K., and Kohler, M, *Uber die Zusammensetzung des boldoblatterols, parf kosm*, **55,** 225, 1975

5.2.6.5.3.3 Aromatic Terpene Aldehyde   In comparison to aliphatic aldehydes, the aromatic aldehydes invariably play a vital role in essential oils. It has been observed that a major portion of certain volatile oils mainly comprise of aromatic terpene aldehydes, such as : **bitter almond** and **cassia.** A variety of such aromatic aldehydes commonly found in essential oils are, namely: anisaldehyde, benzaldehyde, cinnamaldehyde, cuminaldehyde and salicyldehyde.

| *p*-Anisal-dehyde | Benzal-dehyde | Cinnamal-dehyde | Cuminaldehyde | Salicylal-dehyde |

Examples: A few typical examples of aromatic terpene aldehyde are discussed below, for instance: **Cumminaldehyde, Vanillin** etc.

A. Cuminaldehyde

Chemical Structure   4(1-Methylethyl) benzaldehyde.

Cuminaldehyde

Occurrence   It occurs as a constituent of essential oils present in eucalyptus, myrrh, cassia and cumin. Cumin mainly comprises of the dried ripe fruits of *Cuminum cyminum* Linn., (family: *Umbelliferae*).

Isolation   The essential oil obtained from the dried ripe fruits of cumin ranges between 2-4%, the major constituents of which cuminaldehyde (35-60%). The aldehyde may be separated by forming its sodium bisulphite adduct and subsequently regenerating the desired product by treatment with alkaline solution carefully.

Characteristic Features   It is a colourless to yellowish, oily liquid. It possesses a strong persistent odour, acrid and burning taste.

The physical characteristic of **cuminaldehyde** are as follows: d^{20} 0.978; bp_{760} 235-236°C; n_D^{20} 1.5301. It is practically insoluble in water, but freely soluble in ether and ethanol.

Identification   It is identified by forming its **thiosemicarbazone** derivative ($C_{11}H_{15}N_3S$).

Uses   It is extensively employed as an adjunct in perfumery.

B. Vanillin

Chemical Structure   4-Hydroxy-3-methoxybenzaldehyde ($C_8H_8O_3$).

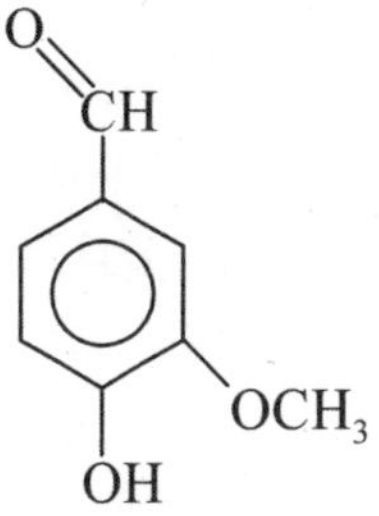

Vanillin

Occurrence   It occurs naturally in vanilla (**vanilla bean**) especially found in cured, fully-grown unripe fruit (pods) of *Vanilla planifolia* Andrews, known in commerce as Bourbon or Mexican vanilla. It is also found in the vanilla pods of *Vanilla tahitensis* J.W. More, usually recognised in commerce as *Tahiti vanilla*. Both these species belong to natural order *Orchidaceae*.

The term *vanilla* has been derived from the spanish word *vania*, meaning sheath like pod and *illa,* meaning small; *planifolia* is derived from the Latin word *planus,* meaning flat, and *follium,* meaning leaf; *tahitensis* refers to Tahiti its adopted home.

It also occurs in small quantities in a variety of essential oils *e.g.*, **clove oil; gums** and **oleoresins** *e.g.*, *benzoin, Peru balsam*. Interestingly, plants do not contain vanillin as such, but they exist in the form of *glycosides,* which upon hydrolysis in the presence of enzymes release **vanillin**.

Isolation   It may be accomplished by any one of the following *five* methods, namely:

(*a*) **From Vanilla Pods:** Vanillin is obtained by the extraction of powdered vanilla pods with ether, by at least three successive extractions, evaporating the combined ethereal fraction (crude vanillin). It is further purified by crystallization of the crude product from ethanol.

(*b*) **From Lignin Waste:** More conveniently, **vanillin** is obtained from the lignin waste, a byproduct in the manufacturer of paper pulp. Lignin is a complex polymeric natural material of woody plants and essentially has the following fragment structural unit:

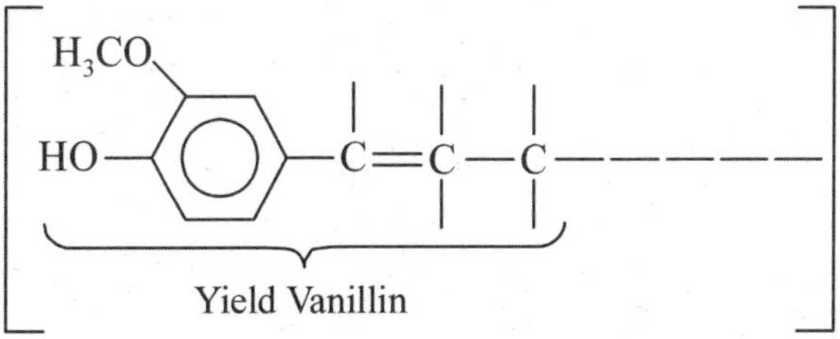

Yield Vanillin

Thus, **lignin** when subjected to oxidation yields **vanillin** in a large extent which ultimately has rendered this process an economically feasible and viable one.

(*c*) **From Eugenol:** It may also be prepared from **eugenol** which is a major constituent of **clove oil** as given below:

Eugenol → Isoeugenol → Acetate Derivative → 4-Acetixy-3-methoxy benzaldehyde → Vanillin

Eugenol on alkaline treatment undergoes intramolecular rearrangement to give rise to **isoeugenol** which on acetylation with acetic anhydride yields the corresponding acetate derivative. The resulting product on oxidation yields 4-acetoxy-3-methoxy benzaldehyde which upon treatment with HCl yields vanillin.

(*d*) **From Guaiacol:** It may be prepared on an industrial scale by the help of **Reimer-Tiemann's reaction,** whereby **o-vanillin** is obtained from guaiacol *i.e.*, **catechol methyl ether** as stated below:

Guaiacol → Vanillin + O-Vanillin

Guaiacol on treatment with sodium hydroxide in the presence of chloroform yields **vanillin** and **o-vanillin.**

(*e*) **From Bisulphite Adduct: Vanillin** may also be isolated from its bisulphite adduct. The ethereal solution containing vanillin is extracted completely with saturated aqueous sodium bisulphite solution. Usually specialized techniques are adopted to ensure pure isolates from its tautomers and closely related isomers.

Characteristic Features It consists of fine, white to slightly yellow, needle-shaped crystals having an odour and taste quite resembling to that of vanilla fruits. It is usually affected by light. On prolonged heating at 105°C, it decomposes with the formation of non-volatile byproducts. It is soluble in hot water (1 g dissolves in 16 ml of water at 80°C), and in glycerol (~ 20 ml of glycerol per 1g of vanillin). It is freely soluble in ethanol, ether, chloroform, carbon disulphide, glacial acetic acid, pyridine, oils and aqueous solutions of alkali hydroxides.

It has the following physical parameters: d 1.056; mp 80-81°C; bp 285°C.

Identification It may be identified by preparing a number of derivatives, such as: semicarbazone (mp 230°C); dinitrohydrazone (mp 271°C); *para*-nitrophenylhydrazone (mp 227°C); benzoate (mp 75°C) and acetyl derivative (mp 77°C).

Uses

1. It is employed as a pharmaceutical aid (flavour).
2. It is extensively used as a flavouring agent in beverages, confectionery, foods and perfumery.
3. It is used in the manufacture of liqueurs.
4. It has been established that 1 part of vanillin equals 400 parts vanilla pods; and 2.5-3 parts equals 500 parts tincture vanilla.
5. It also finds its use as a reagent in analytical chemistry.

5.2.6.5.3.4 Heterocyclic Terpene Aldehyde **Heterocyclic terpene aldehyde** is relatively quite rare as compared to other class of compounds discussed in this context. Example: **Furfural.**

A. Furfural

Chemical Structure 2-Furfuraldehyde ($C_5H_4O_2$).

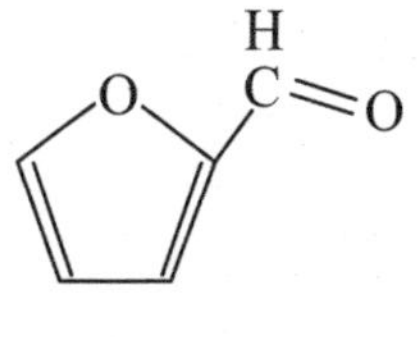

Furfural

Occurrence It occurs in the first fraction of a number of essential oils, belonging to the natural order *Pinaceae*. It is also found in **colophony** (*Pinus paulusteric*); **oil of orris rhizome** (*Iris florentina* Linn., Family: *Iridaceae*); **oil of lavender** (*Lavandula officinalis;* family: *Labiatae*); **oil of cinnamon** (*Cinnamonium cassia* Blums; Family: *Lauraceae*); and **clove oil** (*Eugenia Caryophylus*; Family: *Myrtaceae*).

Isolation It may be accomplished in *two* manners, namely:

(*i*) *Extraction i.e.*, by washing the first fraction of the oil with water, extracting the aqueous layer with ether, and finally evaporating the ether under reduced pressure.

(*ii*) *Addition Compound i.e.*, **furfural** forms an addition compound on being treated with a saturated aqueous solution of sodium bisulphite.

Characteristic Features   It is a colourless oily liquid having a peculiar odour, somewhat resembling the odour of benzaldehyde. The physical characteristic features are: d_4^{20} 1.1563; bp_{760} 161.8°C; mp: -36.5°C; volatile in steam; n_D^{20} 1.5261. It is soluble in ethanol and ether; soluble in 11 parts of water.

Identification

1. It gives an intense red colour with aniline acetate.
2. It is also identified by forming its corresponding oxime and phenyl hydrazone derivatives.
3. It reduces Fehling's solution to give red precipitate of cupric oxide.
4. It also reduces **Tollen's Reagent** (*i.e.*, ammoniacal silver nitrate solution) to give silver mirror.

Uses

1. It is used extensively in the manufacture of furfural-phenol plastics, for instance: *Durite.*
2. It is employed in solvent-refining of petroleum oils.
3. It makes its use as a solvent for nitrated cotton, gums and cellulose acetate.
4. It finds its application for accelerating vulcanization.
5. It is used as insecticide, germicide and fungicide.
6. It is employed in the manufacture of varnishes.
7. It is commonly used as a reagent in analytical chemistry.

5.2.6.5.4 Ketone Volatile Oils   The ketones that invariably occur in volatile oils may be classified in the following *two* categories, namely:

(*i*) Aliphatic ketones, and
(*ii*) Aromatic Ketones.

5.2.6.5.4.1 Aliphatic Ketones   **Aliphatic ketones** do not occur abundantly in volatile oils. However, the relatively lower members of this group originate most probably by virtue of the decomposition of rather more complex compounds during the process of steam distillation. Two such species, for instance *acetone* and *diacetyl* are commonly found in the **'oils of cohobation'** (or the distillation waters) accomplished by redistillation (**cohobation**) of the distillation waters.

Acetone

Diacetyl
(2, 3-Butanedione)

It has been observed that acetone and diacetyl are frequently accompanied by methanol and furfural.

5.2.6.5.4.2 Aromatic Ketones   There are also termed as **'cyclic terpene ketones'.** Generally, the aromatic ketones are classified into two categories, namely:

(*i*) Monocyclic terpene ketones, and
(*ii*) Bicyclic terpene ketones.

These two distinct categories shall be discussed separately in the sections that follows:

A. Monocyclic Terpene Ketones   A few typical examples of this specific class of ketones are: *l*-**menthone; carvone.**

A.1 *l*-Menthone

Chemical Structure   (2S-*trans*)-5-Methyl-2-(1-methylethyl) cyclohexanone. As it has two asymmetric carbon atoms (*i.e.*, chiral centres) it can exist in two pairs of enantiomorphs or four optically active isomers (*d*-; *l*-; ***dl*-menthone** and **isomenthone**).

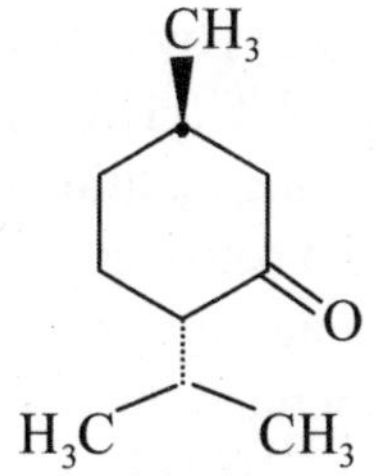

l-Menthone

Occurrence   It is found in a variety of volatile oils, such as: pennyroyal (*Mentha pulegium*, Family-*Lamiaceae*); peppermint (*Mentha piperita* Linn., Family: *Labiateae*); geranium (*Geranium maculatum* L., Family: *Geraniaceae*); and buchu (*Barsoma betulina* (Berg.) Bartl. and Wendel, Family: *Rutaceae*).

Isolation   *l*-Menthone usually occurs in association with **isomenthone.** The former gets solidified at – 6°C whereas the latter at -35°C. In normal practice, the **peppermint oil,** which contains upto 30% of **menthone,** is subjected to its oxime or semicarbazone formation and subsequently the *l*-menthone is regenerated by the aid of dilute sulphuric acid.

Characteristic Features   It is a bitter liquid having peppermint-like odour. It is slightly soluble in water, whereas freely soluble in organic solvents. It has the following physical characteristics: bp 207°C; mp –6°C; d_4^{20} 0.895; n_D^{20} 1.4505; $[\alpha]_D^{20}$ -24.8°.

Identification   The isomeric forms of menthones may be characterized by the preparation of specific derivatives, for instance: oximes, semicarbazones etc.

Uses
  1. It is used extensively in perfume and flavour compositions.
  2. It is also employed in the preparation of artificial essential oils.

A.2 Carvone

Chemical Structure   2-Methyl-5-(1-methylethenyl)-2-cyclohexene-1-one.

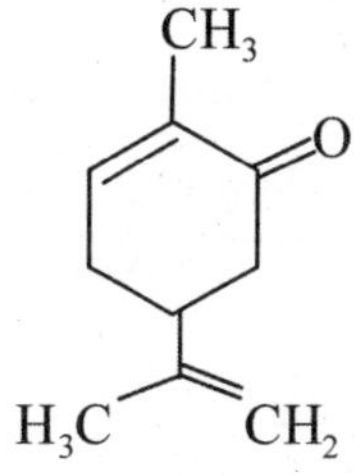

Carvone

Occurrence   It occurs in the **mandarin peel oil** (*Citrus reticulata* Blanco., Family: *Rutaceae*); **spearmint oil** upto 70% (*Mentha spicata* or *Mentha cardiaca*, Family: *Lamiaceae*); **gingergrass oil**

(*Zingiber officinale* Roscoe, Family: *Zingiberaceae*); **oil of caraway** upto 50-60% (*Carum carvi* Linn, Family: *Umbelliferae*).

Isolation   It may be isolated by the following *two* methods:

Method 1: Formation of Sodium Sulphite Adduct. **Carvone** may be conveniently isolated from essential oils (*e.g.*, spearmint oil, oil of caraway) by virtue of the fact that it (a lactone) readily forms the water soluble salt of a hydrosulphonic acid ($C_{10} H_{16} O_7 S_2 Na_2$) on treating with a neutral solution of sodium sulphite, whereby the corresponding addition takes place at the both ethylenic linkages. In order to achieve this, the fraction collected between the boiling range 220-235°C in the case of oil of caraway, is shaken with the requisite quantity of a concentrated aqueous solution of sodium sulphite and the sodium hydroxide thus liberated during the course of reaction is neutralized from time to time with a dilute mineral acid (*e.g.*, HCl) very carefully. As soon as the above process is completed fully, the resulting fractions which have not involved in the above cited reaction may be eliminated by extracting the solution with ether successively (at least three times). At the end, the desired product *carvone* can be regenerated by the action of sodium hydroxide and finally distilled off with steam.

Method 2: Formation of Hydrogen Sulphide Adduct. Alternatively, **carvone** may be separated from the volatile oils by the formation of its hydrogen sulphide adduct [$(C_{10} H_{14} O)_2 . H_2S$]. It is easily accomplished by the passage of a current of hydrogen sulphide (H_2S) gas into an ammoniated alcoholic solution of carvone. Ultimately, the pure ketone *i.e.*, **carvone** may be regenerated from the corresponding separated adduct by careful digestion with alkali.

Characteristic Feature   It is a colourless liquid having a distinct odour typical of **caraway seed.** The various physical parameters of *d-*, *l-* and *dl-*forms are given below:

Form	bp(°C)	d	n_D^{20}	$[a]_D^{20}$
d-Carvone	230 (At 755 mm atmospheric pressure)	0.965 (d_4^{20})	1.4989	+61.2°
l-Carvone	230-231 (At 763 mm atmospheric pressure)	0.9652 (d_{15}^{15})	1.4988	−62.46°
dl-Carvone	230-231 (At 760 mm atmospheric pressure)	0.9645 (d_{15}^{15})	1.5003	–

It is miscible with ethanol but practically insoluble in water. It congeals at very low temperature.

Identification   The different tests for the identification of **carvone** are stated below, namely;

(*a*) **Bromination** of carvone gives rise to a mixture of crystalline derivatives* having distinct melting points:

    d- and *l-*form   : mp 120 and 120-122°C
    *dl-*form   : mp 112-114°C

---

* These are probably the dibromo derivatives because the tetrabromoderivatives are liquids.

(b) **Mono-hydrochloride salt** is formed when it is treated with HCl in acetic acid.

(c) **Hydrobromide salt** is obtained by treating *d*-corvone with HBr (mp 32°C).

(d) **Isomerization of Carvone to Carvacrol.** It undergoes isomerization to form carvacrol with a number of dehydrating agents, such as: H_2SO_4; H_3PO_4; NaOH; $ZnCl_2$.

Carvone   Carvacrol

(e) It is also characterized by the preparation of several compounds, for instance: oxime, semicarbazone, H_2S-derivative, phenylhydrazone.

Uses

1. It is used as **oil of caraway.**
2. It is also used for flavouring liqueurs.
3. It is used extensively in perfumery and soaps.
4. It is employed for flavouring many types of food products and beverages.
5. It finds its enormous applications in *oral hygiene* preparations *e.g.*, toothpastes, gargles, mouth-washes.
6. It is also used in flavouring pharmaceuticals.

B. Bicyclic Terpene Ketones These class of compounds essentially contain two cyclic ring structures fused with each other along with a ketonic function. The two typical examples of pure chemical entities that belong to this group are **camphor** and **d-fenchone,** which have been duly dealt with earlier in this chapter under **'monoterpenoids'** and **'bicyclic monoterpenes'** respectively.

5.2.6.5.5 Phenol Volatile Oils The important drugs containing phenol volatile oils are, namely: **Clove oil, Myrcia oil (Bay oil), Organum oil, Pinetar, Thyme** etc., In fact, they essentially owe their value in the pharmaceutical domain almost exclusively by virtue of their antiseptic and germicidal properties of their *phenolic constituents*. A good many of them are employed as popular flavouring agents, for instance: **oil of anise, clove** and **sassafras.**

5.2.6.5.5.1 General Methods of Isolation Mostly phenols are weak acids. Hence, they react with dilute alkali solutions (3-5% w/v) to result into the formation of corresponding water-soluble salts known as *'phenolates'*. This specific characteristic property usually offers, a convenient method for carrying out the separation of *phenolic components* from the *non-phenolic ones*. To affect the separation, therefore, the volatile oils or fractions are subjected to treatment with dilute alkaline solutions with vigorous shaking. Once the two layers get separated, the water-soluble salts are decomposed by acidification carefully and the phenols thus generated (or liberated) are isolated either by means of steam-distillation or by extraction with ether.

Note

1. **Thymol** and **carvacrol** may be steam-distilled from alkaline solution without previous acidification.
2. Several phenols may be isolated by chilling the oil as such or its fraction to a very low temperature (−20 to −30°C) whereby these compounds normally separate in crystalline form.

5.2.6.5.5.2 General Properties of Terpene Phenols   There are several characteristic features of **terpene phenols** which not only help them in their separation but also aid in their identification as stated below:

1. **Bromine Reaction:** Phenols react with bromine evolving the corresponding HBr. The resulting bromides are usually *crystalline* in nature and sparingly water-soluble. Hence, they may be separated easily and identified accordingly.
2. **Reaction with Ferric Chloride:** Phenols react with dilute aqueous solutions of ferric chloride ($FeCl_3$) (0.1-0.2% w/v) to give rise to intense coloured reactions, which attributes to the *specific colour-tests.*
3. **Formation of Phthaleins:** Several phenols react with phthalic anhydride to form their corresponding phthaleins.
4. Most phenols react with specific reagents, such as: acetic anhydride, benzoyl chloride, phenyl isocyanate and *p*-nitrobenzoyl chloride to give characteristic reaction products that also help in their identifications.

5.2.6.5.5.3 **Classification**   The **terpene phenols** are classified into the following categories, namely:

(*i*) Monohydric phenols and
(*ii*) Dihydric phenols.

The above categories of phenols shall be discussed briefly as under:

5.2.6.5.5.3.1 Monohydric Phenols   The typical examples of monohydric phenols are: **carvacrol, eugenol, thymol.**

A. Carvacrol

Chemical Structure   2-Methyl-5-(1-methylethyl)-phenol.

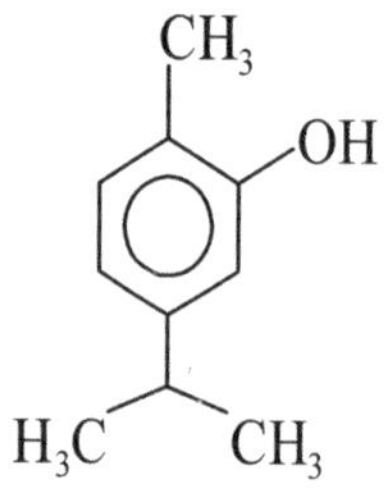

Carvacrol

Occurrence   It occurs in the essential **oil origanum** (*Origanum vulgare* Linn., Family: *Labiatae*); **oil of thyme** (*Thymus serphyllum* Linn., and *T. vulgaris* Linn., Family: *Labiatae*); **oil of marjoram** and **oil of summer savory.**

Characteristic Features   It is a liquid oil having strong thymol odour. Its physical properties are as follows: d_4^{20} 0.976; bp_{760} 237-238°C; mp ~ °C; n_D^{20} 1.52295.

It is practically insoluble in water and freely soluble in alcohol and ether.

Uses

1. It is mostly employed as a disinfectant.
2. It is also used as an anthelmintic (Nematodes).

B. Eugenol   Please see section 5.2.6.1.4.3 in this chapter.

C. Thymol   Please see section 5.2.1.4 in this chapter.

5.2.6.5.5.3.2 Dihydric Phenols   The various dihydric phenols found in natural products are namely: **Catechin (catechol)**. A few of these constituents shall be dealt with here under:

A. Catechin (Catechol)

Chemical Structure   (2R-*trans*)-2-(3, 4-Dihydroxyphenyl)-3, 4-dihydro-4H-1-benzopyran-3, 5, 7-triol.

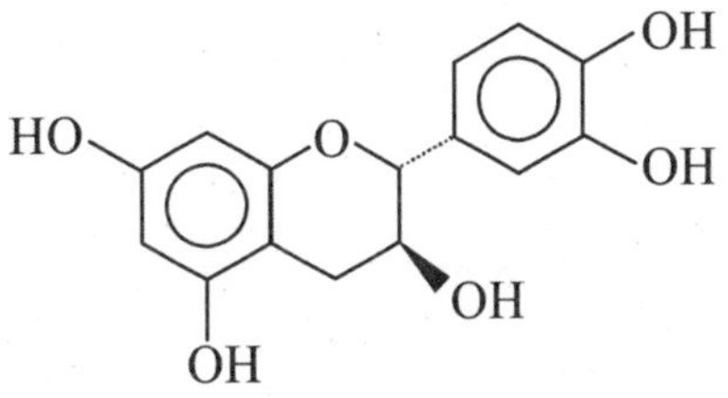

Catechin

Occurrence   It is a flavonoid found primarily in higher woody plants as **(–)-catechin** along with **(–)-epicatechin** (*cis*-form). It is also found in catechu (gambir and acacia), mahogany wood etc. Besides, it occurs in a variety of medicinal-plants, such as: *Argimonia eupatoria* L., (*Rosaceae*)-agrimony; *Areca catechu* L., (*Arecaceae*)-areca-nut, betel-nut palm; *Camellia sinensis* (L.) Kuntze (*Theaceae*)-tea; *Catha edulis* Vahl (*Celastaceae*)-khat; *Cola acuminata* (Beauv.) Schott & Endl. (*Sterculaceae*)-kola nuts, cola, guru; *Caratadegus oxyacantha* L. (*Rosaceae*)-hawthorn; *Ephedra gerardiana* Wall. ex Stapf (*Ephedraceae*)-Paskistani ephedra; *Eucalyptus globulus* Labill. (*Myrataceae*)-eucalypt, tasmanium bluegum; *Leonurus cardiaca* L., (*Lamiaceae*)-motherwort; *Malus sylvestris* Mill., (*Rosaceae*)-apple; *Paullinia cupana* Kunth. ex H.B.K. (Sapindaceae)-guarana, ubano, Brazilian cocoa; *Polygonum aviculare* L., (*Polygunaceae*)-prostrate knotweed; *Rheum officanale* Bail. (*Polygonaceae*)-Chinese rhubarb, Canton rhubarb, Shensi rhubarb; *Santolina chamaecyparissus* L. (*Asteraceae*)-Lavendar-cotton; *Solidago virgaureae* L. (*Asteraceae*)-European goldenrod, woundwort; *Uncaria gambir* (Hunter) Roxo. (*Rubiaceae*)-gombir, pale catechu; *Vanilla planifolia* Andr. (*Orchidaceae*)-vanilla.

Isolation   The areca nut or kola nut is cut into small chips mechanically and filled into the extractors. The steam is passed through the drug profusely to affect maximum extraction. The crude extract is filtered and concentrated under vacuum. The concentrated extract is chilled in deep-freezer when catechin separates as its hydrated product (mp: 93-96°C) and its anhydrous product (mp: 175-177°C).

Characteristic Features Its needles obtained from water and acetic acid give rise to its hydrate form having m.p. 93-96°C, whereas its anhydrous form registers mp 175–177°C, and $[\alpha]_D^{18} + 16°$ to $+ 18.4°$.

The physical parameters of *l*-form and *dl*-form are stated below.

S. No.	l-Catechin	dl-Catechin
1.	Needles from water and acetic acid mp 93-96°C (hydrated form); mp 175-177°C (anhydrous form)	Needles from water and acetic acid mp 212-216°C
2.	$[\alpha]_D$ - 16.8°	–
3.	Solubility in aqueous medium.	Practically insoluble in benzene, chloroform, pet, ether; soluble in hot water, alcohol, acetons, glacial acetic acid; and slightly soluble in cold water and ether.

Note   **Catechin is called catechol (flaran) to distinguish it from catechol (pyrocatechol q.v).**

Identification

1. **Catechin** on being treated with HCl yields phluroglucinol, that burns along with lignin to produce purple or magnata colour. The *tannin extract* is taken on the tip of a match-stick, dipped in HCl and burnt in the blue-flame of the Bunsen-burner.

2. It reacts with vanillin and HCl to produce a pink or red colour.

Uses

1. It is used as an antidiarrheal agent.

2. It is also employed for dycing and tanning.

B. Protocatechuic Acid

Chemical Structure   3,4-Dihydroxybenzoic acid.

Protocatechuic Acid

Occurrence   It is found in the dried fruit of *Illicium verum* Hook. f. (*Magnoliaceae*)-**star anise, Chinese anise;** in the leaves and seeds of *Perilla frutescens* (L.) Britt. (*Lamiaceae*)-**beef-steak plant, perilla, wild coleus;** and in the timbers of *Tabebuia Spp.* (*Bignoniaceae*)-Pao D'Arco. However, minute amounts are found in wheat grains and also in wheat seedlings.

Characteristic Features   It is white to brownish crystalline powder. It undergoes discolouration on exposure to air. Its mp ~ 200°C and d 1.54. It is soluble in 50 parts of water and freely soluble in ether and alcohol.

5.2.6.5.6 Phenolic Ether Volatile Oils   A good number of volatile oils essentially contain phenolic ethers which attribute powerful aromatic ou·ur and flavour. Because of their distinct characteristic aroma they are used extensively as pharmaceutical aids, perfumery and confectionery. A few typical examples of phenolic ether volatile oils are, namely: **Anethole; Safrole; Myristicin; Apiole; Cineole** and **Ascaridole.**

General Properties of Phenolic Ether Volatile Oils There are certain characteristic general properties of phenolic ether volatile oils that help in their identifications:

1. They are very stable *neutral compounds* which are sparingly water-soluble. They do not react with alkalies.
2. Phenolic ethers, in general, yield the corresponding phenols on treatment with HBr or HCl.
3. They form crystalline derivatives on account of various reactions, such as: bromination, nitration and oxidation.
4. Phenolic ethers give rise to the formation of **sulphonamides** in a two-step reaction depicted below:

Step 1: It react with chloro sulphonic acid to yield the corresponding sulphonyl chloride together with a molecule each of hydrochloric acid and sulphuric acid.

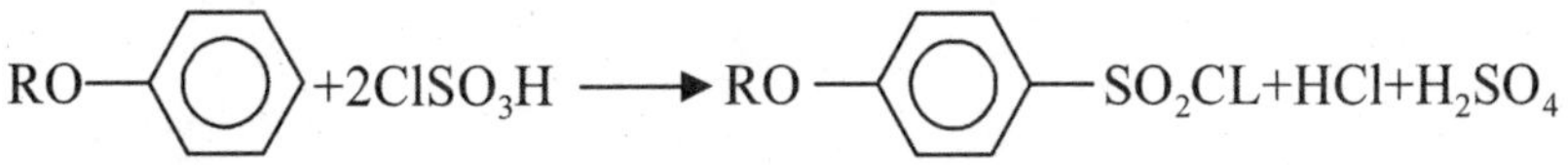

$$RO-\langle\bigcirc\rangle+2ClSO_3H \longrightarrow RO-\langle\bigcirc\rangle-SO_2CL+HCl+H_2SO_4$$

A phenolic ether Chloro-sulphonic   A Sulphonyl
acid   Chloride

Step 2: The resulting sulphonyl chloride (**Step 1**) on reaction with ammonium carbonate gives rise to the desired **sulphonamide** and a mole each of ammonium chloride, carbon dioxide and water.

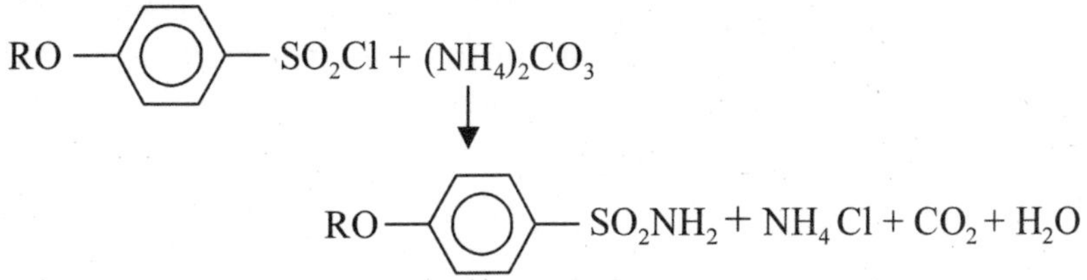

$$RO-\langle\bigcirc\rangle-SO_2Cl + (NH_4)_2CO_3$$

$$\downarrow$$

$$RO-\langle\bigcirc\rangle-SO_2NH_2 + NH_4Cl + CO_2 + H_2O$$

These chemical constituents shall be discussed individually in the sections that follows:

A. Anethole (**Synonym** Anise camphor, Monasirup)

Chemical Structure 1-Methoxy-4-(1-propenyl) benzene.

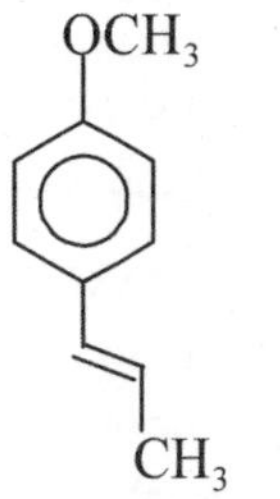

Anethole

It has a monohydric phenolic ether function.

Occurrence   It is the chief constituent of *anise* **(anise fruit, aniseed)** *i.e.*, the dried ripe fruits of *Pimpinella anisum* Linn' (Family: *Umbelliferae*); *star anise* **(star anise fruit, Chinese anise** *i.e.*, the dried ripe fruits of *Illicium verum* Hoop (Family: *Magnoliaceae*); and *fennel* **(fennel fruits finnocchio),** *i.e.*, the dried ripe fruits of *Foeniculum vulgare* Mill (Family: *Apiaceae*). It is also found in *Ocimum basilicum* L. (Family: *Lamiaceae*)-**Sweet Basil, Garden Basil;** *Pinus elliottii* Engelm. (Family: *Abiataceae*)-**Slash Pine;** *Sassafras albidum* (Nutt.) Nees (Family: *Lauraceae*)-**sassafras;** and *Syzygium aromaticum* (L.) Merr & Perry (Family: *Myrtaceae*)-**cloves, clavos.**

Isolation   It may be isolated from the volatile oils by first subjecting the oil to fractionation and then cooling the corresponding fraction to a very low temperature and recrystallization. However, it may also be obtained directly from the **anethole-rich oils,** such as: **oil of anise, oil of fennel** by simply chilling it to $-30°C$ in a deep freezer.

     Commercially, anethole may be synthesized in its purest form from anisole as shown below:

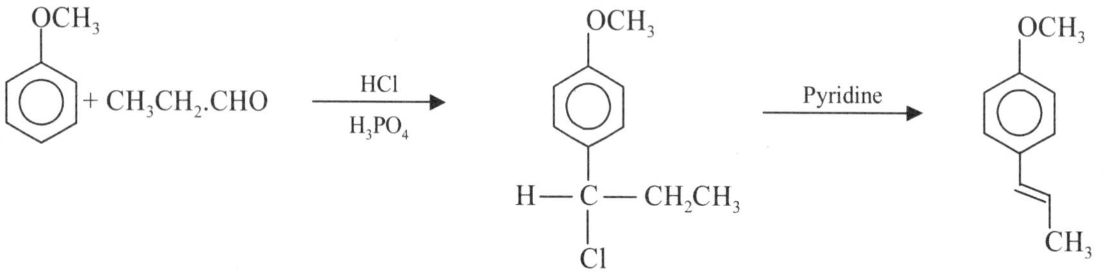

Anisole   Propionaldehyde   Anisole-p-(1-chloropropane)   Anethole

     Anisole on reacting with propionaldehyde in the presence of HCl and H_3PO_4 yields an intermediate anisole-p-(1-chloropropane) which finally with pyridine yields **anethole.**

Characteristic Features   It exists in *two* isomeric forms namely: *trans*-and *cis*-isomer, having physical parameters as stated below:

Forms	Nature	mp(°C)	d_4^{20}	$bp_{2.3}$	n_D^{20}	λ_{max} (EtOH)
trans- Anethole	Crystalline mass at 20-21°C	21.4 (Liquid above 23°)	0.9883	81-81.5°	1.56145	259 nm (ε 22300)
cis- Anethole	–	–	0.9878	79-79.5	1.55455	253.5 nm (ε 18500)

     It is a white crystalline substance with an intense sweet odour. It possesses a characteristic taste similar to anise fruit. It is practically soluble in most organic solvents but insoluble in water.

Formation of 'Photoanethole' (or p, p′-dimethoxystilbene)   **Anethole** on exposure to air (oxygen), light or heat undergoes structural modifications to yield **photoanethole** which is a viscid yellow coloured mass having a disagreeable taste and odour with a poor solubility in solvents. Perhaps the conversion of anethole to photoanethole lakes place *via* the formation of **anisaldehyde** as given below:

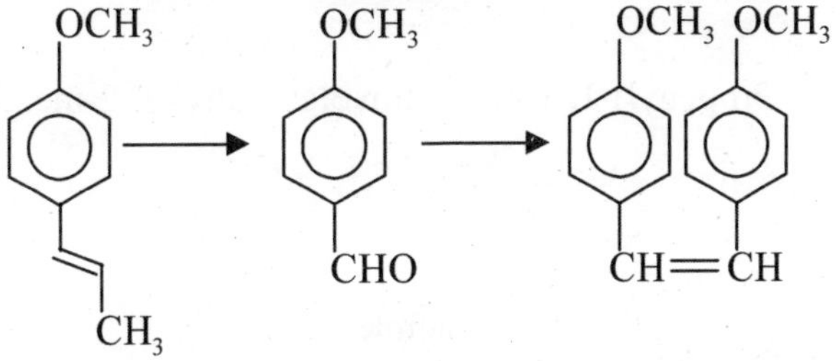

Anethole   Anisaldehyde   Photoanethole
(or *p*-Methoxy-   (or p,pODimethoxy-
benzaldehyde)   stilbene)

Identification

1. **Anethole** undergoes oxidation with $K_2Cr_2O_7$ in two steps; *first step*-yields anisaldehyde (*para*-methoxy benzaldehyde), and *second step*-gives rise to *para*-methoxy benzoic acid (mp 184°C) as depicted below:

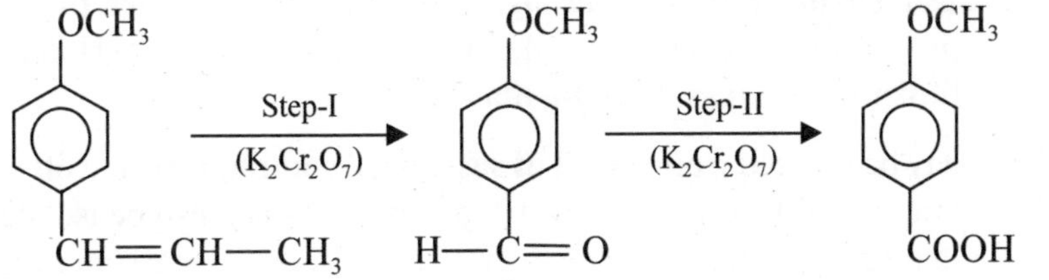

Anethole   Anisaldehyde   p-Methoxy benzoie acid

2. It gets condensed with maleic anhydride to yield a condensation product having mp 310°C as shown below:

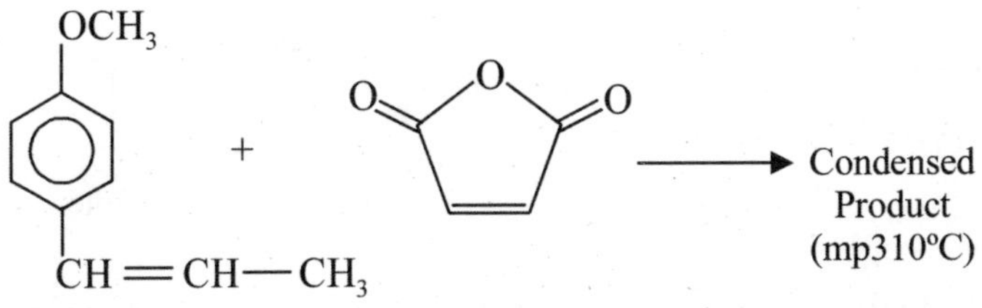

Anethole   Maleic anhydride

3. It gives rise to the formation of nitroso derivative having mp 126°C.

Uses

1. It is used as a flavouring agent in perfumery particularly for soap and dentifrices.
2. It is also employed as a pharmaceutical and (flavour).
3. It finds its application as an imbedding material in microscopy.
4. It is employed as a flavouring agent in alcholic, non-aleoholic beverages and confectionaries.
5. It is used as a sensitizer in bleaching colours in colour photography.

B. Safrole

Chemical Structure 5-(2-Propenyl)-1, 3-benzodioxole; 4-allyl-1, 2-methylenedioxybenzene.

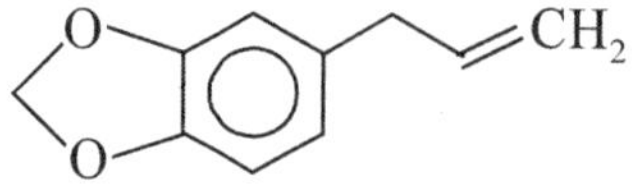

Safrole

Occurrence It is the constituent of a number of volatile oils, notably of *sassafras i.e.*, the dried dark of the roots of *Sassafras albidum* Nees, belonging to the family *Lauraceae,* in which it is present to the extent of 75%.

It is extensively found in a variety of other plant sources, namely: *Acorus calamus L., Araceae* **(sweet flag, flagroot, calamus);** *Angelica polymorpha* Max., *Apiaceae* **(dong quai);** *Cananga odorata* (Lam.) Hook. f. & Thoms., *Annonaceae* **(cananga, ylang-ylang);** *Cinnamomum comphora* (L.) J.S. Presl., *Lauraceae* **(camphor, hon-sho);** *Illicum verum* Hook. f. *Magnoliaceae* **(Star-anise, Chinese anise);** *Myristica fragrans* Houtt. *Myristicaceae* **(mace, nutmeg);** *Ocimum basilicum* L. *Lamiaceae* **(sweet basil, garden basil);** *Piper nigrum* L. *Piperaceae* **(black pepper);** *Theobroma cacao* L. *Sterculiaceae* (chocolate, cocoa, cacao); *Umbellularia california* (Hook. and Arn.) Nutt. **(California bay, California sassafras, (California laurel).**

Isolation **Safrole** may be isolated from the **oil of sassafras, comphor oil** and **oil of star-anise** and also the safrole-rich fraction of the oil to about –10 to –15°C. It may also be isolated by subjecting the above safrole containing oils to fractional distillation under reduced pressure, chilling the fraction and finally crystallization.

Characteristic Features It is colourless or slightly yellow liquid having a specific sassafras odour. Its physical properties are: d^{20} 1.096, mp ~ 11°C, bp 232-234°C and n_D^{20} 1.5383. It is insoluble in water, very soluble in alcohol and freely miscible with ether and chloroform.

It undergoes isomerization on being heated with alkalies to yield **isosafrole** as shown below:

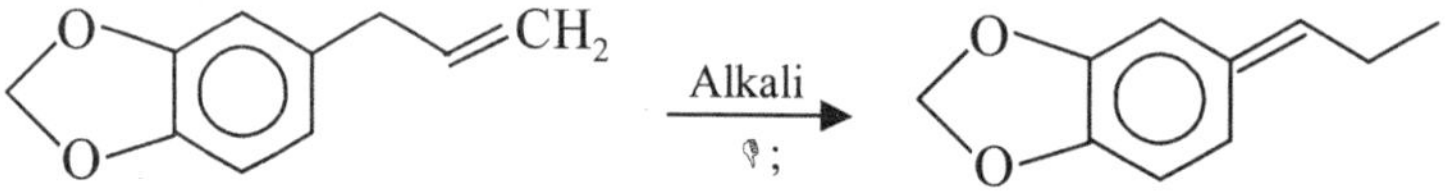

Safrole   Isosafrole

Identification

1. *Bromination:* **Safrole** on bromination yields the corresponding pentabromosafrole (mp 169-170°C).
2. *Oxidation:* **Safrole** on oxidation with $K_2Cr_2O_7$ and dilute H_2SO_4 (6 N) gives rise to the aldehyde derivative piperonol as shown below:

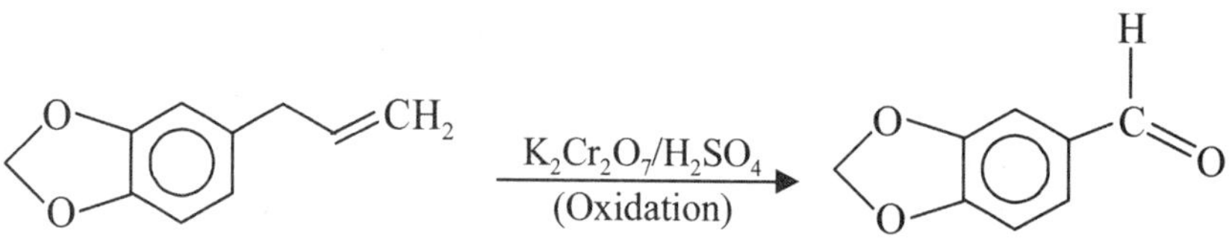

Safrole

Piperonal
(Heliotropin)

3. *Colour test:* Both **safrole** and **isosafrole** on treatment with concentrated sulphuric acid instantly produces an intense red colouration.

Uses

1. It is widely used as a flavouring agent for a variety of products, such as: beverages, pharmaceuticals chewing gums, toothpastes, in perfumery and scenting soaps.
2. It is also used in denaturing fats in soap manufacturing process.
3. It is mostly employed for the conversion to isosafrole and the manufacture of **heliotropin.**

C. Myristicin

Chemical Structure   4-(Methoxy)-6-(2-propenyl)-1, 3-benzodioxole.

Myristicin

Occurrence   The aromatic ether is extracted from nutmeg, mace, French parsley, carrots and **dill oils.**

The botanical sources of **myristicin** are as follows: *Anethum graveolens* L. (*Apiaciae*) **(Dil, Dill Seed, Garden Dill);** *Daucus Carota* subsp. Sativus (Hoffm.) Arcang [*Apiaceae*] **(Cultivated carrot,** Queen Anne's Lace (Wild));* *Myristica fragrans* Houtt. [*Myristaceae*] **(Mace, Nutmeg);** *Petroselinum crispum* (Mill) Nym. [*Apiaceae*] **(Parsley);** *Piper nigrum* L. [*Piperaceae*] **(Black Pepper);** *Sassafras albidum* (Nutt.) Nees [*Lauraceae*] **(Sassafras).**

Isolation   The rich source of volatile oil containing **myristicin** is subjected to fractional distillation under reduced pressure when the latter is collected as a colourless oily liquid.

Characteristic Features   It is an oily liquid having a characteristic aromatic odour. It does not congeal at low-temperature.

Myristicin on being treated with either metallic sodium or boiled with alcoholic KOH undergoes isomerism to yield **isomyristicin** as given below:

Myristicin   Isomyristicin

i.e., the allyl group in the former gets converted to the propenyl group in the latter.

It has the following physical parameters:

bp_{40} 173°C; n_D^{20} 1.54032; d_{20}^{20} 1.1437.

Identification

1. On oxidation with $KMnO_4$ it gives rise to *two* products, namely:

(*a*) Myristicin aldehyde (mp 130°C); and

(*b*) Myristinic acid (mp 208-210°C).

2. On interaction with bromine it yields the corresponding dibromoderivative having mp 130°C.

Uses   It is used as a flavouring agent in food products and confectioneries.

D. Apiole

Synonym   Dill; Dill apiole; Parsley comphor.

Chemical Structure   4,5-Dimethoxy-6-(2-propenyl)-1, 3-benzodioxole.

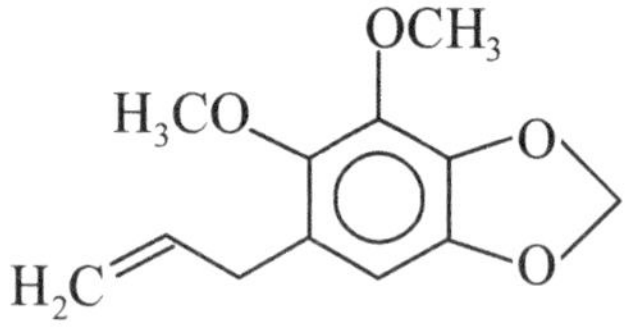

Apiole

Occurrence   It occurs abundantly in **dill oil** *Anethum graveolus* L., belonging to the natural order *Umbelliferae*. It is also found in the **Parsley seed oil** *Petroselinum crispum* (Mill.) Nym. (Family: *Apiaceae*). The volatile oil of *Sassafras albidum* (Nutt.) Nees (Family: *Lauraceae*) contains **apiole.**

Isolation   It is obtained by chilling the volatile oil to a very low temperature in a deep-freezer and finally recrystallizing it either from ethanol or petroleum ether (mp 29.5°C).

Characteristic Features   **Apiole** crystallises usually in the shape of long colourless needles with a faint specific odour of *Parsley.* Its physical parameters are: mp 29.5°C, bp 285°C; n_D^{17} 1.5305; d_{15}^{15} 1.1598. It is practically insoluble in water, but soluble in ethanol, ether and in fatty oils.

Apiole on boiling with alcoholic KOH undergoes isomerisation to yield isoapiole (mp 55-56°C) whereby the allyl group in the former gets isomerized to the propenyl function in the latter as given below:

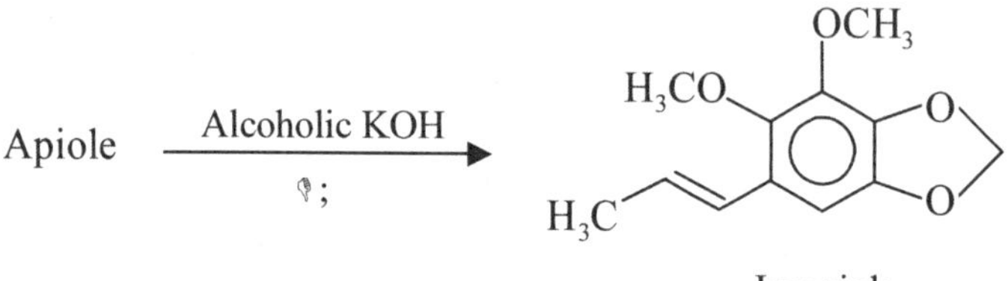

Isoapiole

Apiole on treatment with bromine yields a monobromide (mp 51°C), a dibromide (mp 75°C) and also a tribromide (mp 120°C) as depicted below:

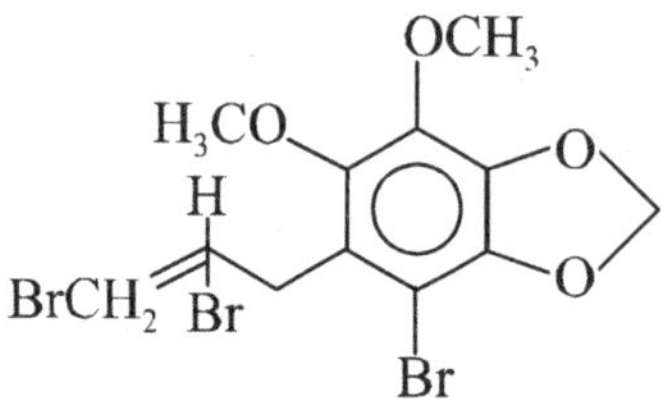

Apiole Tribromide

On oxidation with $KMnO_4$ both **apiole** and **isoapiole** yield the corresponding **apioaldehyde** and **apiolic acid.**

Identification

1. It may be identified by forming its bromoderivatives as stated above having a specific melting point.
2. It may also be identified by preparing its oxidative products with $KMnO_4$, such as: opioaldeyde (mp 102°C) and apiolic acid (mp 173°C).

Uses

1. It exerts a synergistic activity with insecticides.
2. Dill is frequently employed as an aromatic stimulant, carminative and flavouring agent.
3. **Dill oil** is an important ingredient of **'Gripe Water'** which is given to infants to relieve them from flatulence.

E. Cineole

Synonyms   Eucalyptol; Cajeputol.

Chemical Structure   1, 8-Epoxy-p-menthane.

Cineole

Occurrence   It is the chief constituent of **oil of eucalyptus** obtained from the leaves of *Eucalyptus globulus* Labill (Family: *Myrtaceae*) and other species of *Eucalyptus.* It also occurs largely in a variety of plants, namely: *Acorus calamus* L., (*Araceae*); *Aloysia triphylla* Britton (Family: *Verbenaceae*)-**Lemon Verbena;** *Artemisia vulgaris* L., (Family: *Asteraceae*)-**Mugwort, Carline Thistle;** *Chamaemelum nobile* (L.) All (Family: *Asteraceae*)-**Roman Camomile, English Camomile, Camomile,** *Cinnamomum verum* J.S. Presl (Family: *Lauraceae*)-**Ceylon Cinnamon;** *Crocus sativus* L., (Family: *Iridaceae*)-**Saffron,** *Saffron crocus*; *Croton eleutheria* Sw. (Family: *Euphorbiaceae*-Cascarilla; *Illicium verum* Hook. f. (Family: *Magnoliaceae*)-**Star-Anise, Chinese Anise;** *Juniperus communis* L. (Family: *Cupressaceae*)-Common Juniper; *Juniperus sabina* L. (Family *Cupressaceae*)-Sabine, Savin; *Laurus nobilis* L., (Family: *Lauraceae*)-Bay, Grecian Laurel, **Green Bay;** *Melaleuca leucadenron* L. (Family: *Myrtaceae*)-**Cajeput;** *Pimenta diocia* (L.) Merr. (Family: *Myrtaceae*)-**Allspice, Jamaica Pepper, Clove Pepper;** *Rosmarinus officinalis* L. (Family: *Lamiaceae*)-**Rosemary;** *Salvia sclarea* L., Family: *Lamiaceae*)-Clary, **Muscatel Sage;** *Tanecetum vulgare* L., (Family: *Asteraceae*)-**Tansy;** *Umbellularia californica* (Hook and Arn.) Nutt.-**California Bay, California Laurel, California Sassafras.**

Isolation   **Cineole** may be isolated from **Eucalyptus oil,** which contains this ingredient to the extent of 80% by any one of the following *four* methods, namely:

Method I: Fractional Distillation. It may be obtained from fractional distillation under vacuo and the colourless liquid is collected over powdered anhydrous sodium sulphate. The clear oily substance is obtained finally in the pure crystalline form by chilling it (mp + 1.5°C).

Method II: Addition Products with Halogen Acids (HCl, HBr). It forms addition compounds with HCl and HBr as: $C_{10}H_{18}O$. HCl and $C_{10}H_{18}O$. HBr, from which the pure cincole may be regenerated conveniently.

Method III: Addition Product with Resorcinol. It forms an addition compound with 50% (w/v) solution of pure resorcinol as $[(C_{10}H_{18}O)_2 . C_6H_6O_2]$ having mp 80-85°C, from which cineole may be regenerated easily.

Note   **This reaction may eater for the separation of cineole from essential oils having a high cineole content (more than 50-60%), otherwise the volatile oil must first be fractionated.**

Method IV: Addition Product with Phosphoric Acid. Cineole readily forms addition product with phosphoric acid as: $[C_{10}H_{18}O . H_3PO_4]$ having mp 84°C, that may be decomposed by hot water.

Note   **This method is also utilized for the estimation of cineole in volatile oils in v/v percentage.**

Characteristic Features   It is a colourless liquid having a camphor-like odour. It possesses a spicy and cooling taste. Its physical characteristics are: d_{25}^{25} 0.921-0.923, bp 176-177°C, mp + 1.5°C, n_D^{20} 1.455-1.460, flash point (closed-up) 48°C. It is almost insoluble in water but miscible with alcohol, chloroform, ether, glacial acetic acid and oils.

    Cineole forms addition compounds with resorcinol and phosphoric acid, that are found to be fairly stable, having mp 80-85°C and 80°C respectively.

    It is not attacked by ordinary reducing agents, such as: glucose etc.

Identification

1. **Cineole** may be characterized by a host of derivatives/addition compounds obtained from pure chemical substances, for instance: halogen acids, resorcinol, phosphoric acid, *orthocresol* etc.

2. **Microchemical Test of Cineole:** A drop of pure cineole or a drop of Eucalyptus oil or a few drops of an alcoholic extract of eucalyptus leaf, is made to react with a drop of 5% (w/v) solution of *hydroquinone* on a microscopic slide and subsequently examined under a low-power microscope one may observe either colourless prisms or rhomboid crystals.

    However, an identical treatment with a 50% (w/v) solution of *resorcinol* gives rise to beautiful leaf-like crystals.

Uses

1. It is used quite extensively in pharmaceutical preparations both meant for internal and external utilities, such as:
   Internal usage—as a stimulating expectorant in cases of chromic bronchitis
   External usage—as a mild antiseptic, anaesthetic in cases of inflammatory conditions.
2. It is also employed in room-sprays, hand lotions and all types of cosmetic formulations.
3. It is invariably used as a pharmaceutical aid *i.e.*, flavouring agent.

F. Ascaridole (Synonym Ascarisin)

Chemical Structure   1, 4-Peroxido-p-menthene-2. It is an organic peroxide which constitutes 60-80% of **oil of chenopodium.** It is the only naturally occurring **terpenoid peroxide.**

Ascaridiole

Occurrence   **Ascaridiole** is the major constituent (65-70%) in the **chenopodium oil,** *i.e.,* a volatile oil, obtained by the steam distillation from the fresh flowing and fruiting plants (except roots) of the botanical species *Chenopodium ambrosioides* var *anthelminticum* Linn., belonging to the family *Chenopodiaceae.*

Isolation   It is isolated by the repeated fractional distillation of the volatile oil of chenopodium (**American wormseed oil**) *under vacuo* and collecting the fraction boiling at 95-98°C.

Characteristic Features   **Ascaridiole** is a viscid yellow oily liquid having a very peculiar and most disagreable odour and flavour. It is highly unstable and is prone to explode when either subjected to heat or when treated with organic acids, *e.g.,* acetic acid; and with inorganic acids, *e.g.,* sulphuric, nitric; hydrochloric and phosphoric acids. It being a peroxide liberates I_2 from KI in acetic acid solution.

It is soluble in hexane, pentane, ethanol, toluene, benzene and castor oil. Its physical characteristics are: mp + 3.3°C; $bp_{0.2}$ 39-40°C; $[\alpha]_D^{20}$ 0.00; d_4^{20} 1.0103;

Prepared Synthetically   **Ascaridiole** may be synthesized from ∝-terpinene by treatment with oxygen, chlorophyll and light as given below:

⊘-Terpinene   Ascaridiole

Identification   As **ascaridiole** does not produce any crystalline derivative, therefore, it is usually characterized by the help of the following **two specific reactions:**

1. **Formation of cis-1:4-Terpin [$C_{10} H_{18} (OH)_2$]: Ascaridiole** on reduction with H_2 and Pd as a catalyst gives rise to the formation of ***cis*-1, 4-terpin** as follows:

    The resulting *cis*-1, 4-terpin is *optically inactive* and also it is not identical with 1, 8-terpin, although the two compounds have similar melting points *i.e.*, 116–117°C.

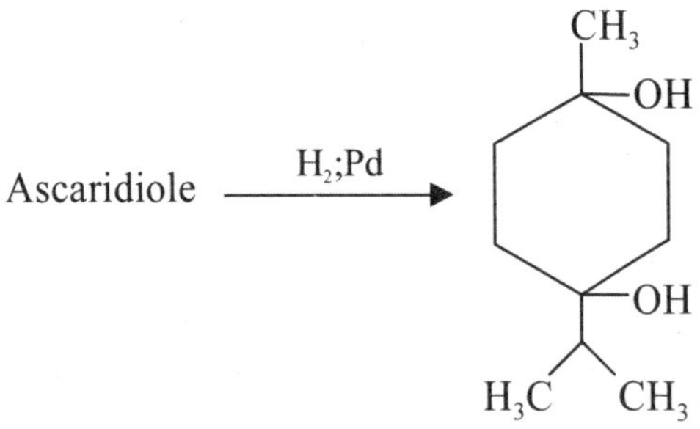

Ascaridiole $\xrightarrow{\text{H}_2;\text{Pd}}$

cis-1,4-Terpin

2. **Formation of Ascaridole Glycol: Ascaridole** upon oxidation with $FeSO_4$ yield chiefly a '*glycol*' which is not steam-volatile *viz.*, **ascaridole glycol.** Consequently, this glycol may be further characterized by the formation of its monobenzoate (mp 136-137°C) and dibenzoate derivatives (mp 116.5°C).

Uses

1. It has been used as an anthelmintic (Nematodes).
2. It is also employed for eliminating hookworms and roundworms.
3. It is used most frequently in large number of medical and veterinary formulations.

Note   Estimation of Ascaridole* Ascaridole may be determined quantitatively by the method described in the Extra Pharmacopoea, which is developed by Cocking and Hymas and based upon the oxidizing property of the 'peroxide function' exclusively present in it on the strongly acidified solution of KI (with HCl and glacial acetic acid). Thus, the liberated I_2 is titrated with sodium thiosulphate ($Na_2S_2O_3$) using freshly prepared starch solution as an indicator (colour change from blue to colourless) under the specified experimental parameters.

Precautions

1. Addition of oxygenated constituents must be avoided in the assay procedure that may give rise to eroneous results.
2. As the liberated iodine is capable of being absorbed by unsaturated components present in the volatile oil, it is absolutely necessary to carry out the assay at low temperature so as to maintain such secondary reactions at the lowest level.

5.2.6.5.7 Oxide Volatile Oils The various chemical constituents containing oxide function present in naturally occurring volatile oils are namely: **Safrole, Myristicin, Apiole, Cineole and Ascaridole.** These compounds have already been discussed under section *Phenolic Ether Volatile Oils* (5.2.6.5.6) in this chapter.

---

* *Analyst*, **55**, 180, 1930.

5.2.6.5.8 Ester Volatile Oils The '**Ester Volatile Oils**' essentially attribute their flavouring characteristics, odour, aroma and specific perfume by virtue of the presence of a good number of naturally occurring esters, most common among which are the acetates of borneol, geraniol and terpineol. However, it is an age-old practice to allow the maturation or ageing of such ester-containing perfumes in order to enhance the process of esterification *in situ* thereby ultimately improving the overall aroma and bouquet of the volatile oil. Incidentally, there are certain exceptions, such as: the '**Oil of Wintergreen**' which contains upto 99% of **methyl salicylate** (an ester).

Classification The ester volatile oils may be classified conveniently into *three* categories as follows:

(*i*) Esters of Aliphatic Acids,
(*ii*) Esters of Aromatic Acids, and
(*iii*) Esters containing Nitrogen.

These different categories of ester volatile oils shall be discussed along with their typical examples as under:

5.2.6.5.8.1 Esters of Aliphatic Acids The typical examples of esters of the aliphatic acids are, namely: **Geranyl acetate, Linalyl acetate.**

A. Geranyl Acetate

Chemical Structure 3, 7-Dimethyl-2, 6-octadien-8-acetate; ($C_{12} H_{20} O_2$). It is an olefenic terpene acetate mostly found in a number of essential oils.

Geranyl Acetate

Occurrence The ester is very widely distributed in a variety of essential oils, such as: **oil of citronella, petit grain, lemon-grass, coriander, lavender** etc. It is also found in *Satureja montana* L. (*Lamiaceae*)-**Winter Savory, White Thyme, Spanish Savory;** and *Tilia europaea* L. (*Tiliaceae*)-**Lime Tree** (Europe), **Linden Tree** (America).

Isolation It may be obtained from the rich source of volatile oil containing **greanyl acetate** by fractional distillation under vacuum.

Characteristic Features It is a colourless liquid having a pleasant aromatic fragrance resembling to that of rose. It boils at 242-245°C with decomposition at atmospheric pressure.

Identification The ester on saponification with alcoholic KOH yields geraniol and acetic acid as the products of reaction. The former may be identified by examining its physical parameters, for instance: bp_{757} 229-230°C; bp_{12} 114-115°C; d_4^{20} 0.8894; n_D^{20} 1.4766; uv_{max} 190-195 nm (ε 18000).

Uses
1. It is used abundantly in perfumery.
2. It is also employed in making cosmetics and various types of toilet soaps.

B. Linalyl Acetate

Synonym   Bergamot.

Chemical Structure   3, 7-Dimethyl-1, 6-octadien-3-yl acetate; ($C_{12} H_{20} O_2$). It is also an olefinic terpene acetate and regarded as the most valuable constituent of bergamot and lavender oils.

Linalyl Acetate

Occurrence   It is found in a number of volatile oils, namely: *Lavandula angustifolia* Mill. (*Lamiaceae*)-**Lavender, True or Common Lavender;** *Salvia selarea* L. (*Lamiaceae*)-**Clary, Cleareye, Muscatel Sage;** *Satureja montana* L. (*Lamiaceae*)-**Winter Savory, White Thyme, Spanish Savory;** *Thymus vulgaris* L. (*Lamiaceae*)-**Common Thyme;** *Tilia europaea* L. (*Tiliaceae*)-**Linden Tree** (America), **Lime Tree** (Europe).

Isolation   It may be obtained from **lavender oil** or **bergamot oil** by subjecting it to distillation under very high vacuum, because on distillation at atmospheric pressure or with steam distillation linalyl acetate gets hydrolysed rapidly and decomposed eventually.

Characteristic Features   It is a colourless oily liquid having a very pleasant fruity odour of **bergamot oil.** Its physical properties are: d_4^{20} 0.885; bp 220°C; n_D^{20} 1.4460. It is almost insoluble in water but miscible freely with ether and alcohol.

Identification   Linalyl acetate upon saponification with alcoholic KOH yields **linalool (linalol)** and acetic acid. The *dl*-form of **linalool** has a bp_{720} 194-197°C.

Uses   It is used extensively in perfumery.

5.2.6.5.8.2 Esters of Aromatic Acids   The various esters that are associated with aromatic acids and found in volatile oils are: **Benzyl benzoate, Cinnamyl Cinnamate; Methyl Salicylate.**

A. Benzyl Benzoate

Synonyms   Ascabin; Venzonate; Ascabiol.

Chemical Structure   Benzoic acid phenyl methyl ester; ($C_{14}H_{12}O_2$).

Benzyl Benzoate

Occurrence   It is contained in **Peru and Tolu balsams.** It is also found in a variety of volatile oils, such as: *Cananga odorata* (Lam.) Hook. f. & Thomas (*Annonaceae*)-**Ylang-Ylang, Cananga;** *Cinnamonum verum* J S Presl (*Lauraceae*)-**Ceylon Cinnamon;** *Myroxylon balsamum* Var. *Pereirae*

(Royle) Harms. (*Fabaceae*)-**Balsam of Peru**; *Peumus boldus* Molina (*Monimiaceae*)-**Baldo;** *Vanilla planifolia* Andr. (*Orchidaceae*)-**Vanilla**.

Isolation   Benzyl benzoate may be isolated by cooling the corresponding fraction to a very low temperature when it gets separated as a solid (mp 21°C). It may also be further recrystallized from chloroform or ether.

Characteristic Features   It is an oily liquid or leaflets, having a faint, pleasant aromatic odour. It possesses a sharp burning taste. Its physical characteristics are: mp 21°C; d_4^{20}1.118; bp 323-324°C; bp_{16} 189-191°C; $bp_{4.5}$ 156°C, and n_D^{21} 1.5681. It is sparingly volatile with steam. It is insoluble in water or glycerol, but miscible with alcohol, chloroform, ether and oils.

Identification   The benzyl benzoate on saponification yields the two products of reaction *i.e.,* benzoic acid and benzyl alcohol that may be identified by carrying out specific tests for these compounds.

Uses
1. It is used extensively as a diluent and solvent of solid aromatics *e.g.*, artificial musk.
2. By virtue of its low volatility benzyl benzoate is employed as a fixative in perfume composition.
3. It is used as a solvent for cellulose acetate and nitrocellulose.
4. It serves as a substitute for camphor in celluloid and plastic pyroxylin compounds.
5. It is also employed in confectionery and chewing gum flavours.

B. Cinnamyl Cinnamate

Synonyms   Cinnyl cinnamate; Styracin.

Chemical Structure   3-Phenyl-2-propenoic acid 3-phenyl-2-propenyl ester.

Cinnamyl Cinnamate

Occurrence   It occurs in the buds of *Populus balsamifer* L., (Family: *Salicaceae*)-Goris; *Lavanga scandens* Buch-Ham., *Lavangalata*-Baslas; and *Styrox Benzoin* Dryander (Family: *Styracaceae*)-**Benzoin, Sumatra Benzoin, Styrax**.

Isolation   It may be obtained from the volatile oil fraction by chilling it to low temperature and collecting the solids having mp 44°C.

Characteristic Features   The characteristic features of the ***trans-trans*-cinnamyl cinnamate** are: mp 44°C; uv_{max} (95% ethanol): 216, 223 nm (log ε 3.45, 3.25). It is practically insoluble in water but sparingly soluble in cold ethanol and soluble in ether (1 g in 3 ml).

Identification   On saponification with alcoholic KOH this ester gives rise to cinnamic acid and cinnamyl alcohol which may be further identified by performing their specific tests.

Uses

1. It is used in perfumery.
2. It is also employed in making toilet soaps etc.

C. Methyl Salicylate

Synonyms   Winter green oil; Betula oil; Sweet birch oil; Teabery oil.

Chemical Structure   2-Hydroxybenzoic acid methyl ester; ($C_8 H_8 O_3$)

Methyl Salicylate

Occurrence   It is largely found in a variety of medicinal plants, namely: Flowers of *Acacia farnesiana* (L.) Willd. (Family: *Fabaceae*)-**Cassie, Huisache;** *Cananga odorata* (Lam.) Hook. f. & Thoms (Family: *Annonaceae*)-**Cananga, Ylang-Ylang;** Leaves of *Chenopodium ambrosioides* L. (Family: *Chenopodiaceae*)-**Wormseed;** *Erythroxylum coca* Lam. (Family: *Erythroxylaceae*)-**Coca;** Flowerbuds of *Filipendula ulmaria* (L.) Maxim (Family: *Rosaceae*)-**Meadowsweet, Queen of the Meadow;** Twigs of *Gaultheria procumbens* L. (Family: *Ericaceae*)-**Wintergreen, Teaberry, Boxberry;** Bark of *Betula lenta* L. (Family: *Betulaceae*)-**Sweet Birch.** However, **oil of wintergreen** contains upto 99% **methyl salicylate.**

It is pertinent to mention here that in several aromatic medicinal plants, for instance: *Wintergreen,* the active chemical constituent *i.e.,* **methyl salicylate** does not occur as such, but is present in the form of a *glucoside* known as **Gaultherin** which upon enzymatic hydrolysis gives **methyl salicylate** and **primeverose (glucoxylose)** as shown under:

Gaultherin   Methyl   Primeverose
                             Salicylate

Isolation   **Methyl salicylate** may be obtained from gaultherin by enzymatic hydrolysis and then subjecting the resulting products of reaction to very low temperature when the former gets solidified at − 8.6°C and hence may be separated easily.

Characteristic Features   It is a colourless, yellowish or reddish, oily liquid. Its odour and taste resembles to that of gaultheria. Its physical parameters are: mp − 8.6°C; bp 220-224°C; d$_{25}^{25}$ 1.184; d of the natural ester is ~ 1.180; and n$_D^{20}$ 1.535-1.538. It is very sparingly soluble in water (1 g in 1500 ml), but freely soluble in chloroform and ether. It is, however, miscible with alcohol and glacial acetic acid.

Identifications

1. It develops a red-violet colouration on being treated with cold saturated aqueous solution of $FeCl_3$, that lasts for about 15 minutes.
2. **Methyl salicylate** readily forms a soluble ester-salt with a moderately concentrated aqueous solution of KOH as *potassium methyl salicylate.*
3. Upon saponification the ester yields salicylic acid (mp 158°C) and methanol respectively.
4. **Methyl salicylate** may also be identified by the formation of several derivatives as stated below:
    (*i*) Methylo-acetoxy benzoate (mp 52-52.5°C)—with Acetic Anhydride,
    (*ii*) Methyl-o-benzoxy benzoate (mp 92°C)—with Benzoyl Chloride,
    (*iii*) o-Cabomethoxyphenyl-N-phenyl urethane—with Phenylisocyanate.

Uses

1. **Methyl salicylate** has local irritant, antirheumatic and antiseptic properties. It is an important ingredient of **Iodex$^{(R)}$** ointment for relief of pain in several conditions like, pulled muscle, muscular pain, pain in joints, etc.
2. It also finds its extensive usage in a variety of products, such as: flavouring of food products, beverages, candies, confectionery, toothpastes, mouth washes, gargles, and pharmaceutical preparations.
3. It is also used in perfumery.

5.2.6.5.8.3 Esters Containing Nitrogen The specific example of an ester containing *nitrogen* is **Methyl Anthranilate** which is present in several volatile oils. It is described below:

A. Methyl Anthranilate

Synonyms   Neroli Oil (Artificial).

Chemical Structure   2-Aminobenzoic acid methyl ester, $(C_8 H_9 NO_2)$.

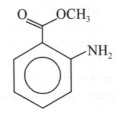

Methyl Anthranilate

Occurrence   It occurs in a good number of medicinal herbs, for instance: Flowers of *Robinia pseudoacacia* L. (Family: *Fabaceae*)-**Black Locust, False Acacia**; *Citrus sinensis* (Linn.) Osbeck. (Family: *Rutaceae*)-**Sweet Orange**; *Cananga odorata* (Lam.) Hook. f. & Thoms. (Family: *Annonaceae*)-**Ylang-Ylang, Cananga**; *Jasminum officinale* Linn. var *grandiflorum* Bailey., (Family: *Oleaceae*)-**Jasmine.** It is also found in bergamot, other essential oils and in grape juice.

It is also obtained synthetically by carrying out the esterification of anthranilic acid with methanol in the presence of HCl.

Isolation   **Methyl anthranilate** may be isolated from the essential oils very conveniently by shaking the volatile oil with cold dilute sulphuic acid (2 N) *i.e.*, 1 ml of conc. H_2SO_4 dissolved slowly in

17 ml of distilled water. The resulting methyl anthranilate sulphate thus obtained gets crystallized in the cold, which may be further purified by recrystallization from alcohol. Finally the pure desired ester is regenerated by treatment with dilute NaOH solution (2 N) carefully.

Characteristic Features   It is a crystalline mass having a powerful pleasant taste. It has a peculiar odour that mostly resembles to orange blossoms and certain varieties of grape. It gives an inherent blue-violet fluorescence which is distinctly visible in any volatile oil containing it. **Methyl anthranilate** has the following physical parameters, namely:

d 1.168; mp 24-25°C; bp_{15} 135.5°C.

It is slightly soluble in water, but freely soluble in ethanol and ether.

Identification   It may be identified by preparing its derivatives, such as: Picrate (mp 104°C); Benzoate (mp 100°C).

Uses
1. It is used frequently as a perfume for ointments.
2. It is also employed for the manufacture of synthetic perfumes.

5.2.7   Resins and Resin Combinations

Resins, in general, are amorphous solid or semisolid substances that are invariably water insoluble but mostly soluble in alcohol or other organic solvents. However, physically they are found to be hard, translucent or transparent and fusible *i.e.*, upon heating they first get softened and ultimately melt. But chemically, they are complex mixtures of allied substances, such as: **resin acids, resin alcohols** (or **resinols**), **resinotannols, resin esters, glucoresins** and the like.

Another school of thought considers **Resins** as amorphous products having an inherent complex chemical entity. These are normally produced *either* in schizogenous or in sehizolysigenous ducts or in carities and are regarded as the end products of metabolism. The physical general characteristic features of resins are namely: hard, transparent, or translucent and, when heated they yield usually complex mixtures that comprise of resin acids, resin alcoholds, resinotannols, esters and resenes. Some researehers do believe that the resins are nothing but the oxidation products of the **terpenes.** They are found to be mostly insoluble in water, but soluble in ethanol and organic solvents. They are electrically non-conductive and combustible in nature.

Resins shall now be discussed at length in their various aspects as enumerated here under:

(*a*) Distribution of Resins in Plants
(*b*) Occurrence in Plants
(*c*) Physical Properties of Resins
(*d*) Chemical Properties of Resins
(*e*) Solubility
(*f*) Preparation of Resins
(*g*) Chemical Composition of Resins
(*h*) Classification of Resins.

5.2.7.1   *Distribution of Resins in Plants*

Interestingly, the **resins** and resinous substances are more or less extensively distributed throughout the entire plant kingdom, specifically the *Spermatophyta i.e.*, the seed plants. Notably, their presence is almost rare and practically negligible in the *Pteridophyta i.e.*, the ferns and their allies. However, the resins have not been reported in the *Thallophyta i.e.*, the sea-weeds, fungi etc.

Therefore, all these findings and observations lead one to the fact the *resins* are the overall and net result of metabolism in the *higher plants,* since the majority of them belong to the phyllum *Angiosperum i.e.*, seed-enclosed flowering plants, and *Gymnosperm i.e.*, naked-seed non-flowering plants.

In general, the most important and extensively studied resin-containing families are, namely: *Pinaceae* (*Colophory* or *Rosin*); *Leguminosae* (*Tolu Balsam* and *Balsam of Peru*); *Dipterocarpaceae* ('*Garijan*'—a Balsam substitute for copaiba); *Burseraceae* (Myrrh) and *Umbelliferae* (Asafoetida).

5.2.7.2 *Occurrence in Plants*

In the plants resins usually occur in different secretory zones or structures. A few typical examples of such plant sources along with their specific secretary structures are given below:

(*i*)	**Resin Cells**	: *Ginger–Zingiber officinale* Roscoe (Family: *Zingiberaceae*);
(*ii*)	**Schizogenous Ducts**	: *Pine Wood–Pinus polustris* Miller.
	or Schizolysogenous	(Family: *Pinaceae*).
	Ducts	
	or Cavities	
(*iii*)	**Glandular Hairs**	: *Cannabis–Cannabis sativa* Linne'.
		(Family: *Moraceae*)

The formation of **resins** in the plant is by virtue of its normal physiological functions. However, its yield may be enhanced in certain exceptional instances by inflicting injury to the living plant, for instance: *Pinus*. Furthermore, many resisnous products are not formed by the plant itself unless and until purposeful and methodical injuries in the shape of incisions are made on them and the secretions or plant exudates are tapped carefully, such as: **Balsam of Talu** and **Benzoin**. In other words, these resins are of pathological origin. One school of thought has categorically termed the secretion exclusively obtained from the naturally occurring secretory structure as the *Primary Flow,* whereas the one collected through man-made-incisions on the plant *i.e.*, abnormally formed secretary structures, as the **Secondary Flow.**

In normal practice, it has been observed evidently that resins are invariably produced in ducts as well as cavities; sometimes they do not occur in the so called specialized-secretory structures, but tend to get impregnated in all the elements of a tissue, for example: **Guaiacum Resin**—is obtained from the heartwood of *Guaiacum officinale* Linn. and *G. sanctum* Linn., (Family: *Zygophyllaceae*) *i.e.*, it is found in the vessels, fibres, medullary ray cells and wood parenchyma. In this particular instance, the resins occur as **tyloses,** achieved by chopping off the conduction in these areas so as to enhance the effective usage of root pressure and the capillaries in forcing both the nutritive contents and forcing water to reach the top end of these tall trees.

It is pertinent to mention here that in some exceptionally rare instances the resin occurs as a result of sucking the juice of the plant by scale insects and converting the sucked-juice into a resinous substance that ultimately covers the insect itself and twigs of the plant as well, for instance: *Laccifer lacca* (Family: *Coccidae*)-**Shellac.**

5.2.7.3 Physical Properties of Resins

The various physical properties of **resins** can be generalized as detailed below:

1. **Resins,** as a class, are hard, transparent or translucent brittle materials.
2. They are invariably heavier than water having the specific gravity ranging from 0.9-1.25.
3. **Resins** are more or less amorphous materials but rarely crystallisable in nature.
4. On being heated at a relatively low temperature **resins** first get softened and ultimately melt down thereby forming either an adhesive or a sticky massive fluid, without undergoing any sort of decomposition or volatilization.
5. On being heated in the air *i.e.*, in the presence of oxygen, resins usually burn readily with a smoky flame by virtue of the presence of a large number of C-atoms in their structure.
6. On being heated in a closed container *i.e.*, in the absence of oxygen, they undergo decomposition and very often give rise to **empyreumatic products** *i.e.*, products chiefly comprising of hydrocarbons.
7. Resins are bad conductors of electricity, but when rubbed usually become negatively charged.
8. They are practically insoluble in water, but frequently soluble in ethanol, volatile oils, fixed oils, chloral hydrate and non-polar organic solvents *e.g.*, benzene, n-hexane and petroleum ether.

5.2.7.4 Chemical Properties of Pesins

The various chemical properties of **resins** may be summarized as stated below:

1. Resins, in general, are enriched with carbon, deprived of nitrogen and contain a few oxygen in their respective molecules.
2. Majority of them undergo slow atmospheric oxidation whereby their colour get darkened with impaired solubility.
3. Resins are found to be a mixture of numerous compounds rather than a single pure chemical entity.
4. Their chemical properties are exclusively based upon the functional groups present in these substances.
5. Consequently, the resins are broadly divided into **resin alcohols, resin acids, resin esters, glycosidal resins** and **resenes** (*i.e.*, inert neutral compounds).
6. Resins are regarded as complex mixtures of a variety of substances, such as: **resinotannols, resin acids, resin esters, resin alcohols and resenes.**
7. One school of thought believes that resins are nothing but **oxidative products of terpenes.**
8. They may also be regarded as the end-products of *destructive metabolism.*
9. The acidic resins when treated with alkaline solutions they yield soaps (or **resin-soaps**).

Note **The solutions of resins in alkalies distinctly differ from ordinary soap solutions by virtue of the fact that the former cannot be easily 'salted-out' by the addition of NaCl, unless it is used in large excess quantity.**

5.2.7.5 Solubility

The solubility of various types of **resins** are as follows:

1. Majority of **resins** are water-insoluble and hence they have practically little taste.

2. They are usually insoluble in petroleum ether (a non-polar solvent) but with a few exceptions, such as: colophory (freshly powdered) and mastic.

3. Resins mostly got completely dissolved in a number of polar organic solvents, for instance: ethanol, ether and chloroform, thereby forming their respective solutions which on evaporation, leaves behind a thin-varnish-like film deposit.

4. They are also freely soluble in many other organic solvents, namely: acetone, carbon disulphide, as well as in fixed oils and volatile oils.

5. Resins dissolve in chloral hydrate solution, normally employed for clarification of certain sections of plant organs.

5.2.7.6 Preparation of Resins

So far, no general method has either been suggested or proposed for the preparation of resins. In fact, there are *two* categories of resinous products, namely: (*a*) **Natural Resins;** and (*b*) **Prepared Resins,** have been duly accepted and recognized. Therefore, this classification forms the basis of the methods employed in the preparation of the *two* aforesaid resins.

A. Natural Resins: These resins usually formed as the exudates from various plants obtained either normally or as a result of pathogenic conditions (*i.e.*, by causing artificial punctures), such as: mastic, sandarac. These are also obtained by causing deep incisions or cuts in the trunk of the plant, for instance: **turpentine.** They may also be procured by hammering and scorching, such as: **balsam of Peru.**

B. Prepared Resins: The resins obtained here are by different methods as described below:

(*i*) The crude drug containing resins is powdered and extracted with ethanol several times till complete exhaustion takes place. The combined alcoholic extract is either, evaporated on a electric water-bath slowly in a fuming cup-board or poured slowly into cold distilled water. The precipitated resin is collected, washed with cold water and dried carefully under shade or in a vacuum desiccator,

   Examples: **Podophyllum; Scammony** and **Jalap.**

(*ii*) In the case of *alco-resins*, organic solvents with lower boiling points are normally employed *e.g.*, solvent ether (bp 37°C); acetone (bp 56.5°C), for their extraction. However, the volatile oil fraction can be removed conveniently through distillation under vacuo.

(*iii*) In the instance of **gum-resins,** the resin is aptly extracted with 95% (v/v) ethanol while leaving the insoluble gum residue in the flask (or soxhlet thimble).

5.2.7.7 Chemical Composition of Resins

The copious volume of information with regard to the **'chemistry of resins'** is mainly attributed by the meaningful research carried out by Tschirch and Stock, who advocated that the proximate constituents of resins may be classified under the following heads, namely:

(*i*) *Resin Acids*

(*ii*) *Resin Esters and their Decomposition Products i.e., Resin Alcohols* (*Resinols*) and *Resin Phenols* (*Resinotannols*).

---

* Tschirch. A, and L. Stock: *Die Harze, Borntraegr*, Berlin, Vols. 1 & 2, 1933-36.

(*iii*) *Resenes i.e.*, the chemical inert compounds.

However, it has been observed that in majority of the known **resins** these *three* aforesaid categories evidently predominates and thus the resulting product consequently falls into one of these groups. It is worth mentioning here that representatives of all the three said groups are rarely present in the same product.

Given below are some typical examples of resin substances that predominates the *three* classes suggested by Tschirch and Stock, namely:

A. **Resin-Esters**   : *Examples:* Ammoniacum; Asafoetida; Benzoin; Balsam of Peru and Tolu; Galbanum; Storax;

B. **Resin-Acids**   : *Examples:* Colophony; Copaiba; and

C. **Resenes**   : *Examples:* Bdellium; Dammar; Mastic; Myrrh; Olibanum.

A few important and typical chemical constituents that have been duly isolated and characterized from various **naturally occurring resins** are discussed below:

1. Resin Acids

Synonyms   Resinolic Acid.

The **resin acids** essentially contain a large portion of carboxylic acids and phenols. However, they occur both in the *free state* and as their *respective esters*. They are usually found to be soluble in aqueous solutions of the alkalies, thereby forming either soap like solutions or colloidal suspensions. **Resinates,** *i.e.*, the metallic salts of these acids find their extensive usage in the manufacture of inferior varities of soaps and varnishes.

A few typical examples of resin acids are enumerated below:

S. No.	Name	Chemical Structure	Source(s)
1	**Abietic Acid**	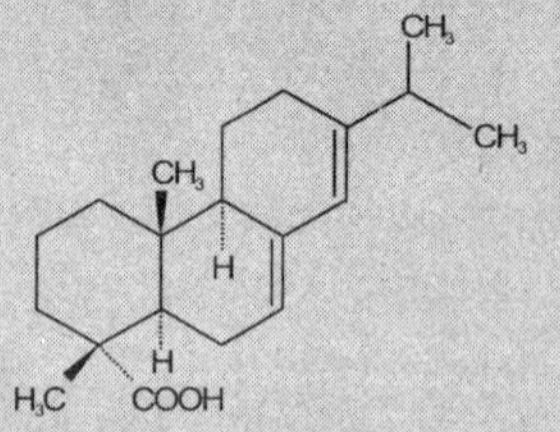	Colophony, Rosin
2	**Copaivic Acid and Oxycopaivic Acid**	—	Copaiba
3	**Guaiaconic Acid**	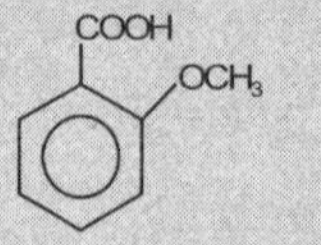	Guaic
4	**Pimaric Acid**	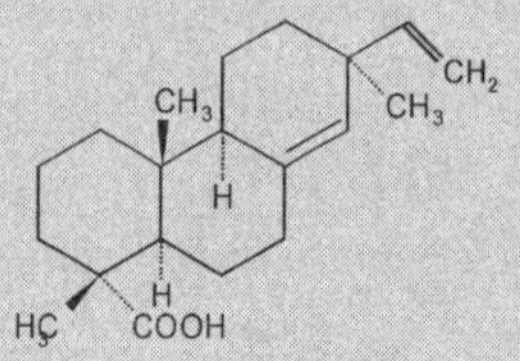	Burgandy Pitch, Fankicense
5	**Sandracolic Acid**	—	Sandarac
6	**Commiphoric Acid**	—	Myrrh

Out of all the six commonly found resin acids *Abietic Acid* shall be discussed here under:

Abietic Acid   (Synonym   Sylvic Acid)

Chemical Structure   13-Isopropylpodocarpa-7, 13-dien-15-oic acid; $(C_{20} H_{30} O_2)$.

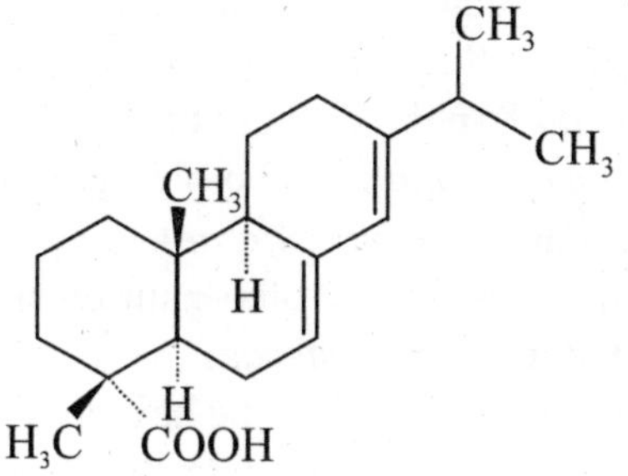

Abietic Acid

It is a **tricyclic diterpene** embedded with four isoprene units. It is studded with four methyl moieties and a carboxylic acid function. Besides, it also has two double bonds one each in ring-B and ring-C of the phenanthrene nucleus.

Preparation   It is a widely available organic acid, prepared by the isomerization of **rosin.*** It may also be synthesized from **dehydroabietic acid.****

The commercial grade of abietic acid is normally obtained by heating either rosin alone or with mineral acids. The product thus achieved may be glassy or partly crystalline in nature. It is usually of yellow colour and has a mp 85°C *i.e.*, much lower than the pure product (mp 172-175°C).

Characteristic Features   It is obtained as monoclinic plates from alcohol and water. Its physical parameters are: mp 172-175°C; $[\alpha]_D^{24}$ -106° (c = 1 in absolute alcohol); uv_{max} 235, 241.5, 250 nm (ε 19500, 22000, 14300). It is practically insoluble in water, but freely soluble in ethanol, benzene, chloroform, ether, acetone, carbon disulphide and also in dilute NaOH solution.

Identification   It readily forms the corresponding methyl ester as methyl abietate $(C_{21} H_{32} O_2)$, which is colourless to yellow thick liquid bp 360-365°C, d_{20}^{20} 1.040, and n_D^{20} 1.530.

Uses
1. It is used for manufacture of esters (ester gums), such as: methyl, vinyl and glyceryl esters for use in lacquers and varnishes.
2. It is also employed extensively in the manufacture of 'metal resinates' *e.g.*, soaps, plastics and paper sizes.
3. It also assists in the growth of butyric and lactic acid bacteria.

2. Resin Alcohols   In general, resin alcohols are complex alcohols having higher molecular weight. These are of *two* types, namely:

---

* Harris, Sanderson, *Org. Syn. Coll. Vol. IV*, 1 (1963); and Fieser and Fieser, *The chemistry of Natural Products Related to Phenanthrene* (New York, 3rd. edn., 1949).
** A.W. Burgastahler, and L.W. Worden., *J. Am. Chem. Soc.*, **83**, 2587, (1961) E. Wenkert *et al., ibid,* **86**, 2038, (1964).

(*a*) **Resinotannols:** The resin alcohols which give a specific tannin reaction with iron salts are termed as **resinotannols.**

A number of **resinotannols** have been isolated from the plant kingdom. It is an usual practice to name them according to the resins in which they are found, such as:

Alocresinotannol — From *Aloe* species viz., *Aloe barbedensis* Miller, (Curacao Aloes); *Aloe perryi* Baker, (Socotrine Aloes); *Aloe* ferrox Miller, *Aloe africana* Miller, *Aloe spicata* Baper. All these belong to the natural order *Liaceae*.

Ammoresinotannol — From *Ammoniacum i.e.,* the oleo-gum-resin from *Dorema ammoniacum* D. Don. (Family: *Umbelliferae*).

Galbaresinotannol — From *Galbanm i.e.,* the oleo-gum-resin from *Ferula galbaniflua* Boiss et Bubse (Family: *Unbelliferae*).

Peruresinotannol — From Balsam of Peru *i.e.,* the balsam obtained from *Myroxylon balsamum* var Pereirae (Royle) Harms (Family: *Fabaceae*);

Siaresinotannol — From Sumatra Benzoin (Benzoin, Styrax) *i.e.,* the gum exuded from *Styrax benzoin* Dryander (Family: *Styracaceae*).

Toluresinotallol — From Balsam of Tolu *i.e.,* the Balsam obtained from *Myroxylon balsamum* (Linn.) Harms. (belonging to the family. *Leguminosae*).

(*b*) **Resinols:** The resin alcohols that fail to give a positive reaction with tannin and iron salts are known as *resinols. The following* are some typical examples of *resinols*, for instance:

Benzoresinol — From Benzoin which is purely a pathological product obtained either from *Styrax benzoin* Dryander and *Styrax paralleloneurus* Brans. (*Sumatra Benzoin*) or from *Styrax tonkinensis* Craib. (*Siam Benzoin*) belonging to family *Styraceae.*

Storesinol — From storax which is the balsamic resin usually obtained from the trunk of *Liquidamber orientalis* Mill. family *Hamamelidaceae.*

Gurjuresinol — From Gurjun Balsam that is the aleo-resin obtained from *Dipterocarpus turbinatus* Gaertn. F. belonging to family: *Dipterocarpaceae.*

Guaiaresinol — From Guaiacum Resin obtained from the heartwood of *Guaiacum officinale* Linn. and *Guaiacum sanctum* Linn. belonging to family: *Zygophyllaceae.*

3. Resenes These are oxygenated compounds, but are not affected either by alkalies or acids. In fact, they are more or less neutral substances being devoid of characteristic functional groups, and, therefore, do not exhibit any characteristic chemical properties. Interestingly, they are immune to oxidizing agents and variant climatic conditions, a fact which essentially attributes the resins containing them one of their major plus points for the manufacture of **varnishes.** A few important examples of *resenes are* as follows:

Dracoresene — Derived from the scales of the fruit of Dragon's Blood *i.e., Daemonorops draco* Bl. (and other species) belonging to the natural order (*Arecaceae*).

Masticoresene — Derived from Mastic-an oleo-resin obtained from *Pistacia lentiscus* Linn belonging to family: *Anacardiaceae.*

Fluavil — Obtained from **Gutta-percha** and also from the bark of various trees. Gutta-percha is hard and has a very low elasticity. X-ray diffraction studies have revealed that rubber is composed of long chains built up of isoprene units arranged in the *cis*-form, whereas gutta-percha is the *trans*-form as shown below:

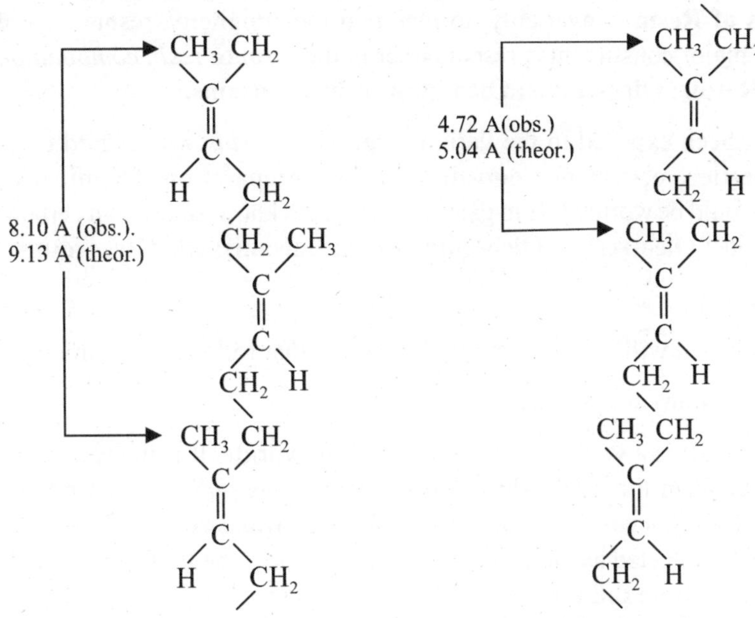

Rubber
cis-form

Gutta-percha
trans-form

5.2.7.8 Classification of Resins

The *resins* are broadly classified under *three* major categories, namely:

A. Taxonomical Classification   The resins are grouped together according to their botanical origin exclusively, such as:

Coniferous Resins	– *e.g.*, Colophony; Sandarac;
Berberidaceae Resins	– *e.g.*, Podophyllum; and
Zygophyllaceae Resins	– *e.g.*, Guaiacum.

In this particular instance, it has been observed that the resins that usually occur in plants of the same natural order (*i.e.*, family), may exhibit more or less related characteristic features.

B. Chemical Classification   The resins may also be classified as per the presence of the predominating chemical constituents for instance:

Acid Resins	– *e.g.*, Colophony (Abietic acid); Sandarac (Sandracolic acid); Shellac (Alleuritic acid); Myrrh (Commiphoric acid);
Ester Resins	– *e.g.*, Benzoin (Benzyl benzoate); Storax (Cinnamyl cinnamate);
Resin Alcohols	– *e.g.*, Balsam of Peru (Peruresinotannol) Guaiacum resin (Guaicresinol); Gurjun balsam (Gurjuresinol);
Resene Resins	– *e.g.*, Dragon's Blood (Dracoresene); Gutta-percha (Fluavil);

Glycoresins   – *e.g.*, Jalap Resin from Jalap *i.e.*, *Ipomea purga* Hayne; (Family: *Conrulvulaceae*) Podophylloresin from the dried roots and rhizomes of *Podophyllum hexandrum* (*P. emodi*) Royle. (Family *Berberidae*).

C. Constituents of Resin   Invariably, to maintain the simplicity, resins may also be classified according to the major constituents present either in the *resin* or *resin combinations*.

   Examples: **Resins; Oleo-resins; Oleo-gum resins; Balsams.**

After having been exposed to the various aspects of *resins* with regard to their physical and chemical, properties, occurrence and distribution, preparation, chemical composition and classification, it would be worthwhile to gain some in-depth knowledge about certain typical examples belonging to Resins; **Oleo-resins; Oleo-gum-resins; Balsams;** and **Glycoresins.**

5.2.7.8.A   *Resins*

The various **resins** that will be discussed in the section that follows are, namely:

1. Colophony   (**Synonym**   Rosin)

Biological Source   It is a yellow resin, and abietic anhydride. It is the residue left after distilling off the volatile oil from the **oleoresin** obtained from *Pinus palustris* and other species of *Pinus* belonging to family *Pinaceae*. Generally, it is offered as **wood rosin** obtained from southern pine stumps, **gum rosin** collected as the exudate from incisions in the living tree *viz.*, *P. palustris* and *P. caribaea,* and finally from **tall oil rosin.** It is chiefly produced in the USA.

Characteristic Features   Colophony fuses gradually at 100°C and at a higher temperature it burns with a smoky flame, while leaving not more than 0.1% of ash as a residue. The alcoholic solution of colophony turns into milky-white on addition of water. When fragments of rosin are heated with water, they first melt then flow together and ultimately forms a sticky-mass.

   It is a pale yellow to amber, translucent fragments, brittle fracture at ordinary temperature. It has a slight turpentine-like odour and taste.

   Its acid number is not less than 150 and d 1.07-1.09. It is almost insoluble in water, but freely soluble in ethanol, benzene, ether, glacial acetic acid, oils, carbon disulphide and also soluble in dilute solutions of fixed alkali hydroxides.

Chemical Constituents
1. **Colophony** contains 90% resin acids known as abietic acid (see Section 5.2.7.7). The remaining 10% as resene-an inert substance and esters of fatty acids.
2. It also contains a mixture of dihydroabietic acid ($C_{20}H_{30}O_2$) and dehydroabietic acid ($C_{20}H_{28}O_2$).
3. On being heated at 300°C, abietic acid undergoes further molecular rearrangement to produce neo-abietic acid.

Chemical Tests
1. Dissolve 0.1 g of powdered **colophony resin** in 10 ml of acetic anhydride, add one drop of sulphuric acid and shake well. The appearance of a purple colour which rapidly changes to violet colour.
2. The alcoholic solution of **colophony** is acidic to litmus paper *i.e.*, it turns blue litmus paper to red.

3. Dissolve 0.2 g of **colophony** with 5 ml of petroleum ether (60-80°C) and filter to discard the undissolved resin, if any. Shake the resulting clear solution with twice its volume of 0.1% (w/v) cupric acetate solution. The petroleum ether layer attains an *emerald-green colouration* due to the formation of the copper salt of abietic acid.

Uses

1. **Colophony** is used in pharmacy for the preparation of zinc oxide plasters, ointments and other adhesive plasters.
2. It is widely used in the manufacture of printing inks, rubber, dark varnishes, sealing wax, linoleum and thermoplastic floor tiles.
3. It also finds its application as varnish and paint dries, cements, soaps, wood polishes, paper, plastics, fireworks, tree wax, sizes, rosin oil
4. It is used for waterproofing cardboard, walls etc.

2. Eriodictyon

Synonyms   Yerba Santa; Consumptive's weed; Bear's weed; Mountain balm; Gum plant.

Biological Source   It is obtained from the dried leaves of *Eriodictyon californicum* (H. & A.) Greene belonging to family: *Hydrophyllaceae*.

The plant is an evergreen shrub indigenous to the mountains of California (USA) and northern Mexico. The Indians of California have been using this as a drug since many years.

Chemical Constituents   It contains a volatile oil, **eviodictyol** *i.e.*, the aglycone of **eriodictin, homoeriodictyol, chrysoeriodictyol, xanthoeriodictyol, eriodonol, eriodictyonic acid, ericolin,** formic acid, butyric acid, tannin and a *resin*.

Uses

1. It is used as a pharmaceutic flavouring aid to disguise the bitter taste of quinine formulations.
2. It has also been employed as a stimulating expectorant.

3. Guaiac

Synonyms   Guaiacum resin; Gum guaiac; Resin guaiac.

Biological Source   **Guaiac** is obtained from the heartwood of *Guaiacum officinale* L. or *G. sanctum* L., belonging to family: *Zygophyllaceae*.

Preparation   The **resin** is obtained by cutting the tree and the log is suspended horizontally. The either ends of the log are set on fire and the resin which oozes out is collected carefully in earthen or metallic cups and allowed to harden in shade.

Characteristic Features   The **guaiac resin** is brown or greenish-brown irregular lumps. It has an aromatic odour. The fracture is brittle and splintery and the exposed surface is usually glossy. It melts at 85-90°C. It is insoluble in water, but freely soluble in ethanol, ether, chloroform, creosote, solution of chloral hydrate and alkalies. It is, however, slightly soluble in carbon disulphide and benzene.

It is found to be incompatible in liquid preparations containing **acacia,** mineral acids, ferric chloride, gold chloride, water, spirit nitrous ether and permanganates.

Chemical Constituents   A few of the major resinous constituents belong to the group of **'lignans'**. These are essentially phenolic compounds with a C_{18} structure and made up from two C_6-C_3 units. About 10% of the **guaiac** is *guaiaretic acid* which is nothing but diaryl butane. It also contains both **α-and β-guaiaconic acids** (70%) and **guaiacie acid.** Besides, it contains traces of vanillin, saponin and volatile oil.

Chemical Tests   When a small quantity of the resin is oxidised it gives rise to a distinct blue colouration (*guaiac blue*) due to the oxidation of **α-guaiacic acid.**

Uses
1. It is mostly employed as a diaphoretic and an expectorant.
2. It is used as a clinical reagent for the testing of blood and haemoglobin.
3. An ethanolic solution of guaiac is used for the detection of oxidase enzymes and cyanogenetic glycosides.

4. Cannabis

Synonyms   Indian Hemp; Indian cannabis; Marihuana; Marijuana; Pot; Grass; Weed; Bhang; Ganja; Charas, Hashish.

Biological Source   **Cannabis** consists of the dried flowering tops of pistillate plants of *Cannabis sativa* L., (*C. satira* var. *indica* Auth.), belonging to family: *Moraceae*.

Preparation   After years of intensive and extensive research carried out on the selective cultivation of *Cannabis,* two of its *genetic types* have been evolved, namely: (*i*) Drug Type, and (*ii*) Hemp Type. These *two* distinctly separate genetic types of **Cannabis** shall be described briefly as stated below:

A. Drug type (Cannabis): It is, in fact, the rich (upto 15%) in the psychoactive constituent (–)-Δ^9-*trans*-tetra-hydrocannabinol (Δ9-THC) as shown below:

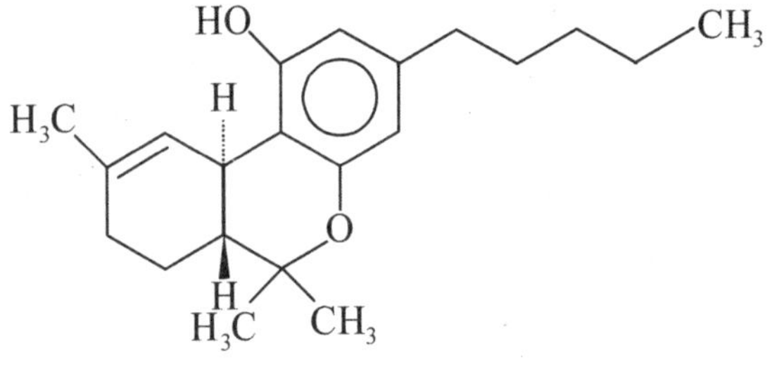

(–)-Δ^9-*trans*-Tetrahydrocannabinol (Δ^9-THC)

The Δ^9-THC is usually concentrated into a **resin** that is secreted right into the *trichomes* located on the small leaves (bracts) and *bracteoles* (*i.e.*, the leaf-like structure which encloses the ovary) of the flowering tops of the *female plant*. Interestingly, for the specific drug usages either the resin (*hashish*) is employed or the flowering tops of the female plant (*marijiana*). Nevertheless, the male plant also generates an equivalent quantity of the active constituents; however, it is not concentrated into a resin but found throughout the entire plant.

B. Hemp Type (Cannapis): It contains surprisingly very little active principal. **Cannabidiol** is the predominant **cannabinoid** present in it as given below:

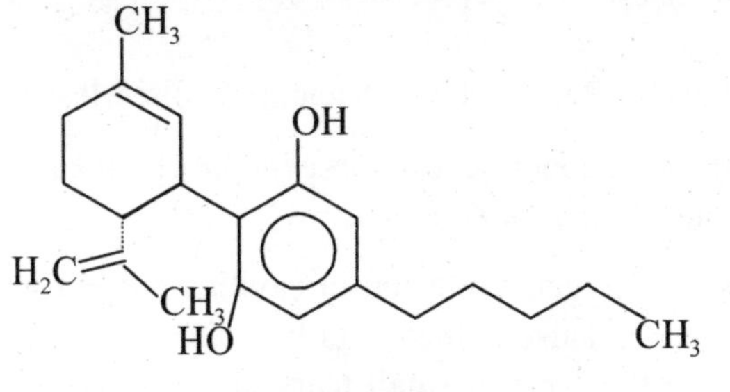

Cannabidiol

The hemp-type cannabis also possesses the elongated **bast*** fibers which is very much desired in the manufacture of ropes.

Chemical Constituents The chemical constituents Δ^9 THC and cannabidiol present in the drug-type and hemp-type cannabis have already been discussed above. Besides, the resin contains several active constituents, such as: **cannabinol, cannin, cannabol, tetrahydrocannabinol, cannabigerol, cannabichromene** and **Δ^8-tetrahydrocannabinol.**

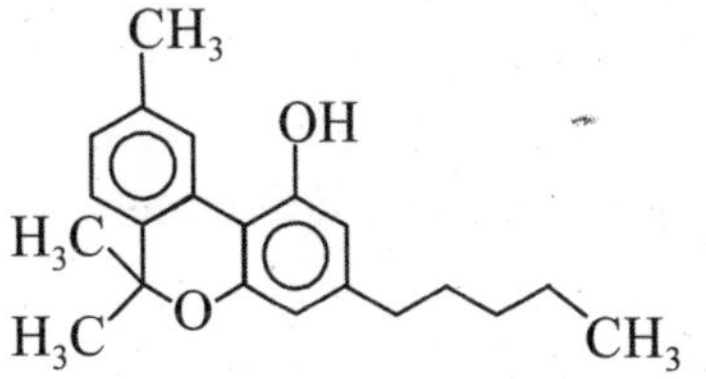

Cannabinol 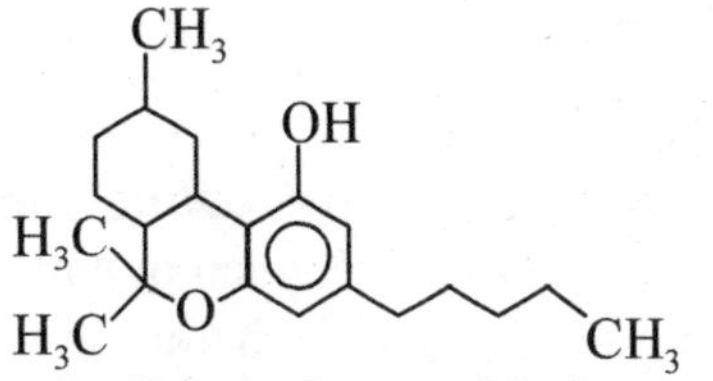   Tetrahydrocannabinol

It also contains choline, volatile oil and **trigonelline.** However, the Indian Hemp seeds contain 20% of fixed oil.

Chemical Tests

1. Shake 0.1g of resin with 5 ml petroleum ether (60-80°C) and filter. To 1 ml of the filtrate, add 2 ml of 15% solution of HCl gas in ethanol, when a red colouration appears at the junction of the two layers. However, after shaking, the upper layer becomes colourless while the lower one attains a distinct orange pink colour, which finally vanishes upon addition of water.

2. Extract 1g of resin with methanol, filter and evaporate to complete dryness. Again extract the resulting residue with petroleum ether (60-80°C), filter directly into a separating funnel and extract the ethereal layer successively with 5% (w/v) Na_2CO_3 and 5% (w/w) H_2SO_4. Wash the ethereal layer with distilled water, decolourise with powdered activated carbon, if necessary, and evaporate the filtrate. Add to the residue a few drops of N/10 alcoholic KOH solution, wen a purple colouration is obtained.

Uses It has been used as a sedative in equine colic.

---

* **Bast:** Fibrous material obtained from the pholeum of jute, flax etc., used for making rope, matting etc.,

5. Mastic

Synonyms   Mastiche; Mastich; Balsam Tree; Pistachia Galls; Mastix; Lentisk; Mastisol;

Biological Source   **Mastic** is the concrete resinous exudate obtained from *Pistacia lentiscus* Linne' belonging to the natural order *Anacardiaceae*.

Preparation   The resinous juice gets collected in cavities present in the inner bark. Fairly long incisions are made in the trunk and also in the larger branches, through which the resin exudes. The resin finally gets collected in the form of small tears on the outside. These are hand-picked and stored in dry place.

Characteristic Features   It is a pale yellow or greenish yellow, globular, elongated or pear-shaped tears. It has a slightly balsamic odour and a **terebene*** taste. It is practically insoluble in water, but completely soluble in ethanol, chloroform (1g/0.5 ml), ether (0.1g/0.5 ml), partially soluble in **oil of turpentine.**

Chemical Composition   **Mastic** contains 90% of a resin, comprising of **masticchic acid (α-resin),** which is soluble in ethanol and **masticin (β-resin),** which is insoluble in ethanol, and a volatile oil, 1 to 2.5%, that has the specific balsamic odour of the drug and largely contains **(+)-pinene.** A **bitter principle** is also present.

Uses
1. It is employed as an '*enteric coating*' material in the formulation of tablets.
2. It is also used as a microscopical mountant.
3. It is widely used in the manufacture of varnishes.
4. Mastic is used in the form of a 'dental varnish' in dentistry to seal off cavities.
5. It is also used in tooth cements, plasters, lacquers, chewing gums and incense.
6. It is employed for retouching negatives.

6. Podophyllum

Synonyms   Podophyllum resin; May apple; Mandrakes Root; Indian apple; Vegetable calomel.

Biological Sources   **Podophyllum** is the dried rhizomes and roots of *Podophyllum peltatum* L., family: *Berberidaceae,* known as *American Podophyllum;* and from *Podophyllum hexandrum* Royle (*Syn. P. emodi* Wall. ex Hook. f. & Th.) usually called *Indian Podophyllum*.

Preparation   Extract powdered **podophyllum** (1 killo) by means of slow percolation until it is almost exhausted of its resin content, using ethanol as the menstruum. Carefully concentrate the percolate by evaporation until the residue attains the consistency of a thin syrup. Pour the resulting syrupy liquid with constant stirring into 1 L of distilled water containing 10 ml of concentrated HCl and previously cooled to a temperature less than 10°C. Allow the precipitate to settle down completely, decant the clean supernatant liquid and wash the precipitate with two 1000 ml portions of cold distilled water slowly, dry the resin and powder it.

---

* **Terebene:** A mixture of hydrocarbons prepared from oil of turpentine and sulphuric acid, used to make paints and varnishes and medicinally as an expectorant and antiseptic.

Characteristic Features   It is a light brown to greenish-yellow powder, or small, yellowish, bulky, fragile lumps usually becoming darker in shade on exposure to either heat (> 25°C) or light (uv-rays). It has a characteristic faint odour and a bitter acrid taste. It is freely soluble in ethanol, usually with a slight opalescence. It is also soluble in dilute alkaline solution. It is found to be not less than 65% soluble in chloroform and 75% soluble in ether.

Chemical Constituents   Podophyllum contains 3.5 to 6% of a resin whose active principles are **lignans,** which are essentially C_{18}-compounds related biosynthetically to the **flavonoids,** and are derived by dimerisation of two C_6-C_3 units. The most important ones present in the **podophyllum resin,** are **podophyllotoxin** (20% in *American Podophyllum*) and in much higher quantum almost upto 40% in *Indian Podophyllum.* Besides, it also contains **α-peltatin** (10%) and **β-peltatin** (5%). It is pertinent to mention here that a host of **lignan glycosides** are also present in the plant, but by virtue of their water-soluble properties, they are almost eliminated during the normal preparation of the resin.

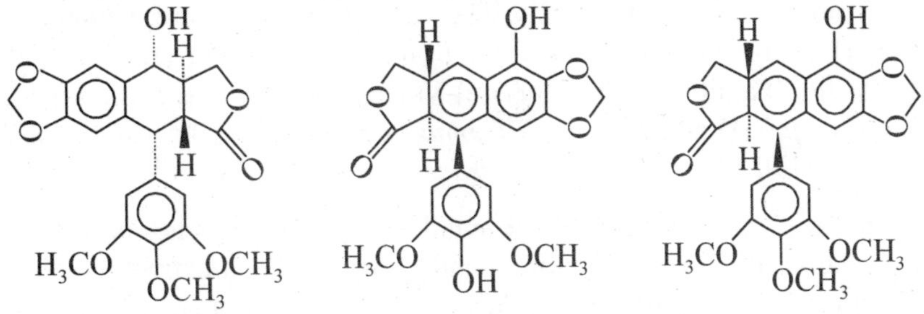

Podophyllotoxin   ∝-Peltatin   β-Peltatin

Interestingly, all the three above mentioned chemical constituents are present both in free state and as their respective glycosides. The Indian Podophyllum is devoid of **α-and β-peltatins.** The resin also comprise of the closely related **dimethylpodophyllotoxin** and its glycoside; and **dehydropodophyllotoxin,** as well as **quercetin**-a tetra-hydroxy flavonol.

Chemical Tests
1. **Podophyllotoxin** (*active lactone*) present in the resin when dissolved in alkali, cooled to 0°C and subsequently treated with an acid it yields an unstable gelatinous *podophyllic acid.*
2. The resulting **podophyllic acid** when treated with dehydrating agents easily loses a molecule of water and gives rise to **picropodophyllin** (*inactive lactone*), which being an isomer of **podophyllotoxin.**

The resins obtained from the American and Indian podophyllum are not quite identical and these two drugs of the trade may be distinguished chemically as given below:

(*a*) Prepare an alcoholic extract from *each* resin and filter. Add a few drops of strong solution of cupric acetate 5% (w/v) to each of the above two filtrates. The **American podophyllum** containing α-and β-peltatin produces an instant bright green colouration, while the **Indian podophyllum** (devoid of peltatin) fails this test.
(*b*) An alcoholic solution of **Indian podophyllum** resin readily gelatinizes on being treated with alkali hydroxide, while the American resin does not gelatinize. This is due to the fact

that the former contains **podophyllic acid** and it gives the alkali salt of this acid which is gelatinous in nature.

Uses

1. It is used as a drastic but slow-acting purgative.
2. Podophyllotoxin possesses anti-tumour (antineoplastic) properties and may be used in the treatment of cancer.
3. It is invariably prescribed with other purgatives, henbane or belladonna to prevent gripping in infants.

7. Shellac

Synonyms   Lacca; Lac.

Biological Sources   Shellac is the resinous excretion of the *insect Laccifer* (Tachardia) *lacca* Kerr, order *Homoptera* belonging to family: *Coccidae*. The insects usually suck the juice of the tree and exerete '*stick-lac*' more or less continuously. The various host trees are, namely: *Butea frondosa* Koen. ex. Roxb. (Family: *Leguminosae*) and *Butea monosperma* (Lam.) Kuntze; *Aleurites moluccanna* (L.) Willd. (Family: *Euphorbiaceae*)-**Varnish Tree;** *Ficus benjamina* Linn., (Family: *Moraceae*); *Zizyphus jujuba* (Lam.) (Family: *Rhamnaceae*). However, the *whitest shellac* is produced while the **Kusum tree** is the host *i.e.*, *Schleichera trijuga* (Willd.) (Family: *Sapindaceae*).

Preparation   The resin which is stuck on the smaller twigs and branches is normally serapped by means of knives. The resulting resin is subsequently powdered and extracted either with water or with alkaline solution so as to remove the colouring matter. The residual product is dried, melted in narrow bags suspended over a fire. The contents of the bags *i.e.*, the molten shellac, are squeezed out mechanically so as to force the liquid shallac through the cloth on to a previously cleaned surface of tiles to obtain the product as flat cakes. The product may also be obtained as thin sheets by streching the semi-cooled product on the tiles with the help of a scrapper (or spreader). The thin sheets thus obtained get hardened after cooling and are subsequently broken up to obtain the flakes of shellac for the commercial market.

Characteristic Features   Shellac is a brittle, yellowish, transparent/translucent sheets or crushed pieces or powder. It does not has any specific odour and taste. Its mp is 115-120°C and d 1.035-1.140. Its solubility in alcohol is 85-95% (w/w) (very slowly soluble); in ether 13-15%; in benzene 10-20% and in petroleum ether 2-6%. It is sparingly soluble in **oil of turpentine.** It is practically insoluble in water, but soluble in alkaline solutions, in aqueous solution of ethanolamines and in borax solutions with slightly purple colouration.

Chemical Constituents   The major component of **shellac** is a resin that on being subjected to mild hydrolysis yields a complex mixture of aliphatic and alicyclic hydroxy acids and their polyesters respectively. Interestingly, the composite of the resultant hydrolysate solely depends on the source of shellac and the time of collection.

The major component of the aliphatic fraction is **aleuritic acid,** while the major component of the alicyclic fraction is **shellolic acid.** *

---

* *Notes Field* Tetrahedron, **26**, 3135 (1970)

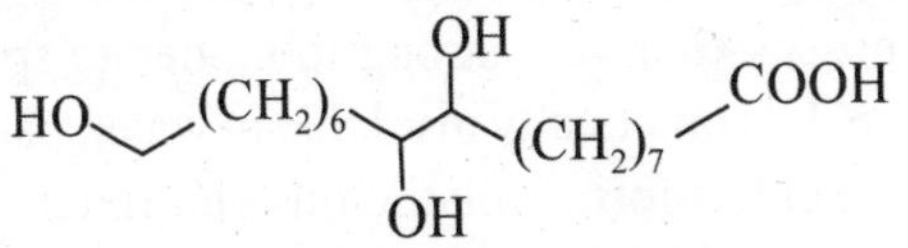

Aleuritic Acid
(9, 10, 16-Trihydroxy palmitic Acid)

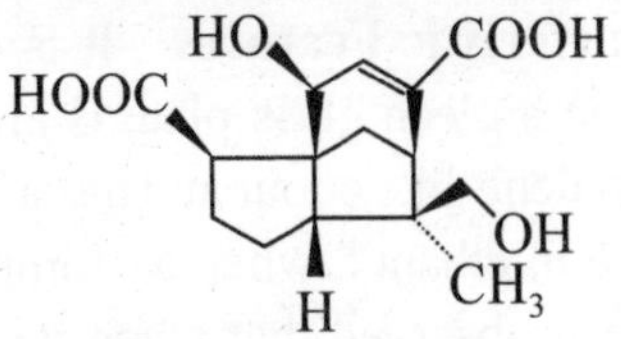

Shellolic Acid
(10β, 13-Dihydroxycedr-8-ene-
12, 15-dioic acid)

However, it also contains the isomers of **shellolic acid** along with small amounts of **kerrolic acid** and **butolic acid.** The colouring matter is due to the presence of **laccaic acid,** which is water-soluble, as given below:

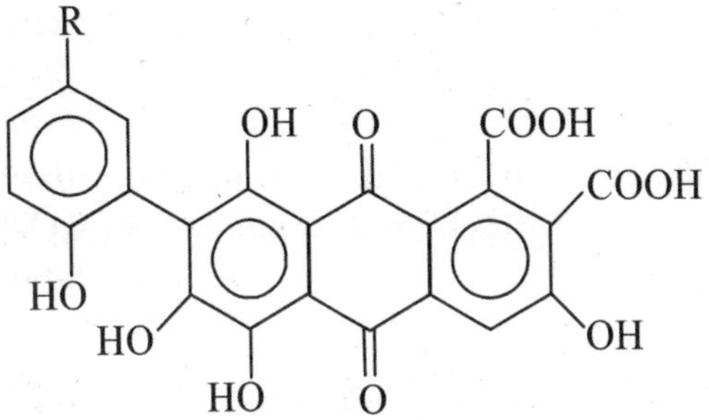

Laccaic Acid -A: R == CH₂CH₂NHCOCH₃
Laccaic Acid -A: R == CH₂CH₂OH
Laccaic Acid -A: R == CH₂CH(NH₂)COOH

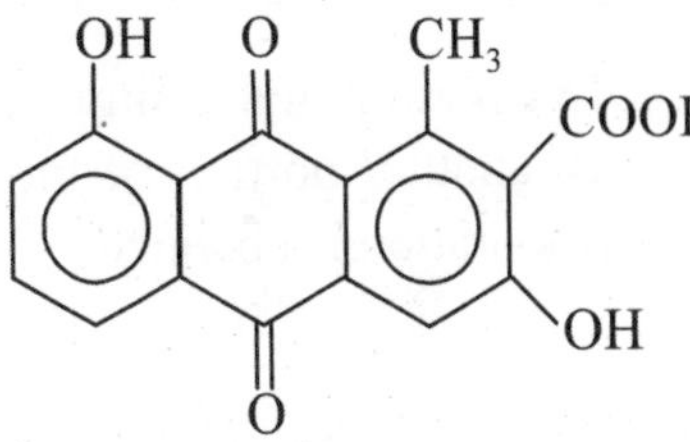

Laccaic Acid-D

Note   **Laccaic acid-A is the major component while the rest are present in relatively smaller quantities.**

Uses
1. It is used chiefly in laquers and varnishes.
2. It is also employed in the manufacture of buttons, sealing wax, cements, inks, grinding wheels, photograph records, paper.
3. It also finds its use in electrical machines and for stiffening hats.
4. It is also used for finishing leather.
5. It is extensively used for coating tablets and confections.
6. It has also been used for preparing *sustained release medicament* formulations.

8. Tar

Synonyms   Chair Tar; Pine Tar; Stockholm Tar.

Biological Source   **Tar** is a bituminous liquid obtained from the wood of various species of the natural order *Pinaceae,* such as: *Pinus longifolia* Roxb. [*Pinus roxburghii* Sargent. It is also present in *Pinus elliotth* (Engelm.) belonging to family *Abietaceae* (Slash Pine).

Preparation   It is usually obtained by the destructive distillation of the wood cuttings from the various species of *Pinus* as stated above.

Characteristic Features   It is dark brown or sometimes black viscous liquid, but its very thin layer on a clean glass plate is almost transparent. It possesses a very strong to moderate specific naphthalene-like odour and has a bitter and pungent taste. It is practically insoluble in water, partially soluble in ethanol, whereas completely soluble in ether, chloroform, volatile oils and fixed oils. It has been observed that when tar is stored for a longer duration, it separates into a layer which is granular in nature by virtue of the fact that minute and critical crystallization of resin acids and catechol take place. **Tar** is found to be *acidic* in reaction.

Chemical Constituents   Tar contains a good number of chemical constituents in various proportions depending upon the particular species of *Pinus* and its geographic location, such as: hydrocarbons, resin acid, resinous matter, and includes phenols, phenolic ethers, cresols, catechol, methyl cresols, guaiacol, benzene, toluene, xylene and styrene.

Chemical Tests
1. Shake 1g of drug in 20 ml of water and filter:

   (*a*) To a portion of the filtrate dip a blue-litmus paper which turns red showing acidic reaction.

   (*b*) To another portion of the filtrate add 2-3 drops ferric chloride solutions (0.1%) a red colouration is obtained.

Uses
1. It serves as an expectorant when used in the form of a syrup.
2. Pine tar is frequently employed as antipruritic and antibacterial.
3. It is used largely in ointments externally for the treatment of chronic skin diseases and eczema.

Note   **This 'Pine Tar' distinctly differs from the 'Coal Tar' in the following aspects, namely:**

(*a*) **Coal tar** is obtained by the destructive distillation of bituminous coal at a temperature less than 1000°C.

(*b*) **Coal tar** mostly contains, benzone, naphthalene, phenols and pyridine.

(*c*) It is alkaline to litmus paper.

(*d*) It has more disinfectant and irritating properties to pine tar.

(*e*) It becomes more viscous on exposure to air.

9. Kava

Synonyms   Kava-Kava; Ava-ava; Kawa.

Biological Source   It is the dried rhizome and roots of *Piper methysticum* Forst. belonging to the natural order *Piperaceae*.

Chemical Constituents   Besides, an appreciable quantity of starch present in it, the drug also comprises of about 5 to 10% of a resin from which six different and closely related *styrylpyrones* have been duly isolated and characterized, namely: **Yangonin, Desmethoxy yangonin, Kawain, Dihydrokawain, Methysticin** and **Dihydromethysticin.**

Kawain	Yangonin	Methysticin
mp 105-106°C	155-157°C	132-134°C
uv$_{max}$ In methanol 210, 245, 282 nm (log ε 4.38, 4.44, 2.81)	In ethanol 360 nm (log ε 4.33) Ethanol (hot), acetone,	In ethanol 226, 267, 306n (log ε 4.40, 4.14, 3.93) Ethanol (hot), acetone,
Soluble Acetone, ether, **in** methanol	Ethyl acetate, glacial acetic acid.	Ethanol, ether, acetone

Uses

1. The drug (**kava pyrones**) acts as potent centrally acting skeletal muscle relaxants.
2. It also possesses antipyretic and local anaesthetic properties.
3. Its underground parts have been used extensively by the natives (Oceania Islands) in the preparation of an intoxication drink prepared from the roots of this plant.

5.2.8 Oleoresins

Oleoresins are homogenous mixtures of resins and volatile oils. These are, in fact, the vegetative secretions obtained as natural products and composed of resin(s) dissolved in essential oils.

Nevertheless, based on the presence of the relative quantum of volatile oil in the naturally occurring mixture, the **oleoresins** may be either liquid, or semisolid, or solid. In normal practice, there exists a small amount of "natural" exudate from **oleoresin** containing trees attributed to insect damage, traces of broken twigs, and other similar injuries, but the commercial supplies are invariably accomplished by deliberate methodical and artificial incisions made on the bark and even into the wood.

A few important **oleoresins** shall be discussed in the Sections that follow, namely: **Capsaicin, Capaiba, Male Fern, Ginger, Turpentine.**

1. Capsaicin

Synonyms   Axsain; Mioton; Zostrix.

Biological Sources   It is the pungent principle present in fruit of various species of *Capsicum,* namely: *Capsicum annuum* L. (Family: *Solanaceae*)-**Paprika, Chili, Sweet Peppers;** *Capsicum frutescens* Linn., [*Synonyms   C. minimum* Roxb.]-**Bridchilli.**

Preparation   Capsaicin, the **oleoresin** from capsicum is prepared by extracting the crushed fruit with either hot acetone or hot ethanol by the method of percolation. The solvent *i.e.,* hot ethanol or acetone is evaporated on an electric-water bath in a fume-cupboard. The resulting residue is once again subjected to successive extraction with cold acetone or ethanol until the residue is free from the pungent odour. The solvent is removed and the **capsaicin** collected is not less than 8%.

Characteristic Features It has a monoclinic and rectangular plates, or scales from petroleum ether. Its mp is 65°C, $bp_{0.01}$ 210-220°C (air-bath temperature), uv_{max} 227, 281 nm (ε 7000, 2500). It has a burning taste, one part in 100,000 can be detected easily by tasting. It is practically insoluble in cold water. It is freely soluble ethanol, ether, benzene, chloroform and slightly soluble in CS_2.

Chemical Constituents The capsicum contains 8-12% of an oleoresin **capsaicin** and a red colouring principle known as **capsanthin** as given below:

Capsaicin

Capsanthin

However, the pungency of **capsaicin** is not affected by dilute alkali, but is destroyed almost completely by subjecting it to oxidation with either $KMnO_4$ or $K_2Cr_2O_7$.

Uses
1. It is used as a tool in neurobiological research.
2. Pretreatment with capsaicin induces long-lasting desensitization of airway mucosa to various mechanical and chemical irritants.

2. Copaiba

Synonyms Balsam copaiba; Balsam capivi; Jesuit's Balgar.

Biological Source Copaiba is the oleoresin obtained from the South American species of *Copaifera* (*Copaiba*) belonging to family: *Leguminosae*.

Preparation The **oleoresin** is collected by incisions made on the trunk of various species of *Copaifera* Linn., (a method similar to **colophony** described under Section 5.2.7).

Characteristic Features It is a transparent, viscid to pale-yellow to brownish-yellow liquid. It has a peculiar odour and bears a nauseating, bitter and acrid taste. Its acid number in 28-95 and d 0.930-0.995. It is practically insoluble in water, but soluble in benzene, chloroform, ether, oils, CS_2, absolute ethanol, petroleum ether and partly soluble in 95% ethanol. It is incompatible with mineral acids, magnesia and water. **Capaiba** is found to contain a volatile oil, **resin acids** (*e.g.*, **capaivic acid** and **illurinic acid**), besides a small quantity of a **bilter principle** and a fluorescent substance. The major constituents of the *volatile oil* are **cryophyllene, isocaryophyllene** and that of the *resin acid* is **β-metacapaivic acid** as given below:

Caryophyllene   Isocaryophyllene

Uses

1. It is used in varnishes.
2. It is also employed for removing old oil varnish from oil paintings.
3. It is used in the manufacture of photographic paper.

3. Male Fern

Synonyms   Aspidium; Filix mas (B.P.); Male shield-fern; Male fern rhizome.

Biological Source   **Male fern** comprises of rhizomes and stipes of Dryopteris filix-mas (L.) Schott.; *D. marginata* (Wall.) Christ; *D. odontolma* (Hochst.)C. Chr., and other species of Dryopteris belonging to family: *Polypodiaceae.*

Preparation   The **male ferns** are prepared by first collecting the rhizomes in the autumn, washed, roots and the stipes except their bases are removed. Finally, the trimmed rhizomes are dried by applying a moderate heat very carefully.

Characteristic Features   The rhizomes are dark brown or reddish brown externally and surrounded by **stipes bases.** The stipes bases are covered with membranous scales (ramenta). It has a slight and characteristic odour. It gives initially a sweetish taste, followed by bitter, astringent and nauseous taste. The rhizomes are cylindrical to conical in shape.

Chemical Constituents   The main active constituents of male fern are derivatives of **phloroglucinol** and **butyric acid.**

It has been observed that two or more molecules of simple *monocyclic derivatives,* such as: **aspidinol, filicinic acid** and **acylfilicinic acid** may get condensed to give rise to *bicyclic derivatives,* for instance; **albaspidin, flavaspidic acid** and **filicic acid** as given here under:

Aspidinol   Filicinic Acid   Acylfilicinic Acid

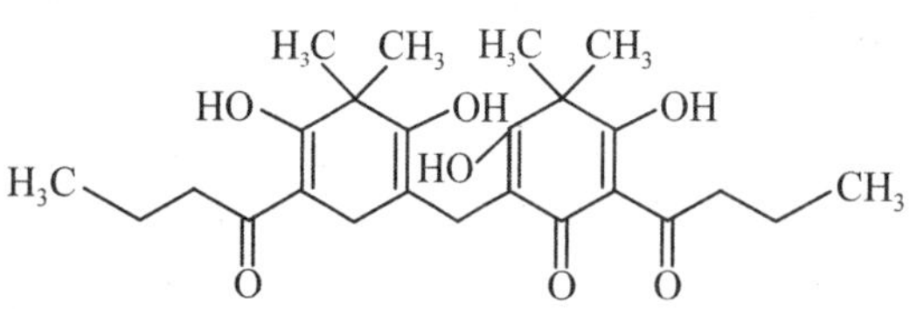

Albaspidin

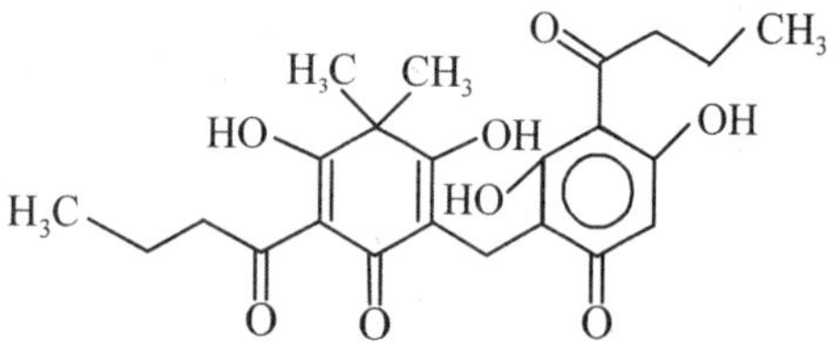

Flavaspidic Acid

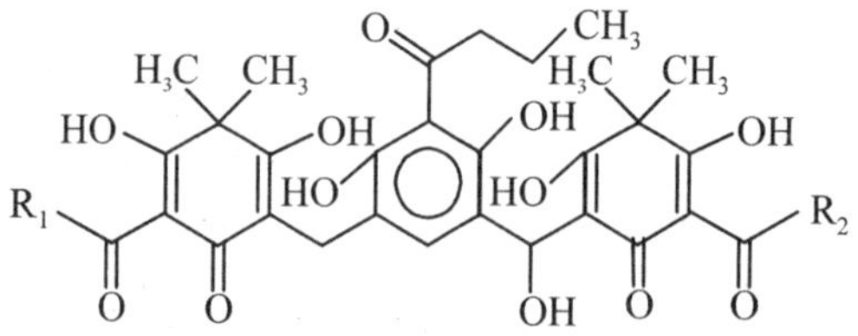

Filicic Acid

BBB : $R_1 = R_2 = C_3 H_7$; mp 172-174°C;
PBB : $R_1 = C_2 H_5$; $R_2 = C_3 H_7$; mp 184-186°C;
PBP : $R_1 = R_2 = C_2 H_5$; mp 192-194°C;

Crystals from ethylacetate

Note: **Filicic acid is a mixture of six homologues, the three main components (i.e., BBB, PBB, PBP) which are obtaine by recrystallization from ethyl acetate.**

Filicin is the lactone of **filicic acid,** which occurs as granular sediment in all male fern extracts and may be obtained by collecting it and subsequently washing with ether-ethanol mixture (1 : 1). The insoluble portion is dissolved in ethyl acetate or methanol and allowed to crystallize slowly when it yields yellow flakes.

Uses

1. Male fern **oleoresin** is an anthelmintic, specifically a taeniafuge.
2. It is also used as its extract for the expulsion of tapeworms.

4. Ginger

Synonyms   Gingerin.

Biological Source   It is the **oleoresin** obtained by the method of percolation of the powdered rhizomes of *Zingiber officinale* Roscoe, belonging to the Family: *Zingiberaceae.*

Preparation   The rhizomes are sliced, dried and powdered. The powdered ginger is extracted either with acetone or ether or ethylene dichloride by the method of cold percolation repeatedly till the gingerin is no longer present in the marc. The solvent is removed by distillation under reduced pressure. Ethanol gives the max yield of the oleoresin. The average yield of the **oleoresin** is 6.5% but it may range between 3.5 to 9.0% based solely upon the source of the plant product and to a great extent on the technique adopted in the course of preparation.

Characteristic Features   It is a dark brown, aromatic and pungent viscous liquid.

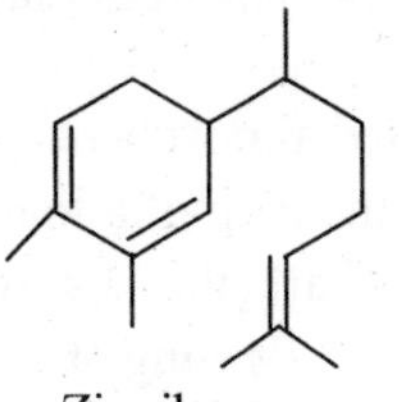

Zingiberene
(a)

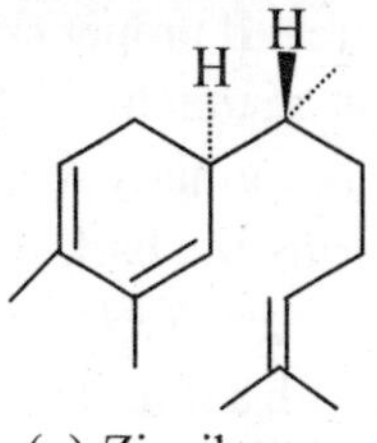

(–)-Zingiberene
(b)

Chemical Constituents **Ginger** contains volatile oil (1-3%), which comprises of **zingiberene,** **α-curcumene, β-sesquiphellandrene** and **β-bisabolene. Zingiberene** (*a*) has two chiral centres. The *acyclc chiral centre* has been stereochemically related to that in **(+)-citronellal,** and the *cyclic chiral centre* to that in **(–)-phellandrene.** Hence, **(–)-zingiberene** has the absolute configuration (*b*). The **oleooresin** contains the pungent **gingerols** and **shogaols.**

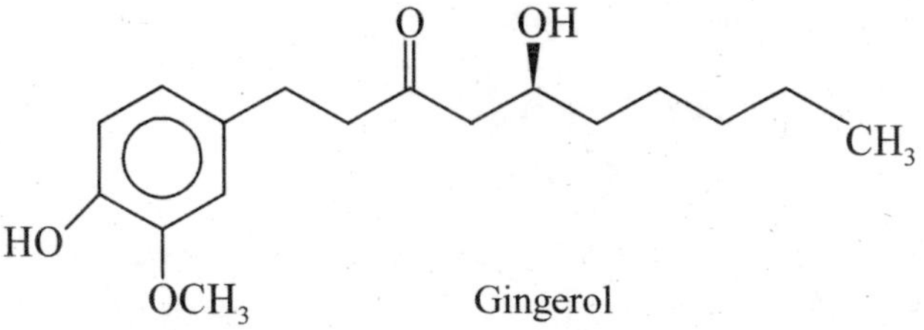

Gingerol

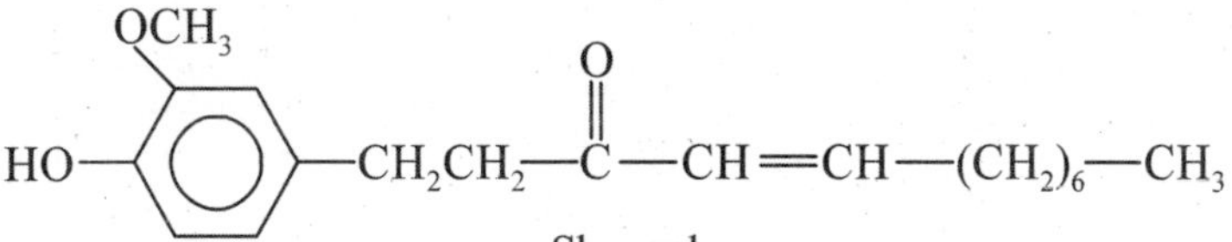

Shogaol

Uses

1. It is used as a flavouring agent, carminative, aromatic and stimulant to gastrointestinal tract (GIT).
2. **Ginger** finds its wide applications in soft drinks, beverages, ginger beer and wine.
3. It is extensively used for culinary purposes in ginger-bread, biscuits, puddings, cakes, soups and pickles.

5. Turpentine

Synonyms Gum turpentine; Gum thus.

Biological Source **Turpentine** is the **oleoresin** obtained from *pinus palustris* Miller and from other species of *Pinus,* belonging to the natural order *Pinaceae.*

Preparation **Turpentine** is usually collected from the slash pine *i.e., Pinus elliottii* Engelmann var. eliotti, and *Pinus palustris* Miller, which grow in abundance in the Northern Florida, Georgia, and North and South Carolina. However, the yield of **turpentine** exclusively depends on the treatment and the size of the tree. If proper skill and expertise are practiced the pine trees may yield turpentine for 15 to 20 years at a stretch.

The **oleoresin** is normally secreted in the ducts that are situated almost beneath the cambium in the sapwood. In spring the bark is neatly cut from the tree with the help of a long-handled cutting knife known as the "*bark-hack*". After the removal of the chipped bark, the freshly exposed surface is quickly sprayed with a solution of 50% (w/w) sulphuric acid.* The flowing **oleoresin** is guided by galvanized metal gutters right into the various containers tied close to the tree-trunk. The thick-liquid thus collected is removed as **turpentine** by pot-still distillation periodically.

Characteristic Features   The **gum turpentine** is an yellowish, opaque, sticky mass having a characteristic odour and taste. It is almost insoluble in water, but soluble in ether, ethanol, chloroform and glacial acetic acid.

Chemical Constituents   The **gum-turpentine** when subjected to steam-distillation yields 15 to 30% of a volatile oil known in the trade as **"turpentine oil"**. It contains mainly the terpenes, such as: *dextro-* and *laevo*-α-pinene, β-pinene and **camphene.**

α-Pinene   β-Pinene   Camphene

Uses

1. It is employed externally as a counterirritant.
2. It is also used as a rubefacient.
3. It is used as a constituent of stimulating ointments.
4. It is employed industrially as an insecticide.
5. It is used as a solvent for waxes.
6. It is utilized extensively in the production of synthetic comphor.
7. It is used in making various types of polishes, such as: shoe polish, furniture polish and stove polish.

5.2.9   Oleo-Gum-Resins

The **oleo-gum-resins** are the naturally occurring mixture of resin, gum, volatile oil, and mostly small quantities of other substances.

---

* Acid treatment collapses the thin-walled parenchymal cells which line the resin ducts. Thus, the duct channels get enlarged thereby allowing a faster uninterrupted flow of oleoresin and minimising the chances of hardened secretions blocking the outlets.

There are some potent **oleo-gum-resins** which exhibit remarkable medicinal values. A few such drugs shall be discussed briefly here under: **Asafoetida; Ammoniacum; Turmeric; Myrrh; Indian Bdellium** etc.

1. Asafoetida

Synonyms Asafetida; Asant; Devil's dung; Food of the Gods; Gum Asafoetida.

Biological Sources **Asafoetida** the oleo-gum-resin is obtained as an exudation of the decapitated rhizome on roots of *Ferula assafoetida* L.; *Ferula foetida* Regel, and some other species of *Ferula,* belonging to the nature order *Umbelliferae.*

Preparation **Asafoetida** is generally present as a milky liquid in the large schizogenous ducts and lysigenous cavities. However, these ducts and cavities are located more intensively in the cortex region of the stem and root. The drug is obtaining chiefly from the stem.

The fully grown plants are usually cut down to the crown region during the spring. The exposed surface is protected by a dome-like covering made up of twigs and leaves. After about a month, the hardened resinous substance is collected by scrapping. Likewise, the stems are also cut off and thereby additional collections of **asafoetida** are made frequently at an interval of 10 days unless and until the exudation ceases to ooze. Furthermore, it is also collected from the root by exposing its crown and excising the stem. The oleo-gum-resin exudes from the cut surface of the root and the former is collected soonafter it gets dried. Thus, the entire collection of **asafoetida** from the various portions of the plant are mixed together and dried in the sun.

Characteristic Features The drug occurs normally as soft mass or irregular lumps or 'tears' or agglomeration of tears. The tears are brittle and tough. **Asafoetida** has a strong, alliaceous, persistent garlic-like odour and having a bitter acrid taste. This **oleo-gum-resin** when triturated with water it gives a milky emulsion.

Chemical Constituents **Asafoetida** contains volatile oil (8-16°C) gum (25%) and resin (40-60%). The volatile oil essentially consists of some organic sulphides solely responsible for attributing the characteristic garlic-like odour. The resin cousists of **notannol, asaresinotannol** *i.e.,* the **resin alcohols,** which are present partially in the free state and partially in the combined form with **ferulic acid.** It also contains **umbellic acid** and **umbelliferone;** the latter is found combined with ferulic acid, but it gets generated on being treated with dilute HCl.

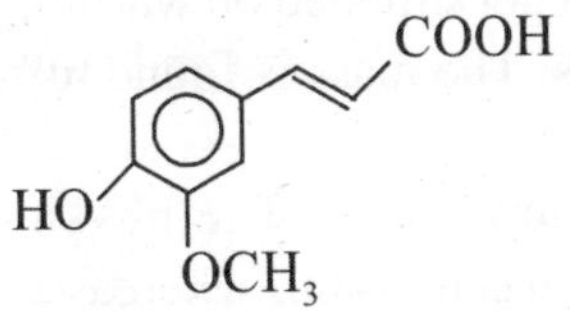

| *trans*-Ferulic Acid | Umbellic Acid | Umbelliferone |

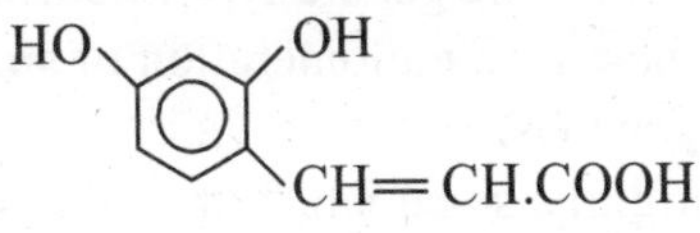

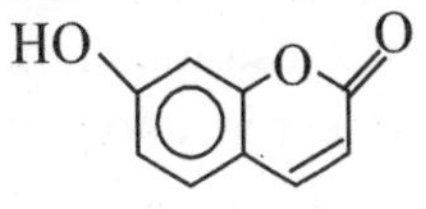

There are *three* sulphur-compounds that have been isolated from the **asafoctida resin,** namely:

(*a*) 1-Methylpropyl-1-propenyl disulphide,
(*b*) 1-(Methylthio) propyl-1-propenyl disulphide, and
(*c*) 1-Methylpropyl-3-(methylthio)-2- propenyl disulphide.

Interestingly, the latter two (*i.e.*, '*b*' and '*c*') have pesticidal properties.

Chemical Tests

1. It forms an instant milky-white emulsion when triturated with water owing to the presence of gum.
2. The freshly fractured surface when treated with a drop of sulphuric acid (conc.), it gives rise to a reddish-brown colour which on being washed with water changes to violet colouration.
3. Likewise, when the freshly fractured surface is treated with nitric acid (50%), it produces a green colour readily.
4. Boil 1 g asafoetida powder with HCl (50%), filter and make the filtrate strongly alkaline with NH_4OH (conc.), it gives a blue fluorescence. It is also known as the **Umbelliferone Test.**

Uses

1. It is abundantly used in India and Iran as a common condiment and flavouring agent in food products.
2. It is also an important ingredient in *Worcestershire Sauce.*
3. It is used as a repellant [2% (w/v) suspension] against dogs, cats, deer, rabbits etc.
4. It is used seldomly as an antispasmodic, carminative, expedorant and laxative.
5. It is still employed in veterinary externally to prevent bandage chewing by dogs.
6. It is also used as a powerful nerving stimulant especially in nervous disorders related to hysteria.

2. Ammoniacum

Synonym   Gum ammoniac.

Biological Source   It is a **oleo-gum-resin** exuded from the flowering and fruiting stem of *Dorema ammoniacum,* D. Don. and probably other species belonging to family: *Umbelliferae.*

Preparation   The exudation of the milky-secretions obtained in the form droplets is usually caused by the *beetles* that puncture the fruiting stem of *D. ammoniacum*. While quite a few of these milky-droplets get hardened on the stem itself, and the rest falls on the ground. The solidified **oleo-gum-resins** are scrapped from the stem with a plant-knife and also collected from the droppings on the ground.

Characteristic Features   The drug has an irregular, rounded tears, that are yellowish or browish outside and whitish from within; these are generally brittle when cold, but get softened on warming. It is also found, in the form of mass *i.e.*, agglomeration of small droplets. The mass is found to be darker in colour and less homogeneous.

It has a peculiar odour, slightly sweetish, bitter and somewhat acrid taste. The physical characteristics are: mp 45-55°C and d 1.207. Its acid number varies between 60-80, whereas the saponification number ranges between 97-114. It is partly soluble in water, ethanol, ether, vineger, or alkaline solution. It readily forms an emulsion with water.

Chemical Composition   Ammoniacum-the **oleo-gum-resin** consists of volatile oil (0.1-1.0%), resin (65-70%), gum (20%), moisture (2-12%), insoluble residue (3.5%) and ash (1%). **Ammoresinol,** a phenolic substance is the main constituent of the resin, which is a colourless crystal, mp 110°C. It also contains traces of salicylic acid.

Chemical Tests

1. **Ammoniacum** when triturated with water, it forms a white emulsion.
2. A portion of the above emulsion when treated with a solution of chlorinated soda gives a deep orange-red colouration.
3. A portion of the emulsion on being treated with a potash solution yields a yellow colour.
4. A portion of the emulsion when treated with a 0.1% (w/v) solution of $FeCl_3$, it gives an instant violet colouration due to the presence of traces of salicylic acid.

Uses

1. It is an important ingredient of porcelain cements.
2. It is a stimulant, and secreted by the bronchial mucous surface, thereby disinfecting the secretions.
3. It is used in plaster-of-paris (POP) plasters as a stimulant to the skin.
4. It is also used as a disinfectant expectorant in chronic bronchitis amalgamated with excessive discharge.

3. Turmeric

Synonyms   Curcuma; Indian Saffron; Tumeric.

Biological Source   **Turmeric** is obtained from the rhizome of *Curcuma longa* Linn. (*Curcuma domestica* Valeton) belonging to the natural order *Zingiberaceae*.

Preparation   The plant is normally harvested after 9-10 months when the lower leaves start becoming yellow. The rhizome is carefully dug out from the soil with a blunt knife without damaging it. The fibrous roots are discarded. The raw green **turmeric** is cured and processed by boiling the rhizomes with water for a duration ranging between 12-14 hours. Subsequently, the cooked rhizomes are dried in the sun for 5-7 days. Cooking process helps in achieving *two* objects, namely:

   (*a*) Gelatinization of starch, and
   (*b*) Yellow colouration, due to *curcumin,* spreads over the entire rhizome.

Characteristic Features   **Turmeric** has an aromatic pepper-like but somewhat bitter taste. It gives curry dishes their characteristic yellowish colouration.

Chemical Constituents   It contains volatile oil (5-6%), resin and substantial quantity of **zingiberaceous starch grains.** The marked and pronounced yellow colour in **turmeric** is due to the presence of **curcuminoids** which essentially contains **curcumin** as given below:

Curcumin
(Orange-yellow crystalline powder, mp 183°C)

The **curcuma oil*** obtained from turmeric contains **(±)-ar-turmerone** as given below:

---

* H. Rupe *et. al. Helv. Chim. Acta,* **17**, 372 (1934).

(±)–ar–Turmerone

The volatile oil contains a host of chemical substances, such as: *d-α-phellandene, d-sabinene,* **cineol, borneol, zingiberene,** and **sesquiterpenes.**

Turmeric also contains some other chemical constituents, namely: ***p,p*-dihydroxy** **dicinnamoylmethane;** *p-α*-**dimethy benzyl alcohol;** *p*-**hydroxy-cinnamoylferuloylmethane; 1-** **methyl-4-acetyl-1-cyclohexene;** and **caprylic acid.**

Chemical Tests

1. **Turmeric** powder when triturated with alcohol it imparts a deep yellow colour to the resulting solution.
2. The powdered drug when treated with sulphuric acid it imparts a crimson colour.
3. The aqueous solution of turmeric with boric acid gives rise to a reddish-brown colouration which on subsequent addition of dilute alkali changes instantly to greenish-blue.
4. **Turmeric** powder when reacted with acetic anhydride and a few drops of concentrated sulphuric acid (36 N), it readily gives a violet colouration. Interestingly, the resulting solution when observed under the ultraviolet light (preferably in a **uv-chamber**), it exhibits an intense red fluorescence, which is due to the presence of **Curcumin.**

Uses

1. It is extensively used across the globe as a condiment as curry powder.
2. It is employed as a colouring agent for ointments.
3. It is used medicinally as a tonic, as a blood purifier, as an anthelmintic and finally as an aid to digestion.
4. It is used extennally in the form of a facial cream to improve complexion and get rid of pimples.
5. A small quantity of turmeric when boiled with milk and sugar; it helps to cure common cold and cough symptoms.

4. Myrrh

Synonyms   Gum Myrrh, Myrrha.

Biological Source   Myrrh is an **oleo-gum-oresin** obtained from the stem and branches of *Commiphora obyssinica* (Berg) Engler or from other species of *Commiphora* belonging to family *Burseraceae.*

Preparation   The plants usually exude yellow coloured resin after proper incisions are made in the bark of a tree. It gradually hardens and becomes dark or reddish-brown in appearance. The mass is collected by the native tribals of Somalia for trading.

Characteristic Features   Myrrh normally occurs either in the form of isolated irregular, rounded tears of 2.5 cm in diameter or as masses duly formed by the agglomeration of these tears. The tears are dull, rough and reddish-brown in appearance. It has a strong aromatic odour and possesses an acrid, bitter taste.

Chemical Constituents **Myrrh** contains volatile oil (7-17%), resin (20-25%), gum (57-61%), and bitter principle (3 to 4%). The volatile oil consists of **eugenol, *m*-cresol** and **cuminaldehyde.** The resin is found to consist of a mixture of **α-, β-, and γ-commiphoric acids (resin acids).** Besides, it also contains two phenolic resins **α- and β-heerabomyrrholic acids** which are ether insoluble. The oleo-gum-resin yields alcohol-soluble extract not less than 30%. It also contains phenolic compound such as: **pyrocatechin** and **protocatechuic acid.** The crude alcohol-insoluble fraction *i.e.*, '*gum*, comprises of protein (18%) and carbohydrate (64%) made up of **arabinose, galactose** and **glucuronic acid.** However, the gum is found to be associated with an oxidase enzyme.

Protocatechuic Acid

Chemical Tests

1. **Myrrh** when triturated with water produces an yellow-emulsion.
2. When **myrrh** (0.1 g) is triturated with 0.5 g of pure washed sand (SiO_2) in the presence of ether, filtered and evaporated on an electric water-bath, it forms a thin film of violet colour on being exposed to bromine vapours in a closed dessicator.

Uses

1. It is used chiefly in perfumes and incense.
2. It is frequently employed as an antiseptic and stimulant.
3. **Myrrh** acts as an astringent to the mucous membrane and hence it find its application in oral hygiene formulations, such as: gargles, mouth-washes.
4. It is also used as a carminative.

5. Indian Bdellium

Synonym Scented bdellium.

Biological Sources **Indian bdellium** is the oleo-gum-resin obtained from the bark of the naturally occurring plant *Commiphora mukul* Engler., *Balsamodendron mukul* Hook. ex. Stocks., and *Commiphora weightii* (*Arn*) Bhand, belonging to family: *Burseraceae*.

Preparation The **oleo-gum-resin Indian bdellium** is obtained by the incision made on the bark and the exudates are collected. Each fully grown plant produces about 0.5 to 1 kg of the product which is normally collected from January through March every year.

Characteristic Features The **oleo-gum-resin** from **Indian bdellium** has a brown to pale yellow or sometimes dull green colour. It has an agreeable balsamic and aromatic odour with a typical bitter taste. The drug is usually obtained as irregular mass, rounded or agglomerated cluster of tears. The tears are found to be transparent, having a waxy surface and quite brittle in nature. It is sticky in touch and has a fractured surface. It is partially alcohol soluble; but when triturated with water it usually gives rise to a white emulsion.

Chemical Constituents This **oleo-gum-resin** mostly comprises of resin (60%), gum (30%), volatile oil (1–1.5%) moisture (5%) and foreign organic substances (3-4%). The volatile oil fraction contains various terpenes, such as: **β-murcene, dimyrcene, polymyrcene, caryophyllene and isocaryophyllene** (Section 5.2.9.2).

$$CH_2$$

$$CH_2$$

$$H_3C \quad CH_3$$
β-Myrcene

5.2.10 Balsams

Balsams are the resinous mixtures that essentially contain large quantum of benoic acid, cinnamic acid or both, or esters of these organic aromatic acids.

A galaxy of typical examples of naturally occurring *balsams* will be discussed in the sections that follow, namely: **Storax; Peruvain Balsam; Tolu Balsam;** and **Benzoin.**

1. Storax

Synonyms   Styrax; Sweet oriental gum; Levant Storax; Purified or prepared Storax; American Storax; Liquid Storax;

Biological Source   Storax is the *balsam* obtained from the trunk of *Liquidamber orientalis* Mill., termed as **Levant Storax,** or of *L. styraciflua* L.,known as **American Storax** belonging to the natural order *Hamamelidaceae.*

Preparation   The natural balsam *storax* is a pathological product formed as a result of injury caused to the plant. It generally, exudes into the natural pockets between the bark and the wood and may be located by exerscences on the outside of the bark. These pockets, that may contain upto 4 kg of the balsam, *are* conveniently tapped with the help of strategically positioned gutters, and the product is ultimately allowed to fill into containers. The crude storax, thus collected, is further purified by dissolving in ethanol, filtration and subsequent evaporation of the solvent to obtain the pure storax.

Characteristic Features   The **balsam storax** is a semiliquid grayish, sticky, opaque mass (*Levant Storax*), or a semisolid sometimes solid mass softened by gentle warming (*American Storax*). In general, **storax** is transparent in thin layers, possesses a characteristic agreeable balsamic taste and odour. It is, however, denser than water. It is almost insoluble in water, but completely soluble in 1 part of warm ethanol, ether, acetone and CS_2.

Chemical Constituents   Storax contains the following chemical compounds, namely: **α-and β-storesin** and its **cinnamic ester** (30-50%), **styracin** (5-10%); **phenylpropyl cinnamate** (10%); **free-cinnamic acid** (5-15%); levorotatory oil (0.4%); small amounts of **ethyl cinnamate, benzyl cinnamate,** traces of **vanillin** and **styrene** ($C_6H_5CH=CH_2$).

Besides, *Levant storax* contains free **storesinol, isocinnamic acid, ethylvanillin, styrogenin,** and **styrocamphene.**

In addition to these, **American Storax** contains **styaresin** (*i.e.,* -cinnamic acid ester of the alcohol **styresinol,** an isomer of **storesinol**) and **styresinolic acid.** It also yields upto 7% of a dextrorotatony volatile oil, styrol and traces of vanillin.

Chemical Tests

1. **Benzaldehyde Test**—Treat 1 g of **storax** with 5 ml of $K_2Cr_2O_7$ solution (10% w/v) followed by a few drops of concentrated sulphuric acid (36 N) it produces benzaldehyde, which may be detected easily as the odour of bitter almonds.

2. Mix 1g of **storax** with 3 g of pure sand (SiO_2) and 5 ml of $KMnO_4$ solution (5% w/v) and heat it gently. It gives a distinct odour of benzaldehyde.

Uses

1. It is used in fumigating pastilles and powders.
2. It finds its application in perfumery.
3. It is employed as an imbedding material in microscopy.
4. It is used as an expectorant, antiseptic and stimulant.
5. It is employed as a preservative for fatty substances *e.g.,* lard and tallow.
6. It is also used as a flavouring agent for tobacco.
7. It is a vital ingredient of **"Compound Benzoin Tincture".**

2. Peruvian Balsam

Synonyms   Balsam Peru; Indian balsam; Black balsam; China oil; Honduras balsam; Surinam balsam.

Biological Source   **Balsam Peru** is obtained from *Toluifer pereiare* (Klotzsch) Baill. (*Myroxylon pereiare* Klotzsch) belonging to family: *Leguminosae.*

Preparation   **Peruvian Balsam** is a pathological product and is obtained usually by inflicting injury to the trees. Most of the world's commercial supply comes from El Salvador, although some is also produced in Honduras.

It is prepared by beating the stems of the trees with mallet. After a week the injured areas of the stem are scorched so as to separate the bark from the stem and after a similar duration the bark is peeled off completely. The desired balsam starts exuding freely from all the exposed surfaces, which are then covered carefully with cloth or rags to absorb the exuding balsam. The cloth or rags that are completely soaked with the balsam is then removed and boiled with water in a large vessel slowly. Thus, the balsam gets separated and settles at the bottom of the vessel. The supernatant layer of water is removed by decantation and the residual balsam is dried and packed in the containers.

Characteristic Features   It is a dark brown, viscid liquid having a pleasant aromatic odour. It has a peculiar warm bitter taste and persistent aftertaste which resembles like vanilla. The **Balsam Peru** is transparent in thin films. It does not harden on being exposed to atmosphere. It is brittle when cold. It is almost insoluble in water and petroleum ether but soluble in ethanol, chloroform and glacial acetic acid.

Chemical Constituents   **Peruvian balsam** contains free benzoic and cinnamic acids (12-15%); benzyl (40%); esters of these acids (5.2-13.4% **cinnamein**); and volatile oil (1.5-3%).

The fragrant volatile oil contains toluene, styrol, benzoic and cinnamic acids.

It also contains total **balsamic acids,** which is calculated on the basis of dry alcohol-soluble matter ranging between (35-50%).

Cinnamein
(Benzyl Cinnamate)

The **resins esters** (30-38%) are chiefly composed of **peruresinotannol cinnamate** and benzoate, vanillin, free cinnamic acid and **peruviol** (or **nerolidol**).

Peruviol (Nerolidol)

Uses

1. **Peru balsam** is a local protectant and rubefacient.
2. It also serves as a parasiticide in certain skin disorder.
3. It is used as an antiseptic and **vulnerary*** and is applied externally either as ointment or alone or in alcoholic solution.
4. It acts as an astringent to treat hemorrhoids.

3. Tolu Balsam

Synonyms   Thomas balsam; Opobalsam; Resin Tolu; Balsam of Tolu.

Biological Source   **Tolu Balsam** is a balsam obtained from *Toluifera balsamum* L., (*Myroxylon toluiferum* H.B.K.), belonging to family: *Leguminosae*. It is also obtained from *Myroxylon balsamum* (Linne') Harms. Family: *Fabaceae.*

Preparation   Tolu Balsam is considered to be a pathological product produced in the new wood formed as a result of inflicted injury. For its preparation, it is an usual practice to make 'V' shaped incisions deep into the body of the main trunk. The exudate thus produced is collected either in cups or gourds held strategically just at the base of each incisions. **Balsam of Tolu** is collected from these cups, mixed and packed in air-tight sealed tins.

Characteristic Features   It is a yellowish-brown or brown semifluid or nearly solid resinous mass. It has a characteristic aromatic vanilla-like odour and slightly pungent taste. It is usually brittle when cold. It is found to be transparent in thin layers, and shows numerous crystals of cinnamic

---

* **Vulnerary:** A folk remedy or herb to promote wound healing.

acid. It is almost insoluble in water and petroleum ether, but freely soluble in ethanol, benzene chloroform, ether, glacial acetic acid and partially in CS_2 or NaOH solution.

Chemical Constituents   The drug contains **resin esters** (75-80%) *viz.*, **toluresinotannol cinnamate** along with a small proportion of the benzoate; volatile oil (7-8%)-containing chiefly **benzyl benzoate;** free cinnamic acid (12-15%); free **benzoic acid** (2-8%); **vanillin** and other constituents in small quantities. It also contains **cinnamein** (5-13%).

Chemical Tests
1. An alcoholic solution of **Tolu Balsam** (0.2% w/v) where treated with a $FeCl_3$ solution (0.5% w/v), the appearances of a green colour takes place.
2. Treatment of 1 g of the drug with 5 ml of 10% w/v $KMnO_4$ solution when subjected to gentle heating yields benzaldehyde.

Uses
1. It is used extensively in perfumery, confectionery and chewing gums.
2. It is used widely as an expectorant in cough mixture.
3. It also finds its application as an antiseptic in the form of its tincture.

4. Benzoin

Synonyms   Bitter-almond-oil camphor.

Biological Source   **Benzoin** in the **balsamic resin** obtained from *Styrax benzoin* Dryander and *Styrax paralleloneurus* Perkins, generally known in trade as **Sumatra Benzoin;** whereas, *Styrax tonkinensis* (Pierre) Craib ex Hartwich, or other species of the section Anthostyrax of the genus *Styrax,* known commonly in the trade as **Siam Benzoin** both belong to the family: *Styraceae.*

Preparation   **Benzoin** is also a pathological product that is obtained by incising a deep-cut in the bark. It has been observed that after a span of about eight weeks, the exudating **balsamic resin** tends to become less sticky in nature and firm enough to collect. The entire exudate is usually collected in *two* stages, namely:

Stage 1: *First tapping*-yields *almond tears*, and

Stage 2: *Second tapping*-yields a more fluid material.

Characteristic Features

Sumatra Benzoin: It is pertinent to mention here that in pharmacy, only the **Sumatra Benzoin** is used. It occurs as blocks or irregular masses of tears having variable sizes usually imbedded either in an opaque or translucent matrix. It is rather brittle, and from within the tears are milky white in appearance. It generally becomes soft when warmed and gritty when chewed. The matrix is grayish brown to reddish in colour. Its taste is quite agreeable, balsamic and resembles to that of **storax.** It has a resinous and aromatic taste.

Siam Benzoin: The smaller tears of **Siam Benzoin** are darker in colour. It occurs largely in separate concavo-convex tears which are yellowish brown to rusty brown externally, whereas milky white internally. The tears are fairly brittle but normally become soft and plastic like on being chewed. It has a vanilla-like fragrance.

Chemical Constituents   The chemical constituents of the *two* types of **Benzoin** are given below:

(*a*) **Sumatra Benzoin:** It contains free balsamic acids, largely cinnamic acid (10%), benzoic acid (6%)-along with their corresponding ester derivatives. Besides, it also contains **teriterpene acids,** namely: **19-hydroxyloleanolic** and **6-hydroxyoleanolic acids, cinnamyl cinnamate, phenyl propyl cinnamate, phenylethylene** and lastly the traces of vanillin. It yields not less than 75% of alccohol-soluble extractives.

(*b*) **Siam Benzoin:** It chiefly comprises of **coniferyl benzoate** (60-70%), benzoic acid (10%), **triterpene siaresinol** (6%) and traces of vanillin. It yields not less than 90% of alcohol-soluble extractives.

$$CH=CH-CH_2-C=O$$

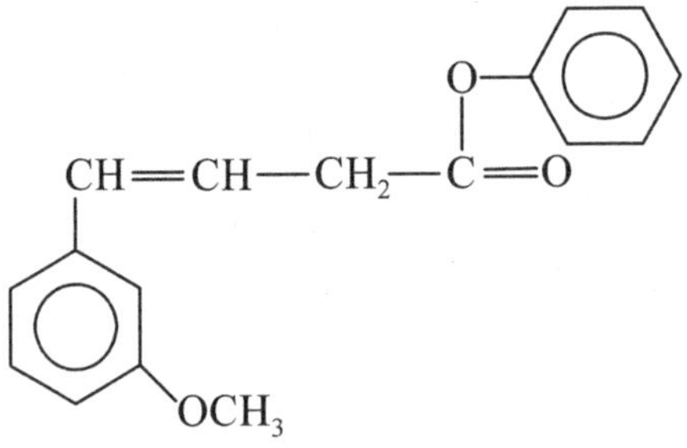

Coniferyl Benzoate

Chemical Tests

1. When 0.5 g of **Sumatra Benzoin** powder is warmed with 10 ml of $KMnO_4$ solution (5% w/v) in a test tube, a faint and distinct odour of benzaldehyde is developed. **Siam Benzoin** gives a negative test.

2. When 0.2 g of **Siam Benzoin** powder is digested with 5 ml of ether for 5 minutes and filtered; 1 ml of the filtrate is poured into a clean china-dish containing 2-3 drops of concentrated H_2SO_4 and mixed carefully, a deep purplish red colouration is developed instantly. **Sumatra Benzoin** gives a negative test.

Uses

1. Compound benzoin tincture is frequently employed as a topical protectant.
2. It is valuable as an expectorant when vapourized.
3. It finds its usage as a cosmetic lotion usually prepared from a simple tincture.
4. **Siam Benzoin** has been proved to be a better preservative for lard than the **Sumatra Benzoin.**

FURTHER READING REFERENCES

1. Agurell, S., Dewey, W.L., Willette, R.E., eds.: **The Cannabinoids: Chemical, Pharmacologic and Therapeutic Aspects,** Academic Press Inc., Orlando, Florida, (1984).

2. Atal, C.K. and Kapoor, B.M., eds., **'Cultivation and Utilization of Medicinal Plants',** Regional Research Laboratory, Jammu-Tawi, India, (1982).

3. Brown, R.G., and Brown, M.L., **'Woody Plants of Maryland',** Port City Press, Baltimore, (1972).

4. Council of Scientific and Industrial Research, **The Wealth of India,** 11 vols., New Delhi, (1948-1976).

5. Cutler, S.J., and Cutler, H.G. eds, 'Biologically Active Natural Products: Pharmaceuticals', CRC Press, London, (1999).

6. Duke, J.A., 'Handbook of Legumes of World Economic Importance', Plenum Press, New York, (1981).

7. Duke, J.A., 'Handbook of Medicinal Herbs', CRC Press, New York, (2001).

8. Dewick, P.M., 'Medicinal Natural Products: A Biosynthetic Approach', John Wiley & Sons, Ltd., 2nd, edn., New York, (2001).

9. Earle, F.R. and Jones, Q., *Analyses of Seed Samples from 113 Plant Families, Econ. Bot.* **16** (4), (1962).

10. Erichsen-Brown, C., 'Use of Plants for the Past 500 Years', Breezy Creeks Press, Aurora. Can., (1979).

11. Guenther, E., 'The Essential Oils', Vol. 1-6, Van Nostrand, New York, (1948-1952).

12. Hagen-Smit, A.J., 'Progress in the Chemistry of Natural Products', Vol. 1-12, Springer, Vienna, (1955).

13. Harborne, J.B., Tomas-Barberan, F.A., eds.: 'Ecological Chemistry and Biochemistry Plant Terpenoids', Oxford, Clarendon Press,. London, (1991).

14. Herbert RB: *The biosynthesis of plant alkaloids and nitrogenous microbial metabolites, Nat. Prod. Rep,* **18**, 50-65, 2001; **Earlier Reviews:** 1999, **16**, 199-208; 1997, **14**, 359-372.

15. Hibino S., and Choshi T., *Simple indole alkaloids and those with a nonrearranged monoterpenoid unit. Nat Prod Rep.* **18**, 66-87, **Earlier Review:** Lounasmaa M and Tolvanen A, **17**, 175-191, 2000.

16. Irvine, F.R., 'Woody Plants of Ghana', Oxford University Press, London, (1961).

17. Keys, J.D., 'Chinese Herbs: Their Botany, Chemistry and Pharmacodynamics', Chas. E. Tuttle, Tokyo, (1976).

18. Kirtikar, K.R., Basu, B.D., and I.C.S. 'Indian Medicinal Plants', Vol. 1-4, 2nd. edn. reprint, Jayyed Press, New Delhi, (1975).

19. Kutchan T.M., **Molecular Genetics of Plant Alkaloid Biosynthesis**, In: The Alkaloids, Chemistry and Pharmacology (ed. Cordell GA). Vol. 50, Academic, San Diego, pp 257-316, 1998.

20. Misra N., Luthra R., Singh K.L., and Kumar S., **Recent Advances in Biosynthesis of Alkaloids,** In: **Comprehensive Natural Products Chemistry,** Vol. 4, Elsevier, Amsterdam, pp 25-59, 1999.

21. Purseglove, J.W., Brown, E.G., Green, C.L., and Robbins, S.R.J., 'Spices', Vol. 1-2, Longman, London, (1981).

22. Ramstad, E., 'Modern Pharmacognosy', McGraw Hill, London, (1956).

23. Robinson, R., 'The Structural Relation of Natural Products', Oxford-Clarendon Press, London, (1955).

24. Stöckigt J. and Ruppert M., **Striclosidine—the biosynthetic key to monoterpenoid indole alkaloids,** In: **Comprehensive Natural Products Chemistry,** Vol. 4, Elsevier, Amsterdam, pp 109-138, 1999.

25. Teranishi, R., Buttery, R.G., Sugisawa, H., Eds., 'Bioactive Volatile Compounds from Plants', Washington, DC, American Chemical Society, (1993).

26. Tyler, V.E., 'The Honest Herbal—A Sensible Guide to the Use of Herbs and Related Remedies', George F. Stickely, Philadelphia, (1982).

6

Phenylpropanoids

- Introduction
- Classification
- Biosynthesis of Phenylpropanoids
- Further Reading References

6.1 INTRODUCTION

Phenylpropanoids represent a large conglomerate of naturally occurring phenolic compounds essentially derived from the aromatic amino acids **phenylalanine** and **tyrosine** or in certain specific instances the intermediates obtained from **Shikimic Acid Biosynthetic Pathway.** In other words, these compounds comprise of a phenylring to which is attached a 3C-side chain; and may also contain one or more C_6—C_3 residues.

Interestingly, the unique combination of the phenyl-propane side chain (*i.e.*, 3C-atom) evidently present in **'phenylpropanoids'** are absolutely devoid of nitrogen atom, which is observed to be in contradiction to such other vital class of natural products, namely: **alkaloids, cyanogenic glycosides, and glucosinolates.** Obviously, the **phenylpropanoids** are distinctly phenolic in character by virtue of the presence of one or several hydroxyl groups attached to the aromatic ring ($C_6 H_6$), they are more often known among the phytochemists as **'plant phenolics'.**

6.2 CLASSIFICATION

The **phenylpropanoids** may be classified on the basis of their basic chemical moieties as enumerated below:

- (*i*) Hydroxycinnamic Acids
- (*ii*) Phenylpropenes
- (*iii*) Coumarins
- (*iv*) Abridged phenylpropanoids
- (*v*) Biphenylpropenoid derivatives
- (*vi*) High molecular weight phenylpropanoids

The above different categories of compounds belonging to the **phenyl propanoids** shall be discussed separately with the help of certain important examples of natural products in a systematic manner in the sections that follow:

6.2.1 Hydroxycinnamic Acids

The typical examples of **hydroxycinnamic acids** are, namely: *p*-**coumaric acid, caffeic acid, ferulic acid,** and **sinapic acid,** which shall be enumerated in the sections that follow:

6.2.1.1 Para-Coumaric Acid

Synonym *p*-Hydroxycinnamic acid.

Chemical Structure

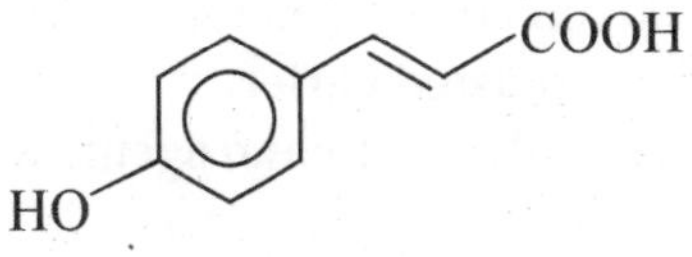

para-Coumaric Acid

Biological Sources It is present in a variety of medicinal plant, namely: *Aloe barbadensis* Mill. (*Liliaceae*)-**Barbados Aloe**, Mediterranean Aloe, Curaeao Aloe; *Euphorbia lathyris* L. (*Euphorbiaceae*)-**Mole plant**, Petroleum plant **Caper spurge**; *Hedra helix* L. (*Araliaceae*)-Ivy; *Hura crepitans* L. (*Euphorbiaceae*)-**Sandhox Tree**; *Malus sylvestris* Mill. (*Rosaceae*)-**Apple**; *Melilotus officinalis* Lam. (*Fabaceae*)-**Yellow Sweetelover**; *Trifolium pratense* L. (*Fabaceae*)-**Red Clover, Pavine Clover, Cowgrass.**

Characteristic Features It occurs as needles having mp 210-213°C. It may be crystallized in its anhydrous form from concentrated hot aqueous solution, but as the monohydrate from dilute aqueous solution on gradual chilling. Its uv_{max} (in 95% ethanol) are 223 and 286 nm (ε 14,450, 19,000). It is practically insoluble in ligroin and benzene, slightly soluble in cold water, and freely soluble in ethanol, ether and hot water.

6.2.1.2 Caffeic Acid

Synonym 3, 4-Dihydroxycinnamic acid.

Chemical Structure

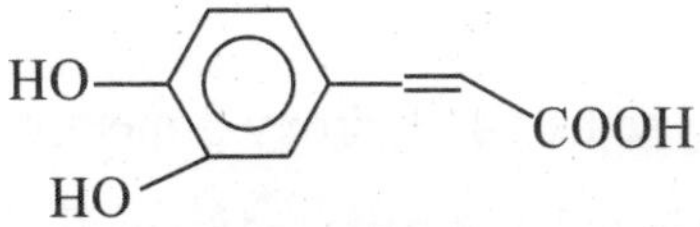

Caffeic Acid

Biological Source It occurs widely in more than twenty different species of plants as detailed below: *Aconitum napellus* L. (*Ranunculacea*)-**Aconite, Monkshood, Blue Rocket**; *Arctium lappa* L. (*Asteraceae*)-**Edible Burdock, Great Burdock, Lappa**; *Arnica montana* L. (*Asteraceae*)-**Mountain Tobacco, Leopard's-bane**; *Cinnamonum camphora* (L.) J.S. Presl. (*Lauraceae*)-**Camphor, Hon-Sho**; *Citrullus coloeynthis* (L.) Sehrad. (*Cucurbitaceae*)-**Colocynth, Bitter Apple, Wild Gourd** *Clematis vitalba* L. (*Ranunculaceae*)-**Traveler's Joy**; *Coniun maculatum* L. (*Apiaceae*)-Hemlock; *Convalaria majalis* L. (*Liliaceae*)-**Lily of the Valley**; *Crataegus oxycantha* L. (*Rosaceae*)-Howthorn; *Digitalis purpurea* L. (*Serophulariaceae*)-**Common Foxglove, Digitalis**; *Equisetum hyemale* L.

(*Equisetaceae*)-Shavegrass, **Great Scouring Rush;** *Euphorbia pulcherrima* Wild ex Klotsch (*Euphorbiaceae*)-**Poinsettia;** *Euphrasia officinalis* L. (*Scrophulariaceae*)-**Eyebright;** *Gaultheria procumbens* L. (*Ericaceae*)-**Wintergreen, Teaberry, Boxberry;** *Leonurus cardiaca* L. (*Lamiaceae*)-Motherwort, *Santolina charnaecyparissus* L. (*Asteraceae*)-**Lavender-Cotton,** *Seopolia carniolica* Jacq. (*Solanaceae*)-**Seopolia;** *Solanum tuberosum* L. (*Solanaceae*)-**Potato;** *Solidago virgaurea* L. (*Asteraceae*)-**European Goldenrod, Woundwort;** *Stachys officinalis* (L.) Trevisan (*Lamiaceae*)-Betony; *Trifolium pratense* L. (*Fabaceae*)-**Red Clover, Pavine Clover, Cowgrass;** *Valeriana officinalis* L. (*Valerianaceae*)-**Valerian;** and *Viscum album* L. (*Loranthaceae*)-**European Mistletoe.**

Preparation It occurs in plants only in conjugated forms *e.g.*, **chlorogenic acid.** It has also been isolated from **green coffee,*** and from **roasted coffee.****

It can also be prepared by the hydrolysis of **chlorogenic acid** in an acidic medium as shown below:*******

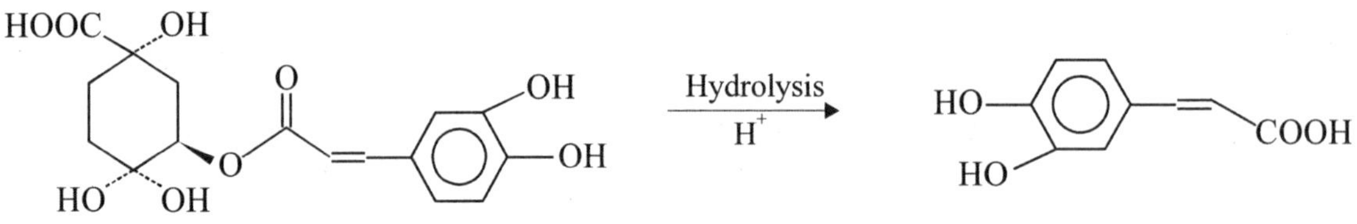

| Chlorogenic Acid | | Caffeic Acid |

Characteristic Features **Caffeic acid** has yellow crystals obtained from concentrated aqueous solutions and the corresponding monohydrate from dilute solutions. It gets softened at 194°C and decomposes at 223-225°C. It is sparingly soluble in cold water, but freely soluble in cold ethanol and hot water.

Chemical Tests

1. It changes colour from yellow to orange in an alkaline medium.
2. It readily forms the methyl ester ($C_{10}H_{10}O_4$) which are obtained as colourless crystals from water (mp 152-153°C).

6.2.1.3 Ferulic Acid

Synonyms Caffeic acid 3-methyl ether; 4-Hydroxy-3-methoxycinnamic acid.

Biological Sources **Ferulic acid** is widely distributed in small amounts in a variety of plants, namely: seeds of *Citrullus colocynthis* (L.) Schrad. (*Cucurbitaceae*)-**Colocynth, Bilter Apple, Wild Gourd;** flowers of *Convallaria majalis* L. (*Liliaceae*)-**Lily-of-the-Valley;** leaves of *Digitalis purpurea* L. (*Scrophulariaceae*)-**Common Foxglove, Digitalis;** young shoots of *Equisetum hyemale* L. (*Equisetaceae*)-**Shavegrass, Great Scouring Rush;** leaves of *Euphorbia lathyris* L. (*Euphorbiaceae*)-

---

* Wolfrom *et al. J. Agr. Food Chem.*, **8**, 58 (1960).

** Krasemann, *Arch. Pharm*, **293**, 721 (1960).

*** Fiedler, *Arzneimittel–Forseh*, **4**, 41 (1954); Whiting, Carr, *Nature* **180**, 1479 (1957), Guren, *Chemical Abstracts*, **61**, 9965h (1964).

Mole Plant, Petroleum Plant, Caper Spurge; dried herb of *Euphrasia officinalis* L. (*Scrophulariaceae*)-**Eyebright;** gum-resin of *Ferula assafoetida* L. (*Apiaceae*)-**Asafoetida;** volatile oil of *Gaultheria procumbens* L. (*Ericaceae*)-**Wintergreen, Teaberry, Boxberry;** twigs of *Hedera helix* L. (Araliaceae)-**Ivy;** leaves of *Hura crepitans* L. (*Euphorbiaceae*)-**Sandbox Tree;** leaves of *Plantago major* L. (*Plantaginaceae*)-**Plantain;** volatile oil of *Rheum officinale* Baill. (*Polygonaceae*)-**Chinese Rhubarb, Canton Rhubarb, Shensi Rhubarb;** shrubs of *Serenoa repens* (Bartel.) Small (*Arecaceae*)-**Saw Palmetto.**

Preparation   It has been isolated from *Ferula foetida* Reg. (*Umbelliferae*)* and from *Pirus laricio* Poir. (*Abietineae*)**.

It may also be prepared by the interaction of vanillin, malonic acid and piperidine in pyridine for three weeks and then precipitating **ferulic acid** with dilute HCl.

Chemical Structure

trans-Ferulic Acid

Characteristic Features

cis-form   : Yellow oil; uv_{max} (in ethanol): 316 nm.

trans-form   : Orthorhombic needles obtained from water; mp 174°C uv_{max} (in ethanol): 236, 322 nm. It is soluble in hot water, ethanol and ethyl acetate; moderately soluble in ether; and sparingly soluble in benzene and petroleum ether.

Identification Test   It forms the corresponding sodium salt by treatment with NaOH solution whereby the solubility gets enhanced appreciably.

Uses   It is used as a preservative of food products.

6.2.1.4 *Sinapic Acid*

Biological Source   It is obtained from the leaves and twigs of *Viscum album* L. (*Loranthaceae*)-**European Mistletoe.**

Preparation   It may be prepared by the hydrolysis of **sinapic acid choline ester** obtained from the **black mustard seeds** of *Brassica nigra* Koch (*Cruciferae*) either in acidic medium or by enzymatic hydrolysis as given below:

---

* H. Hlasiwetz, L. Barth, *Ann.,* **138**, 61 (1966)
** M. Bamberger, *Monatsh.,* **12**, 441 (1891).

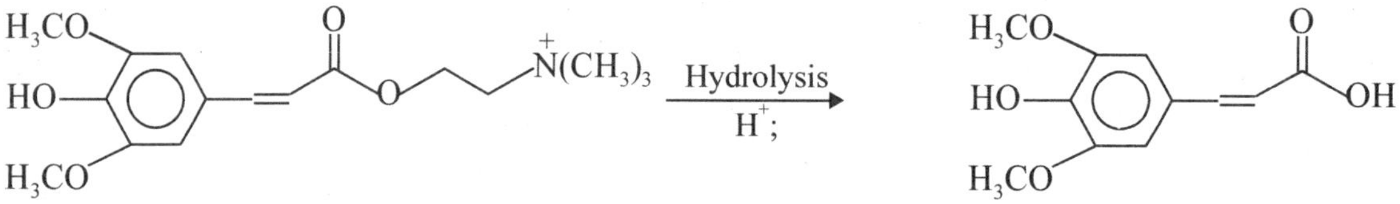

Sinapine
(Sinapic Acid Choline Ester)

Sinapic Acid

Uses

1. It is used as an antiseptic, antispasmodic and emetic.
2. It is also employed for arteriosclerosis, cardiac stimulant, cancer, hepatosis and hypertension.
3. It also finds its use in epilepsy, hysteria and nervous debility.

6.2.2 Phenylpropenes

Phenylpropenes have gained their legitimate cognizance in **phytochemistry** by virtue of their vital contributions to the volatile oil flavours and aroma of medicinal plants. In general, the **phenylpropenes** are normally isolated in the *volatile oil* component of plant tissues, along with the volatile terpenes. It is pertinent to note here that these are evidently lipid-soluble, a distinct deviation from a majority of other phenolic compounds.

A few typical examples of important members of **phenylpropenes** are, namely:

(*a*) **Eugenol :**   A major constituent of oil of cloves;
              (Section 5.2.6.1.4.3 Chapter 5)
(*b*) **Anethole:**   A principle of anise and fennel;
              (Section 5.2.6.5.6A. Chapter 5)
(*c*) **Myristicin:** A component of nutmeg;
              (Section 5.2.6.5.6C. Chapter 5)

Synonyms   Cinnamal; Phenylacrolein; Cinnamic aldehyde;

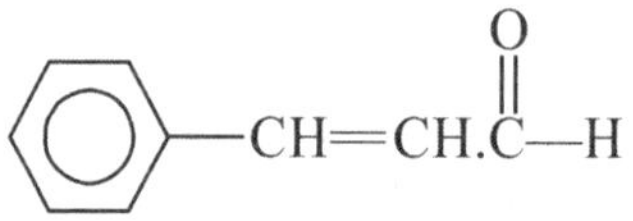

Cinnamaldehyde

Biological Sources   It is obtained from **ceylon cinnamon oil** *Cinnamomum verum* J.S. Presler (*Lauraceae*)-**Ceylon Cinnamon;** *Myroxylon balsamum* var. Pereirae (Royle) Harms. (*Fabaceae*)-**Balsam of Peru;** and *Syzygium oromaticum* (L.) Merr. & Perry (*Myrtaceae*)-**Clovers, Clavos.**

Preparation   Cassia oil (*Cinnamomum cassia* Blume., family: *Lauraceae*) contains volatile oil (1-2%). This volatile oil contains **cinnamaldehyde** (80-85%) which is isolated by subjecting it to fractional distillation under vacuo.

Characteristic Features **Cinnamaldehyde** is a yellowish oily liquid having a strong odour of cinnamon. Its physical parameters are: d_{25}^{25} 1.048-1.052; bp_{100} 177.7°C, bp_{200} 199.3°C and bp_{760} 246°C, n_D^{20} 1.618-1.623. It dissolves in about 700 parts of water and in about 7 volumes of 60% ethanol. It is, however, miscible with ethanol, ether, chloroform and oils.

Chemical Test On addition of a drop of $FeCl_3$ (1% w/v) solution to a few drops of **cinnamaldehyde** a distinct brown colour is produced.

Uses
1. It is used extensively in the perfume industry.
2. It is employed for flavouring foods and beverages.

Interestingly, it has been observed that the pairs of the allyl (CH_2=CH—CH_2—) and propenyl (CH_3CH=CH–) isomers, such as: *eugenol* and *isoeugenol* invariably occur together in the same medicinal plant as stated below:

(*i*) *Cananga odorata* (Lam.) Hook. f. & Thoms. (*Annonaceae*)-Cananaga, **Ylang-Ylang;** and

(*ii*) *Myristica fragrans* Houtt. (*Myristicaceae*)-**Mael, Nutmeg**

Note **Isomerization of the allyl to the propenyl form may also be accomplished in the laboratory, but only under very drastic and specific experimental parameters i.e., in the presence of strong alkali. However, such isomerization rarely takes place under normal conditions of isolation from natural products, such as: solvent extraction with ether etc.**

6.2.3   Coumarins

Coumarin and its derivatives, such as: **hydroxy-coumarins** and **furanocoumarins** are present in a plethora of medicinal plants. However, the most common and the most widespread plant coumarin is the parent compound *i.e.*, coumarin itself, which is reported to occur in more than twenty-seven plant families *viz.*, *Caprifoliaceae, Leguminosae, Oleaceae, Rubiaceae, Solanaceae, Umbelliferae*-to name a few such families.

In a broader sense, the **coumarins** may be classified into *three* major categories, namely:

(*a*) Coumarins,

(*b*) Hydroxycoumarins, and

(*c*) Furanocoumarins.

All these *three* classes of drugs shall be described with the help of some important examples from each class individually as below:

6.2.3.1 Coumarins

The chemistry of **coumarin** may be understood more vividly with the help of geometrical isomers of *o*-**hydroxycinnamic acids,** one of which instantly yields the **lactone coumarin** (or **benzopyran**), whereas the other fails to do so. Therefore, the former is the *cis*-isomer called **coumarinic acid,** and the latter the *trans*-isomer known as the **coumaric acid** as given below:

Coumaric Acid	Coumarinic Acid	Coumarin
(*trans*-isomer)	(*cis*-isomer)	

Coumarin

Synonyms   *cis-o*-Coumarinic acid lactone; Cumarin; Coumarinic anhydride; Tonka bean comphor.

Biological Sources   Coumarin is present in a large number of medicinal herbs, such as:
Acacia farnesiana (L.) Willd (*Fabaceae*)-**Cassie, Huisache;** *Apium graveolens* L. (*Apiceae*)-**Celery;** *Artemisia dracunculus* L. (*Asteraceae*)-**Tarragon;** *Chamaemelum nobile* (L.) All. (*Asteraceae*)-**Roman Camomile, English Camomile, Camomile;** *Cinnamomum verum* J.S. Presler (*Lauraceae*)-**Ceylon Cinnamon;** *Dipteryx odorata* (Aubl.) Willd (*Fabaceae*)-**Tonka Bean, Tonga, Cumaru;** *Hyoseyamus niger* L. (*Solanaceae*)-**Henbane, Henblain, Jusquaime;** *Myroxylon balsamum* var. Pereirae (Royle) Harms. (*Fabaceae*)-**Balsam of Peru;** *Peumus boldus* Molina (*Monimiaceae*)-**Boldo;** *Pimpinella anisum* L. (*Apiaceae*)-**Anise;** and *Trilisa odoratissima* (J.F. Gemel.) Cass (*Asteraceae*)-**Deertongue, Deer's Tongue.**

Characteristic Features   **Coumarin** crystals have an orthorhombic and rectangular plates. They have a pleasant, fragrant odour resembling to that of the vanilla beans and a burning taste. The physical characteristics are, namely: mp 68-70°C and bp 297-299°C. Its solubility in water is very poor, viz., 1g dissolves in m 400 ml of cold and 50 ml of boiling water. However, it is freely soluble in ethanol, chloroform, ether, oils and also in alkaline solutions of NaOH or KOH.

Uses   It is used extensively as a flavouring agent in pharmaceutical formulations.

6.2.3.2 *Hydroxycoumarins*

Hydroxycoumarins are invariably found in a large number of plant families. However, the relatively more common ones are based upon the following substances, such as: *umbelliferone* (**7-hydroxy coumarin**), *aesculetin* (**6, 7-dihydroxy-coumarin**) and *scopoletin* (**6-methoxy-7-hydroxy coumarin**) as given below.

Umbelliferone : R = H;
Aesculetin   : R = OH;
Scopoletin   : R = OCH_3;

Interestingly, some rarer **hydroxycoumarins** are, namely, **dephentin** (7, 8-dihydroxy coumarin) and **fraxetin** (6-methoxy, 7-8-dihydroxy coumarin) are both obtained from plant sources.

A few typical examples of **hydroxycoumarins** shall be described in the sections that follow, *e.g.*, **Umbelliferone, Esculetin,** and **Scopoletin.**

6.2.3.2.1 Umbelliferone

Synonyms Hydrangin; Skimmetin.

Biological Sources **Umbelliferone** is present in a variety of medicinal plants, for instance: *Apium graveolens* L. (*Apiaceae*) **Celery;** *Artemisia abrotanum* L. (*Asteraceae*)-**Southernwood, Old Man;** *Daphne mezereum* L. (*Thymelaeaceae*)-**Mezereon;** *Dipteryx odorata* (Aubl.) Willd. (*Fabaceae*)-**Tonka Bean, Tonga, Cumaru;** *Ferula sumbul* Hook. (*Apiaceae*)-**Sumbul, Mask Root;** *Hydrangea paniculata* Seib. (*Saxifragaceae*)-**Peegee;** *Lavandule angustifolia* Mill. (*Lamiaceae*)-**Lavender;** *Matricaria chamomilla* L. (*Asteraceae*)-**Hungarian Camomile, German Camomile, Manzanilla;** and *Pimpinella anisum* L. (*Apiaceae*)-**Anise.**

Preparation **Asafoetida** contains resin (40-65%) which consits of chiefly a resin-alcohol **asaresinotannol** both in the free or combined form with ferulic acid, and of course, free **umbelliferone** is totally *absent* in the drug. Thus, umbelliferone is prepared by treating **ferulic acid** with HCl which gets converted to **umbellic acid** and the latter loses a molecule of water to give rise to **umbelliferone** as given below:

trans-Ferulic Acid   Umbellic Acid

Umbelliferone

Umbelliferone may also be obtained by distillation of resin from **Umbelliferae.***

Characteristic Features It is obtained as needles from water. It develops the characteristic odour of coumarin on heating. Its mp is 225-228°C. It usually sublimes. Its solubility in water is very poor *i.e.,* it dissolves 1 g in nearly 100 ml of boiling water. It is freely soluble in ethanol, chloroform, acetic acid and dilute alkaline solution. It is sparingly soluble in ether and the solutions exhibit a distinct blue fluorescence.

Identification Test When 0.5 g of **umbelliferone** is triturated with pure sand (SiO_2) and 5 ml of HCl, added 5 ml of water, filtered and to the filtrate added an equal volume of ammonia solution, it gives a beautiful blue fluorescence.

Uses
1. It is an important ingredient in most sunscreen lotions and creams.
2. It is most importantly used as an intracellular and pH sensitive fluorescent indicator and blood-brain-barrier (BBB) probe.

---

* Z wenger, *Ann.*, **115**, 1, 15 (1860).

6.2.3.2.2 *Esculetin*

Synonyms Aesculetin; Chicorigenin; 6, 7-Dihydroxy-coumarin.

Biological Source It is the *aglucon* of **esculin** and **cichorlin:** Esculin is derived from two different plant sources, namely: (*a*) the barks of *Crataegus oxycantha* L. (*Rosaceae*)-**Hawthorn;** and (*b*) the flowers of *Centarea cyanus* Linn., (*Compositae*). It is a glucoside which upon hydrolysis gives the aglucon **esculetin**.

    Esculetin is also obtained from **cichorlin**, which is a glucoside and found to be isomeric with esculin. **Cichorlin** is present in the flowers of the **chicory plant** (*Chichorium intybus* L., family: *Compositae*).

Preparation It is obtained by the hydrolysis of the following *two* glucosides, namely:

(*a*) **From Esculin:**

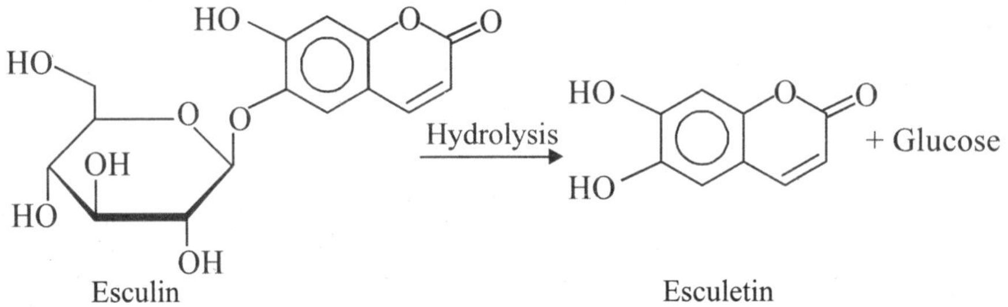

Esculin   Hydrolysis   Esculetin   + Glucose

(*b*) **From Cichorlin:**

Cichorlin   Hydrolysis   Esculetin   + Glucose

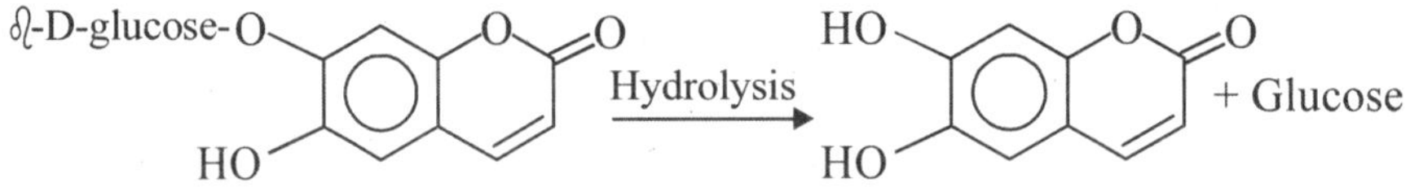

Characteristic Features It is obtained as prisms from glacial acetic acid and as leaflets by vacuum sublimation. Its mp is 268-270°C. It is soluble in dilute alkalies (2M solution) with the emission of blue fluorescence. It is almost insoluble in ether and in boiling water, but moderately soluble in hot ethanol and in glacial acetic acid.

Uses It is mostly in filters for absorption of uv-light

6.2.3.2.3 *Scopoletin*

Synonyms Chrysatropic acid; Gelseminic acid; 6-Methoxyumbelliferone; β-Methylesculetin; 7-Hydroxy 6-methoxycoumarin.

Biological Sources It is the *aglucone* of **scopolin. Scopoletin** occurs in the roots of *Arnica montana* L. (*Asteraceae*)-**Mountain Tobacco, Leopard's-bane;** leaves of *Artemesia abrotanum* L. (*Asteraceae*)-**Southernwood, Old Man;** roots and leaves of *Atropa belladona* L. (*Solanaceae*)-**Belladonna, Deadly Nightshade;** barks of *Brunfelsia uniflorus* (Phol.) D. Don. (*Solanaceae*)-**Manaca, Manacan;** fruits of *Capsicum annuum* L. (*Solanaceae*)-**Chili, Sweet Peppers, Paprika;**

oil of the plant *Chamaemelum nobile* (L.) All. (*Asteraceae*)-**Roman Comomile; English Camomile, Comomile;** and roots of *Withania somniferum* (L.) Dunal (*Solanaceae*)-**Ashwagandha.**

Preparation   It is obtained by the hydrolysis of the glucoside scopolin *i.e.*, 7-(β-D glucopyranosyloxy)-6-methoxy-2H-1-benzopyran-2-one as follows:

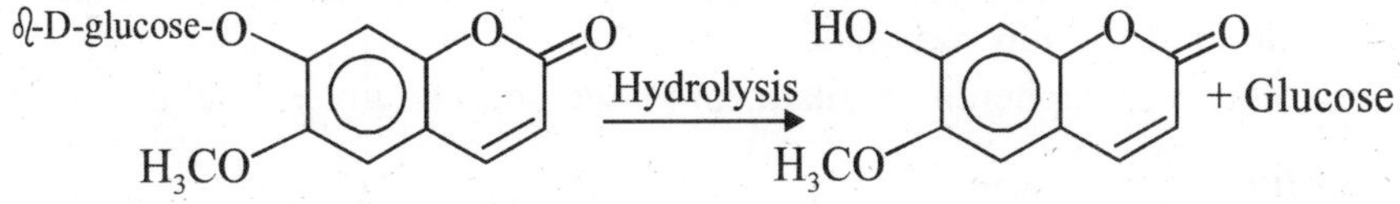

Scopolin   Scopoletin

Characteristic Features   **Scopoletin** occurs as prisms or needles from either acetic acid or chloroform. It melts at 204°C and has a uv_{max}: 230, 254, 260, 298, 346 nm (log ε 4.11, 3.68, 3.63, 3.68, 4.07). It is slightly soluble in water or cold ethanol and quite soluble in hot ethanol and hot glacial acetic acid. It is moderately soluble in chloroform, but practically insoluble in the non-polar solvent benzene.

Identification Tests

1. Dissolve 0.1 g in ethanol and warm it in an electric water-bath to affect dissolution. The resulting solution gives a blue fluorescence.
2. A solution of 0.1 g in 3 ml of hot ethanol reduces the Fehling's solution thereby leaving behind a brick-red precipitate of cupric oxide (CuO).

It is pertinent to mention here that there exists some rarer species of hydroxycoumarins, such as: **daphentin** and **fraxetin,** which shall now be discussed in the sections that follows:

6.2.3.2.4 *Daphentin*

Synonyms   7, 8-Dihydroxycoumarin;

Biological Sources   It is the aglucon of **daphnin.** It is obtained from the seeds and fruits of *Daphne mezereum* L. (*Thymelaeaceae*)-**Mezereon**; and the seeds of *Euphorbia lathyris* L. (*Euphorbiaceae*)-**Mole Plant, Petroleum Plant, Caper Spurge.**

Preparation   **Daphentin** is prepared conveniently from its glucoside known as **daphnin** *i.e.*, 7, 8-dihydroxycoumarin 7-β-D-glucoside by treating the latter in *three* different ways, namely: (*i*) By boiling with dilute mineral acids; (*ii*) By enzymatic hydrolysis; and (*iii*) By sublimation as given below:

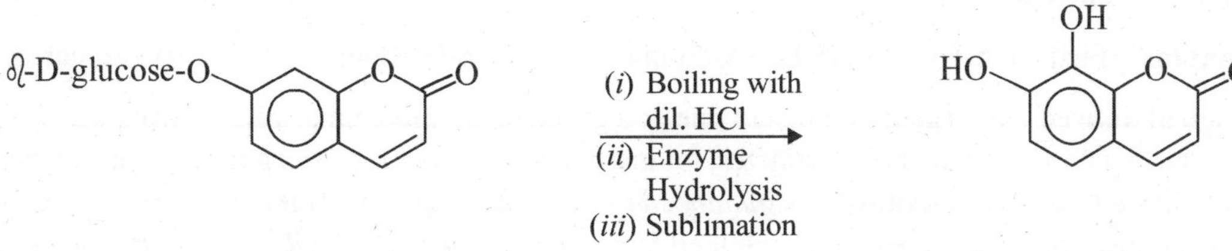

(*i*) Boiling with dil. HCl
(*ii*) Enzyme Hydrolysis
(*iii*) Sublimation

Daphnin   Daphentin

Characteristic Features   The crystals obtained from dilute ethanol has a mp 256°C (decomposes). It undergoes sublimation on heating. It is soluble in boiling water, hot dilute alcohol and hot glacial acetic acid. It is found to be sparingly soluble in ether, CS_2, chloroform, and benzene.

Identification Tests
1. An aqueous solution of daphentin gives a green colouration with $FeCl_3$ solution, which turns red on the addition of sodium carbonate.
2. An alkaline solution of daphentin in alkali carbonate or alkali gives a yellow colour.

6.2.3.2.5 Fraxetin

Synonyms   7, 8-Dihydroxy-6-methoxycoumarin.

Biological Source   It is the aglucon of **fraxin**. **Fraxin** is present in the seeds of *Acsculus hippocastanum* L. (*Hippocastanaceae*)-**Horse Chestnut**.

Preparation   Fraxetin is obtained by heating **fraxin** with dilute sulphuric acid to affect the hydrolysis of glucoside and get the desired aglucon residue as shown here under:

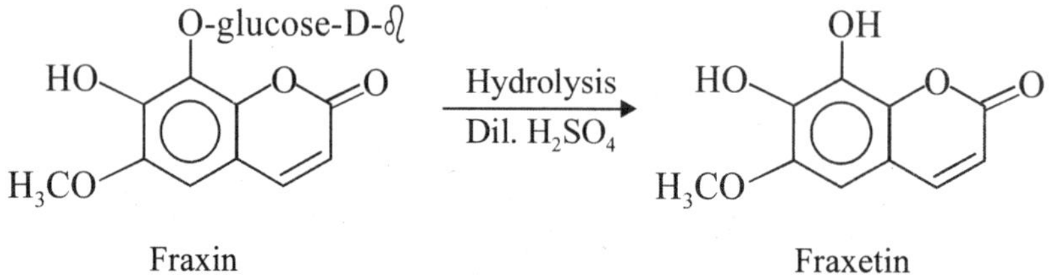

Fraxin   Fraxetin

Characteristic Features   **Fraxetin** is obtained as plates from ethanol having mp 228°C. It has been observed that it turns first yellow at 150°C and subsequently brown at mp. It is soluble in 10 L of cold water, but in 300 ml of boiling water. It is somewhat more soluble in alcohol and practically insoluble in ether.

Identification Tests   It forms the corresponding dimethyl ether termed as 6,7,8-trimethoxycoumarin ($C_{12}H_{12}O_5$) which has a mp 104°C and $bp_{0.2}$ 90-100°C.

6.2.3.3 Furanocoumarins

Furanocoumarins, represent a class of relatively more complex coumarins that occur in various natural plant products. A few important members of this particular class are, namely: **Psoralen; Methoxsalen; Bergapten;** and **Imperatorin,** which shall be discussed below in an elaborated manner.

6.2.3.3.1 Psoralen

Synonyms   Ficusin; 6-Hydroxy-5-Benzofuranacrylic acid δ-lactone; Furo (3, 2-δ)-coumarin.

Biological Source   **Psoralen** belongs to one of a group of furanocoumarins occurring naturally in more than two dozen different plant sources, for instance: *Rutaceae* (*e.g.*, **Bergamot, Limes, Cloves**); *Umbelliferae* (**Celery; Parsnips**); *Leguminosae* (*e.g.*, **Psoralen coryfolia**); and *Moraceae* (*e.g.*, **Figs**). It is also found in the **Rue Oil** obtained from *Ruta graveolens* L. (*Rutaceae*)-known as **Rue, Garden Rue** or **German Rue**. It is obtained from the leaves of *Ficus carica* Linn. (*Moraceae*)-**Figs, Anjir.**

Chemical Structure

Psoralen

Characteristic Features **Psoralen** crystals from ether have two sets of melting points *e.g.*, 163-164°C and 169-179°C (Spath). It is very soluble in chloroform, less soluble in alcohol, sparingly soluble in ether and practically insoluble in petroleum ether (60-80°C).

Identification Tests

1. Dissolve 1 mg of **psoralen** is 5 ml of ethanol and add to it 15 ml of a mixture made up of 3 parts of propylene glycol, 5 parts of acetic acid and 43 parts of water. The resulting mixture on being exposed to the uv-light in a uv-chamber, gives a distinct *blue-fluorescence*.
2. When 1 mg is dissolved in 2 ml ethanol, mixed with two drops of NaOH solution (0.1 M) and the resulting solution is subjected to uv-light, it emits a yellow fluorescence.

Uses

1. It is used in the treatment of leucoderma patches.
2. Psoralens have also exhibited photosensitizing and phototoxic effects in animals and human beings and, hence have been employed extensively in *photochemotherapy* for the treatment and management of **vitiligo***, **psoriasis*** and **mycosis fungoides.*****

6.2.3.3.2   Methoxsalen

Synonyms Xanthotoxin; Meloxine; Ammoidin; Meladinine; 8-Methoxypsoralen; 8-MOP; 8-MP; Oxsoralen.

Biological Source **Methoxsalen** is a naturally occurring analogue of **psoralen,** found in various species of *Rutaceae, Leguminosae,* and *Umbelliferae*. It is obtained from the fruits of *Fragara xanthoxyloides* and the fruits of *Ammi majus* belonging to the natural order *Umbelliferae*. It is also found in the herb *Ruta graveolens* (*Rutaceae*).

Chemical Structure

Methoxsalen

9-Methoxy-7H-furol [3,2-g][1] benzopyran-7-one; ($C_{12} H_8 O_4$).

---

* T.F. Anderson, J.J. Voorhees, *Ann. Rev. Pharmacol. Toxicol.*, **20**, 235 (1980); *Vitiligo*: An acquired cutaneous disorder characterised by white patches, surrounded by areas of normal pigmentation.

** A. Kornhauser *et al., Science*, **217**, 733 (1982); *Psoriasis*: A common chronic disease of the skin consisting of erythematous papules that coalesce to form plaques with distinct borders.

*** B.J. Parsons, *Photochem. Photobiol.*, **32**, 813-821 (1980); *Mycosis Fungoides*: A non-Hodgkin's form of cutaneous T-cell lymphoma of unknown etiology caused by a fungus.

Isolation   The various steps involved are as under:

1. The *A. majus* fruits are dried, powdered, sieved and extracted with petroleum ether to complete exhaustion.
2. The petroleum ether extract is filtered and concentrated to obtain a dark green semi-crystalline solid mass (crude methoxalen) crystallizes out.
   Note: The petroleum ether layer is carefully deeanted off while hot and reserved separately for the isolation of imperatorin.
3. The residual dark-green solid mass is dissolved in minimum quantity of ethanol and boiled over an electric water-bath for 45-60 minutes. The contents are filtered immediately and the filtrate is concentrated under vacuo. It is cooled in a refrigerator overnight when pale-green crystals separate out. The crystals of **methoxsalen** thus obtained are purified first by washing with boiling water and finally recrystallizing from ethyl acetate.

Characteristic Features

1. It is obtained in two forms: *first*—as silky needles either from hot water or benzene + petroleum ether; *secondly*—as long rhombic prisms from ethanol + ether, having mp 148°C.
2. It is odourless *but* has a distinct bitter taste followed by tingling sensation.
3. It has uv$_{max}$: 219, 249, 300 nm (log ε 4.32, 4.35, 4.06).
4. It has a pH 5.5.
5. *Solubility Profile*: It is practically insoluble in cold water; sparingly soluble in boiling water, liquid petroleum, ether; soluble in boiling ethanol, acetone, acetic acid, vegetable fixed oils, propylene glycol, benzene; freely soluble in chloroform; and soluble in aqueous alkalies with ring cleavage, but is reconstituted upon neutralization.

Identification Tests   These are as follows:

1. A few crystals of **methoxsalen** on being triturated with little sulphuric acid in a porcelain dish produces an orange-yellow colour that gets changed to light green finally.
2. **Wagner's Reagent Test: Xanthotoxin** gives an instant precipitate with **Wagner's Reagent** $(I_2 + KI)$.
3. **HNO$_3$ Test:** It gives a distinct yellow colouration with dilute HNO_3, which on rendering to alkaline with KOH or NaOH, changes to crimson colour.

Uses

1. It is used extensively in the treatment of leukoderma.
2. It is employed as a pigmentation agent.
3. It is also used in the treatment of psoriasis and mycosis fungoides.

6.2.3.3.3   Bergapten (e)

Synonyms   Bergapten; Heraclin; Majudin; Psoraderm; 5-Methoxypsoralen; 5-MOP.

Biological Source   **Bergapten** is the naturally occurring analogue of psoralen and an isomer of **methoxsalen**, mostly found in a wide variety of plants, such as: roots and fruits of *Angelica archangelica* L. (*Apiaceae*)-**Angelica, Garden Angelica, European Angelica;** seeds of *Apium* *graveolens* L. (*Apiaceae*)-Celery; leaves, stems and fruits of *Petroselinum crispum* (Mill.) Nym. (*Apiaceae*)-Parsley; **Rue Oil** of *Ruta graveolens* L. (*Rutaceae*)-**Rue, Garden Rue, German Rue.**

Preparation   Bergapten was first isolated from the oil of bergamot from *Citrus bergamia* Risso., belonging to the natural order *Aurantiodiae**. It was also isolated from *Fagara xanthoxyloides* Lam., belonging to family *Rutaceae.***

Chemical Structure

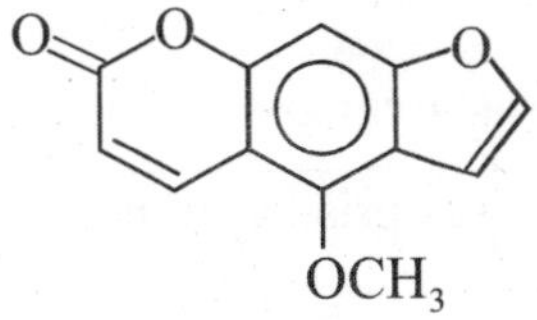

Bergapten

Characteristic Features   The crystals obtained from ethanol are needle-shaped having mp 188°C. It sublimes on heating. It is practically insoluble in boiling water, slightly soluble in glacial acetic acid, chloroform, benzene, and warm phenol. It is soluble in absolute ethanol (1 part in 60).

Identification Test   It gives a distinct yellow-gold colouration when its solution is treated with a few drops of concentrate H_2SO_4.

Uses

1. It is used in photochemotherapy of psoriasis.
2. It has been used to promote tanning in *suntan preparations e.g.*, creams and lotions.

6.2.3.3.4   Imperatorin

Synonyms   Ammidin; Pentosalen; Marmelosin;

Biological Sources   It is obtained from the roots and fruits of *Angelica archangelica* L. (*Apiaceae*) (**Angelica, Garden Angelica, European Angelica**); from the roots of *Imperatoria osthruthium* L. (*Umbelliferae*); from fruit of *Pastinaea sativa* L. (*Umbelliferae*); and also in the fruits of *Ammimajus* (*Umbelliferae*). However, the seed oil of *A. archangelica* is said to contain upto 0.5% **imperatorin.**

Chemical Structure

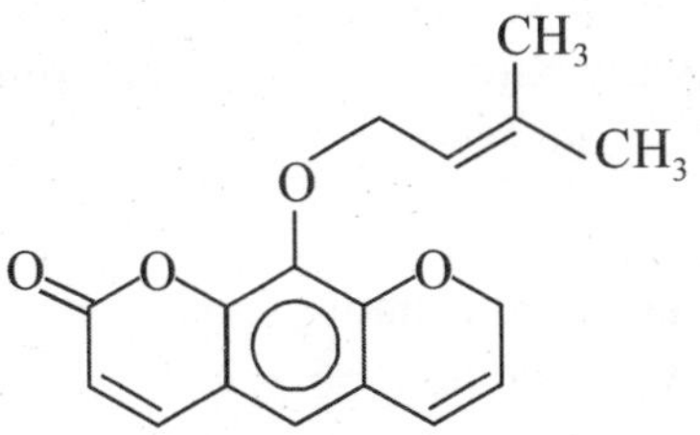

Imperatorin

9-[(3-Methyl-2-butenyl)oxy]-7H-furo [3, 2-g] [1] benzopyran-7-one; ($C_{16} H_{14}O_4$).

---

 * Pomeranz, *Monatsh*, **12**, 379 (1891), **14**, 28 (1893).
** H. Thoms., E. Baeteke, *Ber.*, **44**, 3326 (1911).

Isolation The various steps involved are as follows:

1. The petroleum ether mother liquor left after the separation of **methoxsalen (Xanthotoxin)**, is concentrated under vacuo and allowed to cool in a refrigerator overnight when the crude imperatorin separates out.
2. The crude product is collected, dissolved in ether, filtered and concentrated under reduced pressure. It is kept in a refrigerator, and the crystals separating out are purified subsequently by recrystallization from ethanol.

Characteristic Features These are as given below:

1. It is obtained in *two* forms: *First*—as prisms from ether, and *secondly*—as long fine needles from hot water, having mp 102°C.
2. It has uv$_{max}$: 302, 265, 250 nm (log ε 3.95, 4.00, 4.24).
3. *Solubility Profile*: It is practically insoluble in cold water; very sparingly soluble in boiling water; freely soluble in chloroform; and soluble in benzene, ethanol, ether, petroleum, ether alkali hydroxides.

Identification Tests These are as stated below:

1. **Sulphuric Acid Test:** Imperatorin gives an intense deep orange colouration with a few drops of sulphuric acid which ultimately changes to brown colour.
2. **Marqui's Reagent:** It gives an orange colouration with Marqui's Reagent that rapidly changes to brown.
3. **Tollen's Reagent (Ammoniacal AgNO$_3$):** It reduces Tollen's Reagent to produce a silver mirror.
4. **Fehlings Test:** It reduces Fehling's solution to give a brick-red precipitate of cupric oxide.
5. **Nitric Acid Test:** It gives a distinct yellow colour on boiling with dilute HNO$_3$, and this colour changes to purple on being treated with strong alkali *e.g.* NaOH or KOH.

6.2.4 Abridged Phenylpropanoids

Abridged phenylpropanoids are invariably acids and phenols, and quite rarely alcohol and aldehydes, which are attributed due to the β-oxidation of the C$_3$-side chain of: (*a*) *para*-**Coumaroyl CoA,** and (*b*) *para*-**Cinnamoyl CoA** followed by oxidative decarboxylation.

The various **abridged phenylpropanoids** present in a large number of **medicinal herbs** are usually classified into *three* major heads, namely:

(*a*) With no side-chain,
(*b*) With side-chain having one C-atom, and
(*c*) With side-chain having two C-atoms.

All these *three* classes of compounds occurring in natural plants shall be discussed separately with the help of certain appropriate examples as stated below:

6.2.4.1 With No side-Chain

The most glaring example of an **abridged phenylpropenoid** that has no side-chain is **catechol** which shall be treated more explicitly as follows:

Catechol

Synonyms   Pyrocatechol; Pyrocatechin; 1, 2-Dihydroxybenzene; 1, 2-Benzenediol.

Biological Sources   It occurs naturally in various plant species, such as: whole plant of *Anandenathera peregrina* L. Speg. (*Mimosaceae*)-**Niopo, Cohoba, Yope, Yupa;** cortex of *Melia azedaraeh* L. (*Meliaceae*)-Chinaberry; and plant of *Rumex crispus* L. (*Polygonaceae*)-**Yellow Dock.**

Chemical Structure

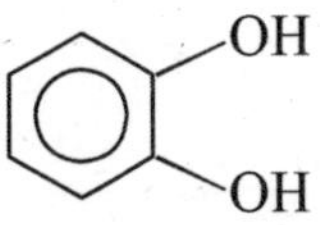

Catechol

Preparation   Being phenolic in character the aqueous extract may be treated with dilute alkalies carefully, and the resulting sodium salts are neutralized to yield the desired **catechol** from the natural plant sources.

It may also be obtained by several other methods as stated below:

(*a*) **Decarboxylation of Protocatechuic Acid:** Protocatechuic acid is found in minute quantities in wheat grains, in wheat seedlings and in many other plants.

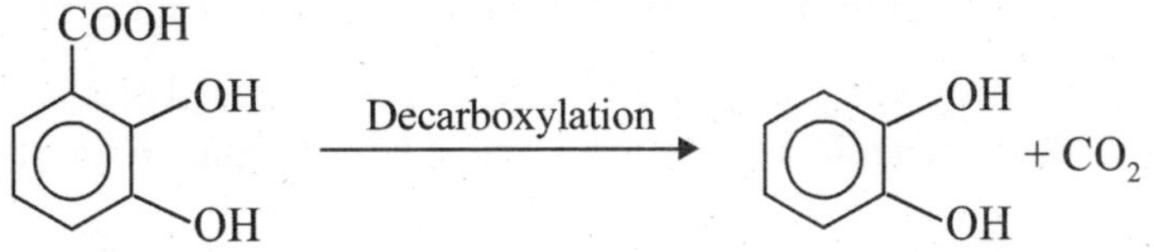

Protocatechuic acid   Catechol

(*b*) **From Salicylaldehyde:** Catechol is also obtained by the interaction of salicylaldehyde with hydrogen peroxide as follows:

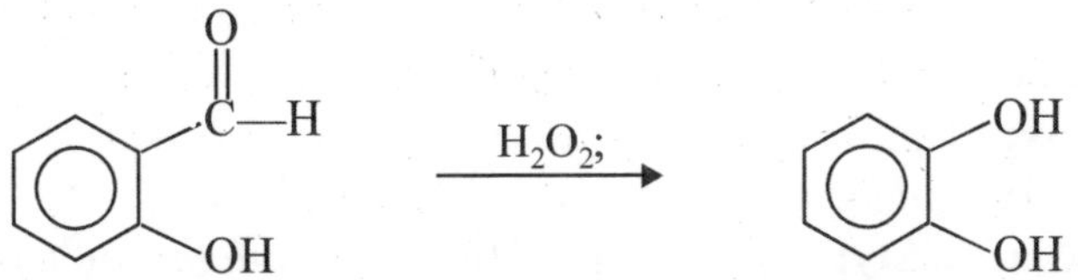

Salicylaldehyde   Catechol

(*c*) **From Guaiacol:** It may also be prepared by treating guaiacol with hydro bromic acid as given below:

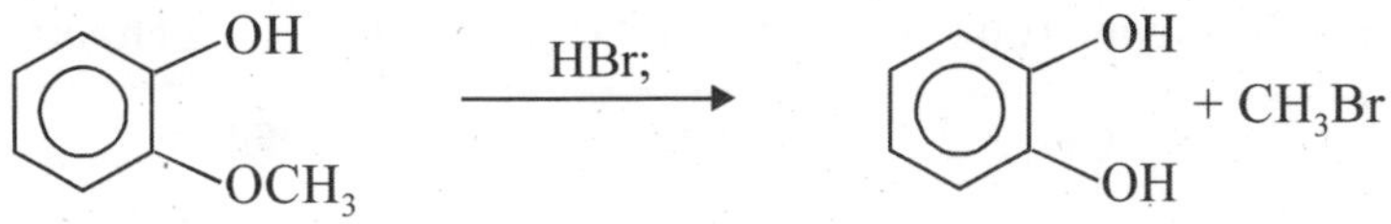

Guaiacol   Catechol

Characteristic Features   **Catechol** is obtained as the monoclinic tablets or prisms from toluene. It usually undergoes discolouration on exposure to air or light. Its physical characteristics are: mp

105°C, d 1.344, bp$_{760}$ 245.5°C, bp$_{100}$ 176°C, bp$_{40}$ 150.6°C. It is steam volatile and sublimes on heating. Its dissociation constant K at 18° = 3.3 × 10^{-10}. It is soluble in 2.3 parts of water, ethanol, benzene, chloroform and ether; and very soluble in aqueous alkali solutions and pyridine. It has been observed that its aqueous solution soon turns brown.

Identification Test   Dissolve 0.2 g of **catechol** in water and add to it a few drops of FeCl$_3$ (0.1% w/v) aqueous solution. The appearance of a green colour confirms the presence of catechol.

Uses

1. It is used as an antiseptic agent.
2. It finds its application in photography.
3. It is also employed for dyeing fur.

6.2.4.2 *With Side-Chain Having One Cabon Atom*

The **abridged phenylpropenoids** having a side chain with one carbon atom represent an important group of naturally occurring plant products, such as: **Benzoic acid, Gallic acid, Methyl salicylate, Salicin** and **Vanillin.**

These compounds shall be discussed here under in a concise descriptive manner.

6.2.4.2.1 **Benzoic Acid**

Synonyms Dracyclic acid: Phenylformic acid, Benzene carboxylic acid.

Biological Source   It mostly occurs in nature in free and combined forms. **Gum benzoin** may contain as much as 20% of **benzoic acid,** whereas most berries contain appreciable amounts *i.e.,* upto 0.05%.

Benzoic acid is found in a large number of medicinal herbs, namely: plant of *Aeacia farnesiana* (L.) Willd. (*Fabaceae*)-**Cassie, Huisache;** oil of *Cananga odorata* (Lam.) Hook. f. & Thoms. (*Annonaceae*)-**Cananga, Ylang-Ylang;** latex of *Daemonorops draco* bl. (*Arecaceae*)-**Dragon's Blood;** tubers of *Gloriosa superba* L. (*Liliaceae*)-**Glory Lilly;** plant of *Illicium verum* Hook. f. (*Magnoliaceae*)-**Star-Anise, Chinese Anise;** volatile of *Narcissus tazetta* L. (*Amaryllidaceae*)-Daffodil, **Chinese Sacred Lilly, Polyanttus Narcissus;** roots of *Paeonia officinalis* L. (*Ranunculaceae*)-**Peony;** Plant of *Piper methysticum* Forst. (*Piperaceae*)-**Kava-Kava;** leaves of *Plantago major* L. (*Plantaginaceae*)-**Plantain;** gum of *Styrax benzoin* Dryander (*Styracaceae*)-**Benzoin, Sumatra Benzoin, Styrax;** and pods of *Vanilla planifolia* Andr. (*Orchidaceae*)-**Vanilla.**

Preparation   The alcoholic extract of the plant is concentrated cooled and treated with dilute mineral acid. The solid residue thus obtained is further recrystallized from hot alcohol.

It is also obtained synthetically in several ways as stated below:

(*a*) **Oxidation of Toluene:** Toluene when oxidized by air, it yields **benzoic acid:**

Toluene   Benzoic Acid

(b) **Decarboxylation of Phthalic Anhydride:** The decarboxylation of phthalic anhydride gives rise to **benzoic acid:**

Pathalic Anhydride   Benzoic Acid

Characteristic Features **Benzoic acid** has been obtained as monoclinic plates or tablets or leaflets. Its density ranges between 1.266-1.321. It has mp 122.4°C; and it sublimes at nearly 100°C. Its bp_{760} 249.2°C, bp_{100} 186.2°C, bp_{40} 162.6°C. It is found to be steam-volatile. It has a flash point ranging between 121-131°C and dissociation constant K at 25°C = 6.40×10^5. The pH of its saturated solution is 2.8. Its solubility in water at 25°C is 3.4 g/L and at 95°C is 68 g/L. Its solubility in other organic solvents are: cold ethanol 1 g/2.3 ml; boiling ethanol 1 g/1.5 ml; chloroform 1 g/4.5 ml; ether 1 g/3 ml; acetone 1 g/3 ml; carbon tetrachloride 1 g/30 ml; benzene 1 g/10 ml. carbon disulphide 1 g/30 ml. It is also soluble in fixed oils and volatile oils. It is slightly soluble in petroleum ether. The solubility of **benzoic acid** is enhanced by the presence of alkaline substances *e.g.*, trisodium phosphate (Na_3PO_4) and borax.

Identification Test The corresponding calcium benzoate trihydrate salt gives an orthorhombic crystal or powder having a density of 1.44. It is highly soluble in boiling water but sparingly soluble in cold water *i.e.*, 1 g/25 ml.

Uses
1. It has been used in conjunction with salicylic acid in creams and ointments as an effective topical antifungal agent.
2. It is used extensively for the preservation of foods, fats, fruit juices, alkaloidal solutions.
3. It is employed as a *mordant* in calico printing.
4. It is also used for curing tobacco.

6.2.4.2.2 Gallic Acid

Synonym 3, 4, 5-Trihydroxybenzoic Acid.

Biological Sources **Gallic acid** is present in a very large cross-section of medicinal plants. A few such species are as follows, namely: seeds of *Abrus precatorius* L. (*Fabaceae*)-**Jequerity;** berries of *Aretostaphylos uva-ursi* (L.)-Spreng. (*Ericaceae*)-**Bearberry;** seeds of *Cimicifuga recemosa* (L.) Nutt. (*Ranunculaceae*)-**Black Cohosh, Black Snakeroot;** fruits of *Coriaria thymifolia* Humb. & Bonpl. (*Coriariaceae*)-**Shanshi;** resinoid substance (cypripedin) obtained from the rhizome of *Cypripedium sp.* (*Orchidaceae*) **Yellow Lady-slipper;** green branches of *Ephedra geradiana* Wall. ex Staph (*Ephadraceae*)-**Pakistani Ephedra;** plant of *Eupatorium pertolatum* L. (*Asteraceae*)-Boneset, Ague Weed; roots of *Geranium maculatum* L. (*Geraniaceae*)-**Cranebill;** plant of *Juniperus sabina* L. (*Cupressaceae*)-**Sabine, Savin;** leaves of *Lawsonia inermis* L. (*Lythraceae*)-Henna, **Egyptian Privet, Mignonette;** root bark of *Quassia amara* L. (*Simaroubaceae*)-**Surinam Quassia, Bitterwood;** leaves of *Tanacetum vulgare* L. (*Asteraceae*)-**Tansy**; and plant of *Tussilago farfara* L. (*Asteraceae*)-**Coltsfoot, Coughwort, Horse-Hoof.**

Preparation   The *two* important methods of preparation of **gallic acid** from natural sources are given below:

(*a*) **From Tannings of Nutgalls:** It is obtained either by alkaline or acid hydrolysis of the tannins from Nutgalls.

(*b*) **From Spent Broths of Penicillium glaucum or Aspergillus niger:** It may also be prepared by carrying out the enzymatic hydrolysis from the spent broths of *P. glaucum* and *A. niger* which contains the enzyme *tannase*.

Chemical Structure

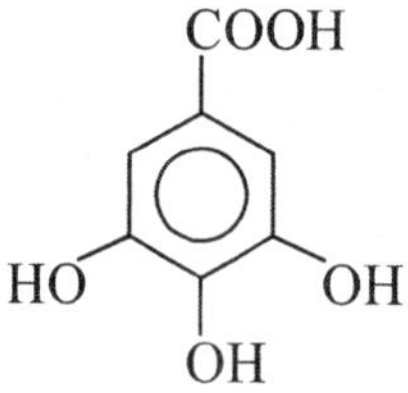

Gallic Acid

Characteristic Features   **Gallic acid** is obtained as needles either from methanol or chloroform. It sublimes at 210°C that yields a fairly stable form which melts at 258-265°C (decomposed) and also an unstable form having mp 225-230°C. Its solubility in water in 1 g/87 ml, boiling water 1 g/3 ml, ethane 1 g/6 ml, ether 1 g/100 ml, glycerol 1 g/10 ml, and acetone 1 g/5 ml. It is found to be practically insoluble in benzene, chloroform and petroleum ether.

Identification Tests

1. **Gallic acid** is first converted to pyrogallol by means of the decarboxylation of the latter, which gives a distinct blue colour with $FeCl_3$ solution (0.1% w/v).

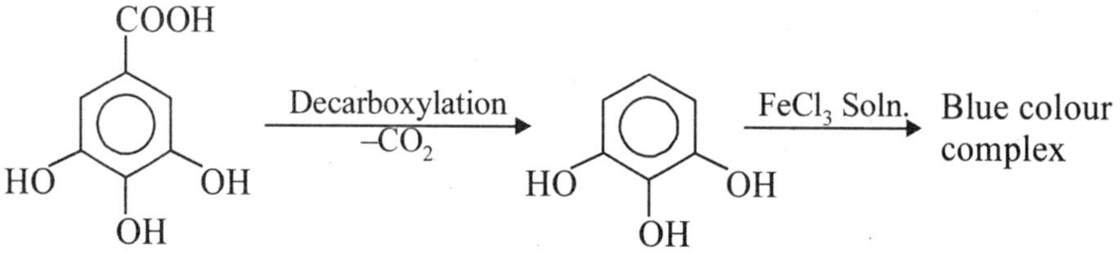

Gallic Acid   Pyrogallol

2. It forms its corresponding methyl ester with methanol which gives a sharp mp 202°C.

Uses   It was used formerly as an astringent and styptic.

6.2.4.2.3 Methyl Salicylate   It has been discussed in details under section 5.2.6.5.8.2 (c) in Chapter-5 on **'Terpenoids'.**

6.2.4.2.4 Salicin

Synonyms   Salicoside; Salicyl alcohol glucoside; Saligenin-β-D-glucopyranoside; 2-(Hydroxymethyl) phenyl-β-D-glucopyranoside.

Biological Sources It is obtained from the volatile oil of *Filipendula ulmaria* (L.) Maxim. (*Rosaceae*)-**Meadosweet, Queen-of-the Meadow.** It is also found in leaves and female flowers of the willow (*Salix*).

Preparation Salicin is prepared by several methods, such as:

(*a*) **Bark of Poplar (Populus):** It is usually prepared by making the hot water extracts obtained either from the ground barks of poplar or willow.

(*b*) **Root Bark of Viburnum prunifolium** L. *(Caprifoliaceae)*: It may also be isolated from the root barks of *V. prunifolium* by means of the hot water extracts.*

Chemical Structure

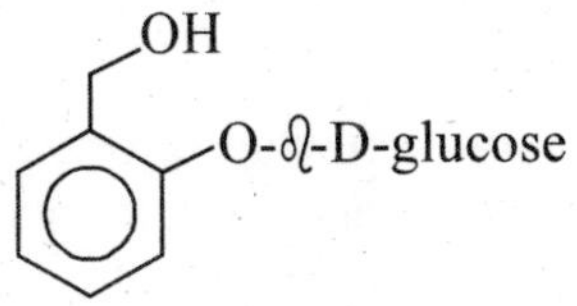

Salicin

Characteristic Features Salicin has orthorhombic crystals from water with mp 199-202°C. Its physical parameters are: $[\alpha]_D^{25} - 62°C$ to $- 67°C$ (c = 3) and $[\alpha]_D^{20} - 45.6°C$ (c = 0.6 in absolute ethanol). It is soluble in water at ambient temperature 1 g/23 ml, in boiling water 1 g/3 ml, in cold alcohol 1 g/90 ml and in alcohol at 60°C (1 g/30 ml). It is freely soluble in alkaline solutions, pyridine, and glacial acetic acid. It is found to be practically insoluble in chloroform and ether. The aqueous solutions are neutral to litmus and possesses a distinct bitter taste.

Uses
1. It is widely used as an analgesic
2. It is employed as a standard substrate in evaluating enzyme preparations containing β-glucosidase.

6.2.4.2.5 Vanillin

Synonyms Vanillic aldehyde; 3-Methoxy-4-hydroxybenzaldehyde; 4-Hydroxy-3-methoxy benzaldehyde.

Biological Sources Vanillin is found in a plethora of medicinal herbs, such as: fruits of *Ananas comosus* (L.) Merr. (*Bromeliaceae*)-**Pineapple**; volatile oil of *Croton eleutheria* Sw. (*Euphorbiaceae*)-**Cascarilla**; oleo-gum-resin of *Ferula asafoetida* L. *(Apiaceae)*-**Asafbetida**; flowerbuds of *Filipendula* ulmaria (L.) Maxim. (*Rosaceae*)-**Meadow-sweet, Queen of the Meadow;** leaves of *Ilex paragua-riensis* St. Hil. (*Aquifoliaceae*)-**Yerba Mate, Paraguay tea, South American Holly;** seeds of *Myroxylon balsamum* var. Pereirae (Royle) Harms. (*Fabiaceae*)-**Balsam of Peru;** essential oil of *Serenoa repens* (Bartel.) Small (*Arecaceae*)-**Saw Palmetto;** leaves of *Tilia europaea* L. (*Tiliaceae*)-**Linden Tree** (America), **Lime Tree** (Europe), and beans of *Vanilla planifolia* Andr. (*Orchidaceae*)-**Vanilla.**

Preparation Vanillin is prepared by the hydrolysis of the aldehyde glycoside *vanilloside* obtained from the unripe vanilla fruit to give rise to the desired aglycone residue (vanillin) as given below:

---

* Evans *et al., J. Am. Pharm. Assoc.,* **34**, 207 (1945).

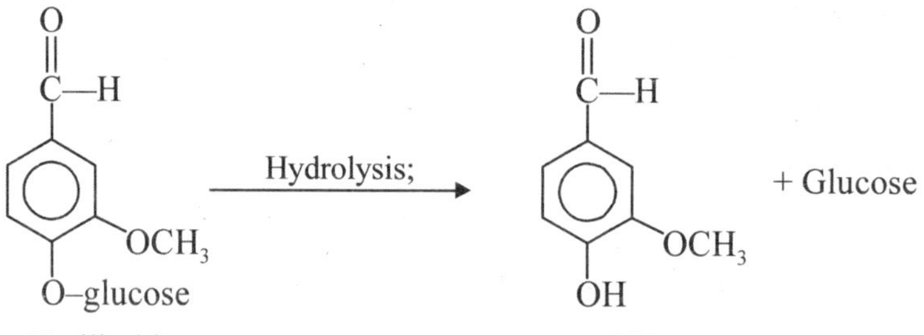

Vanilloside   Vanillin

It may also be obtained synthetically from eugenol or guaiacol; and also from the waste (lignin) of the wood-pulp industry.

Characteristic Features   Vanillin has either a white or very slightly yellow needle-like appearance. It possesses a pleasant aromatic vanila odour and taste. It undergoes gradual oxidation on exposure to humid and moist air. It gets affected by uv-light. Its physical characteristics are: mp 80-81°C; d 1.056 and bp$_{760}$ 285°C. Its solubility in water at ambient temperature is very low (1 g/100 ml), in hot water at 80°C (1 g/16 ml), in glycerol (1 g/20 ml); but freely soluble in ethanol, chloroform, ether, carbon disulfide, glacial acetic acid, pyridine and also soluble in oils and aqueous solutions of alkali hydroxides (NaOH, KOH). The aqueous solution of **vanillin** is acidic to litmus. It must be stored in air-tight and light-resistant containers.

Chemical Test   Vanillin reduces the Tollen's Reagent (*i.e.*, ammoniacal silver nitrate solution) to give rise to the silver-mirror on warning in a water-bath thereby showing the presence of aldehyde moiety present in it.

Uses
1. It is used extensively as a pharmaceutical aid for flavouring pharmaceutical formulations *e.g.*, cough mixture, syrups and elixirs.
2. It is also used as a flavouring agent in beverages, malted-milk-foods, confectionery and in perfumery.
3. It is also employed in manufacture of 'liqueurs'.
4. It has more or less replaced *Vanilla pod* and *tincture vanilla* by virtue of the fact that 1 part of vanillin equals 400 parts of the former and 2.5-3 parts of vanillin equals 500 parts of the latter.
5. It is also used as a reagent in *Analytical Chemistry*.

6.2.4.3 With Side-Chain Having Two Carbon Atoms

The most glaring example of an **abridged-phenylpropanoid** is that of phenyl ethanol which shall be discussed here under:

6.2.4.3.1 Phenyl Ethanol

Synonyms   2-Phenylethanol; β-Phenylethyl alcohol; Benzyl carbinol; β-Hydroxyethylbenzenc; Benzeneethanol.

Biological Sources   Phenyl ethanol is present in variety of essential oils in medicinal plants, namely: *Tillia europaea* L. (*Tiliaceae*)—**Linden Tree** (America), **Lime Tree** (Europe) and other volatile oils of *viz.*, rose, carnation, hyacinth, aleppo pine, orange blossom, geranium Bourbon, champaea and neroli.

Preparation It is obtained by the fractional distillation of volatile oils stated above and collecting the fractions at 219-221°C. It may also be prepared by the reduction of ethylphenyl acetate in the presence pure sodium metal and absolute alcohol in a perfectly dry reaction flask as shown below:

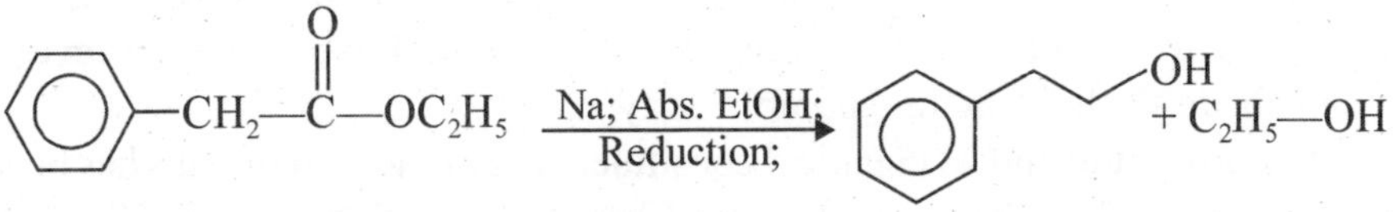

Ethylphenyl Acetate   Phenyl Ethanol

Characteristic Features Phenyl alcohol is a colourless liquid having floral odour resembling to that of rose. Its physical characteristics are, namely: mp $-27°C$; d_{25}^{25} 1.017-1.019; bp_{14} 104°C and n_D^{20} 1.530-1.533. Its solubility in water is very low *i.e.*, 2 ml gets dissolved in 100 ml water after thorough shaking; 1 ml is rapidly soluble in 1 ml of 50% ethanol; and completely miscible with ether and ethanol.

Uses
1. It is used in flavouring foods and beverages.
2. It is extensively employed in perfumery especially for making *rose perfumes*.
3. It is used as a *pharmaceutical aid* to combat microbial infections.

6.2.5 Biphenylpropanoid Derivatives

In this particular class of compounds, the side chains from two **phenylpropanoids** interact with each other to yield **biphenylpropanoid derivatives** that are commonly termed as *Lignans* or *Neolignans*.

(*i*) **Lignans: Lignans**, the plant products with *low molecular weight* that are accomplished by the oxidative coupling of *para*-hydroxyphenylpropene units wherein the two units may be linked by an oxygen bridge. Furthermore, the monomeric precursor units are, namely: cinnamic acid, cinnamyl alcohol, propenylbenzene and allylbenzene. However, the terminology *Lignan* or more precisely **Haworth Lignan** is generally applied to such compounds that are derived by coupling acid and/or alcohol exclusively; whereas, the compounds which are derived by coupling propenyl and/or allyl derivatives are known as **Neolignans.***

Biological Source Lignans occur widely and have been obtained from roots, heart wood, foliage, fruit and resinous exudates of plants. They represent the dimer stage intermediate between the monomeric propylphenol units and lignin. However, the naturally occurring trimers and tetramers have not so far been reported. Nevertheless, the occurrence of **lignans** both in man and animal

---

* Gottlieb, O.R., *Fortschr. Chem. Org. Naturst*, **35**, 1-72 (1978)

species have been reported.* The α-lignan has been found in the roots and rhizomes of *Podophyllum hexandrum* Royle. (*Berberidaceae*).

Preparation   Generally, the **lignans** are formed by the reduction of ferulic acid to coniferyl alcohol as its first and foremost step; and subsequently *via* the oxidative dimerization of the coniferyl alcohol units and the establishment of linkage through the β-carbon atom of the C_3 side-chain.

Characteristic Features   **Lignans** are typically found as single enantiomeric forms *i.e.*, either as *d*-or *l*-isomers. However, these also occur as their racemic products *i.e.*, *dl*-forms. It has been observed that the **lignans** vary to a large extent with regard to their respective oxidation levels, degree of substitution, and above all the structural complexicity.

   Examples: **Podophyllum** and its chemical constituent *podophyllotoxin*. This has been discussed at length under Section 5.2.7 related to '*resin*' in Chapter 5 on '**Terpenoids**'. The two important examples of **lignan** are that of **etoposide** and **teriposide** which shall be discussed in details below:

A. Etoposide

Synonyms   Lastet, Vepesid, VP-16-213, NSC-141540, EPEG, 4′-Demethy-lepipodophyllotoxin 9-[4, 6-O-ethylidene-β-D-glucopyranoside.

Chemical Structure

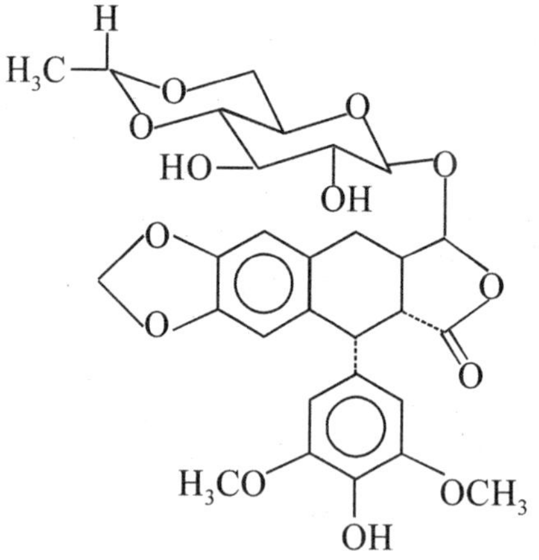

Etoposide

Characteristic Features   **Etoposide** is a semisynthetic **podophyllotoxin** structural analogue used as an '*antineoplastic agent*'. It essentially *differs* structurally from **podophyllotoxin** in the following manners, namely:

   (*a*) It has an ethylidene glucoside moiety attached at the C—1 position.
   (*b*) It has a epimeric configuration at the C—4 position of ring C, and
   (*c*) It possesses a hydroxyl function at the C—4′ position rather than a methoxy moiety.

   However, the hydroxyl (-OH) moiety at C-4′ position exerts *two* important properties to *Etoposide*, namely:

---

* Stitch S.R. *et al.*, *Nature*, **287**, 238 (1980); Setehel K.D.R, *ibid.*, 740

(*i*) It is associated with etoposide's ability to induce *single-stranded DNA breaks*, and

(*ii*) The ethylidene glucoside function is associated with eutopsied's inability to *inhibit microtubule assembly,* an important specific property that may decrease the inherent toxic effects associated with **podophyllotoxin.**

Characterstic Features **Etoposide** is obtained as crystals from methanol having mp 236-251°C. Its physical parameters are $[\alpha]_D^{20} - 110.5°C$ (c = 0.6 in chloroform), uv_{max} (in absolute methanol) is 283 nm (ε 4245) and pKa 9.8.

Uses

1. It is employed in combination with other chemotherapeutic agents for refractory testicular tumours.
2. It is also used as a first line treatment in small cell lung cancer.
3. It has also been used extensively in the treatment of acute nonlymphocytic leukemias, non-Hodgkin's lymphomas, Hodgkin's disease, Kaposi's sarcoma, and neuroblastoma.

B. Teniposide

Synonyms Vumon, ETP, VM-26, Vehem-Sandoz, NSC-122819, 4'-Demethy-lepipodophyllotoxin-β-D-thenylidene glucoside.

Chemical Structure

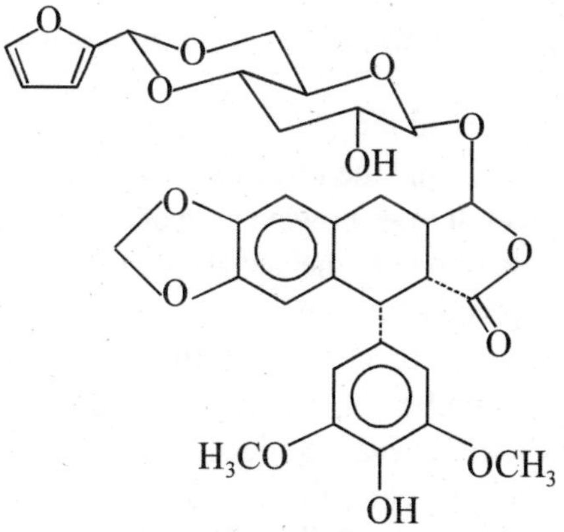

Teniposide

Characterstic Features The characteristics features of the semi-synthetic derivative of podophyllotoxin are as follows the crystals obtained from absolute ethanol has mp 242-246°C. $[\alpha]_D^{20}$- 107° (in 9 : 1 chloroform/methanol), pKa 10.13 and uv_{max} (in methanol): 283 nm ($E_{1cm}^{1\%}$ 64.1).

It differs from **etoposide** in the following respects:

(*i*) It has an additional thenylidene ring on the glucopyranoside ring.
(*ii*) Its pKa value is higher than that of **etoposide.**

Uses It is used as component of multiple-drug antineoplastic regimens for induction therapy in childhood acute lymphoblastic leukemia that is refractory to induction with other therapy.

(*ii*) **Flavonoids:** Interestingly, the *second* important class of the **biphenylpropanoid derivatives** is known as the **Flavonoids.** In general, **flavonoids** are amongst the most abundantly distributed natural product compounds from the medicinal herbs having an enormous range of more than 2000 different compounds reported to be present either in the *free state* or as the *glycosides*. However, the **'flavonoid glycosides'** have been described explicitly under Section 4.2.4 of Chapter 4 on **'Glycosides'.**

Mixed Biogensis in Flavonoids **Flavonoids,** the aromatic compounds occurring in plants are usually biosynthesized by *three* different routes namely: (*a*) **acetate-malonate pathway;** (*b*) **acetate-mevalonate pathway;** and (*c*) **shikimic acid pathway.** Flavonoids have a mixed biogenesis, as evidenced by the fact that they are obtained from products of two or more of the main pathway.

The **flavonoid** and **isoflavonoid** ring structures are of mixed biosynthetic origin as depicted below in Fig. 6.1.

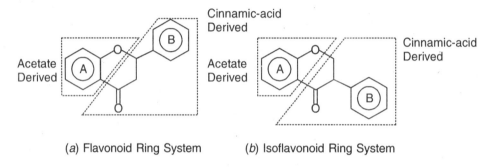

(*a*) Flavonoid Ring System   (*b*) Isoflavonoid Ring System

Fig. 6.1   Derivation of Flavonoid and Isoflavonoid Ring Systems.

From Figure 6.1, it may be observed that the ring A has been derived from *three* acetate units joined head-to-tail, whereas the ring B and the three carbon atoms of the pyran ring (*i.e.*, the central ring) are derived from cinnamic acid. It may, however, be observed that the acetate units are first and foremost get converted to CoA, wherein both the acetate-malonate and the **shikimic acid pathways** contribute to **flavonoid biosynthesis** exclusively.

Chalcones may be regarded as the precursors of all other classes of **flavonoids.** In fact, they have been isolated from a large number of plants, particularly members of the *Acanthaceae, Compositae, Gesneriaceae, Liliaceae, Oxalidaceae,* and *Scrophulariaceae,* wherein their presence can be aparently observed by their bright-yellow colouration to flower pigmentation. Fig. 6.2 represents the biogenetic relationship of the flavonoids.

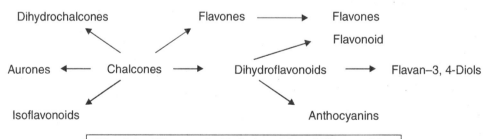

Fig. 6.2   Biogenetic Relationship of Flavonoids.

---

* Hansel et al. *Deut Apotheken Ztog.*, **108**, 198 (1968).

Silybin is the active chemical constituent belonging to the **flavonoids,** which shall be discussed in details here under:

Silybin

Synonyms   Silymarin, Apihepar, Laragon, Pluropon, Silarine, Silepan, Silirex, Silliver, Silmar.

Biological Source   **Silybin** is obtained from the seeds of milk thistle, *Silybum marianum* (L.) Gaertn. (*Carduus marianus* L.) belonging to the natural order *Asteraceae.*

Chemical Constituents   The seeds of milk thistle is chiefly comprised of *three* isomers, namely: **silidianin, silicristin** and the major component **silybin** (formerly known as **silymarin**). It has been recently characterized as a new class of substances termed as the **flavonolignans.** It has been more or less established beyond any reasonable doubt that **silybin** is produced in the plant by means of a radical **coupling of a flavonoid and coniferyl alcohol.***

Chemical Structure

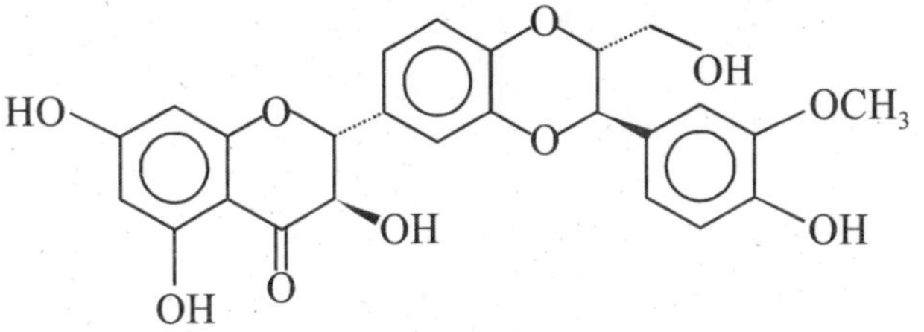

Silybin

Isolation   A crude mixture of antihepatotoxic principle was first isolated from the plant (milk thistle) and designated as **silybin**.

Characteristic Features   The anhydrous **silybin** has mp 158°C and it decomposes at 180°C. Its physical characteristics are as follows: $[\alpha]_D^{20} + 11°$ (c = 0.25 in acetone + alcohol) . Its uv$_{max}$ (in methanol): 288 nm (log ε 4.33). It is soluble in acetone, ethyl acetate, methanol, ethanol and found to be sparingly soluble in chloroform. It is practically insoluble in water. It also occurs as the monohydrate crystals from a mixture of acetone and petroleum ether having mp 167°C (decomposes at 180°C); and from a mixture of methanol and water having mp 180°C.

Uses
1. **Silybin** is most importantly and widely employed as a therapeutic agent for protecting liver cells *in situ* or cell not yet irrerersibly damaged by acting directly on the cell membranes (*i.e.* the targetted site) so as to prevent the entry of toxic substances.
2. It also augments and stimulates the 'protein synthesis' *i.e.,* anabolism of protein, thereby accelerating the process of regeneration and the production of *hepatocytes.*
3. It has also been experimentally proven that **silybin** binds specifically to a *regulative subunit of the DNA-dependent RNA polymerase I* at a particular site ley mimicking a natural steroidal effector and thereby causing an activation of this enzyme. Consequently, the synthetic rate of ribosomal RNAs is increased considerably, thus leading to an enhanced formation of intact ribosomes that ultimately gives rise to an increased protein synthesis.

---

* Wagner *et al. Arzneimittel-Forsch* **18**, 688 (1968); and **24**, 466 (1974).

4. **Silybin** may also be employed as a supportive treatment for the management and cure of chronic inflammatory liver conditions and cirrhosis.*

General Biosynthesis of Flavonoids

The general biosynthesis of **flavonoids** essentially comprises of the interaction amongst the central intermediate *para*-coumaroyl CoA and three malonyl CoA units to elongate the side chain of the initial and original **phenylpropanoid** unit. It has been observed that the closure of the ring A yields the chalcone structure, while the follow up reaction ultimately closes the ring B as shown below in Fig. 6.3.

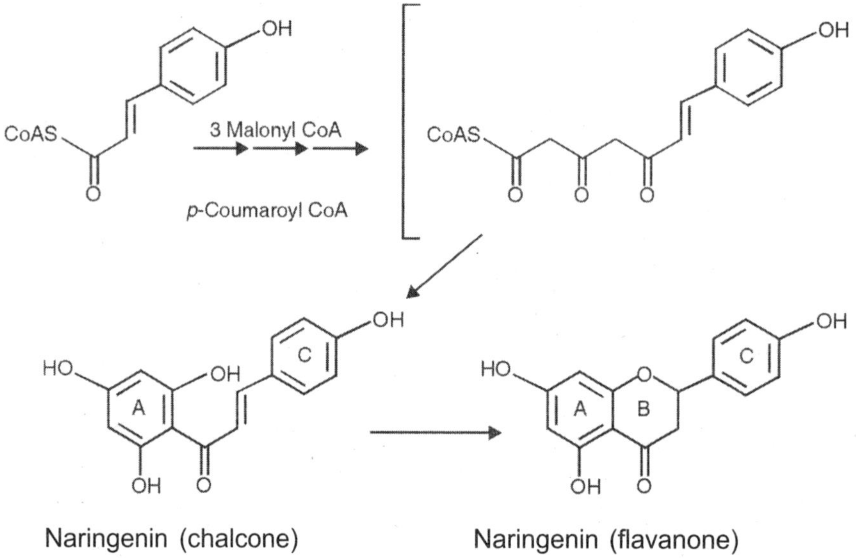

Naringenin (chalcone)   Naringenin (flavanone)

Fig. 6.3   General Flavonoid Biosynthetic Pathway

(Adapted from Robbers, J.E., *et al. Pharmacognosy and Pharmacobiotechnology*, Williams and Wilkins, London, 1996.)

6.2.6 High Molecular Weight Phenylpropanoids

Nevertheless, **phenylpropanoids**, play a vital role as building units in the formation of high-molecular weight polymers in plants. In general, these polymers are broadly classified into *two* major heads, namely:

(*i*) Lignins, and
(*ii*) Tannins

These two different categories of a **high-molecular weight phenylpropanoids** shall be discussed in details as under.

---

* It is marketed in the form of capsules which contains a concentrated extract equivalent to 140 mg of **silybin.**

6.2.6.1 Lignins

Lignins are the most abundant natural aromatic organic polymers found in virtually all vascular plants. It has been observed that the lignins together with cellulose, *q.v.*, and hemicellulose, *q.v.*, are the major cell wall components of the fibers of all *wood* and *grass* species in the plant kingdom. In fact, the **lignins** are sequestered in the secondary layer of the cell wall in close association with the cellulose matrix wherein the *phenolic hydroxy moieties* present in the lignins may be either hydrogen bonded or covalently attached to hemicellulose. **Lignin** is considered to be a sole factor in the contribution towards the strengthening of the cell-wall, and consequently for its synthesis. It is further regarded as a decisive factor in the adaptation of plants to a terrestrial habit in the process of evolution. It could only be possible by virtue of the fact that the lignified cell walls help to build the rigid and strong stems of the woody plants and the tress in general.

Composition   **Lignin** is usually composed of coniferyl, *p*-coumaryl and sinapyl alcohols in varying proportion in a variety of plant species.

Uses
1. It is used as a source of vanillin, syringic aldehyde and dimethyl sulphoxide.
2. It is also employed as an extender for phenolic plastics.
3. It is used to strengthen rubber for shoe-soles.
4. It is used as an oil mud additive.
5. It also finds it application as a stablizer for asphalt emulsions.
6. It is employed to precipitate proteins.

6.2.6.2 Tannins

Synonyms   Tannic Acid; Gallotannin; Gallotannic acid; *Acidum tannicum*.

Biological Sources   **Tannic acid** usually occurs in the bark and fruit of a large number of plants, such as: roots of *Cimicifuga racemosa* (L.) Nutt. (*Ranunculaceae*)-**Black Cohosch, Black Snakeroot;** dried beans of *Coffea arabica* L. (*Rubiaceae*)-**Arabica Coffee, Arabian Coffee, Abyssinian Coffee;** barks of *Carnus florida* L. (*Cornaceae*)-**Dogwood, American Boxwood;** fresh forage (fodder) of *Equisetium arrense* L. (*Equisetaceae*)-**Field Horsetail;** leaves of *Eupatorium perfoliatum* L. (*Asteraceae*)-**Boneset, Ague Wood;** seeds of *Frangula alnus* Mill. (*Rhamnaceae*)-**Buckthorn;** roots of *Glycyrrhiza glabra* L. (*Fabaceae*)-**Common Licorice, Licorice Root, Spanish Licorice Root;** roots of *Paeonia officinals* L. (*Ranunculaceae*)-Peony; leaves of *Pilacarpus spp.* (*Rutaceae*)-**Jaborandi;** weeds of *Polygonum aviculare* L. (*Polygonaceae*)-**Prostrate Knotweed;** juice of the plant of *Rhamnus purshianus* DC. (*Rhamnaceae*)-**Cascara Sagrada, Cascara buckthorn;** flowers of *Tussilago farfara* L. (*Asteraceae*) **Coltsfoot, Coughwort, Horse-Hoof;** and plants of *Verbena officinalis* L. (*Verbenaceae*)-**Vervain, Verbena.**

Preparation   **Tannic acid** is produced from Turkish or Chinese Nutgall usually formed by an aphis, *Schlechtendalia chinensis* found on the trees of *Rhus chinensis* belonging to family *Anacardiaceae*.

It may also be obtained by extraction from specially fermented oak **galls*** that are normally

---

* **Galls:** These are formed by virtue of the deposition of eggs by *gall-wasp viz., Adleria gallaetinctorial*.

grown on the young and tender twigs of *Quercus infectoria* (Oak Tree), belonging to the natural order *Fagaceae*.

Chemical Structure

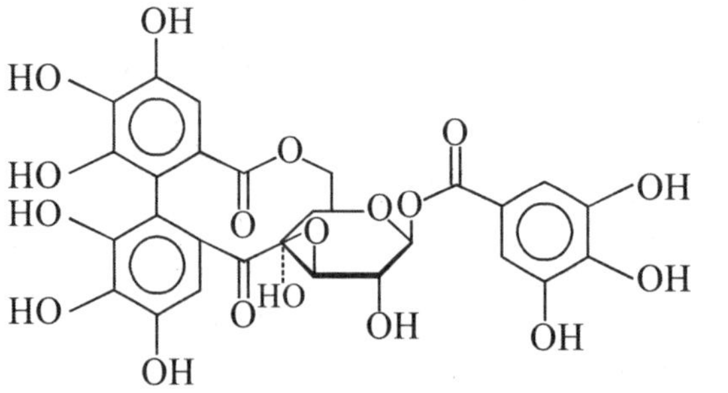

Corilagin
(A Tannic Acid)

Characteristics Features   **Tannic acid** is a yellowish-white to light brown, amorphous bulky powder or flakes, or spongy masses. It has a faint characteristic odour with a distinct astringent taste. It has a tendency to darken gradually on being exposed to air and light. It decomposes at 210-215°C mostly into pyrogallol and CO_2. It is highly soluble in water (1 g in 0.35 ml of water), 1 g in 1 ml of warm glycerol, and very soluble in acetone and ethanol. It is practically insoluble in chloroform, benzene, ether, petroleum ether, carbon disulphide and carbon tetrachloride.

Identification Tests

1. **Tannic acid,** when heated to 210-215°C, gets decomposed to yield **pyrogallol** and CO_2. The evolution of CO_2 may be confirmed when it turns freshly prepared lime-water milky.

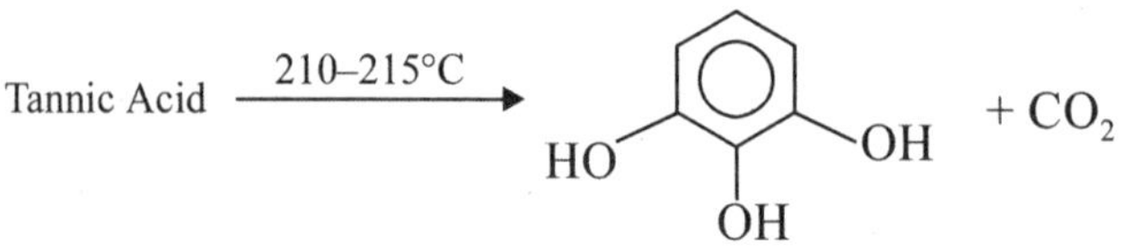

Pyrogallol

2. It instantly gives rise to insoluble precipitates with albumin, starch, gelatin and a host of alkaloidal and metallic salts.
3. It readily forms a bluish-black colour or precipitate with ferric salts *e.g.*, $FeCl_3$.

Storage   **Tannic acid** must be kept in well closed and protected from light containers.

Uses

1. Tannic acid with ferric salts are invariably used in the manufacture of inks.
2. It is used for tanning *i.e.*, making leather from hides of cow, goat, sheep and buffalo skin.
3. It is employed as a *pharmaceutical aid* due to its astringent and antiseptic actions.
4. It is used as a mordant in dyeing.
5. It is employed for sizing paper and silk.

6. It is also used for printing fabrics.

7. It finds its application to make imitation horn and tortoise shell when mixed with gelatin and albumin.

8. It is invariably employed to clarify beer and wine.

9. It is also used in 'photography'.

10. It is employed as a coagulant in the manufacture of rubber.

11. It is used in the large scale production of **gallic acid** and **pyrogallol**.

12. It is employed as a reagent in **'analytical chemistry'**.

6.3   BIOSYNTHESIS OF PHENYLPROPANOIDS

It has been observed that there are **two major precursors** for the **biosynthesis of phenylpropanoids,** namely: (*a*) **cinnamic acid,** and (*b*) **p-hydroxy-cinnamic acid (or p-coumaric acid).** However, in plants these two chemical compounds are exclusively produced from the two aromatic amino acids phenylalanine and tyrosine, respectively, which are subsequently synthesised *via* the **Shikimic Acid Pathway** as depicted in Fig. 6.4.

Salient Features   The salient features of the **biosynthesis of phenylpropanoids** *via* the **shikimic acid pathway** are enumerated below:

1. The biosynthetic pathway has been described explicitly in microorganisms by employing **auxotropic mutants** of *Escherichia coli* and *Enterobacter aerogenes* which essentially require the aromatic amino acids for their normal growth.

2. Two *glucose metabolites*, namely: *erythrose 4-phosphate* and *phosphoenolpyruvate*, are found to react to give rise to a phosphorylated 7-carbon keto sugar, called 3-deoxy D-arabinoheptulosonic acid 7 phosphate (DAHP).

3. DAHP gets cyclized to 3-dehydroquinic acid, which is subsequently converted to **shikimic acid**.

4. The resulting **shikimic acid**, *via* a series of phosphorylated intermediates, gives rise to *chorismic acid*, which represents a vital branch-point-intermediate.

5. One of the branches leads to the formation of anthranilic acid and finally to tryptophan (an aromatic amino acid).

6. The second branch leads to the production of **prephenic acid**, which represents the last non-aromatic compound in the sequence.

7. **Periphenic acid** may be aromatized in *two* different manners, namely:
   (*a*) First proceeds by dehydration and simultaneous decarboxylation to produce **phenylpyruvic acid,** which is the direct precursor of phenylalanine.
   (*b*) Second takes place by dehydrogenation and decarboxylation to produce *p*-**hydroxy-phenylpyruvic acid,** which is the precursor of tyrosine.

8. **Cinnamic acid,** the phenylpropanoid precursor, is produced by the direct enzymatic deamination of phenylalanine.

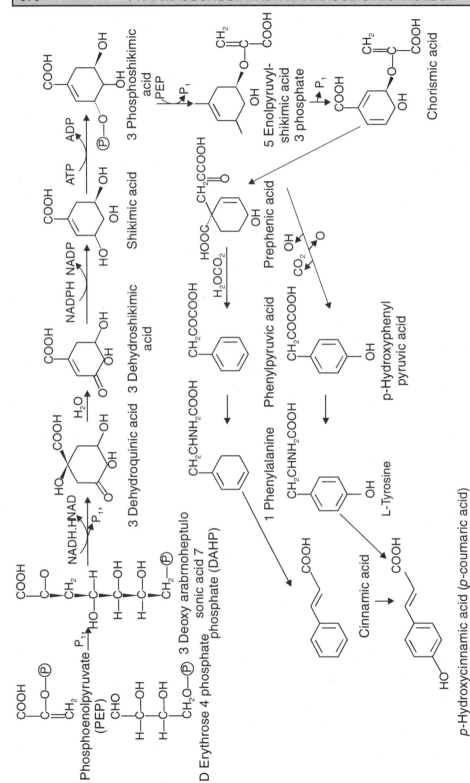

Fig. 6.4 Biosynthesis of Phenylpropanoids via the Shikimic Acid Pathway (Adapted from Rebbers, J.E. et al. Pharmacognosy and Pharmacobiotechnology, Williams & Wilkins, London, 1996.)

9. *para*-**Coumaric acid** may be obtained in two different ways, namely:

(*a*) By hydroxylation of cinnamic acid at the *para*-position, and

(*b*) By an analogous manner from tyrosine.

FURTHER READING REFERENCES

1. Canel C. *et al.*: **Molecules of Interest: Podophyllotoxin,** *Phytochemistry,* **54:** 115-120, 2000.

2. Cheeke, P.R., (ed.): **Toxicants of Plant Origin,** Vol. IV, Bica Raton, Florida, CRC Press Inc., 1989.

3. Davin L.B. and Lewis N.G.: **Dirigent Proteins and Dirigent Sites Explain the Mystery of Specificity of Radical Precursor Coupling in Lignan and Lignin Biosynthesis,** *Plant Physiol,* **123:** 453-461, 2000.

4. Forkmann G. and Heller W.: **Biosynthesis of Flavonoids,** *Comprehensive Natural Product Chemistry,* Vol. 1, Elsevier, Amsterdam, pp. 713-748, 1999.

5. Hahlbrock, K., School, D.: **Physiology and Molecular Biology of Phenylpropanoid Metabolism,** *Annu. Rev. Plant Physiol. Plant Mol. Biol.,* **40:** 347, 1989.

6. Haslam, E.: **Plant Polyhenols: Vegetable Tannins Revisited.** Combridge, Great Britain, Combridge University Press, 1989.

7. Harborne, J.B., Mobry, T.J. (eds.): **The Flavonoids: Advances in Research Since 1980,** Chapman and Hill, Ltd., London, 1988.

8. Harborne J.B. and Williams C.A.: **Advances in Flavonoid Research Since 1992,** *Phytochemistry,* **55:** 481-504, 2000.

9. Hemingway, R.W., Lake, P.E., (eds.): **Plant Polyphenols: Synthesis Properties, Significance,** Plenium Press, New York, 1992.

10. Lewis, N.G., Davin, L.B., **Evolution of Lignan and Neolignan Biochemical Pathways: In: Isopentenoids and other Natural Products: Evolution and Function,** Nes, W.D., (ed.) American Chemical Society, Washington, D.C., 1994.

11. Lewis N.G. and Davis L.B.: **Lignans: Biosynthesis and Function,** *Comprehensive Natural Products Chemistry,* Vol. 1, Elsevier, Amsterdam, pp. 639-712, 1999.

12. Matern U. *et al.*: **Biosynthesis of Coumarins, Comprehensive Natural Products Chemistry.** Vol. 1, Elsevier, Amsterdam, pp. 623-637, 1999.

13. Murray, R.D.H., Mendez, J., Brown, S.A, **The Natural Coumarins.** John Wiley & Sons Ltd., Chichester, England, 1982.

14. Stafford, H.A., Ibrahim, R.K. (eds.): **Recent Advances in Phytochemistry,** Vol. 26, **Phenolic Metabolism in Plants,** Plenium Press, New York, 1992.

7 Alkaloids

- Introduction
- Classification of Alkaloids
- Alkaloids in Tissue Cultures
- Alkaloids in Chemosystematics
- Further Reading References

7.1 INTRODUCTION

The term **alkaloids** (or alkali-like) was first and foremost proposed by the pharmacist, W. Meissner, in 1819, for the basic nitrogen-containing compounds of plant origin.

Ladenburg defined **alkaloids,—'as naturally occurring plant compounds having a basic character and containing at least one nitrogen in a heterocyclic ring.'**

With the advent of recent advanced knowledge in the chemistry of various alkaloids *two* more inevitable characteristic features were logically and justifiably added to the definition of **alkaloids,** namely:

(*a*) Complex molecular structure, and
(*b*) Significant pharmacological activity.

Furthermore, it was broadly observed that the basic properties of the **alkaloids** is solely by virtue of the presence of N-atom embedded into the *five*-or *six*- membered ring.

Therefore, the **alkaloids** are now generally defined as,—**'physiologically active basic compounds of plant origin, in which at least one nitrogen atom forms part of a cyclic system.'**

Even this definition has a few anomalies as stated below, namely:

(*i*) **Cholines and Betaines:** These two substances have the N-atom in the side chain and not in the aromatic ring as shown below:

$HOCH_2CH_2N^+(CH_3)_3$ — Choline

$(CH_3)3N^+CH_2-COO^-$ — Betaine

The **cholines** and **betaines** are regarded as simple alkylamines and not classified as **alkaloids.** They are designated by some school of thoughts as **'biological-amines'** or **'proto-alkaloids'**.

(*ii*) **Ephedrine:** It has the N-atom only in the side chain and not embedded in the aromatic ring as given below:

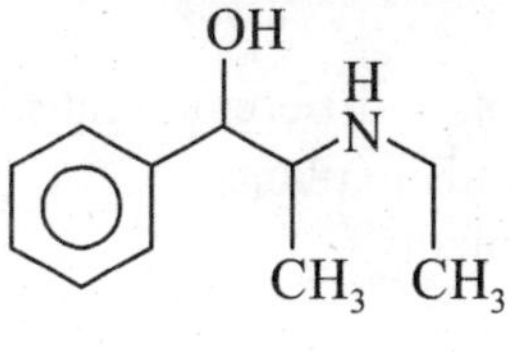

Ephedrine

(*iii*) **Piperidine:** It is obtained *Piper nigrum* (**Black Pepper**) and does not possess any pharmacological activity, but has a N-atom in a heterocyclic ring as given below:

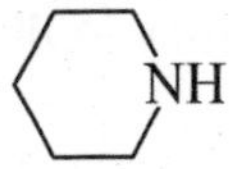

Piperidine

(*iv*) **Colchicine:** It is found to be neither basic nor it contains the N-atom in a heterocyclic ring, whereas it is considered as an alkaloid due to the fact it possesses distinct pharmacological activity as shown below:

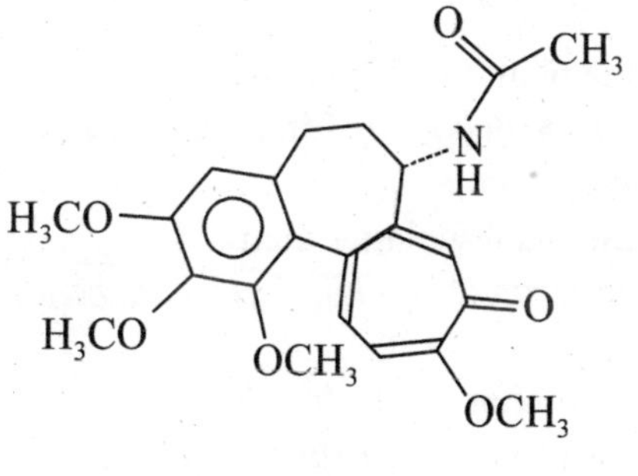

Colchicine

(*v*) **Thiamine (Vitamin B$_1$):** It confines to the definition of **alkaloids** but is not regarded as an 'alkaloid' because of its almost universal distribution in living matter.

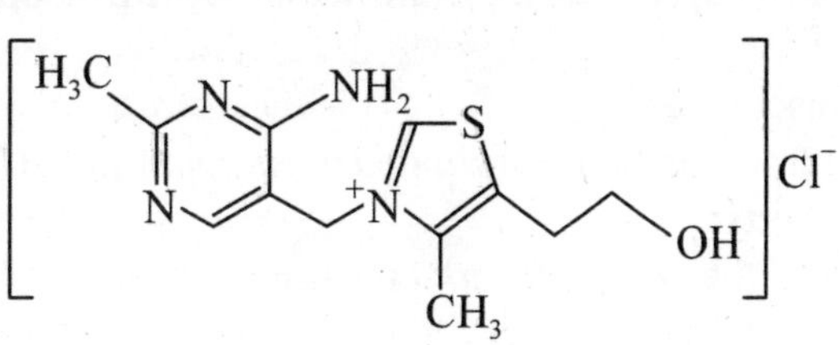

Thiamine Monochloride

Interestingly, **alkaloids** represent one of the most important group of chemical constituents occurring in the entire plant kingdom which exert extremely potent and vital physiological and pharmacological activities in the human beings. Therefore, it will be worthwhile to study the **alkaloids** with regard to the following aspects, namely:

(*i*) Nomenclature

(*ii*) Occurrence and distribution in different organs of the plant

(*iii*) Site of formation of alkaloids in plants

(*iv*) Functions of alkaloids in plants

(*v*) Isomerism

(*vi*) General characteristic features of alkaloids:

    (*a*) Physical characteristics

    (*b*) Chemical characteristics

(*vii*) General methods of extraction and isolation of alkaloids.

These various aspects of **alkaloids** shall now be discussed adequately in a sequential manner so as to have a better in-depth of knowledge.

7.1.1   Nomenclature

The major characteristic of the nomenclature of **alkaloids** is the lack of any agreed systematic prevailing system. Therefore, by a general agreement, the chemical rules designate that the names of all alkaloids must end with the *suffix* (*–ine*). The latin names end with (*–ina*). Thus, the names of the **alkaloids** are usually obtained in a number of ways, namely:

(*a*) From the *generic name* of the plant producing them:

    Examples: Atropine from *Atropa belladona* Linn., (*Solanaceae*); and **Hydrastine** from *Hydrastis canadenisis* L. (*Ranunculaceae*).

(*b*) From the specific name of the plant yielding them:

    Examples: Belladonine from *Atropa belladona* L. (*Solanaceae*); and **Cocaine** from *Erythroxylum coca* Lam. (*Erythroxylaceae*).

(*c*) From the common name of the drug producing them:

    Example: Ergotamine from *Claviceps purpurea* (Er.) Tul. (*Hypocreales*) commonly known as **ergot.**

(*d*) From their specific physiological activity:

    Examples: Emetine from *Hedera helix* L. (*Araliaceae*) called **Ivy; Narcotine** from *Papaver somniferum* L. (*Papaveraceae*) known as **Opium Poppy;** and **Morphine** from *P. somniferum* L.

(*e*) From the name of the discoverer:

    Example: Pelletierine from the barks of *Puniea granatum* Linn., (*Punicaceae*).

(*f*) From their physical property:

    Example: Hygrine from the roots of *Withania somniferum* (L.) Dunal (*Solanaceae*) called **Ashwagandha** (Hygro = moist).

7.1.2   Occurrence and Distribution in Different Organ's of Plant

McKee* (1962) reported that about 1000 **alkaloids,** which are known, belong to almost 100 families, 500 genera and spread over 1200 species. However, it has been observed beyond reasonable doubt

---

* Mckee, H.S., *Nitrogen Metabolism in Plants*, (1962).

that the **alkaloids** are not evenly distributed amongst the plant kingdom. They have been found to be absent in *Algae* and in the lower groups of plants with the exception of one or two families of the fungi. The glaring examples of fungal alkaloids include those of ergot alkaloids.

The seeds of **papaya**, *Carica papaya* L. (*Caricaceae*), yield 660 to 760 mg BITC which is a bactericidal aglycone of **glucotropaeolin benzyl isothiocyanate.**

However, in the plant kingdom, the alkaloids generally, seem to get confined to a certain families and genera with regard to their distribution. For instance, amongst the angiosperms the families which have been recognized as outstanding for alkaloidal-yielding plants are, namely: *Apocynaceae*, *Berberidaceae*, *Papaveraceae*, *Ranunculaceae*, *Rubiaceae* and *Solanaceae*.

Monocotyledons, generally do not produce alkaloids, but investigation have revealed that *two* of the most promising families *viz.*, *Amaryllidaceae* and *Liliaceae* do contain alkaloid-containing plants.

Dicotyledons, mostly contain the **alkaloids.** It has been observed that neither *Labiatae* nor *Rosaceae* contain any alkaloid. Furthermore, almost 15% of all vascular plants contain alkaloids.

Alkaloids may occur in various parts of the plant. It may, however, be pointed out that in a particular species, normally only one or two specific organs and not all organs, essentially afford the function of alkaloidal formation. For instance, the **alkaloids** of the **tobacco plant**, *Nicotiana tabacum* Linn., (*Solanaceae*), are produced in the root and are subsequently translocated to the leaves where they usually accumulate, whereas the seeds are completely devoid of alkaloid. In another glaring example the **opium poppy**, *Papaver somniferum*, the alkaloids solely occur in the fresh latex of the fruit, while the seeds of poppy are virtually devoid of alkaloids. Likewise, the **colchicum*** corm. *Colchicum autumnale* Linn. (*Liliaceae*), the alkaloids are found both in the seed and in the corm. Interestingly, the bark of cinchona tree, *Cinchona officinalis* Linn., (*Rubiaceae*) contain the alkaloids (*viz.*, **quinine**) exclusively.

In some instances, there are noticeable fluctuations in the alkaloidal content in various organs of the plant during the different stages of its growth, during different seasons, and lastly between day and night. In certain perennials, the localization and accumulation of the alkaloids in one or two particular organs, appears to be more marked and pronounced with the advancement in the age of the plant.

In a broader sense, the particular **alkaloids** of complex structures are normally confined to specific plant families, such as: **hyoscyamine** in *Solanaceae*; and **colchicine** in *Liliaceae*. More importantly, a specific family may also contain several structurally non-related alkaloids *i.e.*, the basic-structure of alkaloids are altogether different, as examplified under.

Salts of Alkaloids   It has been found that a plethora of **alkaloids** occurring in various plant species are in the form of salts of organic acids, such as: acetic acid, malic acid, oxalic acid, succinic acid, tartaric acid, tannic acid or some other specific plant acids. In certain instances, the **alkaloids** are found to be in combination with **special plant acids,** for examples:

---

* **Colchicum:** It is derived from *Colchiss*, a port on the Black Sea where the plant was first found to be growing.

Family	Common Name	Botanical Name	Chemical Structure
Solanaceae	**Nicotine**	*Nicotiana tabacum*, or *N.rustica*	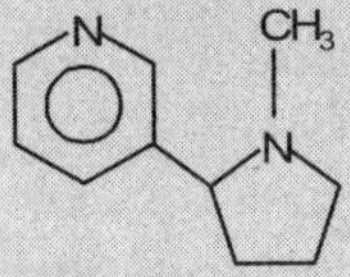
	Hyoscyamine	*Hyoscya mus niger* L.; *Atropa belladona* L.; *Datura Stramonium* L.,	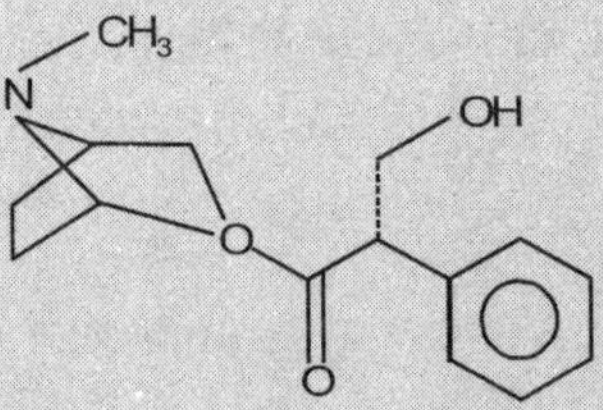
	Solanine	*Solanum tuberosum* L., (potato); *S. nigrum* L., *Lycopersicon eseulentum* Mill. (tomato)	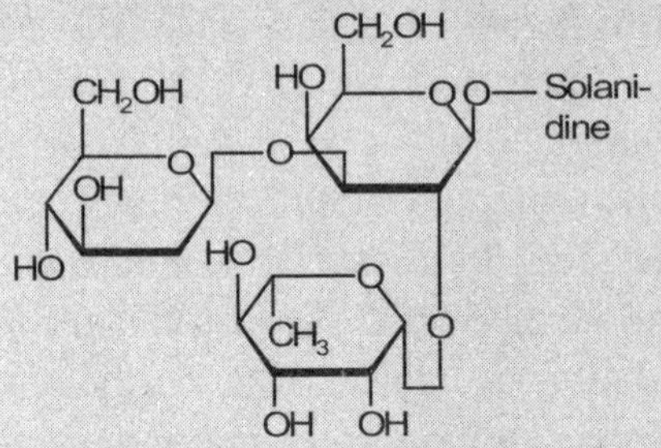
	Capsaicin	*Capsicum annum* Linn, var (Chillies)	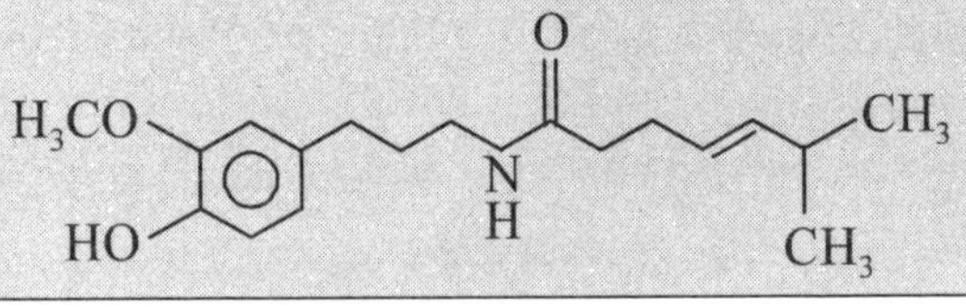

Aconitine   associated with

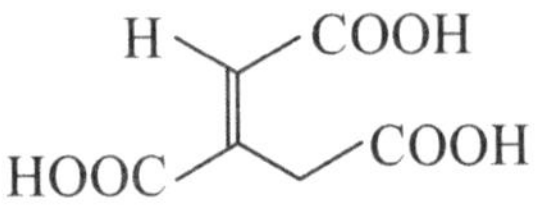

trans–Aconitic acid

Morphine   associated with

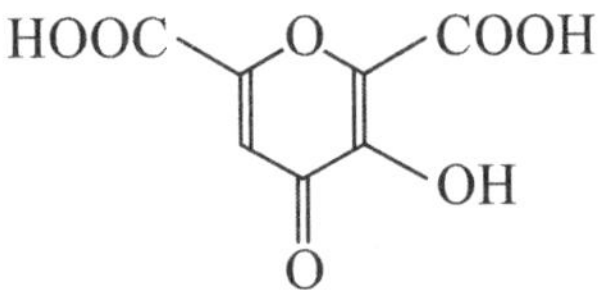

Meconic acid

Quinine   associated with

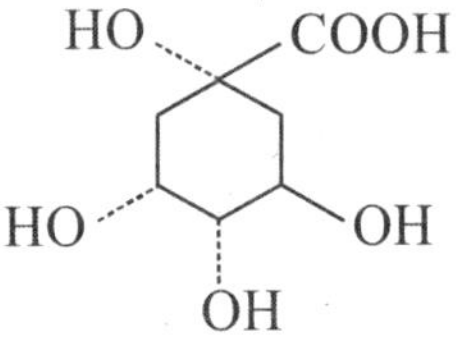

Quinic acid

Chelidonine   associated with

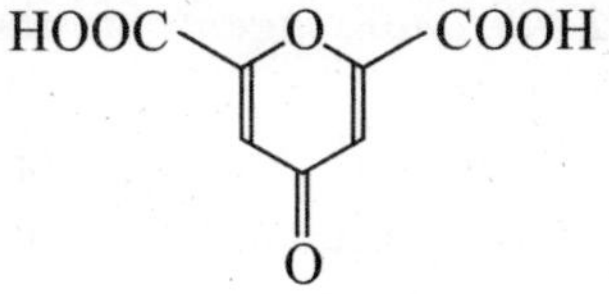

Chelidonic acid

Rarely, alkaloidal salts with inorganic acids may also be present in plant products, such as: **morphine** sulphate in **opium poppy.**

Gluco-Alkaloids   A few typical **alkaloids** are found in glycosidal combination with sugar moieties there by yielding the **gluco-alkaloids.**

Example: Solanidine (aglycone) obtained from the hydrolysis of the toxic glycoside **solanine** found in sprouts of potato tubers as given below:

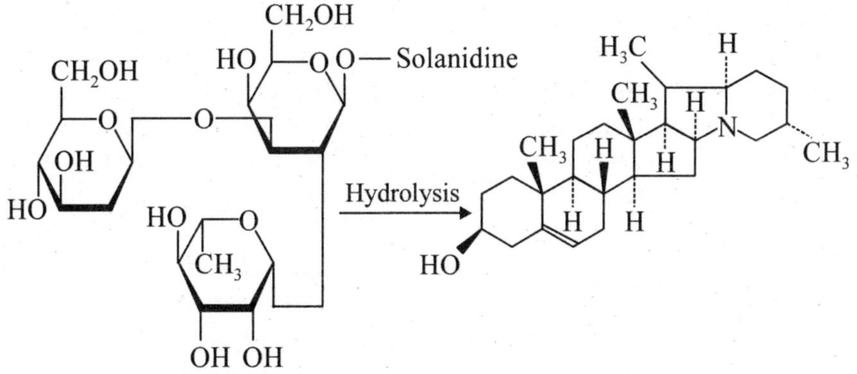

Solanine
(Gluco-Alkaloid)

Solanidine
(Alkaloid)

7.1.3 Site of Formation of Alkaloids in Plants

The naturally occurring **alkaloids** that are found to be present in particular organs or parts of a specific plant, it does not logically suggest that they are either synthesized or formed in those particular organs. It may be further expatiated by the typical example of the **alkaloids** found in several **Datura** species and **Nicotiana** species, already discussed earlier, are invariably formed in the roots, but are rapidly translocated to the leaves. This glaring fact has been legitimately and explicitly demonstrated by the help of various experimental techniques innovated by researchers, namely: grafting techniques, labelling with radio-isotopes. Consequently, the leaves of such medicinal herbs, where the alkaloids usually get accumulated, is the ideal and vital part (organ) to be used for the subsequent extraction and isolation of relatively appreciable quantities of the alkaloids.

7.1.4 Function of Alkaloids in Plants

A good number of logical explanations, theories and principles have been put forward with regard to the possible function of **alkaloids** in plants or the probable reasons why they are present in them. It would be worthwhile to have a closer look and perhaps a better insight about certain possibilities that have gained cognizance over the years are described below along with their functions, namely:

(*a*) As strategically located *poisonous agents* in plants thereby protecting them either against herbivorous animals or insects,

(*b*) As probable by-products of various detoxification reactions representing a metabolic locking-up of compounds, otherwise harmful or detrimental to the plant,

(*c*) As pronounced regulatory growth factors, and

(*d*) As reserve substances in plant capable of supplying nitrogen or other necessary elements to its economy.

7.1.5 Isomerism

Generally, **isomerization** is the process of involving the change of one structure into another having the same emperical formula but with different properties in one or more respects.

A plethora of **alkaloids** contain one or more asymmetric carbon atoms in the molecule, and hence exhibit **optical activity**. It has been observed that in the majority of instances only the (–)-isomer (*i.e.*, the *levorotatory* component) has appreciable and distinct pharmacological activity than the corresponding (+)-isomer (*i.e.*, the *dextrorotatory*, component) of the same alkaloidal species.

At this juncture, one needs to understand clearly the traditional designations *l*- and *d*- for the *levo*- and *dextro*- rotatory isomers respectively; and these are to distinguished from the designations L- and D- which refer not to the *optical activity*, but to the *steric configuration* with regard to a conventionally accepted reference compound.

In fact, the optical activity is invariably associated with the **alkaloids** and their respective salts. However, the optical activity and the specific rotation usually varies with the solvent used, the temperature, the wave length of light and other minor factors.

There are quite a few typical and glaring examples that may serve to illustrate the considerable difference in the pharmacological activity observed amongst the different isomers of an **alkaloid.**

Examples

(*a*) Showing *d*- and *l*-isomers with distinct pharmacological activities, such as:

(*i*) **Relative pressor activities* of D(–)-ephedrine and D(+) ephedrine:** The relative pressor activities of **D(–)-ephedrine** is found to be 36 with regard to its **D(+)-ephedrine** isomer at ll *i.e.*, the former is almost 3½ times more active than the latter as shown below:

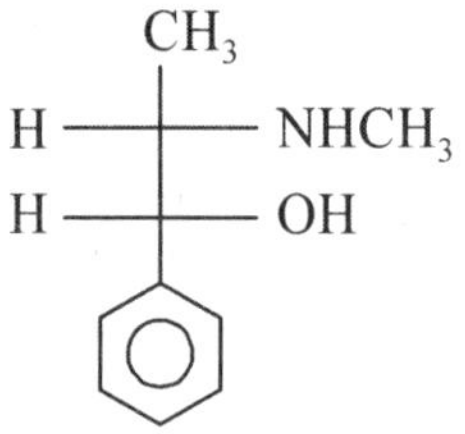

D (–)-Ephedrine
(Relative pressure
activity = 36)

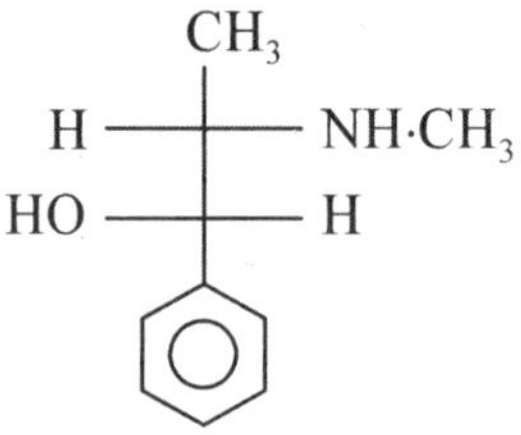

D (+)-Ephedrine
(Relative pressure
activity = 11)

---

* Increase of arterial blood-pressure.

(*ii*) **Antimigraine activity of (–)-ergotamine and (+)-ergotamine:** It has been observed that the antimigraine activity of **(–)-ergotamine** possesses 3-4 times more activity than its corresponding (+)-ergotamine isomer:

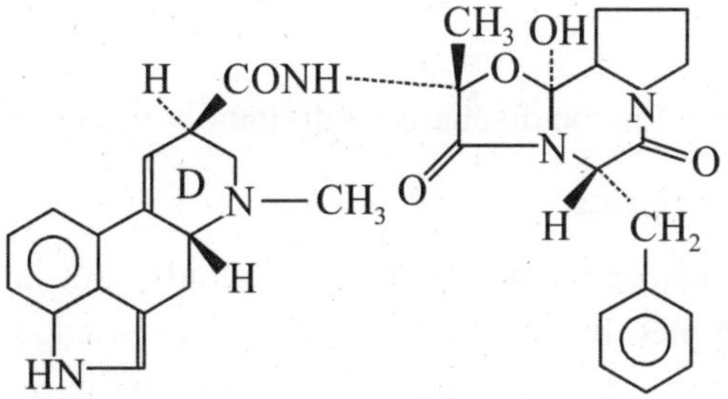

(–)-Ergotamine

(*b*) **Showing both (–)-and (+)-forms active pharmacologically:** In certain alkaloids, the (–) form as well as the (+) form are medicinally useful. **Examples:** The (–)-Quinine is primarily employed as a potent antimalarial agent; whereas the (+)-Quinine, also known as **quinidine**, is solely used in restoring cardiac arrythmia to normal rythm, as given below:

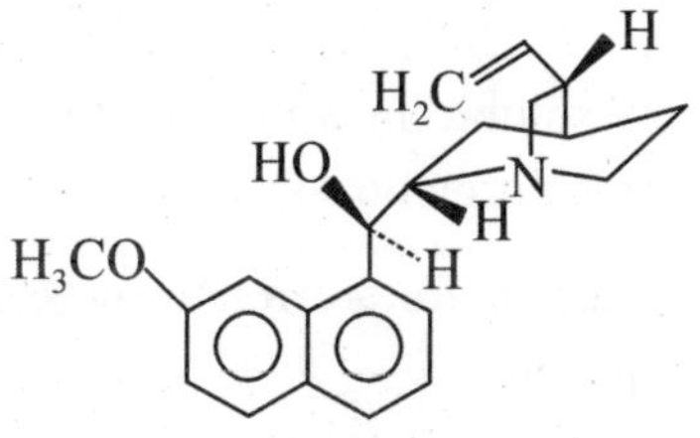

(–)–Quinine

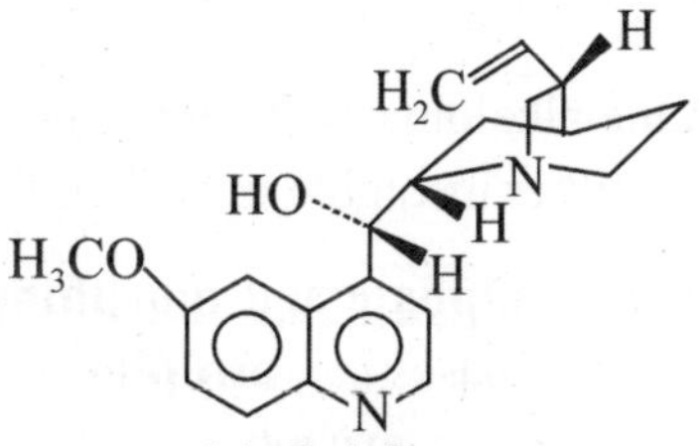

(–)–Quinine
(Quinidine)

(*c*) **Exception:** The (+) (+)–*d*-tubocurarine of *d*-tubocurarine is the only isomer that exhibits muscle relaxant properties, as shown below:

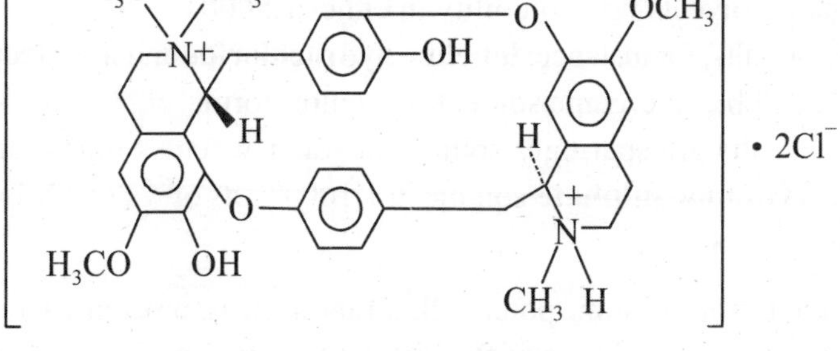

(+)–d-Tubocurarine Chloride

7.1.6　General Characteristics of Alkaloids

The general characteristics of **alkaloids** may be grouped together in *two* categories, namely:

(*a*) Physical characteristics, and

(*b*) Chemical characteristics.

These *two* categories shall now be discussed individually in the sections that follows:

7.1.6.1　Physical Characteristics

First and foremost, let us consider the solubility of alkaloids both in water and organic solvents along with some typical examples. In fact, a comprehensive knowledge of the solubility of complete range of alkaloids and their corresponding salts is of utmost pharmaceutical importance because of their extremely specific and potent pharmacological actions.

It is pertinent to mention here that in general the solubilities of different alkaloids and their respective salts usually exhibit considerable variation, which may be attributed from their extremely complex and varied chemical structures. However, it has been observed that the free alkaloid bases as such are invariably found to be fairly soluble in organic solvents, such as: either, chloroform, relatively non-polar solvents (hexane, benzene, petroleum ether), immiscible solvent, lower alcohols (methanol, ethanol); but they are either practically insoluble or very sparingly soluble in water.

Interestingly, the alkaloidal salts are almost freely soluble in water, relatively less soluble in alcohol and mostly either insoluble or sparingly soluble in organic solvents:

Examples　Atropine sulphate and **morphine hydrochloride** are much more soluble in water than their corresponding bases *i.e.*, **atropine** and **morphine.**

However, there are a few exceptions to the above stated generalizations, namely:

(*i*)　Certain **alkaloid** bases are water soluble, but these may be solely regarded as exceptions rather than any specific rule, such as: **ephedrine, colchicine, pilocarpine;** the **quaternary alkaloid-base** like **berberine** and **tubocurarine; caffeine-base** readily extracted from tea with water.

(*ii*)　**Narceine** and **pilocarpine** are insoluble in organic solvents, whereas morphine is sparingly soluble in organic solvents *viz.*, solubility in either 1:5000.

(*iii*)　Certain alkaloidal salts, for instance: **lobeline hydrochloride** and **apoatropine hydrochloride** are found to be soluble in organic solvent like chloroform.

(*iv*)　Some alkaloidal salts are sparingly soluble in water whereas others are extremely water-soluble, such as: **Quinine sulphate**-soluble in 1:1000 parts of water, **Quinine hydrochloride**-soluble in 1:1 part of water.

The physical characteristics of some potent **alkaloids,** such as: mp, optical rotation and solubility are enlisted below so as to have a glimps of the distinct variation in the observed parameters:

S.No.	Alkaloid	mp (°C)	Optical rotation	Solubility
1.	Ajmaline	150-160	$[\alpha]_D^{20} + 144°$	Chloroform, ether, ethanol, methanol
2.	Atropine	144-116	–	Benzene, chloroform, ether
3.	Berberine	145	–	Water
4.	Colchicine	142-150	$[\alpha]_D^{17} - 429°$	Water, chloroform, ethanol
5.	Ephedrine	79	–	Water, ethanol, ether, chloroform, oils
6.	Hyoscyamine	108.5	$[\alpha]_D^{20} - 21.0°$	Ethanol, dilute acids
7.	Morphine	197	$[\alpha]_D^{25} - 132°$	Sparingly soluble in ethanol, chloroform, amyl alcohol,
8.	Physostigmine	105-106	$[\alpha]_D^{25} - 120°$	Benzene, chloroform, oils
9.	Quinine	177	$[\alpha]_D^{17} - 117°$	Chloroform, ether
10.	Reserpine	264-265 (dec.)	$[\alpha]_D^{23} - 118°$	Chloroform, ethyl acetate, benzene.
11.	Strychnine	275-285	$[\alpha]_D^{18} - 104.3°$	Chloroform, methanol, benzene
12.	Taxol	213-216 (dec.)	$[\alpha]_D^{20} - 49°$	Methanol
13.	Vinblastine	211-216	$[\alpha]_D^{20} + 42°$	Chloroform, ethanol
14.	Yohimbine	234	$[\alpha]_D^{20} + 108°$	Chloroform, ethanol, benzene

7.1.6.2 Chemical Characteristics

The general chemical characteristics of the **alkaloids** are so broadly spread out, therefore, they shall be treated individually under the following heads, namely.

[A] N-in the Molecule Besides, the other normal elements *e.g.*, carbon, hydrogen, oxygen, the alkaloids must essentially contain at least one N-atom. The number of N-atoms vary from the bear minimum one in a molecule *e.g.*, **cocaine**, to even five in a molecule *e.g.*, **ergotamine**. It has been observed that these N-atoms are normally present as a part of the **heterocyclic ring** in the alkaloid molecule *e.g.*, **quinine, reserpine, strychnine, vinblastine** and **yohimbine;** whereas there are certain alkaloids that contain the N-atom in the aliphatic side chain *e.g.*, **ephedrine, mescaline.**

Invariably, the alkaloids contain the N-atom in the **tertiary-amine form** (R_3N) *e.g.*, **morphine, reserpine;** lesser in the **secondary-amine form** (R_2NH) *e.g.*, **ephedrine;** and very rarely in the **primary-amine form** (RNH_2) *e.g.*, **nor-pseudo-ephedrine.** Furthermore, whenever N-atom occurs either in the *tertiary-* or *secondary-*form, it essentially constitutes as an integral part of the ring-system, precisely the heterocyclic ring system.

Noticeably, the tertiary N-atoms wherein only two of the bonds are involved in a ring, the methyl moiety is usually found as the third component, for instance: N-methyl group in **morphine, cocaine, colchicine, dextro methorphan, codeine, physostigmine, vinblastine, vindesine** etc.

Hence, methyl moiety seems to be the only **alkyl group** that has been found to be substituted on the **N-atom.**

However, in some very specific cases, the N-atom occurs in the **quaternary ammonium form** $(R_4N^+ \cdot X^-)$ *e.g.,* **tubocurarine chloride** [see section 7.1.5 (c)]. Nevertheless, the quaternary ammonium compounds are logically and technically not regarded as alkaloids by virtue of the following *two* particular reasons, namely:

(*i*) N-atom does not possess a H-atom, and
(*ii*) Chemical properties are quite different.

As a matter of convenience, they are legitimately grouped along with the *alkaloids.*

[B] O-in the Molecule In addition to the common elements C, H and N, a variety of **alkaloids** normally contains O-atom. Invariably, these specific alkaloids are found in the solid state, with a few exceptions where the oxygenated alkaloids usually occur as non-volatile liquids, such as: **pilocarpine.**

[C] Basicity (Alkalinity) In general, the **alkaloids** are basic (alkaline) in reaction, by virtue of the presence of N-atom present in the molecule. Hence, these are prone to the formation of their respective salts with various acids.

Pilocarpine (Liquid, mp34°C)	Morphine (Solid, mp197°C)	Strychnine (Solid, mp 268–270°)

Degree of Basicity: The degree of basicity of the **alkaloids** mostly depends upon the prevailing influence caused due to the electrostatic status of the N-atom present in the alkaloid molecule, for instance, the number of N-atom present in the alkaloid, whether the N-atom is located in the ring or in the side-chain, the presence of alkyl group (*e.g.,* methyl) to the N-atom etc.

Another vital factor, which establishes the degree of basicity of an alkaloid, is the presence of *pri-, sec-, tert-,* or *quaternary* N-atom or atoms in it. In fact, such apparent differences in the degree of basicity arising from the various structural features, are eventually reflected by the different dissociation constant values (*i.e.,* pKa values) with regard to various alkaloids as stated below:

S.No.	Alkaloid	pKa Values
1	Berberine	$2.47 \ (K = 3.35 \times 10^{-3})$
2	Colchicine	12.35 (at 20°C)
3	Emetine	$pK_1 = 5.77; pK_2 = 6.64$
4	Morphine	9.85
5	Papaverine	8.07 (at 25°C)
6	Physostigmine	$pKa_1 = 6.12; pKa_2 = 12.24;$
7	Quinine	$pK_1 = 5.07 \ (at \ 18°C); pK_2 = 9.7;$
8	Reserpine	6.6
9	Vinblastine sulphate	$pKa_1 = 5.4 ; pKa_2 = 7.4;$
10	Vincristine	5.0 ; 7.4 (in 33% DMF)

Salient Features

1. The weaker bases, *i.e.*, **alkaloids** having low pKa values, shall require a more acidic medium to form their respective salts with the corresponding acid.

2. The strongly basic **alkaloids** *i.e.*, those possessing high pKa values, shall require comparatively low acidic medium to form their respective salts with the acid.

   Note: In a medium at a weakly acidic pH certain strongly basic alkaloids would be easily converted to their respective salt by interaction with the corresponding acid, whereas the alkaloids which are relatively weaker bases having lower pKa values shall still remain in their free-base form. Such a critical situation is skillfully exploited for the separation of a specific alkaloid or a group of alkaloids having closely identical pKa values, from other alkaloids that essentially possess either very low or very high pKa values.

3. The **alkaloids** are usually neutrallized with acids to form salts that may be converted to the corresponding **free-base** by the cautious addition of selective weak bases, such as, ammonia, calcium hydroxide or sodium carbonate. The usage of either NaOH or KOH solutions must be avoided so as to prevent the decomposition or destruction of highly sensitive alkaloids.

4. **Amphoteric alkaloids:** There are some **alkaloids** which are amphoteric in nature *i.e.*, they are neither acidic nor basic in character; this is due to the presence of phenolic (–OH) moiety in **Morphine,** or the presence of carboxylic (–COOH) function in **Narceine,** as shown below:

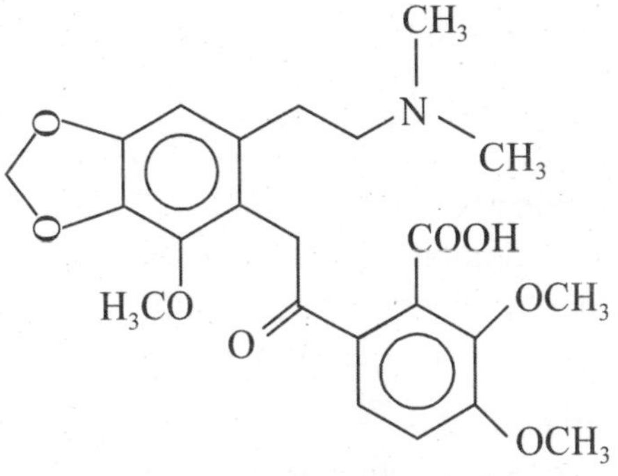

Narceine

5. **Unstable alkaloidal salts:** There exists some specific **alkaloids** that inherently possess *weak-basic properties* and their salts are not so stable, for instance: **piperine, papaverine, narceine, narcotine,** and **caffeine.**

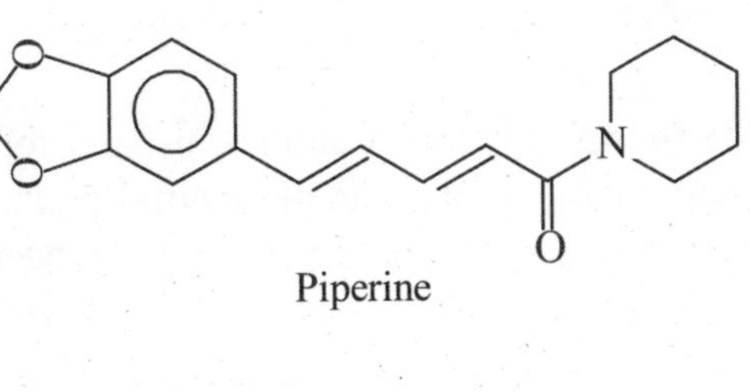

Piperine 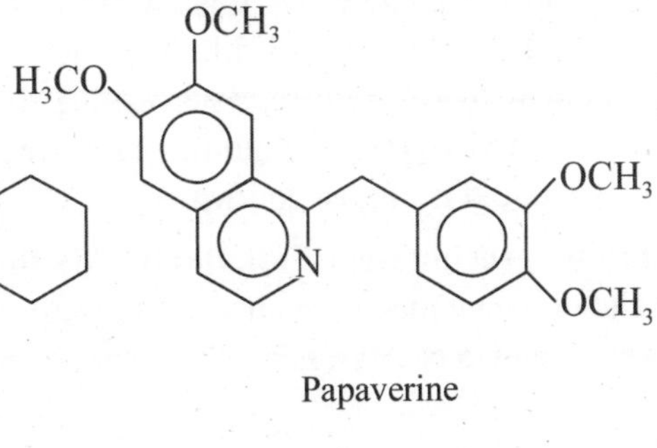   Papaverine

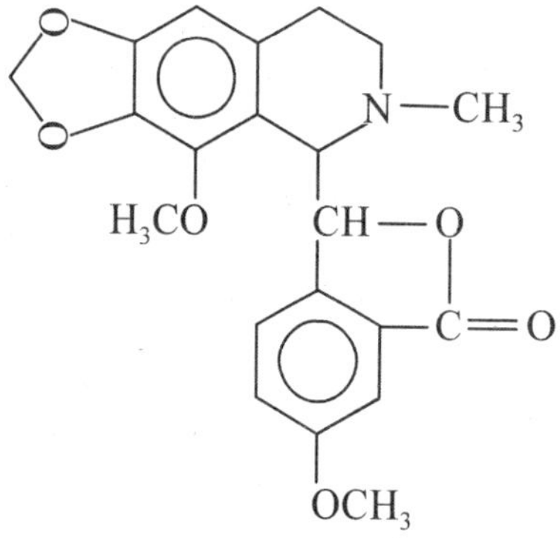

Narcotine 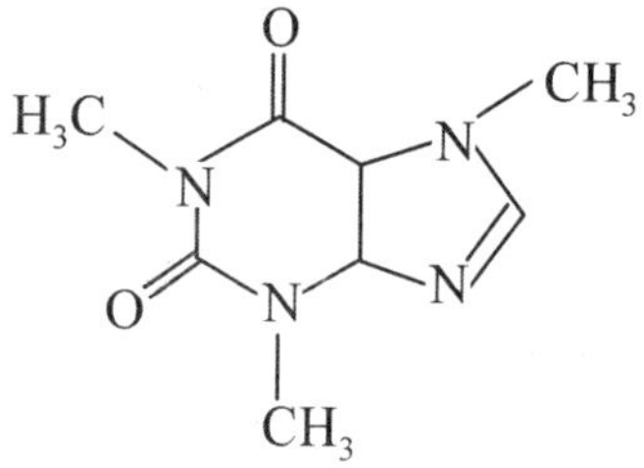　　　　　　　　　　Caffeine

6. **Neutral or slightly acidic alkaloids:** There are a few typical naturally occurring **alkaloids** that almost behave as either neutral or slightly acidic character, namely: ricinine and theophylline, as depicted below:

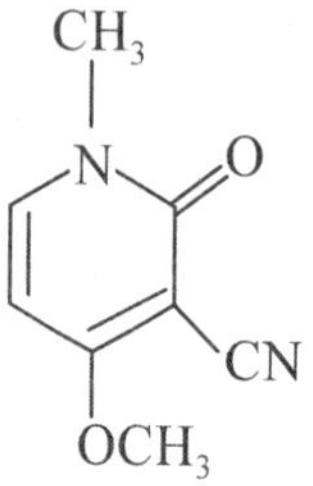

Ricinine 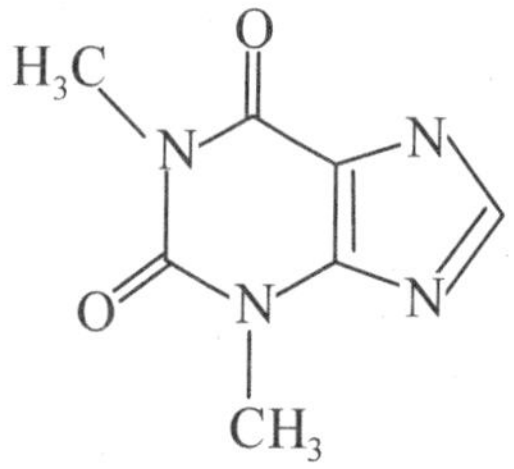　　　　　　　　Theopylline

[D] Precipitation by Specific Reagents　A good number of **alkaloids** obtained from various plant sources invariably give a distinct precipitate with certain specific reagents to an extent as small as *one microgram.* Based on these observations, these **alkaloid-precipitating reagents** are sometimes employed for either detecting the presence or absence of alkaloids in:

(*a*) Crude extracts or plant materials, and
(*b*) For ascertaining whether a specific extraction procedure has exhausted completely the alkaloidal contents or not.

However, a negative test *i.e.*, the absence of precipitation, may infer that the alkaloids are absent. It is pertinent to mention here that a positive test may not always indicate the presence of alkaloids, but may also be due to the presence of other plant constituents, such as: purines, proteins, betaines and ammonium salts etc. Therefore, it is always desired to rule out the possibility of a *false-test* by alkalifying the acidic solution with dilute ammonium hydroxide and subsequently extracting the liberated alkaloid with chloroform. The residue thus obtained, after the removal of the solvent (chloroform), is tested with the **alkaloid-precipitating reagents.** Now, if the test is positive, the presence of an alkaloid is almost confirmed.

Microcrystalline precipitates of alkaloids: Alkaloids, alike other amines, usually form *double-salts* with salts of heavy metals, such as, gold (Au), mercury (Hg) and platinum (Pt). The resulting double salts are found to be possessing characteristic microcrystalline structures. It has been observed that under controlled and specific experimental parameters *viz.*, profile of mixing and gradual evaporation, a drop of an alkaloidal solution reacting with a drop of an appropriate alkaloidal-precipitating reagent, such as: chloroplatinic acid (H_2PtCl_6) or chlorauric acid ($HAu . Cl_4$), on a microscopic-glass slide, gives rise to microcrystalline products having specific and characteristic shapes and structures solely based upon the manner of aggregation.* It may, however, be exploited skillfully as a convenient means of rapid-microscopical identification of an **alkaloid**.

The various reagents that are invariably used either for the testing of **alkaloids** by precipitation or by the formation of microcrystalline complexes (salts) are as stated below along with their individual compositions, namely:

(*i*) **Mayer's Reagent (Potassium-Mercuric Iodide Test Solution):**

Mercuric chloride	=	1.36 g
Potassium Iodide	=	3.00 g
Distilled water to make	=	100.00 ml

(*ii*) **Wagner's Reagent (Potassium Triiodide):**

Iodine	=	1.3 g
Potassium	=	2.0 g
Distilled water to make	=	100.00 ml

(*iii*) **Kraut's Reagent (Modified Dragendorff's Reagent or Potassium Bismuth Iodide):**

Bismuth Nitrate	=	8.0 g
Nitric Acid	=	20.0 ml
Potassium Iodide	=	27.2 g
Distilled water to make	=	100.00 ml

(*iv*) **Marme's Reagent (Potassium-Cadmium Iodide Reagent):**

Cadmium Iodide	=	10.0 g
Potassium Iodide	=	20.0 g
Distilled water to make	=	100.00 ml

(*v*) **Scheibler's Reagent (Phosphotungstic Acid Reagent):**

Sodium Tungstate	=	20.0 g
Disodium Phosphate	=	70.0 g
Distilled water to make	=	100.00 ml

Note: Acidify with nitric acid to litmus paper.

(*vi*) **Hager's Reagent:**
A saturated solution of *Picric Acid.*

(*vii*) **Sonnenschein's Reagent (Phosphomolybdic Acid):**
A 1% (w/v) solution of phosphomolybdic acid in ethanol.

(*viii*) **Bertrand's Reagent (Silicotungstic Acid):**
A 1% (w/v) solution of silicotungstic acid in distilled water.

(*ix*) **Reineckate salt solution:**

Ammonium Reineckate	=	1.0 g

$NH4 [\dot{C}r (NH_3)_2 (SCN)_4$

---

* A whole combination of several components.

Hydroxylamine HCl	=	0.3 g
Ethanol	=	100.00 ml

Note: Filter and store in a refrigerator.

[E] Colour Reactions with Specific Reagents Broadly speaking the colour reactions of the **alkaloids** are rather unspecific; however, they are certainly very sensitive so much so that even alkaloids present in microgram quantities invariably afford immediate and instant response. The ultimate development of a characteristic colour reaction is solely dependent upon either the dehydration or the oxidation of the alkaloid. Generally, a large number of these reagents essentially consist of concentrated sulphuric acid along with certain specific added compounds, such as, sulphomolybdic acid, formaldehyde, sulphovanadic acid, potassium arsenate, hydrogen peroxide, and selenious acid.

A number of such **specific reagents** shall be described in the section that follows:

(*a*) **Froehd's reagent:** Dissolve 5 mg of molybdic acid or sodium molybdate in 5 ml of pure concentrated H_2SO_4.

Note: The reagent should be freshly prepared before use.

(*b*) **Erdmann's reagent:** A mixture of 10 drops of concentrates HNO_3, and 100 ml of water are added to 20 ml of pure concentrated H_2SO_4.

(*c*) **Marqui's reagent:** A mixture of 2-3 drops of formaldehyde solution (40%) with 3 ml of concentrated H_2SO_4.

(*d*) **Mandalin's reagent:** Dissolve 1 g of finely powdered ammonium vanadate in 200 g of pure conc. H_2SO_4.

(*e*) **Mecke's Reagent:** Dissolve 1 g of selenious acid in 200 g of pure concentrated H_2SO_4.

(*f*) **Modified Dragendroff's reagent:** Dissolve 1.6 g of bismuth subnitrate in 60 ml of 20% glacial acetic acid, add to it 5 ml of 40% aqueous solution of KI, 5ml of glacial acetic acid and make up the volume to 100 ml of water.

(*g*) **Rosenthaler's reagent:** Dissolve 1 g of potassium arsenates in 100 g of pure concentrated H_2SO_4.

(*h*) **Schaer's reagent:** Mix carefully 1 volume of pure 30% H_2O_2 with 10 volumes of concentrated H_2SO_4.

Note: The reagent is always prepared afresh, before use.

Interestingly, there are some instances where in the intensity of the colour so produced is in *linear proportion* under standardized experimental parameters. Therefore, such specific colour reactions may be used exclusively for the quantitative determination of certain groups of **alkaloids**, such as:

(*i*) **For Ergot Alkaloids:** The blue colour produced by the ergot alkaloids with the **Van Urk Reagent** (or **Ehrlich Reagent**) *i.e.*, *para*-dimethylaminobenzaldehyde in 65% H_2SO_4, is employed for the quantitative estimation of **ergot alkaloids.**

(*ii*) **For Belladona Alkaloids:** The violet colour caused by the belladona alkaloids with fuming HNO_3 and alcoholic KOH solution is employed for their assay.

[F] Stability of Alkaloids **Alkaloids**, in general, are not very stable. They normally undergo degradation or decomposition on being exposed to air, light, moisture and heat, besides chemical reagents. A few typical examples of alkaloids *vis-a-vis* their stability are stated below, namely:

(*i*) Ergotamine gets destroyed by prolonged treatment with alkali, whereas strychnine can stand such vigorous action.

(*ii*) An aqueous solution of alkaloids undergo rapid decomposition or degradation as compared to their solid forms.

(*iii*) Storage of **alkaloids** in pure form or their dry extracts is usually done in a vacuum desiccator over a dehydrating agent *e.g.*, phosphorous pentoxide (P_2O_5) or calcium chloride ($CaCl_2$) anhydrous for their better stability.

(*iv*) During the course of extraction of **alkaloids** followed by isolation, the solvent is preferably removed effectively by distillation under vacuum* (or reduced atmospheric pressure) or by subjecting it to evaporation in a Rotary Thin-Film Evaporator under vacuum so that the desired product is not exposed to excessive heat, thus avoiding decomposition.

(*v*) **Alkaloids**, are stored in amber-coloured glass bottles preferably in a vacuum desiccator.

[G] Acid salts of Alkaloids A plethora of **alkaloids** are strongly alkaline in nature and most of them form well-defined salts. However, in certain instances the basicity of an **alkaloid** is quite weak and feeble, and hence the formation of the corresponding salts with either acetic or other weak acids is practically insignificant and rare. The salts formed with stronger acids *e.g.*, HCl, H_2SO_4 etc., get decomposed in the presence of water to liberate the free base and the acid. It has been observed that only a few of the alkaloids form carbonates, and consequently either the alkali carbonates or the alkali hydrogen carbonates are invariably used to liberate them from the aqueous solutions of their corresponding salts.

Alkaloids, in general, containing either one or more than one N-atom usually behave as **monoacidic bases;** and, therefore, form only one series of salts with acids as designated by '*BA*' (where: B = base; and A = acid). It is pertinent to mention here that **quinine** in particular and the **cinchona alkaloids** in general are an exception to the earlier concept and found to behave as *diacidic bases*. Besides, a number of alkaloids to behave as monoacidic bases, even though they contain two N-atoms in their molecule. It is worthwhile to mention here that the basicities of the alkaloids is of utmost importance with regard to their quantitative volumetric estimation.

In common practice the salts of alkaloids are prepared by using cold and dilute solutions of the mineral acid specifically, *e.g.*, **morphine hydrochloride, atropine sulphate, quinine sulphate, ephedrine hydrochloride** etc. It may be pointed out that the use of concentrated mineral acids, or heating an alkaloid even with a dilute acid under pressure may ultimately lead to profound changes in them. Noticeably, the concentrated mineral acids invariably give rise to characteristic colour changes, that are usually used as a means of identification and characterization of the alkaloids. In addition to the complete decomposition of **alkaloids** by strong acids to result the various colour changes, the chemical changes caused by the mineral acids on them may be categorized into *three* different types, namely:

---

* Under vacuum (or reduced atmospheric pressure) the boiling point of solvent is lowered significantly *e.g.*, alcohol pp 78.5°C boils in vacuum at 40°C.

(*a*) **Dehydration:** Dehydration of **alkaloids** give rise to either *anhydro-* or *apo-* alkaloids, such as:
  Apomorphine obtained from **Morphine**
  Apoatropine obtained from **Atropine**

(*b*) **Demethoxylation:** The removal or elimination of the methoxyl groups from the alkaloids by treatment with either concentrated HCl or HI to produce methyl chloride (CH_3Cl) or methyl iodide (CH_3I) while giving rise to the corresponding *hydroxy base*. The methoxyl group (s) are present in a variety of alkaloids, for instance: **codeine, quinine, narcotine** and **papaverine.**
Example:

$$NARCOTINE + 3HI \longrightarrow NORNARCOTINE + 3CH_3I$$

(*c*) **Hydrolysis:** A good number of **naturally occurring alkaloids** are obtained as *esters*. They easily undergo hydrolysis on being heated with either alkalies or mineral acids thereby resulting into the formation of the corresponding acids along with respective alcohols or phenols of the alkaloids. A few typical examples are as give below:

  (*i*) $ATROPINE + H_2O \longrightarrow TROPINE + TROPIC\ ACID$
  (*ii*) $COCAINE + 2H_2O \longrightarrow ECGONINE + BENZOIC\ ACID$
  $+ METHANOL$

[H] Action of Alkalies   The action of alkalies *e.g.*, NaOH and KOH on the **alkaloids** are found to be varying in nature as enumerated below:

(*a*) Dilute alkaline solutions of KOH or NaOH normally decompose most alkaloidal salts and finally liberate the free alkaloids.
(*b*) Certain alkaloids containing phenolic hydroxyl groups *e.g.*, **morphine,** on being treated with alkaline solutions yield, their corresponding soluble sodium or potassium salts.
(*c*) The ester alkaloids usually undergo hydrolysis on being treated with dilute alkalies, such as: atropine, cocaine.
(*d*) **Racemic Isomeride:** The action of alkali hydroxides on **hyoscyamine** in alcohol gives rise to the racemic isomeride atropine.
(*e*) Fusion of alkaloids with dry KOH or NaOH by the application of heat ultimately leads to drastic decomposition of the former thereby yielding ultimately the simple heterocyclic bases, for instance: pyridine, quinoline, pyrrolidine etc.
(*f*) Simple fusion of **alkaloids** with alkali hydroxides may give rise to distinct and visible colour changes.

[I] Pharmacological Activity   The **alkaloids** exhibit a wide-spectrum and complete diversity of complex structures which ultimately is responsible for their extra ordinary broad-range of pharmacological activities covering both the cardio-vascular and central nervous system. It has been observed beyond any reasonable doubt that most alkaloids usually exert certain specific and definite pharmacological action. Moreover, a small quantity of an alkaloid (0.1–1.0 mg) may bring about a marked and pronounced pharmacological action on various organs and tissues both of animal and human origin. However, the potency of an individual alkaloid varies from one another widely and profusely.

A few typical pharmacological actions of some **alkaloids** are stated below showing their broad-spectrum of activities, namely:

S.No.	Alkaloid	Pharmacological Action
1	Morphine	Narcotic analgesic
2	Codeine	Expectorant, analgesic
3	Brucine	CNS-Stimulants
4	Strychnine	CNS-Stimulants
5	Ergotamine	Uterine muscle contractions
6	Atropine	Mydriatics
7	Homotropine	Mydriatics
8	Pilocarpine	Myotics
9	Physostigmine	Myotics
10	Ephedrine	Hypertensive
11	Reserpine	Hypotensive
12	Quinine	Antimalarial
13	Caffeine	CNS-stimulant
14	Tubocurarine	Neuromuscular blocking action
15	Emetine	Antiprotozoal action
16	Hyoscyamine	Relief of spasms of urinary tract
17	Cocaine	CNS-stimulant
18	Colchicine	Anti-gout
19	Lobeline	Treatment of asthma
20	Arecoline	Parasympathomimetic action
21	Protoveratrine A	For management of hypertension in pregnancy
22	Conessine	Antiprotozoal and antiamoebic
23	Vasicine	Expectorant and bronchodilator
24	Vinblastine	Antineoplastic
25	Vincristine	Antineoplastic
26	Piperine	Carminative, stomachic
27	Heroin	Narcotic analgesic
28	Hyoscine	Motion sickness (sedation)
29	Theophylline	Smooth musele relaxant
30	Aconitine	Treatment of neuralgia, sciatica, rheumatism and inflammation.

7.1.7 General Methods of Extraction and Isolation of Alkaloids

The general methods of extraction and isolation of the alkaloids from the plant sources one has to take into consideration the following steps in a sequential manner, namely:

(*i*) Separation of the alkaloid(s) from the main bulk of the non-alkaloidal substances,

(*ii*) Most of the alkaloid-containing plants, several alkaloids having closely related chemical structures are normally present, such as: the cinchona alkaloids consist of more than twenty-five alkaloids. There is hardly any known plant source that contains only one alkaloid exclusively,

(*iii*) Separation of each individual alkaloid from the mixture of alkaloids obtained from a particular plant source (*e.g.*, **cinchona bark**) using latest separation techniques, for instance, preparative **high-performances liquid chromatography, (HPLC)** column chromatography, by the help of chromatotron, and **high-performance thin-layer chromatography (HPTLC).**

Nevertheless, the general methods of isolation of alkaloids largely depend upon several vital factors, for instance: (*a*) the alkaline nature of most alkaloids, (*b*) the ability and ease of formation of alkaloidal salts with acids, and (*c*) the relative solubilities of the resulting alkaloidal salts either in polar organic solvents *e.g.*, ethanol, chloroform, isopropanol etc., or in aqueous medium.

The general methods of **extraction of alkaloids** from the plant sources solely depend upon the purpose and scale of the operation (*e.g.*, pilot scale or commercial scale). It is also based on the quantum and bulk of the raw material to be employed in the operation. Of course, for research purposes column chromatography using ion-exchange resins have been used successfully and effectively to strip the plant materials of their alkaloidal contents. However, in the commercial scale large volumes of aqueous extracts of plant materials are normally pumped through huge metallic columns packed with cationic resins, which in turn pick up all basic components (cations). Subsequently, the alkaloids (*i.e.*, the basic components are conveniently washed off by flushing the column with a moderately strong acid. The column having the cationic resins can be reused once again for the next drug substances.

By the advent of the latest separation techniques and the copious volume of informations accumulated through the intensive and extensive research carried out with regard to the conventional processes essentially associated with the separation as well as isolation of the hundreds of **alkaloids** from the natural plant sources, the following *five* steps are most important and vital, namely:

(*i*) Sample preparation
(*ii*) Liberation of free alkaloidal base
(*iii*) Extraction of alkaloidal base with organic solvent
(*iv*) Purification of crude alkaloidal extract
(*v*) Fractionation of crude alkaloids

All these *five* steps shall be discussed individually as under:

7.1.7.1 Sample Preparation

The first and foremost step is the sample preparation. The plant material is reduced to a moderately coarse powder by appropriate means using grinders and sieves, to facilitate maximum effective contact of the solvent with the ruptured alkaloid bearing tissues and cells. In the case of plant substances that are rich in oils and fats, such as: seeds, kernels, these non-alkaloidal chemical components need to be eliminated completely by extraction with a suitable non-polar solvent like n-hexane, light petroleum ether, in a soxhlet apparatus, which would not extract the alkaloids in question. However, it is always advisable to shake the light-petroleum ether or n-hexane fraction with a dilute mineral acid and subsequently test the acidic solution for the presence of alkaloids.

7.1.7.2 Liberation of Free Alkaloidal Base

It has been observed that the **alkaloids** invariably occur in the plant sources as the salt of acids, such as: oxalates, tannates etc. Therefore, when the plant substance is exposed to an alkaline medium, the alkaloidal salts are readily converted to the corresponding alkaloid bases.

Choice of Alkali   Indeed, the choice of a suitable *mineral base* (alkali) for the ease of liberation of the alkaloid from the salts is not only very vital but also equally significant and largely depend on the following factors, namely:

(*a*) **Natural state of the alkaloids:** It has been observed that the salt of a *strongly basic alkaloid* with a mineral acid usually tends to undergo cleavage under the influences of a stronger base. Likewise, the corresponding salt of a *weakly basic alkaloid* and a relatively weak organic acid shall require a rather weaker base for its cleavage.

(*b*) **Chemical characteristics of the alkaloidal base:** The usage of strong alkali *e.g.*, NaOH or KOH should be avoided as far as possible by virtue of the fact that certain alkaloids undergo hydrolysis on prolonged contact with a strong base.

Example

   (*i*) **Hydrolysis of ester-alkaloids,** *e.g.*, **cocaine, hyoscyamine;**

   (*ii*) **Phenolic alkaloids** *e.g.*, **cephaeline, morphine.** These **alkaloids** normally get solubilized while in contact with a strong alkali and, therefore milder alkaline reagents *e.g.*, dilute ammonia solution are necessary for their liberation.

(*c*) **Presence of fatty substances:** The usage of strong alkali is strictly prohibited in the case of fat containing plant materials because of the formation of saponified products causing troublesome emulsions. In such cases, it is always preferred to defat the plant substance before proceeding for the liberation of free alkaloids.

Ammonium Hydroxide Solution   Dilute aqueous ammonium hydroxide solution is one of the choicest alkali most frequently used for the liberation of alkaloids from the plant sources. It enjoys a two-fold advantage. First, being its adequate alkalinity to liberate most of the common alkaloids, and second by, its volatile nature so that it may be removed by evaporation of the solvent. As it has a tendency to be extracted by solvent ether from the aqueous solution, therefore, it is almost necessary to get rid of it by evaporation and subsequent washing repeatedly. In normal practice, usually even the last traces of ammonia are removed when the combined ethereal extract is reduced to half of its original volume under vacuum.

NaOH or KOH Solution   The **alkaloids** that occur naturally as their tannate salts specially require either NaOH or KOH solution for their subsequent liberation. In certain typical instance even the use of KOH or NaOH fails to cleave the tannate salts because of their intimately strong bondage with the alkaloid and extremely insoluble nature.

Example

(*i*) **Cinchona Bark:** It has got to be treated first by heating with dilute HCl so as to decompose the salts and liberate the alkaloids in the form of water soluble hydrochlorides, and

(*ii*) **Pomegranate Bark:** It does not have the tannin so tenaciously bound to the alkaloids as in the case of cinchona bark. Hence, NaOH solution is strong enough to cause on effective split of the alkaloidal salts. It also acts to control the solubility of the water-soluble pomegranate alkaloids by preventing their dissociation.

7.1.7.3 *Extraction of Alkaloidal Base*

The extraction of alkaloidal base may be accomplished by *three* different types of solvents that are discussed below, namely:

[A] Extraction with Water-Miscible Solvents   A plethora of **alkaloids** and their respective salts are soluble in alcohols, such as: methanol, ethanol, isopropanol; therefore, these very solvents may also be employed for the extraction of the plant substances. The usual pretreatment of the crude drug with alkali may be avoided completely, because alcohol appears to affect dissolution of not only the *alkaloidal salts* but also the *free bases* found in the plant substances. It is, however, believed that alcohol predominantly exerts a *hydrolyzing effect* upon the alkaloidal tannates and other salts. In actual practice, neither pretreatment of the crude drug with an alkali nor acidification of the alcohol with a small amount of a mineral acid or an organic acid is required.

Note

1. The penetration and hence the subsequent extraction of the crude drug is almost complete with the help of four successive extractions with an alcohol. Further, the loss of solvent is comparatively less than the chlorinated solvents e.g., chloroform.

2. The extraction of total alkaloids with alcohol is highly recommended because of its maximum efficiency and economical viability.

[B] Extraction with Water-Immiscible Solvents In reality, the most widely used water-immiscible solvents for the extraction of alkaloids are: chloroform, diethyl ether (solvent ether) and isopropyl ether. However, a few other specific organic solvents, namely: ethylene chloride, carbon tetrachloride and **benzene*** may be employed with an evident advantage for certain specific alkaloids. Interestingly, *chloroform* is regarded as the choicest water-immiscible solvent for a broad-spectrum of alkaloids present in the plant kingdom and extracts them with varying degrees of ease.

Note: Chloroform is not suitable for the extraction of quaternary alkaloids e.g., tubocurarine.

[C] Extraction with Water The crude drug is subjected to extraction with water previously acidified with dilute solution of HCl, H_2SO_4 or CH_3COOH, which is subsequently rendered alkaline, preferably with dilute NH_4OH solution and finally extracted with a water-immiscible solvent as stated in [B] above.

Undoubtedly, water being an excellent and absolutely inexpensive polar solvent for the extraction of alkaloids, but if offers an enormous volume of disadvantages because it carries along with it a large number of other plant components, for instance: sugar, pigments (*e.g.*, **chlorophylls**), starches, tannins, proteins etc., which ultimately puts across a collosal waste of time, energy and chemicals. Hence, its usage has been resulting to a bear minimum level.

In general, the alkaloids may be extracted by any of the following *three* well-defined and widely accepted processes, namely:

(*a*) Soxhlet Extraction Process

(*b*) Stas-Otto Process, and

(*c*) Kippenberger's Process.

All these three processes shall now be discussed briefly in the sections that follows:

(*a*) **Soxhlet Extraction Process:** The soxhlet assembly is a continuous extractor which is generally suitable for the extraction of alkaloids from powdered plant materials with the help of organic solvents. In this instance, the powdered drug is usually moistened with dilute ammonia solution and then packed loosely in the thimble of the Soxhlet apparatus; and the organic solvent affords a deep penetration of the moist drug thereby allowing the greatest possible extraction of the alkaloids from the exposed surfaces of the cells and tissues of the crude drug. Once, the extraction is ascertained to have completed, the solvent is filtered and evaporated in a **Rotary Thin-Film Evaporator** and the residue is treated further for the isolation of individual alkaloids.

---

* **Benzene:** It is a carcinogenic chemical and hence its use may be avoided or done in a highly efficient fume cupboard.

(*b*) **Stas-Otto Process:** The **Stas-Otto process** essentially consists of treating the powdered and sieved drug substance with 90–95% (v/v) ethanol, previously acidified with tartaric acid. The proportion of crude drug to solvent should be maintained as 1 Kg to 1 L. The alcohol is distilled off under vacuum and the resulting aqueous residue is treated with petroleum-ether (60-80°C) to remove the fatty components completely. If any alkaloid is removed by the petroleum ether, it must be recovered by treating it with dilute mineral acid. Thus, the resulting aqueous extract is mixed with the main bulk of aqueous extract. The combined aqueous extract is filtered and evaporated to dryness preferably in a **Rotary *Thin*-Film Evaporator** under vacuum. The residue is extracted with absolute ethanol thereby dissolving the total alkaloids.

(*c*) **Kippenberger's Process:** In Kippenberger's process the powdered and sieved plant substance is first and foremost digested with solution of tannin (100 g) in glycerol (500 g) at a constant temperature of 40°C for a duration of 48 hours. The resulting mixture is further heated to 50°C so as to help in the complete coagnlation of proteinous substances, cooled to ambient temperature and finally filtered. The resulting filtrate is thoroughly shaken with petroleum ether to get rid of faulty materials (oils, fats and waxes), and the last traces of petroleum ether is removed from the extract by heating either on a water-bath (electric) or exposure to Infra-Red Lamp. The fat-free crude plant extract is subsequently acidified and shaken with chloroform, successively to remove the bulk of the alkaloids, namely, atropine, codeine, colchicine, narcotine, nicotine, papaverine, spartenine and thebaine.

The resulting residual extract may still contain narceine, curarine and morphine. However, narceine and morphine may be isolated by passing freshly generated CO_2 directly into extract so as to convert the alkali hydroxide into their corresponding carbonate, which is then ultimately subjected to solvent extraction using a mixture of alcohol and chloroform. Finally, the third alkaloid, curarine, may be extracted by agitation with a mixture of equal volumes of ether and chloroform.

However, a combination of **Kippenberger's process** and **Stas-Otto process** by its application to the final alcoholic extract obtained by the latter process is found to give better separation of alkaloids.

7.1.7.4 *Purification of Alkaloidal Extract*

The main bulk of the **crude alkaloidal extract** is invariably subjected to further purification by means of either anyone or combination of the following methods:

(*a*) **Extraction with Acid Solution**   The extraction of the **alkaloid** from the bulk of the crude alkaloid solution in immiscible organic solvent is invariably carried out by shaking with an acid solution. In usual practice, the use of HCl is restricted when chloroform remains as the solvent because of the fact that quite a few alkaloidal hydrochlorides are distinctly soluble in the latter. However, dilute H_2SO_4 is always preferred over HCl for general use in the extraction of alkaloids. Subsequently, the acid solution is rendered alkaline with dilute NH_4OH solution to liberate the alkaloids which is then extracted with an organic solvent. The solvent is removed under reduced pressure and the traces of moisture is removed with anhydrous sodium sulphate.

Note: The following two precautions may be observed, namely

  (*i*) **To avoid the formation of stubborn and troublesome emulsions a solution of gum-tragacanth is often added to the aqueous-phase. In case, it still persists the two phases may be got separated by centrifugation, and** (*ii*) **To discard the presence of foreign interfering extractive components present in plant substances, such as: pigments, resins, waxes, oils and fats, the use of a 2.5-5% (w/v) solution of lead acetate is made to the alkaloidal extract which precipitates them effectively. The excess of lead present in the filtrate is removed by either passing H_2S gas through the Kipp's Apparatus or by adding sodium phosphate.**

(*b*) **Precipitation of Alkaloid with Precipitating Reagent** The usual precipitation of the **alkaloid** as a complex compound is accomplished by the addition of a suitable precipitating reagent. The resulting alkaloidal complex is further purified by filtration, recrystallization and ultimately decomposed to obtain the desired free alkaloid(s).

Example

(*i*) **Tannic-acid Complex:** It is normally decomposed by treatment with freshly prepared $Pb(OH)_2$ or $Pb(CO_3)_2$.

(*ii*) **Precipitates obtained with $HgCl_2$, $AuCl_3$, $PtCl_4$, Mayer's Reagent:** These precipitates are decomposed by passing a stream of H_2S gas through its suspension.

(*iii*) **Precipitates with Double Salts:** The double salt obtained with Dragendorff's Regent is quickly boiled with 5% (w/v) $BaCO_3$ solution.

(*iv*) **Precipitates with Nitrogenous Acids:** The precipitates obtained with nitrogenous acids like picric acid and picrolonic acid are normally decomposed by treatment with either NH_4OH or NaOH.

Picric acid · Picrolonic acid

(*v*) **Reineckate Complex:** The complex obtained from alkaloid with *Reinecke Salt*, $NH_4[Cr(NH_3)_2(SCN)_4]$, is normally decomposed by treating its solution in a mixture of acetone and water (1:1) with a silver sulphate solution.

It is pertinent to mention here that the **free liberated alkaloid** from the complexes stated above, (*i*) through (*v*), may be further extracted for its final recovery with an appropriate organic solvent, such as: chloroform.

(*c*) The purification of **alkaloids** may also be accomplished by the formation of its crystallised alkaloidal salt by the addition of an appropriate mineral or organic acid, such as: hydrochloric, hydrobromic, perchloric, sulphuric, oxalic and tartaric acids.

(*d*) Various known **separation techniques,** namely: **partition, ion-exchange** and **column chromatography** are invariably used for the purification of a host of alkaloids.

Besides, various physical parameters like: specific rotation, melting point, solubility are frequently used as a definite criteria of ascertaining the purity of alkaloids.

7.1.7.5 *Fractionation of Crude Alkaloids*

It has been observed largely that most of the alkaloid-bearing plant materials usually contain a mixture of closely-related alkaloids. Therefore, it has become almost necessary to carry out an effective fractionation of crude alkaloids from the extract or solution of total crude alkaloids.

However, the traditional and orthodox methods of separation are not only difficult but also tedious and cumbersome. The commonly employed techniques of separation that were found to the reliable and dependable may be short-listed as follows:

(*i*) Fractional crystallization,

(*ii*) Fractional distillation, and

(*iii*) Derivatization with low solubility products.

The latest methods employed for the separation of **alkaloids** are the preparative **high performance liquid chromatography (HPLC), high performance thin-layer chromatography (HPTLC),** chromatotron, counter-current distribution and other chromatographic techniques including column chromatography, ion-exchange chromatography.

Following are some of the typical situations whereby the mixture of **alkaloids** may be separated effectively, such as:

(*a*) A larger section of the **alkaloids** are easily soluble in chloroform and relatively less soluble in other organic solvents. In general, the order of solubility is as stated below chloroform > acetone > ethanol > methanol > ethyl acetate > ether > n-hexane. Keeping in view the above solubility profile of alkaloids in organic solvents, if one of the alkaloids is much less soluble in ethanol than chloroform, the fractional crystallization of this alkaloid is possible. In this particular instance the chloroform-fraction is concentrated to an appropriate level, and hot ethanol added in small proportions at intervals. Thus, upon cooling the alkaloid, which is less soluble in ethanol, separates out conveniently.

(*b*) In case, the fractional crystallization of the mixture of closely related alkaloids become tedious and ineffective, one may try to form their respective salts,* and then carry out the separation indicated above.

(*c*) The various acids, namely: HCl, HBr, HI, $HClO_4$, HNO_3, $C_2H_2O_4$, and $C_6H_3N_3O_7$, may either be employed in aqueous or methanolic solution. Thus, from the resulting methanolic solution, the salts of the respective alkaloids may be precipitated by the addition of ether. The precipitated crude alkaloidal salts may be further recrystallized from hot acetone containing a small proportion of methanol.

(*d*) In certain other specific instances, the salts of the respective oxalates, picrates and perchlorates may be precipitated from their solutions in acetone, by the addition of ethyl acetate.

7.2 CLASSIFICATION OF ALKALOIDS

The **alkaloids,** as an important and enormously large conglomerate of naturally occurring nitrogen-containing plant substances having very specific as well as most diversified pharmacological properties may be classified in a number of modes and means.

---

* **Salts of Alkaloids:** that are used frequently are hydrochloride, hydrobromide, hydroiodide perchlorate, nitrate, oxalate and picrate.

Hegnauer* (1963) conveniently classified alkaloids into *six* important groups, corresponding to the six amino-acids legitimately considered as the starting points for their biosynthesis, such as: anthranilic acid, histidine, lysine, ornithine phenylalanine and tryptophan. Price* (1963) further took a leading clue from the earlier observation and considered in details the alkaloids present in one of the families, (*Rutaceae*) and logically placed them in the following *nine* chemical-structural categories, namely: **acridines, amides, amines, benzylisoquinolines, canthinones, imidazoles, indolquinazolines, furoquinolines,** and **quinazolines.**

Another school of thought classifies **alkaloids** in the following *four* heads, namely:

(*a*) **Biosynthetic Classification**   In this particular instance the significance solely lies to the precursor from which the alkaloids in question are produced in the plant biosynthetically. Therefore, it is quite convenient and also logical to group together all alkaloids having been derived from the same precursor but possessing different taxonomic distribution and pharmacological activities.

Examples
- (*i*) Indole alkaloids derived from *tryptophan*.
- (*ii*) Piperidine alkaloids derived from *lysine*.
- (*iii*) Pyrrolidine alkaloids derived from *ornithine*.
- (*iv*) Phenylethylamine alkaloids derived from *tyrosine*.
- (*v*) Imidazole alkaloids derived from *histidine*.

(*b*) **Chemical Classification**   It is probably the most widely accepted and common mode of classification of **alkaloids** for which the main criterion is the presence of the basic heterocyclic nucleus (*i.e.*, the **chemical entity**).

Examples
- (*i*) Pyrrolidine alkaloids *e.g.*, **Hygrine;**
- (*ii*) Piperidine alkaloids *e.g.*, **Lobeline;**
- (*iii*) Pyrrolizidine alkaloids *e.g.*, **Senecionine;**
- (*iv*) Tropane alkaloids *e.g.*, **Atropine;**
- (*v*) Quinoline alkaloids *e.g.*, **Quinine;**
- (*vi*) Isoquinoline alkaloids *e.g.*, **Morphine;**
- (*vii*) Aporphine alkaloids *e.g.*, **Boldine;**
- (*viii*) Indole alkaloids *e.g.*, **Ergometrine;**
- (*ix*) Imidazole alkaloids *e.g.*, **Pilocarpine;**
- (*x*) Diazocin alkaloids *e.g.*, **Lupanine;**
- (*xi*) Purine alkaloids *e.g.*, **Caffeine;**
- (*xii*) Steroidal alkaloids *e.g.*, **Solanidine;**
- (*xiii*) Amino alkaloids *e.g.*, **Ephedrine;**
- (*xiv*) Diterpene alkaloids *e.g.*, **Aconitine.**

(*c*) **Pharmacological Classification**   Interestingly, the **alkaloids** exhibit a broad range of very specific pharmacological characteristics. Perhaps this might also be used as a strong basis for the general classification of the wide-spectrum of alkaloids derived from the plant kingdom, such as:

---

* Swain, T. (ed), **'Chemical Plant Taxonomy'**, Academic Press, London, (1963).

analgesics, cardio-vascular drugs, CNS-stimulants and depressants, dilation of pupil of eye, mydriatics, anticholinergics, sympathomimetics, antimalarials, purgatives, and the like. However, such a classification is not quite common and broadly known.

Examples

   (*i*) **Morphine** as Narcotic analgesic;

  (*ii*) **Quinine** as Antimalarial;

 (*iii*) **Strychnine** as Reflex excitability;

 (*iv*) **Lobeline** as Respiratory stimulant;

   (*v*) **Boldine** as Choleretics and laxatives;

  (*vi*) **Aconitine** as Neuralgia;

 (*vii*) **Pilocarpine** as Antiglaucoma agent and miotic;

(*viii*) **Ergonovine** as Oxytocic;

  (*ix*) **Ephedrine** as Bronchodilator;

   (*x*) **Narceine** as Analgesic (narcotic) and antitussive.

(*d*) **Taxonomic Classification**   This particular classification essentially deals with the **'Taxon'** *i.e.*, the **taxonomic category.** The most common *taxa* are the genus, subgenus, species, subspecies, and variety. Therefore, the taxonomic classification encompasses the plethora of alkaloids exclusively based on their respective distribution in a variety of **Plant Families,** sometimes also referred to as the **'Natural order'.** A few typical examples of plant families and the various species associated with them are stated below, namely:

   (*i*) **Cannabinaceous Alkaloids:** *e.g.*, *Cannabis sativa* Linn., (**Hemp, Marijuana**).

  (*ii*) **Rubiaceous Alkaloids:** *e.g.*, *Cinchona Sp.* (**Quinine**); *Mitragyna speciosa* Korth (**Katum, Kratum, Kutum**); *Pausinystalia johimbe* (K. Schum) (**Yohimbe**).

 (*iii*) **Solanaceous Alkaloids:** *e.g.*, *Atropa belladona* L., (**Deadly Nightshade, Belladona**); *Brunfelsia uniflorus* (Pohl) D. Don (**Manaca, Manacan**); *Capsicum annuum* L., (**Sweet Peppers, Paprika**); *Datura candida* (Pers.) Saff. (**Borrachero, Floripondio**); *Duboisia myoporoides* R. Br. (**Corkwood Tree, Pituri**); *Hyoscyamus niger* L. (**Henbane, Henblain, Jusquaime**); *Mandragora officinarum* L. (**Mandrake, Loveapple**); *Nicotiana glauca* R. Grah. (**Tree Tobacco**); *Seopolia carniolica* Jacq. (**Scopolia**); *Solanum dulcamara* L., (**Bittersweet, Bitter Nightshade, Felonwood**); *Withania somniferum* (L.) Dunal (**Ashwagandha**), etc.

Invariably, they are grouped together according to the name of the *genus* wherein they belong to, such as: **coca, cinchona, ephedra.**

Some **'phytochemists'** have even gone a step further and classified the **alkaloids** based on their **chemotaxonomic classification.**

In the recent past, the **alkaloids** have been divided into *two* major categories based on the analogy that one containing a *non-heterocyclic nucleus*, while the other having the *heterocyclic nucleus*. These *two* classes of alkaloids shall be discussed briefly as under.

(*a*) **Non-heterocyclic Alkaloids**   A few typical **alkaloids** having non-heterocyclic nucleus are erumerated below:

S.No.	Basic Ring Structure	Alkaloid	Botanical Origin	Family
1	Phenylethylamine	Ephedrine	*Ephedra vulgaris*	*Gnetaceae*
		Hordenine	*Hordeum vulgare*	*Graminae*
		Capsaicin	*Capsicum annunum*	*Solanaceae*
		Mescaline	*Laphophora williamsii*	*Cactaceae*
		Narceine	*Papaver somniferum*	*Papaveraceae*

(*b*) **Heterocyclic Alkaloids**   A large number of specific **alkaloids** possessing heterocyclic nucleus are stated below:

S.No.	Basic Ring Structure	Alkaloid	Botanical Origin	Family
1	**Pyrrolidine**	Hygrine	*Erythroxylon coca*	*Erythroxylaceae*
		Stachydrine	*Stachys tuberifera* .	*Labiatae*
2	**Pyrindine**	Arecoline	*Areca catchu*	*Palmaceae*
		Ricinine	*Ricinus communis*	*Euphorbiaceae*
		Trigenelline	*Trigonella foenumgraecum*	*Leguminosae*
3	**Piperidine**	Connine	*Conium maculatum*	*Umbelliferae*
		Lobeline	*Lobelia inflata*	*Lobeliaceae*
		Pelletierine	*Punica granatum*	*Punicaceae*
4	**Tropane [Piperidine- Pyrrolidine (N-Methyl)]**	Atropine	*Atropa belladone*	*Solanaceae*
			Datura stramonium	*Solanaceae*
		Cocaine	*Erythroxylon coca*	*Erythroxylaceae*
		Hyoscyamine	*Atropa belladona*	*Solanaceae*
5	**Quinoline**	Quinine, Quinidine	*Cinchona officinalis*	*Rubiaceae*
		Cuspareine	*Cusparia trifoliata*	*Rutaceae*
6	**Isoquinoline**	Papaverine	*Papaver somniferum*	*Papaveraceae*
		Berberine	*Hydrastis canadensis*	*Berberidaceae*
		Emetine	*Uragoga ipecacuanha*	*Rubiaceae*
		Corydaline	*Corydalis aurea*	*Fumariaceae*
			Corydalis solida	*Fumariaceae*
		Tubocurarine	*Chondodendron tomentosum*	*Menispermaceae*

(*Contd.*)

(Contd.)

7	**Aporphine** **Isoquinoline** **Phenanthrene**	Boldine	*Peumus boldus*	*Monimiaceae*

8	**Norlupinane**	Sparteine	*Lupinus lutens,* *Lupinus niger,* *Cytisus scoparius,* *Anagyris boetida*	*Leguminosae*
		Lupinine	*Lupinus luteus* *Anabasis aphylla*	*Leguminosae* *Chenopodiaceae*

9	**Indole** **(Benzopyrrole)**	Ergotamine, Ergometrine	*Claviceps purpurea*	*Hypocreales*
		Physostigmine	*Physostigma Venenosum*	*Leguminosae*
		Reserpine	*Rauwolfia serpentina*	*Apocynaceae*
		Yohimbine	*Coryanthe johimbe*	*Rubiaceae*
			Rauwolfia serpentina	*Apocynaceae*
		Vinblastine (Vincaleukoblastine)	*Vince rosea*	*Apocynaceae*
		Strychnine	*Strychnos nux-vomica*	*Loganiaceae*

10	**Imidazole** **(Glyoxaline)**	Pilocarpine	*Pilocarpus jaborandi*	*Rutaceae*

11	**Purine** **(Pyrimidine-Imidazole)**	Caffeine	*Thea sinensis* *Camellia sinensis* *Coffea arabica* *Theobroma cacao*	*Ternstroemiaceae* *Rubiaceae* *Sterculiaceae*

(Contd.)

12	**Tropolone**	Colchicine	*Colchicum autumnale*	*Liliaceae*
13	**Steroid**	Connesine	*Holarrhena anti-dysenterica*	*Apocynaceae*
		Funtumine	*Funtumia latifolia*	*Apocynaceae*
		Solanidine	*Solanum spp.*	*Solanaceae*
		Veratramine	*Veratrum grandiflorum, Veratrum viride*	*Liliaceae*
14	**Terpenoid (Diterpene)**	Aconine	*Aconitum napellus*	*Ranunculaceae*
		Aconitine (Glycoside)	–do–	–do–
		Atisine	*Aconitum heterophyllum, Aconitum anthora,*	*Ranunculaceae*
		Lycoetonine	*Aconitum lycoctonum,*	*Ranunculaceae*
15	**Pyrrolizidine**	Sennecionine	*Senecio vulgaris*	*Compositae*
		Senneciphylline	*Senecio platyphllus*	*Compositae*

It is, however, pertinent to mention at this juncture that the enormous volume of authentic information accumulated so far with regard to the isolation of **alkaloids** from a variety of plant species and their subsequent characterization by the help of latest analytical techniques they may be classified as follows:

A. **Alkaloids derived from Amination Reactions**
    (*i*) Acetate-derived Alkaloids
    (*ii*) Phenylalanine-derived Alkaloids
    (*iii*) Terpenoid Alkaloids
    (*iv*) Steroidal Alkaloids

B. **Alkaloids derived from Anthranilic Acid**
    (*i*) Quinazoline Alkaloids
    (*ii*) Quinoline Alkaloids
    (*iii*) Acridine Alkaloids

C. **Alkaloids derived from Histidine**
    Imidazole Alkaloids

D. **Alkaloids derived from Lysine**
    (*i*) Piperidine Alkaloids

(*ii*) Quinolizidine Alkaloids

(*iii*) Indolizidine Alkaloids

E. **Alkaloids derived from Nicotinic Acid**

   Pyridine Alkaloids

F. **Alkaloids derived from Ornithine**

   (*i*) Pyrrolidine Alkaloids

   (*ii*) Tropane Alkaloids

   (*iii*) Pyrrolizidine Alkaloids

G. **Alkaloids derived** from Tyrosine

   (*i*) Phenylethylamine Alkaloids

   (*ii*) Simple Tetrahydro iso-quinoline Alkaloids

   (*iii*) Modified Benzyl Tetrahydro iso-quinoline Alkaloids

H. **Alkaloids derived from Tryptophan**

   (*i*) Simple Indole Alkaloids

   (*ii*) Simple β-Carboline Alkaloids

   (*iii*) Terpenoid Indole Alkaloids

   (*iv*) Quinoline Alkaloids

   (*v*) Pyrroloindole Alkaloids

   (*vi*) Ergot Alkaloids

I. **Purine Alkaloids**

These broad and elaborated classification of the alkaloids shall now be treated individually at length in the sections that follows:

7.2.1 Alkaloids Derived from Amination Reactions

It has been duly established that the larger section of **alkaloids** are virtually derived from amino acid precursors by the help of certain specific processes that essentially introduce into the final structure not only a N-atom but also an amino acid carbon skeleton or a major part of it. However, a good number of **alkaloids** do not essentially conform with this analogy. They are usually synthesized primarily from non-amino acid precursors having the N-atom inserted into the structure at a comparatively latter stage. Interestingly, such structures are predominantly based on both steroidal and terpenoid skeletons. Besides, a few comparatively simpler **alkaloids** also appear to be derived exclusively with the help of similar late amination processes. An extensive and intensive studies on certain alkaloids it has been observed that the N-atom is specifically donated from an **amino acid source** through a *transamination reaction* using an appropriate ketone or aldehyde.

7.2.1.1 Acetate-Derived Alkaloids

Socrates was made to drink the decoction of the *Hemlock* plant and died soonafter. Thus, the poison present in it is really too dangerous for herbal administration by the uninitiated. The Hemlock plant is comprised of several potent alkaloids, such as: **coniine, γ-coniceine, conhydrine, N-methyl conine** and **pseudoconhydrine**. These **alkaloids** shall now be discussed as under:

A. Coniine

Synonyms   Cicutine, Conicine.

Biological Sources It is obtained from the unripe, fully grown dried fruits of *Conium maculatum* L. (*Umbelliferae*).

It also occurs in the plant *Aethusa cynapium* L. (*Apiaceae*) (Fool's Parsley); *Cicuta maculata* L. (*Apiaceae*) (Water Hemlock).

Chemical Structure

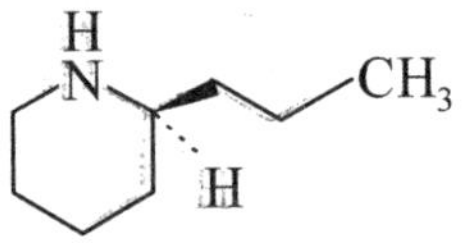

Coniine

(S)-2-Propylpiperidine. It occurs naturally as the (S)-(+)- isomer.

Isolation **Coniine** may be isolated by adopting the various following steps, namely:

(*i*) The powdered unripe, fully grown dried fruits of hemlock are mixed with a dilute solution of KOH and then subjected to stream distillation. The distillate is collected and neutrallized carefully with dilute HCl and evaporated to dryness preferably under vacuum.

(*ii*) The residue obtained as stated in (i) above is extracted with alcohol, filtered and the alcohol evaporated to dryness under vacuum. The alcohol helps in extracting the alkaloidal salts that are dissolved in water; it is then rendered alkaline either with diluted KOH solution or with dilute NH_4OH and finally extracted with ether successively.

(*iii*) The ether from the combined ethereal layer is evaporated completely, when an oily liquid consisting of the free bases remains in the residue.

(*iv*) Finally, the residue is subjected to fractional distillation in a current of H_2-gas when the alkaloids could be broadly separated and a mixture containing *coniine* and **γ-coniceine** shall pars over as the first fraction at 171-172°C. These two alkaloids are consequently made to their corresponding hydrochloride salts, evaporated to dryness and extracted with acetone. Thus, coniine hydrochloride would be separated as an insoluble product, while the **γ-coniceine** may be recovered by evaporating acetone under vacuum.

Note: Coniine enjoys the unique distinction of being the First Alkaloid produced synthetically.

Characteristic Features

(*i*) It is a colourless alkaline liquid.

(*ii*) It darkens and polymerizes on being exposed to air and light.

(*iii*) It has a mousy odour.

(*iv*) Its physical parameters are as follows: mp ~ – 2°C; bp 166-166.5°C; bp_{20} 65-66°C. d_4^{20} 0.844 – 0.848; n_D^{23} 1.4505; $[\alpha]_D^{25}$ +8.4°C (c = 4.0 in $CHCl_3$); $[\alpha]_D^{23}$ +14.6° (heat) pK_a = 3.1.

(*v*) It is steam volatile.

(*vi*) **Solubility:** 1 ml dissolves in 90 ml of water, less soluble in hot water. The base dissolves in about 25% water at room temperature. It is found to be soluble in alcohol, ether, acetone, benzene, amyl alcohol, and slightly soluble in chloroform.

Identification Tests

(*i*) It readily forms the corresponding hydrobromide ($C_8H_{17}N.HBr$), obtained as prisms, mp 211°C, 1 g dissolves in 2 ml water, 3 ml alcohol, and soluble freely in ether and chloroform.

(*ii*) Its hydrochloride ($C_8H_{17}N . HCl$) forms rhomboids, mp 221°C, freely soluble in water, alcohol and chloroform.

(*iii*) It gives a red colouration with sodium nitroprusside slowly, which on addition of acetaldehyde changes to violet or blue.

Caution **It exhibits potential symptoms of over exposure as: weakness, drowsiness, parasthesias, ataxia, nausea, excessive salivation, and bradycardia followed by tachycardia.***

Uses Externally, the coniine salts are used as ointments and infrequently employed for their local analgesic action in the symptomatic relief of pruritis, hemorrhoids and fissures.

B. γ-Coniceine

Biological Source It is obtained from the seeds of *Conium maculatum* L. (*Umbelliferae*).

Chemical Structure

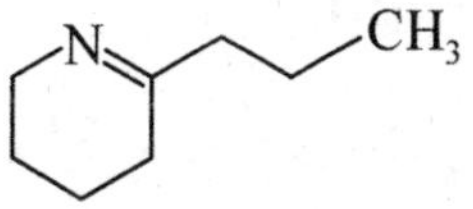

γ-Coniceine

2, 3, 4, 5-Tetrahydro-6-propylpyridine.

Characteristic Features

(*i*) It is a colourless liquid alkaloid.

(*ii*) It possesses a distinct mousy odour.

(*iii*) It is steam volatile.

(*iv*) Its physical parameters are: bp 171°C; d_4^{15} 0.8753; n_D^{16} 1.4661.

(*v*) It is slightly soluble in water, but freely soluble in ethanol, chloroform and ether.

Identification Test

(*i*) **γ-Coniceine** when subjected to reduction, it gives rise to a racemic mixture of *dl*-coniine.

(*ii*) It forms **γ-coniceine hydrochloride** ($C_8H_{15}N.HCl$) which gives hygroscopic crystals from ether mp 143°C.

C. Conhydrine

Biological Source It is obtained from the seeds of *Conium maculatum* L. (*Umbelliferae*).

---

* Gosselin *et al.* Eds. **Clinical Toxicology of Commercial Products,** Williams and Wilkins, Baltimore, 5th ed., Sec-II., pp. 249-250 (1984).

Chemical Structure

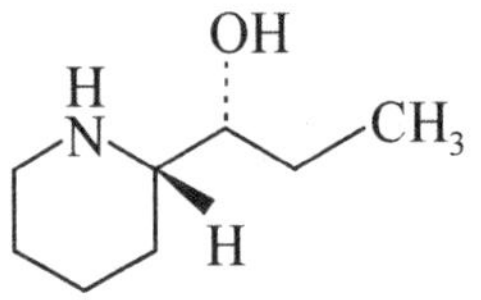

Conhydrine

[R-(R*, S*)-α-Ethyl-2-piperidine methanol.

Characteristic Features

(*i*) The crystals obtained from ether has mp 121°C, bp 226°C and [α]$_D$ + 10°C.

(*ii*) It is slightly soluble in water, but easily soluble in ethanol, ether and chloroform.

D. N-Methylconiine

Biological Source   It is same as for (C) above.

Chemical Structure

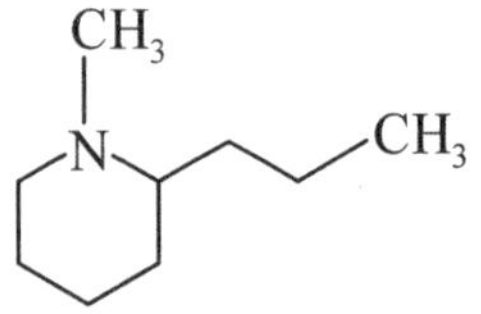

N-Methylconiine

1-Methyl-2-propylpiperidine.

Isolation   The *d*-form is stated to occur in Hemlock in small quantities, while the *l*-form may be isolated from residues left in the preparation of **coniine** by crystallization of the hydrobromides.

Characteristic Features   The physical characteristic features of *dl*, *d*- and *l*-forms are given below:

Form	Nature	bp (°C)	d^{24}	$[\alpha]_D^{24}$	n_D^{13}	Solubility
dl-	–	bp 10.5 56.6	–	–	–	–
d-	Oily liquid	173-174	0.8318	+ 81°	1.4538	Slightly in water, soluble in organic solvents
l-	–	–	0.8318	– 84°	1.4538	Slightly in water, soluble in organic solvents

E. Pseudoconhydrine

Biological Source   Its biological source is same as for (A) through (D) above.

Chemical Structure

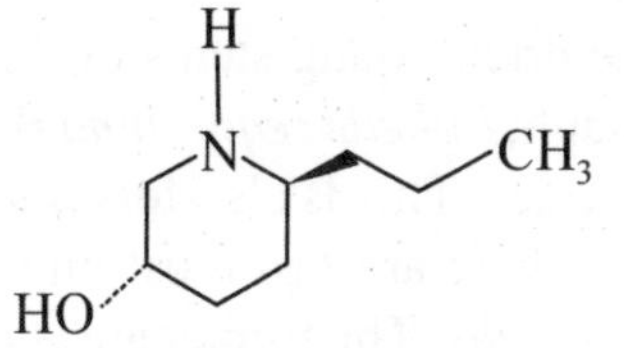

Pseudoconhydrine

(3S-*trans*)-6-Propyl-3-piperidinol.

Characteristic Features

(*i*) It gives hygroscopic needles from absolute ether.
(*ii*) Its mp stands at 106°C, whereas its monohydrate, scales, gives mp 60°C from moist ether.
(*iii*) Its physical parameters are: bp 236°C ; $[\alpha]_D^{20} + 11°$ (c = 10 in alcohol); pK (18°C): 3.70
(*iv*) It is soluble in water and

Identification Tests   It readily forms the hydrochloride salt ($C_8H_{17}NO.HCl$) as the crystals from ethanol having mp 213°C.

Biosynthesis of γ-Coniceine and Coniine   A fatty acid precursor **octanoic acid (capric acid)** is employed, which is subsequently transformed into the ketoaldehyde through successive oxidation and reduction steps. The resulting ketoaldehyde acts as a substrate for a transamination reaction, the amino moiety is derived from L-alanine. The ultimate transformation lead to the formation of imine giving the heterocyclic ring present in **γ-coniceine**, and then reduction the **coniine** as shown below:

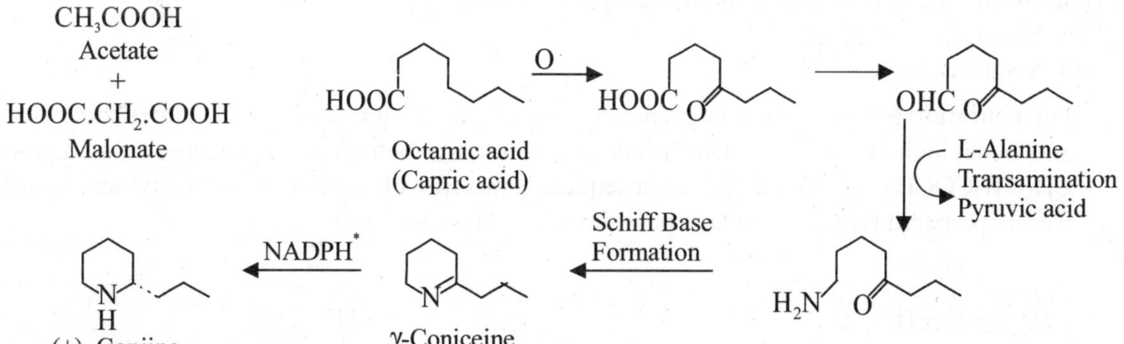

7.2.1.2 Phenylalanine-Derived Alkaloids

It has been observed that the aromatic amino acid **L-tyrosine** is not only a common but also an extremely vital precursor of **alkaloids;** whereas, **L-phenylalanine** is found to be much less frequently employed, and normally it specifically contributes *carbon atoms only*, such as: C_6C_1, C_6C_2 or C_6C_3 units, without making available a N-atom from its amino function *e.g.*, as in the biosynthesis of **colchicine** and **lobeline**.

   The various typical examples of phenylalanine-derived alkaloids are: **ephedrine, norpseudoephedrine (cathine)** and **capsaicin**, which shall be described hereunder:

A. Ephedrine

Biological Source   It occurs in the dried young stems of the Chinese wonder drug **Ma Huang**, *Emhedra vulgaris*, *Ephedra sinica* Stapf., *Ephedra equisetina* Bunge belonging to family *Ginetaceae*, and also in several other Ephedra species. This is also found in *Ephedra geradiana* Wall ex. Stapf. (*Ephedraceae*) (Pakistani Ephedra). There are *two* most important forage ephedras in the United States, namely: *E. nevadensis* and *E. viridis*. The former are is *E. nevadensis* S. Wats (*Ephedraceae*) and known as **Mormon Tea** and **Nevada Jointfir.**

Chemical Structure

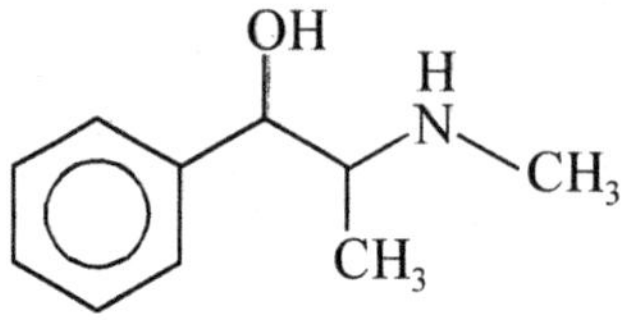

Ephedrine

α-[1-(Methylamino)ethyl] benzene methanol ($C_{10}H_{15}HO$).

Isolation   **Ephedrine** usually exists singly in *Ephedra sinica* (1-3%) and *E. equisetina* (2%). However, it occurs in association with ┼-**Ephedrine** (*i.e.*, **pseudoephedrine**) in *E. vulgaris*.

However, the ephedrine and **pseudoephedrine** may be extracted conveniently from the dried young stems of the plant material by adopting the 'general procedures for alkaloid extraction' (section 1.7.3), by the help of successive benzene and dilute HCl extractions.

Preparation   Ephedrine may be prepared by *two* methods, namely:
   (*i*) Fermentation method, and
   (*ii*) Synthetic method.

(*a*) **Fermentation Method:** It can be prepared commercially by fermenting a mixture of molasses* and benzaldehyde. The reaction product *i.e.*, methyl benzyl alcohol ketone *i.e.*, C_6H_5-$CH(OH)COCH_3$, a keto-alcohol is subsequently mixed with a solution of methyl amine and freshly prepared H_2-gas is made to pass though it. Thus, we have:

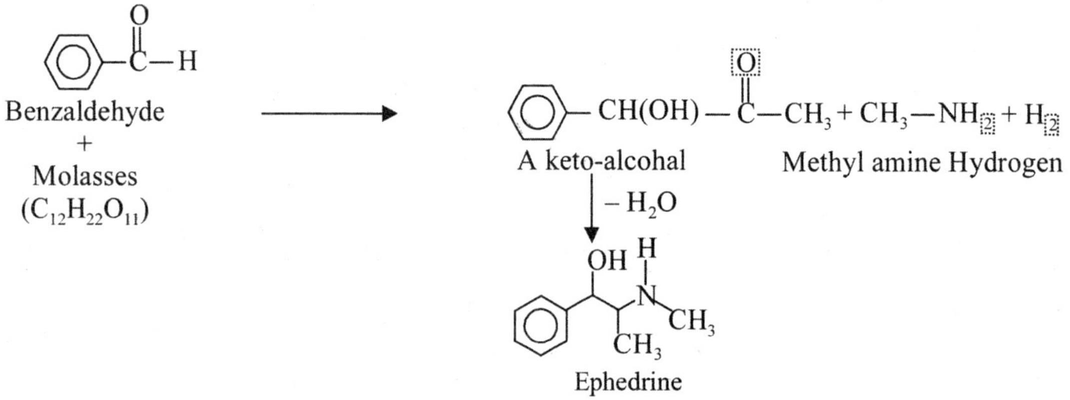

---

* **Molasses:** A thick brown viscous liquid obtained as a by product of '*Sugar Industry*' containing 8-10% cane sugar.

(b) **Synthetic Method:** Manske *et al.** (1929) synthesized **(±)-Ephedrine** by the catalytic reduction of 1-phenylpropane-1, 2-dione (or benzoylacetyl) in the presence of methylamine in methanol solution as given below:

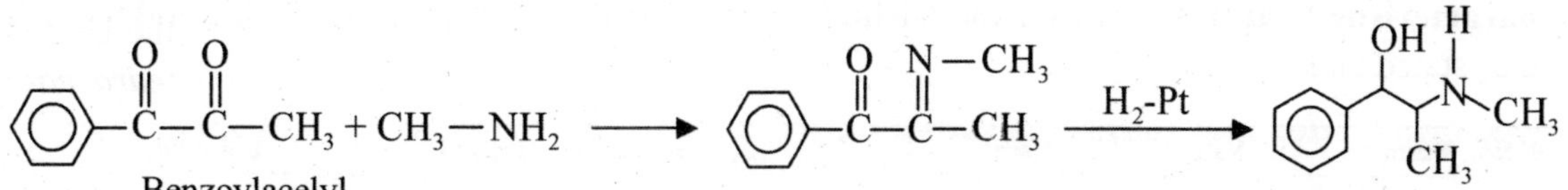

Benzoylacelyl

H_2-Pt

(±)–Ephedrine

Stereochemistry Since the **ephedrine** molecule contains *two* dissimilar chiral centres, four optically active isomers (or two pairs of enantiomers) are possible theoretically. Freudenberg (1932) put forward the following configurations of **ephedrine** and **ψ-ephedrine** (mp 118°C, $[\alpha]_D \pm 51.2°$) are as follows:

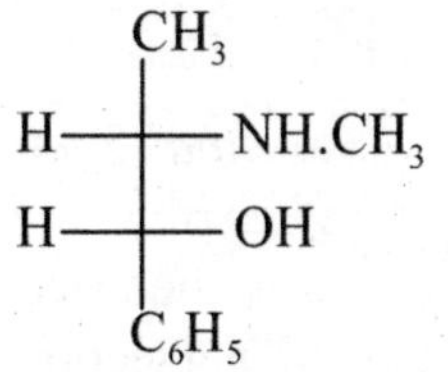

D(–)-Ephedrine 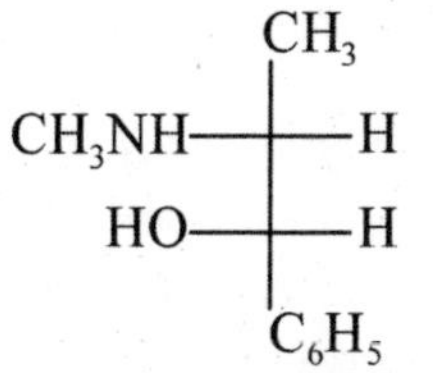   L(+)-Ephedrine 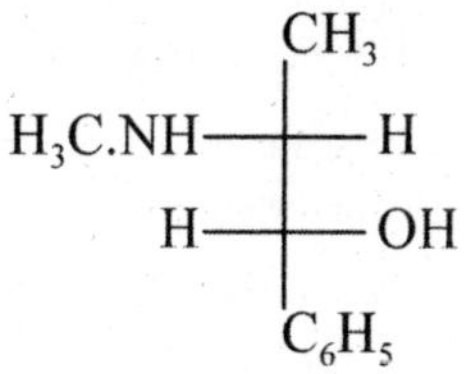   D(–)-ψ-Ephedrine 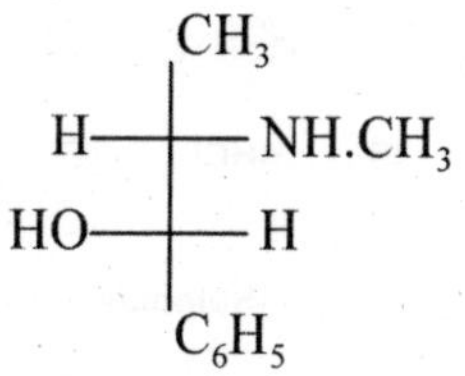   L(+)-ψ-Ephedrine

Foder *et al.* (1949, 1950) confirmed that the ephedrine has the *erythro*-configuration, and ψ-ephedrine the *threo*-configuration as stated below:

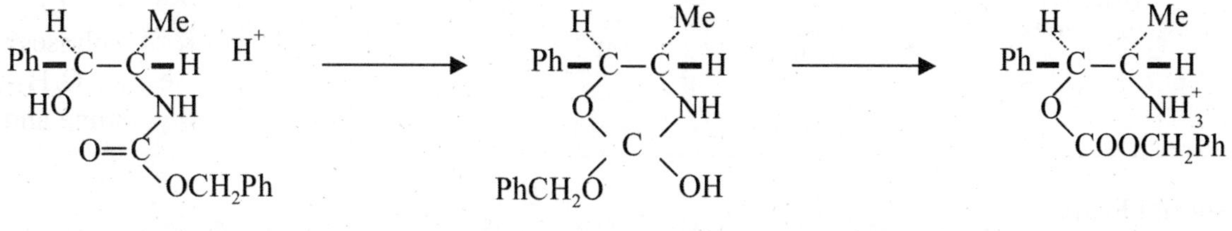

The carbobenzoxy derivative of **nor-Ψ-ephedrine** undergoes intramolecular rearrangement to the *O*-derivative in an acidic medium. In case, **nor-Ψ-ephedrine** possesses the *threo*-configuration, then this ultimately gives rise to the favourable *trans*-orientation of the phenyl and methyl groups in the cyclic intermediate *i.e.*, the **steric repulsions** are at a bear minimum level. Likewise, the **nor-ephedrine** shall, therefore, exhibit essentially the *crythro*-configuration; and it was further revealed that its corresponding N-carbobenzoxy derivative does not undergo any molecular rearrangement whatsoever in an acidic environment to produce the *O*-derivative. Therefore, one may infer that the steric repulsions that would take place between the phenyl and methyl groups in

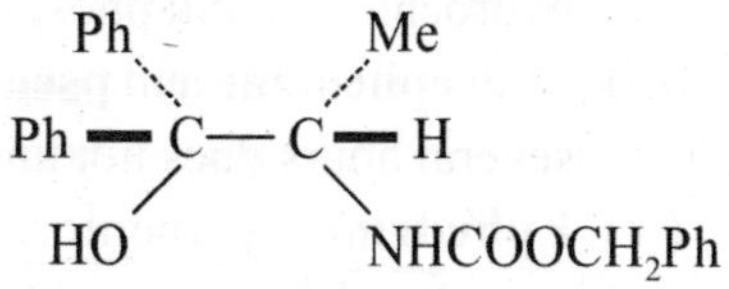

Nor-Ephedrine

---

* Manske and Holmes (eds). **The Alkaloids**, Academic Press. N. York. Vol. 1 (1950)

the cyclic intermediate is evidently too high to allow its subsequent formation. Thus, it is absolutely possible, on this basis, to differentiate and distinguish between the stereoisomers of **ephedrine** and **Ψ-ephedrine.**

Characteristic Features   The characteristic features of various forms of **ephedrine** and its salts are as stated under:

S. No.	Form	Nature	Name	mp (°C)	bp (°C)	[µ]D25	Solubility
1.	*dl-*	Crystals	Racephedrine, Racemic ephedrine	79	–	–	Soluble in waver, ethanol, ether, chloroform, oils.
2.	*dl-*HCl	-do-	Ephetonin, Racephedrine HCl	187–188	–	–	1 g dissolves in 4 ml water, in 40 ml of 95% alcohol at 20°C. Insoluble in ether
3.	*dl-* Sulphate	-do-	Racephedrine Sulphate	247	–	–	Soluble in water and ethanol
4.	*l-*HCl	Crystals, waxy solid, granules	L-Erythro-2-(methylamino)-1-phenylpropan-1-ol.	34	255	–	1 g dissolves in 20 ml H_2O, 0.2 ml ethanol, soluble in chloroform, ether, oils.
5.	*l-*HCl	Ortho-rhombic needles	Ephedral, Sanedrine	216–220	–	–30 to –35.5° (c = 5)	1 g dissolves in 3 ml water, 14 ml ethanol; In soluble in ether and chloroform
6.	*l-*Sulphate	-do-	–	245 (dec.)	–	–29.5 to –32.0° (c = 5)	1 g dissolves in 1.2 ml water, 95 ml ethanol; Freely soluble in hot alcohol.
7.	*d-*Pseudo-ephedrine	Rhombic tablets	*d-*Ψ-ephedrine, *d-*iso-ephedrine	119	–	+51° (c = 0.6 in alc.)	Sparingly soluble in water (differs from *l-*ephedrine). Freely soluble in alc. or ether.
8.	*d-*Pseudo-ephedrine hydrochloride	Needles	Galseud, Novafed, Rhinalair, Otrinol, Sinufed, Sudafed, Symptom-2,	181 to 182	–	+ 62° (c = 0.8)	Soluble in water, alcohol and chloroform

Special Features

   (*i*) **Ephedrine** does not yield a precipitate with Mayer's Reagent except in concentrated solution.

   (*ii*) Ephedrine in chloroform solution after long standing or on evaporation usually forms ephedrine hydrochloride and phosgene.

   (*iii*) Both **ephedrine** and **pseudoephedrine** are fairly stable to heat and when heated at 100°C for several hours does not undergo any decomposition.

   (*iv*) **Ephedrine** hydrochloride on being heated with 25% HCl gets partially converted to **pseudoephedrine**; and this conversion is reversible and soon attains on equilibrium.

Identification Tests

   (*i*) **Colour Test:** Dissolve 0.1 g ephedrine in 1 ml water with the addition of a few drops of dilute HCl. Add to it two drops of $CuSO_4$ solution (5% w/v) followed by a few-drops of NaOH (1N) solution when a reddish colour is obtained. Add to it 2-3 ml of ether and shake vigorously, the ethereal layer becomes purple and the aqueous layer turns blue.

(*ii*) **Formation of Ephedrine Hydrochloride:** Dissolve 0.2-0.3g of ephedrine in 35 ml of chloroform in a stoppered test tube and shake vigorously. Allow it to stand for 12 hours and evaporate the chloroform, when crystals of ephedrine HCl are obtained, and

(*iii*) **Formation of Benzaldehyde Odour:** Take 0.05 g of ephedrine in a small porcelain dish and triturate it with a few crystals of pure potassium ferricyanide, $[K_3Fe(CN)_6]$, add a few drops of water and heat on a water-bath, it gives rise to a distinct odour of *benzaldehyde.*

Biosynthesis of Ephedrine Alkaloids   Interestingly, phenylalanine and ephedrine not only have the same carbon and nitrogen atoms but also have the same arrangement of C and N-atoms *i.e.*, the skeleton of atoms. Noticeably, L-phenylalanine is a precursor, possessing only seven carbons, a C_6C_1 fragment, gets actually incorporated. It has been observed that phenylalanine undergoes metabolism, probably *via* cinnamic acid to benzoic acid; and this perhaps in the form of its coenzyme–A ester, which is acylated with pyruvic acid and undergoes decarboxylation during the addition as shown below.

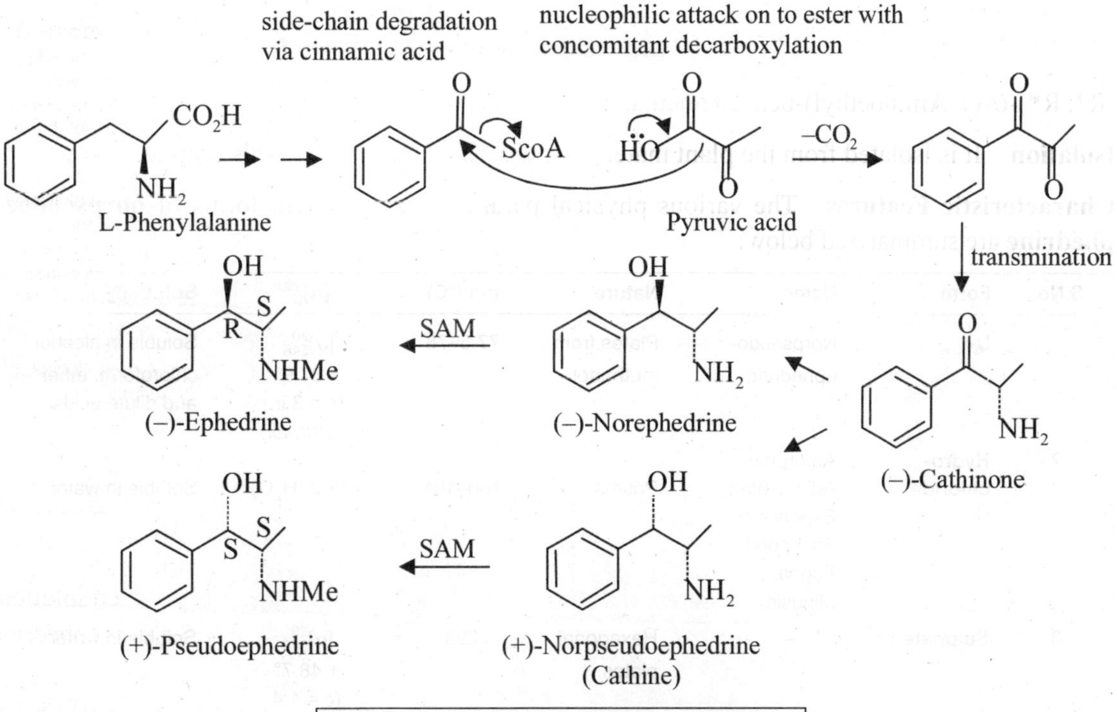

Biosynthesis of Ephedrine Alkaloids

A thiamine PP-mediated mechanism is put forward for the formation of the diketone, and a transamination reaction shall give rise to **cathinone.** Further reduction of the carbonyl moiety from either face yields the diastereomeric **norephedrine** or **norpseudoephedrine (Cathine).** Ultimately, N-methylation would give rise to **ephedrine** or **pseudoephedrine.**

Uses

1. The *l*-**ephedrine** is extensively used as a bronchodilator.
2. The *d*-**psendoephedrine** is employed widely as a decongestant.

B. Norpseudoephedrine

Synonyms   Cathine; Katine; Nor-ψ-ephedrine.

Biological Sources   It occurs naturally as the D-*threo*-form in the leaves of the **khat plant**, *Catha edulis* Forsk. (*Celastraceae*), which is widely found as an evergreen shrub native to Southern Arabia and Ethiopia. It is also found in relatively smaller amounts in the South American tree *Maytenus krukovii* A.C. Smith (*Celastraceae*); and in the mother liquors obtained from **Ma Huang** after the recovery of **ephedrine**.

Chemical Structure

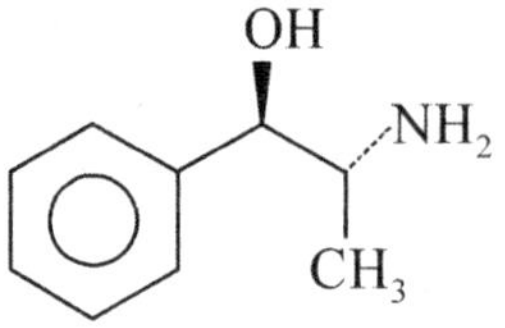

Norpseudoephedrine

(R*, R*)-α-(1-Aminoethyl)-benzenemethanol.

Isolation   It is isolated from the plant material as described under (A) in this section.

Characteristic Features   The various physical parameters of different forms of **norpseudoephedrine** are summarized below:

S.No.	Form	Name	Nature	mp (°C)	$[\alpha]_D^{20}$	Solubility
1.	D-	Norpseudo-ephedrine	Plates from methanol	77.5–78	$[\alpha]_{546}^{20}$ + 37.9° (c = 3 in methanol)	Soluble in alcohol chloroform, ether, and dilute acids
2.	Hydro-chloride	Amorphan, Adiposetten, Exponcit N, Fasupond, Fugoa, Minusin	Prisms	180–181	+43.2 (H₂O)	Soluble in water
3.	Sulphate	–	Hexagonal plates.	298	$[\alpha]_{546}^{20}$ + 48.7° (c = 1.4 in H₂O)	Soluble in water
4.	*dl*-Hydro-chloride	–	Crystals	169–171	–	Soluble in water

Uses

1. It is widely employed as an anorexic.
2. It is also used in the optical resolution of externally compensated acids.

C. Capsaicin

Synonyms   Axsain; Mioton; Zostrix.

Biological Source It is the pungent principle obtained in the fruit of various species of **Capsicum**, *viz.*, *Capsicum annum* L. (*Solanaceae*) (Chilli, **Sweet Peppers, Paprika**).

Chemical Structure

Capsaicin

(E)-N-[4-Hydroxy-3-methoxyphenyl)-methyl]-8-methyl-6-noenamide. It is phenolic in nature.

Isolation The **capsicum fruits** are crushed and extracted with either hot acetone or ethanol by using the method of percolation. The solvent *i.e.*, hot acetone or ethanol is evaporated under vacuum. The residue is extracted once again with successive quantities of warm acetone or ethanol until and unless the marc is completely free from any pungent principles. It contains approximately not less than 8% of **capsaicin**.

Characteristic Features
1. **Capsaicin** gives a distinct burning taste even when diluted to the extent of one part in one million parts of water. However, its pungency is destroyed by oxidation.
2. It is obtained as monoclinic, rectangular plates, scales from petroleum ether, having mp 65°C.
3. It has $bp_{0.01}$ 210-220°C (air-bath temperature).
4. It has uv maximum: 227, 281 nm ($\in$ 7000, 2500).
5. It is freely soluble in ether, benzene, chloroform; slightly soluble in CS_2; and practically in soluble in water.

Identification Tests
1. An alcoholic solution of **capsaicin** gives rise to a distinct bluish green colour upon adding a few drops of $FeCl_3$ solution (0.5% w/v).
2. When capsaicin is dissolved in a few drops of concentrated H_2SO_4 and a few crystals of sucrose is added, it yields a violet colour after a few hours.

Uses
1. It is used as a topical analgesic.
2. It is often employed as a tool in neurobiological research.
3. It is used in creams to counter neuralgia caused by herpes infections and in other pain-relieving formulations.

Biosynthesis of Capsaicin The aromatic fragment of the **capsaicin** molecule is derived solely from phenylalanine through chemical entities, *viz.*, **ferulic acid** and **vanillin**. The later compound, an aldehyde, is actually the substrate for transamination to yield **vanillylamine**. However, the acid part of the resulting amide structure is of polypeptide origin having essentially a branched-chain fatty acyl-CoA which is produced by chain extension of isobutyryl-CoA. The aforesaid source of reactions are as given under:

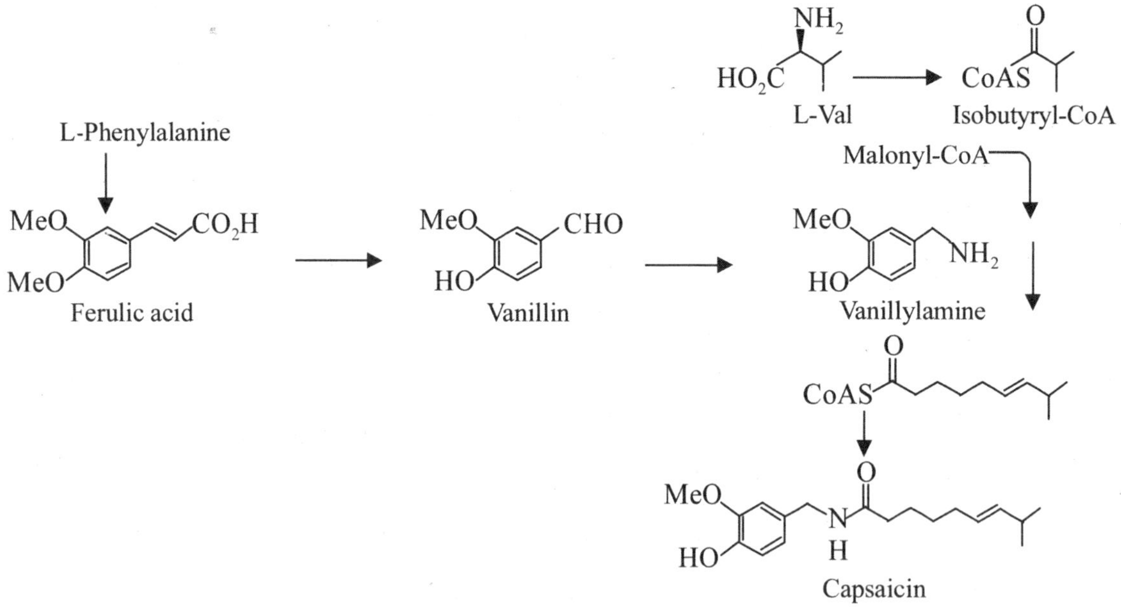

Biosynthesis of Capsaicin

7.2.1.3 Terpenoid Alkaloids

A plethora of **alkaloids** solely based on mono-, sesqui-, di-, and tri-terpenoid skeletons have been isolated and characterized. However, logistic and scientific information (s) with regard to their actual formation in nature is more or less sparse. It has been observed that the monoterpene alkaloids are derived from the structurally related **iridoid materials**, wherein the O-atom in the heterocyclic ring is replaced by a N-containing ring as depicted below.

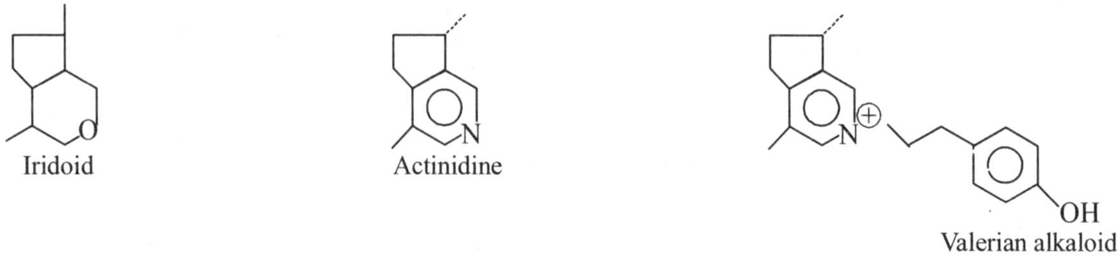

Terpenoid Alkaloids

A few typical examples of the **terpenoid alkaloids** are, namely: **aconine** and **actinitine**, which shall be discussed in the sections that follow:

A. Aconine

Biological Source   **Aconine** is the hydrolyzed product of aconitine which is obtained from the dried roots of *Aconitum napellus* Linn. (*Ranunculaceae*) and other aconites. *A. napellus* in also known as **aconite, blue rocket** and **monkshood**. Usually it contains upto 0.6% of the total alkaloids of aconite, of which approximately one third is the alkaloid **aconitine**.

Chemical Structure   (1α, 3α, 6α, 14α, 15α, 16α)-20-Ethyl-1, 6-16-trimethoxy-4-(methoxy-methyl) aconitane-3, 8, 13, 14, 15-pentol.

Isolation The alkaloid **aconitine** is subjected to hydrolysis which yields benzoyl aconine and acetic acid. The resulting benzoyl aconine is further hydrolyzed to yield aconine and benzoic acid. **Aconine** being very soluble in water may be separated easily from the less water-soluble by product, *i.e.*, benzoic acid.

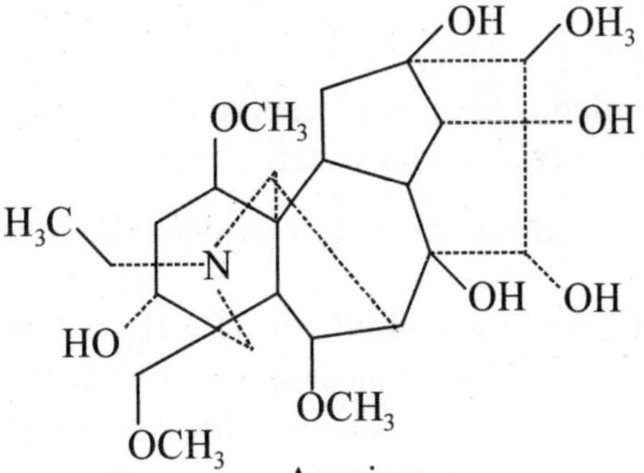

Aconine

Characteristic Features

(*i*) It is an amorphous powder with a bitter taste.

(*ii*) It has mp 132°C, $[\alpha]_D + 23°$ and pK_a 9.52.

(*iii*) It is extremely soluble in water, alcohol; moderately soluble in chloroform and slightly soluble in benzene. It is practically insoluble in ether and petroleum ether.

Identification Tests It forms *two* distinct derivatives as given below:

(*a*) **Aconine Hydrochloride Dihydrate ($C_{25}H_{42}ClNO_9.2H_2O$):** It is obtained as crystals having mp 175-176°C and $[\alpha]_D-8°$.

(*b*) **Aconine Hydrobromide Sesquihydrate ($C_{25}H_{42}BrNO_9 .1½ H_2O$]:** It is obtained as crystals from water with mp 225°C.

Uses

1. It is used in the treatment of neuralgia, sciatica, rheumatism and inflammation.

2. It is employed occasionally as analgesic and cardiac depressant.

B. Aconitine

Biological Source The bolanical source is the same as described under (A) above.

Chemical Structure

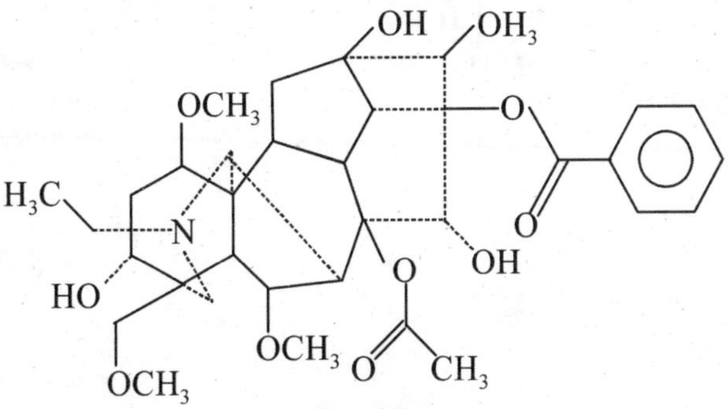

Aconitine

(1α, 3α, 6α, 14α, 15α, 16(β)-20-Ethyl-1, 6,-16-trimethoxy-4-(methoxymethyl) aconitane-3, 8, 13, 14, 15,-pentol 8-acetate 14-benzoate ($C_{34}H_{47}NO_{11}$).

Characteristic Features

1. It occurs as hexagonal plates having mp 204°C.
2. Its pK_a value stands at 5.88.
3. Its specific rotation $[\alpha]_D$ + 17.3° (Chloroform).
4. It is slightly soluble in petroleum ether; but 1 g dissolves in 2 ml chloroform, 7 ml benzene, 28 ml absolute ethanol, 50 ml ether, 3300 ml water.

Identification Tests   **Aconitine** forms specific salts with HBr and HNO_3 having the following physical parameters.

(a) **Aconitine Hydrobromide Hemipentahydrate ($C_{34}H_{47}O_{11}$.HBr.2½ H_2O):** The hexagonal tablets mp 200-207°C and the dried substance mp 115-120°C. Its crystals obtained from ethanol and ether with ½ H_2O has mp 206-207°C. Its specific rotation $[\alpha]_D$ – 30.9°.

(b) **Aconitine Nitrate ($C_{34}H_{47}NO_{11}$.HNO_3):** The crystals have mp about 200°C (decomposes), $[\alpha]_D^{20}$ – 35° (c = 2 in H_2O).

Uses

1. It is exclusively used in producing heart arrythmia in experimental animals.
2. It has also been used topically in neuralgia.

Biosynthesis of Aconitine-Type Alkaloids   **Aconite** is particularly regarded as extremely toxic, due to the presence of **aconitine,** and closely related C_{19} **nonditerpenoid alkaloids.** It has been observed that the species of *Delphinium* accumulate **diterpenoid alkaloids,** for instance: **atisine,** which proved to be much less toxic when compared to aconitine. A vivid close resemblance of their structural relationship to diterpenes, such as: **ent-kaurene,** of course, little experimental evidence is available.

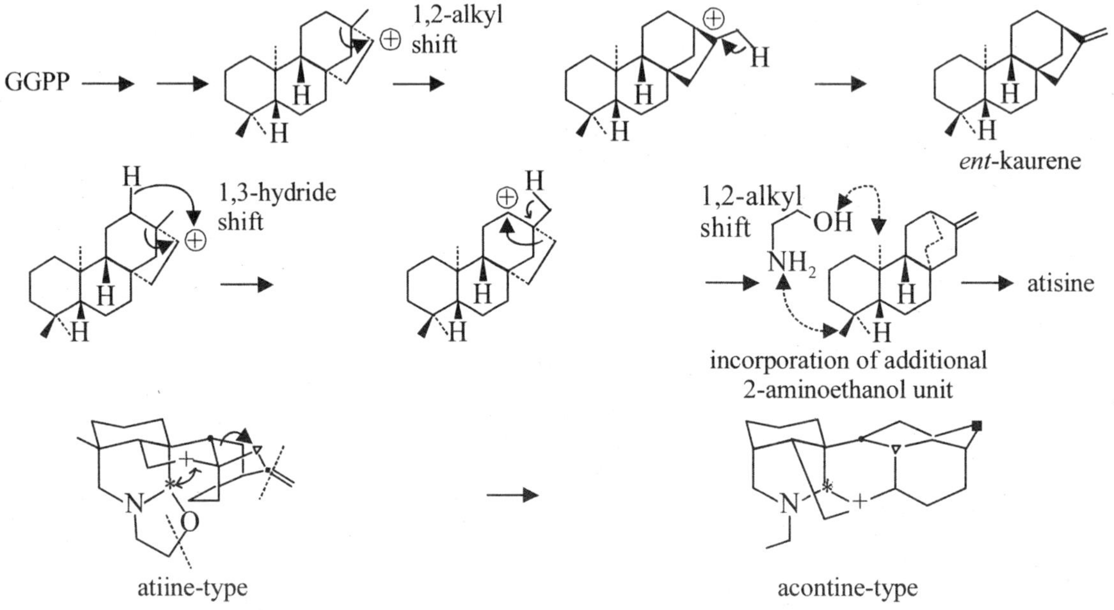

ent-kaurene

atisine

incorporation of additional 2-aminoethanol unit

atiine-type

acontine-type

Biosynthesis of Aconitine-Type Alkaloids

From the above course of reactions it appears quite feasible that:

(*a*) A **pre-*ent*-kaurene** carbocation usually undergoes **Wagner-Meerwein Rearrangements,**

(*b*) The **atisine-skeleton** is produced subsequently by incorporating an N–CH$_2$–CH$_2$–O fragment (*e.g.,* from 2-aminoethanol) to form the resulting heterocyclic rings,

(*c*) The **aconitine-skeleton** is perhaps formed from the **atisine-skeleton** by further modifications as stated above,

(*d*) A rearrangement process converts two fused 6-membered rings into a (7 + 5)-membered bicyclic system, and

(*e*) One carbon from the exocyclic double bond is eliminated.

7.2.1.4 Steroidal Alkaloids

In general, the **steroidal alkaloids** represent an important class of alkaloids that essentially afford a close structural relationship to sterols *i.e.*, they contain a perhydro-1, 2-cyclopentanophenanthrene nucleus. Interestingly, these group of alkaloids invariably occur in the plant kingdom as glycosidal combination with carbohydrate moieties.

The **steroidal alkaloids** may be broadly classified into *two* major groups, namely:

(*a*) Solanum Alkaloids, and

(*b*) Veratrum Alkaloids.

These two class of alkaloids shall now be discussed in an elaborated fashion hereunder:

A. Solanum Alkaloids

A good number of plants belonging to the natural order *Solanaceae* have been found to accumulate favourably several **steroidal alkaloids** based on a C_{27} *cholestane skeleton*, such as: **solasodine, tomatidine, solanidine.** These alkaloids usually occur in a wide variety of the genus *Solanum*, for instance: *Solanum laciniatum; S. dulcamara* Linn.; *S. nigrum* Linn.; *S. torvum* Swartz.; *S. lycopersicum* Linn.; (*Lycopersicon exculentum* Mill); *S. tuberosum*; *S. aviculare* etc. The three above mentioned alkaloids normally occur naturally in the plant as their corresponding glycosides. However, the two species of *Solanum*, namely: *S. laciniatum* and *S. aviculare* are considered to be a rich source of alkaloids (*i.e.*, the aglycone moieties) that are employed exclusively as the starting materials for the synthesis of several hormones and adreno-cortical steroids.

The **solanum alkaloids**, stated above are essentially the nitrogen-analogues of steroidal saponins. Unlike, their *oxygen* counterparts, all these N-containing alkaloids exhibit the same stereochemistry at C-25 (methyl being equatorial always), but C-22 isomers do exist, such as: solasodine and tomatidine.

The above cited *three* members of the **solanum alkaloids** shall be discussed as under:

A.1 Solasodine

Synonyms Solancarpidine; Solanidine-S; Purapuridine.

Biological Sources It is obtained from the fruits of *Capsicum annuum* L. (*Solanaceae*) (**Chili, Paprika, Sweet Peppers**); shoots and berries of *S. dulcamara* L. (*Solanaceae*) (**Bittersweet, Bitter**

---

* GGPP = Geranylgeranyl diphosphate

Nightshade, Felonwood); leaves of *S. nigrum* L. (*Solanaceae*) (**Wonderberry, Black Nightshade, Prairie Huckleberry**).

Chemical Structure

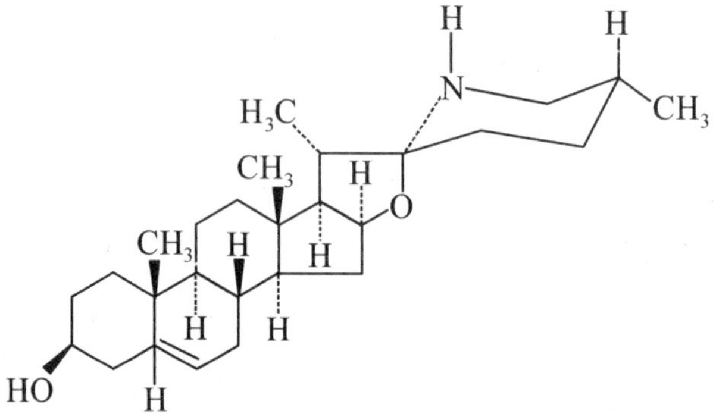

Solasodine

(3β, 22α, 25R)-Spirosol-5-en-3-ol; ($C_{27}H_{43}NO_2$).

Isolation It is obtained by the hydrolysis of **solasonine** which yields **solasodine**, L-rhamnose, D-galactose and D-glucose respectively. It is the dehydrated product.

Characteristic Features

(*i*) It is obtained as hexagonal plates from methanol or by sublimation under high vacuum.

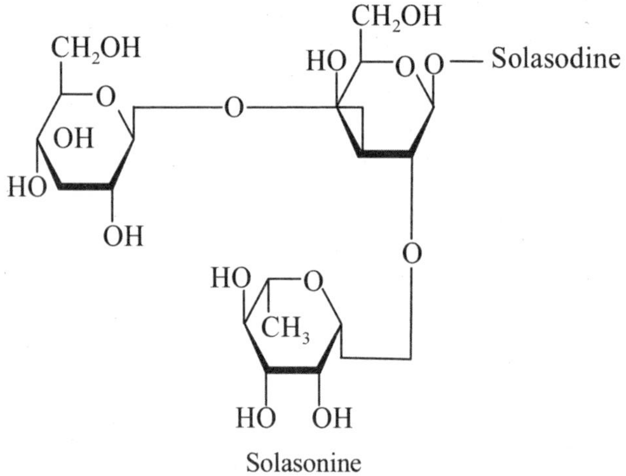

Solasonine

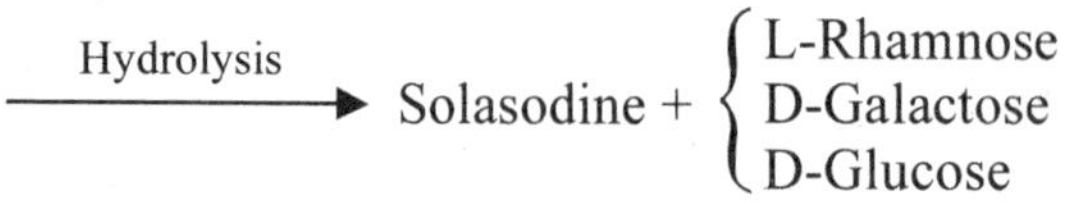

$$\xrightarrow[\text{Hydrolysis}]{} \text{Solasodine} + \begin{cases} \text{L-Rhamnose} \\ \text{D-Galactose} \\ \text{D-Glucose} \end{cases}$$

(*ii*) It has mp 200-202°C; $[\alpha]_D^{25} - 98°C$ [c = 0.14 in methanol); $[\alpha]_D -113°$ ($CHCl_3$); pK_b 6.30.

(*iii*) It is freely soluble in benzene, pyridine, and chloroform; moderately soluble in ethanol, methanol, and acetone; slightly soluble in water and practically insoluble in ether.

Identification Tests (for Solanum Alkaloids)

1. Dissolve 5-10 mg of the alkaloid in a few drops of hot amyl alcohol or ethanol and allow it cool gradually. The appearance of jelly-like product gives the characteristic test of the solanum alkaloids.

2. When a few mg of the alkaloids is treated with antimony trichloride solution in dry chloroform, it gives rise to a distinct red colouration.

3. The **solanum alkaloids**, in general, produces an instant red-violet colour with formaldehyde (HCHO) and sulphuric acid (H_2SO_4). This particular test is so distinct and sensitive that it is used for the quantitative estimation of these alkaloids colorimetrically.

Uses   It is invariably used as a starting material for steroidal drugs.

A.2 Tomatidine

Biological Source   It is obtained from the roots of Rutgers tomato plant [*Lycopersicon esculentum* Mill., cultivar. "Rutgers"] (*Solanaceae*) (Tomato).

Chemical Structure   (3β, 5α, 22β, 25 S)-Spirosolan-3-ol; ($C_{27}H_{45}NO_2$).

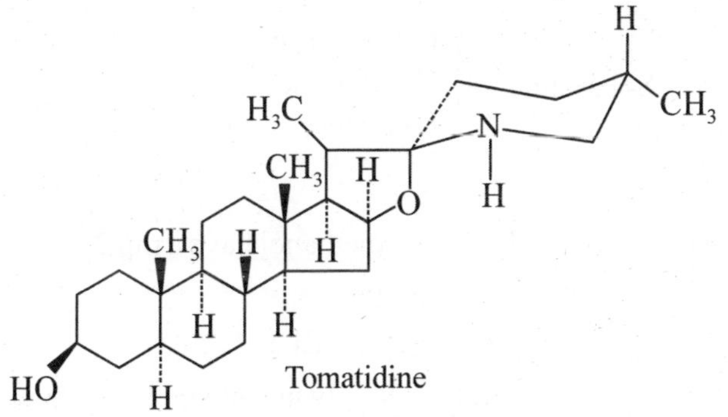

Tomatidine

Characteristic Features

1. It is obtained as plates from ethyl acetate having mp 202-206°C.

2. It specific rotation $[\alpha]_D^{25} + 8°$ (chloroform).

Isolation   It is obtained by the hydrolysis of **tomatine** to yield a molecule of **tomatidine** along with 2 moles of D-glucose, 1-mole of D-xylose and 1-mole of D-galactose as depicted below:

$$\text{Tomatine} \xrightarrow{\text{Hydrolysis}} \text{Tomatidine} + \begin{cases} 2 \text{ moles of D-Glucose} \\ 1 \text{ mole of D-Xylose} \\ 1 \text{ mole of D-Galactose} \end{cases}$$

Identification Test   Its hydrochloride derivative ($C_{27}H_{45}NO_2 . HCl$) is obtained as crystals from absolute ethanol having mp 265-270°C and $[\alpha]_D^{25} - 5°$ (methanol).

A.3 Solanidine

Synonym   Solatubine.

Biological Source   The plant of *Capsicum annuum* L. (*Solanaceae*) (**Chili, Peppers, Paprika**) contains **solanidine**.

Chemical Structure

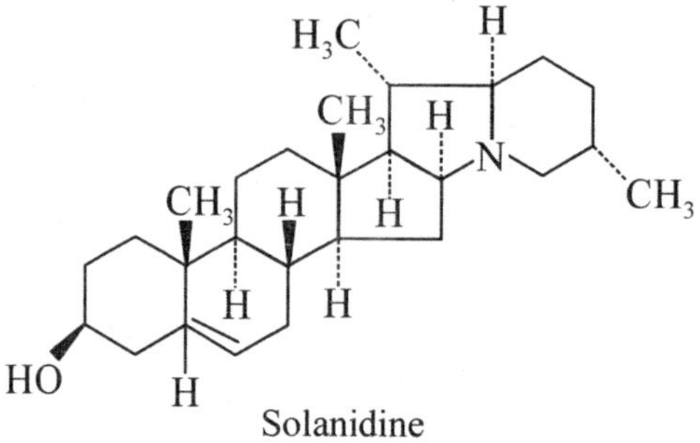

Solanidine

(3β)-Solanid-5 en-3-ol; ($C_{27}H_{43}NO$).

Isolation   It is obtained by the hydrolysis of **solanine** which yields one mole each of L-Rhamnose, D-Galactose, and D-Glucose as shown below.

$$\text{Solanine} \xrightarrow{\text{Hydrolysis}} \text{Solanidine} + \begin{cases} \text{L-Rhamnose} \\ \text{D-Galactose} \\ \text{D-Glucose} \end{cases}$$

Characteristic Features

1. The long needles obtained from chloroform-methanol have a mp 218-219°C. It usually sublimes very close to its mp with slight decomposition.

2. It is specific rotation $[\alpha]_D^{21} - 29°$ (c = 0.5 in $CHCl_3$).

3. It is freely soluble in benzene, chloroform, slightly in methanol and ethanol; and almost insoluble in ether and water.

Identification Tests   The same as described under A.1. earlier in this section. Besides, it has the following specific features for the corresponding derivatives, namely:

(*a*) **Hydrochloride Derivative: ($C_{27}H_{43}NO.HCl$):** Prisms from 80% alcohol and gets decomposed at 345°C.

(*b*) **Methyliodide Derivative: ($C_{27}H_{43}NO.CH_3I$):** Crystals from 50% (v/v) ethanol and decomposes at 286°C.

(*c*) **Acetylsolanidine Derivative: ($C_{29}H_{45}NO_2$):** Crystals obtained from ethanol having mp 208°C.

Biosynthesis of Solasodine, Tomatidine and Solanidine   Like the **sapogenins**, the **steroidal alkaloids** are also derived from *cholesterol*, with suitable side-chain modification during the course of biochemical sequence of reactions as given under.

From the above biochemical sequence of reactions it is evident that:

(*i*) L-arginine seems to be used as a source for N-atom through amination *via* a substitution process upon 26-hydroxycholesterol,

Biosynthesis of Solasodine, Tomatidine and Solanidine

(*ii*) Another substitution affords 26-amino-22-hydroxycholesterol to cyclize thereby forming a heterocyclic piperidine ring,

(*iii*) After 16β-hydroxylation, the secondary amine is oxidized to an imine, and the ultimate *spiro-system* may be envisaged by virtue of a nucleophilic addition of the 16β-hydroxyl on to the imine, and

(*iv*) This specific reaction, however, establishes the configurations, *viz:* 22R-as in the case of **Solasodine,** and 22S-as in the case of **Tomatidine**.

B. Veratrum Alkaloids   The **Veratrum alkaloids** represent the most important and medicinally significant class of steroidal alkaloids. It is, however, pertinent to mention here that the *basic ring systems* present in the Veratrum alkaloids are not quite the same as seen in the usual steroidal nucleus, as present either in the cholesterol or in the aglycone residues of the cardiac glycosides (A). Interestingly, one may observe in the structures of Veratrum alkaloids that the ring 'C' is a five-membered ring while ring 'D' is a six-membered ring (B) which apparently is just the reverse of the pattern in the regular steroidal nucleus as depicted in next page.

(A)   (B)

Examples

(*a*) Alkamine portion of the **ester alkaloids of Veratrum,** *viz.,* **Protoverine, Veracevine, Germine.**

(*b*) **Alkamine aglycones of glycosidic veratrum alkaloids,** *viz.,* **Veratramine.**

In general, the majority of **Veratrum alkaloids** may be classified into *two* categories solely based on their characteristic structural features, namely:

(*i*) Cevaratrum alkaloids, and

(*ii*) Jeveratrum alkaloids

These *two* categories of **Veratrum alkaloids** shall now be discussed individually in the sections that follows:

B.1 Ceveratrum Alkaloids The important alkaloids belonging to this group of alkaloids are, namely: **Protoveratrines; Veratridine, Cevadine, Germine** etc., which shall be treated separately hereunder:

B.1.1 Protoveratrines

Biological Sources It is obtained from the rhizome of *Veratrum album* L. (*Liliaceae*) and *Veratrum viride* Ait. (*Liliaceae*) (**American Hellebore**).

However, the alkaloids present in the rhizomes of *V. viride* are placed in *three* groups, such as:

Group-'A': *Alkamines* (esters of the steroidal bases) with organic acids, including **germidine, germitrine,** most valued therapeutically; besides, **cevadine, neogermitrine, neoprotoveratrine, protoveratrines** and **veratridine,**

Group-'B': (Glycosides of the alkamines), mainly **pseudojervine** and **veratrosine,** and

Group-'C': (Alkamines), **germine, jervine, rubijervine,** and **veratramine.**

Chemical Structure

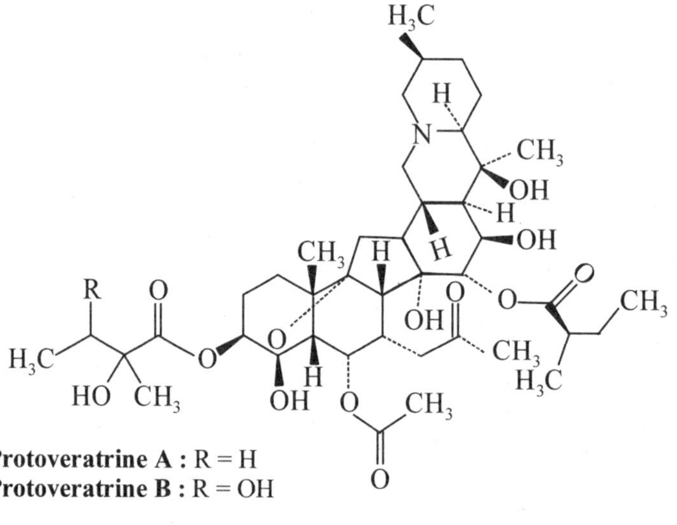

Protoveratrine A : R = H
Protoveratrine B : R = OH

Isolation **Protoveratrine A and B** are usually extracted together and referred to as **'protoveratrines'.** About 2 kg of dried rhizomes of *V. album* is powdered and then extracted with benzene and ammonia. The total alkaloids are purified by extraction with acetic acid, re-extracted into benzene. The solvent is removed under vacuum, the residue is dissolved in ether from which the crystalline powder of the crude protoveratrines separates out. The crude product is recrystallized from alcohol-acetic acid and upon subsequent alkalinization of the solution with dilute ammonia. By this method one may obtain 8-10 g of **protoveratrine** powder from 8 kg of *V. album* rhizomes.

Consequently, **protaverine A and B** may be separated by the help of counter current distribution of the **"protaverine"** between benzene and acetate buffer (pH 5.5) and ultimately subjected to column chromatography on acid aaluminium oxide (Al_2O_3).

Characteristic Features   The characteristic features of the **protoveratrines** are as follows:

(*i*)   The sternutative crystals obtained from ethanol have a slightly bitter taste.

(*ii*) It decomposes at 266-267°C.

(*iii*) Its specific rotation $[\alpha]_D^{25} - 38.6°$ (pyridine), and $[\alpha]_D^{25} - 8.5°$ (C = 1.99 in chloroform).

(*iv*) It is soluble in chloroform, dilute aqueous acidic solutions and slightly soluble in ether. It is practically insoluble in water and petroleum ether.

However, the characteristic features of **protoveratrine A and B** are as stated below:

S. No.	Characteristic Features	Protoveratrine-A (Protalba)	Protoveratrine-B (Veratetrine; Neoprotoveratrine)
1.	Nature	Crystals obtained from acetone	Crystals obtained from acetone
2.	Decomposition temperature/mp	267-269° (dec.)	268-270° (dec.)
3.	Specific rotation	$[\alpha]_D^{25} - 40.5°$ (pyridine); $[\alpha]_D^{25} - 10.5°$ (chloroform);	$[\alpha]_D^{25} - 37°$ (dec.); $[\alpha]_D^{25} - 3.5°$ (chloroform);
4.	Solubility	Soluble in chloroform, hot ethanol and pyridine	Soluble in hot ethanol, pyridine and chloroform
5.	Stability in alkaline medium	Decomposes	Decomposes

Uses

1. It is used as an antihypertensive agent which exerts its action through reflex inhibition of pressor receptors in the heart and carotid sinus.
2. It also possesses emetic action.
3. It is used in the treatment of toxemia of pregnancy.

B.1.2 Veratridine

Biological Sources   It is obtained from the seeds of *Schoenocaulon officinale* (Schelecht. and Cham.) A. Gray and also from the rhizome of *Veratrum album* L. (*Liliaceae*).

Chemical Structure   (3β, 4α, 16β)-4, 9-Epoxycevane-3, 4, 12, 14, 16, 17, 20-heptol 3-(3, 4-dimethoxybenzoate) as given under.

Isolation   Veratridine can be isolated as the commercial **veratrine** (mixture) *i.e.*, the mixture of alkaloids **cevadine, veratridine, cevadiline, sabadine** and **cevine** obtained from the seeds of *S. officinale* stated above, as its sparingly soluble nitrate derivative.*

---

* Blount, *J. Chem. Soc*, 122, (1935); Vejdelek *et. al. Chem. Listy* **153**, 33, (1956); Coll. *Czech. Chem. Commun.*, **22**, 98 (1957).

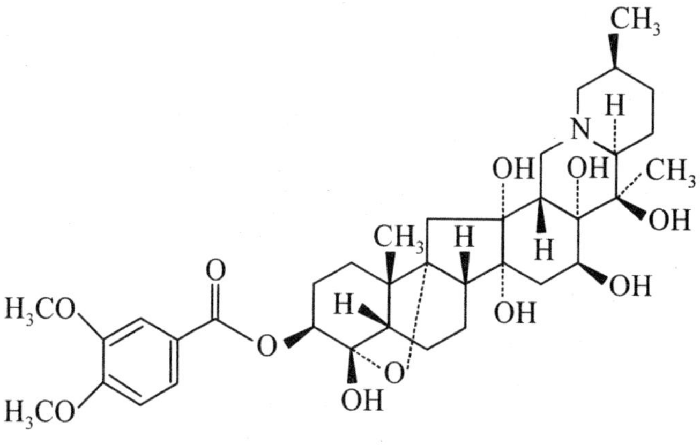

Veratridine

Characteristic Features

1. It is yellowish-white amorphous powder.
2. It tenaciously retains water.
3. It has mp 180°C after drying at 130°C.
4. Its specific rotation is $[\alpha]_D^{20} + 8.0°$ (ethanol) and pK_a 9.54 ± 0.02.
5. It is insoluble in water but slightly soluble in ether.

Identification Tests

1. It readily forms its nitrate derivative which is an amorphous powder and sparingly soluble in water.
2. Its sulphate salt is formed as its needles which happens to be very hygroscopic.
3. It readily forms its perchlorate derivative as long needles from water having mp 259-260°C (after drying at 120°C *in Vacuo*).

B.1.3 Cevadine

Synonym   Veratrine

Biological Source   It is obtained from the seeds of *Schoenocaulon officinale* (Schlecht and Cham.) A. Gray (*Sabadilla officinarum* Brandt.) belonging to family *Liliaceae*.

Chemical Structure   [3β(Z), 4α, 16β]-4, 9-Epoxycevane-3, 4, 12, 14, 16, 17, 20-heptol 3-(2-methyl-2-butenoate) as stated below.

Characteristic Features

1. It gives rise to flat needles from ether which decomposes at 213-214.5°C.
2. It has specific rotation $[\alpha]_D^{20} + 12.8°$ (C = 3.2 in ethanol).
3. *Solubility:* 1 g dissolves in 15 ml ether or ethanol and is very slightly soluble in wager.

Identification Tests

1. It forms **aurichloride derivative** which are obtained as fine yellow needles from ethanol that gets decomposed at 190°C.

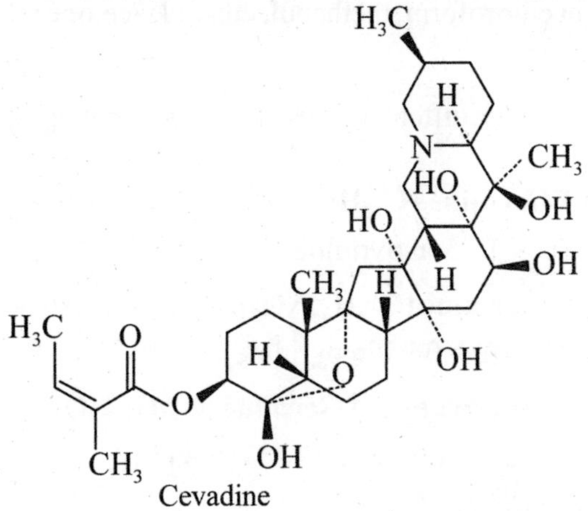

Cevadine

2. It readily produces **mercurichloride derivative** ($C_{32}H_{49}NO_9.HCl.HgCl_2$) as silvery scales which decomposes at 172°C.

Caution   **Cevadine is extremely irritating locally particularly to the mucous membranes. Caution must be used in handling.**

B.1.4 Germine

Biological Source   Germine (an **alkamine**) is present in a plethora of *polyester alkaloids* that occur in *Veratrum* and *Zygadenus* species, such as: *Veratrum viride* Ait. (*Liliaceae*).

Chemical Structure   (3α, 4α, 7α, 15α, 16β)-4, 9-Epoxycevane-3, 4, 7, 14, 15, 16, 20-heptol ($C_{27}H_{43}NO_8$).

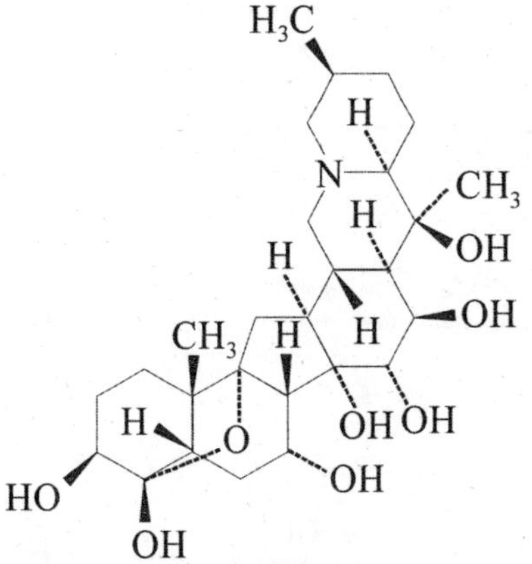

Germine

Characteristic Features

1. It is obtained as crystals from methanol mp 221.5-223 C°.

2. It has specific rotation $[\alpha]_D^{25} + 4.5°$ (95% ethanol) and $[\alpha]_D^{16} + 23.1°$ (C = 1.13 in 10% acetic acid).

3. *Solubility:* It is soluble in chloroform, methanol, ethanol, acetone and water; and slightly soluble in ether.

Identification Tests   It forms *three* different types of '*acetates*' having specific characteristic features as stated below:

1. **3-Acetate derivative of Germine ($C_{29}H_{45}NO_9$):** It forms needles from ether having mp 219-221°C and $[\alpha]_D^{23} + 10°$ (C = 1.05 in pyridine).

2. **16-Acetate derivative of Germine ($C_{29}H_{45}NO_9$):** It forms crystals from chloroform having mp 225-227°C and $[\alpha]_D^{23} - 19°$ (C = 0.93 in pyridine).

3. **3, 4, 7, 15, 16-Pentaacetate derivative of Germine ($C_{37}H_{53}NO_{13}$):** It yields prisms from acetone + petroleum ether which decomposes at 285-287°C and $[\alpha]_D^{23} - 65°$ (C = 0.65 in pyridine).

B.2 Jeveratrum Alkaloids   The **Jeveratrum group of alkaloids** is usually represented by the structure of **veratramine, jervine** and **pseudojervine** etc., which essentially have the following salient features showing the points of difference in comparison to the *Ceveratrum alkaloids:*

The *three* important members of this particular category of alkaloids shall be treated separately in sections that follows:

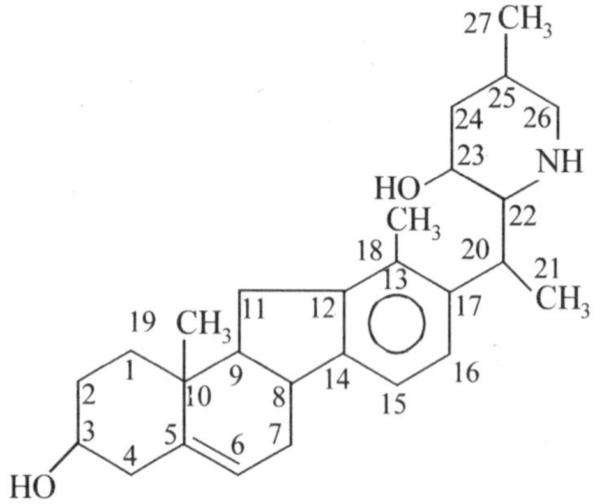

Veratramine
[Jeveratrum Alkaloid]

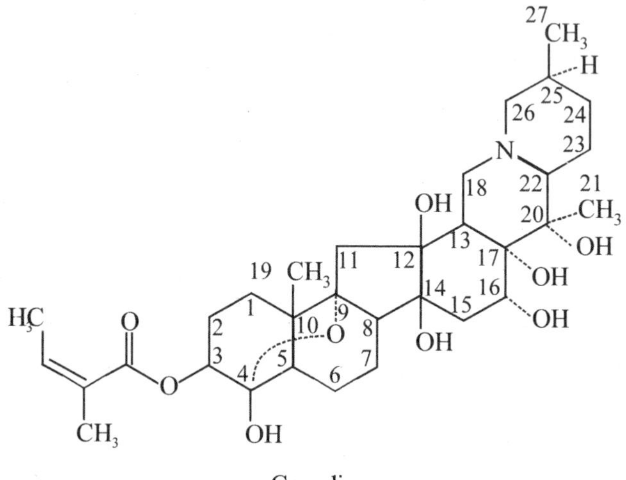

Cevadine
[Ceveratrum Alkaloid]

S.No.	Jeveratrum Alkaloids	S.No.	Ceveratrum Alkaloids
1	The ring system beyond C-17 *i.e.*, the last two of the 6-membered rings, are altogether different from those in the Ceveratrum group of alkaloids	1	The alkamine portion has several –OH groups, (normally 6 to 9 in number), which are linked to various acids *e.g.*, vanillic acid, veratric acid, tiglic acid (angelic acid) to form their corresponding ester alkaloids.
2	The absence of the oxygen-bridge between C-4 and C-9.	2	An oxygen-bridge exists between C-4 and C-9.
3	The absence of several –OH moieties at C-4, C-12, C-14, C-17, C-20.	3	It has a chain of six cyclic rings of which the last two have a common N-atom.
4	The presence of a double-bond between C-5 and C-6.	4	At C-3 the H is replaced by a C_5H_7O moiety.

B.2.1 Veratramine

Biological Sources It is obtained in the rhizomes of *Viratrum viride* Ait. (*Liliaceae*) (**American Hellebore**); and also from *Veratrum grandiflorum* (Maxim.) Loes. F. (*Liliaceae*).

Chemical Structure The chemical structure of **veratramine** has also been referred to as **azasteroid**, wherein the N-atom is present is in one or more side chains.

Veratramine

$(3\beta, 23\beta)$-14, 15, 16, 17-Tetrahydro-veratraman-3, 23-diol ($C_{27}H_{39}NO_2$).

Characteristic Features
1. It is obtained as crystals having mp 206-207°C.
2. It is slightly soluble in water, but soluble in ethanol and methanol.

Identification Tests
1. It forms a complex with digitonin (1:1) that has uv_{mas} : 268 nm and $[\alpha]_D^{25} - 71.8°$ (C = 1.21; $[\alpha]_D^{25} - 70°$ (C = 1.56 in methanol).
2. **Dihydroveratramine Derivative:** The crystals of dihydroveratramine derivative has mp 192.5-194°C ; $[\alpha]_D^{25} + 26°$ (C = 1.26 in acetic acid).

B.2.2 Jervine

Biological Sources It is obtained in the rhizomes of *Veratrum grandiflorum* (Maxim.) Loes F. *Veratrum album* L., and *Veratrum viride* Sol. (*Liliaceae*).

Chemical Structure

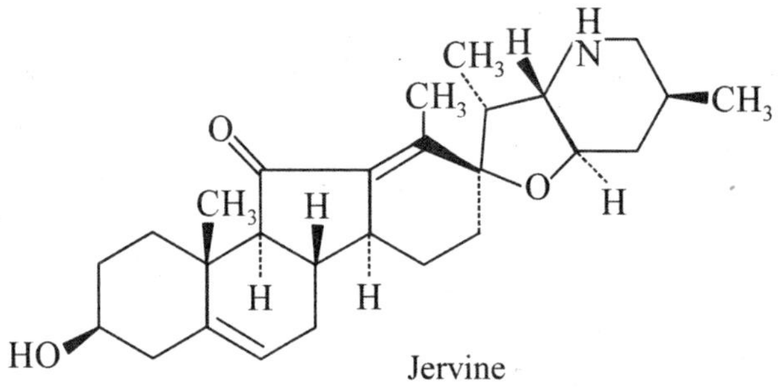

Jervine

(3β, 23β)-17, 23-Epoxy-3-hydroxyveratraman-11-one ($C_{27}H_{39}NO_3$).

Characteristic Features

1. The needles obtained from methanol and water has mp 243.5-244°C (Saito).
2. Its specific rotation $[\alpha]_D^{20} - 150°$ (ethanol) (Saito); and $[\alpha]_D^{20} - 167.6°$ (chloroform) (Poethke).
3. It has uv_{max} : 250, 360 nm ($\in$ 1500, 60).

Identification Tests

1. **Diacetyljervine ($C_{31}H_{43}NO_5$):** The diacetyljervine has mp 173-175°C; $[\alpha]_D - 112°$; uv_{max} (ethanol): 250, 360 nm ($\in$ 16400, 80).
2. **Jervine Hydrochloride** has mp 300-302°C.

B.2.3 Pseudojervine

Biological Sources It is obtained from the rhizomes of *Veratrum viride* Ait (*Liliaceae*) (**American Hellebore**); *V. album* L. (*Liliaceae*); and *V. eschscholtzii* Gray. (*Liliaceae*).

Chemical Structure It is the glucoside of **jervine** as given below.

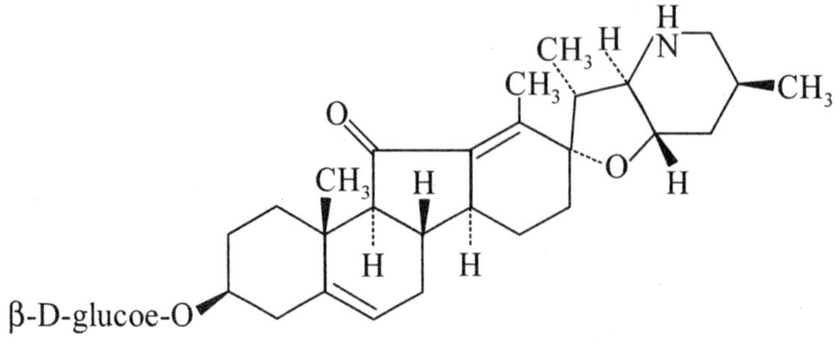

Pseudojervine

(3β, 23β)-17, 23-Epoxy-3-(β-D-glucopyrnosyloxy) veratraman-11-one. ($C_{33}H_{49}NO_8$).

Characteristic Features

1. It is obtained as lustrous leaflets having mp 300-301°C (dec.).
2. It specific rotation $[\alpha]_D^{25} - 133°$ (C = 0.48 in 1.3 ethanol-chloroform).
3. *Solubility:* It is soluble in benzene, chloroform; slightly soluble in ethanol and almost insoluble in ether.

Note: It is, however, pertinent to observe here that the Zygadenus species and the Schoenocaulon species appear to have only the Ceveratrum alkaloids and practically no Jeveratrum alkaloids. Interestingly, the large number of Veratrum species seem to contain both these type of steroidal alkaloids.

7.2.2 Alkaloids Derived from Anthranilic Acid

Anthranilic acid is found to be a key intermediate in the biosynthesis of L-tryptophan. Therefore, it has been established that this biotransformation ultimately is solely responsible to the elaboration of the **indole alkaloids**. In the course of this conversion, the anthranilic acid residue is specifically decarboxylated, thus the C_6N skeleton is further utilized. In general, there are several such instances wherein the anthranilic acid itself serves as an *alkaloid precursor*, by employing various means and processes that essentially retain the full skeleton and further exploit the carboxyl function legitimately. Interestingly, in mammals, L-tryptophan gets degraded back to anthranilic acid. However, this particular route is of least importance in the plant kingdom.

The alkaloids derived from anthranilic acid may be classified into *three* major categories, namely:

(*i*) Quinazoline alkaloids,
(*ii*) Quinoline alkaloids, and
(*iii*) Acridine alkaloids.

The aforesaid categories of alkaloids shall be discussed in an elaborated fashion hereunder individually.

7.2.2.1 Quinazoline Alkaloids

Vasicine is a **quinazoline alkaloid** which will be described below.

A. Vasicine

Synonym   Peganine

Biological Sources   It is obtained from the leaves of *Adhatoda vasica* (L.) Nees (*Acanthaceae*) (**Malabar Nut, Adotodai, Paveltia**); and the seeds of *Peganum harmala* L. (*Rutaceae*) (**Harmel, Syrian Rue, African Rue**).

Chemical Structure

Vasicine

1, 2, 3, 9-Tetrahydropyrrolo [2, 1-b] quinazoline-3-ol; ($C_{11}H_{12}N_2O$).

Isolation   It is isolated from the leaves of *Adhatoda vasica** and also from the seeds of *Peganum harmala*** by adopting the standard methods of isolation described earlier in this chapter.

---

* Sen, Ghosh, *J. Indian Chem.* Soe., **1**, 315 (1924);
** Späth, Nikawitz, *Ber.* **67**, 45, (1934);

Characteristic Features

dl-**Form:** 1. It is obtained as needles from ethanol having mp 210°C.
2. It sublimes on being subjected to high vacuum.
3. It is soluble in acetone, alcohol, chloroform; and slightly soluble in water, ether and benzene.

l-**Form:** 1. It is obtained as needles from ethanol with mp 212°C.
2. Its specific rotation $[\alpha]_D^{14} - 254°$ (C = 2.4 in CHCl$_3$);
$[\alpha]_D^{14} - 62°$ (C = 2.4 in ethanol).

Note: In dilute HCl it is obtained as its dextrorotatory form.

Identification Tests

1. Hydrochloride dihydrate derivative is obtained as needles having mp 208°C (dry).
2. Hydroiodide dihydrate derivative is formed as needles with mp 195°C (dry).
3. Methiodide derivative is obtained as needles from methanol having mp 187°C.
4. Acetyl vasicine derivative ($C_{11}H_{11}N_2O$ COCH$_3$) is formed as crystals having mp 123°C and bp$_{0.01}$ 230-240°C.

Uses

1. It is mostly used as an expectorant and bronchodilator.
2. It also shows oxytocic properties very similar to those exhibited by **oxytocin** and **methyl ergometrine**.
3. **Vasicine** also shows abortifacient action which is due to the release of prostaglandins.

Biosynthesis of Vasicine   Various studies in *Peganum harmala* have evidently revealed **vasicine (peganine)** to be derived from the anthranilic acid, while the remaining portion of the structure comprising of a pyrrolidine ring provided by ornithine. The probable mechanism of **vasicine** skeleton may be explained by virtue of the nucleophilic attack from the N-atom present in anthranilate upon the pyrrolidinium cation, ultimately followed by amide formation. However, interestingly this pathway is not being adopted in *Justicia adhatoda*. Thus, a comparatively less predictable sequence from N-acetylanthranilic acid and aspartic acid is observed as shown below:

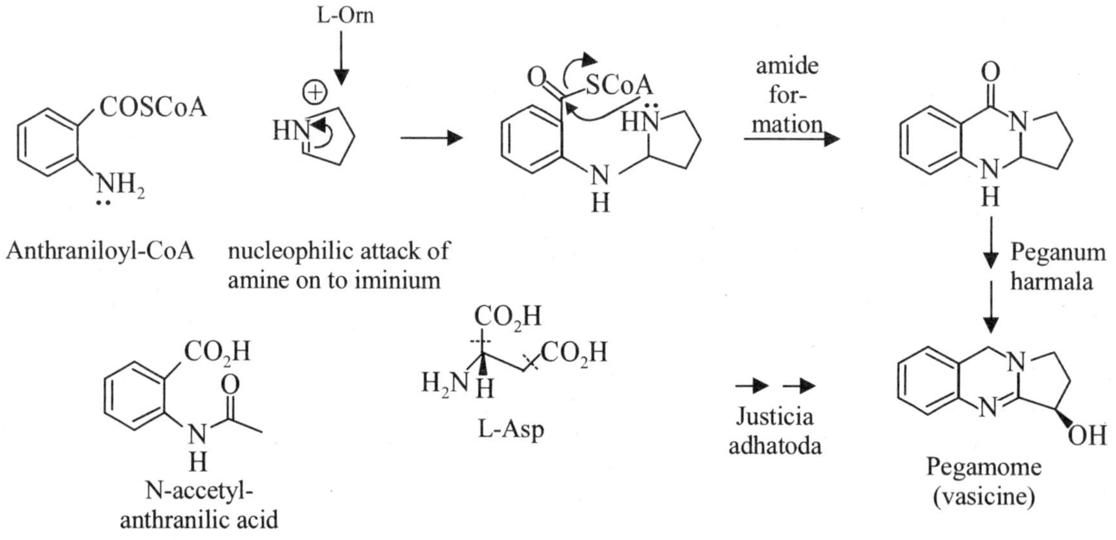

B. Vasicinone

Biological Source   The plant source remain the same as described under **vasicine**.

Chemical Structure

Vasicinone

1, 2, 3, 9-Tetrahydropyrrolo [2, 1-b] quinazoline-6-one-3 ol ($C_{11}H_{10}N_2O_2$).

Uses   It is used mainly as an expectorant which action is solely due to stimulation of the bronchial glands.

7.2.2.2 Quinoline Alkaloids

In general, the alkaloids containing essentially the '**quinoline**' nucleus include a series of alkaloids obtained exclusively from the **cinchona bark**, the major members of this particular group are, namely: **quinine, quinidine, cinchonine** and **cinchonidine.** Interestingly, more than twenty five alkaloids have been isolated and characterized either from the *Yellow Cinchona i.e., Cinchona calisaya* Wedd. and *Cinchona ledgeriana* Moens ex Trimen, or from the *Red Cinchona i.e., Cinchona succirubra* Pavon ex Klotzsch (Family: *Rubiaceae*). The aforesaid alkaloids are also found in their hybrids as well as in the *Cuprea Bark* obtained from *Remijia pedunculata* and *Remijia purdieana* belonging to the natural order *Rubiaceae.*

However, it has been revealed that an average commercial yield of the **cinchona alkaloids** in the dry bark materials from the said plant materials are as follows: **quinine** (5.7%); **quinidine** (0.1-0.3%); **cinchonine** and **cinchonidine** (0.2-0.4%). Nevertheless, the other closely related minor alkaloids are present in relatively smaller quantities.

Basic Structures of Cinchona Alkaloids   The various **quinoline alkaloids**, which possess potent medicinal activities are, namely: **quinine, quinidine, cinchonine,** and **cinchonidine.** It is interesting to observe that these alkaloids not only have a closely related structure but also similar medicinal characteristics. These alkaloids possess the *basic skeleton* of 9'-rubanol that is derived from the parent compound known as ruban. Thus, ruban is obtained from the combination of *two* distinct heterocyclic nuclii, namely: (*a*) 4-methyl quinoline nucleus, and (*b*) quinuclidine nucleus. However, this particular nomenclature was suggested by Rabe so as to simplify the naming of such compounds and also to signify its origin from the natural order *Rubiaceae.*

4-Methyl Quinoline
Nucleus

Quinuclidine
Nucleus

Quinuclidine
Nucleus

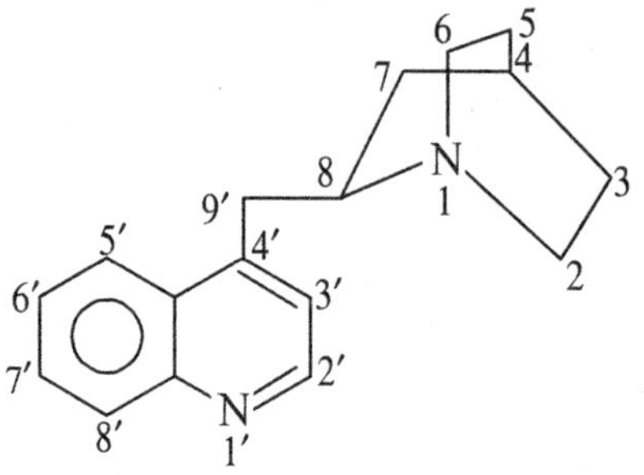

Ruban
[8-9′ Quinuclidyl Methyl
Quinoline nucleus]

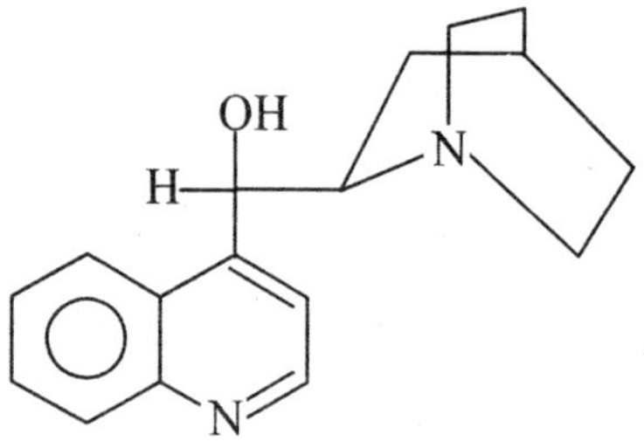

9′-Rubanol

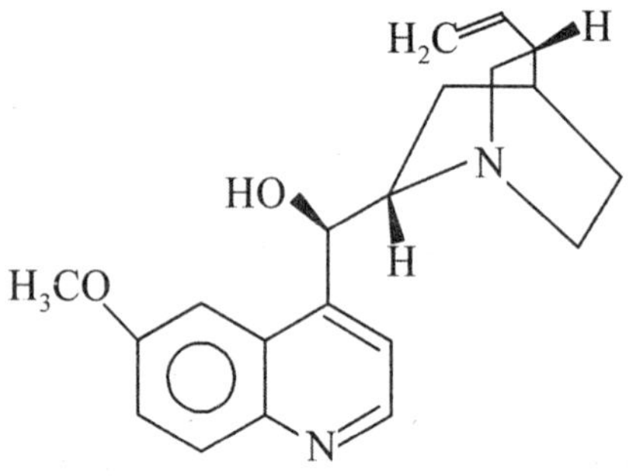

Quinine

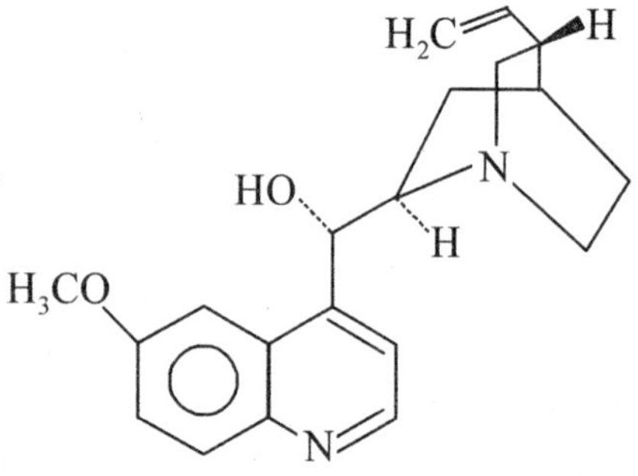

Quinidine

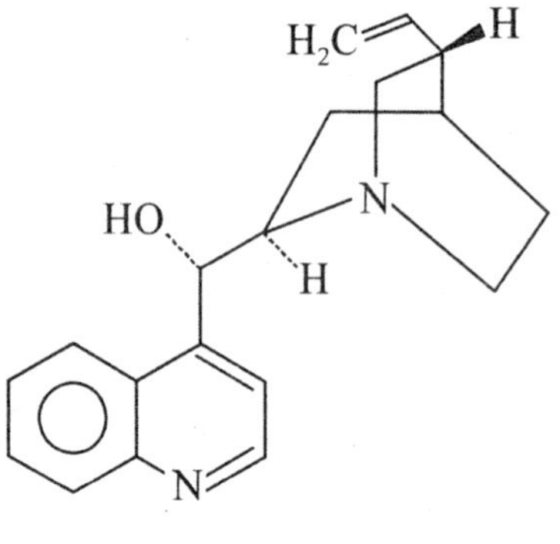

Cinchonine

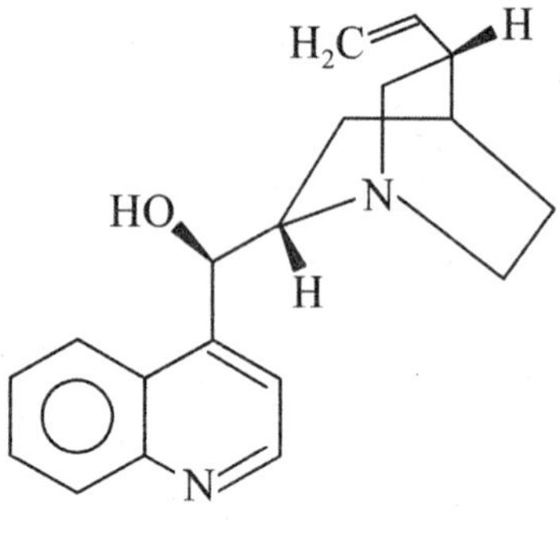

Cinchonidine

In this context, a few important drugs belonging to the **quinoline alkaloids** shall now be discussed in the sections that follows:

A. Quinine

Biological Sources   It is obtained from the bark of *Cinchona calisaya* Wedd; *Cinchona ledgeriana* Moens ex Trimen; *Cinchona officinalis* Linn. f.; *Cinchona robusta* How; and *Cinchona succirubra* Pavon ex Klotzsch belonging to family *Rubiaceae.*

Chemical Structure

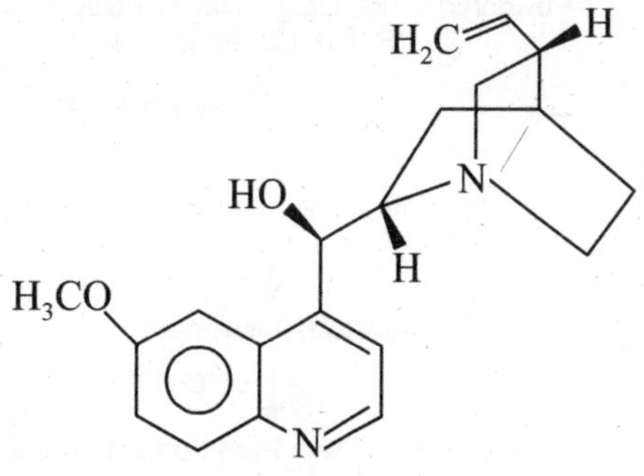

Quinine

(8α, 9R)-6′-Methoxycinchonan-9-ol, ($C_{20}H_{24}N_2O_2$).

Isolation   The schematic method of isolation of the *Cinchona Alkaloids* in general and that of **quinine** in particular has been provided in the following *Flow-chart* in a sequential manner. Hence, this particular flow-chart also includes the method of isolation of other important members of this group *i.e.*, **quinidine, cinchonine** and **cinchonidine** as given under.

Notes
1. Bisulphates of cinchona as alkaloids [$B.H_2SO_4$] are readily soluble in water.
2. **Quinine sulphate** [$Br.H_2SO_4$] is sparingly soluble in water [1:720].
3. **Cinchonine** is practically insoluble in ether.
4. Tartrates of **Quinine** and **Cinchonidine** are insoluble, whereas the tartrates of **Cinchonine** and **Quinidine** are soluble in water.

Characteristic Features
1. The orthorhombic needles obtained from absolute ethanol are triboluminescent and having mp 177°C (with some decomposition).
2. It sublimes in high vacuum at 170-180°C.
3. Its specific rotation is $[\alpha]_D^{15} - 169°$ (C = 2 in 97% ethanol); $[\alpha]_D^{17} - 117°$ (C = 1.5 in chloroform); and $[\alpha]_D^{15} - 285°$ (C = 0.4 M in 0.1 N H_2SO_4).
4. Its dissociation constant pK_1 (18°) is 5.07 and pK_2 9.7.
5. **Neutral Salt of Quinine [$(B)_2.H_2SO_4.8H_2O$]:** It is formed by neutralization from boiling water, which is sparingly soluble in water (*viz.*, 1 in 720 at 25°C). The octahydrate neutral salts of quinine undergoes efflorescence on being exposed to air and gets converted to the corresponding dihydrate salt which is more stable.
6. **Acid Sulphate of Quinine [$(B).H_2SO_4.7H_2O$]:** The quinine bisulphate is soluble in water (1 in 8.5 at 25°C) and in ethanol (1 in 18). The aqueous solution is acidic to litmus.
7. **Tetrasulphate Salt of Quinine [$(B)_2.2H_2SO_4.7H_2O$]:** The tetrasulphate salt of quinine is very soluble in water.

Schematic Method of Isolation of Cinchona Alkaloids

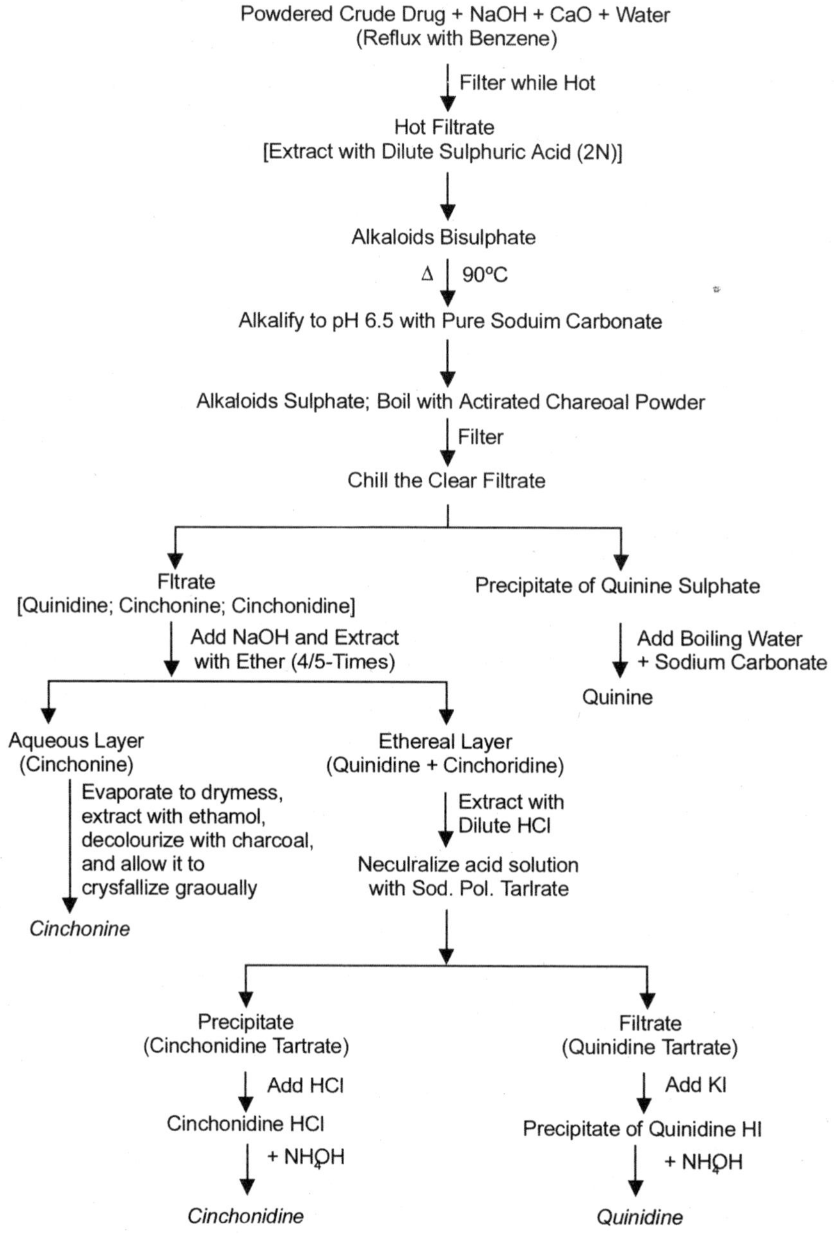

Powdered Crude Drug + NaOH + CaO + Water
(Reflux with Benzene)

↓ Filter while Hot

Hot Filtrate
[Extract with Dilute Sulphuric Acid (2N)]

↓

Alkaloids Bisulphate

Δ ↓ 90°C

Alkalify to pH 6.5 with Pure Soduim Carbonate

↓

Alkaloids Sulphate; Boil with Actirated Chareoal Powder

↓ Filter

Chill the Clear Filtrate

Fltrate
[Quinidine; Cinchonine; Cinchonidine]

↓ Add NaOH and Extract
with Ether (4/5-Times)

Precipitate of Quinine Sulphate

↓ Add Boiling Water
+ Sodium Carbonate

Quinine

Aqueous Layer
(Cinchonine)

↓ Evaporate to drymess,
extract with ethamol,
decolourize with charcoal,
and allow it to
crysfallize graoually

Cinchonine

Ethereal Layer
(Quinidine + Cinchoridine)

↓ Extract with
Dilute HCl

Neculralize acid solution
with Sod. Pol. Tarlrate

↓

Precipitate
(Cinchonidine Tartrate)

↓ Add HCl

Cinchonidine HCl

↓ + NH$_2$OH

Cinchonidine

Filtrate
(Quinidine Tartrate)

↓ Add KI

Precipitate of Quinidine HI

↓ + NH$_2$OH

Quinidine

Identification Tests

1. **Fluorescence Test: Quinine** gives a distinct and strong blue fluorescence when treated with an *oxygenated acid*, such as: acetic acid, sulphuric acid. This test is very marked and pronounced even to a few mg concentration of quinine.

   Note: The hydrochloride and hydroiodide salts of quinine do not respond to this fluorescence test.

2. **Thalleioquin Test:** Add to 2-3 ml of a weakly acidic solution of a quinine salt a few drops of bromine-water followed by 0.5 ml of strong ammonia solution, a distinct and characteristic emerald green colour is produced. The coloured product is termed as **thalleioquin**, the chemical composition of which is yet to be established. This test is so sensitive that quinine may be detected to a concentration as low as 0.005%.

   Notes: Quinidine and cupreine (a Remijia alkaloid) give also a positive response to this test; but cinchoninine and cinchonidine give a negative test.

3. **Erythroquinine Test (or Rosequin Test):** Add to a solution of quinine in dilute acetic acid 1-2 drops of bromine water, a drop of a solution of potassium ferrocyanide $[K_4(FeCN)_6]$ (10% w/v), and to it add a drop of strong ammonia solution, the solution turns red instantly. In case, it is shaken immediately with 1 ml of chloroform, the red colour is taken up by the chloroform layer.

4. **Herpathite Test:** To a boiling mixture containing 0.25 g of quinine in 7.5 ml glacial acetic acid, 3 ml ethanol (90% v/v), 5 drops of conc. sulphuric acid and add to it 3.5 ml of 1% iodine solution in ethanol, the appearance of crystals of **iodosulphate of quinine** (*i.e.*, **sulphate of iodo-quinine**)-is known as **Herpathite** after the name of its discoverer. It has the chemical composition $[(B_4).3H_2SO_4.2HI.I_4.3H_2O]$ which separates out as crystals (on cooling), having a metallic lustre that appears dark green in reflected light and olive green in transmitted light.

Uses

1. It is used as a flavour in carbonated beverages.
2. It is widely used as an antimalarial agent in tropical countries.
3. It is employed as a skeletal muscle relaxant.

Biosynthesis of Quinine   The various steps whereby *Coryanthe-type* indole alkaloids are converted to quinoline derivatives have not yet been elucidated and hence established. Therefore, only a partial biosynthetic pathway may be written for **quinine** as given under.

B. Cinchonine

Biological Source   **Cinchonine** is obtained from a variety of cinchona bark, especially in the bark of *Cinchona micrantha* R. and P. belonging to family *Rubiaceae.*

Chemical Structure   Please see structure under Section 7.2.2.2, (9S-Cinchonan-9-ol) ($C_{19}H_{22}N_2O$).

Isolation   It has already been described under **quinine** Section 'A' above.

Characteristic Features

1. Its prisms, needles are obtained from ether and ethanol having mp 265°C.
2. It begins to sublime at 220°C.
3. Its specific rotation is $[\alpha]_D$ + 229° (in ethanol).
4. One gramme of it dissolves in 60 ml ethanol, 25 ml boiling ethanol, 110 ml chloroform and 500 ml ether. It is practically insoluble in water.

Identification Tests

1. **Cinchonine dihydrochloride ($C_{19}H_{22}N_2O.HCl$):** It is white or faintly yellow crystals or crystalline powder. It is freely soluble in water and ethanol.

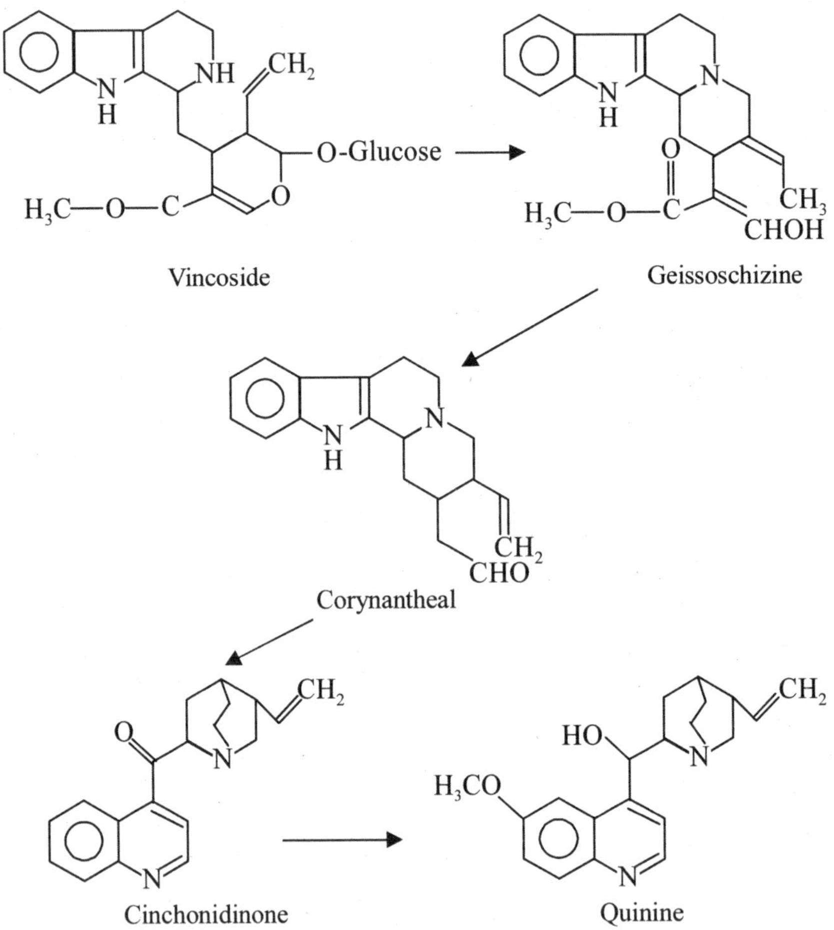

Vincoside   Geissoschizine

Corynantheal

Cinchonidinone   Quinine

Biosynthesis of Quinine

2. **Cinchonine hydrochloride dihydrate ($C_{19}H_{22}N_2O.HCl.2H_2O$):** It is obtained as fine crystals having mp when anhydrous 215°C with decomposition. One g dissolves in 20 ml of water, 3.5 ml of boiling water, 1.5 ml of ethanol, 20 ml of chloroform and slightly soluble in ether.

3. **Cinchonine sulphate dihydrate [$(C_{19}H_{27}N_2O)_2.H_2SO_4.2H_2O$)]:** It occurs as lustrous, very brittle crystals having mp 198°C (when anhydrous). One g dissolves in 65 ml of water, 30 ml of hot water, 12.5 ml of ethanol, 7 ml of hot ethanol, 47 ml of chloroform and slightly soluble in ether.

7.2.2.3 Acridine Alkaloids

The origin of the **acridine-ring-system** is by virtue of an extension of the process that essentially involves the combination of anthranilic acid and acetate/malonate as shown in the following sequence of reactions; whereas, a rather more direct route to the above leads to the **quinoline-ring-system** discussed in Section 7.2.2.2 earlier.

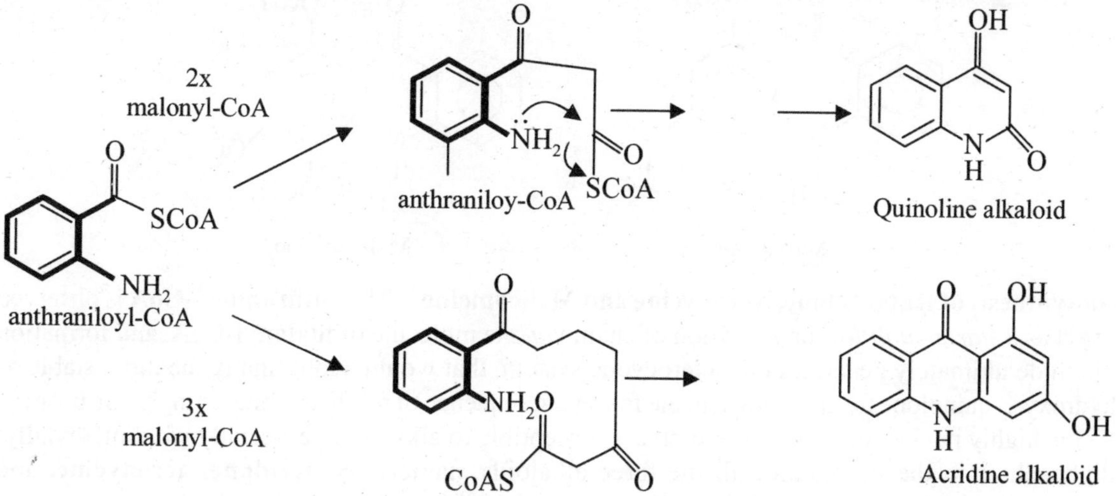

Quinoline alkaloid

Acridine alkaloid

There are a few typical examples of the **acridine alkaloids,** such as: **Rutacridone, Acronycine** and **Melicopicine.**

A. Rutacridone

Biological Source The fresh and dried leaves of *Ruta graveolens* L. (*Rutaceae*) (**Rue, Garden Rue, German Rue**).

Chemical Structure

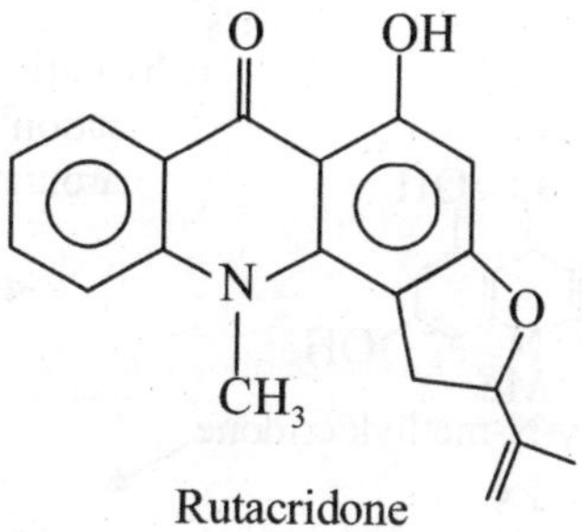

Rutacridone

Uses

1. In Chinese medicine rue is considered as an emmenagogue, hemostat, intestinal antispasmodic, sedative, uterine stimulant, vermifuge, rheumatism, cold and fever.
2. In Poland, it is used as an aphrodisiac and choleretic.
3. The herb is used medicinally as a bitters, an aromatic stimulant, ecbolic and in suppression of the menses.

The chemical structures of **acronycine** and **melicopicine** are given below:

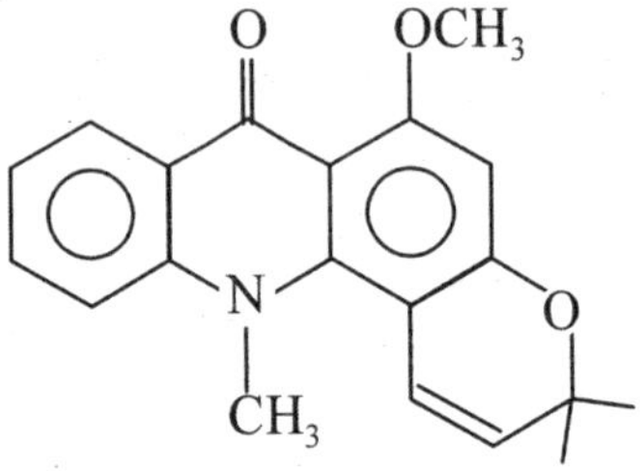

Acronycine

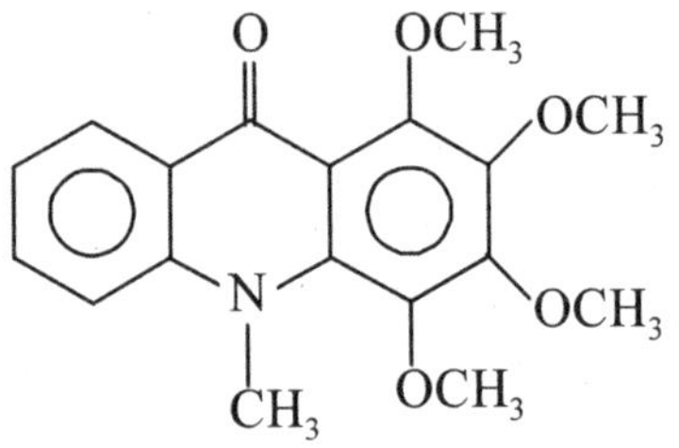

Melicopicine

Biosynthesis of Rutacridone, Acronycine and Melicopicine The **anthraniloyl-CoA** is observed to act as a *starter-unit* for the extension of chain *via* one molecule of **malonyl-CoA**, and formation of amide ultimately generates the heterocyclic system, that would adopt finally the more stable 4-hydroxy-2-quinolone form as shown in the following sequence of reactions. Interestingly, the position C-3 is highly nucleophilic; and, therefore, is susceptible to alkylation, especially *via* dimethylallyl diphosphate in the instance of all the three alkaloids, namely: **rutacridone, acronycine,** and **melicopicine.** This seems to allow the formation of additional six-membered oxygen containing heterocyclic ring system (**acronycine**); and five-membered oxygen containing heterocyclic ring system (**rutacridone**).

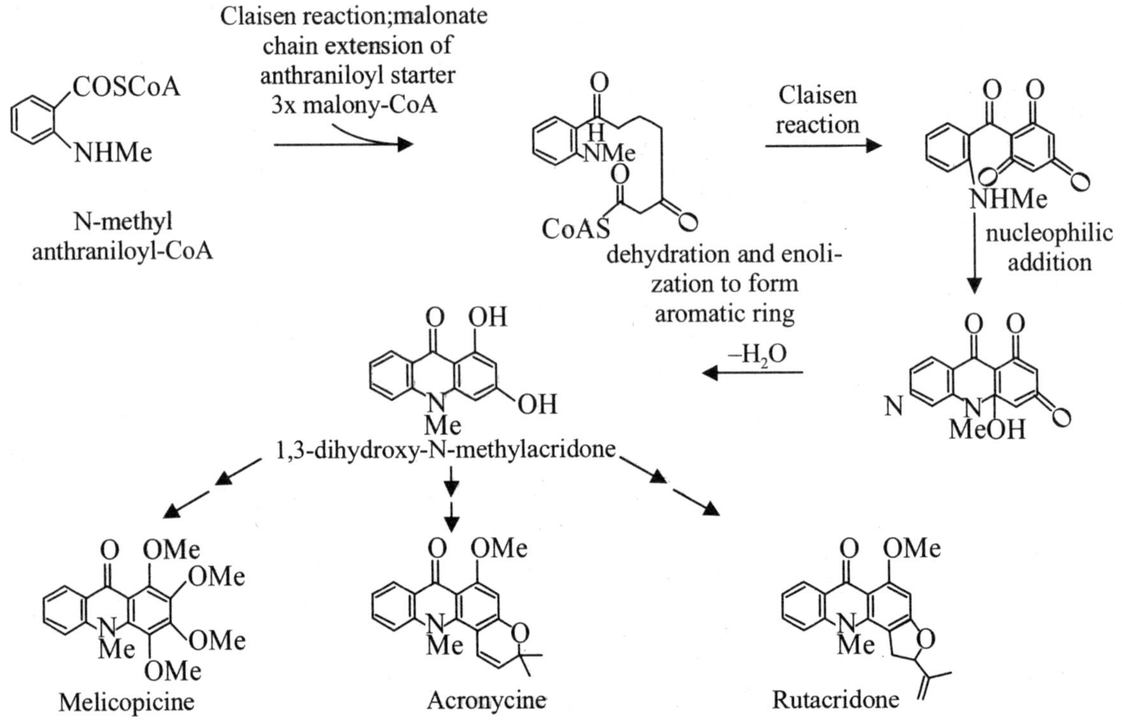

7.2.3 Alkaloids Derived from Histidine

The amino acid *L-histidine*, containing the heterocyclic imidazole ring, is considered to be the right precursor of alkaloids that essentially comprise of this ring-system.

A good number of *Pilocarpus species*, belonging to family *Rutaceae*, found to contain plethora of alkaloids with an *imidazole ring*, namely: **pilocarpine, isopilocarpine,** and **pilosene.** It has been observed that the alkaloids in these species invariably reside in the leaves. **Pilocarpine** constitutes 0.5-1.0% of the dried leaf material. **Isopilocarpine** appears to vary significantly within a range from 5 to 7.5% of the total alkaloids. Further, the alkaloids are located mostly in the upper epidermal leaves of the cells of the leaves, and also in the cells of the mesophyll bordering upon the lower epidermis.

The *three* major alkaloids derived from histidine shall be described in the sections that follows.

7.2.3.1 Pilocarpine

Synonyms   Ocusert Pilo.

Biological Source   **Pilocarpine** is obtained from the leaves of closely related plants of the genus *Pilocarpus,* belonging to the natural order *Rutaceae*. However, the genus comprised of a variety of species commonly known by various names, such as: *Pilocarpus jaborandi* (*Pernambuco Jaborandi*), (*Pilocarpus pennatifolius* (**Paraguay Jaborandi**); *Pilocarpus microphyllus* (**Maranham Jaborandi**); *Pilocarpus selloanus* (**Rio Jaborandi**); *Pilocarpus trachylophus* (**Ceara Jaborandi**); *Pilocarpus spicatus* (**Aracati Jaborandi**); *Pilocarpus heterophyllus* (**Barqui Simento Jaborandi**); and *Pilocarpus racemosus* (**Guadeloupe**).

It is worthwhile to mention here that *P. microphyllus* is the major commercial source of this drug.

Chemical Structure

Pilocarpine

(3S-*cis*)-3-Ethyldihydro-4-[1-methyl-1H-imidazol-5-yl) methyl]-2(3H)-furanone ($C_{11}H_{16}N_2O_2$).

Pilocarpine is a monoacidic tertiary base comprising of a lactone ring and an imidazole nucleus. It is the lactone of **pilocarpic acid,** an acid with a **glyoxaline** nucleus, as given below:

α-Methyl, β-ethyl-   3-Methyl   Pilocarpic Acid
β-Carboxy propanol   Imidazole

Isolation   The finely powdered leaves of **Jaborandi** is first extracted with ethanol (95% v/v) containing 1% HCl. The ethanol is distilled off under vacuo and the residue is taken up with a little water and neutralized carefully by the addition of dilute ammonia. The resins separating out are filtered off and the filtrate is concentrated to a small volume. The resulting concentrated filtrate is alkalified with an excess of ammonia and the liberated alkaloids are shaken out with at least three successive portions of chloroform. The chloroform is removed from the combined extract under vacuo.

The residue is dissolved in a minimum volume of distilled water and neutralized with dilute HNO_3 (6N). The mixture of nitrates of **pilocarpine** and **isopilocarpine** crystallizes out upon cooling; which may be further separated by fractional crystallization from ethanol.

Characteristic Features

1. It is found as oil or crystals having mp 34°C.
2. It boils at bp_5 260°C with partial conversion to its isomer isopilocarpine.
3. Its specific rotation is $[\alpha]_D^{18} + 106°$ (C = 2) and dissociation constant pK_1 (20°C) 7.15; and pK_2 (20°C) 12.57.
4. It is soluble in water, alcohol, chloroform, sparingly soluble in ether and benzene; and practically insoluble in petroleum ether.
5. It exhibits an absorption maximum at 263 nm.
6. It behaves as a monoacidic base.
7. It usually gives distinct precipitates with a number of reagents, such as: **Wagner's Reagent, Mayer's Reagent, Hager's Reagent, silicotungstic acid, phosphomolybdic acid,** gold and platinic halides.
   Note: Some of these precipitates do help in the identification of pilocarpine.
8. **Cessation of Lactone-Ring:** The lactone ring is opened-up (undergoes cessation) by treatment with strong alkalies like NaOH, KOH, which ultimately form salts with the formation of **pilocarpic acid** as given below:

$$\text{Pilocarpine} \xrightarrow[\substack{\text{(Sodium or} \\ \text{Potassium salt)}}]{\text{KOH/NaOH}} \text{Pilocarpine} + \text{Pilocarpic Acid}$$

   Note: The cessation of the lactone-ring absolutely destroys the physiological activity of pilocarpine; and the lactone-ring is not affected by either ammonia or alkali carbonates.
9. **$KMnO_4$-Oxidation:** $KMnO_4$ oxidation destroys the imidazole ring in pilocarpine and yields ammonia, methyl amine, **pilopic acid, homopilopic acids** plus other products.

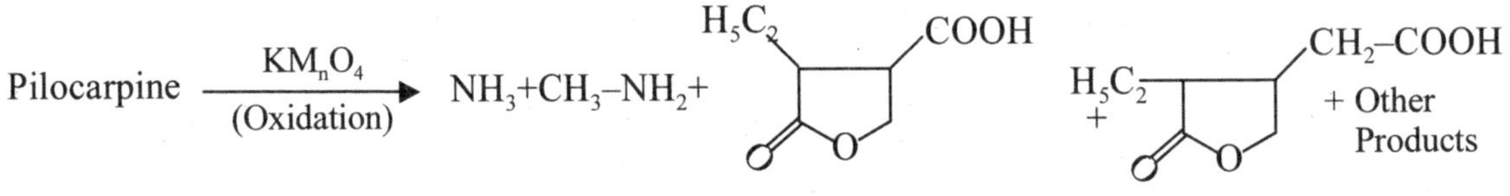

$$\text{Pilocarpine} \xrightarrow[\text{(Oxidation)}]{KM_nO_4} NH_3 + CH_3-NH_2 +$$

| Ammonia | Methyl Amide | Pilopic Acid | Homopilopic Acid |

Isomerism   Pilocarpine and **isopilocarpine** are stereoisomers, that essentially exhibit the stereochemical difference in the **lactone moiety** of the molecule as shown below:

Pilocarpine Isopilocarpine

However, the above observation is based on the experimental evidence, which specifically depicts that the isomerism of the above two alkaloids still persists, even when the **imidazole moiety** undergoes destruction under mild experimental conditions.

Identification Tests

1. **Helch's Violet-Colour Test:** Pilocarpine readily forms a violet coloured compound when a solution of either the base or its salt is first treated with hydrogen peroxide (H_2O_2) and then with potassium dichromate ($K_2Cr_2O_7$) in the presence of few drops of dilute sulphuric acid (Helch, 1902).

   Note:
   (*i*) **The violet-coloured compound (*i.e.*, pilocarpine perchromate) is soluble in chloro-form and benzene. It was further characterized as pilocarpine perchromate by Biedebach (1933).**
   (*ii*) **Shupe successfully employed the Helch's reaction to determine pilocarpine quanti-tatively by the colourimetric assay.**

2. **Ekkert's Colour Tests:** Add to 1 ml of 1% (w/v) solution of pilocarpine hydrochloride ($C_{11}H_{16}N_2O_2$.HCl) 1 ml of sodium nitroprusside solution (2% w/v) and 1 ml of NaOH solution (1N). Allow the reaction mixture to stand for 6-8 minutes and then acidify with dilute HCl when a wine or red colour develops.

   (Note: Isopilocarpine hydrochloride also gives a similar colour test.)

Further, when a few drops of 0.1 N sodium thiosulphate solution are added to the wine or red colour solution, it changes to distinct green colouration.

Note: Elvidge (1947) put forward a method for the assay of the total alkaloids of Pilocarpus leaves based on the Ekkert's colour test.

Uses

1. Pilocarpine possesses miotic and diaphoretic actions.
2. Pilocarpine nitrate is used extensively as an ophthalmic drug having cholinergic action.
3. It is also employed to reduce the intra-ocular pressure in glaucoma patients.

7.2.3.2 Isopilocarpine

Synonym β-Pilocarpine.

Biological Source It is same as stated under Section 7.2.3.1 on **pilocarpine.**

Chemical Structure

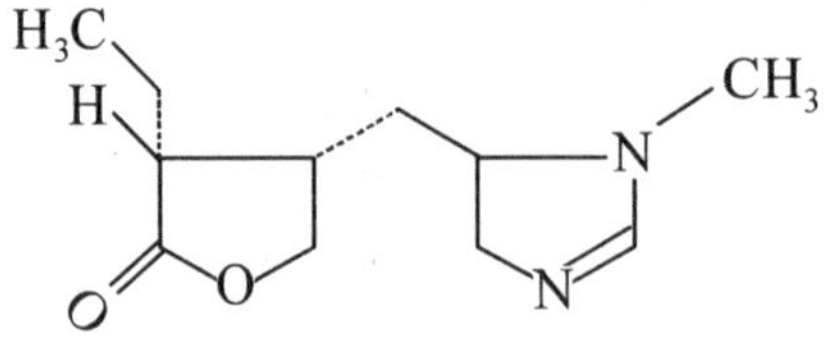

Isopilocarpine

Isolation   It has been discussed under Section 7.2.3.1 above

Characteristic Features
1. It is a hygroscopic oily liquid or prisms.
2. It has the following physical parameters: bp_{10} 261°C; $[\alpha]_D^{18} + 50°C$ (C = 2); pK_1 (18°C) 7.17.
3. It is miscible with water and alcohol; very soluble in chloroform; less soluble in ether and benzene; and almost insoluble in petroleum-ether.

Identification Tests   Its derivatives have the specific physical parameters, namely:

1. **Isopilocarpine hydrochloride hemihydrate ($C_{11}H_{16}N_2O_2$. HCl.½H_2O):** It is obtained as scales from ethanol having mp 127°C; when anhydrous mp 161°C; $[\alpha]_D^{18} + 39°$ (C = 5). It is soluble 0.27 part water and 2.1 parts ethanol.

2. **Isopilocarpine nitrate ($C_{11}H_{16}N_2O$. HNO_3):** It occurs as prisms from water, scales from ethanol, having mp 159°C; $[\alpha]_D^{18} + 39°C$ (C = 2). It is soluble in 8.4 parts of water and in 350 parts of absolute ethanol.

Uses
1. It is used as an antiglaucoma agent
2. It is also employed as miotic.

7.2.3.3   Isopilosine

Synonyms   Carpiline; Carpidine; Pilosine (this compound was originally called pilosine *i.e.*, the *cis-isomer* of isopilosine.

Biological Source   It is obtained from the dried leaflets of *Pilocarpus microphyllus* (*Rutaceae*), which has the total alkaloidal content (0.5-1.%) that consists principally **pilocarpine** along with small portion of **isopilosine, pilosine** and related structures.

Chemical Structure

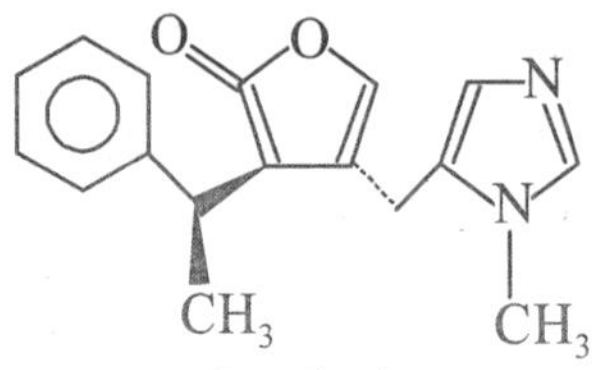

Isopilosine

[3S-[3α (S*), 4β]]-Dihydro-3-(hydroxyphenylmethyl)-4-[(1-methyl-1H-imidazol-5-yl) methyl]-2 (3H)-furanone. ($C_{16}H_{18}N_2O_3$).

Isolation   It is isolated from the leaves of *P. microphyllus* Stapf. (*Rutaceae*) by adopting standard procedures.*

Characteristic Features

1. It is obtained as needles from ethanol mp 182-182.5°C.

2. Its specific rotation $[\alpha]_D^{20} + 83.9°$ (ethanol); uv_{max} (ethanol) : 210 nm (log ∈ 4.10).

Biosynthesis of Imidazole Alkaloids   *L-Histidine*, an amino acid contains an imidazole ring; and is, therefore, the most probable precursor of alkaloids containing this ring system. The **imidazole alkaloids** usually found in Jaborandi leaves (*P. microphyllus* and *P. jaborandi; Rutaceae*) are most likely derived from histidine; however, sufficient experimental data are lacking. Interestingly, the additional carbon atoms may originate from acetate or supposedly from threonine in the case of **pilocarpine,** whereas **pilosine** incorporates a phenylpropane C_6H_3 unit as shown below.

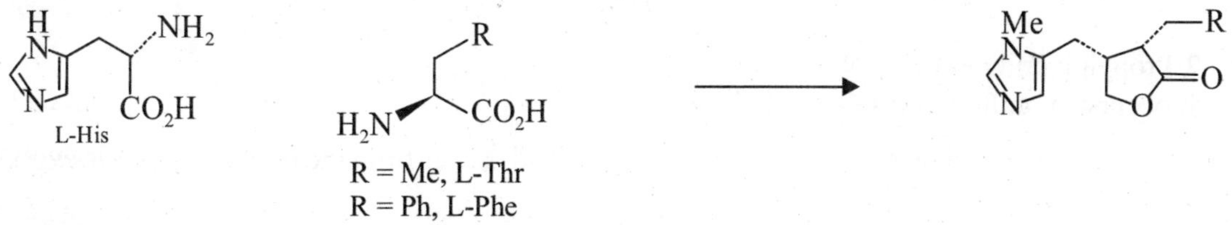

R = Me, L-Thr
R = Ph, L-Phe

7.2.4   Alkaloids Derived from Lysine

The amino acid *L-lysine* happens to be the homologue of L-ornithine, and it also caters as an alkaloid precursor, employing pathways that are analogous to those known for ornithine. The *'additional methylene moiety'* present in lysine affords the formation of six-membered piperidine ring systems, very similar to ornithine that provided five-membered ring systems, as shown below:

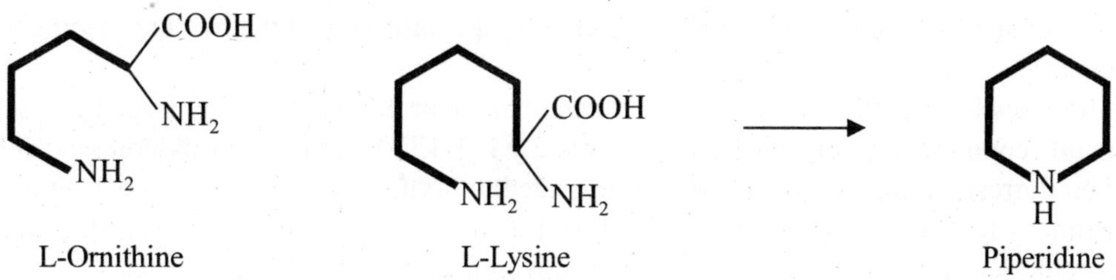

L-Ornithine   L-Lysine   Piperidine

The various alkaloids that are derived from lysine are invariably grouped together under the following categories, namely:

(*a*) Piperidine alkaloids
(*b*) Quinolizidine alkaloids, and
(*c*) Indolizidine alkaloids

The above cited categories of alkaloids shall now be discussed separately here under.

---

* F.L. Pyman *J. Chem. Soc.* **101**, 2260 (1912).

7.2.4.1 Piperidine Alkaloids

The various important alkaloids that essentially have the *piperidine nucleus* are, namely: **Coniine, Lobeline, Lobelanine** and **Piperine,** which shall be discussed individually in the sections that follows:

A. Coniine

Synonyms   Cicutine; Conicine.

Biological Source   It is the toxic principle of poison *Hemlock, Conium maculatum* L. (*Umbelliferae*). It is found in the seeds of *Cicuta maculata* L. (*Apiaceae*) (Water Hemlock).

Chemical Structure

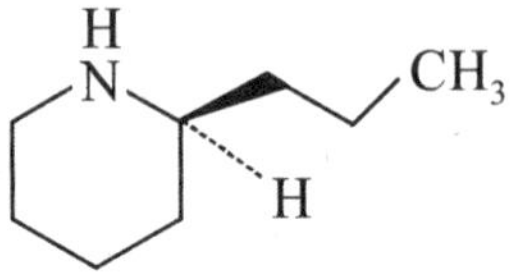

Coniine

(S)-2-Propylpiperidine ($C_8H_{17}N$)
    It occurs naturally as the (S)–(+) isomer.

Isolation   It is isolated by standard procedures described earlier from the pitcher plant *Sarracenia flava**.
    The various steps involved in the isolation of **coniine** are as follows:

1. The powdered Hemlock fruits are mixed with KOH solution and then subjected to steam distillation. The distillate thus obtained is neutralized and evaporated to dryness.
2. The resulting residue is extracted with ethanol successively, filtered and the solvent evaporated under vacuo. The ethanol extracts the alkaloidal salts that are dissolved in water, which is subsequently rendered alkaline with KOH solution and finally extracted with ether at least 3-4 times.
3. Ether is evaporated under vacuo, when an oily liquid comprising of the free bases remains as the residue.
4. The fractional distillation of the oily liquid *under vacuo* or in a current of hydrogen gas, separates them into coniine and γ-coniceine at approximately 171-172°C. These two alkaloids are converted to their corresponding hydrochlorides, evaporated to dryness and extracted with acetone. Thus, coniine hydrochloride will be obtained as the insoluble substance, while the coniceine hydrochloride shall remain in acetone and recovered separately.
    Note: Coniine enjoys the distinction of being the first ever alkaloid prepared synthetically.

Characteristic Features
1. It is a colourless alkaline liquid, which darkens and polymerizes on exposure to light and air.
2. It has a typical mousy odour.
3. It has mp ~ -2°C, and bp 166-166.5°C; bp_{20} 65-66°C.
4. It is a steam-volatile substance.

---

* N.V. Mody *et al. Experientra*, **32**, 829 (1976)

5. Its physical parameters are: d_4^{20} 0.8440-0.848; n_D^{23} 1.4505; $[\alpha]_D^{25} + 8.4°$ (C = 4.0 in chloroform); $[\alpha]_D^{23} + 14.6°$ (neat) and pK_a 3.1.

6. *Solubility:* 1 ml dissolves in 90 ml of water, and less soluble in hot water. The base dissolves about 25% of water of ambient temperature. It is freely soluble in ethanol, ether, benzene, acetone and amyl alcohol; and slightly soluble in chloroform.

Identification Tests

1. **Coniine Hydrobromide Derivative ($C_8H_{17}N$. HBr):** Its prisms have mp 21°C ; 1 g dissolves in 2 ml water, 3 ml ethanol, and freely soluble in ether and chloroform.

2. **Coniine Hydrochloride Derivative** ($C_8H_{17}N$. HCl): It occurs as rhomboids having mp 221°C, freely soluble in water, chloroform and ethanol.

   (R)-(–) Form: It is a liquid, bp_{756} 165°C; $[\alpha]_D^{25} – 8.1°$ (C = 4.0 in chloroform); $[\alpha]_D^{23} – 14.2°$ (neat).

   (±)-Form: It has bp 200-210°C.

Uses

1. It has been used in convulsive and spasmodic diseases, such as: asthma, chorea, epilepsy, pertussis and tetanus.

2. **Coniine** has also been recommended is carditis, delirium, glandular swellings, jaundis, mania, nervous diseases, neuralgia, rheumatism, spasms and ulcers.

B. Lobeline

Synonyms   α-Lobeline; Inflatine;

Biological Sources   It is obtained from the herb and seeds of *Lobelia inflata* L., (*Lobeliaceae*) (**Indian Tobacco, Asthma Weed**); leaves of *Lobelia tupa* L. (*Campanulaceae*) (**Tupa, Devil's Tobacco**).

Chemical Structure

Lobeline

[2R-[2α, 6α (S*)]]-2-[6-(2-Hydroxy-2-phenylethyl)-1-methyl-2-piperidinyl]-1-phenylethanone ($C_{22}H_{27}NO_2$).

Isolation   The various steps are as follows:

1. The powdered **lobelia herb** is moistened with water, acidified slightly with acetic acid and left as such for 3-4 hours. The resulting mass is then pressed and the process of moistening and pressing is repeated subsequently.

2. The acidic solutions thus collected are mixed and rendered alkaline with sodium bicarbonate carefully. The alkaline solution is extracted with ether successively. For purification, the etherial extract is shaken with water, acidified with dilute sulphuric acid. The acidified liquid is again rendered alkaline with sodium bicarbonate solution and shaken with ether.

3. The combined ethereal extract is evaporated and the yellow oily liquid, comprising of the total alkaloids, is dissolved in water, acidified with HCl, filtered and then shaken with chloroform successively. Thus, the chloroform will exclusively extract the lobeline hydrochloride, while leaving the salts of the other alkaloids in the aqueous layer. The chloroform is then evaporated under vacuo to obtain the brownish oily residue.

4. The above residue is then taken up with double its volume of hot water at 80°C. The aqueous solution is kept in a vacuum desiccator over concentrated H_2SO_4 for several hours when lobeline hydrochloride separates out as crystals.

5. To recover the **lobeline** base, the resulting HCl salt is dissolved in warm water, rendered alkaline with dilute NaOH carefully and extracted with ether several times. The ethereal extract is evaporated and the residue is recrystallized from ethanol or benzene.

Characteristic Features

1. Lobeline is obtained as needles from ethanol, ether and benzene having mp 130-131°C, and specific rotation $[\alpha]_D^{15} - 43°$ (ethanol).

2. It is freely soluble in chloroform, ether, benzene and hot ethanol; and very slightly soluble in water and petroleum ether.

Identification Tests

1. **Colour Test: Lobeline** on the addition of a few drops of concentrated sulphuric acid followed by a drop of formalin solution gives rise to a distinct red colouration.

2. **Froehd's Test:** It produces an instant rose red colouration with **Froehd's Reagent** that ultimately changes to blue.

3. **Erdmann's Reagent:** It develops a faint green colour which intensifies on slight warming.

4. **Lobeline Hydrochloride ($C_{22}H_{27}NO_2$.HCl) (Lobron, Zoolobelin):** It is obtained as rosettes of slender needles from ethanol with mp 178-180°C; $[\alpha]_D^{20} - 43°$ (C = 2); and uv_{max} (methanol) 245, 280 nm (log ∈ 4.08, 3.05). Its solubility profile is as follows: 1 g dissolves in 40 ml of water, 12 ml of ethanol, very soluble in chloroform and very slightly soluble in ether. A 1% (w/v) solution in water has a pH of 4.0-6.0.

5. **Lobeline Sulphate [($C_{22}H_{27}NO_2$)$_2$.H_2SO_4] (Lobeton, Unilobin, Bantron, Toban, Lobidan):** Its crystals obtained from ethanol exhibits specific rotation $[\alpha]_D^{20} - 25°$ (C = 2). It is soluble in 30 parts of water and slightly in ethanol.

Uses

1. It is widely used as a respiratory stimulant.

2. Its effects resemble those of **nicotine** and hence used in lozenges or chewing tablets, containing 0.5-1.5 mg of **Lobeline Sulphate,** to help in breaking the tobacco habit, otherwise known as **'smoking deterrants'.**

C. Lobelanine

Biological Source   After **lobeline, lobelanine** is obtained as the most abundant alkaloid of *Lobelia inflata* L. (*Lobeliaceae*). (**Indian Tobacco, Asthma Weed**).

Chemical Structure

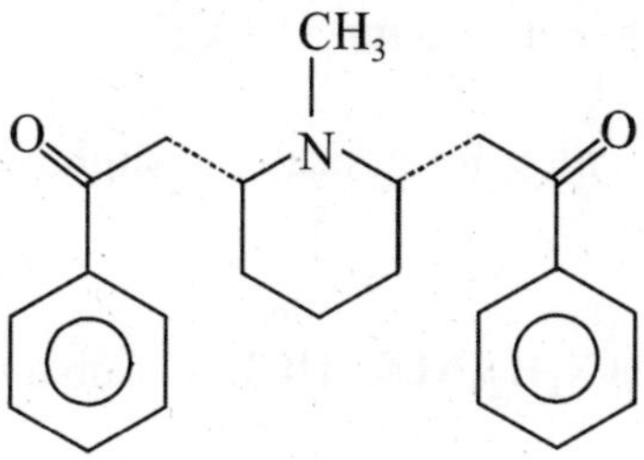

Lobelanine

cis-2, 2′-(1-Methyl-2, 6-piperidine-diyl) bis [1-phenylethanone], ($C_{22}H_{25}NO_2$).

Isolation   The aqueous layer obtained in step (3), as stated under isolation of lobeline, is subjected to column chromatography and the **lobelanine** is collected as one of the major fractions.

Characteristic Features
1. It is obtained as rosettes of needles from ether or petroleum ether having mp 99°C.
2. It is freely soluble in acetone, benzene, ethanol, chloroform; and slightly soluble in water and ether.

Identification Tests
1. **Lobelanine Hydrochloride ($C_{22}H_{25}NO_2$.HCl):** The crystals obtained from dilute ethanol decomposes at 188°C; it is soluble in chloroform; and slightly soluble in absolute ethanol and cold water.
2. **Lobelanine Hydrobromide ($C_{22}H_{25}NO_2$.HBr):** The crystals do not give a sharp mp, but gets decomposed at 188°C.
3. **Lobelanine Nitrate ($C_{22}H_{25}NO_2$.HNO_3):** The crystals obtained from dilute ethanol has mp 153-154°C.
4. If differs from **Lobeline** in lacking OH moiety; and therefore, does not react with nitrous acid nor with benzyl chloride.
5. It being a diketonic compound-forms a dioxime.

D. Lobelanidine

Biological Source   It is same as that of lobelanine.

Chemical Structure

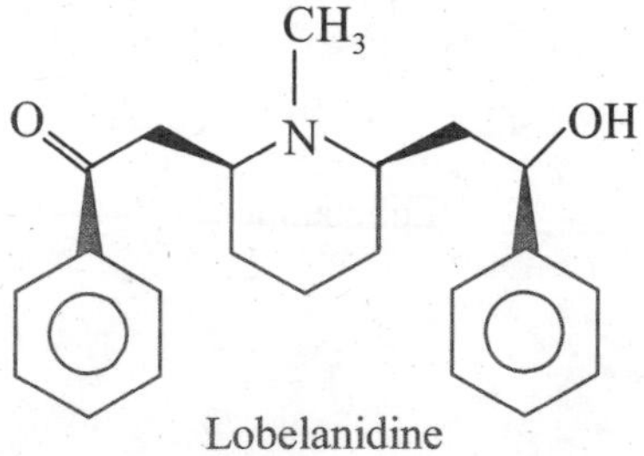

Lobelanidine

[2α(R*), 6α(S*)-Methyl-α, α′-diphenyl-2, 6-piperidine-diethanol ($C_{22}H_{29}NO_2$).

Isolation   It is obtained as one of the fractions obtained from the column chromatography of the aqueous extract from step (3) under isolation of **lobeline**.

Characteristic Features

1. It is obtained as scales from ethanol with mp 150°C.
2. It distils unchanged in vacuo.
3. It is freely soluble in benzene, chloroform, acetone; slightly soluble in ether, petroleum ether; and almost insoluble in water.

Identification Tests

1. **Lobelanidine Hydrochloride ($C_{22}H_{29}NO_2$. HCl):** It is obtained as needles from ethanol having mp 135-138°C.
2. **Lobelanidine Hydrobromide ($C_{22}H_{29}NO_2$.HBr):** Its crystals have a mp 189°C.

Synthesis from Lobeline, Lobelanine and Lobelanidine First of all, **lobelanine** may be synthesized by the interaction of one molecule of glutaric dialdehyde, two moles of benzoyl acetic acid, and one mole of methylamine hydrochloride; allowing the reaction mixture to stand for 40 hours at 35°C and at pH 4.5. Thus, the resulting product **lobelanine** gives rise to:

(*a*) **Lobeline:** When subjected to *partial reduction*, and
(*b*) **Lobelanidine:** On being subjected to *complete reduction*.

All these reactions are summarized as given below.

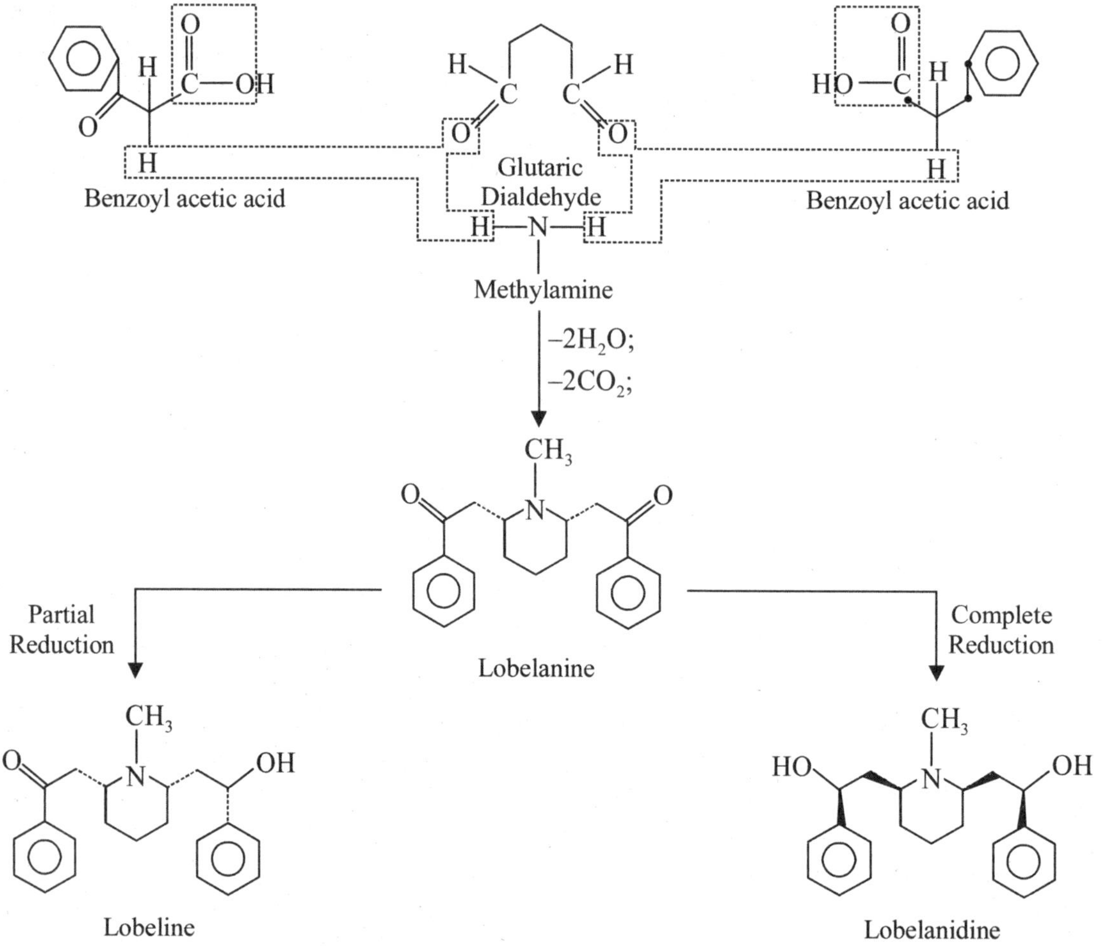

Biosynthesis of Lobeline and Lobelanine   The two above stated alkaloids, namely: **lobeline** and **lobelanine,** commonly found in the antiasthmatic medicinal plant *Lobelia inflata*, found to comprise of the piperidine rings with alternative C_6C_2 side-chains derived from phenylalanine *via* cinnamic acid. In fact, these alkaloids are formed as shown below wherein benzoylacetyl-CoA, an emerging intermediate in the β-oxidation of cinnamic acid helps to cater for the nucleophile engaged in the **Mannich reaction.** Thus, oxidation of the piperidine ring brings forth a new iminium species that can react further with a second mole of **benzoylacetyl-CoA,** again *via* **Mannich reaction.** Both **lobeline** and **lobelanine** are the resulting products obtained from further N-methylation and/or carbonyl reduction reactions.

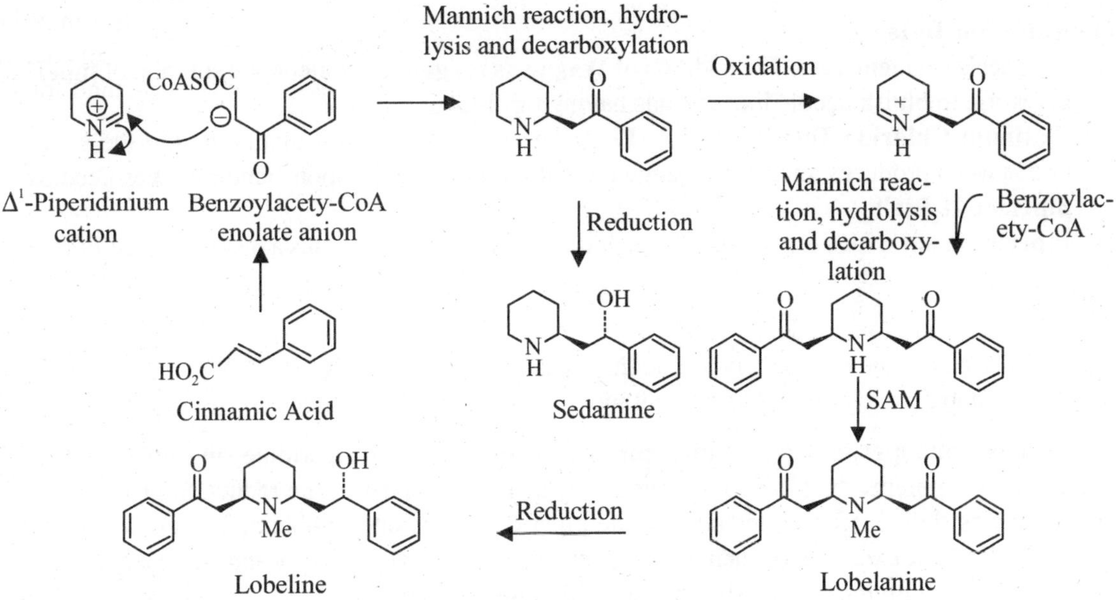

E. Piperine

Biological Source   It is obtained from the dried unripe fruit of *Piper nigrum* L. (Black Pepper), *Piper longum* L., *Piper retrofractum* Vahl. (*Piper officinarum* C.D.C.), and *Piper clusii* C.D.C.; and also in the root bark of *Piper geniculatum*. Sw. belonging to family *Piperaceae*.

Chemical Structure

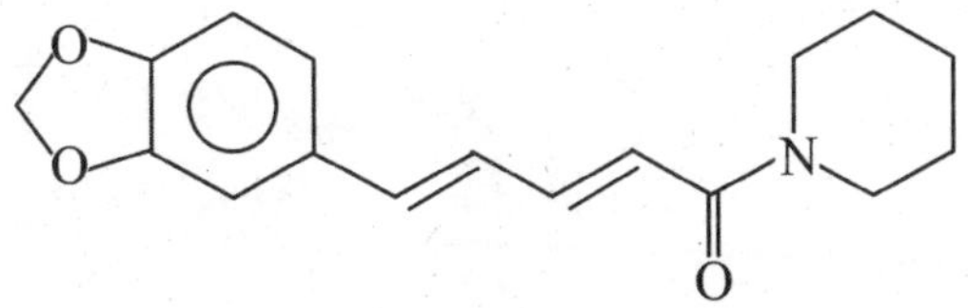

Piperine

(E, E)-1-[5-(1, 3-Benzodioxol-5-yl)-1-oxo-2, 4-pentadienyl] piperidine ($C_{17}H_{19}NO_3$).

Isolation   The dried unripe fruits are extracted with ethanol in a Soxhlet apparatus till extraction is complete. The solvent is evaporated under vacuo in a Rotary Thin Film Evaporator. The residue of the alcoholic extract is digested with dilute alkali to affect saponification, when piperine remains unaffected. The residue, thus obtained is decanted and washed with distilled water several times.

The resulting product is dissolved in hot ethanol and on cooling the crystalline **piperine** separates out.

Characteristic Features

1. Piperine is obtained as monoclinic prisms from alcohol having mp 130°C.
2. It is tasteless at first, but has a burning aftertaste.
3. Its dissociation constant pK (18°C) is 12.22.
4. **Solubility Profile:** 1 g of **piperine** dissolves in 15 ml ethanol, 1.7 ml chloroform, 36 ml ether; freely soluble in acetic acid and benzene; and almost insoluble in water (40 mg/L at 18°C), and petroleum ether.

Identification Tests

1. **Wagner's Reagent Test:** The addition of **Wagner's reagent** to an alcoholic solution of **piperine** gives rise to bluish needle like crystals having mp 145°C.
2. **Platinum Chloride Test [H_2PtCl_6]: Piperine** on treatment with platinum chloride solution (0.5% w/v/) produces an instant orange red colouration, which upon standing gives needles of **piperine-H_2PtCl_6.**
3. **Piperine** reacts with a few drops of concentrated sulphuric acid yields a distinct red colouration.

Uses

1. It is used as an insecticide.
2. It is also employed extensively as condiment in food preparations.
3. It is used to give a *'pungent'* taste to brandy.

Biosynthesis of Piperine   In the **biosynthesis of piperine,** the piperidine ring forms part of a tertiary amide moiety which is incorporated *via* piperidine itself *i.e.*, the reduction product of Δ^1-piperideine as shown under. Interestingly, the piperic acid residue in obtained from a cinnamoyl-CoA precursor. The extension of chain is caused by virtue of acetate/malonate and ultimately combines as its CoA-ester with the previously obtained piperidine nucleus.

Biosynthesis of Piperine

7.2.4.2 *Quinolizidine Alkaloids*

The **quinolizidine alkaloids** comprise of **lupinine, lupanine** and **sparteine** which are responsible for the toxic properties are characterized by a quinolizidine skeleton. The bi-heterocyclic nucleus is closely related to the ornithine-derived pyrrolizidine system, but is believed to be formed from two molecules of lysine.

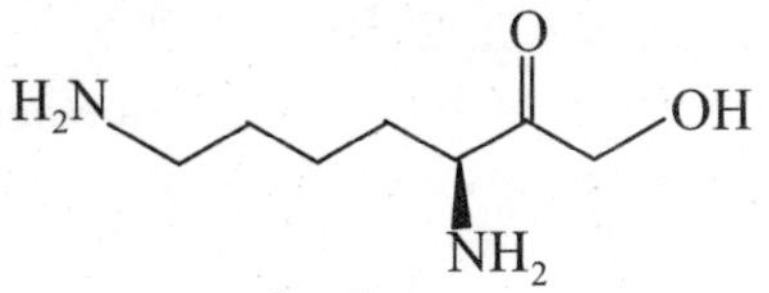

| Lysine | Pyarrolizidine | Quinolizidine |

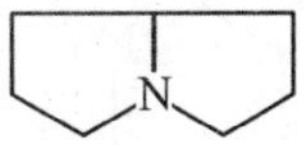

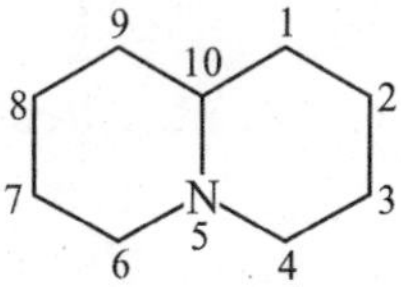

The aforesaid *three* alkaloids shall now be discussed individually in the pages that follows:

A. Lupinine

Synonyms ℓ-Lupinine; (–)-Lupinine.

Biological Source   The naturally occurring ℓ-form is obtained from the seeds and herb of *Lupinus luteus* L. and other *Lupinus* species belonging to the natural order *Lequminoseae*; and also found in *Anabasis aphylla* L. (*Chenopodiaceae*).

Chemical Structure

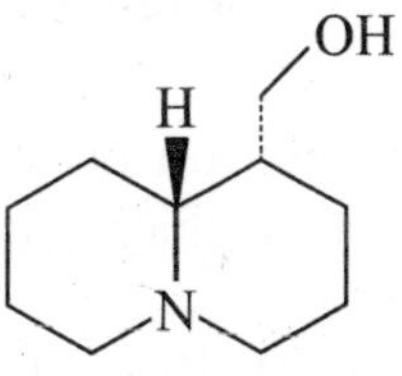

Lupinine

[1R-*trans*]-Octahydro-2H-quinolizidine-1-methanol ($C_{10}H_{19}NO$).

Isolation   The isolation of **lupinine** from the seeds and herb of *Lupinus lutens* may be affected by the method evolved by Couch* (1934).

Characteristic Features
1. **Lupinine** is obtained as stout orthorhombic prisms from acetone having mp 68.5-69.2°C.
2. Its physical parameters are: bp_4 160-164°C; bp_{755} 269-270°C; $[\alpha]_D^{26} - 25.9°$ (C = 3 in water) ; $[\alpha]_D^{28} - 21°$ (C = 9.5 in ethanol);
3. It is soluble in water, ethanol, ether and chloroform.
4. It is a strong base.

Identification Tests
1. **ℓ-Form Lupinine Hydrochloride Derivative ($C_{10}H_{20}ClNO$):** Its orthorhombic prisms have mp 208-213°C, and $[\alpha]_D$–14°.

---

* Couch, J.F., *J. Am. Chem. Soc.,* **56**, 2434 (1934).

2. *dl*-**Form Lupinine:** The crystals obtained from acetone have mp 58.5-59.5°C.

B. Lupanine

Biological Source   It is obtained from the herb of *Genista tinctoria* L. (*Fabaceae*) (**Dyer's Broom**).

Chemical Structure

Lupanine

(7α, 7aα, 14α, 14aβ)-Dodecahydro-7, 14-methano-2H, 11H-dipyridiol [1, 2-a: 1′, 2′-e] diazocin-11-one; ($C_{15}H_{24}N_2O$].

Isolation   The racemic and optical isomers of **lupanine** have been duly isolated from various species of *Lupinus* (*Fabaceae/Leguminosae*) as stated below:

  (±)-**Lupanine**—from white lupins;

  d-**Lupanine**—from blue lupins;

  l-**Lupanine**—from the natural racemic form;

Characteristic Features   The physical parameters of the above *three* forms of **lupanine** are given below:

  dl-**Lupanine:** It is obtained as orthorhombic prisms obtained from acetone having mp 98-99°C; $bp_{1.0}$ 185-195°C; It is soluble in ethanol, ether, chloroform and water; and insoluble in petroleum ether.

  d-**Lupanine (Synonym: 2-Oxosparteine):** It is obtained as syrup crystallizing difficultly in hygroscopic needles having mp 40-44°C; bp_3 190-193°C; n_D^{24} 1.5444; $[\alpha]_D^{25} + 84°$ (C = 4.8 in ethanol). It is found to be freely soluble in water, ethanol, ether and chloroform.

  ℓ-**Lupanine (Synonym: Hydrorhombinine):** It is a viscous liquid having $bp_{1.0}$ 186-188°C; $[\alpha]_D - 61°$ in acetone.

Identification Test   **Lupanine** forms the corresponding lupanine hydrochloride dihydrate ($C_{15}H_{24}N_2O.HCl.2H_2O$) which is obtained as rhombic crystals from water having mp 127°C (dry).

C. Sparteine

Synonyms   *ℓ*-Sparteine; Lupinidine.

Biological Sources   It is obtained from yellow and black **lupin beans** *Lupinus luteus* L., and *Lupinus niger* Hort.; and also found in *Cytisus scoparius* (L.) Link. (*Fabaceae*) (**Scotch Broom**); *Anagyris foetida* L., belonging to natural order *Leguminosae*. Besides, it is also obtained from the roots of *Aconitum napellus* L. (*Ranunculaceae*) (**Aconite, Monkshood, Blue Rocket**); from the herbs of *Chelidonium majus* L. (*Papaveraceae*) (Celandine, Great Celandine, Nipplewort); from leaves of *Peumus boldus* Molina (*Monimiaceae*) (Boldo).

Chemical Structure

Sparteine

[7S-(7α, 7aα, 14α, 14a β]-Dodecahydro-7, 14-methano-2H, 6H-dipyrido [1, 2-a: 1′, 2′-e] [1, 5] diazocine, $(C_{15}H_{26}N_2)$.

Isolation   It is isolated from yellow and black lupin beans by the method put forward by Clemo* (1949).

Characteristic Features

1. It is a viscous oily liquid having bp_8 173°C.
2. It is volatile with steam.
3. Its physical parameters are: $[\alpha]_D^{21} - 16.4°$ (C = 10 in absolute ethanol); n_D^{20} 1.5312; d_4^{20} 1.020; pK_1 at 20°C : 2.24; pK_2:9.46; pH of 0.01 molar solution is 11.6.
4. **Solubility profile:** It is freely soluble in ethanol, ether and chloroform; and 1 g dissolves in 325 ml of water.

Identification Test

Sparteine Sulphate Pentahydrate $(C_{15}H_{26}N_2.H_2SO_4.5H_2O)$: (Synonyms: Depasan; Tocosamine) It is obtained as columnar crystals which loses water of crystallization at 100°C turning brown and ultimately gets decomposed at 136°C. The pH of a 0.05 molar solution is 3.3. It is practically insoluble in ether and chloroform, and 1 g dissolves in 1.1 ml of water, 3 ml of ethanol.

Uses

1. It is used mostly as an oxytocic.
2. It is employed as a cardiac depresant, cathartic, diuretic and for stimulating uterine contractions.
3. Sparteine is used occasionally as a quinidine substitute in stubborn cases of atrial fibrillation.

Biosynthesis of Lupinine, Lupanine and Sparteine   Experimental evidence reveals lysine to be incorporated into **lupinine** *via* **cadaverine**; however, the intermediate related to **homospermidine** is excluded. It has been observed that Δ^1-piperideine happens to be an important intermediate after **cadaverine.** Thus, the proposed pathway given below suggests coupling of two such molecules. In fact, the two tautomers of Δ^1-piperideine, as N-analogues of corresponding carbonyl compounds, are in a position to couple by an aldol-type mechanism. In reality, this coupling takes place in solution at physiological pHs, although the *stereospecific coupling* as shown in the proposed pathway shall evidently require the participation of suitable enzymes. After coupling, the imine system gets hydrolyzed, the resulting primary amine function undergoes oxidation, and ultimately the formation of the **quinolizidine nucleus** is accomplished by Schiff base formation. Thus, **lupinine** is then synthesized by two further reductive steps. Hence, the pathway to **sparteine** and **lupanine** eventually requires participation of another molecule of **cadaverine** or Δ^1-**piperideine.**

---

* Clemo *et al. J. Chem. Soc.* 6.63, (1949)

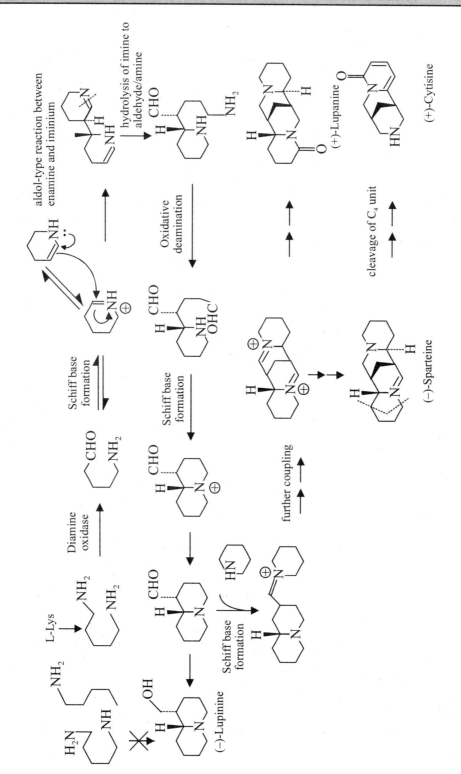

Biosynthesis of Lupinine, Lupanine and Sparteine

7.2.4.3 Indolizidine Alkaloids

The **indolizidine alkaloids** are usually characterized by the presence of a 5-membered and a 6-membered cyclic ring with a N-atom fused in them as shown below:

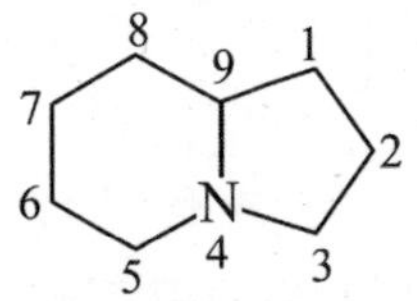

Indolizidine

The two typical examples of **indolizidine alkaloids** are, namely: **castanospermine** and **swansonine,** which shall be discussed hereunder:

A. Castanospermine

Biological Source   It is obtained from the seeds of the **Australian leguminous tree** *Castanospermum australe* A. Cunn. (*Leguminosae*) (**Moreton Bay Chestnut**).

Chemical Structure

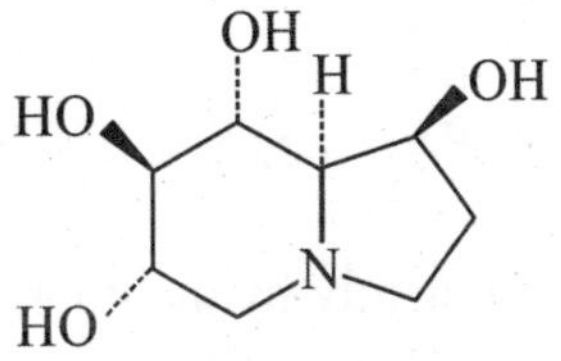

Castanospermine

[1S-(1α, 6β, 7α, 8β, 8aβ]-Octahydro-1, 6, 7, 8-indolizinetetrol; ($C_8H_{15}NO_4$). It is a polyhydroxy alkaloid.

Isolation   The isolation of the naturally occurring (+)-form of **castanospermine** from the seeds of the Australian leguminous tree has been duly accomplished.*

Characteristic Features
  1. The crystals obtained from aqueous ethanol have mp 212-215°C (decomposed).
  2. Its specific optical rotation is $[\alpha]_D^{25} + 79.7°$ (C = 0.93 in water); and dissociation constant pK 6.09.

Uses   Its has demonstrated activity against the AIDS virus HIV, by virtue of their ability to inhibit ghyosidase enzymes involved in glycoprotein biosynthesis. However, the glycoprotein coating seems to be vital for the proliferation of the AIDS virus.

B. Swainsonine

Biological Source   It is obtained from the plant *Swainsona canescens* (*Leguminosae/Fabaceae*).

---

* Hohenschutz *et al. Phytochemistry*, **20**, 811 (1981).

Chemical Structure

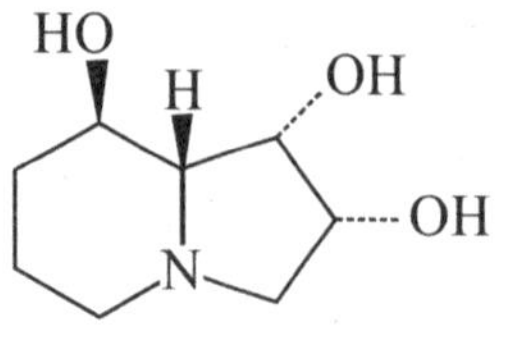

Swainsonine

[IS-(1α, 6β, 7α, 8β, 8aβ)-Octahydro-1, 2, 8-indolizinetriol; ($C_8H_{15}NO_3$).

Biosynthesis of Castanospermine and Swainsonine   These two alkaloids are regarded as a hybrid between the **pyrrolizidine** and **quinolizidine** alkaloids. It is, however, pertinent to mention here that these two alkaloids though are derived from lysine, yet their origin entirely deviates from the usual and common lysine-derived moieties in that **L-pipecolic acid** is found to be an intermediate in the pathway. In fact, there are *two* established routes known to the formation of pipecolic acid in nature, as shown below; wherein the point of difference solely based on whether the N-atom is taken-up either from the α- or the ∈ -amino portion of lysine.

In short, for the **indolizidine-alkaloid biosynthesis** the following salient features may be observed, namely:

- Pipecolic acid is produced *via* the aldehyde and Schiff base by retaining the N-atom from the α-amino function,
- Indolizidine nucleus is formed subsequently by incorporating a C_2-acetate unit through simple reactions,
- The resulting compound leads to the formation of *castanospermine* through a sequential hydroxylation reactions,
- Also a branch point compound results into the formation of **swainsonine** that essentially possess the opposite configuration at the ring fusion.

7.2.5   Alkaloids Derived from Nicotinic Acid

The alkaloids derived from the **nicotinic acid** are commonly known as the **'Pyridine Alkaloids'**.

In general, the alkaloids found in tobacco (*Nicotiana tabacum, Solanaceae*) include a variety of alkaloids, such as: **nicotine, anabasine,** and **niacin (Vitamin B_3, nicotinic acid)**. Interestingly, the *'pyridine unit'* has its origins in **vitamin B_3 (nicotinic acid);** whereas, a combination of a pyridine ring with a pyrrolidine ring gives rise to **nicotine,** or a combination of a pyridine ring with a piperidine unit forms **anabasine.**

7.2.5.1   Pyridine Alkaloids

The *three* above mentioned **pyridine alkaloids,** *viz.*, **nicotine, anabasine** and **niacin,** shall now be discussed individually in the sections that follows:

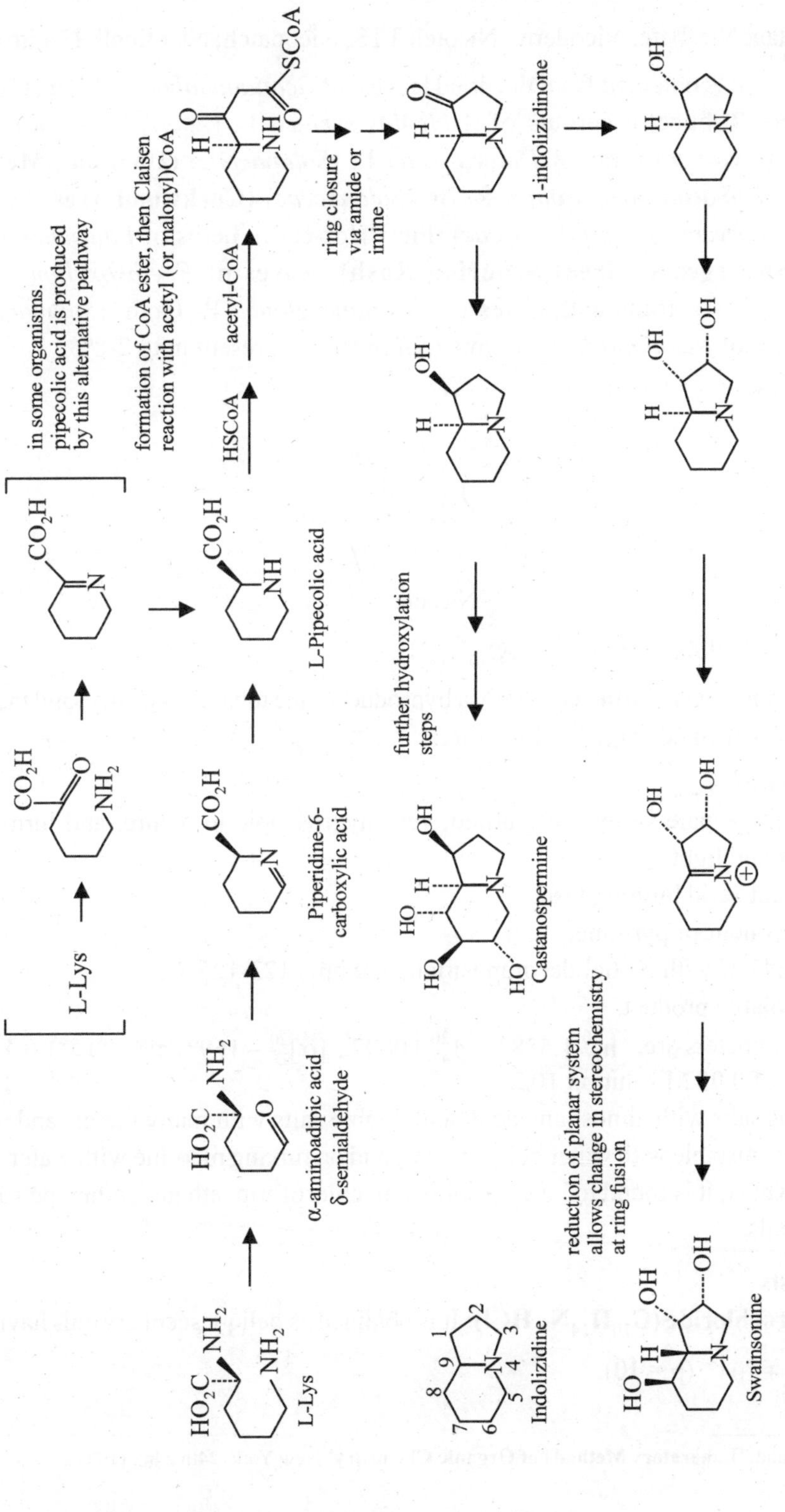

SCoA

in some organisms. pipecolic acid is produced by this alternative pathway

formation of CoA ester, then Claisen reaction with acetyl (or malonyl)CoA

acetyl-CoA

ring closure via amide or imine

1-indolizidinone

HSCoA

L-Lys

CO$_2$H

CO$_2$H

NH

L-Pipecolic acid

further hydroxylation steps

CO$_2$H

L-Lys

α-aminoadipic acid δ-semialdehyde

CO$_2$H

Piperidine-6-carboxylic acid

Castanospermine

reduction of planar system allows change in stereochemistry at ring fusion

Indolizidine

Swainsonine

Biosynthesis of Castanospermine and Swainsonine

A. Nicotine

Synonyms   Nicolan; Nicabate; Nicoderm; Nicotell TTS; Nicopatch; Nicotinell; Habitrol; Tabazur.

Biological Sources   It is obtained from the dried leaves of *Nicotiana tabacum* Linn., (*Solanaceae*) (**Virginia Tobacco; Tobacco**); sprouts of *Asclepias syriaca* L. (*Asclepiadaceae*) (**Common Milkweed**); dried leaves and roots of *Datura metel* L. (*Solanaceae*) (**Unmatal, Metel, Hindu Datura**); leaves of *Duboisia myoporoides* R. Br. (*Solanaceae*) (**Corkwood Tree, Pituri**); fresh forage of *Equisetum arvense* L. (*Equisetaceae*) (Field Horsetail); herbs of *Equisetum hyemale* L. (*Equisetaceae*) (**Shavegrass, Great Scouring Rush**); leaves of *Erythroxylum coca* Lam., (*Erythroxylaceae*) (*Coca*); fruits and leaves of *Nicotiana glauca* R. Grah. (*Solanaceae*) (**Tree Tobacco**); and leaves of *Nicotiana rustica* Linn. (*Solanaceae*)–present upto 2-8%.

Chemical Structure

Nicotine

(S)-3-(1-Methyl-2-pyrrolidixyl) pyridine; ($C_{10}H_{14}N_2$).

Preparation   Commercial **nicotine** is entirely a byproduct of the tobacco industry; and the extraction from-*N. tabacum* has been described in literature.*

Characteristic Features

1. It is a colourless to pale yellow oily liquid, very hygroscopic in nature, and turns brown on exposure to air and light.
2. It has an inherent acrid burning taste.
3. It develops the odour of pyridine.
4. It has a bp_{745} 247°C with partial decomposition; and bp_{17} 123-125°C.
5. It is a steam-volatile product.
6. Its physical parameters are; n_D^{20} 1.5282 ; d_4^{20} 1.0097 ; $[\alpha]_D^{20} - 169°$; pK_1 (15°) 6.16 and pK_2 10.96; and pH of 0.05 M solution 10.2.
7. It readily forms salts with almost any acid; and double salts with many metals and acids.
8. **Solubility:** It is miscible with water below 60 °C; and on mixing nicotine with water the volume contracts. However, it is found to be very soluble in chloroform, ethanol, ether, petroleum ether and kerosene oils.

Identification Tests

1. **Nicotine Hydrochloride ($C_{10}H_{14}N_2.HCl$):** It is obtained as deliquescent crystals having specific rotation $[\alpha]_D^{20} + 104°$ (p = 10).

---

* Gattermann, Wieland, '**Laboratory Methods of Organic Chemistry**' New York, 24th edn., (1937).

2. **Nicotine Dihydrochloride ($C_{10}H_{14}N_2.2HCL$):** The deliquescent crystals are extremely soluble in water and ethanol.

3. **Nicotine Sulphate [($C_{10}H_{14}N_2)_2.H_2SO_4$] (Synonym: Nicotine neutral sulphate):** It is obtained as hexagonal tablets having optical rotation $[\alpha]_D^{20} + 88°$ (p = 70); and is soluble in water and ethanol.

4. **Nicotine Bitartrate ($C_{10}H_{14}N_2.2C_4H_6O_6$) (Synonym: Nicotine Tartrate):** It is obtained as the dihydrate, crystals having mp 90 °C; $[\alpha]_D^{20} + 26°$ (C = 10); and is found to be very soluble in ethanol and water.

5. **Nicotine Zinc Chloride Double Salt Monohydrate ($C_{10}H_{16}Cl_4N_2Zn-H_2O$):** It is very soluble in water; and sparingly soluble in ether and ethanol.

6. **Nicotine Salicylate ($C_{17}H_{20}N_2O_3$): (Synonym: Eudermol):** It is obtained as hexagonal plates having mp 118°C; $[\alpha]_D^{20} + 13°$ (C = 9); and is found to be freely soluble in ethanol and water.

Uses

1. It is used extensively as an insecticide and fumigant.

2. It finds its application as a **'contact poison'** in the form of soap *i.e.*, as its oleate, laurate and naphthenate salts.

3. It is also used as a **'stomach poison'** in combination with bentonite.

4. One of its recent applications nicotine is employed as chewable tablets of lozenges for the treatment of smoking withdrawl syndrome.

5. It possesses a unique action on the autonomic ganglia which it first stimulates and subsequently depresses ultimately leading to *paralysis*.

B. Anabasine

Synonym   Neonicotine;

Biological Sources   It is obtained from the leaves of *Duboisia myoporoides* R. Br. (*Solanaceae*) **(Corkwood tree; Pituri)**; fruits and leaves of *Nicotiana glauca* R. Grah. (*Solanaceae*) **(Tree Tobacco-** claimed to be the richest source of **anabasine** (1.2%); leaves of *Nicotiana tabacum* L. (*Solanaceae*) **(Tobacco, Tabac, Virginia Tobacco)**; and also the leaves of *Anabasis aphylla* L. (*Chenopodiaceae*).

Chemical Structure   3-(2-Piperidixyl) pyridine; ($C_{10}H_{14}N_2$).

Anabasine

Isolation   **Anabasine** is extracted on a large scale in Russia; and the industrial extraction processes have been reported by Sadykov and Timbekov* (1956).

Characteristic Features

1. It is a liquid freezing at 9°C; and boiling at 270-272°C; bp_{14} 145-147°C; bp_2 105°C.

2. Its physical parameters are: d_4^{20} 1.0455; n_D^{20} 1.5430; and $[\alpha]_D^{20} - 83.1°$.

3. It is soluble in most organic solvents and water.

Identification Tests

1. Being a secondary amine it can form a nitroso derivative.

2. **Anabasine Hydrochloride:** Its specific optical rotation is $[\alpha]_D + 16.5°$ (C = 10 in water).

Uses   It is invariably employed as an effective insecticide.

C. Niacin

Synonyms   Nicotinic Acid; Pellagra Preventive Factor (or P.P. Factor); Vitamin B_3; Akotin; Daskil; Nicacid; Niacor; Nicangin; Nicobid; Nicolar; Niconacid; Nico-Span; Wampocap. The term '*niacin*' has also been applied to nicotinamide.

Biological Sources   It is widely distributed in nature; and appreciable quantities are found in fish, yeast, liver, and cereal grains.

Chemical Structure

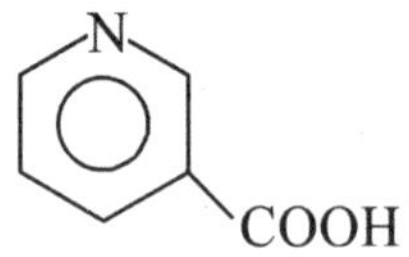

Niacin

3-Pyridinecarboxylic acid; ($C_6H_5NO_2$).

Preparation   It may be prepared by the **oxidation of nicotine**** as given below.

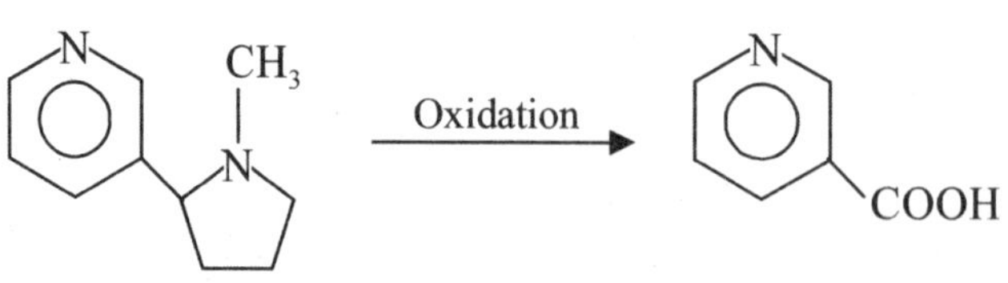

Nicotine   Niacin

Characteristic Features

1. It is obtained as needles from ethanol and water having mp 236.6°C.

---

* Sadykov and Timbekov, **J. Appl. Chem.,** USSR, **29**, 148 (1956).

** MeElvain, S.M., *Org. Synth.* Coll.Vol I, 385 (1941).

2. It sublimes without any decomposition.

3. It is a nonhygroscopic substance and fairly stable in air.

4. It shows uv_{max} : 263 nm; and pH 2-7 of a saturated solution.

5. *Solubility:* 1 g dissolves in 60 ml water; freely soluble in boiling water and ethanol; soluble in propylene glycol; and insoluble in ether.

Identification Test

1. **Niacin Sodium Salt Sesquihydrate ($C_6H_4NNaO_2.1\frac{1}{2}H_2O$) (Synonym: Direktan):** It is obtained as either white crystals or crystalline powder, which is stable in air. Its solubility profile are as follows: 1 g dissolves in ~ 1.4 ml of water, in 60 ml ethanol, in 10 ml glycerol; and insoluble in ether. The pH of aqueous solution is ~ 7.

2. **N-Oxide Derivative (Oxiniacic Acid):** It is obtained as needles mp 254-255°C (dec.) and uv_{max} (0.1 N.H_2SO_4):220, 260 nm ($\in$ 22400, 10200).

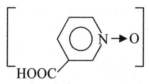

Oxiniacic Acid

Uses

1. It is used as antihyperlipoproteinemic agent.

2. It is a vital vitamin (enzyme cofactor).

Biosynthesis of Nicotine, Anabasine and Niacin Interestingly, plants such as *Nicotiana* make use of an altogether different pathway employing glyceraldehyde 3-phosphate and L-aspartic acid precursors as given under. Thus, the dibasic acid **quinonilic acid** features in the aforesaid pathway which upon decarboxylation gives rise to **nicotinic acid.**

It is pertinent to mention here that the formation of **nicotine** caused by a pyrrolidine ring derived from ornithine, quite possibly as the N-methyl-Δ^1-pyrrolinium cation gets hooked on to the pyridine ring present in nicotinic acid thereby displacing the carboxyl function during the course of reactions as depicted in (B). Further, a **dihydronicotinic acid** intermediate is most likely to be engaged permitting decarboxylation to the enamine 1, 2-dihydropyridine. It, therefore, allows an aldol-type interaction with the N-methylpyrrolinium cation, and ultimately undergoes dehydrogenation of the dihydropyridine ring reversed to a pyridine ring yields *nicotine*. In this fashion, **nornicotine** is derived by the oxidative demethylation of nicotine.

Finally, **anabasine** is generated from nicotinic acid and lysine *via* the Δ^1-piperidinium cation in an effectively analogous sequence as shown in (C) below.

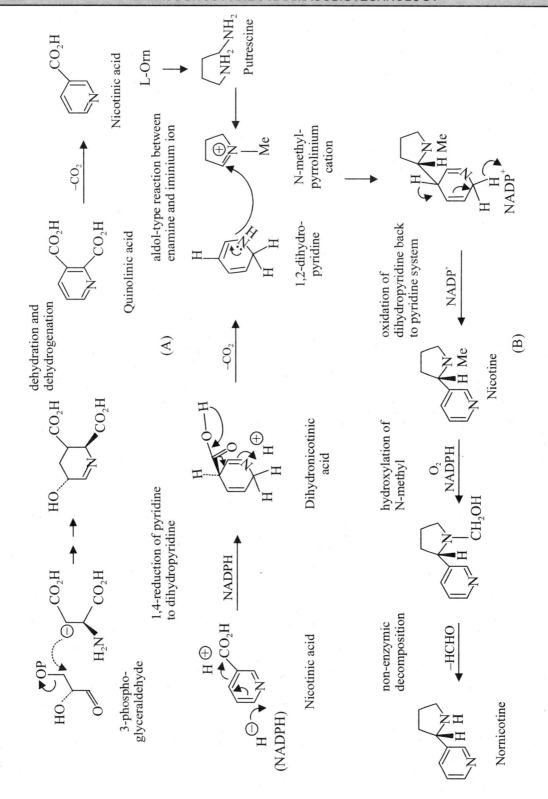

3-phospho-glyceraldehyde

dehydration and dehydrogenation

Quinolinic acid

Nicotinic acid

$-CO_2$

L-Orn

Putrescine

aldol-type reaction between enamine and iminium ion

(A)

1,4-reduction of pyridine to dihydropyridine

NADPH

(NADPH)

Nicotinic acid

$H^{\oplus}$

Dihydronicotinic acid

$-CO_2$

1,2-dihydro-pyridine

N-methyl-pyrrolinium cation

oxidation of dihydropyridine back to pyridine system

$NADP^+$

Nicotine

hydroxylation of N-methyl

O_2
NADPH

non-enzymic decomposition

$-HCHO$

Nornicotine

(B)

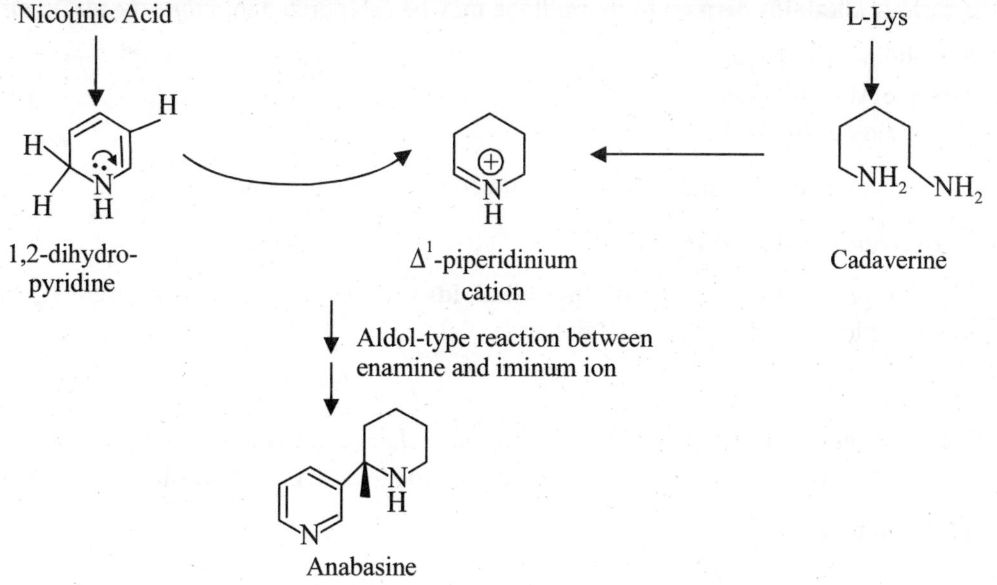

Nicotinic Acid

L-Lys

1,2-dihydro-
pyridine

Δ^1-piperidinium
cation

Cadaverine

Aldol-type reaction between
enamine and iminum ion

Anabasine

(C)

7.2.6 Alkaloids Derived from Ornithine

A non-protein amino acid, *L-ornithine*, usually constitutes an integral part of the '*urea-cycle*' in animals, wherein it is eventually produced from *L-arginine* in a reaction sequence catalyzed by the enzyme *arginase* as given below:

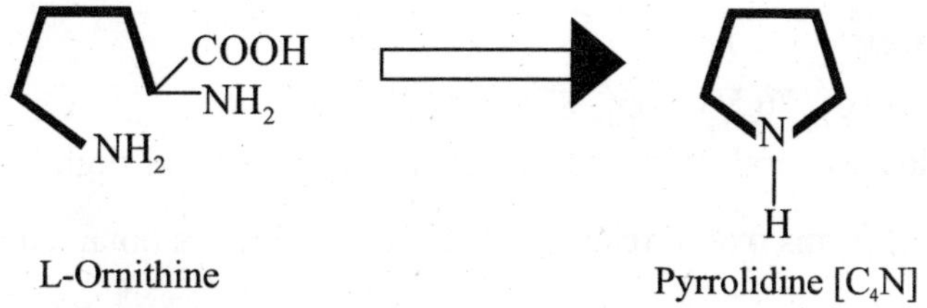

L-Ornithine

Pyrrolidine [C₄N]

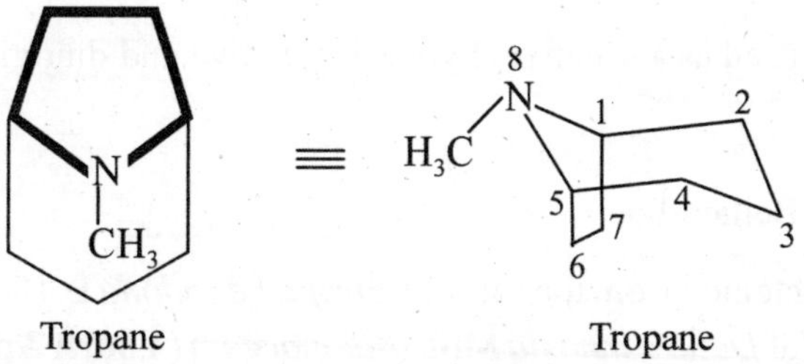

Tropane

Tropane

Evidently, L-ornithine possesses δ-and α-amino moieties, and the N-atom from the former moiety which is eventually incorporated into the alkaloid structures along with the C-chain, except for the carboxyl function. Thus, the L-ornithine exclusively provides a C₄N building block to the alkaloid structure; not only as a **pyrrolidine ring system,** but also as a part of the **tropane alkaloids.** Nevertheless, the reactions of ornithine are fairly comparable to those of lysine, which in turn provides a C₅N unit bearing its ε-amino moiety.

The various **alkaloids** derived from ornithine may be categorized into *three* heads, namely:

(*i*) Pyrrolidine Alkaloids,

(*ii*) Tropane Alkaloids, and

(*iii*) Pyrrolizidine Alkaloids.

The above categories of **alkaloids** shall be discussed separately hereunder.

7.2.6.1 *Pyrrolidine Alkaloids*

The *three* glaring examples of **pyrrolidine alkaloids** are, namely: **hygrine, cuscohygrine** and **stachydrine,** which would be discussed below:

A. Hygrine

Biological Sources   It occurs in the leaves of *Erythroxylon coca* Lam., (*Erythroxylaceae*) (Coca); and the roots of *Withania somniferum* (L.) Dunal. (*Solanaceae*) (**Ashwagandha**).

Chemical Structure

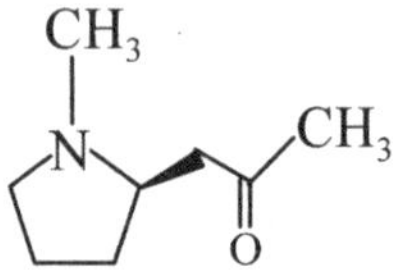

Hygrine

(R)-1-(1-Methyl-2-pyrrolidinyl)-2-propanone; ($C_8H_{15}NO$).

Characteristic Features

1. It is a liquid having bp_{11} 76.5°C; bp_{14} 81°C; n_D^{20} 1.4555.

2. It is soluble in dilute mineral acids, chloroform and ethanol; and slightly soluble in water.

Identification Test   It forms oxime readily ($C_8H_{16}N_2O$) which is obtained as crystals from ether having mp 123-124°C.

Uses   The drug is broadly used as a sedative, hypnotic laxative and diuretic.

B. Cuscohygrine

Synonyms   Cuskhygrine; Bellaradine.

Biological Sources   It is obtained from the roots of *Atropa belladona* L. (*Solanaceae*) (**Belladona, Deadly Nightshade**); roots of *Datura innoxia* Mill. (*Solanaceae*) (**Thorn Apple**) upto 5-30%; seeds of *Datura metal* L. (*Solanaceae*) (**Unmatal, Metel, Hindu Datura**); leaves of *Hyocyamus niger* L. (*Solanaceae*) (**Henbane, Henblain, Jusquaime**); herb of *Mandragora officinarum* L. (*Solanaceae*) (**Mandrake, Loveapple**); rhizome of *Scopolia carniolica* Jacq. (*Solanaceae*) (**Scopolia**); and the roots of *Withania somniferum* (L.) Dunal (*Solanaceae*) (**Ashwagandha**).

Chemical Structure

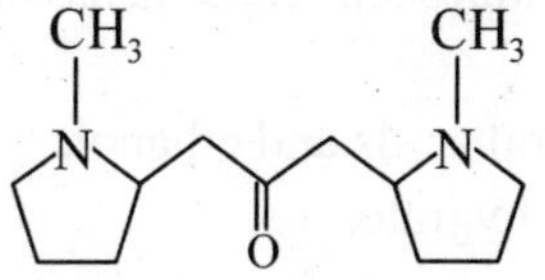

Cuscohygrine

1, 3-Bis (1-methyl-2-pyrrolidinyl)-2-propanone; ($C_{13}H_{24}N_2O$).

Isolation   It is isolated from the naturally occurring plant sources by standard method.*

Characteristic Features

1. It is a oily liquid having bp_{23} 169-170°C; bp_{14} 152°C; bp_2 118-125°C; d_4^{20} 0.9733; n_D^{20} 1.4832.
2. It is found to be miscible with water; and freely soluble in ethanol, ether, and benzene.

Identification Tests

1. Cuscohygrine Hemiheptahydrate: Its needles have mp 40°C.
2. Cuscohygrine Hydrobromide ($C_{13}H_{24}N_2O.2HBr$): It forms prisms from ethanol having mp 234°C.

C. Stachydrine

Synonyms   Methyl hygrate betaine; Hygric acid methylbetaine.

Biological Sources   It is obtained from the forage of *Achillea millefolium* L. (*Asteraceae*) (**Yarrow**); flowers of *Chrysanthemum cinerarifolium* (**Trevir.**) Vis. (*Asteraceae*) (**Pyrethrum, Dalmatian Insect Flower**); branches of *Lagochilus inebrians* Bunge (*Lamiaceae*) (**Intoxicating Mint**); dry plant of, *Leonurus cardiaca* (L.) (*Lamiaceae*) (**Motherwort**); the '*betaine fraction*' of alfalfa *Medicago sativa* L. (*Fabiaceae*) (**Alfalfa**) (0.785%); and herbage of *Stachys officinalis* (L.) Trevisan (*Lamiaceae*) (**Betony**).

Chemical Structure

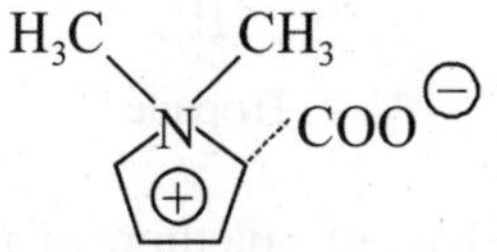

Stachydrine

(S)-2-Carboxy-1, 1-dimethylpyrrolidinium inner salt; ($C_7H_{13}NO_2$).

Isolation   It has been isolated by reported method by Schulze** and Jahns.***

---

* Liebermann, *Ber.*, **22**, 679 (1898)
** Sehulze, *Ber.* **26**, 939 (1893);
*** Jahns, *Ber.* **29**, 2065 (1896);

Characteristic Features

1. It is obtained as monohydrate deliquescent crystals having mp 235°C (anhydrous).
2. It is sweetish in taste.
3. It is soluble in water, dilute mineral acids and ethanol;
4. It isomerizes at the mp to methyl hygrate.

Identification Tests

1. **Stachydrine Hydrochloride ($C_7H_{17}NO_2.HCl$):** Its large prisms are obtained from absolute ethanol which gets decomposed at 235°C. It is very soluble in water and soluble in 13 parts of ethanol.
2. **Stachydrine Acid Oxalate ($C_7H_{13}NO_2.C_2H_2O_4$):** Its needles have mp 106°C. It is practically insoluble in absolute ethanol.
3. **Stachydrine Aurichloride ($C_7H_{13}NO_2.HAuCl_4$):** Its yellow needles have mp 225°C (rapid heating). It is quite soluble in hot water, but practically insoluble in cold water.
4. **Stachydrine Platinichloride Tetrahydrate ($(C_7H_{17}NO_2)_2.H_2PtCl_6.4H_2O$):** It is obtained as orange crystals decomposing at 210-220°C (rapid heating). It is found to be very soluble in dilute ethanol and water. It may also be obtained with two moles of water of crystallization.

7.2.6.2 *Tropane Alkaloids*

Tropane is a bicyclic compound obtained by the condensation of one mole each of **pyrrolidine** and **piperidine** as shown below.

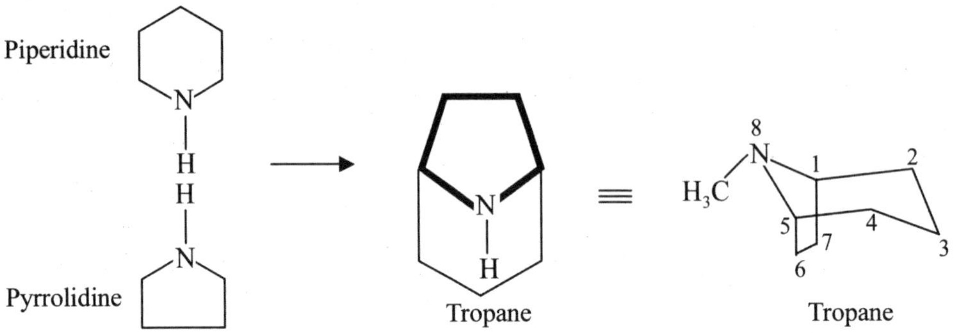

Tropane is regarded as the principle base of a plethora of alkaloids obtained from various members of the natural order, viz., *Solanaceae, Erythroxylaceae, Convolvulaceae,* and *Dioscoreaceae.* It essentially consists of a 7-carbon bicyclic ring with a N-atom strategically bridged between C-1 and C-5 and providing a C_7N unit. It is, however, pertinent to mention here that the tropane base contains two chiral centres (*i.e.*, asymmetric C-atoms), namely: C-1 and C-5, but surprisingly it does not exhibit any optical activity (an exception) by virtue of the fact that *intramolecular compensation* prevails. It happens to be a *meso*-compound.

A few important members belonging to the **tropane alkaloids** are, namely: **atropine, cocaine, cinnamoyl cocaine, ecgonine** and **hyoscyamine.** These alkaloids shall now be treated individually in the sections that follows:

A. Atropine

Synonyms   Tropine tropate; *dl*-Hyoscyamine; *dl*-Tropyl Tropate; Tropic acid ester with Tropine.

Biological Sources   It is obtained from the roots and leaves of *Atropa belladona* Linn. (*Solanaceae*) (**Belladona**); and the seeds and leaves of *Datura stramonium* Linn. (*Syn.: Datura tatula* Linn.) (*Solanaceae*) (**Jimson Weed, Thorn Apple, Stramonium**), besides other species of *Solanaceae*, such as: *D. metel* Linn.; *D. innoxia* Mill., *D. alba* Nees.; and *D. fastuosa* Linn.

Chemical Structure

Atropine

1 α H, 5 α H-Tropan-3α-ol (±)-tropate (ester); ($C_{17}H_{23}NO_3$).

Characteristic Features
 1. **Atropine** is obtained as long orthorhombic prisms from acetone having mp 114-116°C.
 2. It usually sublimes in high vacuum at 93-110°C.
 3. It has a dissociation constant pK 4.35; and the pH of a 0.0015 molar solution is 10.0.
 4. **Solubility:** 1 g dissolves in 455 ml water; 90 ml water at 80°C; 2 ml ethanol; 1.2 ml ethanol at 60°C; 27 ml glycerol; 25 ml ether, 1 ml chloroform; and in benzene.

Identification Tests   It forms various types of salts, namely:
 1. **Atropine Hydrochloride ($C_{17}H_{23}NO_3.CH_3NO_3$):** The granular crystals have mp 165°C. It is soluble in water and ethanol. The pH of 0.05 molar solution is 5.8.
 2. **Atropine Methyl Bromide ($C_{17}H_{23}NO_3.CH_3Br$) (Tropin):** Its crystals have mp 222-223°C. It is soluble in 1 part of water, slightly soluble in ethanol, and practically insoluble in ether and chloroform.
 3. **Atropine Methylnitrate ($C_{17}H_{23}NO_3.CH_3NO_3$) (Methylatropine nitrate, Eumydrin, Metropine, Harvatrate, Metanite, Ekomine):** Its crystals have mp 163°C. It is found to be freely soluble in water or ethanol; and very slightly soluble in chloroform and ether.
 4. **Atropine Sulphate Monohydrate [($C_{17}H_{23}NO_3$)$_2$.H_2SO_4.H_2O] (Atropisol):** It is obtained as either crystals or powder with mp 190-194°C. It is *inactive* optically. It has a very bitter taste. It shows pH ~ 5.4. Its bitterness is threshold 1:10,000. It is found to be incompatible with a host of substances, such as, tannin, alkalies, salts of gold and mercury, borax, bromides, iodides, benzoates and vegetable decoctions or infusions.

Its solubility profile is: 1 g dissolves in 0.4 ml water; in 5 ml cold and 2.5 ml boiling ethanol; in 2.5 ml glycerol; 420 ml chloroform and 3000 ml ether.

Uses

1. It is used in preanaesthetic medication.
2. It is employed as an anticholinergic agent.
3. It is also used as a mydriatic.
4. It is employed as an antidote in opium and chloral hydrate poisoning.
5. It is frequently employed to minimize spasm in cases of intestinal gripping caused due to strong purgatives.
6. It also find its applications to reduce such secretions as: saliva, sweat, and gastric juice.

B. Cocaine

Synonyms   2β-Carbomethoxy-3β-benzoxytropane; *l*-Cocaine; β-Cocaine; Benzoylmethylecgonine; Ecgonine methyl ester benzoate.

Biological Sources   It is obtained from the leaves of *Erythroxylon coca* Lam. and other species of *Erythroxylon*, (*Erythroxylaceae*); and leaves of *Erythroxylon truxillense* Rusby (*Erythroxylaceae*).

Chemical Structure

Cocaine

[IR-(exo, exo]-3-(Benzoyloxy)-8-methyl-8-azabicyclol [3, 2, 1] octane-2-carboxylic acid methyl ester; ($C_{17}H_{21}NO_4$).

Isolation   **Cocaine** is extracted from the plant by digestion either with sodium carbonate solution or with lime water and by subsequent solvent extraction using petroleum ether (bp 160-180°C; or 200-220°C). The combined petroleum ether extract is shaken up with dilute HCl. The solution of hydrochloride thus obtained is concentrated carefully in a thin-film evaporator. In case, the leaves are rich in cocaine content, as in the Peruvian coca leaves, a major portion of cocaine gets separated as crystals.

Characteristic Features

1. **Cocaine** is obtained as the monoclinic tablets from ethanol having mp 98°C.
2. It usually becomes volatile above 90°C; however, the resulting sublimate is *not* crystalline in nature.

3. Its physical parameters are as follows; $bp_{0.1}$, 187-188°C; $[\alpha]_D^{18} - 35°$ (50% ethanol); $[\alpha]_D^{20} - 16°$ (C = 4 in chloroform); pKa (15°C) 8.61 and pKb (15°C) 5.59.

4. **Solubility Profile:** 1 g of cocaine dissolves in 600 ml of water; 270 ml of water at 80°C; 6.5 ml of ethanol; 0.7 ml of chloroform; 3.5 ml of ether; 12 ml of turpentine; 12 ml of pure olive oil; and 30-50 ml of liquid petrolatum. It is also soluble in acetone, carbon disulphide and ethyl acetate.

Identification Tests

1. **Cocaine Permanganate:** The addition of a drop of saturated solution of $KMnO_4$ to a solution of cocaine prepared in a saturated solution of alum gives rise to a violet crystalline precipitate due to the formation of cocaine permanganate. It clearly shows characteristic violet aggregates of plates when examined under the microscope.

2. **Cocaine Hydrochloride ($C_{17}H_{21}NO_4.HCl$) (Cocaine Muriate):** It is obtained as granules, crystals, or powder. It has a slightly bitter taste and usually numbs lips and tongue. Its physical characteristics are: mp ~ 195°C; $[\alpha]_D - 72°$ (C = 2 in aqueous solution); 1 g dissolves in 0.4 ml of water; 3.2 ml cold and 2 ml hot alcohol; 12.5 ml chloroform. It is also soluble in glycerol and acetone; and insoluble in ether or oils.

3. **Cocaine Nitrate Dihydrate ($C_{17}H_{22}N_2O_7.2H_2O$):** Its crystals have mp 58-63°C. It is freely soluble in water or ethanol; and slightly soluble in ether.

4. **Cocaine Sulphate ($C_{17}H_{21}NO_4.H_2SO_4$):** It is obtained as white, crystalline or granular powder, which is soluble in ethanol and water.

Uses

1. It is used as a local anaesthetic as it causes numbness.
2. Its main action is a CNS-stimulant and, therefore, categorized as *'narcotic drugs'*. It is a highly habit-forming drug.

C. Cinnamoyl Cocaine

Synonyms   Ecgonine Methyl Ester; Cinnamoylcocaine; Cinnamoyl-methylecgonine; Ecgonine Cinnamate Methyl Ester.

Biological Source   It is obtained from the leaves of *Erythroxylon coca* Lann. (*Erythroxylaceae*), particularly from the Javanese leaves.

Chemical Structure

Cinnamoylcocaine [(E)-Form]

[1R-(exo, exo)]-8-Methyl-3-[(1-oxo-3-phenyl-2-propenyl)oxy]-8-azabicyclol [3, 2, 1] octane-2-carboxylic acid methyl ester; ($C_{19}H_{23}NO_4$).

Isolation   Instead of the Peruvian leaves the Java leaves of *E. coca* are treated in the same manner and fashion as described under cocaine earlier (section 'B'). It has been observed that the mixed hydrochlorides mostly comprise of cinnamoyl cocaine which gets separated as fine needles.

Characteristic Features

1. It is obtained as fine needles having mp 121°C.
2. Its specific optical rotation is $[\alpha]_D$ – 4.7° (chloroform).
3. It is freely soluble in ether, ethanol and chloroform; and almost insoluble in water.

Identification Tests

1. It reduces an acidic solution of $KMnO_4$ in cold *i.e.*, at ambient temperature, which helps to detect the presence of this alkaloid in an admixture with cocaine.
2. It undergoes hydrolysis when warmed with HCl to yield *l*-ecgonine, cinnamic acid and methanol.

D. Ecgonine

Biological Source   It is also obtained from the leaves of *Erythroxylum coca* Lam. (*Erythroxylaceae*) (**Coca**) as its *l*-form.

Chemical Structure

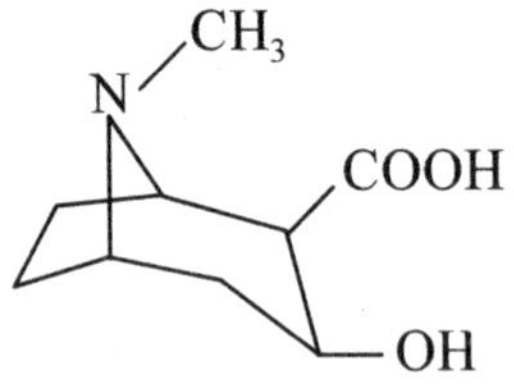

Ecgonine

[1R-(exo, exo)]-3-Hydroxy-8-methyl-8-azabicyclol [3, 2, 1] octane-2-carboxylic acid; ($C_9H_{15}NO_3$).
   It is the principal part of the **cocaine** molecule.

Isolation   Ecgonine may be obtained by the hydrolysis of **cocaine** as given below:

$$\text{Cocaine} \xrightarrow{\text{Hydrolysis}} \text{Ecgonine + Benzoic acid + Methanol}$$

Characteristic Features

1. The *l*-form **ecgonine monohydrate** is obtained as triboluminescent, monoclinic prisms from ethanol having mp 198°C (anhydrous substance gets decomposed at 205°C).
2. Its specific optical rotation $[\alpha]_D^{15}$ – 45° (C = 5); dissociation constants are: pKa 11.11, and pKb 11.22.
3. **Solubility Profile:** 1 g dissolves in 5 ml water, 67 ml ethanol, 20 ml ethanol, 75 ml ethyl acetate; sparingly soluble in ether, acetone, benzene, chloroform and petroleum ether.

Identification Tests

1. **Ecgonine Hydrochloride ($C_9H_{15}NO_3.HCl$):** It is obtained as the triclinic plates obtained from water having mp 246°C; $[\alpha]_D^{15} - 59°$ (C = 10); soluble in water and slightly in ethanol.

2. ***dl*-Ecgonine Trihydrate:** It is obtained as plates from 90% ethanol having mp 93-118°C (anhydrous substance gets decomposed at 212°C).

Uses It is mostly used as a topical anaesthetic.

E. Hyoscyamine

Synonyms *l*-Tropine Tropate; Daturine; Duboisine; *l*-Hyoscyamine; Cystospaz; Levsin; *l*-Tropic acid ester with Tropine; 3α-Tropanyl S-(–)-Tropate.

Biological Sources It is obtained from the roots and leaves of *Atropa bella*-dona L. (*Solanaceae*) (0.21%) (**Thorn Apple**); fruits, roots and leaves of *Datura metel* L. (*Solanaceae*) (**Unmatal, Metel, Hindu Datura**); leaves and seeds of *Datura stramonium* L. (*Solanaceae*) (**Jimson Weed, Thorn Apple, Stramonium**); root bark of *Duboisia myoporoides* R. Br. (*Solanaceae*) (**Pituri, Corkwood Tree**); young plants of *Hyoscyamus niger* L. (*Solanaceae*) (**Henbane, Henblain Jusquaime**); seeds of *Lactuca virosa* L. (*Asteraceae*) (**Bitter Lettuce, Wild Lettuce**); and the herb *Mandragora officinarum* L. (*Solanaceae*) (**Mandrake, Loveapple**).

Chemical Structure

Hyoscyamine

1αH, 5αH-Tropan-3α-ol (–)-tropate (ester); ($C_{17}H_{23}NO_3$).

Isolation **Hyoscyamine** may be isolated from the Belladona leaves by adopting the following steps sequentially:

1. The finely powdered and sieved **Belladona leaves** is extracted with 95% (v/v) ethanol in a Soxhlet Apparatus till no more alkaloids come out from the marc. The ethanolic extract is concentrated to a syrupy residue under vaccuo and subsequently treated with dilute HCl. The resinous matter is separated by filtration and the resulting solution is further purified by shaking out with petroleum ether (40-60°C) several times.

2. The purified acidic solution thus obtained is made alkaline with ammonia solution (dilute) carefully and extracted with chloroform successively. The combined chloroform layer is once

again shaken with dilute HCl, and the acidic solution made alkaline with dilute ammonia solution and extracted with chloroform successively.

3. The combined chloroform layer is removed by distillation under reduced pressure. The crude alkaloids thus obtained is neutralized with oxalic acid. The oxalates of atropine and hyoscyamine may be separated by fractional crystallization from acetone and ether wherein the **hyoscyamine oxalate** being more soluble gets separated as the second crop.

Characteristic Features

1. **Hyoscyamine** is obtained as silky tetragonal needles from evaporating ethanol having mp 108.5°C.

2. The physical parameters are: $[\alpha]_D^{20} - 21°$ (ethanol); and dissociation constant K at 19° is 1.9 × 10^{-12}.

3. **Solubility Profile:** 1 g dissolves in 281 ml water (pH 9.5), 69 ml ether, 150 ml benzene, and 1 ml chloroform. It is freely soluble in dilute mineral acids and ethanol.

Identification Tests   The various identification tests for **hyoscyamine** are, namely:

1. **Gerrard Reaction: Hyoscyamine** (and also **atropine**) responds to the **Gerrard Reaction** wherein about 5-10 mg of it reacts with mereuric chloride solution (2% w/v) in 50% ethanol to give rise to an instant red colouration without warming.

2. **Schaer's Reagent:** A few mg of **hyoscyamine** when made to react with a few drops of the **Schaer's Reagent** i.e., 1 volume of 30% H_2O_2 mixed with 10 volumes of concentrated sulphuric acid, produces a distinct green colouration.

3. **Vitali-Morin Colour Reaction:** A few mg of **hyoscyamine** (and also atropine) is treated with about 0.2 ml of fuming HNO_3, evaporated to dryness on the water-bath. To the residue is then added 0.5 ml of a 3% (w/v) solution of KOH in methanol, it gives a bright purple colouration, that changes to red and finally fades to colourless.

   Note: (*a*) **The 3% solution of KOH must be freshly prepared.**

   (*b*) **The reaction is very sensitive i.e., upto 0.0001 mg of any of the alkaloids viz., strychnine, apomorphine, veratrine, physostigmine etc. give a positive test.**

4. *para*-**Dimethylaminobenzaldehyde Reagent:** [Prepared by dissolving 2 g of *p*-Dimethylaminobenzaldehyde in 6 g of H_2SO_4 to which 0.4 ml of water is added previously]. Add to 5-10 mg of **hyoscyamine** in an evaporating dish 2-3 drops of this reagent and heat on a boiling water-bath for several minutes. A distinct red colouration is produced that ultimately gets changed to permanent cherry red upon cooling.

5. **Hyoscyamine Hydrobromide ($C_{17}H_{23}NO_3$.HBr):** It is obtained as deliquescent crystals having mp 152°C; very soluble in water; 1 g dissolves in 3 ml ethanol; 1.2 ml chloroform and 2260 ml ether.

6. **Hyoscyamine Hydrochloride ($C_{17}H_{23}NO_3$.HCl):** The crystals have mp 149-151°C; and freely soluble in water and ethanol.

7. **Hyoscyamine Methyl Bromide ($C_{17}H_{23}NO_3$.CH_3Br) (N-Methylhyo-scyaminium bromide):** The crystals have mp 210-212°C; and freely soluble in water, dilute ethanol; and slightly soluble in absolute ethanol.

8. **Hyoscyamine Sulphate Dihydrate [$(C_{17}H_{23}NO_3)_2.H_2SO_4.2H_2O$] (Egacene, Peptard, Egazil Duretter):** It is obtained as needles from ethanol having mp 206°C (when dry); $[\alpha]_D^{15} - 29°$ (C = 2); pH 5.3 (1 in 100); 1 g dissolves in 0.5 ml water and about 5.0 ml ethanol; and very slightly soluble in ether and chloroform.

Uses

1. It is mostly employed as an anticholinergic drug.
2. It exerts relaxation of bronchial and intestinal smooth museles (*i.e.*, antispasmodic action).
3. It also inhibits contraction of the iris muscle of the eye to produce mydriasis.
4. It decreases significantly decreases the sweat gland and salivary gland secretions.

Biosynthesis of Hygrine, Cuscohygrine, Cocaine, Cinnamoyl Ecgonine (Methylecgonine) and Hyoscyamine The **pyrrolidine ring system,** present in **hygrine** and **cuscohygrine,** is formed initially as a Δ^1-pyrrolinium cation. The extra C-atoms required for hygrine formation are derived from acetate *via* acetyl-CoA; and the sequence appears to involve stepwise addition of *two* acetyl-CoA units as shown below:

These *two* steps may be explained as under:

(*a*) The enolate anion from acetyl-CoA serves as nucleophile for the pyrrolinium ion in a Mannich-like reaction, that may give rise to products having either R or S stereochemistry.

(*b*) An addition is caused by virtue of a Claisen condensation which essentially extends the side-chain, and the product is 2-substituted pyrrolidine, thereby retaining the thioester moiety of the second acetyl-CoA.

It has been observed that **Hygrine** and most of the naturally occurring **tropane alkaloids** is devoid of this specific C-atom, which is subsequently eliminated by suitable decarboxylation/hydrolysis reactions. Interestingly, the genesis of the bicyclic structure of the tropane skeleton existing in either *cocaine* or **hyoscyamine** is accomplished due to the repeatation of the Mannich-like reaction stated above. These reactions are summarized in the description given under.

7.2.6.2 Pyrrolizidine Alkaloids

The **bicyclic pyrrolizidine nucleus** is formed by the utilization of two moles of ornithine and this pathway is accomplished *via* the intermediate **putrescine.** However, it has been observed that the plant sources usually synthesizing the pyrrolizidine alkaloids seem to be devoid of the *decarboxylase enzyme* that helps in the transformation of ornithine into putrescine; in fact, *ornithine* is really incorporated by way of arginine.

In nature, the **pyrrolizidine alkaloids** have a relatively broad stretch of distribution, but are specifically present in certain genera of the *Leguminosae/Fabaceae* (*e.g.*, **Crotalaria**); the *Compositae/Asteraceae* (*e.g.*, **Senecio**); and the *Boraginaceae* (*e.g.*, **Heliotropium, Symphytum,** and **Cynoglossum**). Broadly speaking the pyrrolizidine bases do not occur in their free form, but are mostly found as esters with rare mono-or di-basic acids, the **necic acids.**

The *two* important alkaloids of this category are, namely: **Retronecine** and **Senecionine,** which shall be discussed as under:

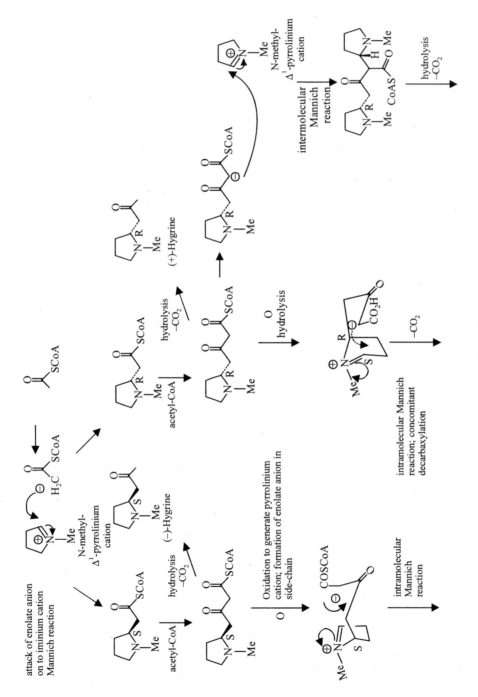

(continued)

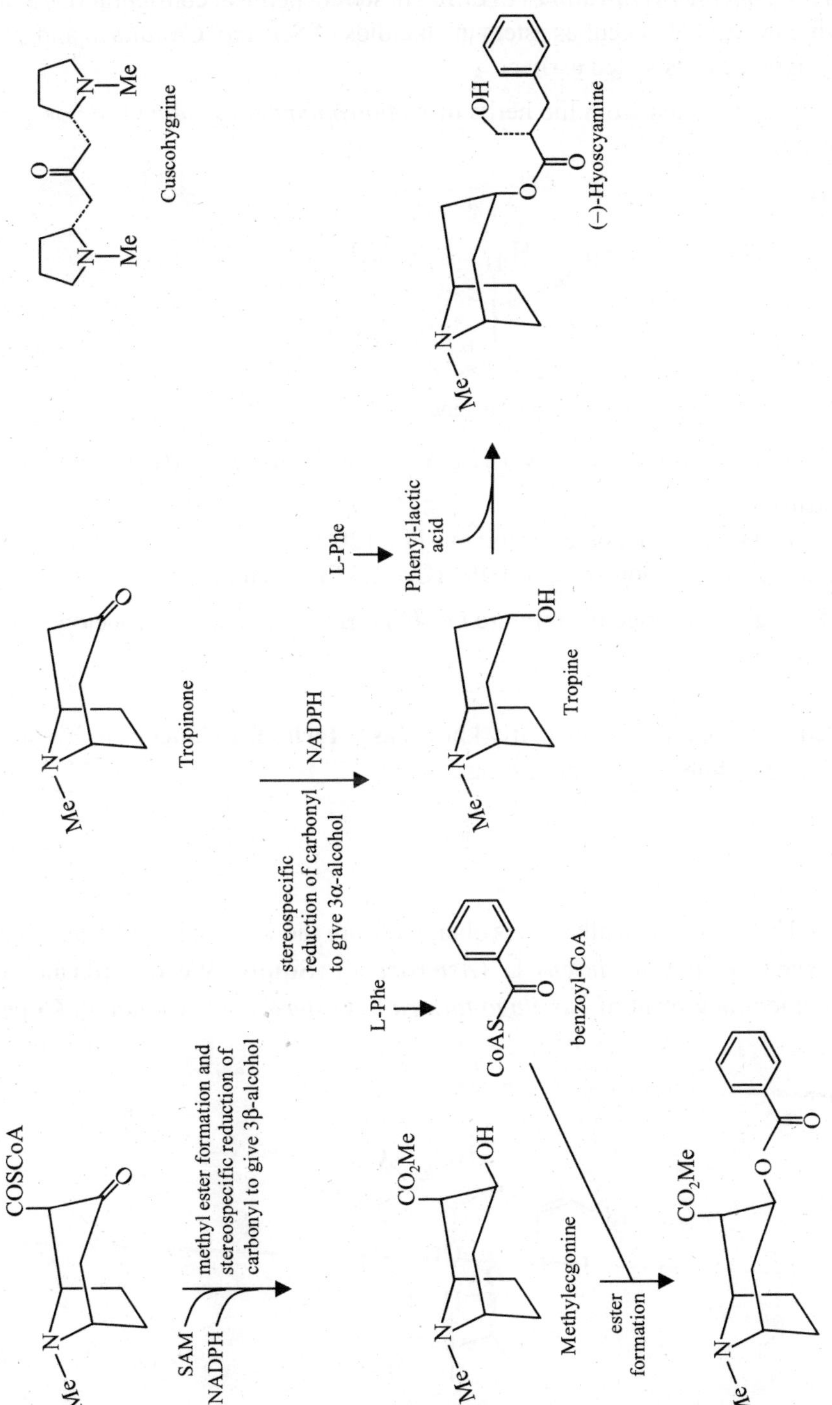

Biosynthesis of Hygrine, Cuscohygrine, Cocaine, Carbamoyl Ecgonine (Methyl-ecgonine) and Hyoscyamine

Cuscohygrine

Tropinone

stereospecific
reduction of carbonyl
to give 3α-alcohol

NADPH

Tropine

L-Phe

Phenyl-lactic
acid

(−)-Hyoscyamine

SAM
NADPH

methyl ester formation and
stereospecific reduction of
carbonyl to give 3β-alcohol

COSCoA

L-Phe

benzoyl-CoA

Methylecgonine

ester
formation

Cocaine

A. Retronecine   The most common base portion of the **pyrrolizidine alkaloids** is **retronecine.** The **'Necine'** *bases are 1-methylpyrrolizidines* of different stereochemical configurations and degree of hydroxylation which invariably occur as esters in alkaloids of *Senecio, Crotalaria* and a plethora of genera of the *Boraginaceae* as stated earlier.

Biological Source   It is obtained from the herbs of *Heliotropium europaeum* L. (*Boraginaceae*) (**Heliotrope, Turnsole**).

Chemical Structure

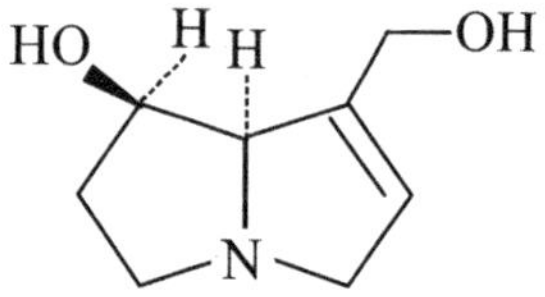

Retronecine

(1R-*trans*)-2, 3, 5, 7, a-Tetrahydro-1-hydroxy-1 H-pyrrolizine-7-methanol; ($C_8H_{13}NO_2$).

Characteristic Features
  1. It is obtained as crystals from acetone having mp 119-120°C.
  2. It has the specific optical rotation $[\alpha]_D^{20} + 4.95°$ (C = 0.58 in ethanol).

Identification Test   It gives the racemic mixture *i.e.,* (±) form as crystals from acetone having mp 130-131°C.

Uses
  1. The plant is used for cancer and is popularly known as **"Herbe Du Cancer"** in Europe.
  2. It is also used for snakebite and scorpion stings.

B. Senecionine

Synonym   Aureine;

Biological Source   The hepatotoxic alkaloid is obtained from the whole plant of *Senecio vulgaris* L. (*Compositae*); weed of *Senecio aureus* L. (*Asteraceae*) (**Squaw Weed, Liferoot, Golden Groundsel**); and preblooming plant of *Tussilago farfara* L. (*Asteraceae*) (**Coltsfoot, Coughwort, Horse-Hoof**).

Chemical Structure

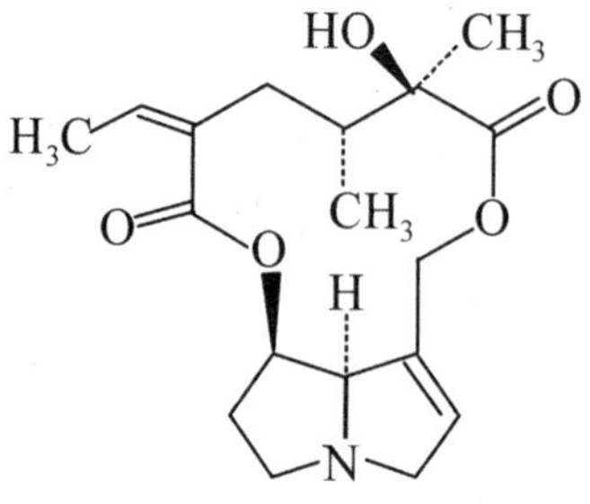

Senecionine

12-Hydroxysenecionan-11, 16-dione; ($C_{18}H_{25}NO_5$): is described by Barger and Blackie (1936).*

Characteristic Features
1. It is obtained as plates having mp 236°C and a bitter taste.
2. Its specific optical rotation $[\alpha]_D^{25} - 55.1°$ (C = 0.034 in chloroform).
3. It is practically insoluble in water; freely soluble in chloroform; and slightly soluble in ether and ethanol.

Uses
1. It is used as an excellent drug to control pulmonary hemorrhage.
2. It is also used to hasten labour and check the pains of parturition.

Biosynthesis of Retronecine and Senecionine It has been observed that the plants synthesizing the above mentioned **pyrrolizidine alkaloids** seem to be devoid of the decarboxylase enzyme transforming ornithine into putrescine; in fact, ornithine is actually incorporated by way of arginine. The various steps involved essentially in the **biosynthesis of retronecine** and **senecionine** are summarized as below:

1. Two moles of putrescine are condensed in an NAD^+-dependent oxidative deamination reaction to yield the corresponding imine, which is subsequently transformed into **homospermidine** by the aid of NADH reduction.
2. The genesis of the creation of the pyrrolizidine skeleton is on account of the **homospermidine** molecule by a sequential series of interactions, such as: oxidative deamination, imine formation, intramolecular **Mannich reaction,** that specifically exploits the enolate anion produced from the aldehyde.
3. The '*pyrrolizidine skeleton*' thus provides a C_4N unit from ornithine, together with an additional four C-atoms from the same amino acid precursor.
4. The **senecionine** is a diester of **retronecine** with **senecic acid.**

These steps have been depicted as under.

7.2.7 Alkaloids Derived from Tyrosine

The pyridoxal phosphate (PLP)-dependent decarboxylation of *L-Tyrosine* yields the simple phenylethylamine *tyramine*, that subsequently undergoes di-N-methylation thereby producing **hordenine. Hordenine** is regarded as a germination inhibitory alkaloid obtained from barely *viz.*, *Hordeum vulgare* (*Graminae/Poaceae*).

There are a number of alkaloids derived from tyrosine which may be classified as stated below:

(*i*) Phenylethylamine alkaloids,
(*ii*) Simple Tetrahydro iso-quinoline alkaloids,
(*iii*) Modified tetrahydro iso-quinoline alkaloids,
(*iv*) Phenylethylisoquinoline alkaloids, and
(*v*) Amaryllidaceae alkaloids.

---

* Barger, Blackie, *J. Chem. Soc.* 743 (1936)

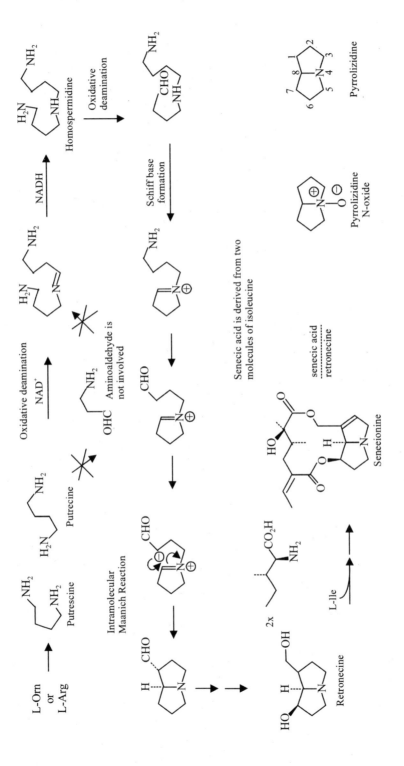

Biosynthesis of Retronecine and Senecionine

The various groups of alkaloids mentioned above shall now be treated individually in the sections that follows:

7.2.7.1 Phenylethylamine Alkaloids

The important alkaloids belonging to this category are, namely: **Ephedrine, Hordenine, Mescaline** and **Narceine,** which shall be discussed as under:

A. Ephedrine

Biological Source   It is obtained from the dried tender stems of the Chinese wonder drug **Ma Huang** which is being used in the Chinese systems of Medicine for more than five thousand years. It occurs in *Ephedra vulgaris* Hook. F. (*E. gerardiana* Wall); *Ephedra sinica* Stapf. (1-3%); *Ephedra equisetina* Bunge. (2%) belonging to the natural order *Gentaceae;* and several other Ephedra species. Besides, it is also found in the roots of *Aconitum napellus* L. (*Ranunculaceae*) (**Aconite, Monkshood, Blue Rocket**); and *Ephedra nevadensis* S. Wats. (*Ephedraceae*) (**Mormon Tea, Nevada Jointfir**).

Chemical Structure

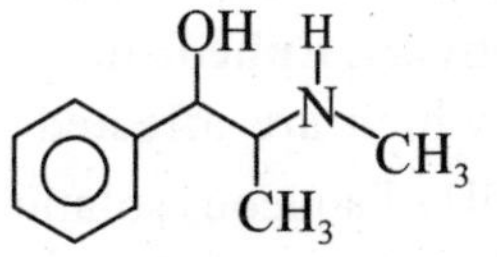

Ephedrine

α-[1-(Methylamino)-ethyl] benzene-methanol; ($C_{10}H_{15}NO$).

Isolation   Both **ephedrine** and **pseudoephedrine** may be extracted from the plant source by general procedures described earlier under alkaloid extraction, through successive and dilute HCl extraction procedures.

However, the separation of ephedrine from **pseudoephedrine** may be accomplished by means of their corresponding oxalate salts; the **ephedrine oxalate** being comparatively less soluble in cold water than **pseudoephedrine oxalate** separates out first.

Note: Chloroform is not ragarded as an appropriate solvent for extraction of ephedrine as it forms its corresponding ephedrine hydrochloride salt after its dissolution in $CHCl_3$ and subsequent evaporation of solvent.

Fermentation Method   **Ephedrine** may be prepared on a commercial scale economically by the process of *fermentation* using a mixture of molasses (a by-product of sugar industry containing 8-10% of cane sugar *i.e.,* $C_6H_{12}O_6$) and benzaldehyde. The resulting keto-alcohol *i.e.,* benzylhydroxy methyl ketone is subsequently mixed with a solution of methylamine and treated with hydrogen gas to yield a racemic mixture of **ephedrine** as given below:

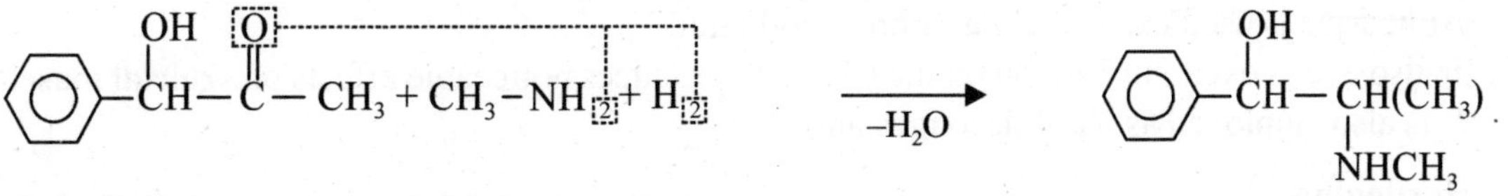

Benzylhydroxy-   Methyl   Hydrogen   (±)-Ephedrine
methylketone   amine   gas

Characteristic Features   The characteristic features of some racemic forms, optical isomers and their respective salts are enumerated below:

1. *dl*-**Ephedrine (Synonyms: Racephedrine; Racemic Ephedrine):** The crystals have mp 79°C; and are soluble in oils, chloroform, ether, water, and ethanol.

2. *dl*-**Ephedrine Hydrochloride (Synonyms: Ephetonin; Racephedrine Hydrochloride) (C$_{10}$H$_{15}$NO.HCl):** The crystals have mp 187–188°C; and pH 6.0. Its solubility profile are: 1 g dissolves 4 ml water, 40 ml of 95% ethanol at 20°C; and practically insoluble in ether.

3. *dl*-**Ephedrine Sulphate (Synonym: Racephedrine Sulphate) (C$_{10}$H$_{15}$NO.H$_2$SO$_4$):** The crystals have mp 247°C, and are soluble in ethanol and water. Its solution has a pH of 6.0.

4. *l*-**Ephedrine [L-Erythro-2(methylamino)-1-phenylpropan-1-ol]:** It is obtained as waxy solid, crystals or granules, having a soapy feel and the substance gradually decomposes on exposure to light. It may contain water upto ½ mole (5.2%). However, the anhydrous product is hygroscopic in nature having mp 34°C. Interestingly, the absorption of water enhances mp to 40°C; and bp 255°C. The pH of aqueous solution (1 in 200) is 10.8. 1 g of it dissolves in 20 ml water, 0.2 ml ethanol; and freely soluble in ether, chloroform and oils.

5. *l*-**Ephdrine Hydrochloride (Synonyms: Ephedral; Senedrine):** It is obtained as orthorhombic needles having mp 216-220°C, which are affected by light. Its specific optical rotation $[\alpha]_D^{25} - 33$ to $-35.5°$ (C = 5). The pH of aqueous solution (1 in 200) is 5.9. 1 g dissolves in 3 ml water, 14 ml ethanol; and is found to be practically insoluble in chloroform and ether.

6. *l*-**Ephedrine Sulphate:** Its orthorhombic needles have mp 245°C (decomposed) and are affected by light. Its specific optical rotation $[\alpha]_D^{25} - 29.5$ to $-32.0°$ (C = 5). 1 g dissolves in 1.2 ml water and 95 ml ethanol; and freely soluble in hot alcohol. Its pH is about 6.

Identification Tests

1. Dissolve 0.01 g of **ephedrine** in 1 ml water by adding a few drops of dilute HCl. To this add two drops of CuSO$_4$ solution (5% w/v) followed by a few-drops of NaOH solution when a reddish colour is developed. Now, add 2-3 ml ether and shake the contents thoroughly; the ethereal layer turns purple while the lower aqueous layer becomes blue.

2. Dissolve 0.2 g of **ephedrine** in 30 ml of chloroform in a stoppered flask and shake the contents vigorously. Allow the mixture to stand for at least 12 hours at room temperature and then remove the chloroform over an electric water bath. The crystals of ephedrine hydrochloride separate out.

3. Triturate 0.05 g of **ephedrine** with a few crystals of [K$_3$Fe(CN)$_6$] *i.e.*, potassium ferricyanide, followed by a few drops of water and heat on a water bath slowly when a distinct odour of benzaldehyde (*i.e.*, similar to the odour of bitter almonds) in given out.

Uses

1. *l*-Ehedrine is used extensively as a bronchodilator.
2. It also exerts excitatory action on the CNS and produces noticeable effects on skeletal muscles.
3. It is also employed as nasal decongestant.

B. Hordenine

Synonyms   Anhaline; Eremursine; Peyocactine.

Biological Sources It is obtained from the plant of *Lophophora williamsii* (Lamaire) Coult. (*Catctaceae*) (**Peyote**) and *Selenicereus grandiflorus* Britt and Rose (*Coctaceae*) (**Night Blooming Cereus**).

Chemical Structure

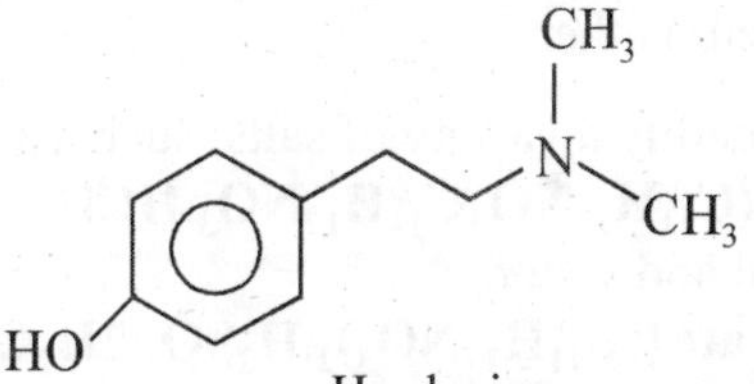

Hordenine

4-[2-Dimethylamino) ethyl] phenol; ($C_{10}H_{15}NO$).

Isolation It is isolated from barley germs by the method suggested by Erspamer and Falconieri* (1952).

Characteristic Features
1. It is obtained as orthorhombic prisms from ethanol or benzene +ether; as needles from water having mp 117-118°C.
2. It sublimes at 140-150°C and has a bp_{11} 173°C.
3. **Solubility Profile:** It is very soluble in chloroform, ethanol and ether; 7 g dissolves in 1 L of water; practically insoluble in petroleum ether; and sparingly soluble in benzene, xylene and toluene.

Identification Test **Hrodenine** readily forms its hydrochloride salt which is obtained as needles from ethanol having mp 177°C; and it is very soluble in water.

Uses It exhibits digitalis-like activity.

C. Mescaline

Synonym Mezcaline

Biological Sources It is obtained from *Peyote* (**Mescal Buttons**) the flowering heads of *Lophophore williamsii* (Lemaire) Coult. (*Coctaceae*) and the cactus *Trichocereus pachanoi* Britton and Rose (*Cactaceae*) (**Achuma, San Pedro Aguacolli**).

Chemical Structure

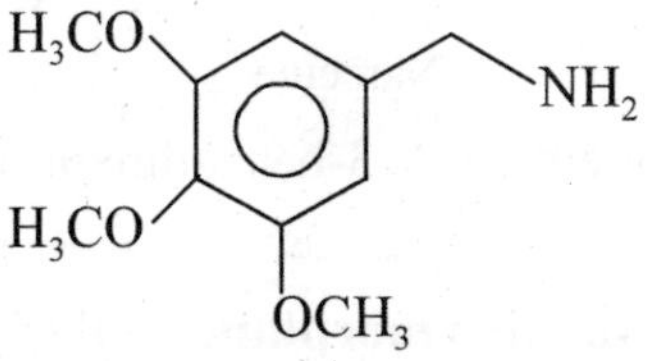

Mescaline

3, 4, 5-Trimethoxybenzeneethanamine; ($C_{11}H_{17}NO_3$).

---

* Erspamer and Falconieri, *Naturniss*, **39**, 431 (1952).

Isolation   Mescaline has been successfully isolated from the plant source by Banholzer *et al*.* (1952).

Characteristic Features
1. The crystals have mp 35-36°C and bp_{12} 180°C.
2. It is moderately soluble in water; freely soluble in ethanol, chloroform and benzene; and practically insoluble in ether and petroleum ether.

Identification Tests   It forms readily a variety of salts, such as:
1. **Mescaline Hydrochloride ($C_{11}H_{17}NO_3C_{11}H_{17}NO_3.HCl$):** The needles have mp 181°C and freely soluble both in ethanol and water.
2. **Mescaline Sulphate Dihydrate [($C_{11}H_{17}NO_3)_2.H_2SO_4.2H_2O$)]:** It is obtained as prisms having mp 183-186°C; soluble freely in methanol and hot water; and sparingly soluble in ethanol and cold water.
3. **Mescaline Acid Sulphate ($C_{11}H_{17}NO_3.H_2SO_4$):** The crystals have mp 158°C.
4. **N-Acetylmescaline:** It mostly occurs naturally, mp 94°C.
5. **N-Methylmescaline:** It occurs naturally, bp 130-140°C.
6. **N-Benzoylmescaline:** It is obtained as needles from aqueous ethanol having mp 121°C; and is found to be very soluble in ether and ethanol.

Note: This is a controlled substance (hallucinogen) listed in the US code of Federal Regulations [Title 21 Part 1308.11 (1995)].

D. Narceine

Biological Source   It is obtained from the dried latex (**opium**) by incision from the unripe capsule of *Papaver somniferum* Linn., (*Papaveraceae*) to the extent of 0.1-0.5%.

Chemical Structure

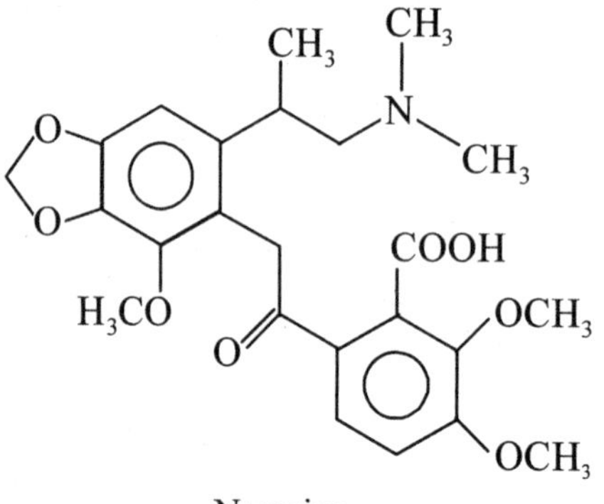

Narceine

6-[[6-[2-(Dimethylamino) ethyl]-4-methoxy-1, 3-benzodioxol-5 yl] acetyl]-2, 3-dimethoxy benzoic .acid; ($C_{23}H_{24}NO_8$).

Isolation   The isolation of **nareceine** from **morphine** mother liquors is tedious.** It may also be prepared from **narcotine** or **gnoscopine.***

---

   * Banholzer *et al. Helv. Chim. Acta*, **35**, 1577 (1952).
  ** Merek, *Chem. Ztg.*, **13**, 525 (1889)
*** Roser, *Ann*. **247**, 167 (1888).

Characteristic Features

1. The anhydrous material is very hygroscopic in nature having mp 138°C; and it: uv_{max} (ethanol) is 270 nm (log $\in$ 3.98).
2. Usually the alkaloid is obtained as the trihydrate.
3. The clusters of silky and prismatic needles are obtained from water having mp 176°C.
4. Its dissociation constants are pK_b at 20° = 10.7; $K_b = 2 \times 10^{-11}$; $pk_a = 9.3$; $K_a = 5 \times 10^{-10}$.
5. Th pH of its saturated solution is 5.8.
6. **Solubility Profile:** 1g dissolves in 770 ml water; 220 ml boiling water; moderately soluble in hot alcohol; almost insoluble in benzene, chloroform, ether, petroleum ether.
7. It forms salts with solutions of alkali hydroxide and also with dilute mineral acids.

Identification Test Ethylnarceine Hydrochloride ($C_{25}H_{32}ClNO_8$) (Synonym: Narcyl): It is obtained as plates from water having mp 208-210°C. It is slightly soluble in cold water, insoluble in ether; and freely soluble in hot water, ethanol and chloroform.

Uses

1. Narcyl is used as a narcotic analgesic.
2. Narcyl is also employed as an antitussive agent.

Biosynthesis of Hordenine and Mescaline   Decarboxylation of L-tyrosine *via* pyridoxal phosphate (PLP) yields the simple phenylethylamine derivative *tyramine*, which an di-N-methylation gives rise to **hordenine.** Besides, phenylethylamine derivatives commonly exhibit either 3, 4-di- or 3, 4, 5-trihydroxylation reactions, and are subsequently derived *via* dopamine *i.e.*, the decarboxylation product obtained from *L-DOPA* (L-dihydroxyphenylalaline). The two variants of **catecholamines,** namely: *first*, a mammalian neurotransmitter **noradrenaline (norepinephrine),** and *secondly*, the most common *'fight or flight'* hormone released in animals from the adrenal gland due to fear phychosis or stress **adrenaline (epinephrine).** Furthermore, these two compounds are formed due to β-hydroxylaton and N-methylation of dopamine.

Lastly, aromatic hydroxylation and O-methylation convert dopamine into *mescaline*. All these reactions have been shown sequentially as given below.

7.2.7.2 Simple Tetrahydro Isoquinoline Alkaloids

The typical representatives of the simple **tetrahydroisoquinoline derivatives** are the closely-related alkaloids occurring along with mescaline are, namely: **anhalamine, anhalonine** and **anhalonidine.**

These *three* alkaloids shall be discussed in the pages that follow:

A. Anhalamine

Biological Sources   It is obtained from the plant *Lophophora williamsii* (Lemaire) Coult. (*Coctaceae*) (*Peyote*), and *Anhalonium lewinii*. Henn. (*Cactaceae*).

Chemical structures

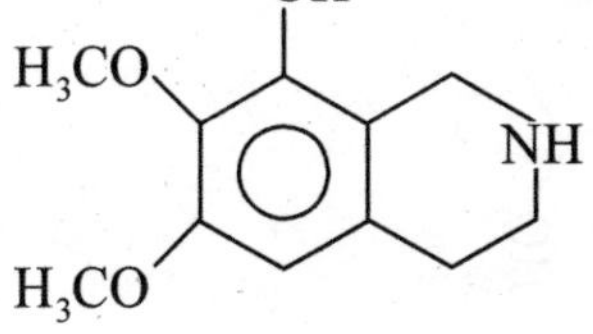

Anhalamine

Biosynthesis of Hordenine and Mescaline

1, 2, 3, 4-Tetrahydro-6, 7-dimethoxy-8-isoquinolinol, $(C_{11}H_{15}NO_3)$.

Characteristic Features
1. The crystals have mp 189-191°C.
2. Its uv_{max} (ethanol) is 274 nm (log $\in$ 2.90).
3. **Solubility Profile:** It is found to be almost insoluble in cold water, cold ethanol, ether and freely soluble in hot water, ethanol, acetone and dilute acids.

Identification Test   Anhalamine Hydrochloride Dihydrate $(C_{11}H_{15}NO_3.HCl. 2H_2O)$: It is obtained as crystals from water having mp 258°C.

Uses   It may play a minor role in causing hallucinatious.

B. Anhalonine

Synonym   Anhalanine

Biological Sources   It is obtained from the **mescal buttons** [*Lophophora williamsii* (Lemaire) Coult. (*Anhalonium lewinii* Henn). *Cactaceae*]; and also in *Ariocarpus*, in *Gymnocalycium gibbosum*.

Chemical Structure

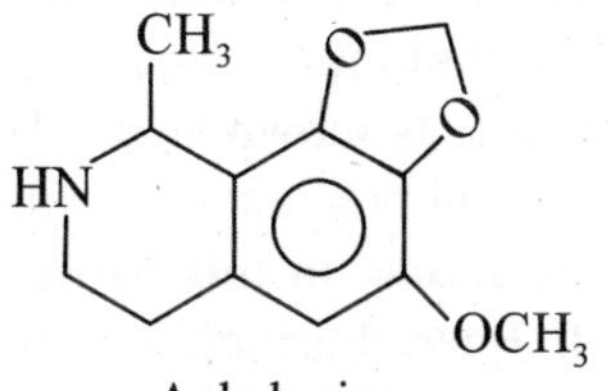

Anhalonine

6, 7, 8, 9-Tetrahydro-4-methoxy-9-methyl-1, 3-dioxolo [4, 5-h] isoquinoline, $(C_{12}H_{15}NO_3)$.

Characteristic Features
1. It is obtained as rhombic needles from petroleum ether having mp 86°C and $bp_{0.02}$ 140°C.
2. Its specific optical rotation $[\alpha]_D^{25} - 63.8°$ (methanol); and $[\alpha]_D^{25} - 56.3°$ (chloroform).
3. It is found to be freely soluble in ethanol, ether, chloroform, benzene and petroleum ether.

Identification Test
Anhalonine Hydrochloride $(C_{12}H_{15}NO_3.HCl)$: It is obtained as orthorhombic prisms decomposing at 255°C. Its aqueous solution is almost neutral. It is found to be freely soluble in hot water.
Uses   It may be employed as a mild hallucinating agent.

C. Anhalonidine

Biological Source   It is invariably obtained from the **mescal buttons,** the buds of *Lophophora williamsii* (Lemaire) Coult. (*Anhalonium lewinii* Henn.) belonging to the natural order *Coctaceae*.

Chemical Structure

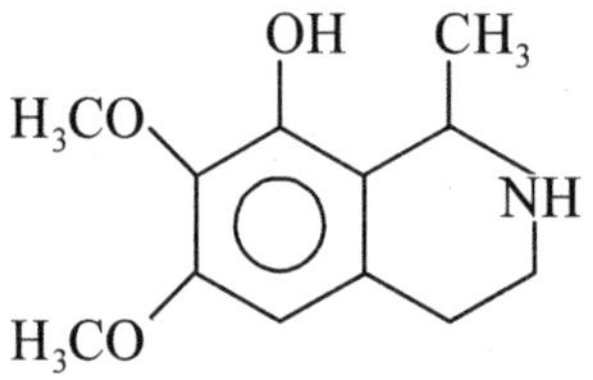

Anhalonidine

1, 2, 3, 4-Tetrahydro-6, 7-dimethoxy-1-methyl-8-isoquinolinol; ($C_{12}H_{17}NO_3$).

Characteristic Features

1. It is mostly obtained as small octahedral crystals from benzene having mp 160-161°C.
2. Its uv_{max} (ethanol) is 270 nm (log $\in$ 2.81).
3. Its aqueous solution acts as a strong base.
4. It is freely soluble in water, ethanol, chloroform and hot benzene; sparingly soluble in ether; and practically insoluble in petroleum ether.
5. It has been observed that the solutions of anhalonidine acquire a reddish colouration on standing.

Uses   It may be used as a mild hallucinogen.

Biosynthesis of Anhalamine, Anhalonine and Anhalonidine   Interestingly, the two additional C-atoms present in **anhalonidine** and **anhalonine** are provided by pyruvate; whereas, the C-atom for **anhalamine** is supplied by glyoxylate, as shown below. However, in each instance, a carboxyl group is lost from this aforesaid additional precursor. The *pyruvate i.e.*, the keto-acid eventually reacts with an appropriate phenylethylamine, in this particular instance the *dimethoxy-hydroxy derivative*, thereby yielding a **Schiff Base.** Further, a **Mannich-like mechanism** helps in the cyclization to produce the heterocyclic isoquinoline nucleus, whereby the mesomeric effect of an oxygen substituent caters for the nucleophilic site on the aromatic ring. Evidently, restoration of aromaticity *via* proton loss yields the tetrahydroquinoline nucleus, thus representing overall a biosynthetic equivalent of the **Pictet-Spengler Isoquinoline Synthesis.** * Subsequently, the carboxyl group is eliminated, not by means of a simple decarboxylation process, but *via* an unusual oxidative decarboxylation process that essentially involves the following steps, namely:

   (*i*)   *First*, producing the intermediate *imine*,
  (*ii*)   *Secondly*, subjecting to *reduction* yielding *anhalonidine*,
 (*iii*)   *Thirdly*, subjecting to *methylation* giving rise to *anhalonine*,
 (*iv*)   *Fourthly*, subjecting phenylethylamine precursor employing the *glyoxylic acid* instead of *pyruvic acid* generating *anhalamine*.

---

   * **Pictet-Spengler Isoquinoline Synthesis:** Formation of tetrahydro-isoquinoline derivatives by condensation of β-arylethylamines with carbonyl compounds and cyclization of the Schiff bases formed:

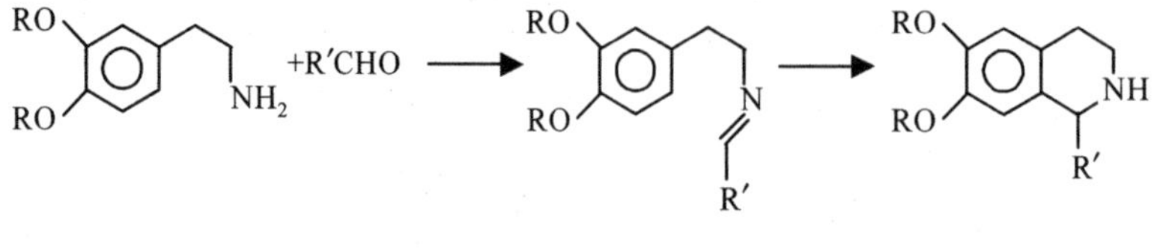

7.2.7.3 Modified Benzyltetrahydroisoquinoline Alkaloids

The modification of *benzyltetrahydroisoquinoline* nucleus to certain other types of alkaloid(s) could be accomplished by virtue of phenolic oxidative coupling.

Benzyltetrahydroisoquinoline

Interestingly, the coupling of two benzyltetrahydroisoquinoline molecules *via* ether bridges result into the formation of two important alkaloids, namely: **tetrandrine** and **tubocurarine,** as given below.

Biosynthesis of Anhalamine, Anhalonine and Anhalonidine

It is, however, pertinent to mention here that the aforesaid mode of coupling is perhaps less frequently found than that involving carbon-carbon bonding between aromatic rings. The major **opium alkaloids** *viz.*, **morphine, codeine** and **thebaine** are obtained through this mode of coupling. (R)-*Reticuline* has been established beyond any reasonable doubt as the precursor of the above *three* **morphinan alkaloids.** Interestingly, there exist an ample evidence to show that the later stages of the proposed biosynthetic pathway undergo *modifications* in certain strains of *opium poppy*. Thus, in such modified strains of opium poppy **thebaine** is being converted to **oripavine** and **morphinone,** whereby the phenolic O-methyl moiety is removed before that of the ether, *i.e.*, the same steps are carried out but in an altogether different order.

The various alkaloids belonging to this category, namely: **morphine, codeine, thebaine, reticuline, oripavine** and **morphinone** shall be discussed separately in the following sections:

A. Morphine

Synonyms   Morphium; Morphia; Dolcontin; Duromorph; Morphina; Nepenthe.

Biological Sources   **Morphine** is obtained from a variety of medicinal plants, such as: *Argemone mexicana* L. (*Papaveraceae*) (**Prickly Poppy**); *Eschscholzia californica* Cham. (*Papaveraceae*) (**California Poppy**); *Papaver bracteatum* Lindl. (*Papaveraceae*) (**Great Scarlet Poppy; Thebaine Poppy**); *Papaver somniferum* L. (*Papaveraceae*) (**Opium Poppy;** and Poppyseed Poppy Keshi).

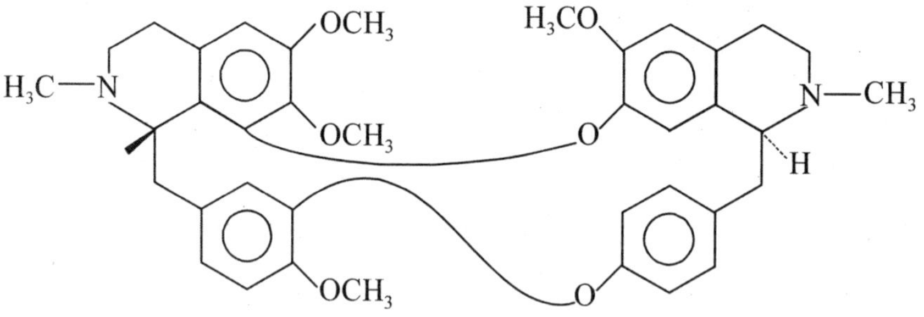

Tetrandrine

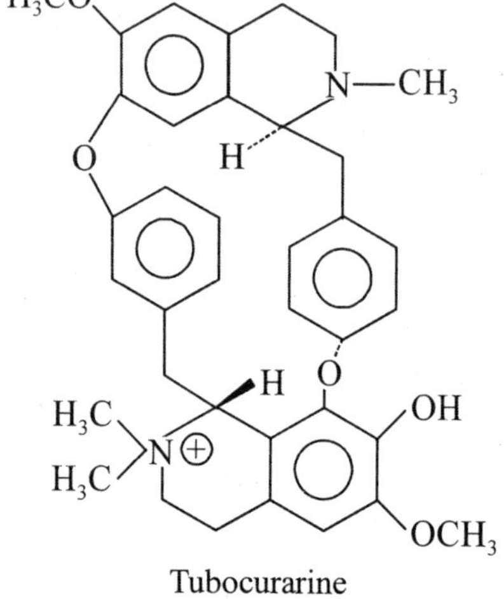

Tubocurarine

Chemical Structure

Morphine

(5α, 6α)-7, 8-Didehydro-4, 5-epoxy-17-methylmorphinan-3, 6-diol; ($C_{17}H_{19}NO_3$).

Isolation   The latex obtained by incision on the unripe capsule of opium poppy is first collected in clean, plastic containers, and the process of incision is repeated at least four times on the same capsule after an interval of two days. Care must be taken to make the incisions on the superficial surface only so as to collect exclusively the external exudation of latex. Subsequently, the latex is dried carefully either by exposing to air on metallic shallow plates or by passing a stream of hot air. Thus the '*opium*' or the dried latex is stored for the isolation of **morphine.** It is found to contain usually 9.5% **morphine** when calculated as anhydrous morphine.

The morphine may be isolated form '**Powdered Opium'** by adopting the following steps sequentially:

Step-1: The powdered opium is shaken with calcium chloride solution and filtered.

Step-2: The resulting filtrate is concentrated and to it is added 10% w/v sodium hydroxide solution carefully *i.e.*, to solubilize morphine, codeine and narceine. It is now filtered.

Step-3: The filtrate containing morphine, codeine and narceine is extracted with chloroform. The resulting mixture is separated.

Step-4: The lower chloroform layer contains codeine, whereas the upper aqueous layer comprises of **morphine** and **narceine.**

Step-5: The aqueous layer is first acidified and subsequently made alkaline with ammonia, whereby morphine gets precipitated and collected as a while solid residue (Yield = 9.5%).

Characteristic Features

1. **Morphine** is obtained as short, orthorhombic, columnar prisms from anisole that gets decomposed at 254°C. It also occurs in its metastable phase having mp 197°C. However, the high melting form sublimes at 190-200°C (0.2 mm pressure at 2 mm distance).

2. It has a bitter taste.

3. **Morphine** (free-base) unlike most other alkaloids in their free-base forms is found to be sparingly soluble in chloroform and nearly insoluble in ether or benzene.

4. **Morphine** gets dissolved in caustic alkalies by virtue of the fact that the OH moiety at C-3 is phenolic in nature and the other OH function at C-6 is a secondary alcoholic group.

5. **Morphine** is a monoacidic base and hence, forms salts that crystallizes rapidly. These are found to be neutral to litmus and methyl orange.

6. The average pH of a saturated solution of morphine salt is found to be 4.68.

7. **Morphine** is levorotatory.
8. **Morphine** upon oxidation converts the secondary alcoholic function to a ketonic group and thus **codeinone** is formed.

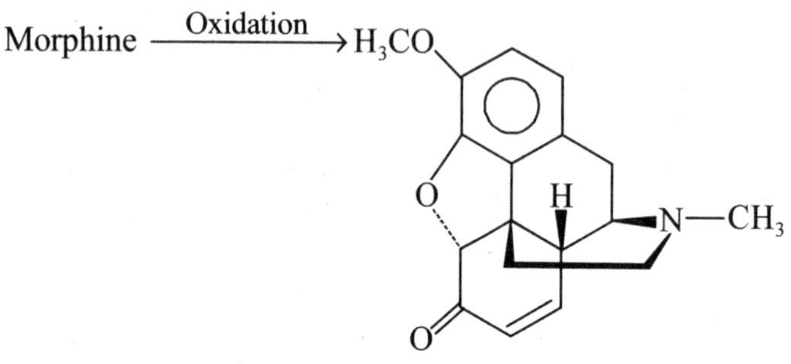

Codeinone

9. **Morphine** upon being heated in a sealed tube with concentrated HCl at 140°C eliminates a molecule of water to yield apomorphine as given below:

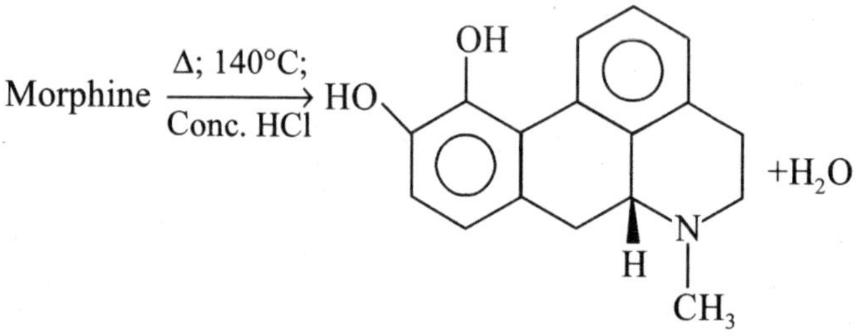

Apomorphine

Identification Tests There are several colour tests that are employed for the identification of **morphine,** namely:

1. **Brouadrel-Boutmy Test:** Add to an aqueous solution of a salt of morphine (*e.g.,* morphine hydrochloride, morphine acetate trihydrate, morphine tartrate trihydrate) a few drops of a mixture of dilute solutions of potassium ferricyanide $[K_3Fe(CN)_6]$ (0.1% w/v) and ferric chloride $[FeCl_3]$ (0.1% w/v) when a deep blue colouration is produced.
   Note: (1) Morphine causes reduction of $K_3Fe(CN)_6$ to $K_4Fe(CN)_6$ i.e., potassium ferro-cyanide which gives a deep blue colouration with $FeCl_3$.
   (2) Codeine fails to give this test; and hence it may be employed to differentiate between morphine and codeine.
2. **Schneider-Weppen Test: Morphine** when mixed with 6 to 8 portions of powdered cane sugar $(C_6H_{12}O_6)$ intimately and treated with a few drops of concentrated H_2SO_4, the development of a purple-red colour takes place. However, the addition of bromine water before the addition of H_2SO_4 renders the test rather more sensitive.
3. **Iodic Acid Test: Morphine** (10 mg) when dissolved in dilute H_2SO_4 (2N) is treated with a solution of pure iodic acid or potassium iodate; and the resulting mixture is shaken with chloroform (5 ml), a distinct violet colouration is imparted to the chloroform layer.

Note: Morphine reduces iodic acid and potassium iodate.

4. **Sodium Nitrite Test:** To a solution of **morphine** in dilute HCl add a few drops of sodium nitrite solution (1% w/v). Allow the reaction mixture to stand for 5-8 minutes and then make it alkaline with dilute ammonia solution, the development of a red colour confirms the presence of morphine.

   Note: (1) It is a non-specific test for morphine and is also given by other phenolic substances.

   (2) It legitimately distinguishes morphine from codeine.

5. **Nitric Acid Test: Morphine** readily gives an orange-red colouration when a few mg of it is treated with a few drops of concentrated nitric acid.

   (a) The resulting orange-red colouration rapidly changes to yellow on heating.

   (b) The orange-red colouration gets easily disappeared on the addition of a few drops of stannous chloride solution ($SnCl_2$) (1% w/v).

6. **Ferric Chloride Test:** When a neutral solution of **morphine** is treated with a few drops of ferric-chloride solution (1% w/v), a greenish-blue colour is produced.

Derivatives of Morphine A number of derivatives of morphine are produced that essentially have distinct characteristic features as enumerated below:

1. **Morphine Monohydrate ($C_{17}H_{19}NO_3.H_2O$):**
   (i) It is obtained as orthorhombic, sphenoidal prisms, or needles from methanol that gets decomposed at 254-256°C with rapid heating.
   (ii) It darkens on exposure to light and also loses water of crystallization at 130°C.
   (iii) Its physical parameters are: d_D^{20} 1.32 ; $[\alpha]_D^{25}$ – 132° (methanol); pK_b at 20°C = 6.13, pK_a 9.85; pH of a saturated solution 8.5; and uv_{max} in acid: 2.85 nm, in alkali: 298 nm.
   (iv) **Solubility Profile:** 1 g dissolves in about 5000 ml of water, 1100 of boiling water, 210 ml of ethanol, 98 ml of boiling ethanol, 1220 ml of chloroform, 6250 ml of ether, 114 ml of amyl alcohol, 10 ml of boiling methanol, 525 ml of ethyl acetate; freely soluble in solutions of fixed alkali and other alkaline earth hydroxides, in phenols, cresols; moderately soluble in mixtures of chloroform with alcohols; and slightly soluble in ammonia benzene.

2. **Morphine Acetate Trihydrate ($C_{19}H_{23}NO_5.3H_2O$):**
   (i) It is a yellowish-white powder.
   (ii) It has a slight acetic odour.
   (iii) It specific optical rotation $[\alpha]_D^{15}$ – 77° (water).
   (iv) It dissolves 1 g in 2.25 ml of water, 2 ml of boiling water, 22 ml of ethanol, 2 ml of ethanol at 60°C, 4.5 ml of glycerol, 4.75 ml of chloroform; and practically insoluble in ether.

3. **Morphine Tartrate Tihydrate [($C_{17}H_{19}NO_3)_2.C_4H_6O_6.3H_2O$)]:** It is obtained as a crystalline powder. It is soluble in 11 parts of water; slightly soluble in alcohol; and practically insoluble in ether, chloroform and carbon disulphide.

Uses

1. It is used as a potent narcotic analgesic.
2. It is usually given in severe pains and also in such instances where patient fails to show positive response to other analgesics.

3. It exerts a biphasic action on the CNS.

4. It is found to sedate the respiratory centre, emetic centre and the cough centre through its action in the medulla.

5. It stimulates the chemoreceptor-trigger-zone located in the medulla that ultimately causes nausea and vomilting; and this is perhaps regarded as a side-effect.

6. It also exerts sedative and hypnotic actions.

Note: Morphine and its salts are habit forming drugs. Hence, its use must be done under the strict observation of a physician.

B. Codeine

Synonyms   Codicept; Morphine monomethyl ether; Morphine 3-methyl ether; Methylmorphine.

Biological Sources   It is obtained from the plant *Argemone mexicana* L. (*Papaveraceae*) **(Prickly Poppy)**; *Eschscholzia california* Cham. (*Papaveraceae*) **(California Poppy)**; *Papaver bracteatum* Lindl. (*Papaveraceae*) **(Great scarlet poppy, Thebaine Poppy)**; and *Papaver somniferum* L. (*Papaveraceae*) **(Opium Poppy, Poppyseed Poppy Keshi).**

Chemical Structure

Codeine

(5α, 6α)-7, 8-Didehydro-4, 5-epoxy-3-methoxy-17-methyl-morphinan-6-ol; ($C_{18}H_{21}NO_3$).

Preparation   It is invariably present in opium from 0.7 to 2.5% depending on the sources of plant substances. However, mostly it is prepared by carrying out the methylation of **morphine.**

Characteristic Features

1. It is obtained as monohydrate orthorhombic sphenoidal rods or tablets (octahedra) from water or dilute ethanol having mp 154-156°C (after drying at 80°C).

2. It is found to sublime (when anhydrous) at 140-145°C under 1.5 mm reduced pressure.

3. It is observed to melt to oily drops when heated in an amount of water is sufficient for complete solution, and subsequently crystallizes on cooling.

4. Its physical parameters are: d_4^{20} 1.32; $[\alpha]_D^{15} - 136°$ (C = 2 in ethanol); $[\alpha]_D^{15} - 112°$ (C = 2 in chloroform); pK (15°) 6.05; pH of a saturated solution 9.8.

5. **Solubility Profile:** 1 g dissolves in 120 ml water, 60 ml water at 80°C, 2 ml ethanol, 1.2 ml hot ethanol, 13 ml benzene, 18 ml ether, 0.5 ml chloroform; freely soluble in methanol, dilute acids and amyl alcohol; and almost insoluble in solutions of alkali hydroxides and in petroleum ether.

Identification Test   It forms various types of salts, namely:

1. **Codeine Acetate (C$_{20}$H$_{25}$NO$_5$):** The dihydrate is obtained as crystals having an acetic acid odour. It is found to be soluble in water and ethanol. It loses acetic acid on keeping and subsequently turns into a product which is incompletely soluble in water.

2. **Codeine Hydrobromide (C$_{18}$H$_{21}$NO$_3$.HBr):** The dihydrate is obtained as crystals and the anhydrous product shows a mp 190-192°C; $[\alpha]_D^{22}$ − 96.6° ; 1 g dissolves in 60 ml water, 110 ml ethanol; and pH about 5.

3. **Codeine Hydrochloride (C$_{18}$H$_{21}$NO$_3$.HCl):** Its dihydrate salt is obtained as small needles having mp ~ 280°C with some decomposition; $[\alpha]_D^{22}$ − 108° ; 1 g dissolves in 20 ml of water, 1 ml boiling water, 180 ml ethanol; and pH about 5.

4. **Codeine Salicylate (C$_{25}$H$_{27}$NO$_6$):** It is obtained as white crystalline powder; slightly soluble in water; and freely soluble in ethanol or ether.

5. **Codeine Phosphate (C$_{18}$H$_{24}$NO$_7$P) (Galcodine):** The hemihydrate salt (USP) is obtained as fine, white, needle-shaped crystals or crystalline powder. It is odorless and affected by light. The solution is acidic to litmus. It is freely soluble in water; very soluble in hot water; slightly soluble in ethanol; and more soluble in boiling ethanol.

6. **Codeine Sulphate (C$_{36}$H$_{44}$N$_2$O$_{10}$S):** The trihydrate is obtained as crystals or crystalline powder; 1 g dissolves in 30 ml water; 6.5 ml water at 80°C; 1300 ml ethanol; insoluble in chloroform or ether; pH 5.0.

7. **Codeine Methyl Bromide (C$_{19}$H$_{24}$Br-NO$_3$) (Eucodin) :** Its crystals have mp ~ 260°C; soluble in 2-3 parts of water, in hot methanol; sparingly soluble in ethanol; and insoluble in chloroform and ether.

Uses

1. It is mostly used as a narcotic analgesic.
2. It is invariably employed as an antitussive.

C. Thebaine

Synonym Paramorphine;

Biological Sources It is obtained from the fresh capsule latex (0.125%), dried 0.25 to 0.26% of *Papaver bracteatum* Lindl. (*Papaveraceae*) (**Great Scarlet Poppy, Thebaine Poppy**); and the air-dried milky exudation obtained from excised unripe fruits of *Papaver somniferium* L. (*Papaveraceae*) (**Opium Poppy, Poppyseed Poppy Keshi**).

Chemical Structure

Thebaine

(5α)-6, 7, 8, 14-Tetrahydro-4, 5-epoxy-3, 6-dimethoxy-17-methylmorphinan; ($C_{19}H_{21}NO_3$).

Isolation   **Thebaine** may be isolated from opium by means of the following steps, namely:

Step-1: Opium (dried latex) is treated with calcium chloride solution and then extracted with warm water. Allow it to remain as such for 24 hours.

Step-2: Filter the resulting product and collect the residue and filtrate separately.

> *Residue*— contains the salts of calcium as lactate, sulphate, resinate and meconate (To be discarded).
>
> *Filtrate*— contains the hydrochloride of various alkaloids present in opium.

Step-3: Add dilute NaOH solution (2N) carefully to the resulting filtrate and allow it to stand for 4-6 hours. Filter the contents of the flask:

> *Filtrate*— contains morphine, codeine and narceine
>
> *Residue*—contains thebaine, papaverine and narcotine

Step-4: Dissolve the residue or precipilate in dilute ethanol (50% v/v), make slightly acidic with the addition of dilute glacial acetic acid and finally add to it approximately *three volumes* of boiling distilled water.

Step-5: Filter the above reaction product:

> *Filtrate*— contains thebaine
>
> *Residue*—contains papaverine and narcotine

Step-6: Concentrate the filtrate obtained in Step-5 under reduced pressure and add to it dilute NH_4OH solution to make it alkaline; and extract the liberated alkaloid thebaine successively with chloroform. Thebaine is obtained after evaportion of chloroform under vaccuo.

Characteristic Features

1. It is obtained as orthorhombic, rectangular plates by sublimation at 170-180°C under atmospheric pressure and a 1 mm distance mp 193°C (rapid heating).
2. Its physical parameters are: $[\alpha]_D^{15} - 219°$ (p = 2 in ethanol); $[\alpha]_D^{23}$ (p = 5 in chloroform); pK at 15°C = 6.05; and pH of a saturated solution is 7.6.
3. **Solubility Profile:** 1 g dissolves in 1460 ml water at 15°C, in about 15 ml hot ethanol, 13 ml chloroform, 200 ml ether, 25 ml benzene, 12 ml pyridine; and not very soluble in petroleum ether.

Identification Tests   **Thebaine** forms a number of salt derivatives which have specific characteristic features, such as:

1. **Thebaine Salicylate ($C_{19}H_{21}NO_3.C_7H_6O_3$):** It is obtained as crystals which are soluble in 750 parts of water. Thus, thebaine may be separated from other major alkaloids of opium by forming its salicylate derivative which is sparingly soluble in water.
2. **Thebaine Hydrochloride Monohydrate ($C_{19}H_{21}NO_3.HCl.H_2O$):** It is obtained as orthorhombic prisms from alcohol having $[\alpha]_D^{23} - 164°$ (p = 2). It is found to be soluble in about 12 parts of water and in ethanol. The pH of a 0.05 molar solution is 4.95.
3. **Thebaine Oxalate Hexahydrate ($2\ C_{19}H_{21}NO_3.C_2H_2O_4.6\ H_2O$):** It is obtained as prisms. It is soluble in 10 parts of water and also in ethanol; and is almost insoluble in ether.
4. **Thebaine Binoxalate Monohydrate ($C_{19}H_{21}NO_3.C_2H_2O_4.H_2O$):** It is obtained as prisms and found to be soluble in 45 parts of water.

5. **Thebaine Bitartrate Monohydrate ($C_{19}H_{21}NO_3.C_4H_6O_6.H_2O$):** It is obtained as prisms, soluble in 130 parts of water, quite soluble in both hot water and hot ethanol.

6. It gives a red colour on the addition of a few drops of cold sulphuric acid which ultimately changes to orange yellow.

Uses   It is an opiate analgesic.

D. Reticuline

Synonym   Coclanoline.

Biological Sources   It is obtained from the plant *Hydratis canadensis* L. (*Ranunculaceae*) (Goldenseal); the leaves of *Laurus nobilis* L. (*Lauraceae*) (**Bay, Grecian Laurel, Green Bay**); the air-dried milky exudation obtained from excised unripe fruits of *Papaver somiferum* L. (*Papaveraceae*) (**Opium Poppy, Poppyseed Poppy Keshi**); and the leaves of *Sassafras albidum* (Nutt.) Nees (*Lauraceae*) (**Sassafras**).

Chemical Structure

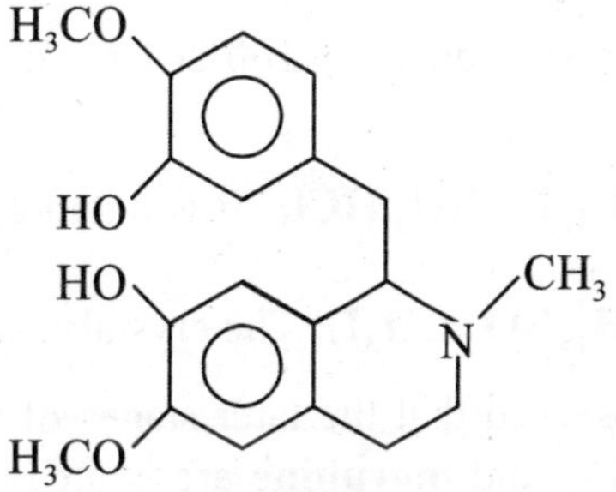

Reticuline

1, 2, 3, 4-Tetrahydro-1-[(3-hydroxy-4-methoxyphenyl) methyl]-6-methoxy-2-methyl-7-isoquinolinol; ($C_{19}H_{23}NO_4$).

Isolation   Gopinath *et al.*,* has described the isolation of *d*-form of reticuline from *Anona reticulata* Linn., (*Annonaceae*).

Characteristic Features
1. The *dl*-form of **reticuline** is obtained as pink crystals having mp 146°C.
2. The uv_{max}: 284 nm (log $\in$ 3.85).
3. *Solubility Profile:* It is soluble in aqueous buffer of pH < 7.5 or > 11; and is practically insoluble in water at pH 8-10.

Identification Tests
   (S)-Form Reticuline Perchlorate ($C_{19}H_{23}NO_4.HClO_4$): It is obtained as colourless prisms from ethanol having mp 203-204°C. Its specific optical rotation $[\alpha]_D^{18}$ + 88.3° (C = 0.21 in ethanol).

E. Oripavine

Synonym O^3-Demethylthebaine.

---

* Gopinath *et al.*, *Ber.* **92**, 776 (1959).

Biological Sources   It is obtained from the plant *Papaver bracteatum* Lindl. (*Papaveraceae*) (**Great Scarlet Poppy, Thebaine Poppy**); and *Papaver orientale* Linn. (*Papaveraceae*).

Chemical Structure

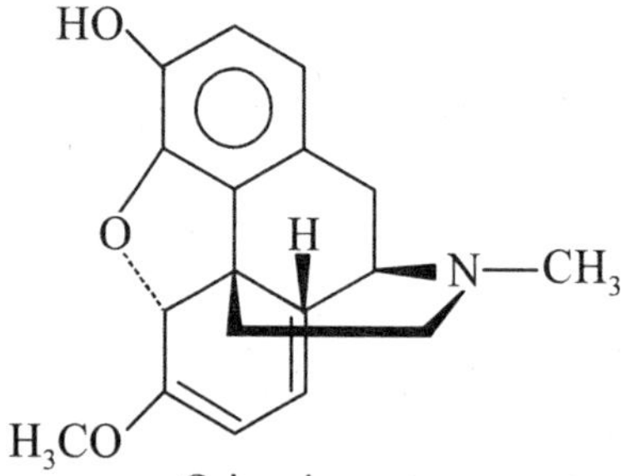

Oripavine

(5α)-6, 7, 8, 14-Tetrahydro-4, 5-epoxy-6-methoxy-17-methyl-morphinan-3-ol; ($C_{18}H_{19}NO_3$).

Isolation   It has been isolated from plant source by Kiselev and Konovalova.*

Characteristic Features   The crystals have mp 200-201°C; and $[\alpha]_D^{20} - 211.8°$.

Identification Tests

1. **Oripavine Hydrochloride ($C_{18}H_{19}NO_3.HCl$):** It is obtained as crystals which decompose at 244-245°C.
2. **Oripavine Methiodide ($C_{18}H_{19}NO_3.CH_3I$):** The crystals decompose at 207-208°C.

F. Morphinone   It has been observed that the later stages of the biosynthetic pathway starting from reticuline leading to **thebaine** and **morphine** are strategically modified in some strains of opium poppy. Therefore, in such strains, thebaine is converted by way of **oripavine** and **morphinone**. In this pathway the phenolic *O*-methyl function is removed before that of the enol ether, *i.e.,* accomplishing the same steps but in a different order. In other words, **morphinone** is obtained by the demethylation of **oripavine** as shown below:

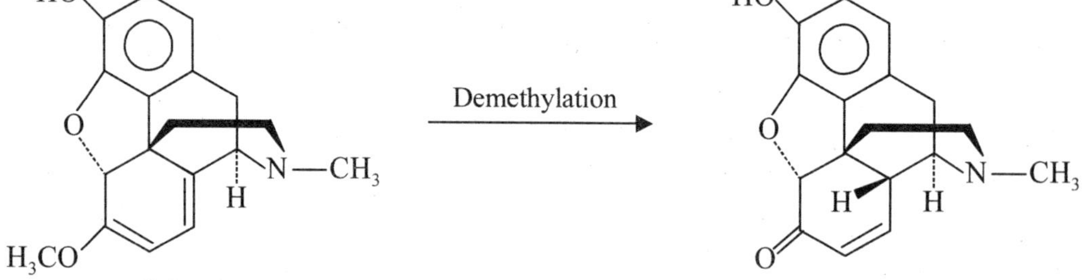

Oripavine   Demethylation   Morphinone

Biosynthesis of Morphine, Codeine, Thebaine, Oripavine and Morphinone The various steps involved are as follows:

* Kiselev and Konovalova *J. Gen. Chem.* USSR, **18**, 142 (1948).

1. **(R)-Reticuline,** may be redrawn as shown in page 495 following pathway is found to be the substrate for one-electron oxidation *via* the phenol moiety present in each ring thereby yielding the diradical.

2. Subsequent coupling *ortho* to the phenol group in the tetrahydroisoquinoline nucleus, and *para* to the phenol in the benzyl substituent, gives rise to **salutaridine**—a *dienone* which is found as minor alkaloidal component in the **opium poppy** *Papaver somniferum.*

3. **Thebaine** is achieved *via* **salutaridinol** produced from salutaridine by means of the stereospecific reduction of the carbonyl group.

4. In **thebaine** the ring closure to form the ether linkage is caused due to the nucleophilic attack of the phenol moiety on the dienol system followed by a displacement of the hydroxyl group.

5. Future reactions essentially involve conversion of **thebaine** into *morphine via codeine* by virtue of a process that exclusively modifies the oxidation state of the diene ring, but apparently removes *two O*-methyl groups.

6. One is evidently present as an enol ether, removal of which yields *neopinone*, that subsequently gives rise to **codeinone** and then **sodeine** by the help of allylic isomerisation and reduction respectively.

7. In certain specific strains of **opium poppy, thebaine** is changed to **oripavine** and **morphinone** by virtue of the pathway that essentially removes the phenolic *O*-methyl function before that of the enol ether.

7.2.8 Alkaloids Derived from Tryptophan

L-Tryptophan is a neutral heterocyclic amino acid containing essentially an indole ring system. It has been observed that it serves as a precursor for a wide spectrum of indole alkaloids. However, there exists an ample concrete evidence that major rearrangement reaction may convert the predominant **indole-ring system** into a **quinoline-ring system** thereby enhancing further the overall ability of tryptophan to act broadly as an alkaloid precursor.

The various alkaloids derived from tryptophan are conveniently classified into the following categories, namely: (*i*) **Simple Indole Alkaloids;** (*ii*) **Simple β-Carboline Alkaloids;** (*iii*) **Terpenoid Indole Alkaloids;** (*iv*) **Quinoline Alkaloids;** (*v*) **Pyrroloindole Alkaloids;** (*vi*) **Ergot Alkaloids.**

These aforesaid categories of alkaloids shall be discussed separately with typical important examples followed by the possible biosynthetic pathways, wherever necessary.

7.2.8.1 Simple Indole Alkaloids

L-Tryptophan (*i.e.,* α-aminoindole-3-propanoic acid) on decarboxylation yields *tryptamine*. The N-methyl and N, N-dimethyl derivatives of the latter are broadly distributed in the plant kingdom as *serotonin*—a simple hydroxylated derivative. Sequential biotransformation *viz.,* decarboxylation, N-methylation and hydroxylation gives rise to the formation of **psilocin;** whereas, phosphorylation of the OH group in psilocin yields *psilocybin.*

The *three* alkaloids, namely: **serotonin, psilocin** and **psilocybin** shall be discussed in the sections that follow:

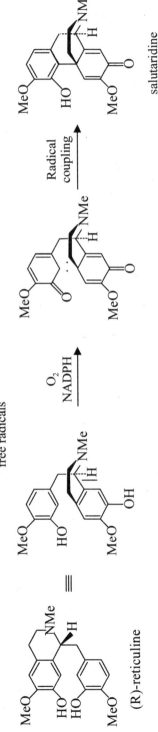

One-electron oxidation of phenol groups to give resonance-stablilized free radicals

Radical coupling

salutaridine

NADPH

stereospecific reduction of carbonyl

salutaridinol

O₂ NADPH

CH₃COSCoA

Esterification provides better leaving group

S_N2' nucleophilic attack with acetate as leaving group

(R)-reticuline

Thebaine

Demethylation

Demethylation of thebaine via hydroxylation, cleaving off methyl as formaldehyde

Biosynthesis of Morphine, Codeine, Thebaine, Oriparine and Morphinone (contd.)

Biosynthesis of Morphine, Codeine, Thebaine, Oriparine and Morphinone

A. Serotonin

Synonyms   5-Hydroxytryptamine; 5-HT; Enteramine; Thrombocytin; Thrombotonin;

Biological Sources   The root bark of *Gossypium hirsutum* L. (*Malvaceae*) (**American Unplanted Cotton**) contains serotonin.

Chemical Structure

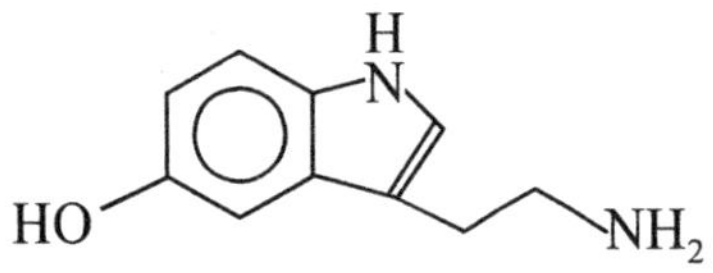

Serotonin

3-(2-Aminoethyl)-1H-indol-5-ol; ($C_{10}H_{12}N_2O$).

Identification Tests

1. **Serotonin Hydrochloride ($C_{10}H_{12}N_2O.HCl$)**   It is obtained as hygroscopic crystals, sensitive to light having mp 167-168°C. It is water soluble and the aqueous solutions are found to be stable at pH 2-6.4.
2. **Serotonin complex with Creatinine Sulphate Monohydrate ($C_{14}H_{21} N_5O_6S.H_2O$) (Antemovis)**   It is obtained as plates which decomposes at 215°C. Its uv_{max} (water at pH 3.5): is 275 nm (ε 15,000). It has two dissociation constants $pK_1' = 4.9$ and $pK_2' = 9.8$. The pH of a 0.01 molar aqueous solution is 3.6. It is found to be soluble in glacial acetic acid; very sparingly soluble in methanol and ethanol (95%); and insoluble in absolute ethanol, acetone, pyridine, ethyl acetate, chloroform, benzene and ether.

Uses

1. It is a potent vasoconstrictor.
2. It is also a neurotransmitter in the CNS and is important in sleep-walking-cycles.

B. Psilocin

Synonyms   Psilocyn.

Biological Sources   It is obtained from the sacred mushroom of Mexico known as **Teonanacatl**. It is also found in the fruiting bodies of *Psilocybe maxicana* Heim, (*Agaricaceae*).

Chemical Structure

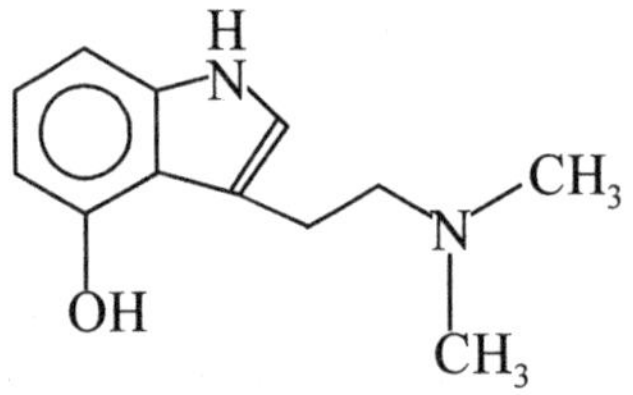

Psilocin

3-[2-(Dimethylamino) ethyl]-1H-indol-4-ol; ($C_{12}H_{16}N_2O$);

Isolation   It has been successfully isolated in trace amounts from the fruiting bodies of *Psilocybe mexicana**.

Characteristic Features

1. It is obtained as plates from methanol having mp 173–176°C.
2. It is an amphoteric substance.
3. It is unstable in solution, more precisely in an alkaline solution.
4. It is very slightly soluble in water.
5. Its uv$_{max}$: 222, 260, 267, 283, 293 nm (log ε 4.6, 3.7, 3.8, 3.7, 3.6).

Uses   It is a hallucinogenic substance

Note   It is a controlled substance listed in the U.S. Code of Federal Regulations, Title 21 Part 1308, 11 (1995).

C. Psilocybin

Synonym   Indocybin;

Biological Sources   These are same as mentioned in **psilocin 'B'** above.

Chemical Structure

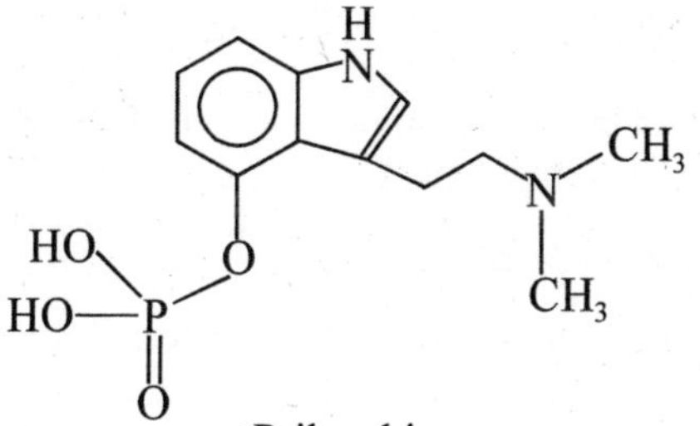

Psilocybin

3-[2-(Dimethylamino) ethyl]-1H-indol-4-ol dihydrogen phosphate ester; ($C_{12}H_{17}N_2O_4P$).

Isolation   The method of isolation of **psilocybin** is the same as stated under **psilocin.**

Characteristic Features

1. **Psilocybin** is obtained as crystals from boiling water having mp 220-228°C; and from boiling methanol mp 185-195°C.
2. It has uv$_{max}$ (methanol): 220, 267, 290 nm (log ε 4.6, 3.8, 3.6).
3. The pH of a saturated solution in 50% aqueous ethanol is 5.2.
4. **Solubility Profile:** It is soluble in 20 parts of boiling water, 120-parts of boiling methanol; sparingly soluble in ethanol; and practically insoluble in chloroform, benzene.

Uses   It is a hallucinogenic substance and exerts its action at a dose level of 6-20 mg.

Biosynthesis of Serotonin, Psilocin and Psilocybin   The different steps involved in the biosynthesis of **serotonin, psilocin** and **psilocybin** may be summarized as stated below:

---

* Hofmann *et al., Experientia,* **14,** 107 (1958); Heim *et al., Helv. Chim. Acta,* **42,** 1557 (1959).

1. L-Tryptophan upon oxidation gives rise to the corresponding hydroxylated derivative known as 5-hydroxyl-L-tryptophan, which further undergoes decarboxylation to yield **serotonin** also termed as **5-hydroxytryptamine (or 5-HT).**
2. L-Tryptophan undergoes decarboxylation to yield the tryptamine, which affords N-Methylation and N,N-dimethylation in the presence of S-adenosylmethionine (SAM). The resulting dimethyl derivative upon oxidation gives rise to the product **psilocin** another hydroxylated derivative.
3. Phosphorylation of the hydroxyl function in psilocin affords **psilocybin.**
4. Interestingly, both **psilocin** and **psilocybin** are solely responsible for attributing the hallucinogenic properties of the so-called '*magic mushrooms*', that include species of **Psilocybe, Panaeolus** and the like.

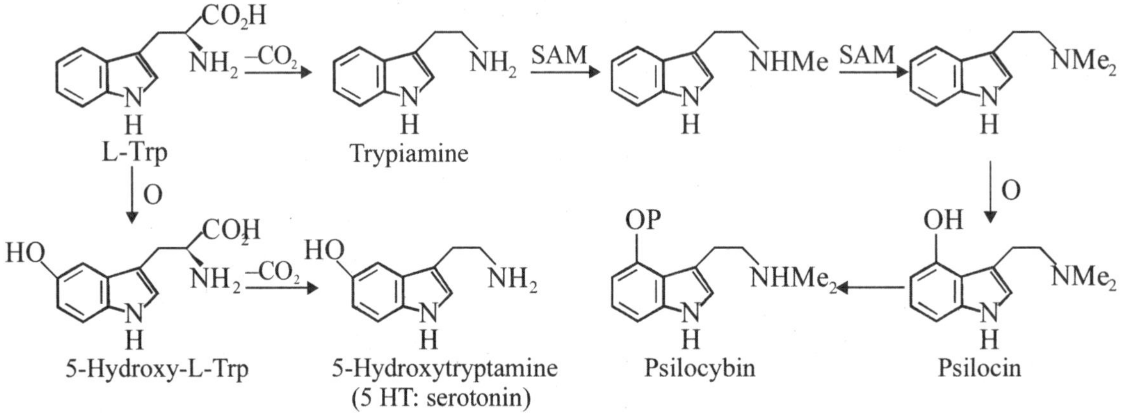

L-Trp   Trypiamine

5-Hydroxy-L-Trp   5-Hydroxytryptamine (5 HT: serotonin)   Psilocybin   Psilocin

7.2.8.2   Simple β-Carboline Alkaloids

The alkaloids based on the **β-carboline ring system** obviously suggest the formation of a new six-membered heterocyclic ring employing the *ethylamine side-chain present in tryptamine* exactly in the same manner to the evolution of tetrahydroisoquinoline alkaloids (see Section 7.2.7.2). The exact mechanism whereby the above rearrangement is accomplished may be explained by virtue of the fact that C-2 of the indole nucleus is *nucleophilic* due to the adjacent nitrogen atom. Therefore, C-2 can conveniently participate in a **Mannich/Pictet-Spengler type reaction,** thereby enabling it to attack a **Schiff base** produced from tryptamine and either an aldehyde (or keto acid) as given below:

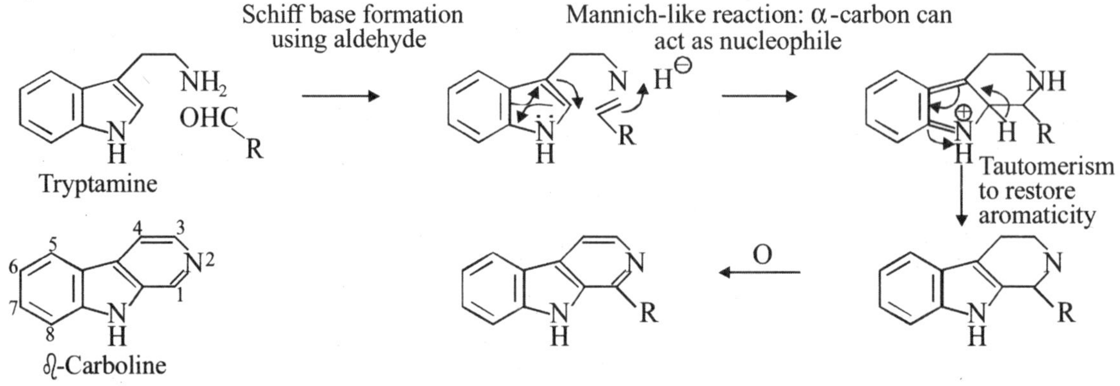

Schiff base formation using aldehyde   Mannich-like reaction: α-carbon can act as nucleophile

Tryptamine

Tautomerism to restore aromaticity

β-Carboline

It has been observed that relatively *simpler structures* make use of *keto-acids*, such as: **harman, harmaline, harmine** and **elaeagnine.** These alkaloids shall be treated individually in the sections that follow.

Interestingly, the comparatively complex carbolines, for instance: the **terpenoid indole alkaloids** *e.g.,* **ajmaline** are usually generated by the help of a pathway that specifically utilize *an aldehyde,* such as: secologanin. This particular section shall be dealt with separately under Section 7.2.8.3.

A. Harman

Synonyms   Aribine; Loturine; Passiflorin; 2-Methyl-β-carboline; 3-Methyl-4-carboline;

Biological Sources   It is obtained from the bark fruit of *Passiflora incarnata* L. (*Passifloraceae*) **(May pop, Passion flower)**; seed of *Peganum harmala* L. (*Rutaceae*) **(Harmel, Syrian Rue, African Rue)**, bark of *Sickingia rubra* (Mart.) K. Schum. (**Arariba rubra Mart.**), (*Rubiaceae*); and bark of *Symplocus racemosa* Roxb. (*Symplocaceae*).

Chemical Structure

Harman

1-Methyl-9H-pyrido [3, 4, b] indole; ($C_{12} H_{10} N_2$).

Isolation   Poindexter and Carpenter* isolated this alkaloid from the cigarette smoke.

Characteristic Features
1. It is obtained as orthorhombic crystals from heptane and cyclohexane having mp 237-238°C.
2. It has a bitter taste.
3. It exhibits distinct bright blue fluorescence in uv light.
4. It pKa's are 7.37 and 144.6.
5. It has uv$_{max}$ (methanol): 234, 287, 347 nm (log ε 4.57, 4.21, 3.66).
6. It is practically insoluble in water and freely soluble in dilute acids.

Identification Test   Harman Hydrochloride ($C_{12}H_{10}N_2$.HCl)   It is obtained as rosettes of needles from a mixture of ethanol + 20% HCl in water which sublimes at 120-130°C.

Uses   It is a narcotic hallucinogen.

B. Harmaline

Synonyms   Harmidine; Harmalol Methyl Ether; O-Methyl-harmalol; 3, 4-Dihydroharmine;

Biological Sources   It is obtained from the seeds of *Peganum harmala* L. (*Zugophyllaceae*); and *Banisteria cappi* Spruce (*Malpighiaceae*). It is also obtained from the fruit of *Passiflora incarnata* L. (*Passifloraceae*) **(Passionflower, Maypop).**

---

* Poindexter and Corpenter, *Chem. & Ind.* (London), **1962**, 176.

Chemical Structure

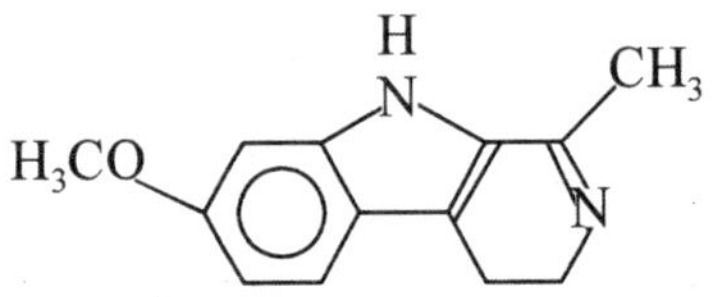

Harmaline

4, 9-Dihydro-7-methoxy-1-methyl-3H-pyridol [3, 4,-b] indole; ($C_{13} H_{14} N_2 O$).

Characteristic Features

1. It is obtained as orthorhombic bipyramidal prisms, or tablets from methanol; and as rhombic octahedra from ethanol having the same mp 229-231°C.
2. Its solutions give a blue fluorescence.
3. Its dissociation constant pK_a 4.2.
4. It has uv_{max} (methanol): 218, 260, 376 nm (log ε 4.27, 3.90 and 4.02)
5. It is found to be slightly soluble in water, ethanol, ether; and very soluble in dilute acids and hot ethanol.

Identification Tests   **Harmaline** forms definite derivatives as shown below:

1. **Harmaline Hydrochloride Dihydrate ($C_{13}H_{14}N_2O.HCl.2H_2O$):** It is obtained as slender, yellow needles that are found to be moderately soluble in ethanol and water.
2. **N-Acetylharmaline:** It is obtained as needles having mp 204-205°C.

Uses

1. It is recognized as a narcotic hallucinogen.
2. It is used as a CNS-stimulant.

C. Harmine

Synonyms   Telepathine; Leucoharmine; Yageine; Banisterine;

Biological Sources   It is obtained from the seeds of *Peganum harmala* L. (*Zygophyllaceae*); *Banisteria caapi* Spruce. (*Malpighiaceae*); and *Banisteriopsis inebrians* Morton. (*Malpighiaceae*). It is also obtained from the fruit of *Passiflora incarnata* L. (*Passifloraceae*).

Chemical Structure

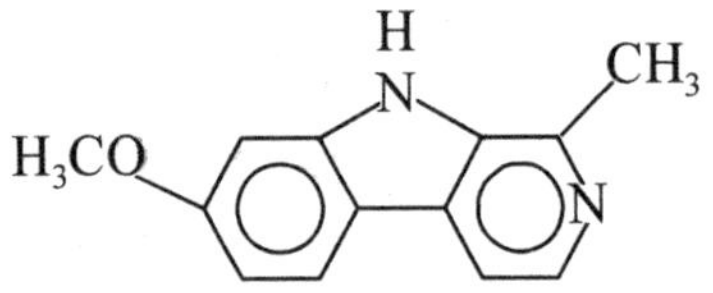

Harmine

7-Methoxy-1-methyl-9H-pyrido [3, 4-b] indole; ($C_{13} H_{12} N_2 O$).

---

* Rainhard *et al. Phytochemistry*, **7**, 503, (1968).

Isolation   Harmin may be isolated from the seeds of *Peganum harmala* L. (*Zygophyllaceae*) by the method suggested by Reinhard *et al*.

Characteristic Features

1. It is obtained as slender, orthorhombic prisms from methanol having mp 261°C (decomposition).
2. It sublimes and has pKa value of 7.70.
3. It as uv$_{max}$ (methanol): 241, 301, 336 nm (log ε 4.61, 4.21, 3.69).
4. It is found to be slightly soluble in water, ethanol, ether and chloroform.

Identification Tests

Harmine Hydrochloride Dihydrate ($C_{13}H_{12}N_2O.HCl.2H_2O$)   It is obtained as crystals having mp 262°C (decomposition), but when anhydrous mp 321°C (decomposition), but when anhydrous mp 321°C. The aqueous solution exhibits a distinct blue fluorescence. It is found to be soluble in 40 parts of water and freely soluble in hot water.

Uses   It finds its usage as a CNS-stimulant and also as a narcotic hallucinogen.

D. Elaeagnine

Biological Source   It is obtained from the bark of *Elaeagnus angustifolia* Linn., (*Synonyms: E. hortensis Bieb.*) (*Elaeagnaceae*).

Chemical Structure

Elaeagnine

Biosynthesis of Elaeagnine, Harman, Harmaline and Harmine   The various steps involved in the biosynthesis of the above mentioned *four* alkaloids are briefly summarized as under:

1. Tryptamine and acetyl carboxylic acid (*i.e.*, keto acid) undergoes a **Mannich-like reaction** to yield a **β-carboline carboxylic acid,** which on oxidative decarboxylation gives rise to 1-methyl β-carboline.
2. The resulting product on subsequent reduction gives rise to the alkaloid **elaeagnine.**
3. The **1-methyl β-carboline** upon mild oxidation yields the alkaloids *harman* with the elimination of a mole of water from the 6-membered heterocyclic nucleus.
4. The **1-methyl β-carboline** upon hydroxylation followed by methylation produces **harmaline.**
5. **Harmaline** on further oxidation generates **harmine** by the loss of a mole of water from the 6-membered pyridine ring at C-3 and C-4 positions.

The these steps are sequentially arranged in the following course of reactions:

Harmine   Harmaline   Tetrahydroharmine   Harman

7.2.8.3 Terpenoid Indole Alkaloids

Terpenoid indole alkaloids is perhaps one of the major groups of alkaloids in the plant kingdom which comprise of more than 3000 recognized alkaloids till date Interestingly, they are found to be confined to *eight* different natural orders (*i.e.*, families), of which the *Apocynaceae,* the *Loganiaceae,* and the *Rubiaceae* are predominantly the best known sources.

However, it is pertinent to mention here that practically in all the structure a *tryptamine residue* is strategically located in the molecule; while the remaining fragment is invariably recognized as a C_9 or C_{10} residue.

The wisdom, relentless efforts and meticulous in-depth studies carried out by numerous groups of researchers dealing with plant substances across the globe ultimately led to *three* main *structural variants* entirely based on their good judgement and understanding namely:

(*a*) *Coryanthe Type e.g.,* **ajmalicine** and **akuammicine,**

(*b*) *Aspidosperma Type e.g.,* **tabersonine,** and

(*c*) *Iboga Type e.g.,* **catharanthine.**

It has since been established beyond any reasonable doubt that the C_9 or C_{10} component present in the aforesaid *three* types of structural variants *i.e., Carynanthe, Aspidosperma* and *Iboga* groups was definitely of the *terpenoid origin.* Besides, it was also confirmed that the *secoridoid secologanin* was duly proclaimed to be the *terpenoid derivative,* which perhaps must have initially combined with the tryptamine residue of the molecule. From these scientific and logical evidences one may safely infer that the *three* above mentioned groups of alkaloids might be not only related but also rationalized in terms of rearrangements taking place exclusively in the *terpenoid portion* of the various structural variants as shown in the pathway given below.

Salient Features   The salient features of the above pathway are as follows:

1. **Secologanin** (a *secoridoid* and a *terpenoid* derivative) is formed through **geraniol** *via* **loganin,** which essentially contains the 10C-framework a typical characteristic feature of the *Coryanthe* moiety.

2. The resulting *Coryanthe* C-skeleton undergoes subsequent rearrangements to give rise to *Aspidosperma* and *Iboga* groups.

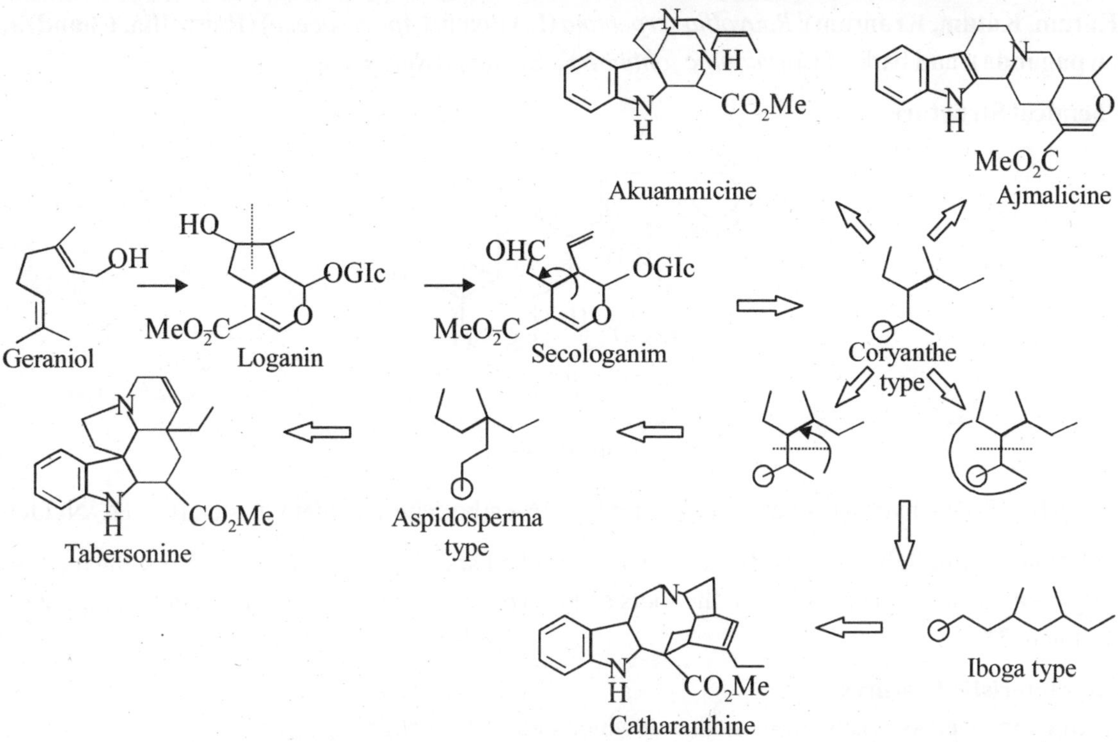

Pathways for Coryanthe, Aspidosperma and Iboga Type Alkaloids

3. This intra-molecular rearrangement may be represented by detachment of a 3C-unit, which is subsequently reunited to the remaining C_7 fragment in one of the two different manners as shown in the pathway.

4. Interestingly, where C_9 terpenoid units are complied with, the alkaloids usually, seem to have lost a C-atom marked in the circle, which exactly corresponds to the carboxylate function of secologanin molecule. Therefore, its ultimate elimination by way of hydrolysis/decarboxylation is now understood without any reasonable doubt.

5. Thus, the *Coryanthe* type of C-skeleton yields *ajmalicine* and *akuammicine.*

6. The *Aspidosperma* type of C-skeleton yields **tabersonine** and **vindoline.**

7. The *Iboga type* of C-skeleton gives rise to *catharanthine.*

A few typical examples of terpenoid indole alkaloids, namely: **Ajmalicine** (Raubasine); Akuammicine; **Vindoline;** and **Catharanthine** shall be discussed below:

A. Ajmalicine

Synonyms   Raubasine; Circolene; Hydrosarpan; Lamuran; Isoarteril;

Biological Sources   It is obtained from the plants of catharanthus lanceus Pichon (Boj.) (*Apocynaceae*) (Lanceleaf Periwinkle); *Catharanthus roseus* (L.) G. Don (*Apocynaceae*) (**Periwinkle, Madagascar** or **Cape Periwinkle, Old Maid**]; leaves of *Mitragyna speciosa* Korth. (*Rubiaceae*)

(**Katum, Kutum, Krantum**); *Rauvolfia scrpentina* (L.) Benth. (*Apocynaceae*) (**Rauvolfia, Chandra, Sarpaganda**); and bark of *Corynanthe johimbe* K. Schum., (*Rubiaceae*).

Chemical Structure

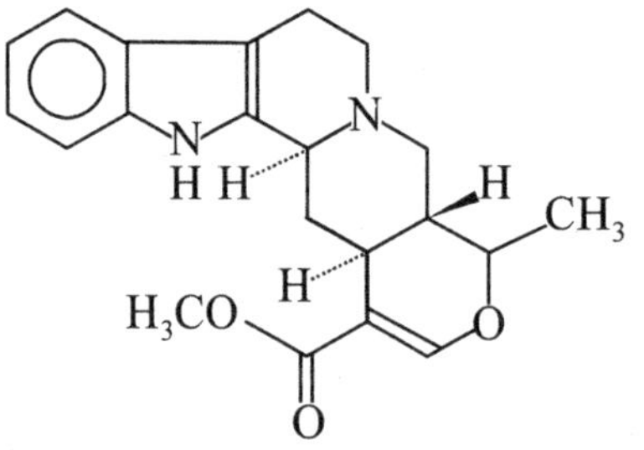

Ajmalicine

(19α)-16, 17-Didehydro-19-methyl-oxayohimban-16-carboxylic acid methyl ester; ($C_{21} H_{24} N_2 O_3$).

Isolation   **Ajmalicine** may be isolated either from the bark of *Corynanthe johimbe* by the method suggested by Heinemann*, or from the roots of *Rauwolfia serpentina* by the procedure adopted by Hofmann.**

Characteristic Features

1. It is obtained as prisms from methanol which decompose at 257°C.
2. It has specific optical rotation $[\alpha]_D^{20} - 60°$ (C = 0.5 in chloroform); $[\alpha]_D^{20} - 45°$ (C = 0.5 in pyridine); and $[\alpha]_D^{20} - 39°$ (C = 0.25 in methanol).
3. It exhibits uv$_{max}$ (methanol): 227, 292 nm (log ε 4.61, 3.79).

Identification Tests

1. **Ajmalicine Hydrochloride ($C_{21}H_{24}N_2O_3$.HCl):** It is obtained as leaflets from ethanol having mp 290°C (decomposed); $[\alpha]_D^{20} - 17°$ (C = 0.5 in methanol); and is sparingly soluble in water or dilute HCl.
2. **Ajmalicine Hydrobromide ($C_{21}H_{24}N_2O_3$.HBr):** It is obtained as diamond-shaped plates from methanol having mp 295-296°C.

Uses

1. It is mostly used as antihypertensive and anti-ischemic agent (both ceretral and peripheral).
2. It has a broad application in the relief of obstruction of normal cerebral blood flow.

B. Akuammicine

Biological Source   It is obtained from the plant substance of *Catharanthus roseus* (L.) G. Don (*Apocyanaceae*) (**Periwinkle, Madagascar** or **Cape Periwinkle, Old Maid**); and also from the seeds of *Picralima klaineana,* Pierre, belonging to the natural order (*Apocyanaceae*).

---

* Heinemann, H., *Ber.* **67**, 15 (1934).

** Hofmann, A, *Helv. Chim. Acta.* **37**, 849, (1954).

Chemical Structure

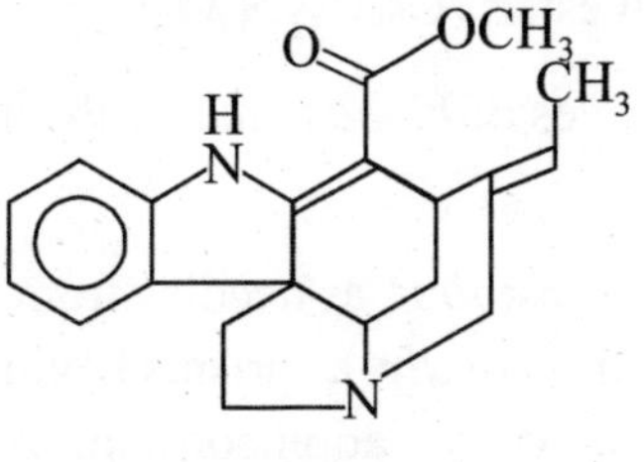

Akuammicine

2, 16, 19-20-Tetradehydrocuran-17-oic acid methyl ster; ($C_{20} H_{22} N_2 O_2$).

Characteristic Features
1. It is obtained as plates from a mixture of ethanol and water having mp 182°C.
2. Its physical parameters are: $[\alpha]_D^{16} - 745°$ (C = 0.994 in ethanol); pKa 7.45; and uv_{max} (ethanol): 227, 330 and 330 nm (log ε 4.09, 4.07, 4.24).

Identification Tests   It forms the following derivatives:

1. **Akuaminicine Hydrochloride Dihydrate ($C_{20}H_{22}N_2O_2$.HCl.2H$_2$O):** It is obtained as leaflets from ethanol or water having mp 171°C; and has $[\alpha]_D^{21} - 610°$ (C = 1.430 in ethanol).
2. **Akuaminicine Perchlorate Monohydrate ($C_{20}H_{22}N_2O_2$.HClO$_4$.H$_2$O):** It is obtained as needles from a mixture of ethanol and water having mp 134-136°C.
3. **Akuammicine Hydroiodide Monohydrate ($C_{20}H_{22}N_2O_2$.HI, H$_2$O):** It is obtained as square plates from water having mp 128°C.
4. **Akuammicine Methiodide:** It is obtained as crystals from water with mp 252°C.
5. **Akuammicine Nitrate:** It is obtained as needles from hot water having mp 182.5°C.

Uses   The drug exhibits a slight digitalis-like reaction; and is, therefore, believed to act as a heart poison.

C. Vindoline

Biological Sources   It is obtained from the plant *Catharanthus roseus* (L.) G. Don (*Apocynaceae*) (**Periwinkle, Madagascar** or **Cape Periwinkle; Old Maid**). It is found to be the major alkaloid from the leaves of *Vinca rosea* Linn. (*Apocynaceae*).

Chemical Structure

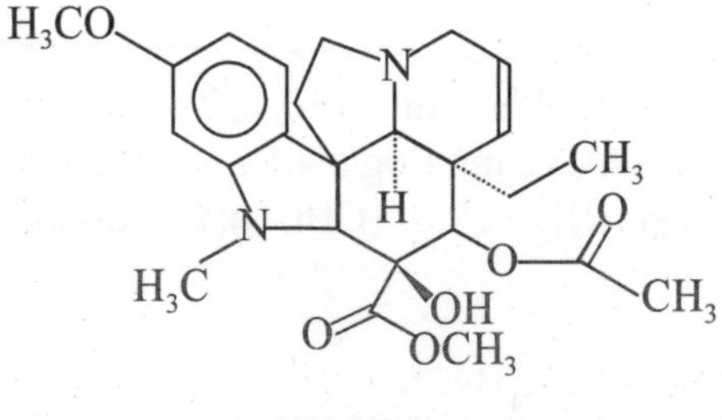

Vindoline

(2β,3β,4β,5α,12β,19α)-4-(Acetyloxy)-6, 7-didehydro-3-hydroxy-16-methoxy-1 methylaspidos-permidine-3-carboxylic acid methyl ester; ($C_{25}H_{32}N_2O_6$).

Isolation It is isolated from the leaves of *Vinca rosea* by the method suggested by Gorman *et al.**

Characteristic Features

1. **Vinodoline** is obtained in two forms: *first*, as needles from a mixture of acetone and petroleum ether having mp 164-165°C; and *secondly*, as prisms having mp 174-175°C.
2. It has $[\alpha]_D^{20}$ - 18° (chloroform) and dissociation constant pKa 5.5 in 66% DMF.
3. It has uv$_{max}$ (ethanol): 212, 250, 304 nm (log ε 4.49, 3.74, 3.57).

Identification Tests It gives specific derivatives as.

1. **Vindoline Hydrochloride ($C_{25}H_{32}N_2O_6$.HCl):** It is obtained as crystals from acetone having mp 161-164°C.
2. **Demethoxy Vindoline ($C_{24}H_{30}N_2O_5$) (Vindorosine, Vindolidine):** It is obtained as needles from benzene and petroleum ether having mp 167°C. It has $[\alpha]_D^{16}$ -31° (Chloroform); and uv$_{max}$ (methanol): 250, 302 nm (log ε 3.98, 3.52).

D. Catharanthine

Biological Sources It is obtained in the plant of *Catharanthus lanceus* Pichon (Boj.) (*Apocynaceae*) (**Lanceleaf Periwinkle**); and *Catharanthus roseus* (L.) G. Don (*Apocyanaceae*) (**Periwinkle, Madagascar** or **Cape Periwinkle, Old Maid**). It is also found in *Vinca rosea* Linn. (*Apocynaceae*).

Chemical Structure

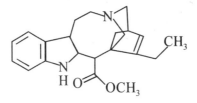

Cathranthine

3, 4-Didehydroibogamine-18-carboxylic acid methyl ester; ($C_{21}H_{24}N_2O_2$).

Isolation It may be isolated from *Vinca rosea* Linn by the method recommended by Gorman *et al.***

Characteristic Feature

1. Its crystals obtained from methanol has mp 126-128°C.
2. It has uv$_{max}$ (ethanol): 226, 284, 292 nm (log ε 4.56, 3.92, 3.88).
3. It has specific optical rotation $[\alpha]_D^{27}$ + 29.8° (CHCl$_3$); and dissociation constant pKa′ 6.8.

---

* Gorman *et al. J. Am. Pharm. Assoc.* **48**, 256, (1959).

** M. Gorman *et al., J. Arn. Pharm. Assoc. Sci.* Ed. **48**, 256 (1959).

Uses

1. Its pharmacological action resembles to that of *R. serpentina*.
2. It also shows beneficial growth inhibition effects in certain human tumors.
3. It is used as a diuretic.

Biosynthesis of Ajmalicine, Vindoline and Catharanthine   The various steps involved in the biosynthesis of **ajmalicine, vindoline** and **catharanthine** are summarized below:

1. Condensation of secologanin with tryptamine in a Mannich-type reaction gives rise to the **tetrahydro-β-carboline system** and generates *strictosidine*.
2. The structural variations involved in converting the *Coryanthe* type skeleton into the corresponding *Aspidosperma* and *Iboga* types are evidently quite complex and are given in the pathway as under.
3. **Preakuammicine** is obtained from **strictosidine** *via* the *enol*-form of **dehydrogeissoschizine.**
4. **Preakuammicine** undergoes intramolecular rearrangement to produce **stemmadenine,** which subsequently gives rise to a hypothetical intermediate.
5. The hypothetical intermediate may be redrawn which undergoes Diel's-Alder type reaction to produce **catharanthine.**
6. Dehydrogeissoschizine yields **ajmalicine.**
7. The hypothetical intermediate gives rise to **vindoline** *via* **tabersonine.**

It is pertinent to mention here that the sequence of alkaloid formation has been proved initially by noting carefully which alkaloids become labelled as a feeding experiment progresses, but more recently it has been confirmed by suitable enzymatic experimental studies.

It is important to mention here that there exists a plethora of structural variants of terpenoid indole alkaloids which may be exemplified with the help of the following specific examples of certain potent alkaloids, namely:

  (*i*) **Yohimbine:** It is a carboxyclic variant related to ajmalicine and appears to arise from dehydrogeissoschizine by an elaborated mechanism.
 (*ii*) **Reserpine:** It is a trimethoxybenzoyl ester of yohimbine-like alkaloid. It has an additional-OCH$_3$ moiety at C.-11 of the indole nucleus.
(*iii*) **Rescinnamine:** It is a trimethoxycinnamoyl ester of yohimbine-like alkaloid. It also contains an additional methoxyl substituent on the indole-system at C-11.
(*iv*) **Vinblastine:** The nucleophilie vindoline, C-5 of the indole nucleous is being activated adequately by the OMe at C-6, besides the N-atom of the indole moiety. The resulting adduct is subsequently reduced in the dihydropyridinium ring by the NADH-dependent 1, 4-addition, giving the substrate for hydroxylation. Its ultimate reduction gives rise to vinblastine.
 (*v*) **Vincristine:** It is the oxidized product of vinblastine whereby the inherent N-formyl group on the indoline fragment is transformed.
(*vi*) **Strychnine:** The loss of one C from a preakuammicine-like structure *via* hydrolysis/decarboxylation followed by an addition of the additional two C-atoms by means of aldol-condensation with the formyl moiety, complexed as a hemiacetal in the well-known **Wieland-Gumlich aldehyde.** The ultimate formation of strychnine from its hemiacetal is by virtue of the formation of both *ether* and *amide* linkages.

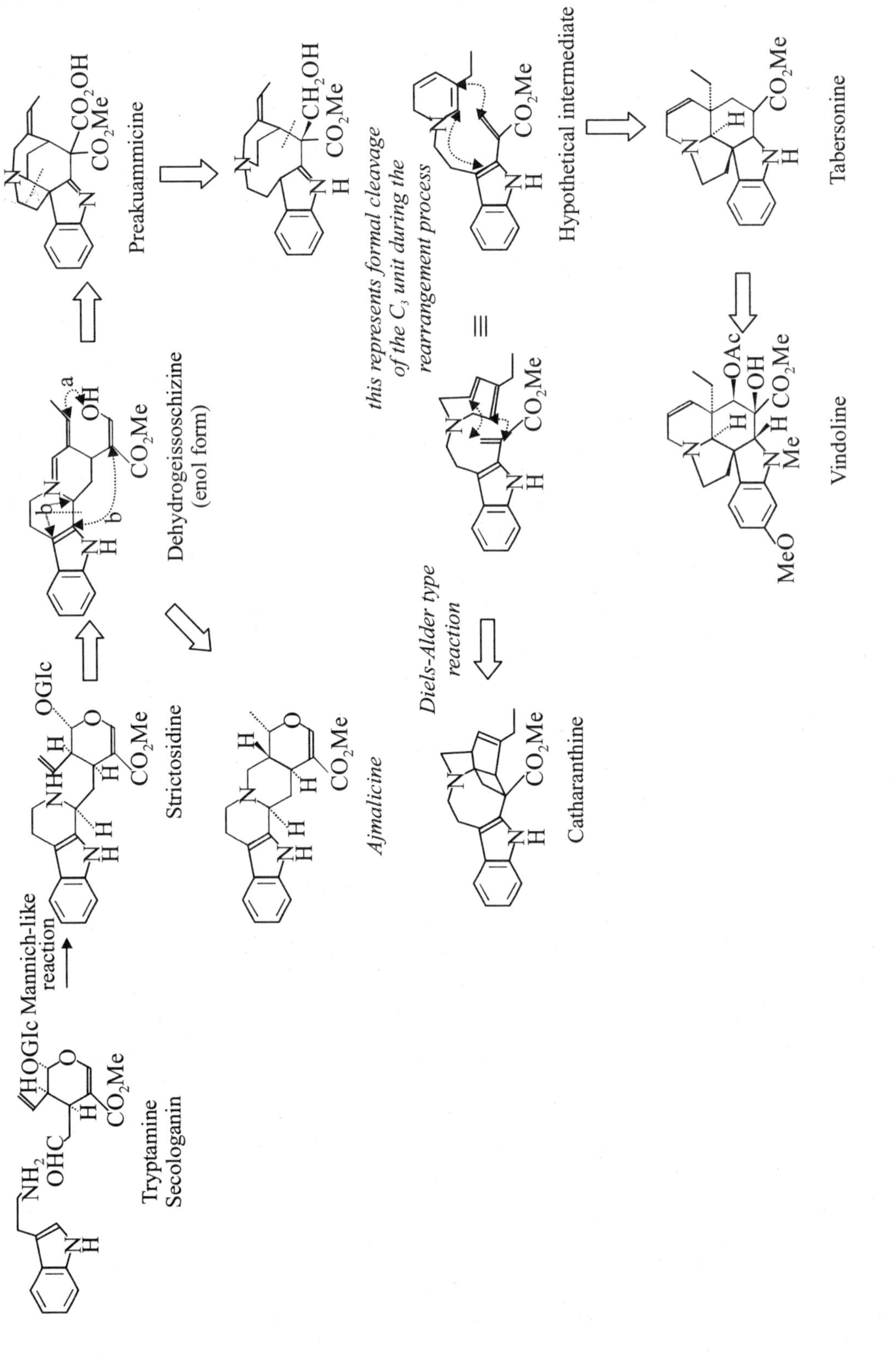

CO_2H

CO_2Me

Preakuammicine

CH_2OH

CO_2Me

H

Hypothetical intermediate

CO_2Me

CO_2Me

H

Tabersonine

OH

CO_2Me

Dehydrogeissoschizine
(enol form)

*this represents formal cleavage
of the C₃ unit during the
rearrangement process*

≡

CO_2Me

H

*Diels-Alder type
reaction*

OAc

OH

H H CO_2Me

Me

MeO

Vindoline

HOGlc

NH H OGlc

CO_2Me

H

OHC

NH₂

Mannich-like
reaction

Tryptamine
Secologanin

Strictosidine

H

O

CO_2Me

H H

Ajmalicine

CO_2Me

H

Catharanthine

Pathways for Ajmalicine, Preakuammicine, Catharanthine and Vindoline

The above mentioned *six* structural variants of the **terpenoid indole alkaloids** shall now be discussed individually in the sections that follow.

A. Yohimbine

Synonyms Quebrachine; Corynine; Aphrodine;

Biological Sources It is found in the root bark of *Alchornea floribunda* Muell. Arg. (*Euphorbiaceae*) (**Niando**); plant* of *Catharanthus lanceus* Pichon (Boj.) (*Apocyraceae*) (**Lanceleaf Periwinkle**); bark of *Pausinystalia johimbe* (K. Schum.) (*Rubiaceae*) (**Yohimbe**); root of *Rauvolfia serpentina* (L.) Benth. (*Apocynaceae*) (**Rauvolfia, Chandra, Sarpaganda**); and plant of *Rauvolfia tetraphylla* L. (*Apocynaceae*) (**Pinque-Pinque**).

Chemical Structure

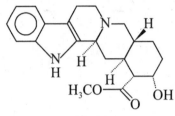

Yohimbine

(16a, 17a)-17-Hydroxyyohimban-16-carboxylic acid methyl ester; ($C_{21}H_{26}N_2O_3$).

Characteristic Features
1. It is obtained as orthorhombic needles from dilute alcohol having mp 234°C.
2. Its specific optical rotations are: $[\alpha]_D^{20} + 50.9°$ to $+ 62.2°$ (ethanol); $[\alpha]_D^{20} + 108°$ (pyridine); and $[\alpha]_{546}^{20} + 129°$ (C = 0.5 in pyridine).
3. It has uv$_{max}$ (methanol): 226, 280, 291 nm (log ε 4.56, 3.88, 3.80).
4. It is freely soluble in ethanol, chloroform, hot benzene; moderately soluble in ether; and sparingly soluble in water.

Identification Tests

Yohimbine Hydrochloride ($C_{21}H_{26}N_2O_3$.HCl) (Aphrodyne, Yocon, Yohimex, Yohydrol): It is obtained as orthorhombic plates or prisms from ethanol which decompose at 302°C. Its specific optical rotation $[\alpha]_D^{22} + 105°$ (water). It is found to be soluble in nearly 120 ml water, 400 ml ethanol, and the aqueous solution is almost neutral.

Uses
1. It is an aderenergic blocking agent, which has been used extensively in angina pectoris and arteriosclerosis.
2. It has been used successfully for the treatment of impotency in patients with vascular or diabetic problems.
3. It is invariably employed as a pharmaiological probe for the study of α_2-adrenoreceptor.

---

* Emboden reported that this plant contains upto 5% **yohimbin.**

B. Reserpine

Synonyms   Crystoserpine; Eskaserp; Rau-sed; Reserpoid; Rivasin; Serfin; Sandril; Sedaraupin; Serpasil; Serpine; Serpasol; Serpiloid.

Biological Sources   It is obtained from the plant *Catharanthus roseus* (L.) G. Don (*Apocynaceae*) (**Periwinkle, Madagascar** or **Cape Periwinkle, Old Maid**); root of *Rauvolfia serpentina* (L.) Benth (*Apocynaceae*) (**Rauvolfia, Chandra, Sarpaganda**); root of *Rauvolfia tetraphylla* L. (*Apocynaceae*) (**Pinque-Pinque**); and from the plant of *Vinca minor* L. (*Apocynaceae*) (**Periwinkle**).

Chemical Structure

Reserpine

(3β, 16β, 17α, 18β, 20α)-11, 17-Dimethoxy-18-[(3, 4, 5-trimethoxy benzoyl)oxy] yohimban-16-carboxylic acid methyl ester; ($C_{33} H_{40} N_2 O_9$);

Isolation   Reserpine may be isolated by adopting the following steps in a sequential manner:

1. The powdered and sieved roots are allowed to swell in a $NaHCO_3$ solution (10% w/v) for a period of 10-12 hours. The resulting solution is extracted with benzene, until the extracts give a weak positive reaction with HgI_2.

2. The combined benzene extracts are concentrated and ether is added to the benzene solution. The resulting mixture is extracted with dilute HCl. The combined acidic solution is washed with ether, filtered and extracted with chloroform in a successive manner.

   Note: The chloroform will specifically extract the weakly basic alkaloids, such as: Reserpine and Rescinnamine.

3. The combined chloroformic extract is washed subsequently with 10% (w/v) sodium carbonate solution and followed by water so as to get rid of any *free acids* present. The resulting extract is finally evaporated to dryness under vacuo.

4. The residue is dissolved in anhydrous methanol and seeded with a pure crystal of **reserpine** and allowed to cool gradually when reserpine will crystallize out.

5. However, **rescinnamine, deserpidine** and other minor weakly basic alkaloids could be obtained from the mother liquor conveniently.

6. The mother liquor is evaporated to dryness, and the residue is dissolved in the minimum quantity of benzene and subjected to column chromatography over a column packed with acid-washed

alumina. The alkaloids are eluted in the different fractions by making use of benzene, chloroform, methanol (10%) in a sequential manner.

Characteristic Features

1. It is obtained as long prisms from dilute acetone which get decomposed at 264-265°C; (decomposes at 277-277.5°C in an evac-tube).
2. Its specific optical rotations are: $[\alpha]_D^{23}$ - 118° (CHCl$_3$); $[\alpha]_D^{26}$ - 164° (C = 0.96 in pyridine; $[\alpha]_D^{26}$ - 168° (C = 0.624 in DMF).
3. It has uv$_{max}$ (CHCl$_3$): 216, 267, 295 nm (61700, 17000, 10200).
4. **Reserpine** is weakly basic in nature, pKa 6.6.
5. It is found to be freely soluble in chloroform (~ 1g/6 ml), glacial acetic acid, methylene chloride; soluble in benzene, ethyl acetate; slightly soluble in acetone, methanol, ethanol (1g/1800 ml), ether, in aqueous solutions of citric and acetic acids; and very sparingly soluble in water.

Identification Tests

1. Most solutions of reserpine upon standing acquire a distant yellow colouration and a marked and pronounced fluorescence; especially after the addition of an acid or upon exposure to light.
2. **Reserpine Hydrochloride Hydrate ($C_{33}H_{40}N_2O_9$.HCl.H$_2$O):** It is obtained as crystals which decompose at 224°C.

Uses

1. It is a hypotensive drug which exhibits strong hypotensive and sedative activity.
2. It is also employed to alleviate mild anxiety conditions *i.e.*, the drug shows a mild tranquillizing effect.

C. Rescinnamine

Synonyms   Reserpinine; Anaprel; Apoterin S; Cartric; Cinnaloid; Moderil;

Biological Sources   It is obtained from the roots of *Rauvolfia serpentina* (L.) Benth. (*Apocynaceae*) **(Rauvolfia, Chandra, Sarpaganda).**

Chemical Structure

Rescinnamine

3, 4 5-Trimethoxy-cinnamic acid ester of methyl reserpate; ($C_{35} H_{42} N_2 O_9$).

Isolation   **Rescinnamine** may be isolated from step (5) onwards as described under **Morphine.**

Characteristic Features

1. It is obtained as fine needles from benzene having mp 238-239°C (under vacuum).
2. Its specific optical rotation is $[\alpha]_D^{24}$ - 97° (C = 1 in chloroform).
3. It has uv_{max} (methanol): 228, 302 nm (log ε 4.79, 4.48).
4. **Solubility Profile:** It is moderately soluble in methanol, benzene, chloroform and other organic solvents; and practically insoluble in water.

Uses   It is mostly used as an antihypertensive.

D. Vinblastine

Synonyms   Vincaleukoblastine; VLB; 29060-LE;

Biological Source   It is obtained from *Vinca rosea* Lin.. (*Apocynaceae*).

Chemical Structure

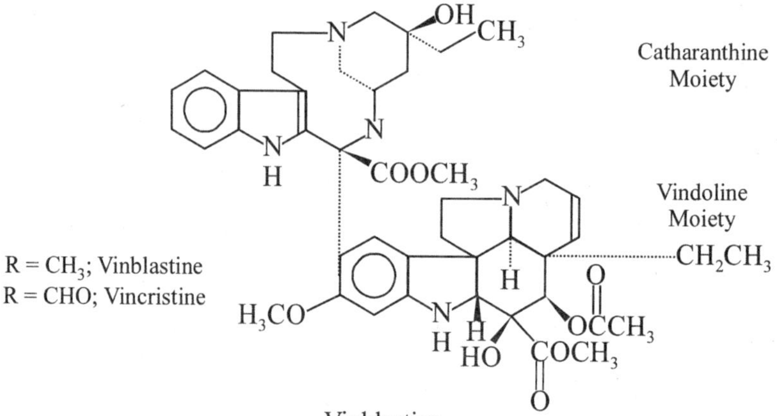

Catharanthine Moiety

Vindoline Moiety

R = CH₃; Vinblastine
R = CHO; Vincristine

Vinblastine

Isolation   It may be isolated from *Vinca rosea* Linn., either by the method suggested by Noble *et al**. or by Gorman *et al.*,**

Characteristic Features

1. It is obtained as solvated needles from methanol having mp 211-216°C.
2. Its specific optical rotation $[\alpha]_D^{26}$ + 42° (chloroform).
3. It has uv_{max} (ethanol): 214, 259 nm (log ε 4.73, 4.21).
4. It is soluble in alcohols, chloroform, acetone, ethyl acetate and is practically insoluble in water and petroleum ether.

Identification Tests   It forms derivatives as given below:

1. **Vinblastine Sulphate ($C_{46}H_{58}N_4O_9.H_2SO_4$) (Exal, Vebe, Velban):** It is obtained as crystals mp 284-285°C. Its physical parameters are: $[\alpha]_D^{26}$ – 28° (C = 1.01 in methanol); pKa₁ 5.4; pKa₂ 7.4. It has uv_{max} (methanol): 212, 262, 284, 292 nm (log ∈ 4.75, 4.28, 4.22, 4.18). One part is

---

* Noble *et al. Ann. N.Y. Acad. Soc.* **76**, Art 3, 892-894 (1958)
** Gorman *et al. J. Am. Chem. Soc.*, **81**, 4745, 4754, (1959).

soluble in 10 parts of water, 50 parts of chloroform; very slightly soluble in ethanol; and practically insoluble in ether.

2. **Vinblastine Dihydrochloride Dihydrate ($C_{46}H_{58}N_4O_9.2HCl.2H_2O$):** It is obtained as crystals that decompose at 244-246°C.

Uses

1. The alkaloid is used for the treatment of a wide variety of neoplasms.
2. It is also recommended for generated Hodgkin's disease, lymphocytic lymphoma, hystiocytic hymphoma, mycosis fungoides, advanced testicular carcinoma, Kaposi's sarcoma, and choriocarcinoma and lastly the breast cancer unresponsive to other therapies.
3. It is effective as a single entity, however, it is normally given along with other neoplastic agents in combination therapy for the increased therapeutic effect without any noticeable additive toxicity.
4. It arrests mitosis at the metaphase.
5. It is found to be effective in the acute leukemia of children.

E. Vincristine

Synonyms   Leurocristine; VCR; LCR.

Biological Sources   It is also obtained from *Vinca rosea* Lin., (*Catharanthus roseus* G. Don) belonging to the natural order *Apocynaceae*.

Chemical Structure   Please see the chemical structure under **Vinblastine**. It may also be named as: 22-Oxovincaleukoblastine.

Isolation   **Vincristine** may be isolated from **Vinca rosea** Linn., by the method suggested by Svoboda.*

Characteristic Features

1. It is obtained as blades from methanol having mp 218-220°C.
2. Its specific optical rotation $[\alpha]_D^{25} + 17°$; $[\alpha]_D^{25} + 26.2°$ (ethylene chloride); pKa: 5.0, 7.4 in 33% DMF.
3. It has uv_{max} (ethanol): 220, 255, 296 nm (log a_m 4.65, 4.21, 4.18).

Identification Tests

Vincristine Sulphate ($C_{46}H_{56}N_4O_{10}.H_2SO_4$) (Vincrex, Oncovin, Vincosid, Kyocrystine): Its crystals are obtained from ethanol and is found to be unstable.

Uses

1. **Vincristine sulphate** is recommended for the treatment of acute lymphocytic leukemia, and in combination therapy in Hodgkin's disease, lymphosarcoma, reticulum cell sarcoma, neuroblastoma, Wilm's tumour and rhabdomyosarcoma.

   Note: **Viucristine sulphate being highly unstable; therefore, its refregerated storage in sealed ampules is absolutely essential.**

2. It is broadly used as an antineoplastic agent.

---

* Svobada, *Lyoydia,* **24**, 173 (1961)

F. Strychnine

Biological Sources   It is abundantly found in the seeds of *Strychnos Nux Vomica* L. (*Loganiaceae*) (**Nux Vomica, Strychnine**); beans of *Strychnos ignatti* Berg. (*Loganiaceae*); roots of *S. cinnamomifolia* Thw.; seeds, bark and wood of *S. colubrina* Linn.; and plant of S. *malaccensis* Benth. (*Syn: S. gautheriana* Pierre).

Chemical Structure

Strychnine

Strychnidine-10-one; ($C_{21} H_{22} N_2 O_2$)

Salient Features

1. **Strychnine** contains *two* N-atoms even then it happens to be a mono-acidic base.
2. **Strychnine** readily forms a variety of salts, such as: nitrate, N_6-oxide, phosphate and sulphate. Interestingly, the N-atom which is specifically involved in the salt formation is the one that is located *farthest* from the aromatic benzene ring.
3. The second N-atom is strategically positioned as an amide nitrogen; and, therefore, it does not exhibit any basic characteristics.

Isolation   **Strychnine** may be isolated from the seeds of *S. nux vomica* by adopting the following steps sequentially:

1. The seeds of nux vomica are dried, ground and sieved which are mixed with an adequate quantum of pure slaked lime and made into a paste by adding a requisite amount of water. The wet mass thus obtained is dried at 100°C and extracted with hot chloroform in a continuous extractor till the extraction is completed.
2. The alkaloids are subsequently removed from the chloroform solution by shaking with successive portions of dilute sulphuric acid (2N). The combined acid extracts are filtered to get rid of any foreign particles or residue.
3. To the resulting acidic filtrate added an excess of ammonia to precipitate the alkaloids (strychnine + brucine).
4. The precipitate is extracted with ethanol (25% v/v) several times which exclusively solubilizes *brucine*, and ultimately leaves *strychnine* as an insoluble residue.
5. The residue containing **strychnine** is filtered off and is finally purified by repeated recrystallization from ethanol.

Characteristic Features

1. It is obtained as brilliant, colourless cubes from a mixture of chloroform and ether having mp 275-285°C, and d^{18} 1.359.

2. Its specific optical rotation $[\alpha]_D^{18}$-104.3° (C = 0.254 in ethanol); $[\alpha]_D^{25}$-13° (C = 0.4 in chloroform).

3. Its dissociation constant pKa (25°) 8.26.

4. It has uvmax (95% ethanol); 2550, 2800, 2900 Å ($E_{1cm}^{1\%}$ 377, 130, 101).

5. **Solubility Profile:** 1g dissolves in 182 ml ethanol, 6.5 ml chloroform, 150 ml benzene, 250 ml methanol, 83 ml pyridine; and very slightly soluble in water and ether.

6. A solution of strychnine containing 1 part in 700,000 parts of water gives a distinct bitter taste.

Identification Tests **Strychnine** may be identified either by specific *colour tests* or by specific *derivatives*:

(a) Colour Tests

1. **Sulphuric Acid-Dichromate Test: Strychnine** (5-10 mg) when dissolved in a few drops of concentrated sulphuric acid and stirred with a crystal of pure potassium dichromate [$K_2 Cr_2 O_7$] it gives an instant reddish-violet to purple colouration.

   Note: Strychnine derivatives will also give this test except strychnine nitrate.

2. **Mandelin's Reagent Test: Strychnine** or its corresponding salt when treated with **Mandelin's Reagent*** it gives rise to a violet to blue colouration.

3. **Ammonium Vanadate (V) Test: Strychnine** or its salt when treated with a saturated solution of ammonium vanadate, it produces a violet to blue colouration.

4. **Nitric Acid Test: Strychnine** on being treated with a trace of HNO_3 (conc.) yields an instant yellow colouration.

   Note: A similar test with Brucine gives an intense orange-red colouration. It may be used to differentiate between strychnine and brucine.

(b) Strychnine Derivatives: The various important strychnine derivatives are as given under:

1. **Strychnine Nitrate ($C_{21}H_{23}N_3O_5$):** It is obtained as colourless, odourless needles or while crystalline powder 1g dissolves in 42 ml water, 10 ml boiling water, 150 ml ethanol, 80 ml ethanol at 60°C, 105 ml chloroform, 50 ml glycerol; and insoluble in ether. It shows a pH ~ 5.7.

2. **Strychnine N_6 Oxide ($C_{21}H_{22}N_2O_3$):** It is obtained as monoclinic prisms from water which decompose at 207°C. It has pK value 5.17. It is found to be freely soluble in ethanol, glacial acetic acid, chloroform; fairly soluble in water; sparingly soluble in benzene; and practically insoluble in ether and petroleum ether.

3. **Strychnine Phosphate ($C_{21}H_{25}N_2O_6P$):** It is usually obtained as its dihydrate salt ($C_{21}H_{25}N_2O_6P.2H_2O$) which is colourless or while crystals or white powder. 1g dissolves in slowly in ~ 30 ml water, more soluble in hot water, and slightly soluble in ethanol. The aqueous solution is acidic to litmus.

4. **Strychnine Sulphate ($C_{42}H_{46}N_4O_8S$):** It normally crystallizes as pentahydrate [$2C_{21}H_{22}N_2O_2.H_2SO_4.5H_2O$]. It is colourless, odourless, very bitter crystals or white crystalline powder. It effloresces in dry air and loses all its water of crystallization at 100°C. It shows mp

---

* **Mandelin's Reagent** Dissolve 0.1g of ammonium vanadate in 10 ml of hot water and add to it 1-2 ml of-conc. H_2SO_4. Filter and preserve the solution.

when anhydrous ~ 200°C with decomposition. 1g dissolves in 35 ml water, 7 ml boiling water, 81 ml ethanol, 26 ml ethanol at 60°C, 220 ml chloroform, 6 ml glycerol, and insoluble in ether. A 1 : 100 solution shows pH 5.5.

5. **Strychnine Gluconate Pentahydrate ($C_{27}H_{34}N_2O_9.5H_2O$):** Its crystals darken above 80°C. It is soluble in 2 parts water ~ 40 parts ethanol. The aqueous solution is found to be neutral.

6. **Strychnine Glycerophosphate Hexahydrate ($C_{45}H_{53}N_4O_{10}P.6H_2O$):** 1g dissolves in ~ 350 ml water, ~ 310 ml ethanol; slightly soluble in chloroform; and very slightly soluble in ether.

7. **Strychnine Hydrochloride Dihydrate ($C_{21}H_{23}ClN_2O_2.2H_2O$):** It is obtained as trimetric prisms which are efflorescent in nature. 1g dissolves in ~ 40 ml water, ~ 80 ml ethanol, and insoluble in ether. The pH of a 0.01 M solution is 5.4.

Uses

1. **Strychinine** is extremely interesting pharmacologically and is regarded as a valuable tool in both physiologic and neuroanatomic research.
2. It is extremely toxic, and functioning as a central stimulant.
3. It causes excitation of all parts of the central nervous system and blocks inhibitory spinal inpulses at the post synaptic level. This may lead to an exaggeration in reflexes ultimately leading to *tonic convulsions.*
4. The drug is rarely used in modern medical practice but is utilized as a *vermin killer i.e.,* animal or insect killer.
5. It is used chiefly in poison baits for rodents.

Biosynthesis of Yohimbine, Reserpine, Rescinnamine, Vinblastine, Vincristine and Strychnine Dehydogeissoschizine (*keto*-form) undergoes isomerization by means of the nucleophilic attack on to carbonyl through a conjugated system, which subsequently forms an onium ion that upon reduction produces **yohimbine** as shown below:

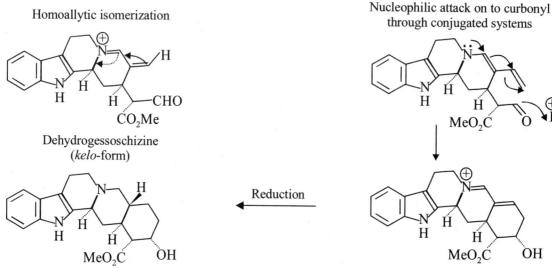

Homoallytic isomerization

Dehydrogessoschizine (*kelo*-form)

Nucleophilic attack on to curbonyl through conjugated systems

Reduction

Yohimbine

Reserpine and **deserpidine** are essentially the trimethoxybenzoyl esters of yohimbine-type alkaloids; whereas, **rescinnamine** is a trimethoxycinnamoyl ester. Interestingly, both **reserpine** and **rescinnamine** contain an additional methoxyl moiety present strategically on the indole ring system at C-11, which is accomplished by virtue of hydroxylation and methylation at a late stage along the pathway. A predominant and characteristic feature of these alkaloids is that they exhibit the *opposite stereochemistry* at C-3 to **yohimbine** and **strictosidine** as depicted below:

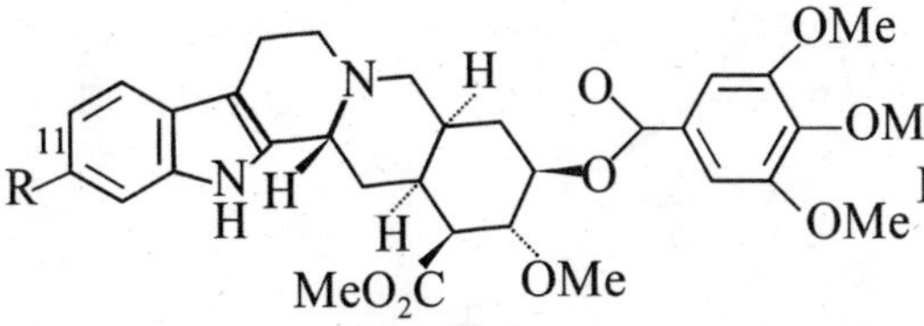

R = OMe, Reserpine
R = H. Deserpindine

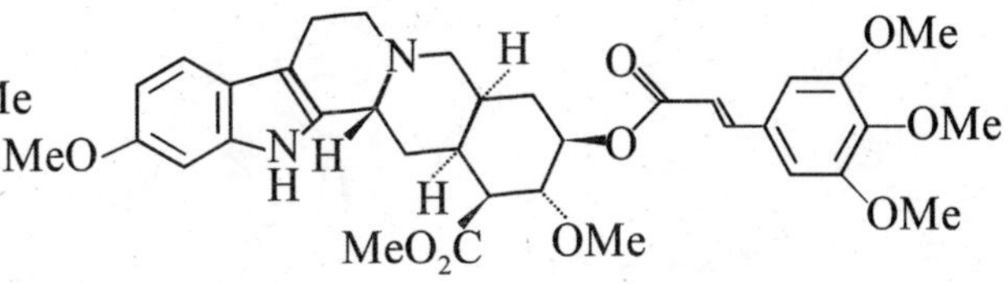

Rescinnamine

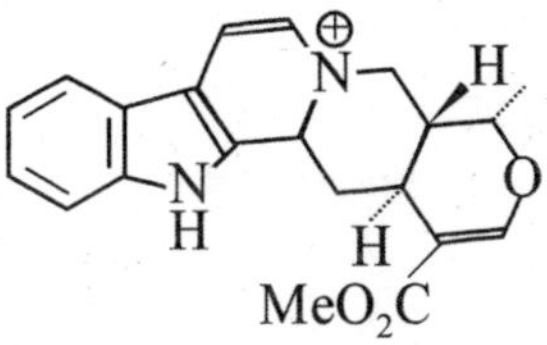

Serpentine

The biosynthetic pathway leading to **vinblastine** and **vincristine** is supposedly involve the following vital steps:

1. An oxidative reaction on **catharanthine**, catalysed by an enzyme peroxidase, thereby producing a peroxide that aptly loses the peroxide as a leaving group, ultimately breaking a carbon-carbon covalent bond as shown in the diagram given below.
2. The intermediate electrophilic ion is attacked on to the conjugated iminium system by the **vindoline,** whereby C-5 of the indole nucleus being appropriately activated by the $-OCH_3$ moiety located at C-6, and also by the N-atom present in the indole ring.
3. The resulting adduct is subsequently reduced in the dihydropyridinium ring by NADH*-dependent 1, 4-addition thereby giving rise to the substrate for hydroxylation.
4. Ultimately, reduction of the above resulting product generates **vinblastine.**
5. The oxidized product from vinblastine, with its N-formyl moiety rather than N-methyl on the vindoline fragment, may finally yield **vincristine.**

The biosynthetic pathway leading to **strychnine** essentially comprise of the following steps, namely:

1. **Preakuammicine** loses one C-atom *via* hydrolysis followed by decarboxylation.
2. Addition of the *two* extra C-atoms is accomplished by means of Aldol-condensation reaction with acetyl-CoA, whereby it yields the **Wieland-Gumlich aldehyde** as a complexed hemiacetal form.

---

* **NADH** = Nicotinamide adenine dinucleotide (reduced form).

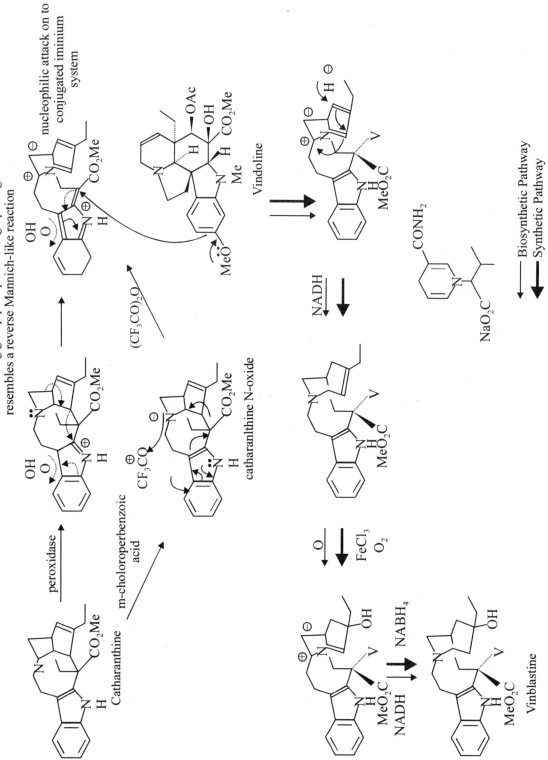

3. The subsequent construction of ether and amide linkages gives rise to the formation of **stryctinine** from the above hemiacetal as shown below.

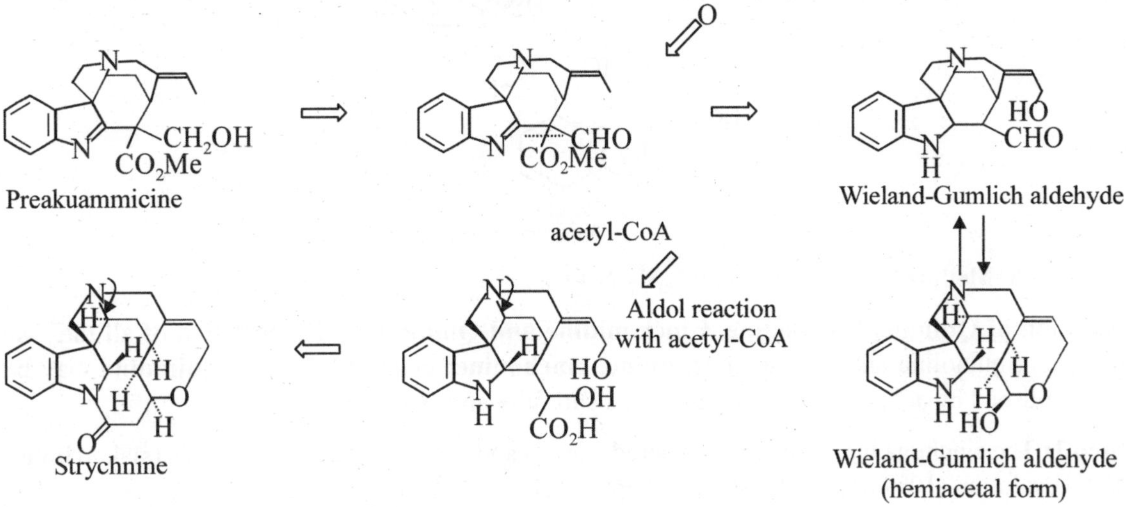

Preakuammicine

Wieland-Gumlich aldehyde

acetyl-CoA

Aldol reaction with acetyl-CoA

Strychnine

Wieland-Gumlich aldehyde (hemiacetal form)

7.2.8.4 Quinoline Alkaloids

A good number of very prominent and remarkable examples of the **'quinoline-alkaloids'** derived from *tryphphan* are nothing but the modifications of the terpenoid indole alkaloids commonly found in the genus *Cinchona* belonging to the natural order *Rubiaceae*.

Interestingly, more than twenty alkaloids have been isolated and characterized from the bark of *Cinchona calisaya* and *Cinchona ledgeriana*, very commonly known across the globe as the **Yellow Cinchona;** besides the other equally well-known species *Cinchona succirubra*, popularly known in trade as the **Red Cinchona.** However, the four long prized and most popular **quinoline alkaloids** known for their antimalarial activities are namely: **quinine, cinchonine, quinidine,** and **cinchonidine.** These alkaloids shall now be described individually in the sections that follow. It is worthwhile to state here that these structures are not only unique but also remarkable wherein the indole nucleus is replaced by a quinoline system through an intramolecular rearrangement as given below:

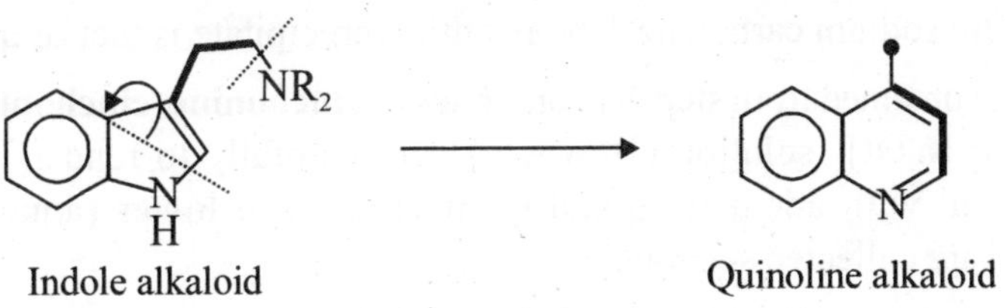

Indole alkaloid

Quinoline alkaloid

A. Quinine

Biological Sources   The *cinchona* species (*Rubiaceae*) specifically contains **quinine** in the bark upto 16% (mostly 6-10%) in a variety of its species, namely: *Cinchona calisaya* Wedd.; *C. ledgeriana* Moens ex Trimen; *C. officinalis* Linn. f.; *C. robusta* How.; and C. *succirubra* Pavon ex Klotzsch. The representative samples of dried **cinchona, cinchona bark** or **peruvian bark** is found to contain nearly 0.4 to 4% **quinine.**

Chemical Structure

Quinine

(8a, 9R)-6′-Methoxycinchonan-9 ol; ($C_{20}H_{24}N_2O_2$).

Isolation of Quinine, Cinchonine, Cinchonidine and Quinidine   The isolation of all the *four* important quinoline alkaloid, such as: **quine, cinchonine; cinchonidine** and **quinidine** may be accomplished by adopting the following steps carefully and sequentially.

Step 1: The cinchona bark is dried, powdered, sieved and treated with calcium oxide (slaked lime), NaOH solution (10% w/v) and water and kept as such for 6-8 hours.

Step II: The resulting mixture is treated with benzene in sufficient quantity and refluxed for 12-16 hours. The mixture is then filtered while it is hot.

Step III: The hot filtrate is extracted successively with 6N. sulphuric acid. The mixture of alkaloidal bisulphate is heated upto 90°C and maintained at this temperature upto 20-30 minutes.

Step IV: The resulting solution is cooled to room temperature and made alkaline by the addition of solid pure sodium carbonate till a pH 6.5 is attained.

Step V: The alkaloidal sulphate solution thus obtained is treated with sufficient quantity of activated charcoal powder (1g per 1L), boil, shake vigorously and filter.

Step VI: Cool the hot filtrate slowly in a refrigerator (2-10°C) overnight and again filter. Collect the residue and the filtrate separately.

Step VII: The residue (or precipitate) of quinine sulphate is boiled with water and made alkaline by adding cautiously solid sodium carbonate. The resulting precipitate is that of **quinine.**

Step VIII: The filtrate obtained from step-VI comprises of **cinchonine, cinchonidine** and **quinidine;** which is treated with NaOH solution (10% w/v) very carefully to render it *just alkaline*. It is successively extracted with adequate quantity of ether. The lower (aqueous layer) and the upper(ethereal layer) are collected separately.

Step IX: The aqueous layer contains **cinchonine.** It is evaporated to dryness in a Rotary Film Evaporator, extracted with absolute ethanol, decolourized with activated charcoal powder and allow it to crystallize slowly in a refrigerator (2-10°C) overnight. The crystals of **cinchonine** are obtained.

Step X: The ethereal layer obtained in step-VIII contains **quinidine** and **cinchonidine.** It is extracted with dilute HCl (2N) several times till a drop of the extract on evaporation does not give a positive test for alkaloids. Neutralize the combined acidic extract by adding solid sodium potassium tartrate *carefully.* Filter the resulting mixture and collect the *precipitate* and the *filtrate* separately.

Step XI: The precipitate of **cinchonidine tartrate** is treated with dilute HCl carefully. The resulting solution of alkaloid hydrochloride is made alkaline by the addition of dilute ammonium hydroxide when **cinchonidine** is obtained as a precipitate.

Step XII: The filtrate obtained from Step-X contains quinidine tartrate which is treated with solid potassium iodide powder carefully till the whole of quinidine gets precipitated as quinidine hydroiodide salt. It is filtered and the solid residue is finally treated with dilute NH_4 OH to obtain the precipitate of **quinidine.**

Characteristic Features

1. It is obtained as triboluminescent, orthorhombic needles from absolute ethanol having mp 177° (with some decomposition).
2. It sublimes in high vacuum at 170-180°C.
3. Its specific optical rotations are: $[\alpha]_D^{15}$ - 169° (C = 2 in 97% ethanol); $[\alpha]_D^{17}$ - 117° (C = 1.5 in chloroform); $[\alpha]_D^{15}$ - 285° (C = 0.4 M in 0.1 N H_2SO_4).
4. Its dissociation constants are: pK_1 (18°) 5.07; and pK_2 9.7.
5. The pH of its saturated solution in 8.8.
6. It gives a distinct and characteristic blue fluorescence which is especially strong in dilute sulphuric acid.
7. **Solubility Profile:** 1 g dissolves in 1900 ml water; 760 ml boiling water; 0.8 ml ethanol; 80 ml benzene; 18 ml benzene at 50°; 1.2 ml chloroform; 250 ml by ether; 20 ml glycerol; 1900 ml of 10% ammonia water; and almost insoluble in petroleum ether.

Identification Tests   **Quinine** may be identified either by a series of **Colour Tests** or by the formation of several known derivatives having characteristic features; and these shall be discussed separately as under:

(*a*) **Colour Tests:** These are, namely

1. **Oxygenated Acids:** Oxygenated acids, such as: sulphuric acid or acetic acid gives a strong blue fluorescence with quinine. This test is very sensitive even in extremely dilute solutions.

   Note: Halogen quinine compounds and hydrochloride salts of quinine do not give fluorescence in solution.

2. **Herpathite Test:** To a boiling mixture of quinine (0.3g) in 7.5 ml glacial acetic acid, 3 ml ethanol (90% v/v) and 5 drops of concentrated H_2SO_4, add 3.5 ml of I_2 solution (1% w/v) in ethanol, crystals of *iodosulphate of quinine* or **Herpathite*** separates out on cooling. The crystals thus obtained exhibit metallic lustre, appears dark in reflected light and alive-green in transmitted light.

3. **Thalleioquin Test:** When a few drops of bromine water are added to 2 or 3 ml of a weakly acidic solution of quinine salt, followed by the addition of 0.5-1.0 ml of strong ammonia solution, it produces a distinct characteristic emerald green colouration. It is an extremely sensitive colour test which may detect quinine even upto a strength as low as 0.005% (w/v). The end coloured product is known as **thalleioquin** for which the exact chemical composition is not yet known.

---

* **Herpathile** The iodo sulphate of quinine (or sulphate of iodo-quinine) is nown as **Herpathitie** after the name of its discover [*Formula*: $B_4 . 3H_2SO_4 . 2HI . I_4 + 3H_2O$]

Note: (*a*) **This test is given by quinidine and also by other Remijia alkaloids e.g., cupreine.**

(*b*) **Both cinchonine and cinchonidine do not respond to the Thalleioquin Test.**

4. **Erythroquinine Test (or Rosequin Test):** Dissolve a few mg of quinine in dilute acetic acid, add to it a few drops of bromine water (freshly prepared), followed by a drop of a 10% (w/v) solution of potassium ferrocyanide $[K_4 Fe(CN)_6]$. Now, the addition of a drop of concentrated NH_4OH solution gives rise to a red colouration instantly. If shaken quickly with 1-2 ml of chloroform, the red colouration is taken up by the lower chloroform-layer.

(*b*) **Derivatives/Salts of Quinine:** These are as follows:

1. **Quinine Trihydrate:** It is obtained as a microcrystalline powder having mp 57°C. It effloresces and loses one mol of water in air, two moles of water over H_2SO_4, and becomes anhydrous at 125°C.

2. **Quinine Bisulphate Heptahydrate ($C_{20}H_{24}N_2O_2.H_2SO_4.7H_2O$)** [*Synonyms:* **Quinbisan, Dentojel, Biquinate**): It is obtained as very bitter crystals or crystalline powder. It effloresces on exposure to air and darkens on exposure to light. 1 g dissolves in 9 ml water, 0.7 ml boiling water, 23 ml ethanol, 0.7 ml ethanol at 60°C, 625 ml chloroform, 2500 ml ether, 15 ml glycerol and having a pH 3.5.

3. **Quinine Dihydrochloride ($C_{20}H_{24}N_2O_2.2HCl$) (*Synonyms:* Quinine dichloride; Acid quinine hydrochloride; Quinine bimuriate):** It is obtained as a powder or crystals having a very bitter taste. 1g dissolves in about 0.6 ml water, 12 ml ethanol; slightly soluble in chloroform; and very slightly soluble in ether. The aqueous solutions are found to be strongly acidic to litmus paper (pH about 2.6).

4. **Quinine Hydrochloride Dihydrate ($C_{20}H_{24}N_2O_2.HCl.2H_2 O$):** It is obtained as silky needles having a bitter taste. It effloresces on exposure to warm air. It does not lose all its water below 120°C. 1 g dissolves in 16 ml water, in 0.5 ml boiling water, 1.0 ml ethanol, 7.0 ml glycerol, 1 ml chloroform, and in 350 ml ether. A 1% (w/v) aqueous solution shows a pH 6.0-7.0.

5. **Quinine Sulphate Dihydrate [($C_{20}H_{24}N_2O_2)_2.H_2SO_4.2H_2O$] (*Synonyms:* Quinamm; Quinsan; Quine, Quinate):** It is obtained as dull needles or rods, making a light and readily compressible mass. It loses its water of crystallization at about 110 °C. It becomes brownish on exposure to light. Optical rotation $[\alpha]_D^{15}$ - 220° (5% solution in about 0.5 N . HCl). 1g dissolves in 810 ml water, 32 ml boiling water, 120 ml ethanol, 10 ml ethanol at 78°C; slightly soluble in ether and chloroform, but freely soluble in a mixture of 2 vols. chloroform and 1 vol. absolute ethanol. Its aqueous solutions are neutral to litmus. The pH of a saturated solution in 6.2.

Uses

1. It is frequently employed as a flavour in carbonated beverages.
2. It is used as an antimalarial agent.
3. It is also employed as a skeletal muscle relaxant.
4. It has been used to treat hemorrhoids and varicose veins.
5. **Quinine** is also used as a oxytocic agent.
6. **Quinine** is supposed to be prophylactic for flu.

Biosynthesis of Quinine A survey of literature reveals that the intrinsic details of the biosynthetic pathways are lacking; however, an assumed biogenetic process essentially involving the following steps:

1. **L-Tryptophan and secologanin yields strictosidine,** which upon hydrolysis and decarboxylation produces **coryantheal.**
2. **Coryantheal** undergoes intramolecular changes, *first*-by cleavage of C-N bond (*via* iminium), and *secondly*-by formation of an altogether new C-N bond (again *via* iminium). This gives rise to an intermediate.
3. The resulting intermediate undergoes further intramolecular changes to yield *cinchoninone* having a quinoline nucleus.
4. **Cinchoninone** in the presence of **NADPH*** reduces the carbony function and generates **quinine:**

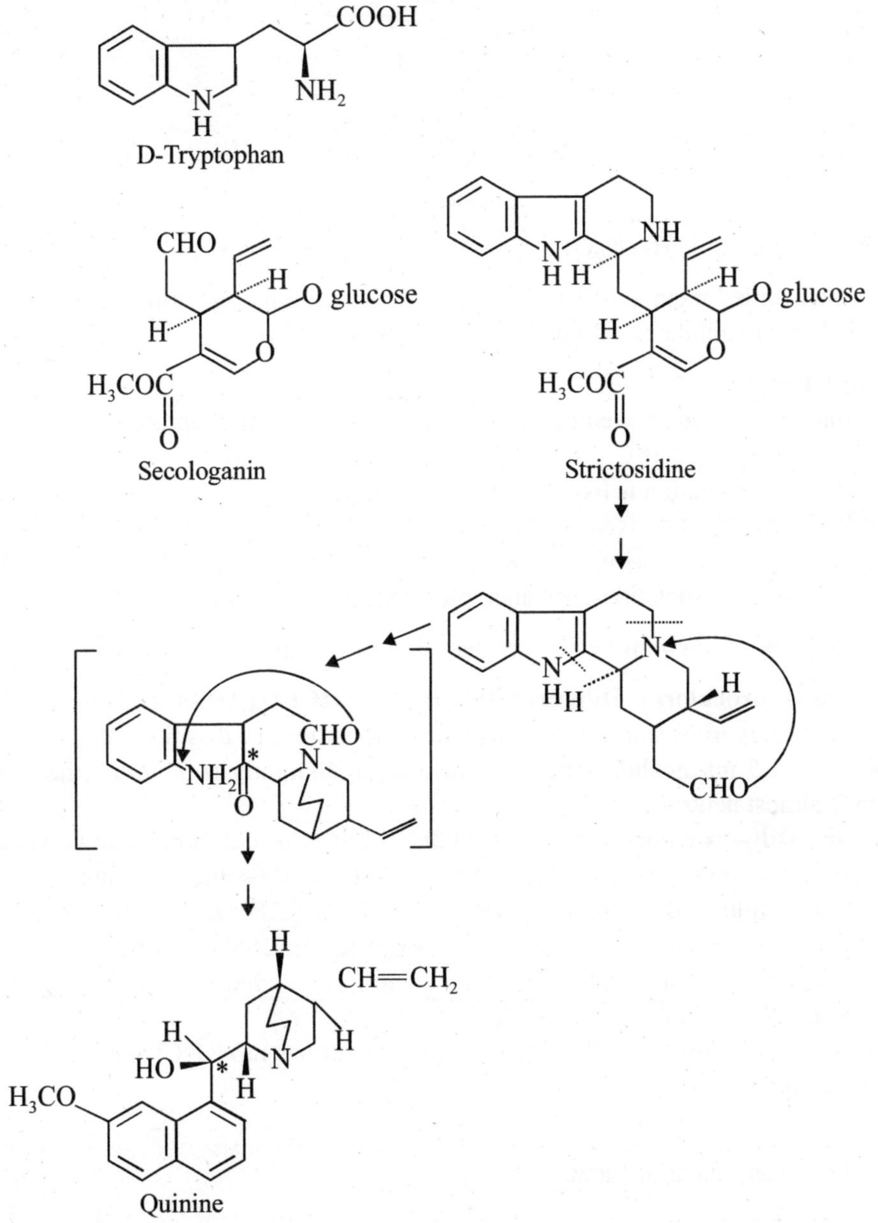

D-Tryptophan

Secologanin

Strictosidine

Quinine

---

* **NADPH** = Nicotinamide adenine dinucleotide phosphate (reduced form).

B. Cinchonine

Biological Sources   It occurs in most varieties of cinchona bark as mentioned under **quinine** (section 'A'). Besides, **cinchonine** especially occurs in the bark of *Cinchona micrantha R & P.* belonging to the natural order *Rubiaceae.*

Chemical Structure

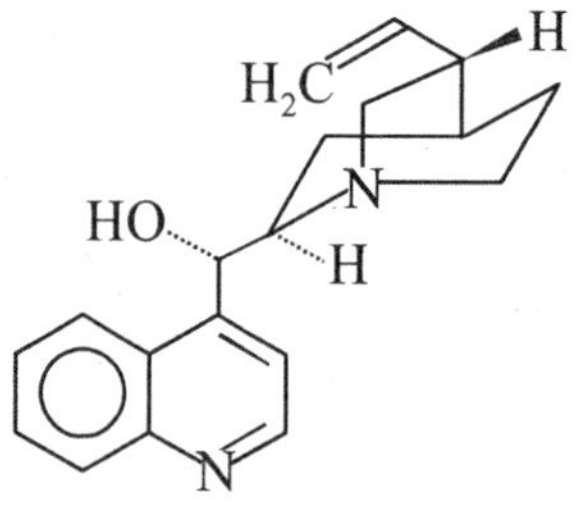

Cinchonine

(9S) - Cinchonan-9-ol; ($C_{19} H_{22} N_2O$)

Isolation   The detailed method of isolation has been given under **quinine** (section 'A'). Besides, Rabe* has put forward another method of isolation of **cinchonine.**

Characteristic Features

1. **Cinchonine** is obtained as needles from ethanol or ether having mp 265°C.
2. It begins to sublime at 220°C.
3. Its specific optical rotation is $[\alpha]_D$ + 229° (in ethanol).
4. **Solubility Profile:** 1g dissolves in 60 ml ethanol, 25 ml boiling ethanol, 110 ml chloroform, 500 ml ether; and practically insoluble in water.
5. It has two distinct dissociation constants: pK_1 5.85 and pK_2 9.92.

Identification Tests   **Cinchonine** may be identified by forming its specific derivatives, namely:

1. **Cinchonine Hydrochloride Dihydrate ($C_{19}H_{22}N_2O.HCl.2H_2O$):** It is obtained as fine crystals. The mp of its anhydrous salt is 215 °C with decomposition. 1g dissolves in 20 ml water, 3.5 ml boiling water 1.5 ml alcohol, 20 ml chloroform; and slightly soluble in ether. The aqueous solution is almost neutral.
2. **Cinchonine Dihydrochloride ($C_9H_{22}N_2O.2HCl$):** It is usually obtained as white or faintly yellow crystals or crystalline powder. It is found to be freely soluble in water or ethanol.
3. **Cinchonine Sulphate Dihydrate [$(C_{19}H_{22}N_2O)_2.H_2SO_4.2H_2O$]:** It is commonly obtained as lustrous extremely bitter crystals. Its anhydrous salt has mp 198°C. 1g dissolves in 65 ml water, 30 ml hot water, 12.5 ml ethanol, 7 ml hot ethanol, 47 ml chloroform; and slightly soluble in ether. The aqueous solution is practically neutral.
4. **Epicinchonine [Synonyms (9R)-Cinchonan-9-ol]:** It has mp 83°C; and $[\alpha]_D^{22}$ + 120.3° (C = 0.806 in ethanol).

Uses

1. It is used as an antimalarial agent.

---

* Rabe, *Ber.* **41**, 63 (1908)

2. It is employed as a tonic in waters, bitters and liqueurs.
3. It is broadly used for febrifuge, schizonticide, stomachic, amebiasis, dysentry, flu, fever, and as a mild stimulant of gastric mucosa.

C. Quinidine

Synonyms   Conquinine; Pitayine; β-Quinine;

Biological Source   **Quinidine** is obtained from the various species of *Cinchona* as described under quinine (section 'A'). It is reported to be present in cinchona barks ranging between 0.25-3.0%.

Chemical Structure   It is the dextrorotatory *stereoisonter* of **quinine**

Quinidine

(9S)-6'-Methoxycinchonan-9-ol; ($C_{20} H_{24} N_2 O_2$).

Isolation   **Quinidine** may be isolated from the cinchona bark by the method stated under **quinine** (section 'A').

Characteristic Features

1. **Quinidine** is obtained as triboluminescent crystals having mp 174-175°C after drying of the solvated crystals.
2. Its specific optical rotations are: $[\alpha]_D^{15} + 230°$ (C = 1.8 in chloroform); $[\alpha]_D^{17} + 258°$ (ethanol); and $[\alpha]_D^{17} + 322°$ (C = 1.6 in 2m HCl).
3. It has two dissociation constants, namely: pK_1 (20°) 5.4; and pK_2 10.0.
4. It gives a distinct and characteristic blue fluorescence in dilute sulphuric acid (2N).
5. The uv absorption spectrum is identical with that of **quinine.**
6. **Solubility Profile:** 1 g gets dissolved in 2000 ml cold water, 800 ml boiling water, 36 ml ethanol, 56 ml ether, 1.6 ml chloroform; very soluble in methanol; and practically insoluble in petroleum ether.

Identification Tests   The various derivatives of **quinidine** have specific characteristic features as enumerated below:

1. **Quinidine Sulphate Dihydrate [$(C_{20}H_{24}N_2O_2)_2.H_2SO_4.2H_2O$] (Synonyms Quinidex; Quinicardine; Quinora; Extentabs; Cin-Quin):** It is mostly obtained as white, very bitter, odorless, fine crystals which is frequently cohering in masses. It does not lose all of its water of crystallization below 120°C. It has been found to darken on exposure to light. It has $[a]_D^{25} \sim +212°$ (in 95% ethanol); and $\sim + 260°$ (in dilute HCl). The pH of a 1% (w/v) solution between

6.0-6.8. Its pKa values are : 4.2 and 8.8. 1 g dissolves in 90 ml water, 15 ml boiling water, 10 ml ethanol, 3 ml methanol, 12 ml chloroform; and insoluble in ether and benzene.

> **Note:** **Quinidine sulphate dihydrate is the salt of an alkaloid obtained either from various species of Cinchona and their hybrids, or from Cuprea bark, obtained from Remijia pedunculata and Remijia purdieana belonging to the natural order Rubiaceae.**

2. **Quinidine Gluconate ($C_{26}H_{36}N_2O_9$) (*Synonyms* Quinaglute; Duraquin; Gluconic acid quinidine salt):** It is obtained as crystals having mp 175-176.5°C; and soluble in 9 parts of water and 60 parts of ethanol.

3. **Quinidine Polygalacturonate ($C_{20}H_{24}N_2O_2 \cdot C_6H_{10}O_7 \cdot H_2O$) [*Synonyms* Galactoquin; Cardioquin; Naticardina):** It is obtained as an amorphous powder mp 180°C (decomposes). The anhydrous substance is found to be insoluble in methanol, ethanol, chloroform, ether, acetone, dioxane; and soluble in 40% methanol or ethanol: 12%; in water at 25°C: ~ 2%.

4. **Quindine Hemipentahydrate:** It is obtained as prisms from dilute ethanol, mp ~ 168°C, and loses 1/2 H_2O on exposure to air.

5. **Quinidine Hydrogen Sulphate Tetrahydrate ($C_{20}H_{24}N_2O_2 \cdot H_2SO_4 \cdot 4H_2O$) (*Synonyms* Kiditard; Kinichron; Kinidin Durules; Quiniduran; Chinidin - Duriles; Quinidine Bisulphate):** It is obtained as rods which is soluble in 8 parts of water and emitting a distinct blue fluorescence.

6. **Neutral Hydroiodide of Quinidine ($C_{20}H_{24}N_2O_2 \cdot HI$):** It is obtained as a crystalline powder when KI is added to a neutral aqueous solution of a quinidine salt. It is very sparingly soluble in water (1 part in 1250 parts at 15°C). It is found to be much less soluble than that of the other cinchona alkaloids.

Quinidine also gives a specific colour test as given below:

Ferrocyanide Test for Quinidine   A small quantum (10-15 mg) of a **quinidine salt** is mixed thoroughly with 0.5-1.0 ml of freshly prepared bromine water in an evaporating dish. The contents are transferred carefully into a test tube with the help of 1 ml of distilled water. To this is added 1 ml of chloroform, contents shaken and then allowed to stay for a few minutes. A few drops of a 10% (w/v) solution of potassium ferrocyanide [K_4 Fe $(CN)_6$] and 3 ml of a 5N. NaOH solution are added with continuous shaking. The chloroform layer attains a red colour.

> **Note: Quinine or its salt under identical treatment gives a negative test, and hence it may be used to distinguish between quinidine and quinine.**

Uses
1. It is used as an antiarrhythmic agent (Class 1A)*.
2. It finds its applications as an antimalarial drug.
3. It is most commonly employed to treat various cardiac arrhythmias, namely: atrial flutter, AV junctional and ventricular contractions, atrial and ventricular tachycardia, atrial fibrillation, and premature atrial condition.

---

* **Class 1A   Antiarrhythmic Agent**   When the antiarrhythmic mechanisms is accomplished through membrane stabilization.

D. Cinchonidine

Synonyms   Cinchovatine; α-Quinidine;

Biological Sources   It is obtained in most varieties of the cinchona bark as described under quinine (section 'A'). It is, however, observed to be present especially in the bark of *Cinchona pubescens* Vahl. (C. *succirubra* Pav.) and *Cinchona pitayensis* Wedd., (*Rubiaceae*).

Chemical Structure

Cinchonidine

(8a, 9R)-Cinchonan-9-ol; (C$_{19}$ H$_{22}$ N$_2$ O).

Isolation   **Cinchonidine** can be conveniently isolated from the bark of various species of *cinchona* as described explicitely under **quinine** (section 'A'). However, it may also be isolated by the method suggested by Leers.*

Characteristic Features
1. It is obtained as orthorhombic prisms or plates from ethanol having mp 210°C.
2. It has specific optical rotation $[\alpha]_D^{20}$ - 109.2° (in ethanol).
3. **Solubility Profile:** It is found to be freely soluble in chloroform and ethanol; moderately soluble in ether; and practically insoluble in water.
4. It has two dissociation constants: pK$_1$ 5.80 and pK$_2$ 10.03.

Identification Tests   **Cinchonidine** may be identified by preparing its specific derivatives that possess characteristic features, such as:

1. **Cinchonidine Dihydrochloride (C$_{19}$H$_{22}$H$_2$O.2HCl):** It is obtained as white or slightly yellow crystals or powder. It is freely soluble in ethanol and water.
2. **Cinchonidine Hydrochloride Dihydrate (C$_{19}$H$_{22}$N$_2$O.HCl.2H$_2$O):** It is obtained as a crystalline powder. It losses all of its water of crystallization at 120°C. It has $[\alpha]_D^{20}$ - 117.5° (in water). It is soluble in 25 parts of cold water, more soluble in boiling water; soluble in chloroform and ethanol; and slightly soluble in ether. The aqueous solution is almost neutral in nature.
3. **Cinchonidine Sulphate Trihydrate [(C$_{19}$H$_{22}$N$_2$O)$_2$.H$_2$SO$_4$.3H$_2$O]:** It is obtained as silky, acicular crystals which effloresce on being exposed to air and get darkened in light. The mp of anhydrous salt is nearly 240°C with decomposition. 1g dissolves in 70 ml water, 20 ml hot water, 90 ml ethanol, 40 ml hot ethanol, 620 ml chloroform; practically insoluble in ether. The aqueous solution is more or less neutral.

** Leers, *Ann.*, **82**, 147 (1952)

4. **Epicinchonidine [Synonyms: (8α, 9S)-Cinchonan-9-ol)]:** It has mp 104°C; and $[\alpha]_D^{20} + 63°$ (C = 0.804 in ethanol).

Uses   It is mostly used as an antimalarial agent.

Totaquine   **Totaquine** is nothing but a mixture of the total alkaloids of the well-known cinchona bark. It is invariably exploited as a '*cheap substitute*' for quinine in an unethecal practice in trade. It is found to contain not less than 7% and not more than 12% of quinine units anhydrous form; and not more than 80% of the total anhydrous crystallizable **cinchona alkaloids.**

The following table summarizes the characteristic features and specific tests for the *four* major **cinchona alkaloids,** namely: **Quinine, Quinidine, Cinchonine** and **Cinchonidine.**

Differences Among Four Major Cinchona Alkaloids

S. No.	Characteristics	Quinine	Quinidine	Cinchonine	Cinchonidine
1	Chemical Formula	Methoxy Vinyl rubanol	Methoxy Vinyl rubanol	Vinyl rubanol	Vinyl rubanol
2	Rotation of Alcoholic solution	(−)	(+)	(+)	(−)
3	Fluorescence in oxygenated acids	Blue	Blue	−	−
4	Thallaioquin Test	+ve	+ve	−ve	−ve
5	Erythroquinine Test	+ve	+ve	−ve	−ve
6	Herrpathite Test	+ve	−ve	+ve	−ve
7	Solubility in (ml):				
	Water	1900	2000	−	−
	Chloroform	1.2	1.6	110	++
	Ethanol	0.8	36.0	60	++
	Glycerol	20.0	−	−	−
	Ether	250	56.0	500	+

Biosynthesis of Cinchonine, Quinidine and Cinchonidine   The various sequential steps involved in the biosynthesis of **Cinchonine, Quinidine** and **Cinchonidine** are stated as under:

1. **Strictosidine** is obtained by the interaction of L-tryptophan and secologanin as already shown in the **Biosynthesis of Quinine.**

2. Strietosidine undergoes a molecular rearrangement to form an aldehyde which upon hydrolysis and decarboxylation yields *coryantheal.*

3. **Coryantheal** generates **cinchoninone** by virtue of *two* transformations; *first:* an intermediate formed due to the cleavage of C-N bond (*via* iminium) then formation of a new C-N bond (again *via* iminium); and *secondly:* cleavage of the indole C-N bond. The resulting product loses a molecule of water to yield **cinchonionone.**

4. **Cinchoninone** undergoes epimerization at C-8 *via* enol to form the stereoisomer, which upon interaction with NADPH gives rise to *chnchonine* and *quindine* respectively.

5. **Cinchonione** with direct interaction with NADPH gives rise to **cinchonidine** and **quinine** respectively.

The outline of the biosynthesis elaborated above from (1) through (5) may be summarized as depicted below:

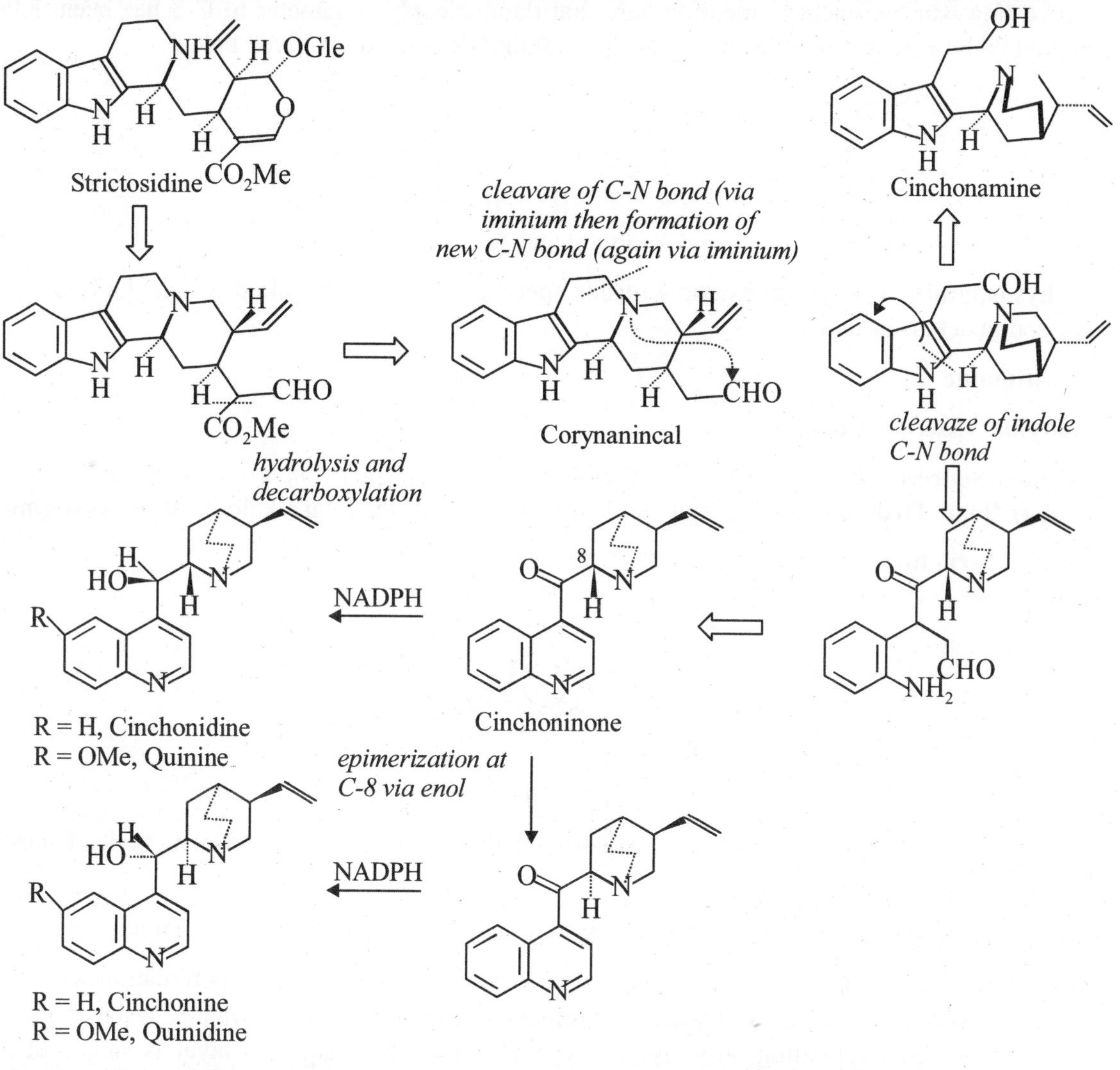

Strictosidine

Corynanincal

Cinchonamine

cleavare of C-N bond (via iminium then formation of new C-N bond (again via iminium)

cleavaze of indole C-N bond

hydrolysis and decarboxylation

R = H, Cinchonidine
R = OMe, Quinine

Cinchoninone

NADPH

epimerization at C-8 via enol

NADPH

R = H, Cinchonine
R = OMe, Quinidine

Biosynthesis of Cinchonine, Quinidine and Cinchonidine

7.2.8.5 *Pyrroloindole Alkaloids*

The *indole* nucleus has two C-atoms in the heterocyclic portion, *viz.*, C-2 and C-3. Interestingly, both C-2 and C-3 may be regarded as nucleophilic in character. However, it has been established beyond any reasonable doubt that the reactions essentially involving C-2 appear to be the most common in **alkaloid biosynthesis.**

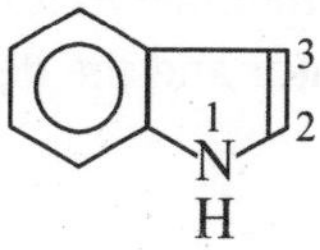

Indole

It is, however, pertinent to mention here that the nucleophic character of C-3 has been duly exploited thereby generating the almost rare **pyrroloindole nucleus** as given below:

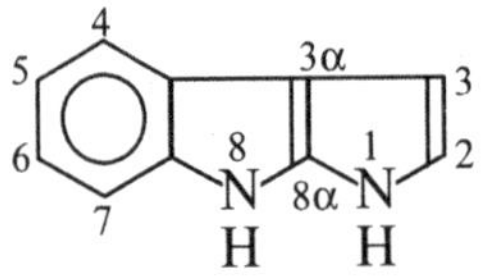

Pyrroloindole

Physostigmine is a typical example of this specific category of alkaloid which shall now be discussed in details as under:

Physostigmine

Synonyms   Eserine; Cogmine;

Biological Sources   It is obtained from the seeds of *Physostigma venenosum* Balf. (*Fabaceae*) **(Calabar Bean, Ordeal Bean)** yielding not less than 0.15% of the total alkaloids of **physostigma.**

Chemical Structure

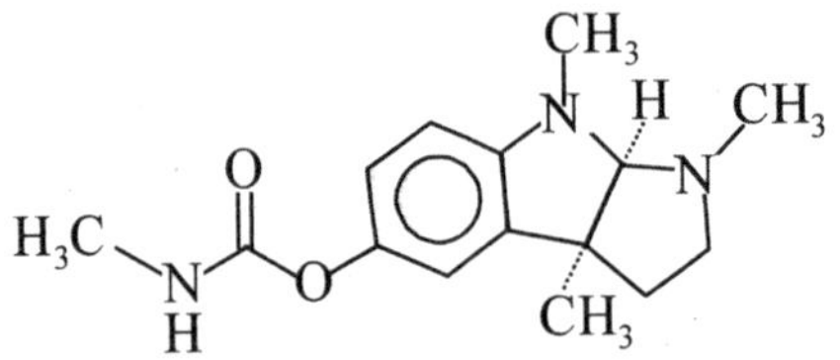

Physostigmine

(3aS-*cis*)-1, 2, 3, 3α, 8, 8α-Hexahydro-1, 3α, 8-trimethylpyrrolol [2, 3-b] indol-5-ol methylcarbamate (ester); ($C_{15} H_{21} N_3 O_2$).

Isolation   **Physostigmine** may be isolated by adopting the following *two* steps, namely:

Step I: The seeds are dried, powdered, sieved and extracted by continuous percolation with hot ethanol (95%) and the solvent is subsequently removed by distillation under vacuo. Water is added to the residue and the floating fatty layer is separated The lower aqueous layer is subjected to alkalinization with sodium carbonate and the liberated alkaloid is then extracted with ether successively.

Step II: The combined ethereal extract is then concentrated to a small volume and washed with 5% (w/v) sulphuric acid repeatedly unless and until the washings give a positive acidic reaction to litmus paper. To this aqueous acidic solution (containing the alkaloids as sulphates) is added an excess of a saturated solution of *sodium salicylate* when the physostigmine salicylate separates out as a crystalline product. The **physostigmine** may be recovered from the resulting salt by treating it with sodium carbonate followed by an immediate extraction with ether successively. The ether is evaporated in a Rotary Thin-Film Evaporator and the desired physostigmine is collected as prisms or clusters.

---

* Schwyzer, *Die Fabrikation Pharmazeutischer and Chemisch-Technischer Produkte* (Berlin, 1931) p 338.

However, **physostigmine** may also be isolated by the methods described by Schwyzer* and Cheminitius.*

Characteristic Features

1. It is obtained as orthorhombic sphenoidal prisms or clusters of leaflets from ether or benzene having mp 105-106°C. It is also available as an unstable, low melting form mp 86-87°C.
2. Its specific optical rotations are: $[\alpha]_D^{17}$ - 76° (C = 1.3 in chloroform); and $[\alpha]_D^{25}$ - 120° (benzene).
3. It has two dissociation constants: pKa_1 6.12, and pKa_2 12.24.
4. **Solubility Profile:** It is slightly soluble in water; soluble in ethanol, benzene, chloroform and oils.

Identification Tests **Physostigmine** may be identified either by specific colour tests or by preparing their derivatives as stated below:

(*a*) *Colour Tests:* These are as follows:

1. **Physostigmine** or its salts, a few mg, when warmed with 1 ml of strong ammonia solution it gives rise to a yellowish-red colouration. On further evaporation to dryness on a steam-bath, a bluish residue (eserine blue) is obtained that is soluble in ethanol forming a blue solution.
2. Both solid and solutions of **physostigmine** eventually turn red on being exposed to heat, light and air; and also on contact with traces of metals. This colour change indicates hydrolysis to **eseroline** and oxidation to **rubreserine.**
3. **Physostigmine** gives an instant blue colouration when treated with potassium ferricyanide [K_3 Fe $(CN)_6$] and a few drops of $FeCl_3$ solution (1% w/v).
4. **Physostigmine** produces a deep-yellow colouration on being heated with 0.5-1 ml of KOH solution (1% w/v).

   Note: (*a*) **This is a very sensitive test and can detect it upto 10 mcg level.**
   (*b*) **Under controlled experimental parameters the intensity of the yellow colour produced may be measured spectrophotometrically at 470 nm and can serve as an assay method.**

5. When a small quantity of **physostigmine** is heated in a porcelain basin on a steam both with a drop or two of fuming HNO_3, a yellow solution is obtained. The resulting solution on evaporation to dryness forms a green residue due to the formation of **chloreserine,** which is readily soluble in ethanol to give a green solution.
6. **Physostigmine** when treated with a solution of phosphomolybdic acid and ammonium meta vanadate in H_2SO_4 it gives rise to an emerald green colour.

(*b*) *Derivatives:* Major derivatives of **physostigmine** are:

1. **Physostigmine Salicylate ($C_{22}H_{27}N_3O_5$) (Antilirium):** It is obtained as acicular crystals having mp 185-187°C. It has uv_{max} (methanol: 239, 252, 303 nm (log ε 4.09, 4.04, 3.78). 1g dissolves in 75 ml water at 25°C. The pH 0.5% (w/v) aqueous solution is 5.8. It is soluble in 16 ml ethanol; 5 ml of boiling ethanol; 6 ml of chloroform; and 250 ml of ether.
2. **Physostigmine Sulphate [$(C_{15}H_{21}N_3O_2)_2.H_2SO_4$]:** It is mostly obtained as deliquescent scales having mp 140°C (after drying at 100°C). 1g dissolves in 0.4 ml ethanol, 4 ml water, 1200 ml

---

* Chemnitius, *J. Prabt. Chem.* **116**, 59 (1927).

ether. The pH of 0.05 M aqueous solution is 4.7. The solutions of the sulphate salt are more prone to change colour than those of the corresponding salt of the salicylate.

3. **Physostigmine Sulphite [$(C_{15}H_{21}N_3O_2)_2.H_2SO_3$]:** The white powder is found to be freely soluble in ethanol and water. The aqueous solution is observed to remain colourless for a long duration.

Uses

1. It possesses a cholinergic (anticholinesterase) and miotic activities.
2. It was used earlier to treat myasthenia gravis; but now it is more frequently used for the eye.
3. It is employed as an antidote for reversing CNS and cardiovascular (*viz.*, arrythmia and tachycardia) effects of excessive dosages with tricyclic antidepressants.
4. It helps in the contraction of the ciliary muscle of eye, and a decrease in the intraocular pressure produced by an increased out-flow of the aqueous humor.
5. Physostigmine is employed frequently in ophthalmology to treat glaucoma.

Biosynthesis of Physostigmine   The various steps involved in the biosynthesis of **physostigmine** are as follows.

1. Tryptamine undergoes C-methylation at C-3 of the indole nucleus due to its nucleophilic character.
2. Formation of the **'third pyrrole'** ring takes place by virtue of the nucleophilic attack of the primary amine function on to the iminium ion.
3. Further substitution on the phenyl ring leads to the formation of physostigmine.

The above *three* steps are summarized as given below:

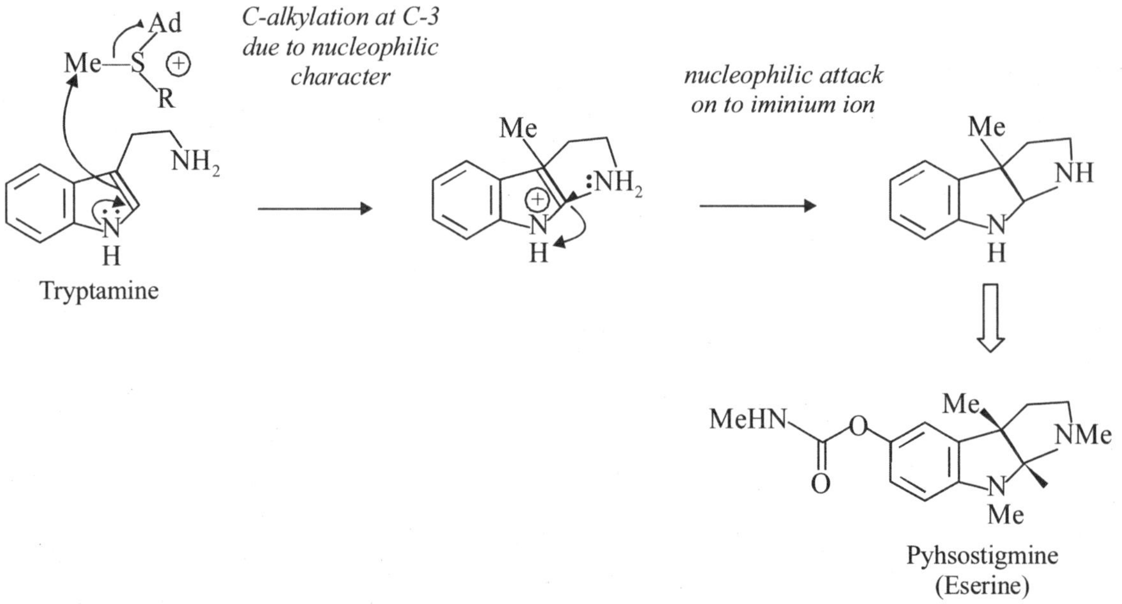

Biosynthesis of Physostigmine

7.2.8.6 *Ergot Alkaloids*

Ergot is a fungal disease very commonly and widely observed on a good number of wild as well as cultivated grasses, and is produced by different species of **claviceps.** This particular disease is usually characterized by the formation of hard and seedlike **'ergots'** in place of the normal seeds. However, these specific structures are frequently termed as **sclerotia,** which represent the **'resting stage'** of the fungus.

The generic name, **'claviceps',** usually refers to the club-like nature of the **sclerotium*,** whereas *purpurea* signifies its purple colour. As these *sclerotia* are elongated and somewhat pointed in shape and appearance, hence the common name of *spurred rye* has been assigned to the drug.

Medicinal **ergot** is the dried sclerotium of the fungus *Claviceps purpurea* (Fries) belonging to the natural order *Clavicipitaceae* developed in the ovary of rye, *Secale cereale* (*Germinae/Poaceae*). There are certain other species of *Claviceps* which have been found to produce ergots in the ovaries of other member of *Graminae* and *Cyperaceae*.

In fact, there exist *four* main categories of **ergot alkaloids** which may be distinguished, namely: (*a*) **clavine alkaloids,** (*b*) **lysergic acids,** (*c*) **lysergic acid amides,** and (*d*) **ergot peptide alkaloids.** There are, in fact, *ten* **ergot peptide alkaloids** which are: **ergotamine, ergosine, ergocristine, ergocryptine, ergocornine, ergotaminine, ergosinine, ergocristinine, ergocryptinine,** and **ergocorninine;** however, the *last five* alkaloids being isomers of the *first five*. The aforesaid alkaloids are beautifully typified by a structure comprising of *four* components, *viz.*, lysergic acid, dimethylpyruvic acid, proline and phenylalanine strategically joined together in amide linkages as depicted below:

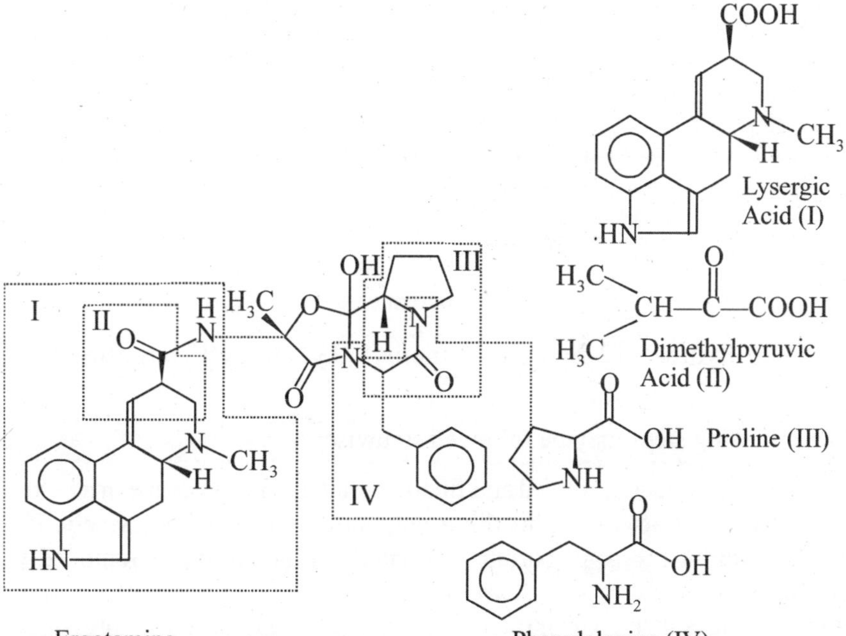

Ergotamine   Phenylalanine (IV)

Interestingly, the poisonous properties of ergots in grain, specifically rye, for animal as well as human consumption, purposefully and unknowingly, have long been recognized. The dreadful causative agents are collectively termed as the **'ergot alkaloids'**, containing essentially an **indole nucleus.** These, group of alkaloids are also referred to as **'ergolines'.**

---

* **Sclerotium** A hardened mass formed by the growth of certain fungi. THe sclerotium formed by ergot on rye is of medical importance due to its toxicity.

The *three* important and typical members of the ergot alkaloids (ergolines), namely: **ergonovine, ergotamine** and **lysergamde (ergine)** shall be discussed individually in the sections that follows:

A. Ergonovine

Synonyms Ergometrine; Ergobasine; Ergotocine; Ergostetrine; Ergotrate; Ergoklinine; Syntometrine.

Biological Sources It is obtained from the seeds of *Ipomea violaceae* Linn. (*Ipomea tricolor* Cav.) belonging to family *Convolvulaceae* (Morning glory, Tlitliltzen, Ololiuqui); and also from the dried seeds of *Rivea corymposa* Hall. F. (*Convolvulaceae*) (Snakeplant).

The percentage of **Ergometrine** and **Ergine** present in the *Rivea* and *Ipomea* species are as given below:

Alkaloids	Rivea (%)	Ipomea (%)
Ergometrine	–	0.005
Ergine	0.0069	0.035

Chemical Structure

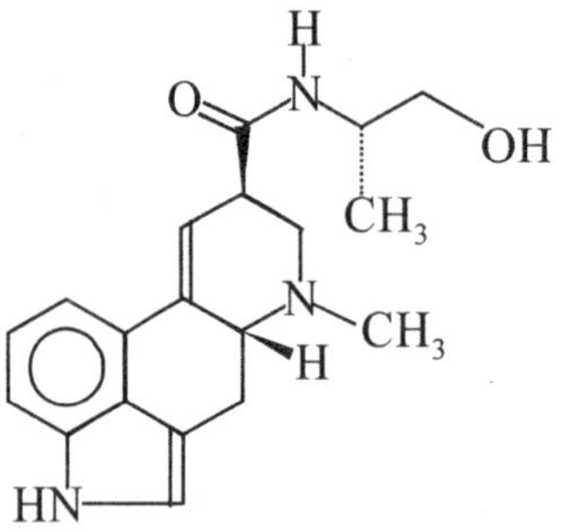

Ergonovine

[8β (s)]-9, 10-Diadehydro-N-(2-hydroxy-1-methylethyl)-6-methylergoline-8-carboxamide; ($C_{19}H_{23}N_3O_2$).

Isolation The following steps may be followed stepwise:

1. The seeds are dried, powdered, sieved and finally defatted with n-hexane in a Soxhlet apparatus.
2. The defatted mare is extracted with hot dilute sulphuric acid (6N) successively. The acid extract is then treated with on excess of barium sulphate, and the barium is removed with CO_2 and subsequent filtration.
3. The resulting filtrate is then concentrated by evaporation under reduced pressure.
4. The concentrated solution is taken up in ethanol, made alkaline with NH_4OH and subjected to extraction with chloroform successively.
5. The resulting chloroform extract is further extracted with dilute H_2SO_4 (6N). The acidic solution is made alkaline with ammonia and saturated with NaCl and then extracted with ether several times.
6. The solvent is removed from the ether extract under vacuo leaving the alkaloidal residue.
7. **Ergonovine** may be recrystallized from acetone.

It may also be prepared from D-lysergic acid and L (+)-2-amino-1-propanol by the method of Stoll and Hofmann.*

Characteristic Features

1. **Ergonovine** is obtained as tetrahedral crystals from ethyl acetate, and as fine needles from benzene. It tends to form solvated crystals having mp 162°C.
2. It has specific optical rotation $[\alpha]_D^{20} + 90°$ (in water).
3. Its dissociation constant is pK_a 6.8.
4. It is found to be freely soluble in lower alcohols, acetone and ethyl acetate; more soluble in water than the other principal alkaloids of ergot; and slightly soluble in chloroform.

Identification Tests   As *per se* the **ergot alkaloids** may be identified either by general precipitation and colour reactions or by preparing their derivatives as stated below:

(a) Precipitation Reactions

(i) The **ergot alkaloids** are readily precipitated by the alkaloidal reagents. However, Mayers reagent is regarded to be the most sensitive test whereby on opalescence in dilutions of 1 ppm can be obtained.

(ii) Iodine solution in KI also gives an instant precipitate with very dilute solutions of **ergot alkaloids.**

(b) Colour Tests: The most vital colour tests are given as under:

(i) **Keller's Test:** To a solution of the alkaloid in glacial acetic acid add a few mg of solid $FeCl_3$ and then add 1-2 ml of concentrated sulphuric acid along the side of the tube. The appearance of an intense blue colouration is accomplished at the junction of the two layers.

(ii) **Van Urk Test:** When a solution containing an **ergot alkaloid** is mixed with **Van Urk Reagent***, it gives rise to a characteristic deep blue colouration.

   Note: (*a*) **Van Urk Reagent may also be used in spraying developed paper chromatograms of the ergot alkaloids, and for this purpose 10% (v/v) HCl is used instead of H_2SO_4.**

   (*b*) **The spectrophotometric assay for total ergot alkaloids is also based on the blue colour given with Van Urk Reagent.**

(iii) **Glyoxylic Acid Reagent Test:** Ergot alkaloids gives a blue colouration with the addition of Glyoxylic acid reagent and a few drops of concentrated H_2SO_4.

(iv) **Fluorescence Test:** The aqueous solution of the salts of ergot alkaloids produce a distinct blue fluorescence.

(c) Derivatives of Ergonovine: The various derivatives of **ergonovine** are as follows:

(i) **Ergonovine Maleate (Ergometrine Maleate) $(C_{19}H_{23}N_2O_2.C_4H_4O_4)$ [*Synonyms* Cornocentin; Ermetrine; Ergotrate Maleate]:** It is obtained as crystals that decompose at 167°C. It has specific optical rotation $[\alpha]_D^{25} + 48°$ to $+ 57°$. 1g dissolves in 36 ml water and 120 ml ethanol. It is almost insoluble in chloroform and ether.

---

* Stoll, A., and Hofmann, A., *Helv. Chim Acta*, **26**, 944 (1943).

** **Van Urk Reagent**   Mix togetehr 0.125g of *para*-dimethylamino. benzaldehyde; 0.1 ml of $FeCl_3$ soln. (5% w/v), and 15% (v/v) H_2SO_4 to make 100 ml.

(*ii*) **Methylergonovine Maleate ($C_{20}H_{25}N_2O_2.C_4H_4O_4$):** It is a semisynthetic homologne of ergonovine and prepared from lysergic acid and 2-aminobutanol. It is obtained as a white to pinkish-tan microcrystalline powder.

(*iii*) **Ergonovine Tartrate Hydrate (Ergometrine Tartrate Hydrate) [($C_{19}H_{23}N_3O_2$)$_2$.$C_4H_6O_6.H_2O$] (Basergin, Neofermergen):** It is obtained as crystals that are slightly soluble in water.

Uses

1. **Ergonovine** is used as an oxytocic.
2. **Ergonovine maleate** also acts as an oxytocic and produces much faster stimulation of the uterine muscles as compared to other ergot alkaloids.
3. **Methylergonovine meleate** is observed to act as an oxytocic whose actions are slightly more active and longer acting than **ergonovine.**

B. Ergotamine

Biological Source   It is obtained from the seeds of *Claviceps purpurea* (Fr.) Tul. (*Hypocreales*) **(Ergot).**

Chemical Structure   The chemical structure of **ergotamine** has been given in Section 7.2.8.6.

Isolation   The method of Stoll* may be adopted as stated below:

1. The powdered dried ergot is first defatted with n-bexane or petroleum ether (40-60°)
2. The marc consisting of the defatted powdered ergot is thoroughly mixed with aluminium sulphate and water so as to fix the alkaloids by converting them into the double salts.
3. The resulting alkaloidal double salts are subjected to continuous extraction with hot benzene that removes the alkaloid exclusively on one hand; and the unwanted substances *e.g.*, **ergot oil,** soluble acid, neutral substances like-phytosterol, colouring matter and organic acids on the other.
4. The benzene is removed under vacuo and the residue thus obtained is stirred for several hours with a large volume of benzene and subsequently made alkaline by passing NH_3 gas.
5. The resulting solution is filtered and the benzene extract is concentrated under vacuo to approximately 1/50th of the original volume, whereupon ergotamine crystallizes out.
6. An additional quantity of ergotamine may also be crystallized from the mother liquour by treatment with petroleum ether.
7. Ergotamine may be further purified by crystallization from aqueous acetone.

Characteristic Features

1. It is obtained as elongated prisms from benzene that get decomposed at 212-214°C.
2. It usually becomes totally solvent-free only after prolonged heating in a high vacuum.
3. It is found to be highly hygroscopic in nature; and darkens and decomposes on exposure to air, heat and light.
4. It has specific optical rotation $[\alpha]_D^{20}$ - 160° (chloroform).
5. It is soluble in 70 parts methanol, 150 parts acetone, 300 parts ethanol; freely soluble in chloroform, pyridine, glacial acetic acid; moderately soluble in ethyl acetate; slightly soluble in benzene; and practically insoluble in petroleum ether and water.

---

* Stoll, *Helv. Chim. Acta* **28**, 1283, (1945)

Identification Tests The precipitation reactions and the colour tests are the same as described under **ergonovine**. However, the specific derivatives of **ergotamine** are as stated below:

1. **Ergotamine Tartrate [(C$_{33}$H$_{35}$N$_5$O$_5$)$_2$.C$_4$H$_6$O$_6$] (Ergomar; Ergate; Ergotartrat; Ergostat; Exmigra; Fermergin; Lingraine; Gynergen; Lingran):** It is normally obtained as solvated crystals *e.g.*, the *dimethanolate;* also occurs as heavy rhombic plates from methanol having mp 203°C (decomposes). It has specific optical rotation $[\alpha]_D^{25} - 125°$ to $- 155°$ (C = 0.4 in chloroform). One gram dissolves in either 500 ml of ethanol or water.

2. **Ergotamine Hydrochloride [C$_{33}$H$_{35}$N$_5$O$_5$.HCl]:** It is obtained as rectangular plates from 90% (v/v) ethanol which get decomposed at 212°C. It is found to be soluble in water-ethanol mixtures; and sparingly in water or ethanol alone.

3. **Dihydroergotamine Mesylate (C$_{33}$H$_{37}$N$_5$O$_5$.CH$_3$SO$_3$H) (Agit;1 Dihydro-ergotamine methane sulphonate; Angionorm; DET MS; Dergotamine; D.H.E. 45; Diergo; Dihydergot; Dirgotarl; Endophleban; Ergomimet; Ikaran; Migranal; Morena; Ergont; Ergotonin; Orstanorm; Tonopres; Verladyn; Seglor):** It is obtained as large prisms from 95% (v/v) ethanol having mp 230-235°C; and moderately soluble in water.

Note: (*a*) **It is the salt of a semisynthetic alkaloid prepared from ergotamine by hydrogenation of the Δ^9 double bond in the lysergic acid nucleus.**

   (*b*) **It is mostly used in the treatment of migraine because it is found to be better in efficacy and more tolerated than the parent alkaloid.**

Uses

1. It is employed as a potent antimigraine drug.
2. **Ergotamine** possesses oxytocic properties, but it is not employed for that effect.
3. **Ergotamine tartrate** is used invariably to prevent or abort vascular headaches, including *migraine* and *cluster headaches.* The mechanism of action is perhaps due to direct vasoconstriction of the dilated carotid artery bed with concomitant lowering in the amplitude of pulsations.
4. **Ergotamine tartrate** is also an antagonist of the serotonin activity.
5. **Ergotamine tartrate** is frequently used along with caffeine for the management and control of migraine headache. Both serve as cerebral vasoconstrictors; while the latter is considered to increase the action of the former.
6. **Methylergonovine maleate** is an oxytocic reported to be longer acting and more active than **ergonovine.**

C. Ergine

Synonyms Lysergamide; Lysergic acid amide;

Biological Sources It is obtained from the immature seeds of *Argyreja nervosa* (Burm.) Bojer (*Convolvulaceae*) (**Wood Rose, Silver Morning Glory**); Beeds of *Ipomea Violaceae* L. (*Convolulaceae*) (**Tlitliltzen, Ololiuqui**); seeds of *Rivea corymbosa* Hall. F. (*Convolvulaceae*) (**Snakeplant**); and also from the seeds of *Ipomea tricolor* Cav (*Convolvulaceae*).

Chemical Structure

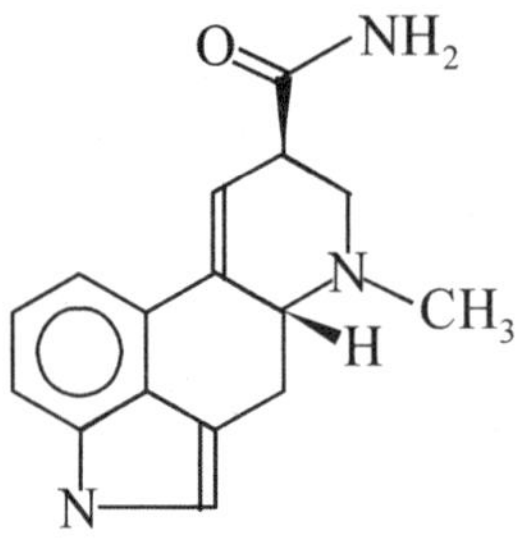

Ergine

9, 10-Didehydro-6-methylergoline-8β-carboxamide; ($C_{16} H_{17} N_3 O$).

Isolation It is isolated from the seeds of *Rivea corymbosa* (L.) and from *Ipomea tricolor* Cav. by the method of Hofmann and Tscherter.*

Characteristic Features
1. It is obtained as prisms from methanol which get decomposed at 242°C.
2. It has a specific optical rotation of $[\alpha]^{20}_{5461}$ + 15° (C = 0.5 in pyridine).

Identification Tests The precipitation reactions and the colour tests are the same as described under **ergonovine** (Section A).

Ergine may also be identified by forming its derivative as stated below:

Ergine Methane Sulphonate ($C_{16}H_{17}N_3O.CH_3SO_3H$) It is obtained as prisms from a mixture of methanol and acetone that get decomposed at 232°C.

Uses It has a pronounced depressant action.

Note: It is a controlled substance listed in the U.S. Code of Federal Regulations. Title 21 Part 1308, 13 (1995).

Biosynthesis of Ergotamine The various steps involved in the biosynthesis of **ergotamine** are as enumerated below:

1. Three amino acids, *viz.*, L-alanine, L-phenylalanine, and L-proline in the presence of ATP and enzyme SH; or D-(+)-lysergic acid in the presence of ATP and enzyme SH undergo two steps: *first*-activation *via* AMP esters, and *secondly*-attachment to the respective enzymes, thereby giving rise to an intermediate. It is worthwhile to observe that the enzyme is comprised of *two subunits* that essentially bind the substrates as indicated in the biosynthetic pathway given below.
2. The comparatively more complex structures comprising of the peptide fragments, such as: **ergotamine** are eventually formed by sequential addition of amino acid residues to the *thioester-bound lysergic acid,* yielding a linear lysergyl-tripeptide covalently attached to the enzyme complex.

---

* Hofmann and Tscherter, *Experientia*, **16**, 414 (1964).

3. The resulting complex undergoes lactam formation followed by release from enzyme. In other words, the cyclized tripeptide residue is rationalized instantly by the formation of a lactam (amide) that releases ultimately the product from the enzyme.

4. This resulting product first affords hydroxylation then followed by generation of a hemeketal-like linkage to give rise to the formation of *ergotamine*.

All these aforesaid steps (1) through (4) have been duly depicted in the following biosynthetic pathway.

Biosynthesis of Ergotamine
(Adapted from - 'Medicinal Natural Products' Dewick P.M.)

Peptide Alkaloids in Ergot   Interestingly, it has been observed critically that three amino acids, namely: alamine, phenylatine and proline, actually from the basis for the various structures which are encountered in the domain of the **'ergot alkaloids'**. Therefore, these known and established structures may be subdivided into *three* major groups which are: ergotamine group, ergoxine group, and ergotoxine group.

The various alkaloids having the peptide linkages found in **'ergot'** are depicted as under.

		Ergotamine group	**Ergoxine group**	**Ergotoxine group**
R = CH$_2$Ph		ergotamine	ergostine	ergocristine
R = CH$_2$CHMe$_2$S		ergosine	ergoptine	α-ergocryptine
R = CH(Me)Et	S	(β-ergosine)	(β-ergoptine)	β-ergocryptine
R = CHMe$_2$		ergovaline	ergonine	ergocornine
R = Et		ergobine	ergobutine	ergobutyrine

( ) Not yet known in nature

7.3   ALKALOIDS IN TISSUE CULTURES

The quantum growth and progress in the past three decades especially with regard to the legitimate utilization of plant **tissue cultures** in the exclusive bioproduction of naturally occurring chemical compounds under specific aseptic conditions through various well established means and methods almost identical to those employed to culture microorganisms has virtually opened up an altogether new and virgin horizon in the latest field of biotechnology. Therefore, the application of tissue culture techniques in the context of the biosynthesis of important secondary metabolites from plants *viz.*, **alkaloids,** not only holds a well-deserved promise for the rational controlled production of plant constituents but also supports the fact that higher plants do provide an important source of medicinally active chemical entities.

Although it has been established beyond any reasonable doubt that most of the work carried but on **'alkaloid biosynthesis'** has been more or less directly concerned with the intact plants or parts thereof, for instance: leaves, roots or shoots, there have been certain evidence and investigations using tissue cultures. This type of work is particularly beneficial in locating and establishing the site of alkaloid synthesis. It is, however, pertinent to mention here that the inferences drawn from various experimental findings that *tobacco stem callus tissue* will not synthesize alkaloids unless and until the root formation has started either spontaneously or by means of chemical stimulation.

Likewise, it has been observed interestingly that the latex isolated from the capsule of the **opium poppy** (*Papaver somniferum*) will synthesize morphine either from dopa or tyrosine, but the latex obtained from the stem will not.

Tissue cultures do not always essentially behave exactly as the **intact plant,** as has been observed with *Catharanthus roseus,* wherein the cultures of either leaf or stem effectively carried out the synthesis of certain alkaloids found in the intact plant, but no **dimeric alkaloids** could either be observed or detected. On the contrary, tissue cultures of tobacoo might convert thebaine to morphine; however, no **benzylisoquinoline alkaloids** have been noticed in *Nicotiana tabacum.*

7.4 ALKALOIDS IN CHEMOSYSTEMATICS

Broadly speaking the alkaloids invariably occur across the entire plant kingdom. In reality, alkaloids are usually found more abundantly in plants specifically belonging to the *Dictoyledones* than in either the *Monocotyledones* or the non-flowering plants. However, it has been observed that amongst the *Pteridophyta* and *Gmnospermae,* only the *Lycopodiaceae* family happens to synthesize these compounds to any reasonable extent. The *Lycopodium* alkaloids are essentially the **quinolizidine derivatives;** and usually have the ring structure as displayed by **Lycopodine** below:

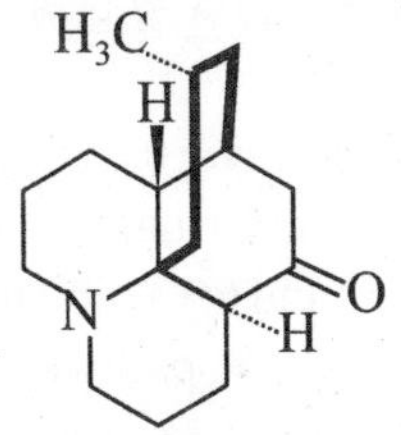

Lycopodine

(15R)-15-Methyllycopodan-5-one; ($C_{16}H_{25}NO$).

One school of thought believes that the alkaloids are confined rarely in dicotyledon orders classified before the Centrospermae, thereby establishing linkage of these simpler flowering plants with the *Gymnospermae.* The distribution and occurrence of alkaloids is found to be quite uneven among the remaining orders. Thus, an order rich in such compounds could be preceded and followed by an order wherein alkaloids are not synthesized at all. Such an erratic distribution may be noticed even more distinctly and apparently in certain plant families also. Therefore, one may safely conclude that alkaloids by themselves are absolutely spinless in establishing phylogenetic relationships either between orders or between families within an order. Of course, there exists some exceptionally few cases, for instance: *Centrospermae* which has been duly illustrated below.

Such natural orders that are found to be rich in **alkaloids** are: Centrospermae, Gentianales, Magnoliales and Ranunculaloes belonging to the class of *Dicotylendones;* and Liliales, and Orchidales belonging to the category of *Monocotylendones.* It has been reported duly tht both *Papaveraceae* and the absolutely unrelated *Apocynaceae* contain the largest number of these secondary metabolites. Surprisingly, each and every species of *Papaveraceae* thoroughly studied till date comprises of *alkaloids;* whereas, the *Apocynaceae* contains a rather more prominent diversity of complex *indole alkaloids.* There are a host of other plant families in which **alkaloids** usually occur more predominantly. and frequently are, namely: *Amaryllidaceae, Compositae, Leguminosae, Liliaceae, Loganiaceae, Orchidaceae, Ranunculaceae, Rubiaceae, Rutaceae* and *Solanaceae.* However, the *Amaryllidaceae* alkaloids are found to be specific only to that family, that contains no other variety.

A broad survey of literature has adequately proved the fact that while applying the chemosystematics to the classification of plants, the biosynthetic pathway is certainly more vital and important than that of the end-product. It may be further examplified by considering, **quinine,** a quinoline derivative obtained in *Rubiaceae,* is biosynthesized from tryptophan by a biosynthetic pathway very similar to that forming the complex **indole alkaloidal** characteristic features of the family. Besides, quinoline derivatives are also found in the *Rutaceae,* but in this particular instance they are biosynthesized from anthranilic acid; and also by a pathway that is very specific to this family.

Lastly, one may draw an inference that the strategic application of alkaloid biosynthesis to classification is made rather complicated by both convergence and divergence. Some typical examples of convergence and divergence are given below:

(*a*) **Examples of Convergence:** The synthesis of the **tropane alkaloids** from hygrine is on account of convergence. It normally occurs in a plethora of unrelated plant families, such as: *Convolvulaceae (Convolvulus* species), *Cruciferae* (*Cochleavia arctica*); *Erythroxylaceae* (*Erythroxylum coca*); *Euphorbiaceae* (*Phyllanthus discoidens*); and *Solanaceae* (includes several genera).

(*b*) **Examples of Divergence:** *Papillionoideae* exhibit several examples of divergence; because, members of this subfamily synthesise virtually a wide spectrum of secondary metabolites. The **Papillionoideae alkaloids** are found to exhibit no apparent relationship either in molecular structure or in their respective biosynthetic pathways. Hence, the **spiroamine alkaloids** found in *Erythrina* species have virtually little structural relationship to the **pyrrolizidine alkaloids** that are characteristic of *Crotolaria* species, and are biosynthesized from tyrosine; whereas, the **pyrolizidine alkaloids** are normally found to originate from ornithine.

FURTHER READING REFERENCES

1. Antkowiak, R. and Autkowiak, W.Z. **Alkaloids from Mushrooms,** *The Alkaloids, Chemistry and Pharmacology,* (ed Brossi A) Vol. 40, Academic, San Diego, pp 189-340, 1991.

2. Atta-ur-Rahman and Choudhary MI: **Chemistry and Biology of Steroidal Alkaloids.** *The Alkaloids, Chemistry and Pharmacology,* (ed Cordell GA), Vol 50, Academic, San Diego, pp 61-108, 1998.

3. Amiya T and Bando H: **Aconitum Alkaloids,** *The Alkaloids Chemistry and Pharmacology* (ed Brossi A) Vol 34, Academic, San Diego, pp 95-179, 1988.

4. Brossi A and Manske RHF., eds: **The Alkaloids,** Vols. XXI-XXV, 26-40, New York, Aeademic Press Inc., 1983-1991.

5. Brossi A and Cordell G A., eds: **The Alkaloids,** Vol 41, San Diego, Academic Press Inc., 1992.

6. Bentley K W: β-**Phenylethylamines and the Isoquinoline Alkaloids.** *nat Prod Rep* **17,** 247-268, Earlier Reviews: 1999, 16, 367-388, 1998, **15,** 341-362, 2000.

7. Bisset NG: **Curare Alkaloids, Chemical and Biological Perspectives** (ed Pelletier S.W.) Vol. 8. Wiley, New York, pp 1-150, 1992.

8. Bosch J, Bonjoch J and Amat M: **The Sytrychnos Alkaloids.** *The Alkaloids, Chemistry and Pharmacology,* (ed Cordell GA). Vol 48, Academic, San Diego, pp 75-189, 1996.

9. Brossi A, Pei XF and Greig NH (1996): **Phenserine, a Novel Cholinesterase Related to Physostigmine: Total Synthesis and Biological Properties,** *Aust J. Chem.,* **49,** 171-181, 1996.

10. Cordell G.A.: **Introduction to Alkaloids: A Biogenetic Approach,** John Wiley Sons. Inc., New York, 1981.

11. Chiara GD and North RA: **Neurobiology of Opiate Abuse.** *Trends Parmacol Sci,* **13**, 185-193, 1992.

12. Cervoni P. Crandall DL and Chan PS: **Cardiovascular Agents-Antiarrhythmic Agents,** Kirk-Othmer Encyclopedia of Chemical Technology, 4th edn. Vol. 5, Wiley, New York, 207-238, 1993.

13. Dey, P.M. and Harborne JB, (eds): **Methods in Plant Biochemistry,** Vol. 8., *Alkaloids and Sulphur Compounds,* Academic Press Ltd., London (1993)

14. Dalton DR: **Alkaloids: Kirk Othmer Encyclopedia of Chemical Technology,** 4th edn., Vol. 1, Wiley, New York, 1039-1087, 1991.

15. Emboden, W.: **'Narcotic Plants',** Mc Millan Publishing Co. Inc. New York (1979).

16. Evans WC: **Datura-a Commercial Source of Hyoscine,** *Pharm. J.,* **244,** 651-653, 1990.

17. Fujii T and Ohba M: **The Ipecac Alkaloids and Related Bases.** *The Alkaloids, Chemistry and Biology* (ed Cordell GA) Vol. 51, Academic San Diego, pp 271-321, 1998.

18. Glasby, J.S.: **Encyclopedia of the Alkaloids,** Vols. 1-4, Plenum Press, New York, 1975, 1977, and 1983.

19. Goodyer L: **Travel Medicine (4): Malaria,** *Pharm. J.,* **264,** 405-410, 2000.

20. Groger D and Floss H: **Biochemistry of Ergot Alkaloids: Achievements and Challenges.** *The Alkaloids Chemistry and Pharmacology* (ed Cordell CA) Vol. 50, Academic, San Diego, pp 171-218, 1998.

21. Herbert, R. B. **The Biosynthesis of Secondary Metabolities,** 2nd ed. Chapman and Hall. New York, (1989).

22. Hibino S and Choshi T: **Simple Indole Alkaloids and those with a Non rearranged Monoterpenoid Unit.** *Nat Prd Rep* **18,** 66-87, 2001. Earlier Review: Lounasmaa M and Tolvanen A **17,** 175-191, 2000.

23. Hartmann T. and Witte L: **Chemistry, Biology and Chemecology of the Pyrrolizidine Alkaloids.** *Alkaloids, Chemical and Biological Perspectives* (ed Pelletier SW) Vol 9, Wiley, New York, 155-233, 1955.

24. Johnson EL and Emcho SSD: **Variation in Alkaloid Content in** *Erythroxylum coca* **Leaves from Leaf-bud to Leaf-drop** *Ann. Bot* **73,** 645-650, 1994.

25. Kutchan TM: **Molecular Genetics of Plant Alkaloid Biosynthesis.** *The alkaloids, Chemistry and Pharmacology.* (ed Cordell GA) Vol. 50, Academic, San Diego, pp. 257-316, 1998.

26. Kutchan TM: **Strictosidine: From Alkaloid to Enzyme to Gene.** *Phytochemistry* **32**, 493-506, 1993.

27. Kutney JP: **Plant Cell Culture Combined with Chemistry: A Powerful Route to Complex Natural Products,** *Account Chem. Res.* **26**, 559-566, 1993.

28. Kren V: **Bioconversions of Ergot Alkaloids.** *Adv. Biochem. Eng. Biotech* **44**, 123-144, 1991.

29. Kalix P: **The Pharmacology of Psychoactive Alkaloids from Ephedra and Catha.** *J. Ethnopharmacol.* **32,** 201-208, 1991.

30. Lee M: **Malaria in Search of Solutions.** *Chem. Brit.* **32,** (8), 28-30, 1996.

31. Leonard J: **Recent Progress in the Chemistry of Monoterpenoid Alkaloids Derived from Secologanin** *Nat Prod Rep* **16,** 319-338, 1999.

32. Lewis JR: **Amaryllidaceae,** *Sealetium,* **Imidazole, Oxazole, Thiazole, Peptide and Miscllaneous Alkaloids.** *Nat Prod Rep* **18**, 95-128, 2001.

33. Misra N, Luthra R, Singh KL and Kumar S: **Recent Advances in Biosynthesis of Alkaloids.** *Comprehensive Natural Products Chemistry,* Vol. 4, Elsevier, Amsterdam, pp. 25-59, 1999.

34. Michael JP: **Indolizidine and Quinolizidine Alkaloids.** *Nat Prod Rep* **17,** 579-602, 2000.

35. Noble RL: **The Discovery of the Vinca Alkaloids-Chemotherapentic Agents against Cancer.** *Biochem Cell Biol* **68**, 1344-1351, 1990.

36. O'Hagan D: **Pyrrole, Pyrrolidine, Pyridine, Piperidine and Tropane Alkaloids.** *Nat Prod Rep* **17,** 435-446, 2000.

37. Pelletier SW (ed) **Alkaloids,** Vols 1-6, John Wiley & Sons. Inc., New York, 1993-1988; Vols 7-8, New York, Springer-Verlag New York Inc., 1991-1992.

38. Philipson JD., Roberts, M.F., Zenk, M.H. eds: **The Chemistry and Biology of Isoquinoline Alkaloids,** Springer-Verlag; Berlin, 1985.

39. Quetin-Leclereq J, Angenot L. and Bisset NG: **South American *Strychnos* species. Ethnototany (except Curare) and Alkaloid Screening.** *J. Ethnopharmacol.* **28,** 1-52, 1990.

40. Ripperger H: **Solanum Steroid Alkaloids: an Update. Alkaloids, Chemical and Biological Perspectives** (ed Pelletier SW) Vol. 12. Elsevier, Amsterdam, pp 103-185, 1998.

41. Robins DJ: **Biosynthesis of Pyrrolizidine and Quinolizidine Alkaloids. The Alkaloids, Chemistry, Pharmacology** (ed Cordell GA) Vol. 46, Academic, San Diego, pp 1-61, 1995.

42. Stockigt, J. and Ruppert M: **Strictosidine-the Biosynthetic Key to Monoterpenoid Indole Alkaloids** *Comprehensive Natural Products Chemistry*, Vol. 4. Elsevier, Amsterdam, pp 109-138, 1999.

43. Schneider MJ: **Pyridine and Piperidine Alkaloids. an Update: Alkaloids, Chemical and Biologial Perspectives** (ed Pelletier SW) Vol 10, Elsevier, Amsterdam, pp 155-299, 1996.

44. Singh, S: **Chemistry, Design, and Structure-activity Relationships of Cocaine Antagonists.** *Chem. Rev.* **100**, 925-1024, 2000.

45. Saxton JE: **The Chemistry of Heterocyclic Compounds: The Monoterpenoid Indole Alkaloids,** Vol 25, Part 4., John Wiley & Sons Inc., New York, 1983.

46. Toyota M. and Ihara M: **Recent Progress in the Chemistry of Non-monoterpenoid Indole Alkaloids** *Nat Prod Rep* **15,** 325-340, 1998, Earlier reviews: Ihara M and Fukumoto K **14,** 413-429, 1997, **13,** 241-261, 1996.

47. Wang FP and Liang XT: **Chemistry of the Diterpenoid Alkaloids: The Alkaloids, Chemistry and Pharmacology** (ed Cordell GA) Vol 42: Academic San Diego, 151-247, 1992.

48. Weiss, R. D., Mirin, SM and Bartel RL: **Coccaine,** 2nd ed., American Psychiatric Press, Inc., Washington DC, 1994.

49. Wills S: **Drugs and Substance Misuse: Plants** *Pharm. J.* **251,** 227-229, 1993.

50. Verpoorte R., Van der Heiden R and Memelink J: **Plant Biotechnology and the Production of Alkaloids: Prospects of Metabolic Engineering:** *The Alkaloids Chemistry and Pharmacology* (ed Cordell GA) Vol 50, Academic San Diegc, pp 453-508, 1998.

8 Bitter Principles

- Introduction
- Classification of Bitter Principles
- Further Reading References

8.1 INTRODUCTION

In general, the **bitter principles** are heterogenous vegetative compounds that neither belong to the class of *alkaloids* nor to the *glycosides,* but they do possess a characteristic bitter taste.

It is, however, pertinent to observe that bitter principles are invariably of vegetative origin and essentially comprise of C, H, and O, but are found to be free from N.

Interestingly, at one point in time the **bitter principles** were frequently and extensively utilized in liquid medicaments to augment and stimulate appetite. It has been established that the bitter constituent particularly stimulate the salivary glands (gustatory-nerves) present in the mouth and cause an enhancement in the psychic secretion of the gastric juice in the stomach. Since the past several decades the extract of the following drugs have been employed both extensively and intensively in various herbal systems of medicine, namely: **calumba, cinchona** (or **quinine**) **gentian, quassia, nux-vomica,** etc.

The **'bitter principles'** are mostly found in a number of plants, and are observed to be present abundantly in certain families, such as: *Compositae Labiatae*, and *Gentiananceae*.

Over the years, considerable research has accelerated the investigation of a number of these **bitter compounds** possibly for other meaningful applications, for instance: the **bitters** (*i.e.*, **bitter principles**) of the *Simaroubaceae* as *antitumour* and *antimalarial* agents.

8.2 CLASSIFICATION OF BITTER PRINCIPLES

Bitter principles have been judiciously classified into *six* categories based on the typical chemical structures present in them, namely:

(*a*) Phenolic Bitter Principles,
(*b*) Lactone Bitter Principles,
(*c*) Chromone Bitter Principles,
(*d*) Coumarin Bitter Principles,
(*e*) Coumarone Bitter Principles, and
(*f*) Miscellaneous Bitter Principles.

All these six different groups of **bitter principles** shall now be discussed at length along with certain important members from each class separately.

8.2.1 Phenolic Bitter Principles

The crystalline **acidic bitter principles** having a phenolic function are found in naturally occurring plant sources, such as: **humulon, lupulon.**

8.2.1.1 Humulon

Synonyms Humulone; α-Lupulic acid, α-Bitter acid.

Biological Source It is obtained as an antibiotic constituent from the strobiles of *Humulus lupulus* L. belonging to the natural order *Moraceae* (Hops).

Chemical Structure

Humulon

(R)-3, 5, 6-Trihydroxy-4, 6-bis (3-methyl-2-butenyl)-2-(3-methyl-1-oxobutyl)-2, 4-cyclohexadien-1-one; ($C_{21}H_{30}O_5$)

Isolation The various steps involved in the isolation of **humulon** from hops strobiles are:

1. Hops strobiles are extracted with ethanol for several hours and the alcoholic extract is filtered.
2. The filtrate is heated with animal charcoal and then cooled. In this manner, the charcoal adsorbs the bitter principles.
3. The charcoal is filtered and the adsorbed bitter principle is extracted with ethanol.
4. The alcoholic extract is evaporated over an water-electric bath and **humulon** is subsequently extracted from the resulting resinous residue by the help of boiling water repeatedly.
5. The combined aqueous fraction is cooled to 20°C and extracted with solvent ether successively.
6. The ethereal layer is filtered and evaporated in a Thin-Film Rotary Evaporator to obtain the bitter principle humulon as a residue.

Characteristic Features
1. The crystals obtained from ether have mp 65-66.5°C
2. It has a distinct bitter taste especially in alcoholic solution.
3. **Humulon** is observed to be more stable to air than lupulon.
4. It is a monobasic acid.
5. It has a specific optical rotation $[\alpha]_D^{20} - 212°$ (1.0 g in 15.5 g 96% v/v ethanol).
6. It has uv_{max} (ethanol): 237, 282 nm (ε 13, 760; 8330).
7. It is found to be soluble in usual organic solvent.

8. It is slightly soluble in boiling water from which it normally separates out as a milky precipitate on cooling.
9. It readily forms a sodium salt which is rapidly soluble in water.
10. **Bacteriostatic Potency: Humulon** suffers no loss of bacteriostatic potency against *Staphylococcus aureus* upon autoclaving 40 ppm in phosphate buffer at pH 6.5 or 8.5. However, the addition of ascorbic acid in low concentrations extends the duration of bacteriostatic action.

Identification Tests   These are as follows:

1. An ethanolic solution of **humulon** gives a reddish-violet colouration with a few-drops of $FeCl_3$ solution (0.5% w/v).
2. A few mg of **humulon** when dissolved in 0.5-1 ml NaOH solution (0.1 N) it produces a yellow colour.
3. **Humulon** reduces Tollen's Reagent (*i.e.*, ammoniaco silver nitrate solution) *in cold* and gives a silver mirror.
4. **Humulon** on being heated with a alcoholic solution of NaOH (0.5 N) undergoes complete decomposition to yield: humulinic acid (an unsaturated acid), acetic acid, isobutyric aldehyde and an unsaturated liquid volatile acid.

Uses
1. **Humulon** exerts bacteriostatic action.
2. It contributes to the bitterness of hops extract used in making beer.

8.1.2.2   *Lupulon*

Synonyms   β-Bitter Acid; β-Lupulic Acid.

Biological Sources   The biological sources of **lupulon** are the same as for humulon given under sections 8.2.1.1.

Chemical Structure

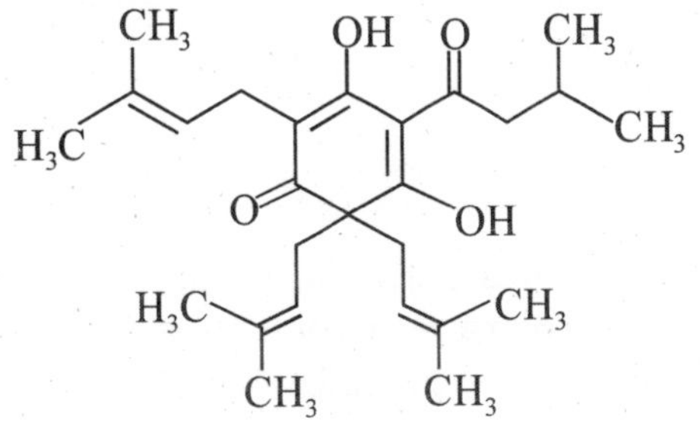

Lupulon

3, 5-Dihydroxy-2, 6, 6-tris (3-methyl-2-butenyl)-4-(3-methy-1-oxobutyl)-2, 4-cyclohexadien-1-one; $(C_{26}H_{38}O_4)$.

Isolation   **Lupulon** may be isolated from the commercial hops *Humulus lupulus* L. (*Moraceae*) by the method suggested by Lewis *et al.**

---

* Lewis *et al.*, *J. Clin. Invest.*, **28**, 916 (1949).

Characteristic Features

1. It is obtained as prisms from 90% (v/v) methanol having mp 92-94°C.
2. It possesses a distinct bitter taste especially in alcoholic solutions.
3. It behaves as a monobasic acid.
4. It is perfectly stable in *vacuo* even upto a temperature of 60°C.
5. It exhibits a slight acid reaction.
6. It is found to be optically inactive.
7. It is freely soluble in ethanol, methanol, hexane, petroleum ether, isooctane; and slightly soluble in either neutral or acidic aqueous solutions.
8. It readily forms a sodium salt which is rapidly soluble in water.
9. The addition of 0.1% solution of ascorbic acid affords a marked and pronounced protective action upon the bacteriostatic activity of **lupulon** steamed or autoclaved at a concentration of 4 ppm in phosphate buffer at pH 6.5 and 8.5.

Identification Tests

1. **Lupulon** turns yellow and amorphous in nature within a few days with the development of a characteristic odour.
2. **Lupulon** on being subjected to oxidation with potassium permanganate solution gives rise to the formation of *valerianic acid*.

Uses

1. **Lupulon** contributes exclusively to the bitterness of hops extract and is employed in the manufacture of beer.
2. It possesses the properties of an aromatic bitter and are said to have a sedative activity.

8.2.2   Lactone Bitter Principles

The **lactone bitter principles** essentially possess a five-membered lactone ring which may be exemplified by the help of *two* glaring potent compounds belonging to this category, namely: **α-santonin** and **picrotoxinin**. These compounds shall now be discussed individually in the sections that follow:

8.2.2.1   α-Santonin

Synonym   *l*-Santonin.

Biological Sources   It is obtained from the dried unexpanded flower heads of *Artemisia maritima* L., sens. lat. (*Compositae*) (**Levant Wormseed**); and other spices of *Artemisia* found mostly in Russia, China and Turkestan besides the Southern Ural Region.

Chemical Structure

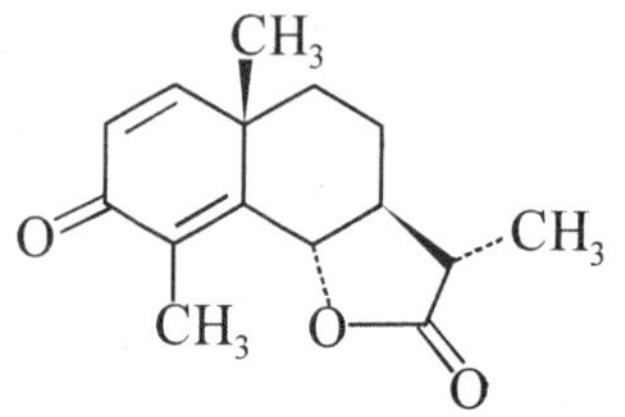

α-Santonin

1, 2, 3, 4, 4α, 7-Hexahydro-1-hydroxy-α, 4α-8-trimethyl-7-oxo-2-naphthaleneacetic acid γ-lactone; ($C_{15}H_{18}O_3$).

Isolation   The dried unexpanded flower heads of **levant wormseed** are treated with milk of lime so as to obtain calcium santoninate. The resulting product is subsequently converted into the corresponding soluble salt of **sodium santoninate** by the careful treatment with either sodium carbonate or sodium hydroxide. A stream of CO_2 is passed through the reaction mixture to get rid of calcium hydroxide as a precipitate of calcium carbonate which is filtered off conveniently. The filtrate is acidified with dilute sulphuric acid (6 N) when the crude **santonin** gets precipitated. The crude product thus obtained is made to dissolve in minimum quantity of ethanol (95%) and treated with activated charcoal powder to decolourize the solution. It is finally filtered off, ethanol is evaporated on an electric water bath and allowed to cool in a refrigerator overnight to obtain the pure α-**santonin.**

Characteristic Features   The *three* different forms of **santonin** have the following characteristic features:

(a) **(–)-Form of Santonin:**

1. It may be obtained either as tabular crystals or as orthorhombic sphenoidal crystals having mp 170-173°C.
2. It is found to be practically tasteless with a positive bitter aftertaste.
3. Its specific optical rotation $[\alpha]_D^{25}$ ranges between $-170°$ to $175°$ (C = 2 in ethanol).
4. It turns yellow on being exposed to light.
5. It causes irritation to the mucous membranes.
6. It has specific gravity d 1.187.
7. **Solubility Profile:** One part dissolves in 5000 parts of cold water, in 250 parts of boiling water, in 280 parts of 55% ethanol at 17°C, in 10 parts of boiling 50%-ethanol, in 44 parts of cold 90% ethanol, in 3 parts of boiling 90% ethanol, in 125 parts of cold ether, in 72 parts of boiling ether, and in 4.3 parts of cold chloroform.

(b) **(+)-Form of Santonin:**

1. It is obtained as colourless plates from methanol having mp 172°C.
2. Its specific optical rotation $[\alpha]_D^{20} + 165.9°$ (C = 1.92 in ethanol).

(c) **(±)-Form of Santonin:**

1. It is obtained as colourless plates from methanol having mp 181°C.
2. It has uv$_{max}$ (ethanol): 241 nm (log ε 4.10).

Identification Tests   The various identification tests for α-**santonin** are as stated below:

1. **Chromosantonin (Photosantonin):** Santonin is fairly stable in air, however, it turns yellow on exposure to *light* whereby it gets converted into its isomeric form chromosantonin, also known as photosantonin. The latter may be regenerated into santonin by simply crystallisation from ethanol.
2. **Santonin** when warmed with ethanolic solution of KOH or NaOH, it first and foremost produces a violet-red colouration, which gradually alters to reddish-yellow.

3. Heat 0.01 g of **santonin** with 2 ml of a mixture of sulphuric acid and water (1 : 1) no colour is produced apparently; but on the addition of 2-3 drops of dilute $FeCl_3$ solution (0.1% w/v) to the hot liquid a violet colouration is produced instantly.

4. **Santonin** when dissolved in a few drops of ethanol containing furfural, 2 ml of concentrated H_2SO_4 and the resulting mixture is heated in a porcelain dish over water-bath it gives a purple-red colouration that gets changed to bluish-violet, to dull blue, and finally to almost black.

5. **Santonin** 0.1 g when dissolved in 5 ml of ethanol (95% v/v) gives a clear solution which being neutral to litmus paper and is levorotatory.

Uses

1. It is mostly used as an anthelmintic (Nematodes).

2. It is very efficient in its action on round worms; but shows less effect on the thread worms and none on taenia.

8.2.2.2 Picrotoxinin

Biological Sources   It is the toxic component of **picrotoxin** obtained from the seed of *Anamirta cocculus* L. Wight & Arn. (*Menispermaceae*); and also found in *Tinomiscium philippinense* Diels.

Chemical Structure

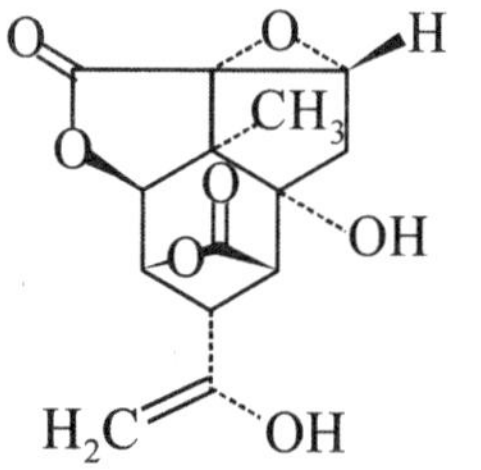

Picrotoxinin

[1aR – (1aα, 2aβ, 3β, 6β, 6aβ, 8aS*, – 8bβ, 9R*)]-Hexahydro-2a-hydroxy-8b-methyl-9-(1-methyl-ethenyl)-3, 6-methano-8H-1, 5, 7-trioxacyclopenta [ij] cycloprop [a] azulene-4, 8 (3H)-dione; $(C_{15}H_{16}O_6)$.

Preparation   **Picrotoxinin** may be prepared from picrotoxin by the method suggested by Horrmann.*

Characteristic Features

1. It is obtained in two different forms: *first*—as large prisms, and *secondly*—as small crystals containing water having mp 209.5°C.

2. Its specific optical rotations are: $[\alpha]_D^{17} + 4.4°$ (C = 4.28 in absolute alcohol); and + 3.49° (C = 7.57 in acetone).

3. It is found to be soluble in hot common organic solvents; and also in cold chloroform and ethanol.

4. Nevertheless it has a very bitter taste.

---

* Horrmann, *Ber.*, **45**, 2090 (1912).

Uses
1. It is employed as a CNS and respiratory stimulant.
2. It may also be used as an antidote to barbiturates.

8.2.3 Chromone Bitter Principles

The following heterocyclic moieties, such as: **chromone, coumarin** and **coumarone** are derived from **γ-pyrone, α-pyrone** and **furan** nucleus respectively in combination with a benzene nucleus.

Chromone

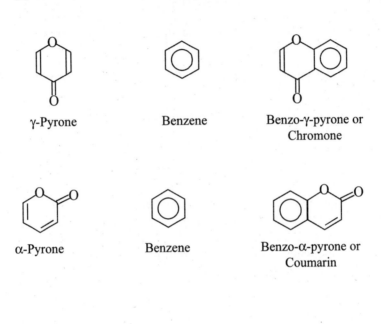

γ-Pyrone   Benzene   Benzo-γ-pyrone or
                                 Chromone

Coumarin

α-Pyrone   Benzene   Benzo-α-pyrone or
                                 Coumarin

Coumarone:

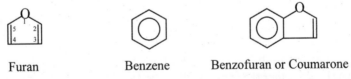

Furan   Benzene   Benzofuran or Coumarone

The important members belonging to the class of **chromone bitter principles** are, namely: **khellin, khellol glucoside** and **visnagin**. These *three* drug substances shall be described as under:

8.2.3.1 *Khellin*

Synonyms Kellin; Kelamin; Kelicor; Keloid; Kelicorin; Khelfren; Gyno khellan; Eskel; Norkel; Amicardine; Ammivisnagen; Viscardan; Visnagen; Visnagalin; Visokellina, Cardio-Khellin; Coronin; Ammivin; Ammipuran; and Ammicardine.

Biological Sources It is the major active chemical constituent obtained from the seeds of *Ammi visnaga* Lam. (*Umbelliferae*) (**Toothpick Ammi; Chellah; Khella**). It is present in the plant substance to the extent of 1%.

Chemical Structure

Khellin

4, 9-Dimethoxy-7-methyl-5H-furo [3, 2-g]-[1]-benzopyran 5-one; ($C_{14}H_{12}O_5$).
   Khellin is a *Furanochromone* compound.

Isolation   The various steps involved in the isolation of **khellin** from the seeds of *A. visnaga* are as stated below:

1. The seeds are dried, powdered, sieved and extracted in Soxhlet apparatus with solvent ether for several hours.
2. The ethereal extract is concentrated in a rotary thin-film evaporator and stored in a refrigerator for a few days.
3. The cold ethereal extract eventually comprise of *three* distinct layers: an upper green oily layer; a middle cream coloured fatty layer; and a lower green crystalline layer. The upper green oil is removed by filtration with gentle suction, the middle cream coloured fatty layer is removed by the help of petroleum ether, and the remaining lower solid residue is duly purified by repeated crystallization from methanol to obtain pure **khellin.**

   Note: The methanol mother liquor is kept aside for the isolation of 'visnagin'.

Characteristic Features
1. The crystals of **khellin** are obtained from methanol having mp 154–155°C.
2. It has a characteristic bitter taste.
3. It boils at $bp_{0.05}$ 180-200°C.
4. It has uv_{max} (ethanol): 250, 338 nm ($E_{1cm}^{1\%}$ 1600, 200).
5. **Solubility Profile:** Its solubility in g/100 ml at 25°C are: water 0.025; acetone 3.0; methanol 2.6; isopropanol 1.25; ether 0.5; and skellysolve B 0.15.
      However, it is found to be much more soluble in hot water and hot methanol.
6. **Khellin** is observed to be significantly stable when mixed with the normal tabletting excipients.

Identification Tests   These are as enumerated below:

1. **Khellin** decolourizes potassium permanganate solution.
2. When 5-8 mg **khellin** is mixed with a small piece of solid KOH or NaOH it produces a distinct rose-red colouration.

   Note: This test is not positive when either K or Na carbonate/bicarbonate used.

3. **Wagner's Reagent Test:** A saturated aqueous solution of khellin yields a precipitate with Wagner's Reagent.*

---

   * **Wagner's Reagent:** It is a solution of iodine with KI.

4. Khellin gives a faint precipitate with tannic acid solution.

Uses
1. **Khellin** is used as a potent vasodilator (coronary).
2. It also finds its application as a potent selective bronchodilator.
3. It is used extensively in the treatment and control of coronary insufficiency, angina pectoris and in chronic bronchial asthma.

8.2.3.2 Khellol Glucoside

Synonyms   Khellinin

Biological Sources   It is obtained from the seeds of *Ammi visnaga* Lam., (*Umbelliferae*); and also from *Eranthis hyemalis* L. (*Ranunculaceae*) upto 0.3%.

Chemical Structure

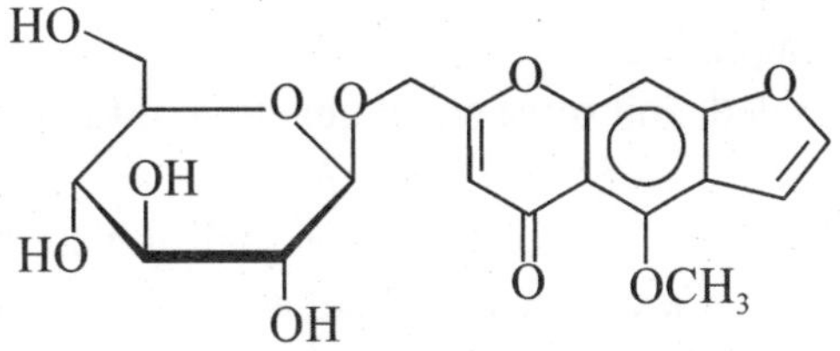

Khellol Glucoside

7-[(β-D-glucopyranosyloxy)-methyl]-4-methoxy-5H-furo [3, 2-g] [1] benzopyran-5-one; ($C_{19}H_{20}O_{10}$).

Isolation   It may be isolated from *Eranthis hyemalis* by the method put forward by Egger.*

Characteristic Features
1. It is obtained as crystals from ethanol having mp 179°C.
2. It has uv$_{max}$ (ethanol): 250, 325 nm.
3. It is found to be soluble in acetic acid, hot ethanol slightly soluble in hot methanol; and almost insoluble in acetone, ethyl acetate, ether, chloroform, cold alkali.

Identification Test   **Khellol glucoside** may be identified by making its following tetraacetate derivative due to the presence of four OH moieties.

Khellol Glucoside Tetracetate   It is obtained as flakes from ethanol having mp 153°C. It is freely soluble in acetone, ethanol, ethyl acetate; and almost insoluble in petroleum ether.

Uses   It is used as a vasodilator.

8.2.3.3 Visnagin

Synonym   Visnacorin.

Biological Sources   It is obtained from *Ammi visnaga* Lam., (*Umbelliferae*).

---

* Egger. Z. *Naturforsch.*, **16B**, 697 (1962).

Chemical Structure

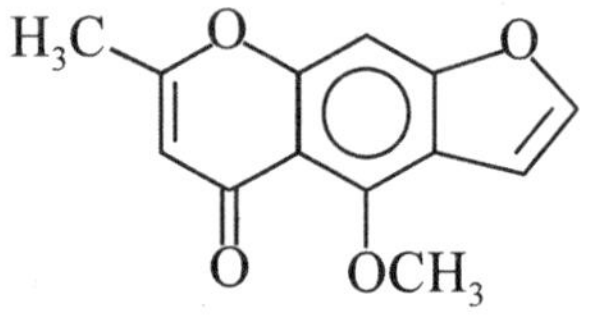

Visnagin

4-Methoxy-7-methyl-5H-furo [3, 2-g] [1]-benzopyran-5-one; ($C_{13}H_{10}O_4$).

Isolation   Various sequential steps involved are as under:

1. The methanol mother-liquor remaining after the isolation of **khellin,** is evaporated to dryness under vacuo.
2. The resulting residue is taken up in benzene and treated subsequently with petroleum ether, until a distinct turbidity is accomplished.
3. The reaction mixture is cooled, and some small quantum of **khellin** shall separate out which is removed by filtration.
4. To the filtrate further addition of petroleum ether shall initiate the process of separation of visnagin as different crops that are removed, dried and subjected to distillation under vacuum carefully.
5. The fraction distilling between 150-155°C is collected and **visnagin** is finally recrystallized from methanol as prigms.

Characteristic Features   These are as follows:

1. **Visnagin** is obtained as thread-like needles from water having mp 142-145°C.
2. It is found to be very slightly soluble in water; sparingly soluble in ethanol; and freely soluble in chloroform.

Identification Tests   **Visnagin** when triturated with a piece of solid KOH or NaOH, it gives rise to a distinct rose-red colour which is certainly lighter in shade than that obtained with **khellin.**

8.2.4   Coumarin Bitter Principles

Coumarin nucleous is generated by the combination of benzene and α-pyrone as already mentioned under section 8.2.3. A good number of *coumarin bitter principles* have been isolated and characterized for their efficacious medicinal values, such as: **psoralen, methoxsalen, bergapten, imperatorin, angelicin and pimpinellin.** Out of these the first four drugs have already been discussed under the chapter on **'Phenylpropanoids'** under Sections 6.2.3.3.1 through 6.2.3.3.4. The remaining *two* drugs shall now be described in the sections that follow:

8.2.4.1   Angelicin

Biological Sources   It occurs in the fruit or root of *Angelica archangelica* L. (*A. officinalis* Moench) (*Umbelliferae*) (**Angelica; Garden Angelica; European Angelica**).

Chemical Structure

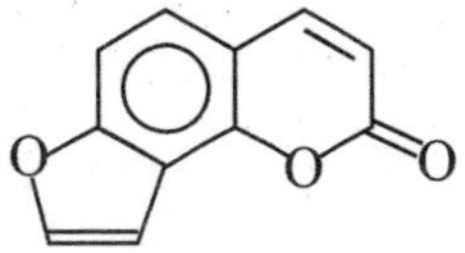

Angelicin

It is an angular furocoumarin.

Uses **Angelica** is useful for dyspepsia, enteritis, flatulance, gastritis, insomnia, neuralgia, rheumatism and ulcers.

8.2.4.2 Pimpinellin

Biological Sources It occurs in the fruits and rhizomes of *Pimpinellin saxifraga* L., *Heracleum spondylium* L.; *H. lanatum* Michx; and *H. panaces* belonging to the natural order *Umbelliferae*.

Chemical Structure

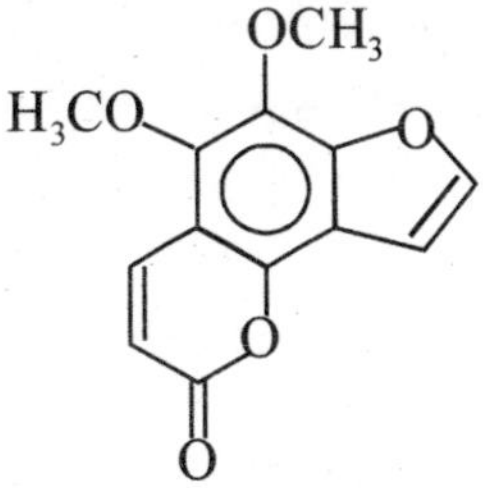

Pimpinellin

5, 6-Dimethoxy-2H-furo [2, 3-h]-1-benzopyran-2-one; $(C_{13}H_{10}O_5)$

Isolation **Pimpinellin** may be isolated by the methods suggested by Fujita and Furuya*, and by Svendsen *et al*.**

Characteristic Features
1. It is obtained as off-white needles from methylene chloride/hexane having mp 119°C.
2. It is found to be practically insoluble in water; and soluble in ethanol.
3. It also undergoes isomerism to give rise to **isopimpinellin** as shown below:

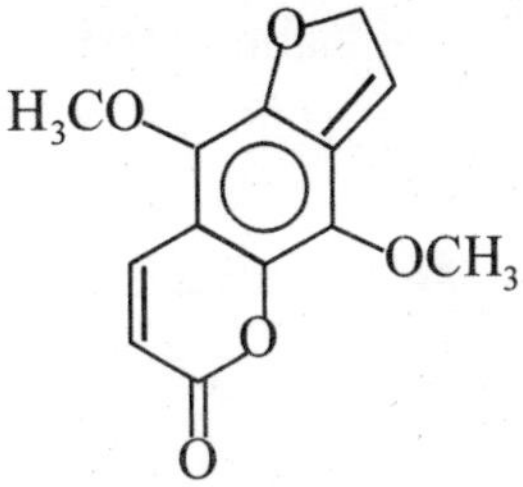

Isopimpinellin

---

  * Fujita, Furuya, *J. Pharm. Soc. Japan*, **74**, 795 (1954); **76**, 535 (1956).
 ** Sevendsen *et al. Planta Med.*, **7**, 113 (1959).

Biosynthesis of Psoralen, Methoxsalen (Xanthotoxin), Bergapten, Angelicin and Isopimpinellin   The various steps that are involved in the *biosynthesis of psoralen, xanthotoxin, bergapten, angelicin and isopimpinellin* are given below in a sequential manner:

1. **Umbelliferone** is first produced by the interaction of an isoprene unit with an appropriate alkylating agent *e.g.*, dimethylallyldiphosphate (DMAPP). Thus, the aromatic ring in the former gets duly activated at positions *ortho* to the hydroxyl group present in it.

2. The newly introduced dimethylallyl function present in *demethyl-suberosin* gets subsequently cyclized, having the phenolic moiety intact, to yield *marmesin*. However, this specific biotransformation is found to be catalyzed by a cytochrome P-450-dependent mono-oxygenase and also essentially requires cofactors such as NADPH and molecular oxygen.

3. It has been suggested appropriately that a *second* cytochrome P-450 dependent mono-oxygenase enzyme then cleaves off the hydroxyisopropyl portion (as a mole of acetone) from marmesin, thus producing the *linear furocoumarin* **psoralen.**

4. **Psoralen** is supposed to act as a precursor for the production of the subsequent series of further **substituted furocoumarins,** namely: **bergapten, xanthotoxin,** and **isopimpinellin** as shown below. Interestingly, such modifications are usually afforded due to steps taking place rather late in the biosynthetic pathway than occurring at the cinnamic-acid stage.

5. **Angelicin**—the so called *angular* furocoumarins, is the outcome of an identical sequence of reactions; however, these steps specifically involve dimethylallylation due to DMAPP at the alternative position *ortho* to the phenol.

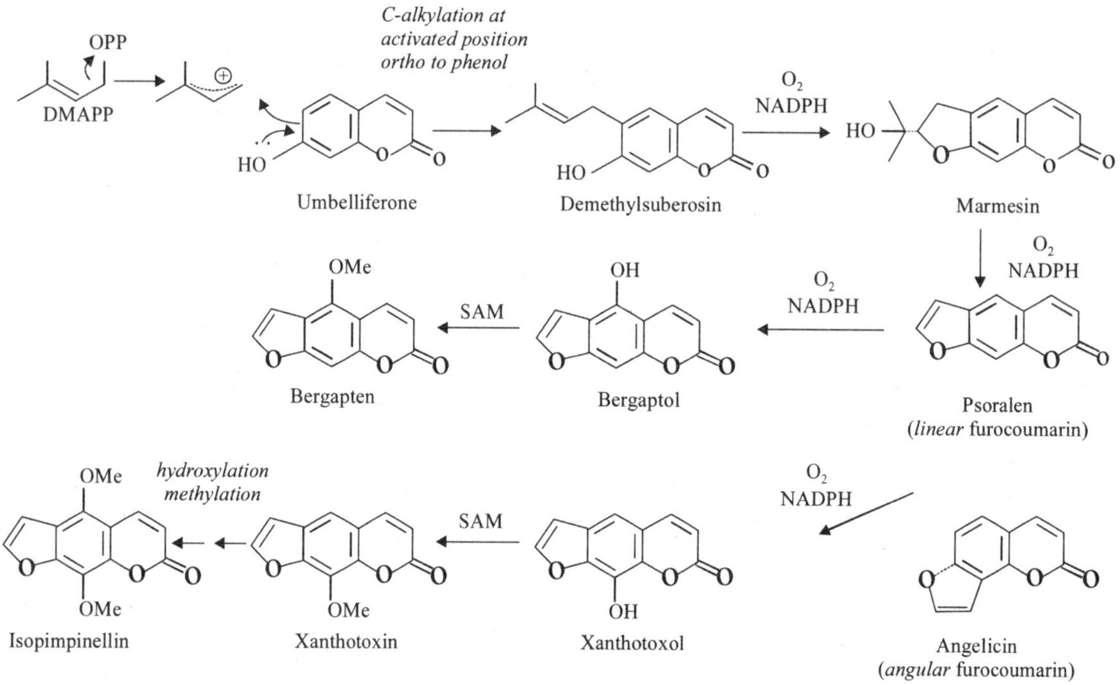

Biosynthesis of Psoralen, Methoxsalen, Bergapten, Angelicin and Isoimpinellin

8.2.5 Coumarone Bitter Principles

The combination of the furan and benzene rings gives rise to the formation of benzofuran nucleus, otherwise termed as **'coumarone'** as already depicted under Section (8.2.3). The most important coumarone based bitter principle is **rotenone** which shall now be discussed in an elaborated fashion in given below.

8.2.5.1 Rotenone

Synonym Canex

Biological Sources The principal insecticidal constituent of the dried **derris roots,** *Derris elliptical* Roxb. and *D. malaccensis* Prain, belonging to family *Leguminoseae*; from **cube roots,** *Lonchocarpus utilis* and *L. urucu*, belonging to the natural order *Leguminoseae*; from *Lonchocarpus nicou* (Aubl.) D.C. (*Leguminoseae*); fruits and plant of *Piscidia piscipula* Sarg. **(Jamaica Dogwood)**; and the roots of *Tephrosia virginiana* (L.) Pers (*Fabaceae*) **(Devil's Shoe String)**.

Chemical Structure

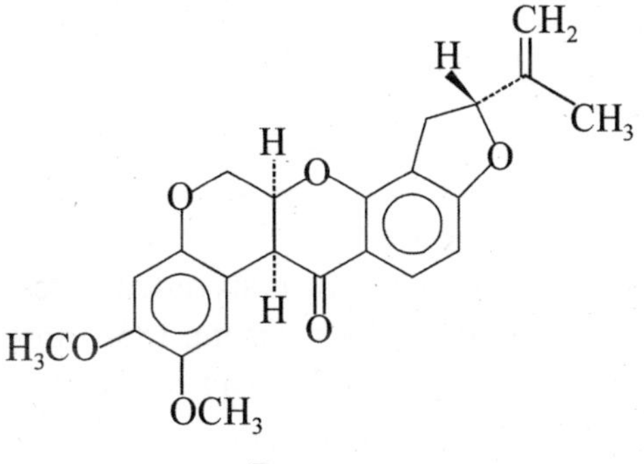

Rotenone

[2R-(2α, 6aα, 12aα)]-1, 2, 12, 12a-Tetrahydro-8, 9-dimethoxy-2-(1-methylethenyl)-[1] benzopyrano [3, 4-6] furo [2, 3-h] [1] benzopyran-6 (6aH)-one; ($C_{23}H_{22}O_6$). It is a *rotenoid*.

Isolation Various steps involved in the isolation of **rotenone** are as follows:

1. The derris roots and rhizomes are dried, powdered, sieved and extracted with carbon tetrachloride in a Soxhlet apparatus for at least 24 hours.
2. The CCl_4 extract is filtered, concentrated under vacuo and allowed to cool at an ambient temperature for 24 hours, when crystals of **rotenone** separate out.
3. The resulting mixture is filtered through a gouche crucible under suction, and the crystals this collected are washed with a little CCl_4; and finally dried in the air.

Characteristic Features Its chemical features are:

1. It is an **'isoflavone compound'** wherein the 2 : 3 double bond has undergone reduction.
2. Its heterocyclic portions are:
   (*a*) A hydrobenzopyran moiety, and
   (*b*) A hydrocoumarone (or 2 : 3-benzofuran) function.

3. **Rotenone** is a derivative of *tubic acid lactone* and is more commonly known as **6, 7-dimethoxy-2, 3-dihydro-benzopyran tubic acid lactone.**

4. Decomposition of **rotenone** yields derric acid and tubic acid; and the latter further gives rise to a '*lactone*' termed as the **tubic acid lactone** as shown below:

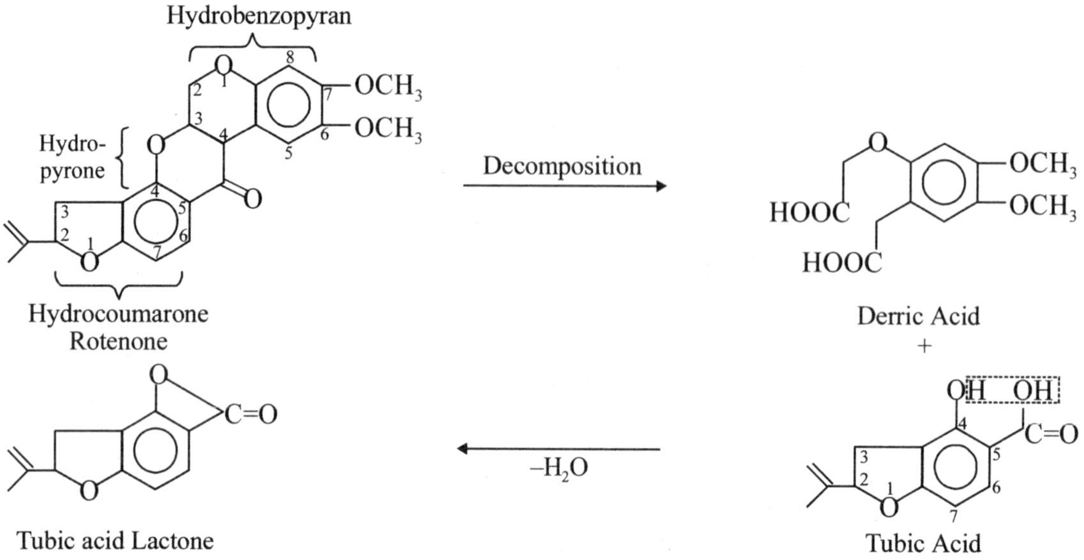

The physical parameters of **rotenone** are:

1. It is usually obtained either as orthorhombic or as six-sided plates from trichloroethylene having mp 165–166°C; however, the dimorphic form has mp 185–186°C.

2. Its specific optical rotation $[\alpha]_D^{20} - 228°$ (C=2.22 in benzene).

3. It gets decomposed upon exposure to air and light.

4. **Rotenone** is almost insoluble in water; and soluble in ethanol acetone, carbon tetrachloride, chloroform, ether, in addition to many other organic solvents.

Identification Tests These are as given below:

1. Dissolve 2-3 mg of **rotenone** in 1 ml acetone and add to it 1 ml dilute HNO_3 (50% v/v), and allow it to stand for about one hour to cause the oxidation. Now, add to it a few drops of NaOH solution (10% w/v) when a distinct blue colour gets developed.

2. Its colourless solutions in organic solvents normally oxidize upon exposure and become yellow, orange and then deep red finally. It may also deposit crystals of **dehydrorotenone** and **rotenonone** that are found to be toxic to insects.

Uses

1. It is mostly used as a potent pesticide.

2. It is widely employed as an acaricide and actoparasiticide in cattles.

3. The action of **rotenone** closely resembles to that of *pyrethrin* in affecting a rapid *knock-down* of the flying insects (*e.g.*, house-flies, mosquitos etc.); and is found to be comparatively harmless to the warm-blooded animals.

4. As **rotenone** does not leave any harmful residue, it may be employed with enormous safety for most delicate and precious garden crops and garden plants.

Note **Interestingly, though the derris roots do contain a natural insecticidal principle (rotenone) they are nevertheless prone to infestation by some specific types of insects obviously unaffected by rotenone.**

Biosynthesis of Rotenone In general, many thousands of wide variety of **isoflavonoids** have been duly isolated, characterised and identified; and subsequently their structural complexity have been resolved logically and methodically by first carrying out the hydroxylation, and secondly by alkylation reactions. These reactions not only helped in varying the oxidation level of the heterocyclic ring, but also produced additional heterocyclic rings.

In the **biosynthesis of rotenone** a simple **isoflavone** called **daidzein** is the starting material which undergoes methylation in the *para* position of the phenyl ring attached to the pyran ring with a covalent bond thereby forming an isoflavone termed as **formononetin.** This undergoes further biotransformations as stated earlier to yield **rotenone.** It contains a C_5 isoprene unit, as could be observed in most of the natural **rotenoids,** * which is afforded *via* dimethyl-allylation of **demethylmunduserone.**

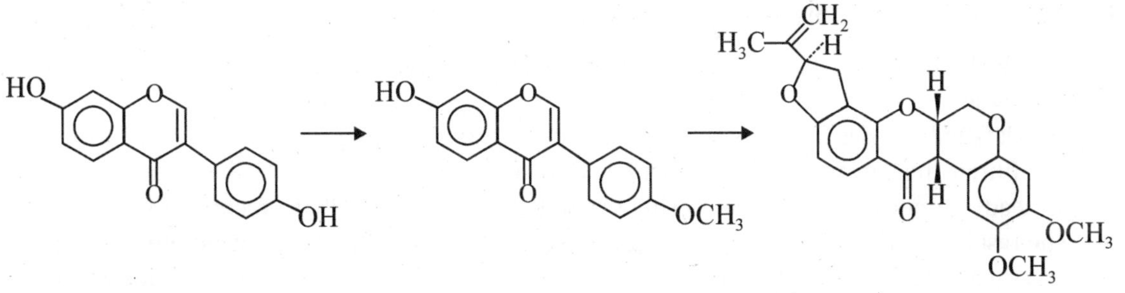

Diadzein	Formononetin	Rotenone
(An Isoflavone)	**(An Isoflavone)**	**(A Rotenoid)**

Biosynthesis of Rotenone

8.2.6 Miscellaneous Bitter Principles

There are some **bitter principles** which normally do not fall into the various categories already discussed from Sections 8.2.1 through 8.2.5. A few important potent drugs used as bitter principles that belong to this group are, namely: **picrotoxin, quassin, cantharidin,** which shall now be described separately as under:

8.2.6.1 Picrotoxin

Synonym Cocculin.

Biological Sources It is obtained as the **bitter principle** from the seed of *Anamirta cocculus* L. Wight & Arn. (*Menispermaceae*); and also found in *Tinomiscium philippinense* Diels.

---

* **Rotenoids:** The rotenoids take their name from the first known example *rotenone* and are usually generated by ring cyclization.

Chemical Structure   **Picrotoxin** is a molecular compound of one mole **picrotoxinin** ($C_{15}H_{16}O_6$), q.v., and one mole **picrotin** ($C_{15}H_{18}O_7$), q.v., into which it is readily separated. Thus, **picrotoxin** may be resolved into the two components by boiling with 20 parts of benzene. In this manner, **picrotoxinin** remains dissolved in benzene whereas *picrotin* that is practically insoluble in benzene can be separated easily. Likewise, this cleavage may also be accomplished by chloroform more efficiently. Thus, we have:

Picrotoxin $\longrightarrow$ Picrotoxinin   +
($C_{30}H_{34}O_{13}$)   ($C_{15}H_{16}O_6$)
                                            [under section 8.2.2.2]

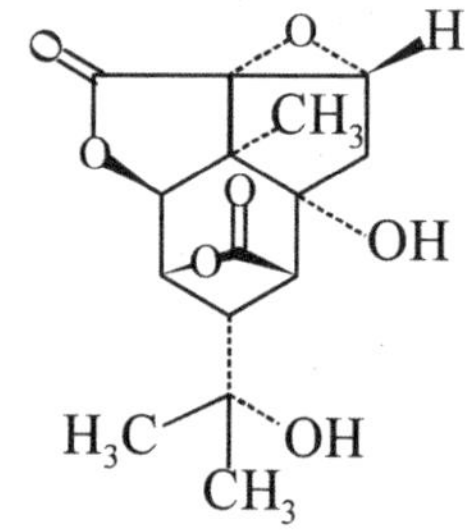

Picrotin
($C_{15}H_{18}O_7$)

Isolation   Various steps involved in the isolation of **picrotoxin** are:

1. The seeds are dried, powdered coarsely, sieved and defatted with petroleum ether in a Soxhlet apparatus.
2. The defatted powder (marc) is subsequently extracted by boiling with ethanol or with water.
3. The filtrate thus obtained is treated with lead acetate solution (5% w/v), filtered and the excess of 'lead' is removed by passing freshly generated H_2S gas (*i.e.*, Pb is precipitated as Pb S).
4. The resulting solution is filtered, residue discarded and the filtrate is concentrated to a syrupy consistency in a Rotary Thin Film Evaporator. The syrupy liquid is kept in a refrigerator overnight.
5. **Picrotoxin** crystallizes out as a crude substance.
6. It may be further purified by treating with ethanol or boiling water and activated charcoal powder to obtain the pure substance.

Characteristic Features
1. It is obtained as shiny rhomboid leaflets mp 203°C.
2. It has an intense bitter taste and is *extremely poisonous*.
3. It has specific optical rotation $[\alpha]_D^{16} - 29.3°$ (C = 4 in absolute ethanol).
4. **Solubility Profile:** 1 g dissolves in 150 ml cold water; 45 ml boiling water, in 13.5 ml 95% ethanol, in 3 ml boiling ethanol; sparingly soluble in ether, chloroform; and readily soluble in aqueous solution of NaOH and in strong NH_4OH.
5. It is highly toxic to fish.
6. It is stable in air, but is affected by light.
7. Picrotoxin is almost neutral to litmus.

Identification Tests   These are as stated below:

1. **Sulphuric Acid Test:** Dissolve 2-3 mg of **picrotoxin** in a few drops of sulphuric acid, a golden-yellow-colour is produced that gets changed to reddish-brown gradually.

2. **Anisaldehyde Test:** Moisten a few crystals of **picrotoxin** with H_2SO_4 and just add 1-2 drops of a solution of anisaldehyde in dehydrated ethanol (1 : 5), a permanent blue colouration is produced.

3. **Potassium-Cupric Tartrate Test:** Add about 5-10 mg of **picrotoxin** to 2 ml of potassium-cupric tartrate solution (0.5%) with 10 ml of water, a red precipitate is formed gradually in the cold, but a little faster on warming.

4. **Vanillin HCl Test:** A few mg of picrotoxin when boiled with vanillin hydrochloride solution (0.1% w/v) it gives rise to a green colouration.

5. **Reduction Tests: Picrotoxin** reduces Fehling's solution to give a brick-red precipitate; and **Tollen's reagent** to give a silver mirror.

6. Mix 0.2 g KNO_3 with four drops of H_2SO_4 in an evaporating dish. Sprinkle a few crystals of **picrotoxin** on the resulting mixture and add dropwise NaOH solution (2N), until it is present in a little excess quantity. The crystals of picrotoxin shall initially acquire a red colouration that fades out slowly.

Uses

1. It is used as a CNS-stimulant. Therefore, it may be employed intravenously as an antidote in barbiturate poisoning and other narcotics also.

2. It also finds its application as an effective respiratory stimulant.

3. Very small quantities of the powdered seeds are sufficient to stupify fish.

8.2.6.2 Quassin

Synonym Nigakilactone D

Biological Sources It is obtained from the wood of *Quassia amara* L., (*Simaroubaceae*) commonly known in commerce as **Surinam quassia.** It is also obtained from the stem wood of *Picrasma excelsa* (Sw.) Planch. (*Aeschrion excelsa* or *Picroena excelsa*) known in commerce as **Jamaican quassia.** All these species belong to the natural order *Simaroubaceae*).

Chemical Structure

Quassin

2, 12-Dimethoxypicrosa-2, 12-diene-1, 11, 16-trione; ($C_{22}H_{28}O_6$).

Isolation The following steps may be adopted in a sequential manner for the isolation of **quassin.**

1. The **quassia wood** is chopped into small pieces and subjected to aqueous decoction, which is filtered and concentrated to the original weight of the wood taken; and finally neutrallized carefully with Na_2CO_3.

2. Tannic acid solution (5% w/v) is added slowly until no more precipitate is obtained.
3. The precipitate thus obtained is filtered, collected and transferred to a pestle and mortar, triturated with solid lead carbonate (or with freshly prepared lead oxide), so as to liberate **quassin** and form lead tannate; and the resulting mass is dried on a water bath.
4. The dried mass is powdered and then subjected to extraction with 80% (v/v) ethanol successively.
5. The combined ethanolic extract is filtered and concentrated under vacuo and left for cooling overnight, when the crystals of **quassin** would separate out.

Quassin may also be obtained by the resolution of the mixture of bitter constituents of **quassia wood** by the method of London *et al.**

Characteristic Features
1. **Quassin** is obtained as rectangular plates from dilute methanol having mp 222°C.
2. Its specific optical rotation $[\alpha]_D^{20}$ + 34.5° (C = 5.0 g in $CHCl_3$).
3. It has uv$_{max}$: ~ 255 nm (ε ~ 11,650).
4. It is extremely bitter; and it has the bitterness threshold 1 : 60,000.
5. It is found to be freely soluble in benzene, acetone, ethanol, chloroform, pyridine, acetic acid, hot ethyl acetate; and sparingly soluble in ether and petroleum ether.

Identification Tests
1. Add to a few crystals of **quassin** 2-3 drops of concentrated, H_2SO_4 and sucrose when a red colouration is produced.
2. **Phloroglucin Test:** Dissolve 2-3 mg **quassin** in 1-2 ml ethanol, and add to it a few crystals of phloroglucin and a few drops of concentrated. HCl, when a crimson red colour is obtained.

Uses
1. It possesses insecticidal properties.
2. The *quassia wood extract* is used as a bitter tonic.
3. **Quassin** exhibits anthelmintic properties, and on being administered as enema *expels thread worms* specifically.

8.2.6.3 Lactucin

Biological Sources It is obtained from the dried milky juice of *Lactuca virosa* L. (*Asteraceae*) (**Bitter Lettuce; Wild Lettuce**); and from the plant of *Cichorium intybus* L. (*Compositae*).

Chemical Structure

Lactucin

* London *et al., J. Chem. Soc.*, 3431, 1950.

[3aR – [3aα, 4β, 9aα, 9bβ)]-3,3a,4,5,9a,9b-Hexahydro 4-hydroxy-9-(hydroxymethyl)-6-methyl-3-methyl-eneazuleno [4, 5-b] furan-2, 7-dione; ($C_{15}H_{16}O_5$).

Isolation   Lectucin may be isolated by the method suggested by Schenck *et al.**

Characteristic Features

1. It is obtained as crystal from methanol which sinters at 218°C and has mp 228-233°C.
2. It exhibits specific optical rotation $[\alpha]_D$ + 49° (C = 0.90 in methanol); and +77.9° (C = 3.44 in pyridine).
3. It has uv_{max}: 257 nm (ε 14,000).
4. It is found to be soluble in water, ethanol, methanol, ethyl acetate, anisol and dioxane.

Identification Tests   It may be identified from its derivative:

Lectucin *para*–hydroxyphenylacetate hydrate ($C_{23}H_{22}O_7$) (Intybin; Lactucopicrin;): It is obtained as crystals from water which get decomposed at 148-151°C. It shows specific optical rotation $[a]_D^{17.5}$ + 67.3° (pyridine).

8.2.6.4 *Erythrocentaurin*

Biological Sources   It is obtained from the plant *Centaurium umbellatum* Gilib. (*Erythraea centaurium* Pers.), *Gentinaceae* or *Swertia japonica* (Maxim.) Makino *Gentianaceae*. It is also accomplished by carrying out the hydrolysis of **swertiamarin** and **erytaurin** with emulsin.

Chemical Structure

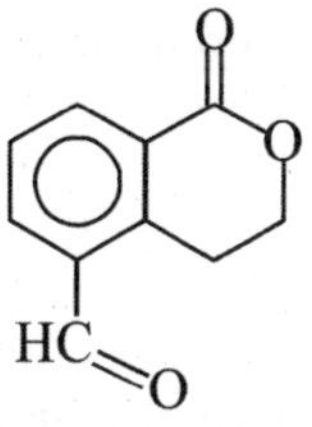

Erythrocentaurin

5-Formyl-3, 4-dihydroisocoumarin; ($C_{10}H_8O_3$).

Isolation   **Erythroceantaurin** may be isolated from *C. umbellatum* by the method of Kariyone and Matsushima.**

Characteristic Features

1. It is obtained as long needles having mp 140-141°C.
2. It turns red on being exposed to sunlight.
3. It has uv_{max}: 223, 290 nm (log ∈ 4.30, 3.13).

Uses   It is mostly employed as a bitter tonic.

---

* Schenck *et. al., Arch. Pharm.,* **294**, 17 (1961).

** Kariyone and Matsushima J., *Pharm. Soc.,* Japan, **47**, 25 (1927).

8.2.6.5 *Gentisin*

Synonyms   Gentianin; Gentiin; Gentianic Acid.

Biological Sources   It is obtained from the roots of *Gentiana lutea* L. (*Gentianaceae*) **(Yellow Gentian)**.

Chemical Structure

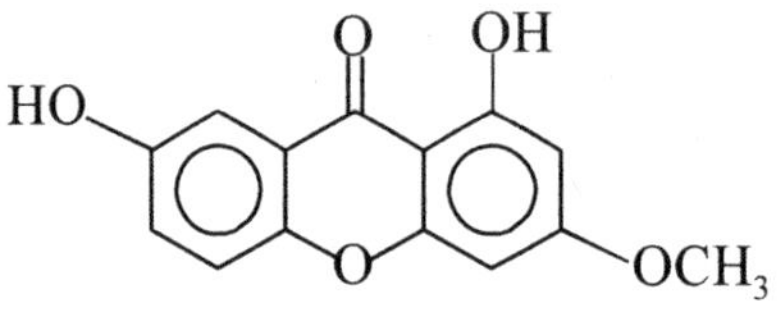

Gentisin

1, 7-Dihydroxy-3-methoxy-9H-xanthen-9-one; ($C_{14}H_{10}O_5$).

Characteristic Features
1. It is obtained as yellow needles from ethanol having mp 266-267°C.
2. It has uv$_{max}$ (methanol): 260, 275, 315, 410 nm (log $\in$ 435, 4.30, 4.10, 3.70).
3. It is observed to be very slightly soluble in water or organic solvents.

Identification Test

Gentisin Diacetate ($C_{18}H_{14}O_7$)   It is obtained as crystals from ethanol having mp 196-197°C. Its absorption max (metanol): 240, 270, 300 nm (log ε 4.58, 4.05, 4.10).

Uses   It may be used to stimulate gastric secretion, improve appetite and digestion, and alleviate debility.

8.2.6.6 *Cantharidin*

Synonym   Cantharides Camphor.

Biological Sources   It is the active vesicating principle of cantharides (q. v) and other insects, in notorious **'Spanish Fly'** aphrodisiac, which essentially comprise of the dried insects (Beetles) *Lytta* (*Cantharis*) *vesicatoria* belonging to the order *Coleoptera*; and family *Meloidae*. It has been found that the soft parts of the insect are the chief seat of **cantharidin.** Besides, cantharidis contain 0.5 to 0.95 of **cantharidin.**

Chemical Structure

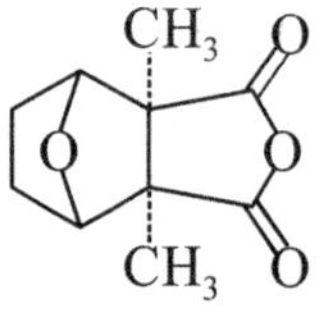

Cantharidin

Exo-1, 2-*cis*-Dimethyl-3, 6-epoxy hexahydrophthalic anhydride; ($C_{10}H_{12}O_4$).

Isolation   The various steps involved in the isolation of **cantharidin** are:

1. The dried insects are collected and powdered. It is now treated with an acid whereby the **cantharidin** gets liberated in the form of its corresponding salts.
2. The resulting product is subjected to extraction, of both **cantharidin** and fat, by the help of ethyl acetate in a Soxhlet apparatus.
3. The solvent is removed carefully under reduced pressure and the crude cantharidin crystallizes out.
4. The fat may be removed by the help of petroleum ether, in which **cantharidin** is only negligibly soluble.
5. Ultimately, the crude defatted **cantharidin** is dissolved in a minimum quantity of hot ethanol and allowed to cool when cantharidin crystallizes out in its purest form.

Charactersitic Features   These are as follows:

1. **Cantharidin** is obtained as orthorhombic plates or as scales having mp 218°C.
2. It sublimes at 110 °C (12 mm Hg, 3-5 mm distances).
3. It is practically insoluble in cold water and somewhat soluble in hot water. 1g dissolves in 40 ml acetone; 65 ml chloroform; 560 ml ether; 150 ml ethyl acetate; and soluble in oils.

Identification Tests

1. **Formaldehyde Test:** Add to a few crystals of **cantharidin** 1-2 drop of dilute formaldehyde solution mixed with H_2SO_4, the development of a brown to black colouration on warming identifies it.
2. A solution of **cantharidin** in olive oil is vesicant to the skin (*i.e.*, sensitive upto an extent of 0.14 mg).

Uses

1. It is mostly used as a vesicant.
2. It is also employed as a rubefacient and counterirritant in veterinary practice.

FURTHER READING REFERENCES

1. Barakat, Z., and Badran, N., **'Identification of Khellin, Visnagin and Khellol Glucoside'**, *J. Pharm. Pharmacol.*, **3**, 576, (1951).
2. Bisset N.G. (Ed.): Max Wichtl—**Herbal Drugs and Phytopharmaceuticals,** CRC Press, London, 1994.
3. Brown, S.A., **Recent Studies on the Formation of Natural Coumarins,** *Lloydia,* **26**, 211, 1963.
4. Dewick, P.M., **'Medicinal Natural Products—A Biosynthetic Approach'**, John Wiley & Sons, Ltd., England, 2nd. edn., 2002.
5. Duke, J.A., **'Handbook of Medicinal Herbs'**, CRC-Press, New York, 2001.
6. Evans, W.C., **Trease and Evan's Pharmacognosy,** W.B. Saunders Company Ltd., London, 14th, edn, 1996.
7. Hostettmann K. *et al.* (eds.), **Phytochemistry of Plants Used in Traditional Medicine,** Proceedings of Phytochemical Society Europe, 37, Oxford Science, New York, 1995.
8. Jisaka M. *et al.*, **Antitumoral and Antibacterial Activities of Bitter Sesquiterpene Lactones of *Vernonia amygdalina*: a possible Medicinal Plant used by Wild Chmpanzees,** *Biosci. Biotech. Biochem.,* **57**: 833-834, 1993.
9. Newall, C.A., Anderson, L.A., and Phillipson, J.D.,: **Herbal Meicines—A Guide for Health care Professionals.** The Pharmaceutical Press, London, 1996.
10. Ramstad, E.: **Modern Pharmaceognosy,** McGraw Hill Book, Co., London, 1959.

9

Antibiotics

9.1 INTRODUCTION

Antibiotics, in today's most up-to-date therapeutic armamentarium, occupy strategically the most coveted and key position during the span of past half-century across the globe. This conglomeration of drugs affords an effective management and critical control of a host of deadly human related pathogenic microorganisms which previously caused pathetic prolonged human sufferings or ultimately leading to death irrespective of the physical condition, age factor or economic status of an individual.

The word **'antibiotic'** has been coined from the term antibiosis that evidently means **'against life'** (*anti*—against and *bios*—life).

Over the years various versions of 'definitions' for an **antibiotic** have been postulated which are enumerated as under.

The most widely accepted definition of an **antibiotic** accepted by the scientific jargons is—**'a chemical substance produced by a microorganism, that has the capacity, in low concentration, to inhibit or kill, selectively, other microorganisms.'** This definition lays particular emphasis on the terminology *'selectivity'* or *'selective toxicity'* that explicitly suggests that the substance either checks the growth of pathogens or exerts a bactericidal action on the microbes without displaying a likewise action on the host organism *i.e..*, the human beings.

The above definition clearly excludes the compounds having the pure synthetic genesis (origin). However, in a rather broader perspective these *'synthetic substances'* are virtually treated at par with the natural compounds along with their corresponding derivatives under the terminology **'antimicrobials'** which may be further categorized into **antifungals** and **antibacterials** based on the particular type of **microbe** undergoing inhibition. Hence, in order to circumvent the practical aspects, both the terminologies *viz.,* **'antibiotic'** and **'antimicrobial'** may be employed interchangeably irrespective of the particular source of the compound.

Even in the ancient and primitive era, dating back to 2500 years, the anti-infective characteristic features of *fungi* and *moulds* usually observed in various food products like: mouldy bread, yoghurt, and soybean curds, and other similar materials to wounds and boils to curb their infection. This sort of age-old treatment one may regard as a **folk-medicine style of antibiotic therapy.**

It is, however, pertinent to mention here that the real impetus and legitimate recognition of the antibiotics in the so called 'modern drugs' was virtually accomplished by the famous french scientist Louis Pasteur. The epoch making introduction of *pyocyanase* interestingly extracted from *Pseudomonas aeruginosa* as a prominent therapeutic agent under the **'antibiotics'** is indeed one of the greatest achievements in the history of medicine. This event was immediately followed by another historic invention of Alexander Fleming for the drug penicillin; and the subsequent antimicrobial activity of *Penicillium notatum* discovered by **Chain Florey and his co-workers.**

In fact, the most effective and wonderful class of life saving antibiotics comprise of a plethora of active substances that are found to be effective on either Gram +ve or Gram –ve micro-organisms; besides the ones that are invariably known as the **broad-spectrum antibiotics.**

In general, the **antibiotics** are produced on a large scale by *three* known methods, namely: (*a*) fermentation process; (*b*) semi-synthetic process; (*c*) synthetic process. Recently, with the advent of a tremendous quantum jump and diversification in the specific field of **'biotechnology'**, the first two processes stated above have not only gained an enormous increase in the rate of production but also improved their yield and purity. Nevertheless, the fermentation process is further categorized into *two* types: (*a*) surface method; (*b*) submerged method. It is worthwhile to mention here that the second method has a much greater efficiency limit and hence used commercially. Over the years, a vast number of altogether newer, purer, and high-yielding **microbial strains** have been developed, tried and tested for evaluating their **antibiotic** yielding strength besides the efficiency in their extraction.

9.2 ANTIBIOTIC DEVELOPMENT

The latest progressive trend in the logistic features of **antibiotic development** may be expatiated by the following sequence of objectives, namely:

(*a*) To screen and evaluate different types of sources of microorganisms for detection of purposeful antagonism.
(*b*) To identify and select modified versions of microbial mutants, establish optimal environmental and nutritional conditions, and to develop appropriate methods for recovering antibiotics from cultures.
(*c*) To induce the production of particular desired metabolites.
(*d*) To improve upon and modify the fermenatative metabolites either by the help of chemical or biological manipulations to accomplish more useful antibiotic products (compounds).
(*e*) To develop detailed methods for **'total synthesis'** of antibiotics from *ab initio* for a feasible economic advantage, and
(*f*) To make use of an adjunct agent to distinctly enhance the impact or availability of an **'antibiotic'**.

9.2.1 Quest for New Antibiotics

In the quest for new **antibiotics,** rather simpler, standardized and quicker procedures have been developed and established for screening viable microorganisms having antibiotic-yielding capability. In actual practice, however, the soil samples are the choicest candidates towards an endeavour to identify the microbes for the simplest logical reason that they are considered as the richest source of antibiotic-producing organisms. Interestingly, majority of these organisms happen to be the bonafide members of a specific class of branching, procaryotic microorganisms which essentially retain a coveted status in their morphologic characteristic features between bacteria and fungi. A survey of literature reveals that between early fifties to late seventies the microbial sources of antibiotics discovered in Japan and USA mainly comprise of actinomycetes (85%), fungi (11%), and bacteria (4%).

The following are the summary of the most prominent **genera** and their **taxonomic relations.**

Genus	Streptomyces	Order	Penicillium
Phylum	–	Eumycophyta (Fungi)	–
Class	–	Ascomycetes	Deuteromycetes (Fungi Imperfecti)
Order	Actinomycetales (Actinomycetes)	Aspergillales	Moniliales
Family	Streptomycetaceae	Aspergillaceae	Moniliaceae

In general, nowadays a great deal of emphasis is being focused upon the pathogens responsible for causing mostly incurable fungal and viral infections, besides the bacterial infections, such as: **methicillin-resistant** *Staphylococcus* and *Pseudomonas* species.

Following are the various steps involved in the so called 'general method' for the methodical screening of **newer antibiotics,** namely:

Step I: Treatment of the soil sample (or sample from other sources) by an antifungal chemical antibiotic, **cycloheximide** which specifically checks the growth of interfering bacteria and fungi but nevertheless affects the *actinomycetes*. Besides, a diluted solution of phenol (1 : 140) may also be used as an antibacterial agent.

Step II: The treated sample, in their varying known dilutions are subsequently streaked on agar plates containing medium (nutrients) which augments and accelerates the growth of actinomycetes.

Step III: The streaked agar plates are incubated for 3 to 7 days between 25-30°C; and examined carefully for their characteristic colonies of actinomycetes. After due physical identification these colonies are selectively transferred onto fresh medium aseptically.

Step IV: Well grown big cluster of colonies of the above selected organisms are cut in such a manner that the '*plugs*' comprise of both the organisms and the underlying agar.

Note: In case, the isolated organisms produces an antibiotic, it must normally diffuse into the agar medium.

Step V: The '**plugs**' are meticulously removed and placed on an agar plate which has already been seeded with a specific '**test organism**' that clearly shows a positive indication of the potential effectiveness and usefulness of the antibiotic in question.

Step VI: All the '**test plates**' are duly incubated for a stipulated temperature and duration required for the maximum (optimum) growth of the '**test organisms**'. In case, there exists a clear zone of inhibition around the '**plug**' of the actinomycete, it may be inferred that an '**antibiotic component**' is present in the '**plug**' which obviously inhibited the growth of the '**test organisms**'.

Step VII: '*Dereplication*' *i.e.*, to establish by appropriate means as to whether the chemical substance (**'antibiotic component'**) which affected the inhibition is either an already known compound* or happens to be a '*new antibiotic*'. In short, if the newly discovered **'antibiotic component'** is really promising and possesses remarkable marked and pronounced **antibiotic activity** only then it will be subjected to further thorough investigation.

<h2>9.2.2   Large-Scale Production</h2>

Always, the ultimate decision to carry out the large-scale production of a '*new antibiotic*' is based on several cardinal qualifying factors, such as: (*a*) its chemical properties, (*b*) its physical characteristics, and (*c*) its detailed biological activities.

However, there are *two* extremely vital requirements for production, namely:

(*i*) The organism should produce the **'new antibiotic'** most preferably, in a submerged culture as opposed to a surface culture, and

(*ii*) The organism should liberate and excrete the **'new antibiotic'** right into the prevailing culture medium.

There are, of course, some other important considerations also for the large-scale production of a **'new antibiotic'** that are of rather minor nature, such as:

(*i*) A few **'antibiotics'** are produced in the cells of the organisms and therefore, requires altogether special cost-involving extraction procedures for their final recovery.

(*ii*) Some other minor but equally important related considerations are, namely: **minimum inhibitory concentration (MIC)** against the strains of pathogenic organisms, chemical stability, activity *in vivo*, and lastly the toxic manifestations in mammals.

The most intricate, diligent and marvellous exploitation of the wisdom of the man in the application of the in-depth knowledge of **microbiology, biotechnology, pharmaceutical chemistry,** and **engineering** has ultimately opened the flood gate towards the development of **'newer antibiotics'** and their commercial production to curtail the existing human sufferings.

The various important sequential procedural steps that are essentially required for the large-scale production of antibiotics are stated as under:

(*i*) Invariably requires growth of the producing organisms in aerated stainless steel tanks with a capacity to hold thousands of gallons of the respective nutrient medium.

(*ii*) The fermentation process is duly initiated with the help of spores or occasionally, vegetative growth from a pure **stock culture**** of the organism.

(*iii*) The inoculation of the huge fermentation tanks are normally accomplished by carrying out successively the transfer of the organism to increasingly greater volumes of nutrient. The major advantages of making use of a large standard inoculum are as stated below:

---

  * Based on the chromatographic, physico-chemical properties, antibiotic spectrum and comparing the same to a database of previously identified compounds.

** **Stock Cultures:** These are maintained very carefully (*e.g.*, by lypholization) that essentially require transfer as infrequently as possible, as repeated transfers may ultimately select only those cells of the organism which are rather poor generators of antibiotic.

(*a*) Considerable reduction in the total incubation time required for the normal production of the antibiotic,

(*b*) Reduces importantly the slightest possible chance for undesired costly contamination by foreign microorganisms, and

(*c*) Caters for the best ever possible scope and opportunity for the entire control and management of subtle nutritional and environmental factors that vitally influence the ultimate yield of the *antibiotic*.

9.2.2.1 Phases in Fermentative Process

In fact, there are *two* important and distinct phases normally encountered in the fermentative process, namely:

(*a*) **Growth Phase of the Organism:** It is also sometimes referred to as the **'trophophase'**; wherein the number of organisms per unit time increases progressively, and

(*b*) **Idiophase of the Organism:** In the idiophase there is a substantial antibiotic production; and hence, invariably termed as the **'antibiotic production phase'**.

The above mentioned *two* phases in the fermentative process may be further explained with the help of the following diagram:

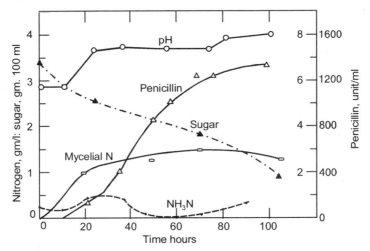

(Adapted from: Robbers, J.E. *et al.* 'Pharmacognosy and Pharmacobiotechnology', Williams & Wilkins, London, 1996)

In this particular instance, both the **growth phase** and the **idiophase** in the course of a typical **'penicillin fermentation'** performed in a culture-medium consisting of:

(*i*) **Source of carbon nutrition:** – *e.g.*, lactose and glucose;

(*ii*) **Nitrogen sources:** – *e.g.*, corn steep liquor; and

(*iii*) **Phosphate buffer:** – to provide *P* in the medium and also to maintain the pH of the medium.

The observations from the above diagram are as follows:

(*a*) The growth of microorganisms is shown in the above diagram by the curve indicating an enhancement of mycelial nitrogen (Mycelial N). This particular phenomenon continues right from the beginning (0 hours) of the culture period to nearly one day (24 hours).

Note: In the 'growth phase', the culture becomes thick by virtue of the formation of 'aggregates of fungal cells' usually known as mycelium.

(b) Glucose is preferentially consumed as compared to lactose specifically in the **'growth phase'**, as it may be employed as a prime source of C directly.

(c) Ammonia (NH_3) gets liberated also in the **'growth phase'** which is caused due to the deamination of various amino acids present in the *corn-steep liquor* (medium).

(d) Release of NH_3 evidently increases the pH of the medium from acidic to almost 7 (neutral). Thus, the ideal and optimum pH necessarily required for the stability of **'penicillin'** is 7, which is maintained by adding adequate 'phosphate buffers' into the medium.

(e) The **'penicillin production'** happens to rise very progressively and rapidly between 24-48 hours.

Note: Just in the initial stage of 'penicillin production', glucose gets fully utilized, and subsequently the fungus makes use of 'lactose' as a source of C.

(f) Interestingly, no additional growth takes place as the lactose cannot be used as such unless and until it gets converted to glucose and galactose *via* hydrolysis. Hence the prevailing decreased availability of C in the medium obviously offers a **'triggering mechanism'** in the production of penicillin.

9.2.2.2 Enhancing Yield in Large-Scale Production

During the past half-a-century an enormous volume of intensive and extensive research has been duly carried out by different groups/individuals across the world to determine and establish the optimal nutritional and environmental parameters required necessarily for antibiotic production. In reality, these conditions are certainly not quite similar to those required for maximum vegetative growth.

The various factors that exert vital impact upon the qualitative and quantitative antibiotic production are enumerated below:

- Sources of nutritional C and N
- Ratio of C/N in nutrients
- Mineral composition of medium
- Temperature of incubation
- Initial pH, control and management of pH during the entire course of fermentation.
- Aeration mode and rate
- Time-phase for addition of special growth and antibiotic enhancing materials.

Empiric Observations   The selection of optimal fermentation parameters is not only based on certain empiric observations but also serve as critical factors.

Examples

1. A few strains of microorganism *Bacillus subtilis* give rise to the maximum yields of **bacitracin***
at a C & N ratio of 1 : 15; but at a lower ratio 1 : 6 it forms **licheniformin*** which happens to
be a structurally related but an undesired commercial antibiotic.

---

* **Bacitracin:** Its antibacterial actions are similar to those of penicillin, including Gram + vc cocci and bacilli and some Gram –ve organisms. Because of its toxicity when used parenterally, it is normally used topically in ointment form.

** **Licheniformins:** These are antibiotic substances usually produced by *Bacillus licheniformis*.

2. **Phenylacetamide** or related substances when added to the culture medium of penicillin production though exhibits a very negligible effect on the yield of penicillin compounds, yet shows a very significant improvement upon the ultimate composition of the penicillin mixture.

3. **Phenylacetic Acid Derivative's** inclusion as a part and parcel in the nutrient mixture composition is observed to influence favourably the production of **Penicillin G;** and this particular vital step has considerably minimised the tedious problems with regard to the use of either unknown or variable composition of mixtures; besides, the significant cost, time and energy involved unnecessarily in separating the individual antibiotic substances.

4. **Acyl Moieties:** The application of different acyl groups so as to achieve the fermentative production of certain other penicillins, for instance: phenoxy-methylpenicillin (or Penicillin V) could not achieve appreciable feasible success in large-scale production; but surprisingly, the various semisynthetic techniques evolved not only superseded this specific line of action but also greatly enhanced the production of specialized penicillins.

5. **Mercaptothiazole:** The incorporation of mercaptothiazole in cultures of *Streptomyces aureofaciens* certainly approves the doctrine that certain 'chemical additives' might be useful without necessarily being introduced into the antibiotic molecule partially or fully.

6. **Effect of Enzyme Induction:** It has been proved beyond any reasonable doubt there are certain **'chemical additives'** that may enhance the antibiotic production by means of an enzyme induction effect.

Example: Methionine when added to a *cephalosporin C* fermentation process, during the growth phase of the organism (*i.e.*, **'trophophase'**) there is an apparent stimulation observed in the actual production of the antibiotic. As methionine does not behave as a precursor to the antibiotic in its biosynthetic process, in comparison to the performance of phenylacetic acid in the biosynthesis of Penicillin G, one may conclude and infer with rather stress and emphasis that methionine stimulates the ultimate production of cephalosporin C biosynthetic enzymes.

7. **Inhibition of Antibiotic Production:** Lysine exhibits an inhibition of penicillin fermentation by its presence in the culture medium which ultimately retards the antibiotic production. This particular phenomenon may, however, be explained by the fact that both lysine and penicillin are the end products of a branched biosynthetic pathway wherein the alpha-amino adipic acid serves as a **'common precursor'.** The production of **'lysine'** is regulated and monitored by two processes, *viz.*, repression or inhibition of the requisite enzymes needed for the production of alpha-aminoadipic acid. Hence, lysine puts a hault of alpha-aminoadipic acid formation which finally causes a decrease in the production of penicillin.

8. **Mutation and Strain Selection: Mutation*** influenced and persuaded by virtue of exposure of the parent-strain to uv-light, X-rays, or a host of mutagenic chemical substances *e.g.*, analogues of purines and pyrimidines, nitrogen mustards (viz., **mechlorethamine hydrochloride, mephalan, cyclophosphamide, chlorambucil)**** is widely recognized as the most virile and versatile means for the selection of **improved strains.**

---

* **Mutation:** A change in a gene potentially capable of being transmilted to offspring.
** Kar, A., **Medicinal Chemistry,** New Age International (Pvt) Ltd, New Delhi, 4th edn, 2006.

It is, however, pertinent to mention here that a constant search across the globe of natural sources for either newer wild-type(s) or various diversified species of organisms that afford to yield the **'antibiotic'** in much higher percentage than the original one. In the particular instance of induced mutations, lethal levels of the mutagen are adjusted in such a manner so that nearly 90-99% of the cells of the organism are destroyed (killed). Thus, the high-antibiotic-yielding mutants are selected meticulously from the remaining surviving cells.

Example: Production of Penicillin: Initially, a penicillin antagonism was noticed from a culture of *Penicillium notatum* Westling, that yielded a meagre 4 mg L^{-1} of penicillin from its culture medium. In other words, no mutation of *Penicillium notatum* were ever observed in the early selection process which could have given a significant yield of penicillin in the submerged fermentation technique. In 1944, there was an unique breakthrough in research whereby through the natural selection, a strain of *Penicillium chrysogenum* Thom was invented that raised the yield of penicillin almost by 10 times *i.e.*, 40 mg L^{-1}. Later on, with the help of vigorous modification of mutation techniques amalgamated with strain-selection, the ultimate yield of penicillin has been successfully enhanced to 21,000 mg L^{-1}.

The recent quantum advancement in the field of **molecular biology** there has been a tremendous expansion with specific reference to the knowledge of molecular regulation related to antibiotic biosynthesis. In this manner perhaps one may accomplish greater heights in the antibiotic production through such measures as:

• Rational manipulation(s) of the antibiotic-producing organisms to enhance its yield significantly.
• Deregulating the particular rate-limiting biosynthetic enzymes.
• Introduction of additional **'copies of genes'** matching the rate-limiting steps.
• Rational implementation of specific genes for parallel/alternate biosynthetic routes.
• Production of **'hybrid-antibiotics'** through the fermentatively-generated structural analogues of the natural antibiotic molecules.

9.2.2.3 *Separation and Isolation of Antibiotics*

Generally, the large-scale-produced antibiotics are released rapidly right into their nearest environment *i.e.*, the nutrient medium, where they get accumulated. However, there are some other instances *e.g.*, the peptide antibiotics, wherein the specific antibiotic is stored endocellularly (within the cells); the fermentation is maintained unless and until the cells accomplish an advanced matured physiologic age, the process of fermentation is arrested (ceased) whereby majority of the cell membranes have either lost their selective retention characteristic property or have undergone lysis—thereby releasing the antibiotic into the surrounding medium. In other words, therefore, the isolation process of various antibiotic substances is nothing but purely a recovery from the culture broth. The various **standard operating procedures (SOPs)** essentially comprise of: selective precipitation, specific adsorption, or finally the chosen extraction with an immiscible solvent.

In fact, in an ideal situation the very first isolation process must be as crisp, selective and efficient as possible so as to achieve the maximum yield, besides to help in subsequent purification without any cumbersome method. However, the particular chemical characteristic feature of an antibiotic shall be the ultimate determining factor, and also their accompanying metabolites to guide and dictate the manipulative procedures which may be adopted effectively in any particular instance.

Obviously, a balanced compromise procedure that is economically viable and feasible shall be the **'ideal procedure'** for all practical purposes.

The various means of extraction and purification of **'antibiotic substances'** may be accomplished through a number laid-down, tested and tried techniques that shall now be discussed briefly as under:

(*a*) **Liquid-Liquid Extraction:** Invariably the application of certain water-immiscible organic solvents *e.g.*, chloroform, solvent ether, carbon tetrachloride etc., are exercised for the extraction of most antibiotics. This particular process has evidently *two* major disadvantages, namely:

     (*i*) Lacks high-degree of selectivity because majority of solvents, which are fairly cheap and hence economical, tend to be employed on a large-scale production, and

     (*ii*) Comparatively inefficient as most of the known *'antibiotic substances'* are generally highly polar molecules.

Interestingly, in most instances the above *two* serious drawbacks are easily circumvented by adopting a **chemical-engineered-flow process;** but even then the highly polar 'antibiotics' fail to separate in which the partition-coefficient obviously favours the aqueous phase.

(*b*) **Recovery through Adsorption:** Extremely polar antibiotics *i.e.*, **the aminoglycoside antibiotics,** such as: **neomycin, streptomycin, paromomycin, kanamycin, amikacin, gentamycin, tobramycin, netilmicin,** are normally recovered from the culture medium through adsorption on certain appropriate adsorbent. It has been observed that—

• Most adsorbents remove highly polar antibiotics from culture media with varying degree of selectivity.

• Selecting a suitable adsorbent offers major limitations by virtue of the fact that while applying reversal of the adsorption process for recovering the antibiotic(s) very careful and moderate conditions be applied so as to avoid its possible denaturation/destruction.

• Ideally, the application of controlled-activity grade charcoal as an adsorbent, and subsequent elution with a dilute mineral acid (H_2SO_4) is normally employed as an universal method of choice.

(*c*) **Chromatography-Recrystallization-Standard Manipulations:** It is, however, pertinent to state here that as soon as one is able to lay hands onto the **'crude antibiotic'** recovered from the culture medium (or nutrient broth), it becomes absolutely necessary to accomplish the said product in its purest form within the permissible attainable limits of purity. In order to achieve this the 'crude product' is subjected to various advanced techniques of chromatography, followed by meticulous recrystallization procedure, and ultimately subjected to the standard manipulative operations using specific skill and wisdom.

Salient Features   Some of the salient features required to cause a suitable extent of purification are:

1. The attempt to achieve a very high degree of *'chemical purity'* is neither practicable nor necessary for therapeutic purposes.

2. Foreign proteins *i.e.*, extraneous metabolites, responsible for undesirable side-effects are excluded automatically through the process of purification.

3. Complete separation/elimination of closely structurally related antibiotic substances is invariably unfeasible.

4. Antibiotics derived from various fermentative procedures most frequently employed in therapy are, in true sense, admixtures of very intimately related chemical entities having one of the metabolites predominantly present in the mixture.

5. Reproducible therapeutic response is of prime importance, which must be attained through permissible practical limits due to the fact that a given antibiotic compound always constitute a major component of the mixture.

6. It also furnishes the economic viability of antibiotic substances in various drug formulative operations by virtue of the fact that the inefficiency and total expenses involved for complete separation of closely related chemical substances having unequal relative concentrations, may be avoided to a great extent.

Example: Chlortetracycline present upto 6% in the commercial *tetracycline* fairly represents an actual realistic and practical approach of such purification considerations.

Note: **The overall accepted standards of purity for antibiotics and other antibiotic formulations (i.e., dosage forms) are strictly controlled and monitored by the pharmacopocia of various countries, such as: USP; B.P.; Eur. P.; Int. P.; Ind. P.; Japanese P., etc.**

(*d*) **Purity of Antibiotic:** The highest attainable purity of an antibiotic is an absolute necessity so as to minimise its undesirable side effects.

Example: Vancomycin is a glycopeptide antibiotic particularly effective for the treatment of **endocarditis*** caused by Gram +ve bacteria. However, its wide application and usefulness was grossly restricted due to its **nephrotoxicity.**** Interestingly, upon much improved purity status of vancomycin not only reduced nephrotoxicity significantly but also raised its position in the therapeutic armamentarium.

(*e*) **Antibiotic Masking of Microbial Contaminants:** The **parenteral preparations** need to be guaranteed for their stringent sterility test(s) in the presence of an antibiotic. Therefore, it has become almost necessary to assess the masking of the very presence of the microbial contaminants by means of the bacteriostatic action exerted by the prevailing antibiotic.

There are, in fact, *three* basic approaches, which are not only vital but also fundamental in nature, that may be employed so as to eliminate as far as possible the **'antibiotic masking'** of microbial contaminants, such as:

1. All antibiotic formulations (dosage forms) which are essentially inactivated promptly either by chemical or biological methods must be suitably treated before carrying out the test for sterility.

   Examples:
   (*a*) Inactivation of the enzyme *penicillinase* by **Penicillin G,** and
   (*b*) Inactivation of hydroxylamine hydrochloride by **Streptomycin.**

---

* **Endocarditis:** Inflammation of the lining membrane of the heart. It may be due to invasion of microorganisms or an abnormal immunological reaction.
** **Nephrotoxicity:** A toxic substance that damages specifically the kidney tissues.

2. Most parenteral antibiotic preparations, particularly those having the relatively more stable ones, may be evaluated conveniently by subjecting the preparations to such a level of dilution so that the **'antibiotic level'** is definitely below the **minimum threshold concentration** for its activity, and

3. Physically removing, at the very first instance, any possible microorganisms by the help of a sterile Millipore filter in such a manipulative manner such that the organisms (undesired) are evidently separated from the antibiotic.

9.2.2.4 *Sophisticated Skillful Antibiotic Preparations*

A lot of wisdom, skill and knowledge has been rightly incorporated in accomplishing fairly stable sophisticated antibiotic preparations. There are various ways and means that have been explored meticulously in order to achieve these objectives, namely:

(*a*) Shielding of relatively less stable antibiotics in gastric juice (acidic) through various chemical and physical approaches,

(*b*) **'Prodrug Approach'**: Usage of rather insoluble corresponding antibiotic analogues so as to get rid of objectionable taste, and thus make it more patient-friendly especially in certain vital oral formulations.

Example: Chloramphenicol Succinate/Palmitate—The bitter taste of chloramphenicol is completely masked by preparing its corresponding esters for use in suitable pareutral preparations.

(*c*) **Soluble/Insoluble Derivatives:** The preparation of various soluble or insoluble derivative of antibiotics are afforded so as to make it convenient for its desired delivery at a particular site *in vivo*.

Example: Gentamycin sulphate, Neomycin sulphate, Tetracycline Hydrochloride, Penicillin G sodium etc. These salts are more readily absorbed *in vivo* and hence enhance their therapeutic efficacy.

It is pertinent to cite here certain **classical examples** highlighting the sophisticated skillful antibiotic preparations, namely:

(*i*) Use of **'buffers'** in oral penicillin G formulations significantly minimise its loss of potency due to gastric juice,

(*ii*) Enteric coating of erythromycin tablets with synthetic polymers, definitely protect the **macrolactone** ring present in it, till it sails through the entire distinctly acidic environment of the stomach (*i.e.*, gastric juice) and subsequently makes it pass into the long small intestinal canal where it eventually gets absorbed.

Example: The two commonly used modified versions of erythromycin are, namely:

(*a*) Erythromycin ethylsuccinate, and

(*b*) Erythromycin estolate (*i.e.* the lauryl sulphate salt of the propionyl ester).

These two salts are very much insoluble than the parent macrolide antibiotic; and provide *dual usefulness* in oral pareteral suspensions viz., *first*, to refrain of their very bitter taste due to poor solubility; and *secondly*, to protect their safe journey till the lower end of the intestine.

(*iii*) Enhancing the solubility characteristics of erythromycin for allowing it to be given intravenously could be accomplished by making its **glucoheptonate** and **lactobionate** salts.

(*iv*) Benzathine penicillin G possesses insoluble property, and this contributes heavily as a stability factor for its usage in oral suspensions.

(v) Penicillins give rise to insoluble procaine and benzathine salts that are used extensively through IM route for prolonged and sustained effects.

(vi) **Probenecid** is invariably employed as an adjunct substance to the *penicillins*; and this affords *two* vital classical plus points: *first,* it checks the tubular excretion of penicillins; and *secondly,* to accomplish significant sustained blood levels of these antibiotics.

(vii) **Amoxicillin and Ticarcillin** supplemented with a **β-lactamase inhibitor,** clavulanic acid, in various preparations usually offers an expanded therapeutic spectrum.

In short, the classical examples enumerated above from (i) through (vii) paints a beautiful rosy picture which further testifies the reality that a constant research in the applications of different aspects of pharmaceutical technology with a very strong bearing on the basic fundamental knowledge of medicinal chemistry shall ever open the limitless boundaries of 'wonderful drug formulations' to save the mankind of its sufferings.

9.3 CLASSIFICATION OF ANTIBIOTICS

Antibiotics are broadly classified on the basis of their inherent chemical structures as stated below:

   (i) Aminoglycosides,
  (ii) Anthracyclines,
 (iii) Cephalosporins,
  (iv) β-Lactams,
   (v) Lincosamides,
  (vi) Macrolides,
 (vii) Penicillins,
(viii) Polypeptide antibiotics,
  (ix) Tetracyclines, and
   (x) Miscellaneous antibiotics.

All these different categories of antibiotics shall now be described individually in the sections that follows:

9.3.1 Aminoglycosides

The **aminoglycosides** each contain one or more amino sugars, for instance: **neosamine** or **glucosamine,** bridged by glycoside linkages to a basic, either amino or guanidino, six-membered carbon ring, such as: streptamine or streptidine as given below:

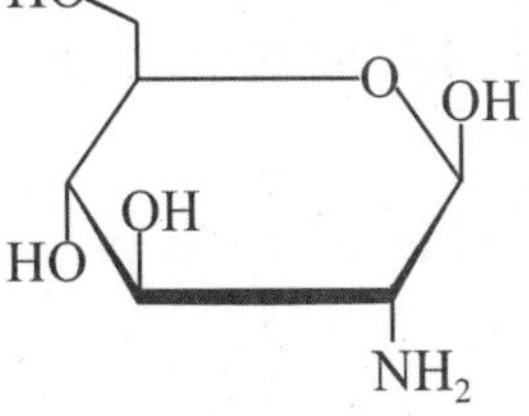

Glucosamine

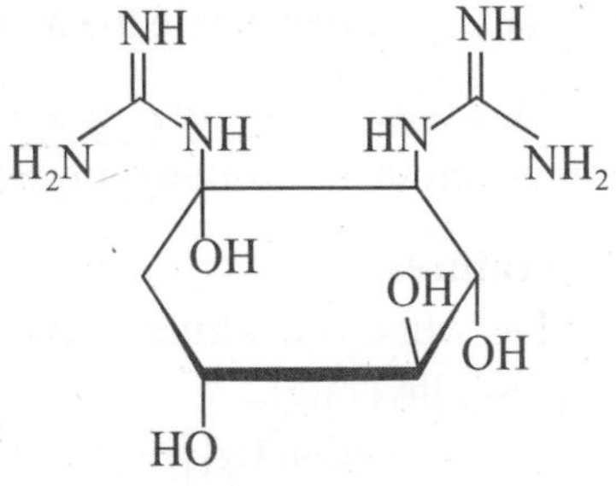

Streptidine

Aminoglycosides occupy a coveted status in the domain of antibiotics exclusively for the control, management and treatment of infections caused by Gram-negative bacilli. However, the overall treatment of most nosocomial Gram negative basillary infections with the aid of third-generation cephalosporins, carbapenems and new fluoroquinolones have made the aminoglycosides more or less as the alternative drugs unless and until resistant strains are suspected invariably amongst the immuno suppressed patients.

It is worthwhile to mention here that the major spectrum of activity of the **aminoglycosides** essentially comprise of aerobic Gram-negative bacilli and *Staphylococcus aureus.*

A few important members of the **aminoglycoside antibiotics** are, namely: **amikacin, gentamycin, paramycin, kanamycin, netilmicin, streptomycin** and **tobramycin** which shall be discussed separately as under:

9.3.1.1 Amikacin

Synonyms   Lukadin.

Biological Source   It is a **semisynthetic aminoglycoside antibiotic** derived from **Kanamycin A.**

Chemical Structure

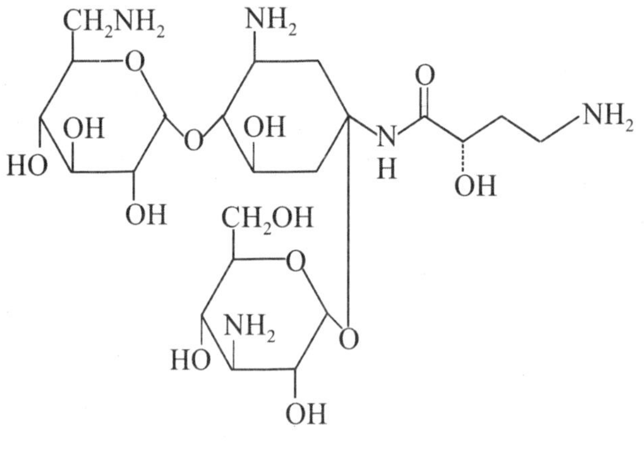

Amikacin

1-N-[L (-)-4-Amino-2-hydroxybutyryl] kanamycin A; ($C_{22}H_{43}N_5O_{13}$).

The presence of the 4-amino-2-hydroxybutyryl moiety protects the antibiotic against the enzymic deactivation at many locations, while the activity of the parent molecule is still maintained.

Preparation   **Amikacin** is obtained by acylation of the C-1 amino function of the 2-deoxystreptamine group of **kanamycin** with L-(-)-4-amino-2-hydroxybutyric acid.

Characteristic Features
1. It is obtained as white crystalline powder from a mixture of methanol-isopropanol having mp 203-204°C (sesquihydrate).
2. Its specific optical rotation $[\alpha]_D^{23} + 99°$ (C = 1.0 in water).

Identification Tests

Amikacin Sulphate ($C_{22}H_{43}N_5O_{13} \cdot 2H_2SO_4$) (Amikin; Amiklin; Biklin; Amikavet; Fabianol; Kaminax; Mikavir; Novamin; Pierami): It is obtained as an amorphous form which gets decomposed at 220-230°C. Its specific optical rotation $[\alpha]_D^{22} + 74.75°$ (water).

Uses

1. **Amikacin** is observed to be fairly stable to most of the aminoglycoside inactivating enzymes, and is, therefore, considered to be valuable for the treatment of serious infections usually caused by Gram –ve bacteria that are resistant to gentamycin or tobramycin.
2. It is mostly employed in a wide range of infections, such as: septicemia, serious infections due to burns, urinary tract, respiratory tract and various soft tissues, meningitis, peritonitis, osteomyelitis, omphalitis in neonates, and other serious surgical infections.

9.3.1.2 Gentamicin

Synonym   Gentamycin.

Biological Sources   It is an antibiotic complex produced by the fermentation of *Micromonospora purpurea* and *M. echinospora;* and a number of variants thereof.

Chemical Structure

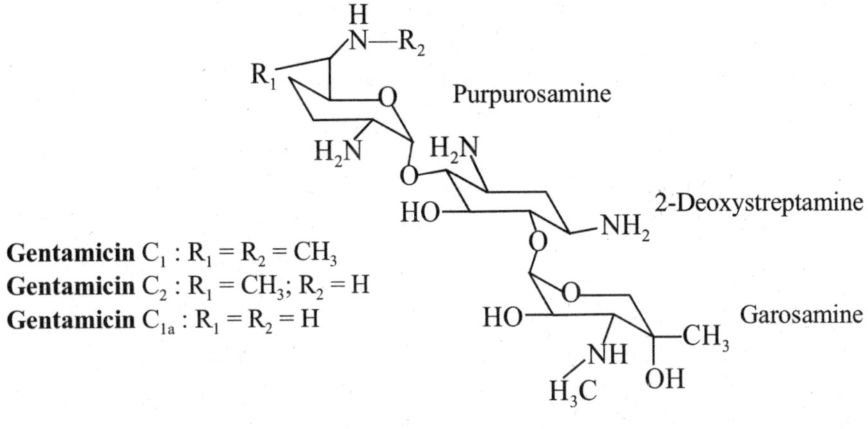

Gentamicin C_1 : $R_1 = R_2 = CH_3$
Gentamicin C_2 : $R_1 = CH_3$; $R_2 = H$
Gentamicin C_{1a} : $R_1 = R_2 = H$

Gentamicin

Preparation   **Gentamycin** is normally recovered from a fermentation broth produced when submerged cultures of two subspecies of *Micromonospora purpurea* are grown in the yeast extract-cerelose medium.

Characteristic Features

1. It is a white amorphous powder having mp 102-108°C
2. It has specific optical rotation $[\alpha]_D^{25} + 146°$.
3. It is found to be freely soluble in water, pyridine, DMF, in acidic media with salt formation; moderately soluble in methanol, ethanol, acetone; and almost insoluble in benzene and halogenated hydrocarbons. Characteristic features of some of its congeners are as follows:

S. No.	Gentamicin Congeners	Molecular formula	mp (°C)	$[\alpha]_D^{25}$
1	Gentamicin C_1	$C_{21}H_{43}N_5O_7$	94-100	+ 158
2	Gentamicin C_2	$C_{20}H_{41}N_5O_7$	107-124	+ 160
3	Gentamicin C_{1a}	$C_{19}H_{39}N_5O_7$	–	–

Identification Tests

1. **Gentamicin Complex Sulphate:** [Synonyms Alcomicin; Bristagen; Cidomycin; Duragentum; Garamycin; Garasol; Genoptic; Gentacin; Gentak; Gentalline; Gentalyn; Gentibioptal; Genticin; Gentocin; Gentogram; Gent-Ophtal; Gentrasul; Lugacin; Nichogencin; Ophtagram; Pangram; Refobacin; Septopal; Sulmycin; and U-Gencin.]

   It is obtained as a white, hygroscopic powder having mp 218-237°C. It has specific optical rotation $[\alpha]_D^{25}$ + 102°. It is soluble in formanide and in ethylene glycol.

2. **Gentamicin Hydrochloride:** It has mp 194-209°C; and specific optical rotation $[\alpha]_D^{25}$ + 113°. It is found to be freely soluble in water, methanol; slightly soluble in ether; and practically insoluble in other organic solvents.

Uses

1. It is currently the most important drug of choice for the treatment of infections caused by most aerobic Gram-negative bacteria, besides several strains of *Staphylococci*.

2. It essentially exhibits a broad-spectrum antibacterial activity.

3. It is found to be specifically effective against *Pseudomonas*, because species of this genus resistant to 'other antibiotics' have proved to be an important cause of **surgical infections.** In the same vein, gentamicin, is also very effective in severe burned-skin patients *i.e.*, third-degree burns; and severe UTI* infections, both caused by *Pseudomonas*.

4. It is employed topically in the treatment of impetigo, infected bed sores, burns and nasal staphylococcal carrier state, pyodermata and also in the infections of external-eye.

Note: Because of gentamicin's systemic toxicity, its present systemic usage is restricted and limited to life-threatening infections produced by Citrobacter, Klebsiella-Enterobacter-Serratia, Proteus and Pseudomonas. To cause an effective control it is invariably combined along with either penicillin or cephalosporin.

9.3.1.3 *Kanamycin*

Biological Sources **Kanamycin** is an **'antibiotic complex'** produced by *Streptomyces kanamyceticus* Okami & Umezawa from the Japanese soil.** The antibiotic complex is comprised of *three* distinct components, namely: **kanamycin A**—representing the *major* component, and usually designated as **kanamycin;** besides two *minor* components (congeners more precisely) usually known as **kanamycins B and C.**

---

* **UTI** = Urinary tract infections.
** Umezawa *et al.*, *J. Antibiot. 10A*, 181 (1957); US patent *2, 931, 798* (1960).

Chemical Structure

	R	R'
Kanamycin A:	NH₂	OH
Kanamycin B:	NH₂	NH₂
Kanamycin C:	OH	NH₂

Interestingly, these *three* antibiotics essentially comprise of *two* aminosugars (*i.e.*, 6-amino-6-deoxy-D-glucose) which are linked individually to one single 2-deoxystreptamine aglycone (*i.e.*, non-sugar) residue.

Characteristic Features   The characteristic features of all the *three* kanamycins and their respective salts shall be discussed as under:

(*a*) **Kanamycin A: [$C_{18}H_{36}N_4O_{11}$];** O-3-Amino-3-deoxy-α-D-glucopyranosyl-(1 → 6)-O-[6-amino-6-deoxy-α-D-glucopyranosyl-(1 → 4)-2-deoxy-D-streptamine.

It is obtained as crystals from a mixture of methanol and ethanol. It has specific optical rotation $[\alpha]_D^{24}$ + 146° (0.1N. H_2SO_4).

Kanamycin A Sulphate   [*Synonyms*: Cantrex; Crystalomicina; Enterokanacin; Kamycin; Kamynex; Kanabristol; Kanacedin; Kanamytrex; Kanasig; Kanatrol; Kanicin; Kannasyn; Kantres; Kantrox; Klebcil; Otokalixin; Resistomycin; Ophthalmokalixan; Kantrexil; Kano; Kanesein; Kanaqua.]

It is obtained as irregular prisms that decompose over a wide range above 250°C. It is freely soluble in water; and almost insoluble in nonpolar solvents and the common alcohols.

Note: USP-requires that Kanamycin A sulphate contains not less than 75% Kanamycin A on an anhydrous basis.

(*b*) **Kanamycin B: [$C_{18}H_{37}N_5O_{10}$]:** [Synonyms: Bekanamycin; Aminodeoxy-kanamycin; NK-1006].

It is obtained as crystals having mp 178-182°C (dec.).

It has specific optical rotations $[\alpha]_D^{18}$ + 130° (C = 0.5 in H_2O); $[\alpha]_D^{21}$ + 114° (C = 0.98 in H_2O). It is found to be soluble in water, formamide; slightly soluble in chloroform, isopropanol; and practically insoluble in the common alcohols and nonpolar solvents.

Kanamycin B Sulphate   [*Synonyms*: Coltericin; Kanendomycin; Kanendos.]

(c) **Kanamycin C: [$C_{18}H_{36}N_4O_{11}$]:** It is obtained as crystals from methanol + ethanol which get decomposed above 270°C. It has specific optical rotation $[\alpha]_D^{20} + 126°$ (H_2O). It is found to be soluble in water; slightly soluble in formamide; and practically insoluble in nonpolar solvents and the common alcohols.

9.3.1.4 Neomycin

Synonyms Fradiomycin; Mycifradin; Neomin; Neolate; Neomas; Pimavecort; Vonamycin Powder V.

Biological Source It is an **'antibiotic complex'** comprised of neomycins A, B and C. It is obtained from *Streptomyces fradiae**.

Chemical Structure

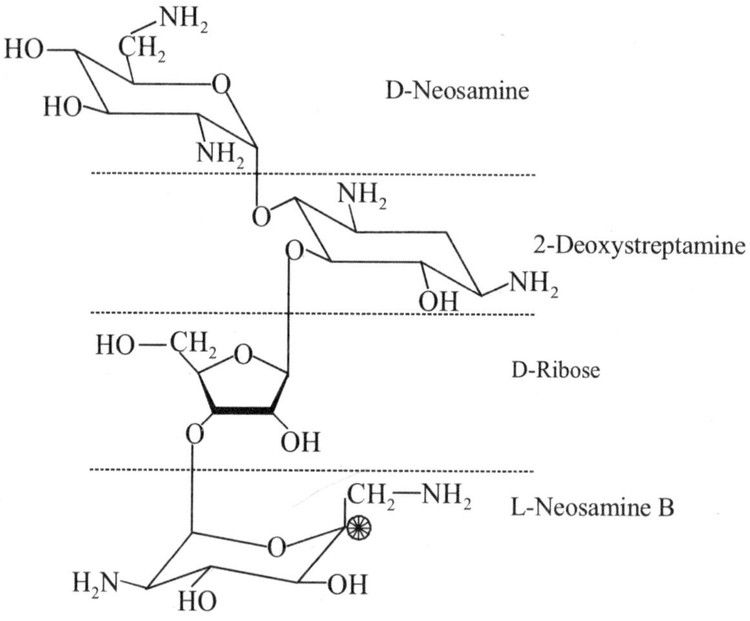

Neomyicin B (Framycetin)
[Neomycin C is Epimer at ✳]

Neomycin is usually obtained as a mixture of neomycin B (*Framycetin*) and its epimer **neomycin C,** the latter constitutes 5-15% of the mixture. Interestingly, in contrast to the other clinically useful aminoglycosides, neomycin is observed to comprise essentially of *three* sugar residues strategically attached to *2-deoxystreptamine* as shown above. One of the three sugars present is the *D-ribose* (a common sugar).

Characteristic Features

(a) **Neomycin Complex:** It is an amorphous base. It is soluble in water, methanol and acidified ethanol; and almost insoluble in common organic solvents.

---

* Waksman and Lechevalier, *Science*, **109**, 305 (1949).

(b) **Neomycin A: [Synonym: Neamine]: $C_{12}H_{26}N_4O_6$:** It is obtained as crystals either from water or aqueous ethanol that get decomposed at 225-226°C. It has specific optical rotation $[\alpha]_D^{25}$ + 112.8° (C = 1)

    Neomycin A Hydrochloride: ($C_{12}H_{26}N_4O_6$.4HCl): It is obtained as an amorphous powder decomposing between 250-260°C. Its specific optical rotation is $[\alpha]_D^{25}$ + 83° (C = 1).

    Neomycin A, N-Acetyl Derivative: [$C_{12}H_{26}N_4O_6$.(CH_3CO)$_4$]: It is obtained as crystals from methanol having mp 334-336°C. It has specific optical rotation $[\alpha]_D^{25}$ + 87°C (C = 1).

(c) **Neomycin B: [Synonyms: Antibiotique EF 185; Framycetin; Enterfram; Framygen; Soframycin; Actilin;] ($C_{23}H_{46}N_6O_{13}$):** It yields on hydrolysis *neomycin A* and *neobiosamine B.*

    Neomycin B Hydrochloride: It is an amorphous white powder having specific optical rotation $[\alpha]_D^{20}$ + 57° (H_2O). Its solubility in mg ml^{-1} at ~ 28°C: water 15.0; methanol 5.7; ethanol 0.65; isopropanol 0.05; isoamyl alcohol 0.33; cyclohexane 0.06; benzene 0.03; and is almost insoluble in acetone, ether, other organic solvents.

    Neomycin B Sulphate: [Synonyms: Biosol, Bykomycin; Endomixin; Fraquinol; Myacine; Neosulf; Neomix; Neobreltin; Nivemycin, Tuttomycin;]. It is an amorphous white powder which is almost tasteless. It has specific optical rotation $[\alpha]_D^{20}$ + 54° (C = 2 in H_2O). Its solubility in mg ml^{-1} ~ 28°C: water 6.3; methanol 0.225; ethanol 0.095; isopropanol 0.05; and almost insoluble in acetone, ether, chloroform. The aqueous solutions are quite stable between a pH 2 to 9. The highly purified preparations are very stable to alkali, but unstable to acids. On being refluxed with Ba (OH)$_2$ for 18 hours it exhibited no loss of activity. On boiling with mineral acids it gives rise to furfural (an aldehyde), and also an organic base.

(d) **Neomycin C: [$C_{23}H_{46}N_6O_{13}$]:** It yields on hydrolysis neomycin A (*i.e.,* neamine) and neobiosamine C.

Uses

1. It has good activity against Gram-positive and Gram-negative bacteria, but is very *ototoxic*. Therefore, its usages has been severely restricted to the oral treatment of intestinal infections.

   Note: It is poorly absorbed from the digestive tract.

2. It also finds its enormous use in topical applications, such as: eardrops, eyedrops, and ointments.

9.3.1.5 Netilmicin

Synonyms   1-N-Ethylsisomicin; Sch-20569.

Biological Sources   **Sisomicin** is known to be the dehydro analogue of **Gentamicin C_{1a}** (see section 9.3.1.2), and is produced by cultures of *Micromonospora inyoensis*. Nevertheless, the semisynthetic N-ethyl derivative, **netilmicin,** is mostly used medicinally because it has an almost identical activity to **gentamicin,** but produces significantly much less ototoxicity.

Chemical Structure

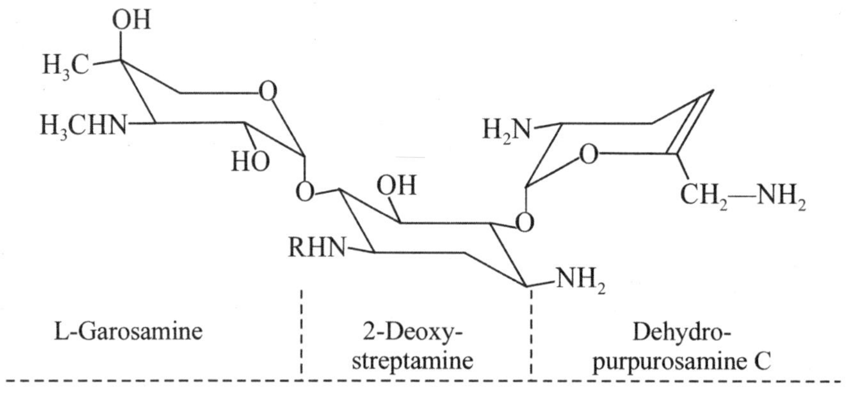

L-Garosamine   2-Deoxy-streptamine   Dehydro-purpurosamine C

Netilmicin : R = C_2H_5
Sisomicin : R = H

Characteristic Features   It has specific optical rotation $[\alpha]_D^{26} + 164°$ (C = 3 in H_2O).

Netilmicin Sulphate [($C_{21}H_{41}N_5O_7$)$_2$.5H_2SO_4] [Synonyms: Certomycin; Nettilin; Netilyn; Netromicine; Netromycin; Nettacin; Vectacin; Zetamicin.]

Preparation   It is a semi-synthetic derivative of sisomycin and is skillfully prepared by ethylation of the amino group in the 1-position of the 2-deoxy-streptamine ring.

Characteristic Features   It is an off-white powder; pH (1 in 25 solution) ranges between 3.5-5.5; and pKa 8.1. It is found to be very soluble in water.

Uses   Its antibiotic profile is very similar to that of **Gentamicin.**

9.3.1.6 *Streptomycin*

Synonym   Streptomycin A.

Biological Sources   After the qualified success and the overwhelming recognition of the therapeutic potential of penicillin an extensive and intensive search for other antibiotic substances gathered a tremendous momentum and stimulation. A major target and goal was the discovery of such antibiotics that are antagonistic to the Gram-negative microorganisms. **Streptomycin** was obtained from a strain of *Streptomyces griseus* (Krainsky) Waksman et Henrici (*Actinomycetaceae*); and produced by the soil Actinomycete.

Chemical Structure

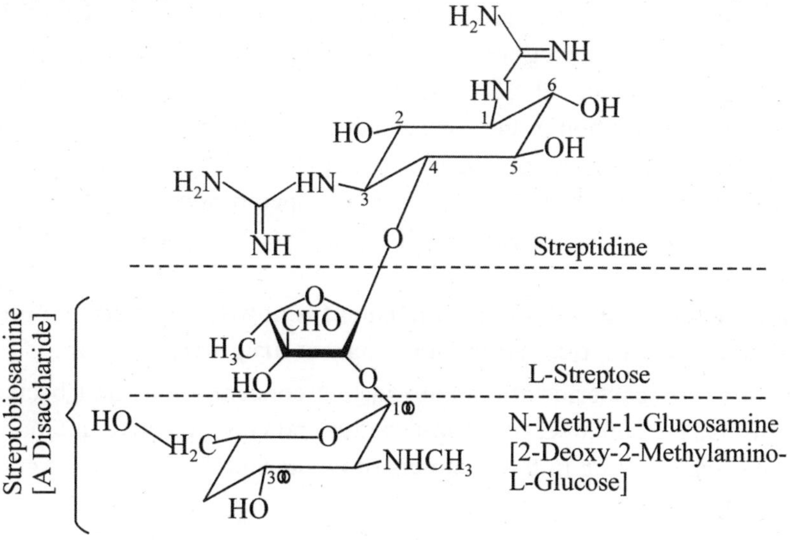

Streptomycin

Streptomycin has essentially *two* sugar components, namely: L-streptose and 2-deoxy-2-methylamino-L-glucose, which are linked to a non-sugar moiety streptidine evidently through *two* ether-linkages.

Characteristic Features **Streptomycin** is normally available as the trichloride, trichloride-calcium chloride double salt, phosphate or sesquisulphate, which invariably occur as powder or granules. It is more or less odourless but possesses a slightly bitter taste. It has been observed that most of its salts are hygroscopic and deliquesce on exposure to air; however, they are not affected by air or light. Nevertheless, the salts are very soluble in water; and practically insoluble in ether, ethanol and chloroform. The solutions of its salts are levorotatory.

(*a*) **Streptomycin Trichloride: [$C_{21}H_{39}N_7O_{12}$·3HCl] [Synonym: Streptomycin Hydrochloride]:** It has specific optical rotation $[\alpha]_D^{25} - 84°$. Its solubilities in mg ml^{-1} at ~ 28°C are: water > 20; methanol > 20; ethanol 0.90; isopropanol 0.12; isoamyl alcohol 0.117; petroleum ether 0.02; ether 0.01; and carbon tetrachloride 0.042.

(*b*) **Streptomycin Trihydrochloride—Calcium Chloride Double Salt: [($C_{21}H_{39}N_7O_{12}$·3HCl)$_2$. CaCl$_2$] [Synonym: Streptomycin hydrochloride-Calcium chloride complex]:** It is prepared from the streptomycin trihydrochloride salt. It is highly hygroscopic in nature, and gets decomposed at ~ 200°C. Its specific optical rotation $[\alpha]_D^{25} - 76°$.

(*c*) **Streptomycin Sesquisulphate: [($C_{21}H_{39}N_7O_{12}$)$_2$·3H$_2$SO$_4$]: [Synonyms: Streptomycin sulphate; Agristrep; Streptobrettin; Vetstrep]:** It is a white to light gray or pale buff powder having faint amine-like odour. It solubilities in mg ml^{-1} at ~ 28°C are: water > 20; methanol 0.85; ethanol 0.30; isopropanol 0.01; petroleum ether 0.015; ether 0.035; and carbon tetrachloride 0.035.

Uses

1. It is a potent antibacterial, and more so as a tuberculosstatic agent. The MIC of streptomycin for *M. tuberculosis* is nearly 0.5 mcg ml^{-1}; whereas many sensitive Gram-negative bacteria have MICs in the range of 2-4 mcg ml^{-1}.

2. **Streptomycin** exerts its action in the control and management of *Yersinia pestis* (*plague*) and *Francisella tularensis* (*tularemia*); and in such typical incidences, it is invariably combined with a **sulphonamide drug.** Mostly hyphenated therapeutic approaches are practised, such as: **streptomycin-penicillin** used for **endocarditis***; and **streptomycin-tetracyclin** employed for **brucellosis.****

Note: The incidence of serious auditory impairment is now recognized and established to be far greater with dihydro-streptomycin than the parent drug streptomycin.

3. **Streptomycin** exerts bacteriostatic action in low concentrations and bactericidal in high concentrations to a good number of Gram-negative and Gram-positive microorganisms.

4. It is an alternate choice drug in the treatment of **chancroid*****, rat-bite fevers (*Spirillum* and *Streptobacillus*).

Biosynthesis of Components of Streptomycin   The so called '**components of streptomycin**' essentially comprise of two major portions, namely: *first*—the *streptidine* moiety; and *secondly* – the **streptobiosamine,** which is, in fact a *disaccharide*, that consists of the two sugar residues *viz.*, **streptose** plus *2-deoxy-2-methylamino-L-glucose.* It has been revealed through an elaborated biosynthetic studies that all the *three* aforesaid '**components of streptomycin**' are derived exclusively from D-glucose. As on date no exact scientific evidence is available which may give an ample proof about the point of attachment of the three different components in the streptomycin molecule. Further, there is scanty and paucity of an elaborated explanation or information with regard to the manner whereby the individual moieties present in an aminoglycoside antibiotic. However, based on the ground realities derived from the metabolic relationships of glucose to the different moieties could be gathered and prevailed, upon directly from the various biosynthetic origins of the '**components of streptomycin**' as shown under.

Sailent Features   The salient features of the biosynthesis of **components of streptomycin** are, namely:

1. **Streptose: D-Glucose** is first converted to 4-hexosulose which on being subjected to transannular rearrangement gives rise to **streptose.**

2. **Streptidine:** D-Glucose upon demethylation yields myoinositol which upon amination produces **streptamine.** The resulting **streptamine** in the presence of L-arginine ultimately affords the formation of streptidine.

---

* **Endocarditis:** Inflammation of the lining membrane of the heart.

** **Brucellosis:** A widespread infection febrile disease affecting mostly cattle, goats, swine, and sometimes humans. In humans, it is called brucellosis or malta fever and is caused by several Brucella species.

*** **Chancroid:** A highly infectious nonsyphlitic ulcer; and is caused by *Haemophilus ducreyi*—a Gram-negative bacillus.

Biosynthetic Pathway of Components of Streptomycin

3. **2-Deoxy-2-methylamino-L-glucose:** D-Glucose through deoxidation and methylamination yields 2-deoxy-2-methylamino-L-glucose.

9.3.1.7 Tobramycin

Synonyms Nebramycin Factor 6; NF 6; Gernebcin; Tobracin; Tobradistin; Tobralex; Tobramaxin; Tobrex;

Biological Sources It is a single factor antibiotic comprising about 10% of nebramycin, previously known as **tenebrimycin, tenemycin;** and the **aminoglycosidic antibiotic complex produced by Streptomyces tenebrarius.**

Chemical Structure

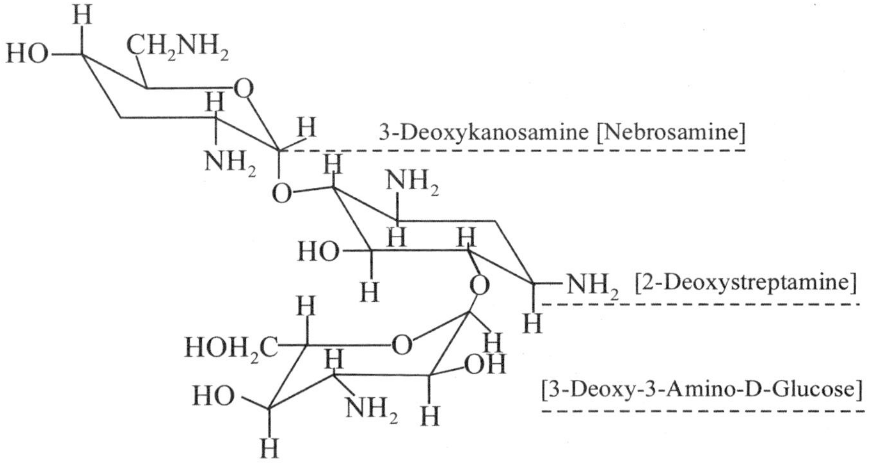

Tobramycin

Tobramycin essentially contains two aminosugar residues namely: nebrosamine and 3-deoxy-3-amino-D-glucose, and a 2-deoxystreptamine moiety. It has been found to be structurally related to **kanamycin B** (section 9.3.1.3); but evidently differs only in the absence of the 3-hydroxyl group present in the **kanasamine residue.**

9.3.2   Anthracyclines

The **anthracyclines** *i.e.*, the **anthracycline antibiotics** essentially contain an anthraquinone moiety fused with a non-aromatic ring:

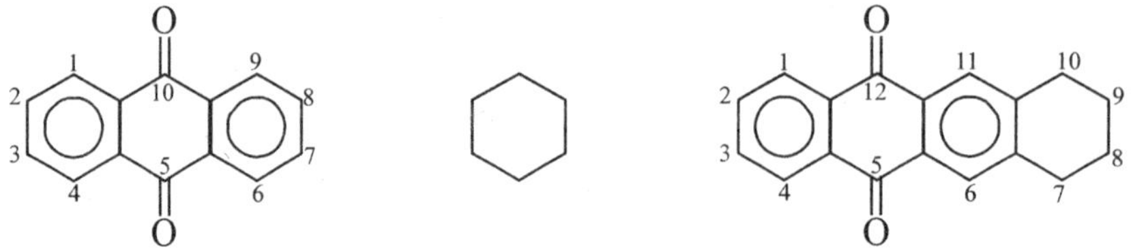

Anthraquinone   Non-Aromatic Ring   Anthracycline

There are quite a few **'anthracycline antibiotics'** which have been isolated, characterized and evaluated for their therapeutic activities, namely: **doxorubicin, epirubicin, aclacinomycin A,** and **idarubicin.** However, **mitoxantrone (mitozantrone),** a synthetic structural analogue of the **anthracyclinones** wherein both the non-aromatic ring and the respective aminosugar have been duly replaced by aminoalkyl side-chains.

All the above mentioned potent compounds shall be described in the sections that follows:

9.3.2.1   *Doxorubicin*

Synonyms   14-Hydroxydaunomycin; NSC-123127; FI-106.

Biological Sources **Doxorubicin,** an anthracycline antibiotic is obtained from the cultures of *Streptomyces peucetius* var *caesius*.

Chemical Structure

Doxorubicin

(8S-*cis*)-10 [(3-Amino-2, 3, 6-trideoxy-α-L-lyxo-hexopyranosyl) oxy]-7, 8, 9, 10-tetrahydro-6, 8, 11-trihydroxy-8-(hydroxyacetyl)-1-methoxy-5, 12-naphthacenedione; [$C_{27}H_{29}NO_{11}$]

Characteristic Feature **Doxorubicin** has mp 229-231°C.

Uses
1. It has one of the broadest spectra of antitumour activity displayed by antitumour drugs.
2. It is extensively employed to treat acute leukemias, lymphomas, and a large number of solid tumours.
3. It has been found to inhibit the synthesis of RNA copies of DNA by virtue of the intercalation of the planar molecule between base pairs on the DNA helix.

Note: The inherent 'sugar moiety' affords an additional strength besides playing a critical role in the sequence-recognition required for the binding.

4. **Doxorubicin** also exerts a few of its cytotoxic effects on account of the inhibition of the enzyme **topoisomerase II,** which is solely responsible for both cleaving and resealing of the double-stranded DNA during the replic-tion process.

Doxorubicin Hydrochloride [$C_{27}H_{29}NO_{11}$·HCl] [*Synonyms* **Adriacin; Adriblastina; Adriamycin**]

1. It is obtained as orange-red coloured thin needles having mp 204-205°C (decomposes).
2. It has specific optical rotation $[\alpha]_D^{20}$ + 248° (C = 0.1 in methanol).
3. It exhibits uv$_{max}$ (methanol): 233, 252, 288, 479, 496, 529 nm.
4. It is found to be soluble in water, methanol, aqueous alcohols; and almost insoluble in acetone, benzene, chloroform, ethyl ether and petroleum ether.
5. The aqueous solutions show different colours at different pH ranges, *e.g.*, at acidic pH yellow-orange; at neutral pH orange-red; and at pH > 9 violet-blue.
6. The aqueous solutions are unstable at higher temperatures or at either alkaline or acidic pHs.

Note: Doxorubicin may reasonably be anticipated to be a carcinogen*.

---

* *Seventh Annual Report on Carcinogen* (PB 95-10978, 1994), p. 86.

9.3.2.2 *Epirubicin*

Synonyms   4′-Epidoxorubicin; 4′-Epiadriamycin; Pidorubicin; 4′-EpiDX; IMI-28.

Biological Source   It has the same biological source as that doxorubicin. It is the structural analogue of the **anthracycline antibiotic doxorubicin,** wherein the only point of difference is in the position of the C-4 hydroxy group of the sugar moiety.

Chemical Structure

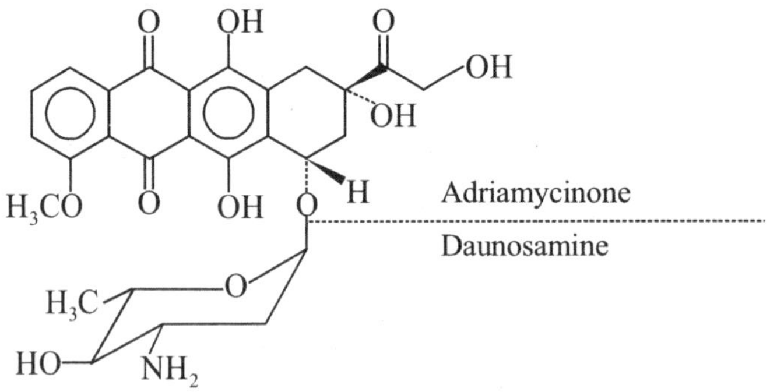

Epirubicin

4′-Epidoxorubicin; $C_{27}H_{29}NO_{11}$

Characteristic Features   **Epirubicin Hydrochloride [$C_{27}H_{29}NO_{11}$.HCl] [Synonyms Farmorubicin; Pharmorubicin].**

1. It is obtained as red-orange crystals having mp 185°C (decomposes).
2. It has specific optical rotation $[\alpha]_D^{20} + 274°$ (C = 0.01 in methanol).

Caution: Its solution should be protected from sunlight.

Uses

1. It is broadly employed as an antineoplastic agent.
2. It is proved to be particularly effective in the treatment of breast cancer, producing much lower side effects than **doxorubicin** itself.

Biosynthesis of Doxorubicin and Epirubicin   The various steps involved in the **biosynthesis of doxorubicin** and **epirubicin** are as follows:

1. The propionyl-CoA is used not only as a 'starter moiety' but also as a chain-extender *via* the methylmalonyl-CoA. The *Actinomycetes* (*e.g.,* **Streptomyces**) has a tendency to use propionate *via* methylation using SAM followed by incorporation of propionate by methylmalonyl-CoA.

Note: It has been observed that the incorporation of propionate by the methyl malonate extender units may undergo unusual frequent interruption, which process may be combated by the addition of further malonate extenders. The said phenomenon usually gives rise to an irregular sequence of methyl side-chains.

2. The alkanonic acid in the presence of S-adenosylmethiorine (SAM) and through aldol condensation yields **aklaviketone.**

3. The resulting **aklaviketone** undergoes reduction of $-\overset{\displaystyle O}{\overset{\|}{C}}-$ at C-7 with NADPH generating the **aklavinone**.

4. Further aklavinone with NADPH in the presence of oxygen causes hydroxylation at C-11 to produce **ε-rhodomycinone**.

5. At this juncture thiamine diphosphate-D-glucose (TDP) yielding thiamine diphosphate-L-daunosamine is introduced. Consequently, a series of *five* sequential reactions, such as: (*i*) glycosylation of 7-hydroxyl moiety; (*ii*) hydrolysis of ester; (*iii*) de-carboxylation 10-carboxylic acid group; (*iv*) oxidation to corresponding 13-ketone; and (*v*) methylation of 4-hydroxyl moiety, ultimately produces **daunorubicin (daunomycin)**.

6. The resulting daunorubicin undergoes hydroxylation at C-14 in the presence of oxygenated NADPH finally yields **doxorubicin (adriamycin)**.

7. Doxorubicin undergoes epimerization at C-4′ (see inset) in the following biosynthetic pathway, to produce **epirubicin**.

Biosynthetic Pathway of Doxorubicin and Epirubicin
[Adapted from: Dewick P.M. *Medicinal Natural Products* 2nd edn, 2001, John Wiley & Sons Ltd., U.K.]

9.3.2.3 *Aclacinomycin A*

Synonyms   Aclarubicin; Antibiotic MA 144 A1; NSC-208734; Jaclacin.

Biological Source   It is obtained from *Streptomyces galilacus*.

Chemical Structure   It is a complex glycoside of **aklavinone ($C_{42}H_{53}NO_{15}$)**.

Aclacinomycin A

Characteristic Features

1. It is obtained as a yellow microcrystalline powder from a mixture of chloroform and hexane having mp 151-153°C (decomposes).
2. It has specific optical rotation $[\alpha]_D^{24}$-11.5° (C = 1 in methylene chloride).
3. It has uv$_{max}$ (methanol): 229.5; 259; 289.5; 431 nm ($E_{1cm}^{1\%}$ 550, 326, 135, 161); (0.1 N HCl) 229.5, 258.5, 290, 431 nm ($E_{1cm}^{1\%}$ 571, 338, 130, 161); (0.1 N NaOH) 239, 287, 523 nm ($E_{1cm}^{1\%}$ 450, 113, 127).
4. It is found to be soluble in chloroform, ethyl acetate; insoluble in ether, n-hexane, petroleum ether.

Identification Tests

1. To an aqueous solution of **aclacinomycin A** add a few-drops of NaOH solution when an intense reddish purple colour is obtained.
2. To a few mg of it add 0.5 ml of pure concentrated HCl when it gives a distinct yellow colouration.

Uses   It shows an enhanced antineoplastic activity with much less cardiotoxicity.

9.3.2.4 *Idarubicin*

Synonyms   4-Demethoxy daunomycin; 4-Demethoxydaunorubicin; DMDR; IMI-30; NSC-256439.

Biological Source   It is an orally active semi-synthetic structural analogue of **daunorubicin** (Section 9.3.2.2).

Chemical Structure

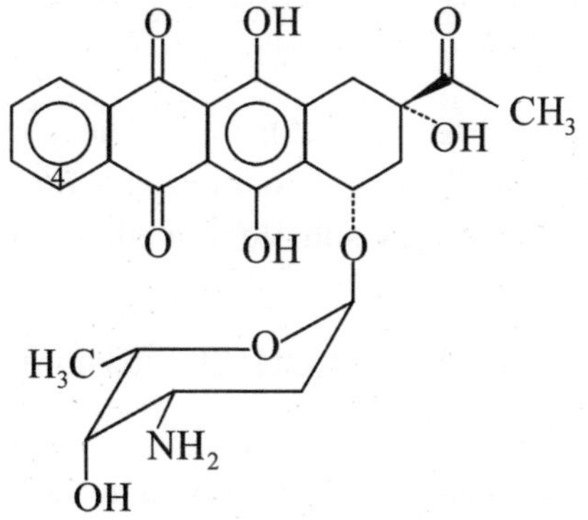

Idarubicin ($C_{26}H_{27}NO_9$]

Characteristic Features Idarubicin Hydrochloride: [$C_{26}H_{27}NO_9$·HCl] [Synonyms: Idamycin, Zavedos]: It is obtained as orange crystalline powder having mp 183-185°C. It has specific optical rotation $[\alpha]_D^{20}$ + 205° (C = 0.1 in methanol).

Uses

1. It is mostly used as an antineoplastic agent.
2. It may show increased activity with comparatively much lesser cardiotoxicity.

Note: The major drawback of structurally related and modified semi-synthetic doxorubicin-type antibiotic is due to their significant cardiotoxicity that invariably comes into being by virtue of the distinct inhibition of cardiac Na^+, K^+-ATpase.

9.3.2.5 Mitoxantrone

Synonyms Mitozantrone; DHAQ; NSC-279836.

Chemical Structure Mitoxantrone is purely a **'synthetic structural analogue'** of the **'anthracyclinones'** wherein *two* important components *viz.*, the *aminosugar* and the **non-aromatic ring** have been strategically replaced with a pair of amino-alkyl side chains *i.e.*, amino-ethyl.

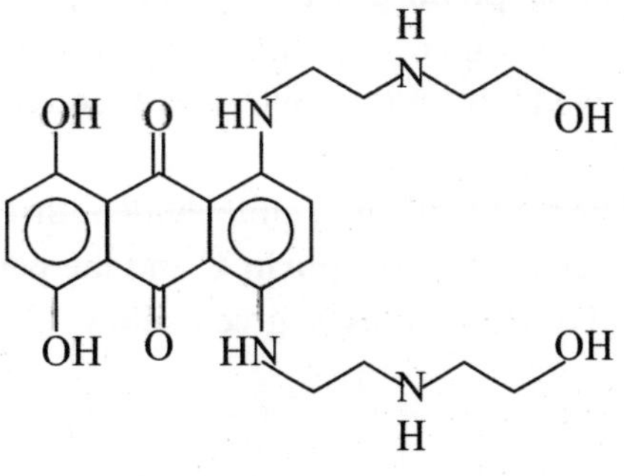

Mitoxantrone

1, 4-Dihydroxy-5, 8-bis [[2-[(2-hydroxyethyl) amino] ethyl] amino]-9, 10-anthracenedione; ($C_{22}H_{28}N_4O_6$).

Characteristic Features

1. It is obtained as crystals from a mixture of ethanol and hexane having mp 160-162°C.
2. It has uv_{max} (ethanol): 244, 279, 525, 620, 660 nm (log ε 4.64, 4.31, 3.70, 4.37, 4.38).
3. It is sparingly soluble in water; slightly soluble in methanol; and almost insoluble in acetone, acetonitrile, chloroform.

Mitoxantrone Dihydrochloride [$C_{22}H_{28}N_4O_6 \cdot 2HCl$]   [Synonyms: Novantrone; DHAD; CL-232315; NSC-301739].

1. It is obtained as a hygroscopic blue-black solid from a mixture of water and ethanol having mp 203-205°C.
2. It has uv_{max} (water): 241, 273, 608, 658 nm (ε 41000, 12000, 19200, 20900).
3. It is found to be sparingly soluble in water; slightly soluble in methanol; and practically insoluble in acetone, acetonitrile, chloroform.

Uses

1. **Mitoxantrone** has a marked and pronounced reduced toxicity as compared to **doxorubicin** (Section 9.3.2.1)
2. It is found to be extremely effective and useful in the treatment of leukemias and solid tumours exclusively.

9.3.3 Cephalosporins

Brotzu*, in 1948, was pioneer in isolating a novel microorganism from the sea water meticulously sampled very close to a sewage outpours off the coast of Sardinia. Interestingly, he noticed its marked and pronounced antagonism to both Gram-positive and Gram-negative microorganisms. Almost after seven years, Abraham** at Oxford first and foremost gave the scientific world the report on the isolation of *three* 'antibiotic substances' from the culture of this specific organism, namely: **cephalosporin P, penicillin N,** and **cephalosporin C.** Out of these three isolated antibiotics, the *first*: **cephalosporin P** has practically accomplished little therapeutic significance; the *second*: **penicillin N** (originally termed as **cephalosporin N**) obtained as the major component and differs significantly from the common penicillin by its antibacterial activity and hydrophilic character; and the *third*: **cephalosporin C** showed low toxicity and *in vitro* activity against the penicillin-resistant *Staphylococci.*

In view of the above statement of facts, it is quite evident that there exist an apparent contrast with regard to the typical features of **cephalosporin C** and the **penicillins** (*viz.,* **benzylpenicillin**) besides other possible structural modifications as given below:

---

* Brotzu, G., *Lav. Ist. Igiene Caligari,* (1948)
** Abraham, Newton, *Nature,* **175**, 548, (1955).

Points of Contrast Between Cephalosporin C and Penicillins

S. No.	Typical Features & Structural Modifications	Cephalosporin C	Penicillins (Benzyl Penicillin)
1	Structure	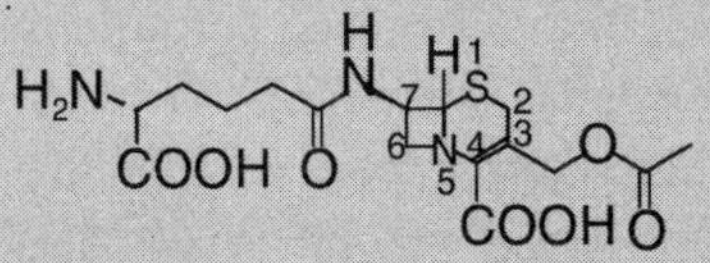	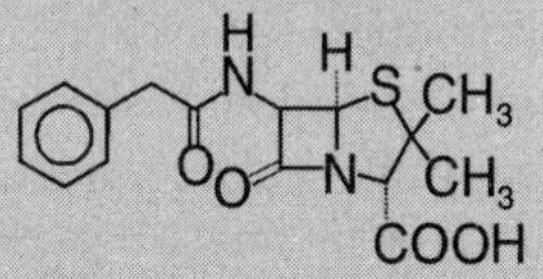
2	Stability	Stable under acidic conditions	Unstable under acidic conditions
3	Effect of Enzyme Penicillinase (β-Lactamase)	Not attacked	Attacked
4	Antibacterial Profile	Low Normal	
5	Absorption after oral administration	Poor	Normal
6	Hydrolysis	Yield 7-ACA (7-Aminocephalosphoranic acid) having a fused dihy-drothiazine β-lactam ring.	Yields 6-APA (6-Aminopenicillanic acid) having a fused thiazo-lidine β-lactam ring.
7	Removal of side-chain at C-7 by enzymes or suitable microorganisms	Afforded fruitful and elusiveresults	—
8	Removal of ester side-chain at C-3	Possible either through (i) Enzymatic hydrolysis by fermentation with a yeast, or (ii) Displacement of acetoxy moiety by nucleophillic reagents.	Possible either through (i) Enzymic removal of side chain, or (ii) Chemical ring expansion
9	Scope for side-chain modifications at C-7.	Ample scope exist	Restricted scope only

In the broader perspective the semi-synthetic cephalosporins may be classified into *three* different manners, namely: (*a*) chemical structure; (*b*) β-lactamase resistance; and (*c*) antibacterial spectrum. However, in usual widely accepted prevailing practice the cephalosporins are logically and legitimately classified by a more arbitrary system, dividing them into '*generations*, such as: **First generation; Second generation;** and **Third generation cephalosporins.**

It is pertinent to mention *two* important points with regard to the **'cephalosporin antibiotics'**, namely:

(*a*) All cephalosporins commence with the prefix *ceph-* or *cef -*; however, the latter spelling now being preferred over the former, though both spellings are usually encountered in certain branded drugs; and

(*b*) The basis for the classification into the said *three* generations depends primarily and solely upon the antibacterial spectrum shown by the drugs, besides the year they were first introduced.

Note: 1. **There are several instances in which the drugs belonging to the 'second generation' may have been introduced after the 'third generation' of drugs had been accomplished.**

2. **Categorically, there is no prevalent practice or demarkation to suggest that the drugs belonging to the 'third generation' automatically supercede second and first genera-**

tion ones. **In fact, cephalosporins from all the three aforesaid categories are still being used across the globe.**

Prodrugs (e.g., cefuroxime-axetil; cefpodoxime-proxetil)   The **prodrugs** of some cephalosporin antibiotics, for instance: cefuroxime-axetile and **cefpodoxime-proxetil** have been duly developed having an additional ester moiety attached to the C-4 carboxyl function. However, these tailor-made 'prodrugs' get duly hydrolyzed to their respective active agents by the aid of esterases.

Cephamycins   These represent another group of **cephalosporin antibiotics** that are characterized by a 7α-methoxy function, and are usually produced by two cosecutive reactions, namely: **hydroxylation** and **methylation.**

Example

Caphamycin C: In this particular instance, the introduction of a carbamate function derived from carbamoyl phosphate on the hydroxymethyl function.

A few important and typical examples of the 'Cephalosporin Antibiotics' belonging to the various recognized groups, such as: first generation, second generation, third generation, prodrugs, and cephamycins have been duly summarized below along with their structural variants, names, synonyms and special remarks:

Cephalosporin Antibiotics: Typical Examples

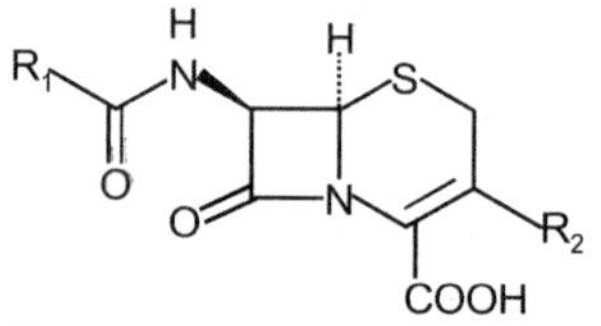

Class	Sl. No.	R_1	R_2	Name (Synonyms)	Special Remarks
First Generation	1	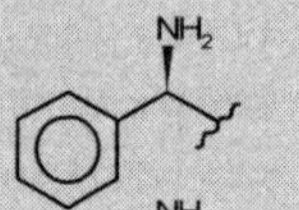	$\{$—CH_3	Cefalexin [Cephalexin]	Orally Active
	2	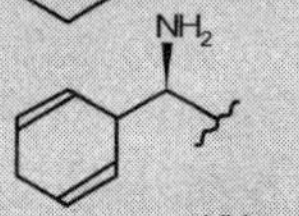	$\{$—CH_3	Cefradine [Cephradine]	Orally Active, superseded generally
	3	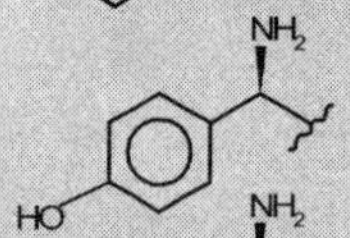	$\{$ —CH_3	Cefadroxil	Orally Active
Second Generation	4	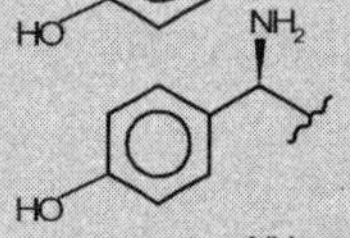	$\{$ —Cl	Cefaclor	Orally Active
	5	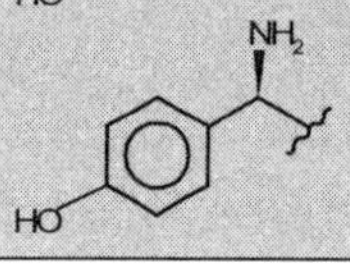	$\{$—CH=CH—CH_3	Cefprozil	Orally Active,

(Contd.)

(*Table contd.*)

Third Generation	6			Cefamandole [Cepha-mandole]	High Resistance to β-lactamases
	7			Caftazidime	Broad-Spectrum Gram-Negative Activity; good Activity against Pseudomonas
	8			Ceftriaxone	Broad-Spectrum Gram-Negative Activity; Longer Half-Life Than Other Cephalosporins
	9		—CH=CH₂	Cefixime	II/III Generation, Orally Active, Long Duration of Action
Prodrugs	10			Cefuroxime -Axetil	II Generation, Orally Active; Hydrolysed by Esterases to Liberate Cefuroxime
	11			Cefpodoxime -Proxetil	II/III Generation, Orally Active; Hydrolysed by Esterases to Liberate Cefpodoxime
Cepha mycins	12		—CH₂—O—C—NH₂	Cefoxitin	Stable to β-Lactamases and Mammalian Esterases

A good number of **cephalosporins** belonging to the three categorized generations are available in the therapeutic armamentarium, besides the cephamycins, which are given as under:

(i) *First generation Cephalosporins:* Cefalotin (Cephalothin); D-Cephalexin (D-Cefalexin); Cephapirin; Cefazolin; D-Cephradine (D-Cefradine); D-Cefadroxil;

(ii) *Second Generation Cephalosporins:* D-Cefactor; D-Cefamandole; Cefuroxime; D-Cefonicid; Ceforanide;

(iii) *Third Generation Cephalosphorins:* Cefotaxime; Ceftizoxime; D-Cefoperazone; Ceftazidime; Ceftriaxone; Cefmonoxime, Moxalactam;

(iv) *Prodrugs:* Cefpodoxime proxetil; Cefuroxime axetil;

(v) *Cephamycins:* Cephamycin C; Cefoxitin.

A few of these important compounds representing the above said categories shall now be discussed individually in the sections that follows:

9.3.3.1 First Generation Cephalosporins

The **first generation cephalosporin** antibiotics are found to be effective against a host of Gram-positive microorganisms, including penicillinase-producing *Staphylococcus*. Besides, being resistant to **penicillinase** they are found to be inactivated by another **cephalosporinase** termed as β-**lactamase**. The Gram-negative organisms that are observed to be highly sensitive to these compounds are, namely: *Escherichia coli; Proteus mirabilis;* and *Klebsiella pneumoniae*. These antibiotics are also found to be less active against *Haemophilus influenzae* as compared to the extended-spectrum penicillins, such as: **ampicillin.**

A. Cephalothin

Synonyms Cefalotin; 7-(Thiophene-2-acetamido) cephalosporanic acid).

Biological Source It is a **semi-synthetic cephalosporin antibiotic** derived from *Cephalosporium acremonium.*

Chemical Structure

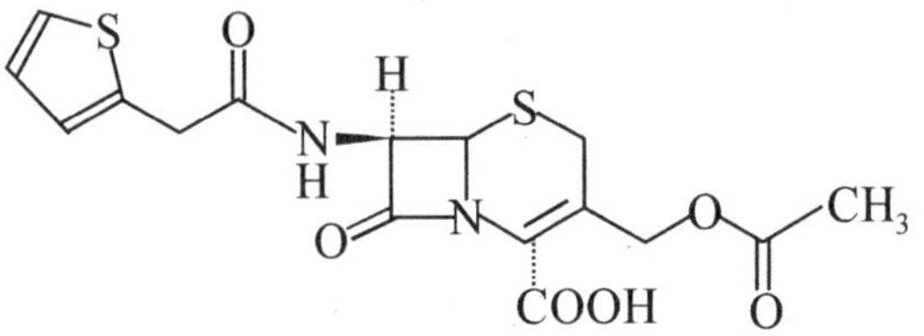

Cephalothin

(6R-*trans*)-3-[(Acetyloxy) methyl]-8-oxo-7-[(2-thienylacetyl) amino]-5-thia-1-azobicyclo [4.2.0] act-2-ene-2-carboxylic acid; ($C_{16}H_{16}N_2O_6S_2$).

Preparation First of all the 7-aminocephalosporanic acid is N-acetylated with 2-thiopheneacetyl chloride in a dehydro-chlorinating environment. The starting acid may be prepared from the natural antibiotic, **cephalosporin C,** either by means of enzymatic hydrolysis or by proton-eatalyzed hydrolysis. The **cephalothin** thus obtained may be purified from acetonitrile.

Characteristic Features
1. It is obtained as a white amorphous powder having mp 160-160.5°C.
2. It has specific optical rotation $[\alpha]_D^{20} + 50°$ (C = 1.03 in acetonitrile).

Cephalothin Sodium $[C_{16}H_{15}N_2NaO_6S_2]$ [*Synonyms* Averon-1; Cefalotin; Cemastin; Cephation; Ceporacin; Cepovenin; Coaxin; Keflin; Lospoven; Microtin; Synclotin; Toricelocin].

1. It is obtained as a white to off-white, crystalline powder, almost odourless, moderately hygroscoic and has mp 204-205°C.
2. It has dissociation constant pKa 2.2.
3. It has specific optical rotation $[\alpha]_D + 135°$ (C = 1.0 in water).
4. It has uv$_{max}$: 236, 260 nm (ε 12950, 9350).
5. **Solubility Profile:** It is freely soluble in water, normal saline or dextrose solution; slightly soluble in ethanol; and practically insoluble in most organic solvents.

Uses
1. It is a potent antibacterial agent.
2. It is a **first-generation cephalosporin** given IM and IV.
3. It is found to be a short-acting antibiotic and exhibits the weakest spectrum of its class.

B. Cephazolin

Synonym   CEZ.

Biological Source   It is also a semi-synthetic antibiotic derived from **7-aminocephalosporanic acid** obtained from *Cephalosporium acremonium.*

Chemical Structure

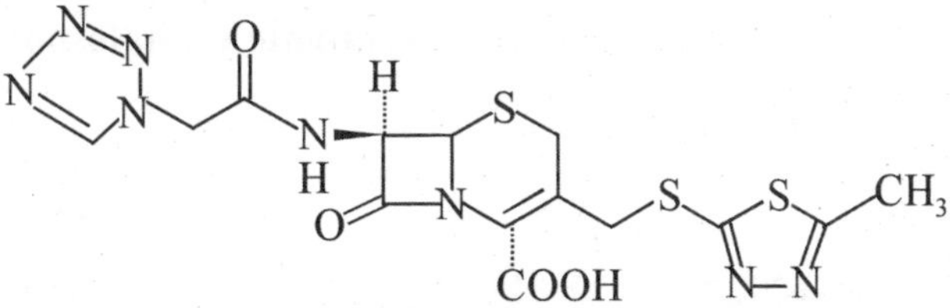

Cephazolin

7-(1-(1H)-Tetrazolyl acetamido)-3-[2-(5-methyl-1, 3, 4-thiadiazolyl) thiomethyl]-Δ^3-cephem-4-carboxylic acid; $(C_{14}H_{14}N_8O_4S_3)$.

Preparation   The sodium salt of **7-aminocephalosporanic acid** is acylated with 1H-tetrazole-1-acetyl chloride. The acetoxy moiety present in the resulting product is then displaced by reaction with 5-methyl-1, 3- 4-thiadiazole-2-thiol to produce the desired product *i.e.,* **cephazolin.** It is then further purified from aqueous ethanol.

Characteristic Features
1. Cephazolin is obtained as needles from aqueous acetone having mp 198-200°C (decomposes).
2. It has uv$_{max}$ (buffer pH 6.4): 272 nm (ε 13150).

3. It is found to be freely soluble in DMF, pyridine; soluble in aqueous acetone, aqueous dioxane, aqueous ethanol, slightly soluble in methanol; and practically insoluble in benzene, chloroform, ether.

Cephazolin Sodium $[C_{14}H_{13}N_8NaO_4S_3]$ **Synonyms Acef; Ancef; Atirin; Biazolina; Bor-Cefazol; Cetacidal; Cefamedin; Cefamezin; Cefazil; Cefazina; Elzogram; Firmacef; Gramaxin; Kefzol; Lampocef; Liviclina; Totacef; Zolicef]:**

1. It is obtained as white to yellowish white, odourless crystalline powder having a bitter salty taste. It crystallizes out in α-, β-, and γ-forms.
2. It is found to be freely soluble in water; slightly soluble in methanol, ethanol; and almost insoluble in benzene, acetone, chloroform.

Uses

1. **Totacef** may be given IV or IM; however, its Gram-negative activity is essentially limited to *E. coli; Klebsiella;* and *Pr mirabilis.*
2. Some Gram-negative organisms and penicillinase-producing staphylococci which are resistant to both **Penicillin G** and **Ampicillin** are found to be sensitive to cefazolin.
3. It may be used to treat infections of the respiratory tract skin, soft tissues, tones, joints and urinary tract and *endocarditis* and septicemia caused by suceptible organisms. However, amongst the UTIs, **cystitis*** specifically responds much better than **pyelonephritis****.
4. It is one of the preferred cophalosporins for most surgical prophylaxis, by virtue of its inherent long half-life (*i.e.*, 1.5 to 2 hours in normal persons but 3 to 42 hours in renal failure).

C. Cefadroxil

Synonyms   BL-S578; MJF-11567-3; Baxan; Bidocef; Cefa-drops; Cefamox; Ceforal; Cephos; Duracef; Duricef; Kefroxil; Oracefal; Sedral; Ultracef.

Biological Source   It is also an orally active **semi-synthetic cephalosporin** antibiotic obtained from the species *Cephalosporium aeremonium.*

Chemical Structure

Cefadroxil

para-Hydroxycephalexine monohydrate; $(C_{16}H_{17}N_3O_5S \cdot H_2O)$.

Characteristic Features   It is obtained as white to yellow white crystals having mp 197°C (decomposes). It is found to be soluble in water, and fairly stable in acidic medium.

---

* **Cystitis:** Inflammation of the bladder usually occurring secondary to ascending urinary tract infections (UTIs).
** **Pyelonephritis:** Inflammation of kidney and renal pelvis.

Uses

1. It is intermediate acting and quite effective against *Staphylococcus* and certain enteric Gram-negative bacilli.
2. Because of its prolonged exeretion criterion, it has an added advantage of catering for more sustained serum and urine concentrations than are usually obtained with other **oral cephalosporins.**
3. Clinical studies have revealed that **cefadroxil** administered, 1g twice daily, is as effective as cephalexin given 500 mg four times daily.

9.3.3.2 *Second Generation Cephalosporins*

Generally, the **'second generation cephalosporins'** exhibit the same spectrum of antibacterial activity as that of the first generation cephalosporins. The glaring exceptions being that these are comparatively much more active against certain specific organisms, namely: *Haemophilus influenzae*, gonococcus, and some enteric Gram-negative bacilli. Interestingly, most of the second generation cephalosporins are adequately absorbed through the oral administration. Some typical examples of **second generation cephalosporins** shall now be described as under:

A. Cefamandole

Synonyms CMT; Compound 83405.

Biological Sources It is a broad-spectrum semi-synthetic cephalosporin antibiotic obtained from *Cephalosporium acremonium.*

Chemical Structure

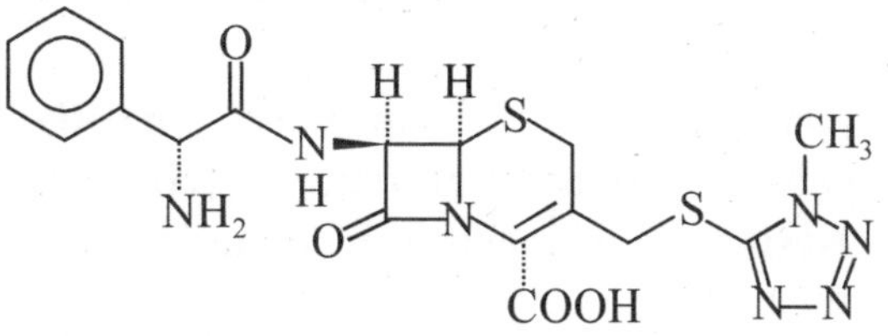

Cefamandole

7-D-Mandelamido-3-[[(1-methyl-1H-tetrazol-5yl) thio]-methyl]-3-cephem-4-carboxylic acid; ($C_{18}H_{18}N_6O_5S_2$).

Characteristic Features

Cefamandole Nafate [$C_{19}H_{17}N_6NaO_6S_2$] [Synonyms Bergacef; Cedol, Cefam; Cefiran; Cemado; Cemandil; Fado; Kefadol; Kefandol; Lampomandol; Mandokef; Mandol; Mandolsan; Neocefal; Pavecef]:

1. It is obtained or white odourless needles having mp 190°C (decomposes).
2. It has uv_{max} (H_2O): 269 nm (ε 10800).
3. Its dissociation constant pKa 2.6-3.0.
4. It is soluble in water, methanol; and almost insoluble in ether, chloroform, benzene, cyclohexane. It is also found to be soluble in saline TS or dextrose solutions.

Uses

1. It is administered effectively through IM and IV.
2. It is found to be short-acting.

B. Cefuroxime

Several antibiotics belonging to the category of '**second generation antibiotics**' are absorbed orally. Interestingly, cefuroxime is available in two different versions; *first*—as its sodium salt and *secondly*— as its *prodrug* cefuroxime axetil that are hydrolyzed once they are absorbed and its absorption rate increased by the intake of food in-take.

Chemical Structure

Cefuroxime

(6R, 7R)-3-Carbamoyloxymethyl-7-[2-(2-furyl)-2-(methoxy-amino) acetamido] ceph-3-em-4-carboxylic acid; ($C_{16}H_{16}N_4O_8S$).

Characteristic Features

1. It is obtained as a white crystalline solid.
2. It has specific optical rotation $[\alpha]_D^{20} + 63.7°$ (C = 1.0 in 0.2 m pH 7 phosphate buffer).
3. It has uv_{max} (pH6 phosphate buffer): 274 nm (ε 17600).

Cefuroxime Sodium [$C_{16}H_{15}N_4NaO_8S$]: [Synonyms Anaptivan; Biociclin; Biofurex; Bioxima; Cefamar; Ceffoprim; Cefumax; Cefurex; Cefurin; Curocef; Curoxim; Duxima; Gibicef; Ipacef; Kefurox; Kesint; Lampsporin; Medoxim; Novocef; Spectrazole; Ultroxim; Zinacef].

It is a white solid; specific optical rotation $[\alpha]_D^{20} + 60°$ (C = 0.91 in water); uv_{max} (water): 274 nm (ε 17400). It is found to be freely soluble in water and buffered solutions; soluble in methanol; very slightly soluble in ether, ethyl acetate, octanol, benzene and chloroform. Its solubility in water in 500 mg/2.5 ml. Its dissociation constant in water pKa 2.5; in DMF 5.1. The stability of cefuroxime sodium salt in water at room temperature stands valid upto 13 hours; and at 25°C for 48 hours nearly 10% decomposition takes place.

Uses

1. Its activity against *H. influenzae* and ability to penetrate into the CSF makes it specifically useful for the treatment, control and management of meningitis caused by this organism. However, it is also recommended to treat meningitis caused by *Strep. pneumoniae, N. meningitidis* and *Staph. aureus*.
2. It exhibits an excellent and super activity against all species of gonococci, hence it is recommended for the treatment of gonorrhea.

3. It may also be employed to treat lower respiratory tract infections normally caused by *H. influenzae* and *parainfluenzae, Klebsiella* species, *E. coli, Strep pneumoniae* and *pyrogenes* and *Staph aureus*.

4. It is also approved for use against UTIs caused by *E. Coli* and *Klebsiella;* of course, a rather more restricted approval as compared to other second-generation drugs.

5. It is also recommended for use in bone infections, septicemias and surgical prophylaxis.

C. Cefonicid

Biological Source   It is essentially an injectable **semi-synthetic cephalosporin** antibiotic related to **cefamandole** which is obtained from *Cephalosporium acremonium*.

Chemical Structure

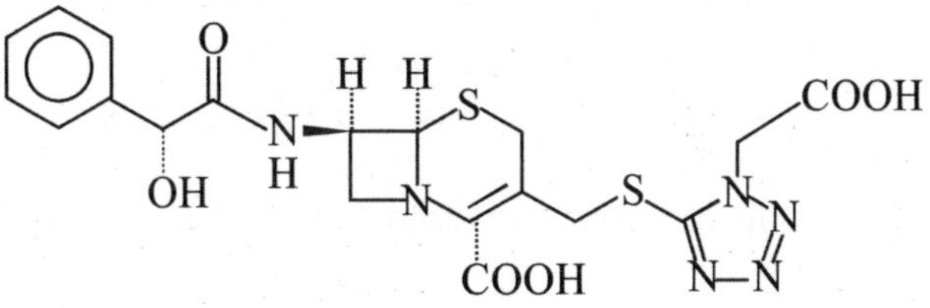

Cefonicid

Characteristic Features

Cefonicid Disodium   [$C_{18}H_{16}N_6Na_2O_8S_3$] [*Synonyms* SKF-75073; Cefodie; Monocid; Monocidur; Praticef;] The pH of 5% (w/v) solution is between 3.5 to 6.5.

Uses

1. It is administered through IV and IM.
2. It is an **intermediate-acting second generation cephalosporin.**

9.3.3.3 Third Generation Cephalosporins

The **'third generation cephalosporins'** are logically differentiated from the first and second generation cephalosporins by virtue of their extended activity against a wide spectrum of **enteric Gram-negative bacillii,** along with the **β-lactamase-producing strains.**

A few potent and typical examples of drugs belonging to this category shall be discussed in the section that follows:

A. Cefotaxime

Biological Source   It is a broad spectrum **third generation cephalosporin** antibiotic derived from *Cephalosporium acremonium*. The name cefotaxime applies to the isomer having a *syn-*methoxyamino moiety.

Chemical Structure   It is the desacetyl active metabolite of **cefotaxime** *i.e.*, another **third generation cephalosporin.**

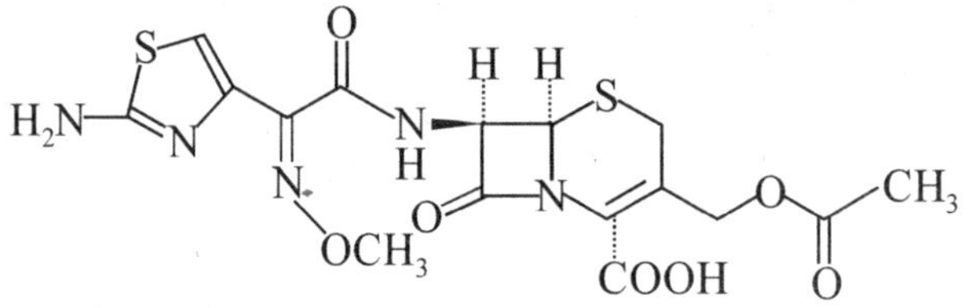

Cefotaxime

7-[2-(2-Amino-4-thiazolyl)-2-methoxyimino acetamido] cephalosporanic acid; ($C_{16}H_{17}N_5O_7S_2$).

Characteristic Features

Cefotaxime Sodium *[syn-Isomer]:* [$C_{16}H_{16}N_5NaO_7S_2$] [*Synonyms: Cefotax; Chemcef; Claforan; Pretor; Tolycar; HR-756; RU-24756]:*

1. It is a white to off-white solid.
2. The pH of a 10% (w/v) solution is approximately 5.5.
3. It has specific optical rotation $[\alpha]_D^{20} + 55° \pm 2$ (C = 0.8 in water).
4. Its pKa (acid) is 3.75.
5. It is found to be freely soluble in water; and almost insoluble in most organic solvents.

Uses

1. It is found to be active against a good number of Gram-negative bacilli and its action is almost equivalent to the **amino glycosides,** except against *Ps aeruginosa, Acinetobacter* and a few *Enterobacter.*
2. It is highly resistant to the β-lactamases.
3. It is found to be less active than either the *first* or the **second generation cephalosporins.**
4. It is a recognized and preferred **third generation cephalosporin** for Gram-negative meningitis and other serious Gram-negative bacillary infections outside the CNS.
5. It is also recommended widely for surgical prophylaxis.
6. **Cefatoxime** has a slightly longer half-life which permits 8 to 12 hour dosing in comparison to 6 to 8 hours for **cefotaxime.**

B. Ceftriaxone

Synonym   Cefatriaxone.

Biological Source   It is a parenteral **third generation cephalosporin antibiotic** obtained from *Cephalosporium acremonium.*

Chemical Structure   [$C_{18}H_{18}N_8O_7S_3$]

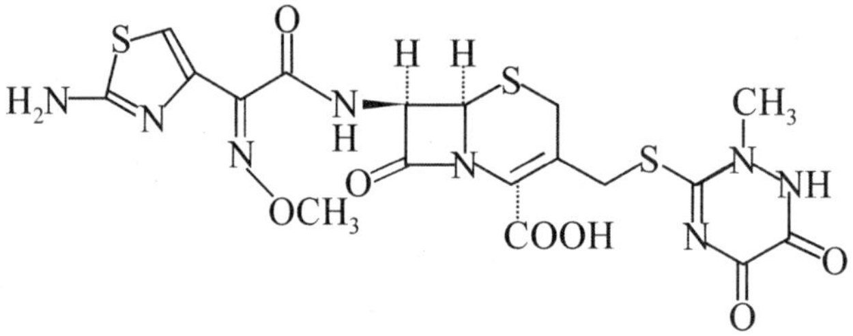

Ceftriaxone

Characteristic Features

Ceftriaxone Disodium Hemiheptahydrate $[C_{18}H_{18}N_8Na_2O_7S_3 \cdot 3\frac{1}{2} H_2O]$: [**Synonyms** *Rocefin; Rocephin(e)*]:

1. It is obtained as white crystalline powder having mp > 155°C. (decomposes).
2. It has specific optical rotation $[\alpha]_D^{25}$-165° (C = 1 in water) (calculated for anhydrous substance).
3. It has uv_{max} (water): 242, 272 nm (ε 32, 300; 29530).
4. It shows dissociation constant pKa : ~ 3 (COOH); 3.2 (NH_3^+), 4.1 (enolic OH).
5. Its solubility in water at 25°C: ~ 40 g/100 ml.
6. The colour of its solution varies from light yellow to amber depending solely on the concentration (g. L^{-1}) and the duration of storage (hrs.)
7. The pH of a 1% (w/v) solution is nearly 6.7.
8. It is found to be sparingly soluble in methanol; and very slightly soluble in ethanol.

Uses

1. **Ceftriaxone sodium** is considered as the drug of choice for uncomplicated and disseminated gonococcal infections.
2. It is also an effective alternative for meningitis in infants essentially caused by *H. influenzae, N. meningitidis* and *Streptococcus pneumoniae.*
3. It is also recommended for Gram-negative bacillary meningitis and some other serious Gram-negative infections, including complications associated with **Lyme disease.***
4. It may also be used for the treatment of bone and joint infections, intra-abdominal infections, lower respiratory tract infections, pelvic infections, skin and urinary tract infections (UTIs).
5. It is also indicated for preoperative prophylaxis, for which its efficiency is almost equivalent to that of **cefazolin.**

C. Ceftazidime

Synonym   GR-20263; Fortaz; Tazicef; Tazidime.

Biological Source   It belongs to the class of third generation cephalosporin antibiotic.

Chemical Structure   The O-substituted oxime function certainly improves upon the potency of the '**third generation cephalosporin**', and ultimately exerts resistance to β-**lactamases.** It is, however, pertinent to mention here that the oximes with *syn* stereochemistry are appreciably more potent and efficient than the corresponding *anti* isomers.

Ceftazidime

---

* **Lyme Disease:** A multisystem disease caused by the tick-transmitted spirochete Borrelia burgodorferi.

1-[[(6R, 7R)-7-[2-(2-amino-4-thiazolyl) glyoxylamido]-2-carboxy-8-oxo-5-thia-1-azabicyclo-[4.2.0] oct-2-en-3-yl] methyl] pyridinium hydroxide inner salt 7^2-(Z)-[0-(1-carboxy-1- methylethyl) oxime]; $(C_{22}H_{22}N_6O_7S_2)$.

Characteristic Features

1. It is obtained as an ivory-coloured powder.
2. Its pKa values are : 1.8, 2.7, 4.1.
3. It has uv_{max} (pH6) : 257 nm ($E_{1cm}^{1\%}$ 348).

Uses

1. **Ceftazidime** is a broad-spectrum antibiotic and is administered IV or IM.
2. It is specifically of great interest because of its distinct high activity against *Pseudomonas* and *Enterobacteriaceae*, but not enterococci.
3. It is an alternative drug for the treatment of hospital-acquired Gram-negative infections especially in immuno-compromised patients when *Ps aeruginosa* is a potential causative organism.
4. It is also recommended for use in the treatment, control, and management of bone and joint infections, CNS-infections, gynecological infections, lower respiratory tract infections, septicemia, skin and UTIs.
5. Its activity is fairly comparable to that of **cefotaxime** and **coftizoxime** *in vitro* but is much more active against *Pseudomonas aeruginosa* and fairly less active against staphylococci and *Bacteroides fragilis*.
6. It is an agent of choice for the **'emperical antibiotic therapy'** when *pseudomonas* happens to be one of the suspected pathogens.

D. Moxalactam

Synonyms   Lamoxactam; Latamoxef.

Biological Source   It is an oxa-substituted **third generation cephalosporin** antibiotic (oxacephalosporin).

Chemical Structure $[C_{20}H_{20}N_6O_9S]$

Moxalactam

Characteristic Features

1. **Moxalactam** is obtained as a colourless powder having mp 117-122°C (decomposes).
2. Its specific optical rotation $[\alpha]_D^{25}$ –15.3 ± 2.6° (C = 0.216 in methanol).
3. It has uv_{max} (methanol): 276 nm (ε 10200).

Moxalactam Disodium $[C_{20}H_{18}N_6Na_2O_9S]$ *[Synonyms* **Festamoxin; Moxalactam; Moxam; Shiomarin; LY-12735; S-6059].**

1. It has specific optical rotation $[\alpha]_D^{22}$-45° (water).
2. It has uv$_{max}$ (water): 270 nm (ϵ 12000).

Uses

1. **Moxalactam** exhibits a spectrum of activity which is almost identical to that of cefotaxime. However, its usage is very much restricted and limited on account of the occurrence of bleeding disorders of serious nature.

   Note: The presence of methyltetrazolethiomethyl moiety may be responsible for causing hypoprothrombinemia; and the α-carboxyl group may attribute to the platelet dysfunction. Perhaps both these vital factors ultimately lead to bleeding disorders.

2. It has an extended Gram-negative spectrum, and are found to be most active against enteric Gram-negative bacilli, but may be less active against certain Gram-positive microorganisms, especially *Staphylococcus aureus*.

9.3.3.4 *Prodrugs*

A major noticeable chief disadvantage of plethora of the current **cephalosporins** is that they are not rapidly and effectively absorbed through oral route. This specific serious drawback is perhaps due to the nature of the side-chain present at C-3. An attempt has been made to design orally active prodrugs, namely: **cefuroxime-axetil** and **cefpodoxime-proxetil,** which have been developed meticulously by providing an additional ester function on the C-4 carboxyl moiety. Nevertheless, these prodrugs are designed in such a manner that they are easily hydrolysed to the active agents *i.e.*, drugs by the *esterases*.

A. Cefpodoxime Proxetil

Synonyms   Banan; Cefodox; Orelox; Otreon; Vantin; CS-807; U-76252;

Biological Source   It is a broad spectrum, orally absorbed third generation cephalosporin, tailor-made ester prodrug of the active-free-acid metabolite, **cefpodoxime.**

Chemical Structure   The skill and wisdom of a pharmaceutical chemist has made it possible to design an ester of the metabolite, **cefpodoxime,** in which the free carboxyl function located at C-4 of the **thiazine ring** *i.e.*, the heterocyclic six-membered ring with one each of S and N atom studded at alternate position in the ring.

Cefpodoxime Proxetil

1-(Isopropyloxy carbonyloxy) ethyl (6R, 7R)-7 [2-(2-amino-4-thiazolyl)-(Z)-2-(methoxyamino) acetamido]-3-methoxymethyl-3-cephem-4-carboxylate; ($C_{21}H_{27}N_5O_9S_2$).

Uses

1. It is a **'third generation cephalosporin'-prodrug** administered orally.
2. It is found to be an **'intermediate acting cephalosporin'**.
3. Its pharmacologic activity is almost similar to that of **cofixime.**

9.3.3.5 Cephamycins

Streptomyces clavuligerus gave rise to the isolation of the natural antibiotic known as *Cephamycin* C, which essentially has an α-methoxy function at C-7 present in the **basic cephalosporin ring system.** It has been observed that the **steric hinderence** caused due to the presence of the additional methoxy moieties, affording thereby a possible resistance to **β-lactamase** hydrolysis, might be solely responsible for the weak antibacterial activity of both **cephamycin C** and other natural **cephamycins.** Various semi-synthetic structural analogues have been designed either:

(*a*) By chemical introduction of the α-methyl moiety at C-7 of the **basic cephalosporin ring system,** or

(*b*) By modification of the side-chains of the naturally occurring **cephamycins.**

A. Cefoxitin

Biological Source   It is a semi-synthetic derived from the **Cephamycin C** through the method 'a' stated above. The synthesis of **Cefoxitin** has been successfully carried out by Karady *et al.**

Chemical Structure

Cefoxitin

3-Carbamoyloxymethyl-7α-methoxy-7-[2-(2-thienyl)-acetamido]-3-cephem-4-carboxylic acid; ($C_{16} H_{17} N_3 O_7 S_2$).

Characteristic Features

1. It is obtained as crystals having mp 148-150°C (decomposes).
2. Its dissociation constant pKa is 2.2.
3. **Solubility Profile:** It is very soluble in acetone; soluble in aqueous $NaHCO_3$; very slightly soluble in water; and almost insoluble in ether and chloroform.

Cefoxitin Sodium   [$C_{16}H_{16}N_3NaO_7S_2$] [*Synonyms* **Betacef; Farmoxin; Mefoxin; Mefoxitin; Merxin; Cenomycin;**]:

1. It is obtained as white crystals with a characteristic odour having mp 150°C.
2. It has specific optical rotation $[\alpha]_{589nm}^{25}$ + 210° (C = 1 in methanol).

---

* Karady *et al. J. Am. Chem. Soc.*, **94**, 1410, (1972).

3. It has dissociation constant pKa 2.2 (acid).
4. **Solubility Profile:** It is found to be very soluble in water; soluble in methanol; sparingly soluble in ethanol or acetone; and practically insoluble in aromatic and aliphatic hydrocarbons.

Uses

1. It is mostly used as an alternative drug for intra-abdominal infections, colorectal surgery or appendectomy and ruptured viscus by virtue of the fact that it is active against most enteric anaerobes including *Bacteroides fragilis.*
2. It is also recommended for use in the treatment of bone and joint infections usually caused by *S. aureus,* gynecological and intra abdominal infections by *Bacteriodes* species
3. It is also approved for lower respiratory tract infections caused by *Bacteroides* species; *E. coli; H. influenzae; Klebsiella* species; *S. aureus* etc.

9.3.4   β-Lactams

The **β-lactam antibiotics** (or **β-lactams**) essentially comprise of the **penicillins, cephalosporins, imipenem, nocardicin A, aztreonam, clavulanic acid, moxalactam,** and **thienamycin.** Interestingly, the β-lactam heterocyclic nucleus consists of a 4-membered cyclic ring with a N-atom. There exist a number of structural variants of β-lactam ring whereby the highly-strained β-lactam nucleus is strategically stabilized by means of the fusion of a variety of either 5-membered or 6-membered heterocyclic moieties to give rise to a wide spectrum of newer antibiotics as enumerated below.

β-Lactam Variants

S. No.	Nomenclature	Chemical Structure (Nucleus)	Notes
1	β-Lactam		Fused skeletons found in penicillins, cep halosporins, imipenem, and aztreonam.
2	Penam		β-Lactam ring fused with a 5-membered dihydrothiazine ring *e.g.,* penicillins (dis-cussed under section 9.3.7).
3	Cephem		β-Lactam ring fused with a 6-membered dihydrothiazine ring eg., cephalosporins (discussed under section 9.3.3).
4	Penem		β-Lactam ring fused with a 5-membered thiazolidine ring having a double bond between C-2 and C-3.
5	Oxapenam		S-Heteroatam in penam nuclei replaced by an O-atom *e.g.,* Clavulanic Acid

(Contd.)

(*Table contd.*)

| 6 | **Oxacepham** | 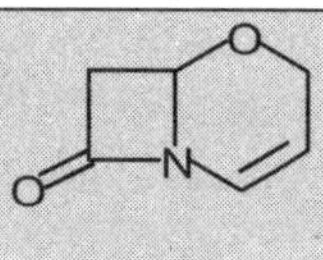 | S-Heteroatom in *cepham* nuclei replaced by an O-atom eg., moxalactam (section 9.3.3.3.D) |
| 7 | **Carbopenem** | | Variant of the penicillin-ring-system wherein the S-heteroatom is replaced by carbon eg., |

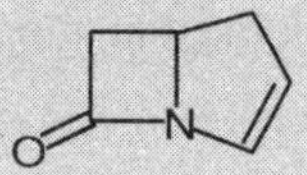

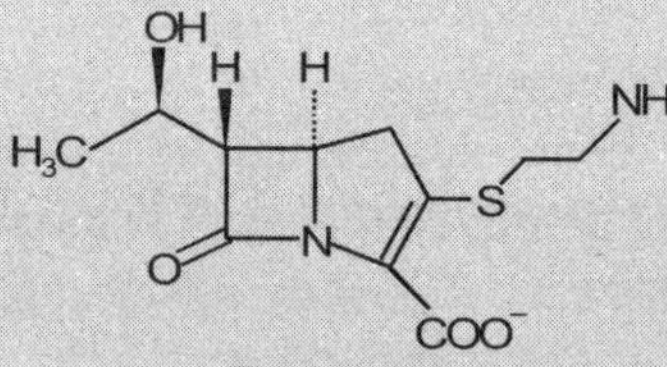

Thienamycin

| 8 | **Monobactam** | | Monocyclic β-lactams *e.g.,* |

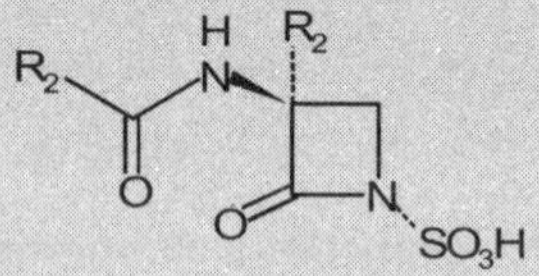

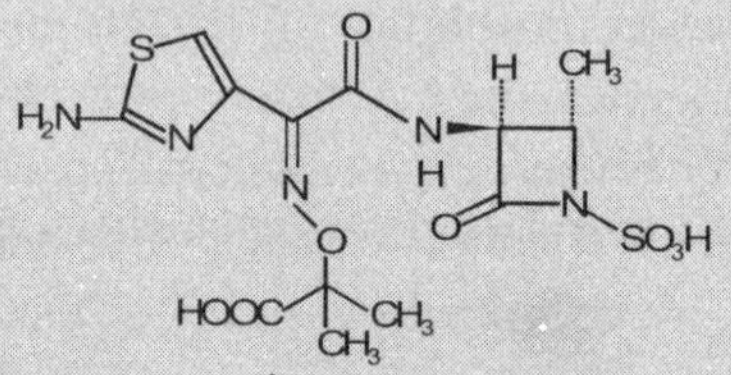

Aztreonam

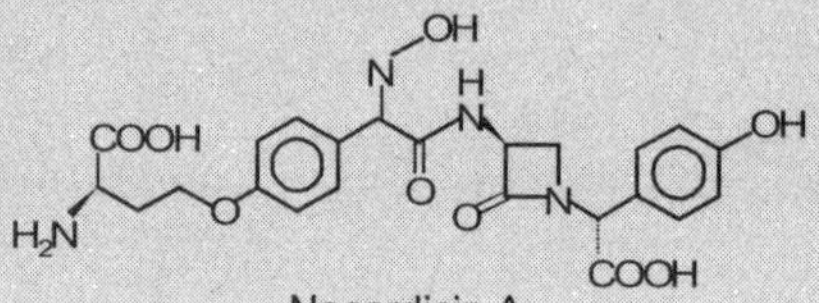

Nocardicin A

A few important compounds belonging to the category of so called '**other β-lactams**', such as: **thienamycin, aztreonam, norcardicin A, imipenem** and **meropenem** shall be treated separately as under:

9.3.4.1 *Thienamycin*

Biological Source   It belongs to the first member of a family of **des-thia-carbapenam nucleus antibiotics** with a thioethylamine side-chain strategically positioned on the enamine portion of the fused 5-membered ring. It is obtained from cultures of *Streptomyces cattleya.*

Chemical Structure

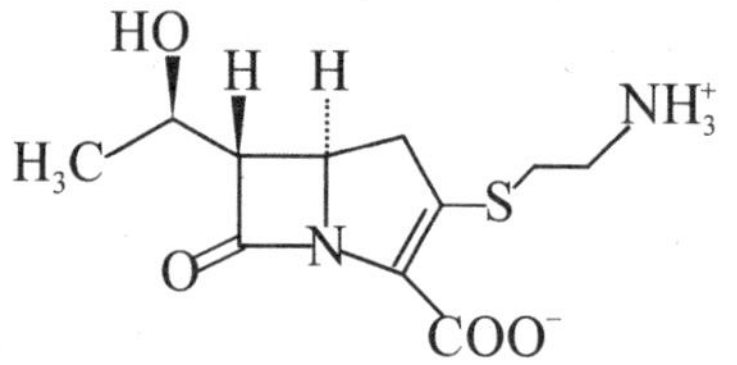

Thienamycin

[5R-[5α, 6α (R*)]]-3 [(2-Aminoethyl) thio]-6-(1-hydroxyethyl)-7-oxo-1-azabicyclo [3, 2, 0]-hept-2-ene-2-carboxylic acid; ($C_{11}H_{16}N_2O_4S$).

Characteristic Features

1. It is obtained as a white hygroscopic solid powder.
2. Its specific optical rotation $[\alpha]_D^{27} + 82.7°$ (C = 1.0 in water).
3. It has uv_{max} (water pH 4.8): 296.5 nm (ε 7900); (pH 2): 309 nm; and (pH 12): 300.5 nm.
4. It is found to be freely soluble in water; and sparingly soluble in methanol.
5. In dilute solution its stability is observed to be optimal between pH 6.7, declining with unusual rapidity above that range.
6. It is found to be susceptible to inactivation by dilute solutions of hydroxylamine and cysteine.

9.3.4.2 Aztreonam

Synonyms Azthreonam; Azactam; Azonam; Aztreon; Nebactam; Primbactam; SQ-26776.

Biological Sources Aztreonam enjoys the reputation of being the first totally synthetic monocyclic β-lactam (monobactam) antibiotic.

Chemical Structure

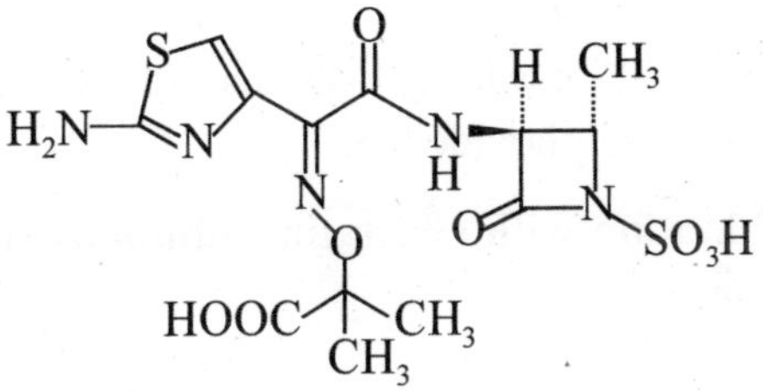

Aztreonam

[2S-[2α, 3β(Z)]]-2-[[[1-(2-Amino-4-thiazolyl)-2-2-methyl-4-oxo-1-sulfo-3-azetidinyl) amino]-2-oxoethylidene] amino]oxy]-2-methylpropanoic acid; ($C_{13}H_{17}N_5O_8S_2$).

Characteristic Features

1. It is obtained as white crystalline odourless powder which decomposes at 227°C.
2. **Solubility Profile:** It is found to be very slightly soluble in ethanol; slightly soluble in methanol; soluble in DMF, DMSO; and almost insoluble in toluene, chloroform, ethyl acetate.

Uses It offers a significantly high degree of resistance to **β-lactamases** and displays specific activity *Vs* aerobic Gram-negative rods.

9.3.4.3 Imipenem

Synonyms Imipemide; N-fomimidoylthienamycin monohydrate; MK-787.

Biological Source **Imipenem** is an extremely broad-spectrum semi-synthetic antibiotic produced by *S. cuttleya*. It is being recognized as the first stable derivative of thienamycin.

Chemical Structure

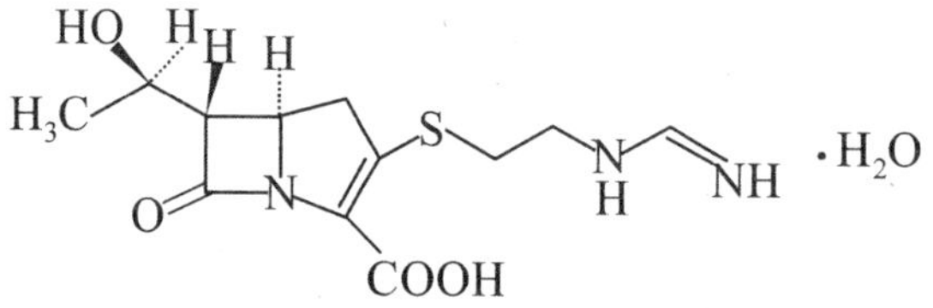

Imipenem

[5R-[5α, 6α (R*)]]-6-(1-Hydroxyethyl)-3[[2-[(iminomethyl) amino] ethyl] thio]-7-oxo-1-azabicyclo-[3, 2, 0] hept-2-ene-2-carboxylic acid monohydrate; ($C_{12}H_{17}N_3O_4S·H_2O$).

Preparation   It is obtained as a crystalline derivative of **thienamycin** by the method suggested by Leanza *et al.**

Characteristic Features
1. It is obtained as crystals from a mixture of water and ethanol.
2. It has specific optical rotation $[\alpha]_D^{25} + 86.8°$ (C = 0.05 in 0.1 M phosphate pH 7).
3. It has dissociation constants $pKa_1 \sim 3.2$, $pKa_2 \sim 9.9$.
4. It shows uv_{max} (water): 299 nm (ε 9670, 98% NH_2 OH ext.)
5. It has a solubility profile (mg . ml^{-1}): water 10, methanol 5, ethanol 0.2, acetone < 0.1, dimethyl formamide < 0.1, and dimethyl sulphoxide 0.3.

Note: It is available in combination with cilastatin sodium as Imipem, Primaxin, Tan Acid, Tienam, Tracix, Zienam.

Uses
1. It exhibits a broader antibacterial spectrum than any other **β-lactams**.
2. It happens to surpass cephalosporins against staphylococci, equals penicillin G against streptococci, equals **third generation cephalosporins** against most aerobic Gram-negative bacilli and is found to be fairly comparable to **ceftazidine** against *Ps aeruginosa*.
3. It is also equally comparable to both **metronidazole** and **clindamycin** against the anaerobes.
4. It is specifically recommended for the treatment, control and management of mixed bacterial infections.

9.3.4.4 Meropenem

Synonyms   Merrem; Meronem; ICI-194660; SM-7338.

Biological Source   It is also another semi-synthetic structural analogue of thienamycin, produced by *S. cuttleya* by the method proposed by Sunagawa *et al.***

---

* Leanza W.J. *et al.*, J. Med. Chem., **22**, 1435 (1979).
** M. Sunagawa *et al.*, *Eur. pat. Appl. 126, 587*; M. Sunagawa, *U.S. Pat. 4, 943, 569* (1984, 1990 both to Sumitomo).

Chemical Structure

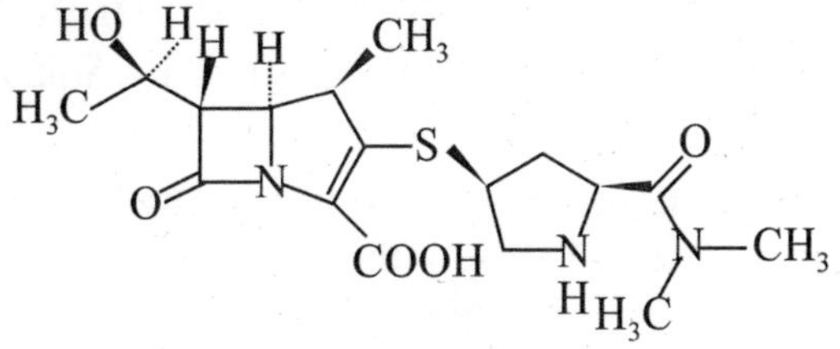

Meropenem

[4R-[3 (3S*, 5S*) 4α, 5β, 6β (R*)]]-3-[[5-[(Dimethylamino) carbonyl]-3-pyrrolidinyl] thio]-6-(1-hydroxyethyl)-4-methyl-7-oxo-1-azabicyclo [3, 2, 0] hept-2-ene-2-carboxylic acid trihydrate; $(C_{17}H_{25}N_3O_5S \cdot 3H_2O)$.

Characteristic Features

1. It is obtained as white to pale yellow crystalline powder.
2. The colour of its solutions vary from colourless to yellow depending on the concentration.
3. **Solubility Profile:** It is found to be sparingly soluble in water; soluble in 5% monobasic sodium phosphate $[H_2NaO_4P]$ solution; very slightly soluble in ethanol; and practically insoluble in acetone or ether.

Uses

1. The resistance of meropenem to most β-lactamases is fairly good.
2. It has a similar distribution as imipenem.
3. It is not degraded by renal dehydropeptidases.
4. It possesses slightly different affinity for specific PBPs* (primary target includes PBPs 2 and 3) depending on the strain of Gram-negative microorganisms.

9.3.4.5 Nocardicin A

Biological Sources   It is a monocyclic β-lactam (monobactam) antibiotic with antimicrobial activity that specifically inhibits bacterial cell wall biosynthesis. In short, **nocardicins A, B, C, D, E, F, G** have been isolated and identified duly. All are produced by *Nocardia uniformis* subspecies *tsuyamenesis*, A being the most important component. However, nocardicin A has also been produced by *Actinosynnema mirum*.**

Chemical Structure

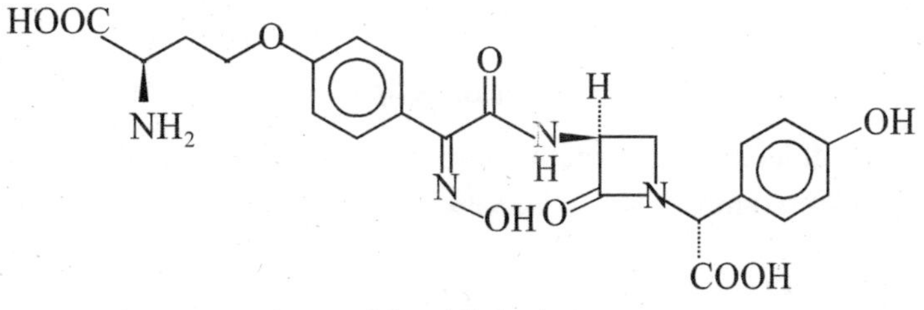

Nocardicin A

---

* Penicillin Binding Proteins.
** K. Watanabe *et al., J. Antibiot.*, **36**, 321 (1983).

[3S-[1(S*), 3R* [Z(S*)]]]-3-[[[4-(3-Amino-3-carboxypropoxy) phenyl] (hydroxy imino) acetyl]-amino]-α-(4-hydroxyphenyl)-2-oxo-1-azetidineacetic acid; [$C_{23}H_{24}N_4O_9$].

Isolation   **Nocardicin A** has been isolated and characterized by Aoki *et al*.*

Characteristic Features

1. It is obtained as colourless needles from acidic water having mp 214–216°C (decomposes).
2. It has specific optical rotation $[\alpha]_D^{25}$-135° (for the sodium salt).
3. Its uv$_{max}$ (1/15 M phosphate buffer); 272 nm (E $_{1cm}^{1\%}$ 310); (0.1 N. NaOH): 244, 283 nm (E$_{1cm}^{1\%}$ 460, 270).
4. It is found to be soluble in alkaline solutions; slightly soluble in methanol; and practically insoluble in chloroform, ethyl acetate, solvent ether.

9.3.5   Lincosamides

Lincosamides essentially comprise of two clinically useful antibiotics, namely: **Lincomycin** and **Clindamycin;** however, their overall general usage has been restricted and limited on account of their inherent potentially fatal side effect called **pseudomembranous colitis.****

These two aforesaid antibiotics shall now be treated individually in the sections that follows:

9.3.5.1   Lincomycin

Synonyms   Lincolnensin; Lincolcina; U-10149; NSC-70731;

Biological Source   It is produced by *Streptomyces lincolensis* var. *lincolensis.*

Chemical Structure   **Lincomycin** has an amide function in its molecule which may have been contributed essentially by an unique strategic combination of amino acid and carbohydrate metabolites. It is also obtained through **stereoselective synthesis** by the method of Knapp and Kukkola.***

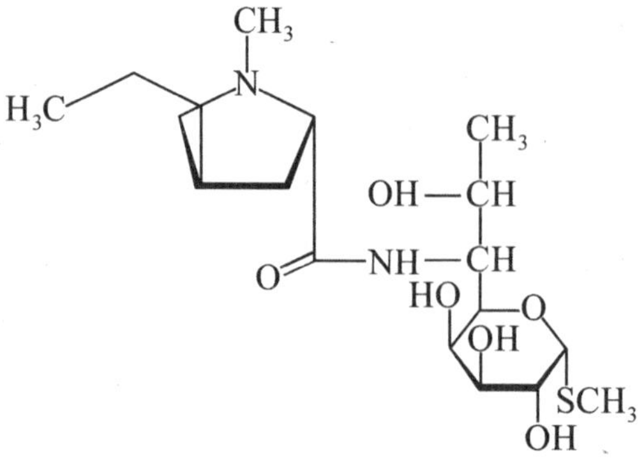

Lincomycin

(2S-*trans*)-Methyl 6, 8-dideoxy-6-[[(1-methyl-4-propyl-2-pyrrodinyl) carbonyl] amino]-1-*thio-p*-erythro-α-D-galacto-octopyranoside; ($C_{18}H_{34}N_2O_6S$).

---

* H. Aoki *et al., J. Antibiot.*, **29**, 492 (1976)
** **Pseudomembranous Colitis:** Colitis associated with antibiotic therapy. It is indicated by formation of a pseudomembrane on the mucosa of the colon. The symptoms are: diarrhaea, abdominal cramps, fever and leukocytosis normally after 4 to 10 days after the start of antibiotic therapy.
*** S. Knapp and P.J. Kukkola, *J. Org. Chem.* **55**, 1637 (1990).

Characteristic Features
1. It is obtained as a free-base invariably.
2. Its dissociation constant is pKa′ 7.6.
3. It is found to be more stable in salt form.
4. It is soluble in methanol, lower alcohols, acetone, ethyl acetate, chloroform; and slightly soluble in water.

Lincomycin Hydrochloride Hemihydrate $(C_{18}H_{34}N_2, O_6S.HCl.\frac{1}{2}H_2O)$: [*Synonyms* **Frademicina; Lincocin; Mycivin; Wayenecomycin;**]

1. It was obtained formerly as needle-like crystals of low specific gravity from aqueous solution by rapid addition of acetone at low temperatures; but nowadays it is mostly obtained as crystals of relatively higher specific gravity, having distinct cubic crystal structure with greater solubility in HCl, by the slow addition of acetone. It has mp 145-147°C.
2. It has specific optical rotation $[\alpha]_D^{25} + 137°$ (water).
3. It is found to be freely soluble in water, methanol, ethanol; and sparingly soluble in most organic solvents other than the hydrocarbons.

Uses
1. It is active against most Gram-positive bacteria, including pneumococci, staphylococci, and streptococci, with the exception of *Enterococcus faecalis*.
2. Its anaerobic spectra (both Gram-positive and Gram-negative) are also recognized as significant and distinctive.
3. Its use is restricted due to its serious side-effects which essentially include: diarrhoea, occasionally serious *pseudomembranous colitis* (caused by overgrowth of resistant strains of *Clostridium difficile*), which may cause serious fatalities especially in aged patients.

Note: Lincomycin inhibits protein biosynthesis due to the blockade of peptidyltransferase site on the 50S subunit of the bacterial ribosomes 70S.

9.3.5.2 *Clindamycin*

Synonyms Antirobe; Cleocin; Dalacin C; Klimicin; Sobelin; Clinimycin (rescinded); 7-Deoxy-7(S)-chloro-lincomycin.

Biological Source **Clindamycin** (7-chloro-7-deoxy-lincomycin) is synthetically derived from **lincomycin,** which is obtained from the cultures of *Streptomyces lincolensis* var *lincolensis*.

Chemical Structure The semi-synthetic derivative is obtained by the chlorination of the *lincomycin* with resultant inversion of stereochemistry.

Clindamycin

(2S-*trans*)-Methyl 7-chloro-6,7,8-trideoxy-6-[[(1-methyl-4-propyl-2-pyrrolidinyl) carbonyl] amino]-1-thio-L-threo-α-galacto-octo-pyranoside; ($C_{18}H_{33}Cl\,N_2O_5S$).

Characteristic Features

1. It is obtained as yellow amorphous solid.
2. It has specific optical rotation $[\alpha]_D$ + 214° (chloroform).

Clindamycin Hydrochloride Monohydrate   [$C_{18}H_{33}Cl\,N_2O_5S.HCl.H_2O$]: [*Synonym Dalacin*]:

1. It is obtained as white crystals obtained from a mixture of ethanol-ethyl acetate having mp 141-143°C.
2. It has specific optical rotation $[\alpha]_D$ + 144° (H_2O).
3. Its dissociation constant is pKa 7.6.
4. It is found to be soluble in water, ethanol, DMF, and pyridine.

Uses

1. It appears slightly more effective quantitatively than its structural analogue lincomycin.
2. It is more readily eliminated from the body. The normal 300 mg dose of lincomycin gives a peak serum level of 2.6 to 3.6 mcg. ml^{-1} in 1-2 hours, and the normal half-life ranges between 2-4 hours.
3. **Clindamycin** is reported to be one of the most effective antibiotics against strains of *Bacteroides fragilis,* the Gram-negative anaerobe that is responsible for a number of abdominal infections.
4. The antianaerobic property of **clindamycin** renders it useful in pneumonias caused by anaerobes.
5. **Clindamycin phosphate** is employed topically for the treatment, control and management of serious acne and vaginally for bacterial vaginosis.

9.3.6   Macrolides

Macrolide antibiotics are typically characterized by macrocyclic lactones having a ring-size ranging between 12-16 atoms and also possess inherent extensive branching through the methyl substituents. However, the macrolactone ring essentially bears a glycosidal linkage to either one or several sugar functions. Exhaustive biosynthetic studies have revealed that the genesis and formation of macrocyclic lactone due to the condensation of either acetate and/or propionate units, evidently *via* malonyl-CoA and 2-methylmalonyl-CoA. Interestingly, the methyl substituents present on the macrolactone ring seem to be contributed exclusively as the residual from incorporation of **propionate units** instead of the so called **terminal biological methylation.** It has been established beyond any reasonable doubt that two or even more 'sugar units' are attached through the glycoside linkages. Further, these sugars are found to be somewhat unusual 6-deoxy structures normally restricted to this particular class of compounds *i.e.*, **macrolides.**

The four 'sugar components' present often in macrolides are, namely: **L-cladinose; L-mycarose; D-mycinose;** and **L-oleandrose,** whose structures are given below:

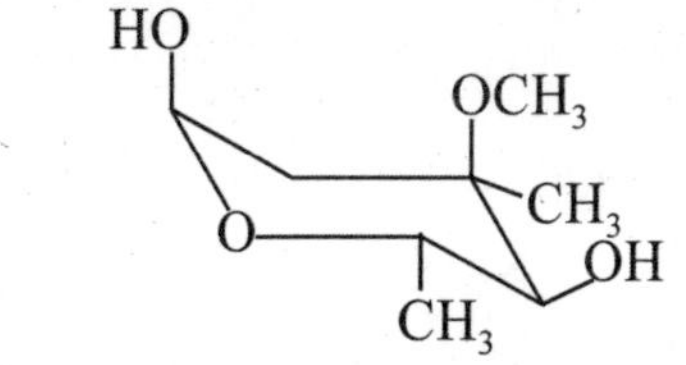

L-Cladinose

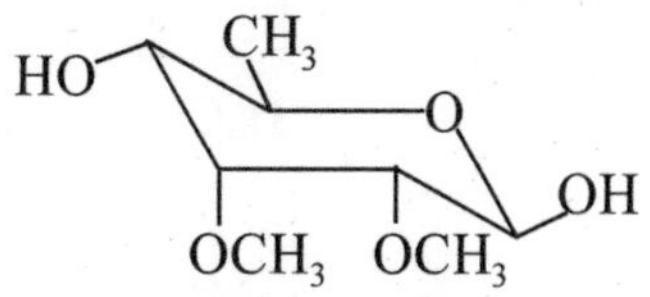

D-Mycinose

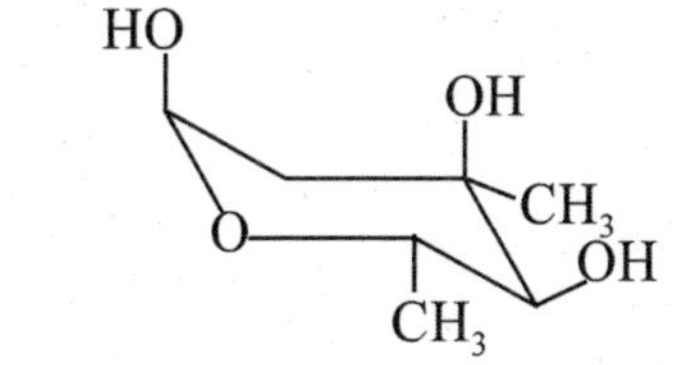

L-Mycarose

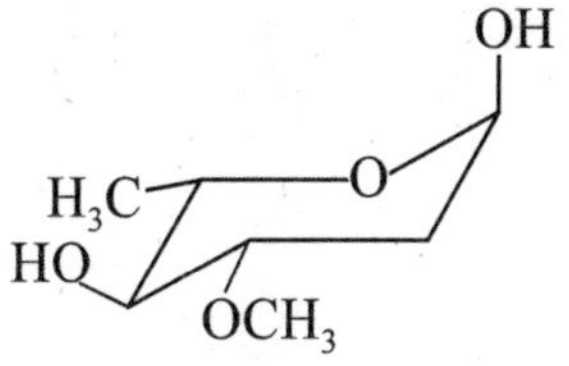

L-Oleandrose

Out of all the 'sugar components' present, at least one sugar is an amino-sugar, such as: D-desosamine; D-forosamine; and D-mycaminose, who structures are as depicted below.

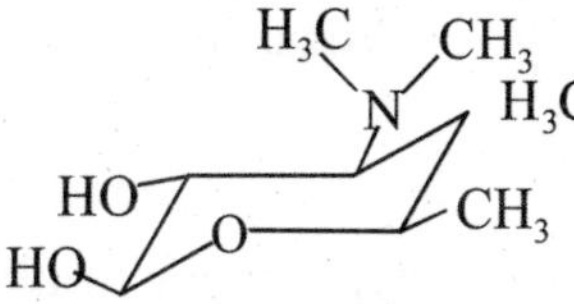

D-Desosamine 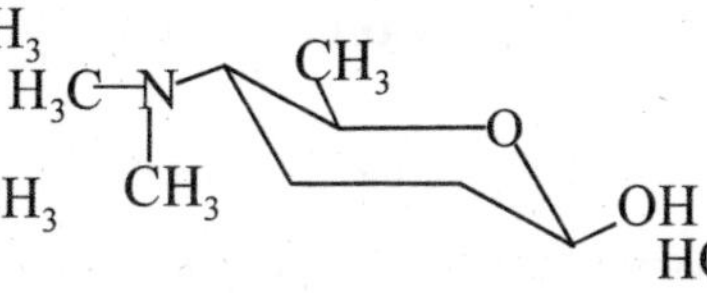   D-Forosamine 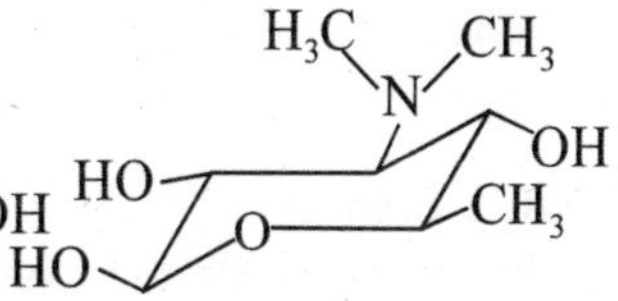   D-Mycaminose

The various important members of 'macrolide antibiotics' are, namely: Erythromycin, Clarithromycin, Arithromycin, Oleandomycin; Troleandomycin; and Spiramycins.

In general, these antibiotics essentially exhibit a narrow spectrum of antibacterial activity, most importantly against the Gram-positive microorganisms. It is, however, pertinent to mention here that the antibacterial spectrum of the aforesaid antibiotics resembles, but is not very much identical to, that of the penicillins; hence, they cater for an extremely valuable alternative or substitute for such patients who are found to be allergic to the penicillins. It is worthwhile mentioning at this point in time that Erythromycin is one of the most important and principal macrolide antibiotics presently employed in medicine.

Some of these antibiotics shall now be treated individually in the sections that follows:

9.3.6.1 Erythromycin

Synonyms   Erythromycin A; Abomacetin; Ak-Mycin; Aknin; E-Base; EMU; E-Mycin; Eritrocina; Ery Derm; Erymax; Ery Tab; Erythromast 36; Erythromid; ERYC, Erycen; Erycin; Erycinum; Ermysin; Ilotycin; Inderm, Retcin; Staticin; Stiemycin, Torlamicina.

Biological Sources   It is produced by cultures of *Saccharopolyspora erythraea* (formerly known as *Streptomyces erythreus*). Waksman and Henrici were the pioneer in finding this antibiotic in a soil sample collected from the Philippine Archipelago.

Erythromycin is, in fact, a mixture containing principally *Erythromycin A*. Together with small quantum of **Erythromycins B and C.**

Chemical Structure

Erythromycin

E-Mycin (3R*, 4S*, 5S*, 6R*, 7R*, 9R*, 11R*, 12R*, 13S*, 14R*)-4-(2, 6-Dideoxy-3-C-methyl-3-0-methyl-α-L-ribo-herapyranosyl) oxy]-14-ethyl-7, 12, 13-trihydrox-3, 5, 7, 9, 11, 13-hexamethyl-6-[[3, 4, 6-trideoxy-3 (Dimethyl-amino)-β-D-xylo-hexopyranosyl] oxy] oxacyelotetradecane-2, 10-dione; ($C_{37}H_{67}NO_{13}$).

Characteristic Features

1. It is obtained as white or slightly yellow-crystals or powder, odourless or practically odourless, slightly hygroscopic in nature, having mp 135-140°C.
2. It is found to get resolidified with second mp 190-193°C.
3. It has specific optical rotation $[\alpha]_D^{25}$-78° (C = 1.99 in ethanol).
4. It has uv_{max} (pH 6.3): 280 nm (ε 50).
5. Its dissociation constant is pKa_1 8.8.
6. It usually shows basic reaction and readily forms salts with acids *e.g.*, acetate, estolate, glucoheptanoate, lactobionate, propionate, stearate and the like.
7. Its solubility in water is nearly 2 mg . ml^{-1}.
8. It is found to be freely soluble in alcohols, acetone, chloroform, acetonitrile, ethyl acetate; and moderately soluble in solvent ether, ethylene dichloride and amyl acetate.

Uses

1. It exhibits a relatively broad spectrum of activity which usually overlaps the activity of penicillin.
2. It is found to be *most effective* against a host of Gram-positive cocci, namely: *Enterococci*, Group A hemolytic streptococci, pneumococci, and *Staphylococcus aureus, N. meningitidis* and *gonorrhoeae, Listeria, Corynebacterium* diphtheria, acnes and certain specific strains of *H. influenzae* are also reported to be sensitive.
3. A low concentration of **erythromycin** also inhibit *mycoplasma* and the agent of Legionnaire's disease*.

---

 * **Legionnaire's Disease:** A severe, often total disease characterized by pneumonia, dry cough, mylagia and sometimes gastrointestinal symptoms. It may occur in epidemic or sporadically and has become an important cause of nosocomial pneumonia. An organism, *Legionella pneumophia*, cause the disease when it is inhaled from aerosols produced by air-conditioning units, shower heads etc.,

4. It inhibits the spirochaete *Treponema pallidum* and is an alternative to penicillin in the treatment of syphilis.
5. It is quite often regarded as the **'drug-of-choice'** for **undiagnosed pneumonias** because it is found to be active against *Streptococcus pneumoniae, Legionella* and *Mycoplasma pneumoniae.*
6. It is extensively employed as an alternative to **β-lactam antibiotics** in soft-tissue infections, skin and in respiratory related diseases particularly in **penicillin-allergic patients.**

9.3.6.2 *Clarithromycin*

Synonyms   Biaxin; Clathromycin; Klacid; Klaricid; Macladin; Naxy; Veclam; Zeclar; A-56268; TE-031.

Biological Source   It is a semi-synthetic derivative of erythromycin which is obtained from *Saccharopolyspora erythraea.*

Chemical Features   **Erythromycin** is fairly unstable under acidic environment whereby it undergoes degradation to inactive molecules through the 6-hydroxyl attacking the 9-carbonyl function to form a **hemiketal** (or **hemiacetal**) as shown below:

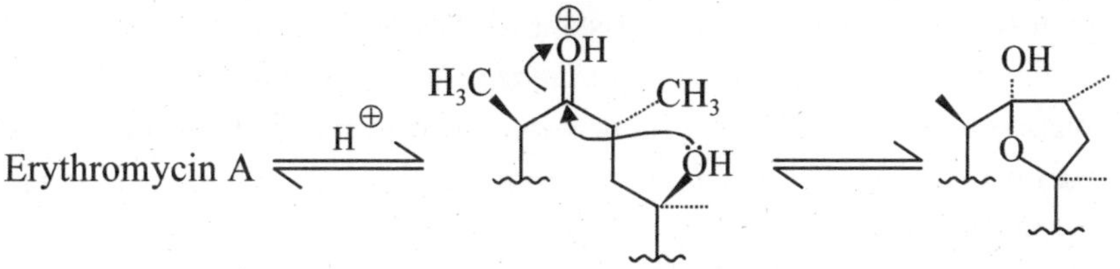

Acid-Catalyzed Formation of Hemiacetal

However, a similar reaction may also take place between the C-12 hydroxyl function and the C-9 carbonyl moiety.

In order to minimise this particular acid-instability semi-synthetic structural analogues of **erythromycin** have been developed by forming the corresponding 6-O-methyl derivative of **erythromycin A,** thereby blocking the possibility of **hemiacetal formation** completely.

Chemical Structure   **Clarithromycin** is nothing but a simple structural variant of **erythromycin A** having a 6-O-methyl substituent.

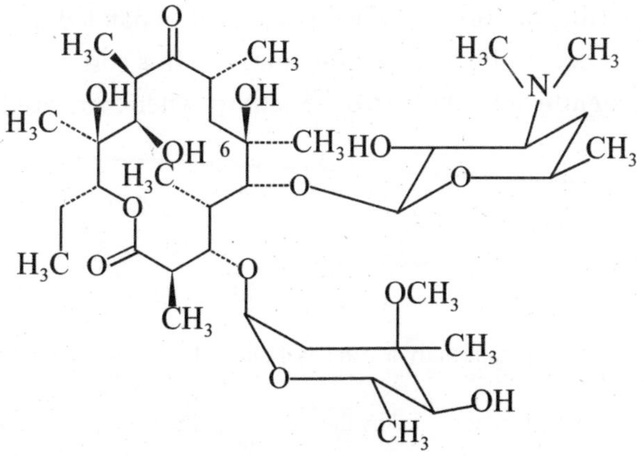

Clarithromycin

6-O-Methylerythromycin; ($C_{38}H_{69}NO_{13}$).

Characteristic Features

1. It is obtained as colourless powder from a (1 : 2) mixture of chloroform and diisopropyl ether having mp 217-220°C (decomposes).
2. It is also obtained as crystals from ethanol with mp 222-225°C (Morimoto).
3. It has uv_{max} (CHCl$_3$) : 288 nm (ε 27.9).
4. It has specific optical rotation $[\alpha]_D^{24}$-90.4° (C = 1 in CHCl$_3$).
5. It is found to be stable at acidic pH.

Uses

1. It is invariably used as an alternative to **erythromycin** for treating streptococcal pharyngitis, community-acquired respiratory tract infections, skin and soft tissue infections and an acute attack of **sinusitis.***
2. It is found to be two-to-four times more active than **erythronycin** itself against a host of *streptococci* and *staphylococci* species; however, certain organisms that are resistant to **erythromycin** are also observed to be resistant to clarithromycin.
3. It exhibits a moderate activity against *H. influenzae* and *N. gonorrhoea*.
4. Clarithromycin is found to be influenced by *Branhamella catarrhalis, Legionella pneumophilia, Mycoplasma pneumoniae, Chlamydia trachomatis* and *pneumoniae* and *Borrelia burgdorferi* (agent of **Lyme's disease****).
5. It also shows activity against *Mycobacterium avium* and *Mycobacterium intracellulare*; and is mostly employed as primary agent for the treatment of disseminated mycobacterial infections.

9.3.6.3 Azithromycin

Synonyms   Azitrocin; Sumamed; Trozocina; Zithromax; Zitromax; CP-62993; XZ-450.

Biological Source   It is a semi-synthetic **macrolide antibiotic** related to **erythromycin A** which is obtained from *Saccharopolyspora erythraae*.

Chemical Structure   **Azithromycin** is a tailor-made ring-expanded aza-macrolide wherein the carbonyl moiety at C-6 has been subjected to reduction; and this sort of minor alternation *vis-a-vis* the complex structure has significantly increased the activity when compared to the parent compound **erythromycin A.**

---

* **Sinusitis:** Inflammation of a sinus, especially a paranasal sinus. It may be caused by various agents, including viruses, bacteria or allergy:
** **Lyme's Disease:** A multisystem disorder caused by the tick-transmitted spirochete *Borhelia burgdorferi.*

Azithromycin

9-Deoxo-9α-methyl-9α-aza-9α-homoerythromycin A; ($C_{38}H_{72}N_2O_{12}$).

Characteristic Features

1. It is obtained as white crystals having mp 113-115°C .
2. It has specific optical rotation $[\alpha]_{20}^{D}$ -37° (C = 1 in $CHCl_3$).

Use

It is found to be active against staphylococci and streptococci but is more active than **erythromycin** against *H. influenzae* and some aerobic Gram-negative bacilli.

9.3.6.4 *Oleandomycin*

Synonyms   Amymicin; Landomycin; Romicil.

Biological Source   It is an **antibiotic** substance produced by fermentation cultures of *Streptomyces antibioticus* no. ATCC 11891.

Chemical Structure

Oleandomycin [$C_{35}H_{61}NO_{12}$]

Characteristic Features

1. It is obtained as white amorphous powder.
2. It has uv_{max} (methanol): 286-289 nm.
3. It is found to be freely soluble in methanol, ethanol, butanol, acetone; and almost insoluble in hexane, carbon tetrachloride, dibutyl ether.

Oleandomycin Hydrochloride $(C_{35}H_{61}NO_{12}\cdot HCl)$:

1. It is obtained as long needles from ethyl acetate having mp 134-135°C.
2. It has specific optical rotation $[\alpha]_D^{25}$-54° (methanol).
3. It is freely soluble in water; and forms various crystalline hydrates.

Oleandomycin Triacetate Ester   [*Synonym* **Troleandomycin; Cyclamycin; Wytrion; Evramycin; Triocetin; TAO; NSC-108166.**]

It is a **semi-synthetic macrolide antibiotic** prepared from oleandomycin wherein the three hydroxyl functions each at C-11, and the two sugar moieties replaced by the acetate groups.

1. It is obtained as crystals from isopropanol that yet decomposed at 176°C.
2. It is practically tasteless.
3. It has specific optical rotation $[\alpha]_D^{25}$-23° (methanol).
4. It shows a dissociation constant pKa 6.6.
5. It is found to be soluble in water < 0.1 g per 100 ml.

Uses   It is useful against a number of Gram-positive bacterial infections.

9.3.6.5 *Spiramycins*

Synonyms   Selectomycin; Revamicina; Rovamycin; RP-5337.

Biological Sources   **Spiramycins** are **macrolides** produced by cultures of *Streptomyces ambofaciens* from the soil of northern France.

Chemical Structure   The mixture of **spiramycins** have been successfully separated into *three* different components termed as: **Spiramycin I, II and III.**

Spiramycin I : R = H
Spiramycin II : R = COCH₃
Spiramycin III : R = COCH₂ CH₃

Characteristic Features

1. It is obtained as an amorphous base.
2. It has specific optical rotation $[\alpha]_D^{20}$-80° (methanol).
3. It has uv_{max} (ethanol): 231 nm.
4. It is found to be slightly soluble in water; and soluble in most organic solvents.

Uses

1. It exhibits activity on Gram-positive organisms and *rickettsiae*.
2. It also shows cross resistance between microorganisms resistant to **erythromycin** and **carbomycin**.

Spiramycin I [$C_{43}H_{74}N_2O_{14}$] [*Synonym* Foromacidin A]: It is obtained as crystals having mp ranging between 134-137°C, and specific optical rotation $[\alpha]_D^{20}$-96°.

Spiramycin II [$C_{45}H_{76}N_2O_{15}$] [*Synonym* Foromacidin B]: It is obtained as crystals having mp 130-133°C, and $[\alpha]_D^{20}$-86°.

Spiramycin III [$C_{46}H_{78}N_2O_{15}$] [*Synonym* Foromacidin C]: It is also obtained as crystals having mp ranging between 140-142°C, and $[\alpha]_D^{20}$-98.4°.

Spetamycin III Diacetate: It is obtained as crystals from cyclohexane having mp 140-142°C; and specific optical rotation $[\alpha]_D^{20}$-90.4°.

Use It is used for the treatment of toxoplasmosis, and also the infections caused by the protozoan *Toxoplasma gondii*.

9.3.7 Penicillins

Alexander Fleming observed in 1928 during the course of examination of certain culture plates in the laboratory of St. Mary's Hospital, London, that the lysis of the staphylococcus organisms takes place by a contaminating mold. Subsequently, the mold was subcultured in a sterile broth under aseptic condition; and it was revealed that it resulted into a powerful, nontoxic antibacterial product. Fleming baptized this substance as '**penicillin**' based on its parent organism *Penicillium notatum* that eventually paved the way for the creation of the so called '**generation of the antibiotic**'—a historic remarkable landmark in the field of medicine derived from the natural products.

'**Penicillin**' categorically symbolizes a host of vital and significantly prominent antibiotic substances produced by the growth of different *Penicillium* species or by various semi-synthetic or synthetic means.

In general, the penicillins are nomenclatured in the literature invariably as the derivatives of: (*a*) (2S-*cis*) -4-thia-1-azabicyclo-(3, 2, 0) heptane-2-carboxylic acid [I]; (*b*) 3, 3-dimethyl-7-oxo-derivative of [I] and also known by its trivial name **penicillanic acid** [II]; and (*c*) α-carboxamido derivative of it [III], here only the '*R*' of the α-carboxamido moiety is identified ultimately, as depicted below:

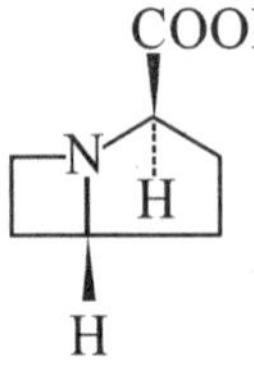

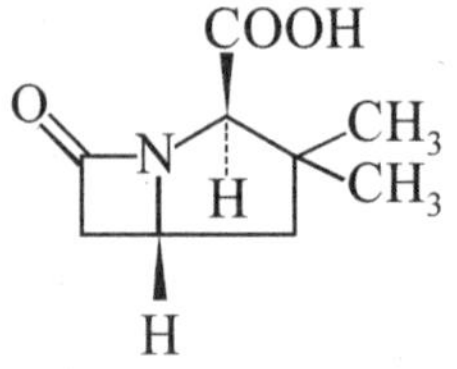

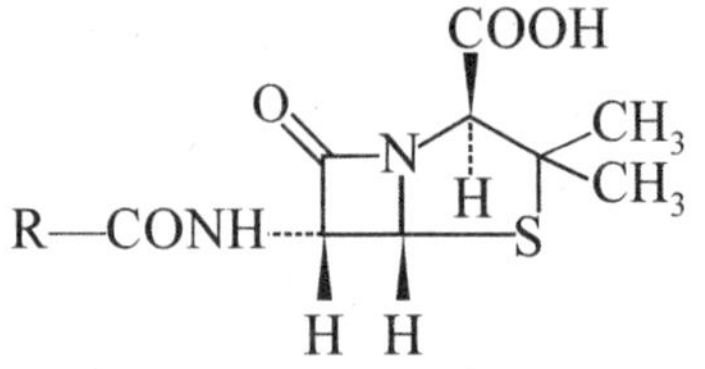

$$\text{I} \qquad \text{II} \qquad \text{III}$$

In actual practice, one comes across *three* different types of **penicillins,** such as:

(*a*) **Biosynthetic Penicillins:** These are usually accomplished by the introduction of various acids, amines or amides directly incorporated into the medium in which the mold is being developed thereby leading to the ultimate production of a spectrum of biosynthetic penicillins which essentially differ only in '*R*' in III. By adopting this unique well-developed and articulated process dozens of **biosynthetic penicillins** have been prepared with a view to obtain newer molecules that have an edge over penicillin G with regard to various physical parameters, microbiological or pharmacological characteristics.

It is pertinent to mention here that in 1958 an altogether new dimension was added to update and boost up the on-going development of penicillins. Methods were devised for modifying the very **'penicillin nucleus'** thereby making it feasible to biosynthesize penicillins which earlier could note be accomplished in a just normal medium. The concerted efforts made by the researchers resulted into the formation of plethora of altogether new series of medicinally potent substances that were often found to be more acid-stable, more-penicillinase resistant or had a wider antibacterial spectrum.

(*b*) **Commercial Penicillins:** In fact, a major portion of the commercial penicillin is pure crystalline penicillin G. It is invariably obtained in the fermentation liquors along with variable quantities of penicillin K and F and relatively smaller amount of others. However, penicillin G is eventually separated from the other congeners during the process of purification. Nevertheless, the commercial process of producing penicillins is observed to suppress, to some extent, the inherent natural tendency of the mold to give rise to penicillins other than the desired **penicillin G** by the introduction of a precursor of G, such as: **phenylacetic acid, phenylacetamide, phenylethylamine** or such other chemical entities containing the **'phenylacetyl'** radical, that is incorporated directly into the **penicillin G** molecule. It is worth while to state here that **penicillin G** enjoys the additional advantage of being crystallized out more easily than K or F.

(*c*) **Salts of Penicillins:** From the figures I, and II and III it is quite evident that penicillin are acids. The potassium salt is more prevalent and hence predominates in actual usage, with the sodium salt next. The inherent acidic moiety may be exploited skillfully and judiciously to combine **penicillins** with various bases, namely: **procaine, benzathine,** to design and evolve rather insoluble salts, for repository application, or for the objective of minimising solubility so as to render the substance more resistant to gastric acid in the stomach.

9.3.7.1 *Classification and Spectrum*

Initially, **penicillins** were classified either on the basis of pseudohistorical categories, or according to various numbered **"generation"**, very much identical to the classification of the **'cephalosporins'** (section 9.3.3). In fact, it is rather more convenient and beneficial as well to classify them according to a well-defined chemical and antimicrobial designations, namely:

(*i*) **Natural Penicillins** (best streptococcal and narrow spectrum)

(*ii*) **Penicillinase-resistant Penicillins** (antistaphylococcal)

(*iii*) **Aminopenicillins** (improved Gram-negative: *H. influenzae, Enterococcus, Shigella, Salmonella*)

(*iv*) **Extended-spectrum (antipseudomonal) penicillins**

(*v*) **Beta Lactamase Combinations** (expand spectrum to staph, beta-lactamase producers)

It will be worthwhile to treat a few **important penicillin drugs** individually from each category in the sections that follow:

9.3.7.1.1 Natural Penicillins

A. Penicillin G Potassium

Synonyms   Crystapen; Cosmopen; Eskacillin; Forpen; Hylenta; Hyasorb; Monopen; Notaral; Pentid.

Preparation   It is prepared by the interaction of 6-amino-penicillanic acid and phenyl acetyl chloride in an inert organic solvent.

Chemical Structure   Please refer to section 9.3.7.1.

Characteristic Features

1. It is obtained as colourless or white crystals, or a white crystalline powder, odourless or practically so; moderately hygroscopic and gets decomposed between 214-217°C.
2. Humidity and moisture accelerates decomposition.
3. It has specific optical rotation $[\alpha]_D^{22} + 285\text{-}310°$ (C = 0.7).
4. It is not appreciably affected either by air or by light.
5. The solutions usually deteriorate at room temperature, but solutions stored lower than 15°C remain stable for several days.
6. It gets rapidly inactivated by acids and alkalies, and also by oxidizing agents.
7. The pH (aqueous solution 30 mg · mL^{-1}) 5 and 7.5.
8. The dissociation constant pKa (acid) 2.8.
9. **Solubility Profile:** It is found to be very soluble in water, saline TS or dextrose solutions; soluble in ethanol (*but is inactivated by this solvent*), glycerol and several other alcohols.
10. **Penicillin G Potassium** 1 mg ≡ 1595 U.S.P. Penicillin Unit or International Unit (IU).

Uses

1. It is still recommended as an important and useful drug for the treatment of many Gram-positive organisms, such as streptococci, pneumococci, gonococci, and meningococci infections.
2. It is mostly destroyed by gastric juice and is, therefore, not given by oral route, and is best administered as IM or IV injection.
3. The K-salt as such has no advantage over the corresponding Na-salt except when high doses are used in patients on sodium restriction *e.g.*, blood-pressure patients.
4. The K-salt also avoids the incidence of *hypokalemic alkalosis* which occasionally takes place during prolonged treatment with high doses of penicillins.
5. The half-life ranges between 0.5 to 0.7 hour; except 2.5 to 10 hour in renal failure or after probenecid.

Penicillins

Class	S.No.	Name (Synonyms)	Chemical Structure	Remarks
I. Natural Penicillins (best streptococcal and narrow spectrum)	1	Penicillins G sodium or Penicillin G potassium [Benzylpenicillin sodium or Benzylpenicillin potassium]	*(structure)*	Best narrow spectrum (streptoeocci), IV, IM.
	2	Penicillin V [Phenoxymethyl-penicillin; Penicillin phenoxy-methyl]	*(structure)*	Same spectrum profile as Penicillin G; Oral only
II. Penicillinase-Resistant Penicillins (antistaphylococcal)	3	Cloxacillin	*(structure)* R = H;	Oral
	4	Dicloxacillin [Maclicine]	R = Cl; in 3 above.	Preferred oral
	5	Methicillin [Dimethoxyphenecillin]	*(structure)*	IV; interstitial nephritis may take place.
	6	Nafcillin [6-(2-Ethoxy-1-naphthamido) penicillin]	*(structure)*	Preferred IV drug for staphylococcus
	7	Oxacillin [Oxazocilline]	*(structure)*	Oral

(Contd.)

Class	S.No.	Name (Synonyms)	Chemical Structure	Remarks
III. Aminopenicillins (Improved Gram-negative H. influenzae, Enterococcus, Shigella, Salmonella.)	8	Amoxicillin [para-hydroxyampicillin; Amoxycillin; Delacillin; Sawacillin; Wide-cillin]		Good oral absorption
	9	Ampicillin [Bonapicillin; Doktacillin; Domicillin; Tokiocillin]		Preferred IV drug; incomplete oral absorption; diarrhoea; rash
	10	Bacampicillin		Oral prodrug converted to ampicillin
IV. Extended-Spectrum (Antipseudomonal) Penicillins	11	Carbenicillin [α-Phenyl (carboxymethyl penicillin)]		IV, high sodium, oral prodrug (Indanyl sodium) available
	12	Tiacarcillin [α-Carboxy-3-thienylmethylpenicillin]		IV, similar to carbenicillin but less sodium
	13	Mezlocillin		IV; similar to piperacillin
	14	Piperacillin [4-Ethyl-2, 3-dioxo piperazine carbonyl ampicillin]		Preferred IV; best Gram-negative spectrum

(Contd.)

Class	S.No.	Name (Synonyms)	Chemical Structure	Remarks
V. β-Lactamase Combination (expand spectrum to staph., β-lactamase producers)	15	Clavulanate Amoxicillin	Clavulanic Acid + Amoxicillin	Oral; more diarrhoea than amoxicillin
	16	Sulbactam-Ampicillin	+ Ampicillin	IV; active vs. staph. and β-lactamase-producing *H. influenzae Strep pneum*
	17	Clavulanate-Ticarcillin	Clavulanic Acid + Ticarcillin	IV; active vs more Gram-negative bacilli
	18	Tazobactam-piperacillin	+ Piperacillin	IV; active vs. more Gram-negative bacilli

(Abstracted from: Remington-The Science and Practice of Pharmacy Vol. II., 20th edn., 2000)

B. Penicillin V

Synonyms   Acipen-V; Distaquaine V; Fenospen; Meropenin; Oracilline; Oratren; V-Cillin.

Biological Source   It is obtained by the addition of phenoxyacetic acid to the *Penicillium chrysogenum* culture using yeast autolyzate as a source of nitrogen, as shown below:

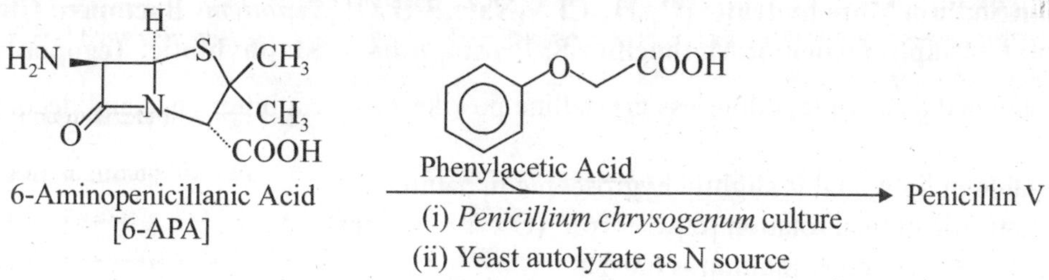

6-Aminopenicillanic Acid
[6-APA]

Phenylacetic Acid
_____→ Penicillin V
(i) *Penicillium chrysogenum* culture
(ii) Yeast autolyzate as N source

Chemical Structure   Please refer to Section 9.3.7.1.

Characteristic Features

1. It is obtained as crystals that get decomposed between 120-128°.
2. It is found to be failry stable in air upto 37°C.
3. It is relatively stable to acid.
4. It has uv_{max}: 268, 274 nm (ε 1330, 1100).
5. **Solubility Profile**   It is found to be soluble in water at pH 1.8 (acidified with HCl) = 25 mg/100 ml; soluble in polar organic solvents; and almost insoluble in vegetable oils and in liquid petrolatum.

Uses

1. **Phenoxymethylpenicillin (Penicillin V)** enjoys the greatest advantage of being recognized as 'acid-resistant, which is solely due to the introduction of an electron-withdrawing heteroatom (*i.e.,* O-atom of phenoxy-moiety) into the side-chain.
2. It is, therefore, suitable for oral administration.
3. It is specifically recommended for respiratory tract infections and tonsilitis.

Penicillin V Potassium Salt [$C_{16}H_{17}KN_2O_5S$]   [*Synonyms* **Antibiocin; Apsin VK; Arcacin; Beromycin; Betapen VK; Calciopen; Cliacil; Compocillin VK; Distakaps V-K; Dowpen VK; Fenoxypen; Ledercillin VK; Penavlon V; Pen-Oral; Stabicilline; Uticillin VK; Vepen; Suspen]**

It is soluble in water; and has specific optical rotation $[\alpha]_D^{25} + 223°$ (C = 0.2).

Uses   It exhibits an antibacterial spectrum very identical to that of **penicillin G** against Gram-positive bacteria but this is less potent and effective against Gram-negative bacteria. Its biological half-life is about 0.5 to 1 hour.

9.3.7.1.2 Penicillinase-resistant Penicillins

A. Cloxacillin

Biological Source   **Cloxacillin** is a **semi-synthetic antibiotic** related to **penicillin;** and is the chlorinated derivative of **oxacilline** which contains an isoxazole group.

Preparation   6-APA is acylated with 3-(o-chlorophenyl)-5-methyl-4-isoxazolecarboxylic acid. The resulting **cloxacillin** is subsequently purified by recrystallization.

Chemical Structure   Please refer to section 9.3.7.1.

Characteristic Features

Cloxacillin Sodium Monohydrate: [$C_{19}H_{17}Cl$ $N_3NaO_5S \cdot H_2O$] [*Synonyms* Bactopen; Cloxapen; Cloxypen; Gelstaph; Orbenin; Methocillin-S; Prostaphlin-A; Staphybiotic; Tegopen]

1. It is obtained as a white, odourless crystalline powder having a bitter taste and decompose at 170°C.
2. It is stable in light; and is slightly hygroscopic in nature.
3. It has specific optical rotation $[\alpha]_D^{20}$ + 163° (C = 1 in water).
4. The pH of 1% aqueous solution is 6.0-7.5.
5. Its dissociation constant pKa (COOH) is 2.7.
6. It is found to be soluble in water, methanol, ethanol, pyridine and ethylene glycol; and slightly soluble in chloroform.

Uses
1. It is **penicillinase-resistant penicillin** (antistaphylococcal) which is administered orally.
2. It is a first-choice agent against penicillin-resistant *Staphylococcus aureus*.

B. Nafcillin

Biological Source   It is a semi-synthetic antibiotic related to penicillin bearing essentially a maphthamido moiety.

Preparation   6-APA is first acylated by treatment with 2-ethoxy-1-naphthoyl chloride in an anhydrous organic solvent containing triethylamine. An aqueous extract of this product is admixed with a water-immiscible solvent and nafcillin is precipitated by the addition of H_2SO_4. The crude product may be recrystallized from chloroform.

Chemical Structure   Please refer to Section 9.3.7.1.

Characteristic Features

Nafcillin Sodium [$C_{21}H_{21}N_2NaO_5S$]: [*Synonyms* Nafcil; Naftopen; Unipen]

1. It is obtained as white to yellowish white powder having not more than a slight characteristic odour.
2. It is freely soluble in water or chloroform; and soluble in alcohol.

Uses
1. It is considered as a preferred drug given through IV for staphylococci.
2. It is a **penicillinase-resistant penicillin,** the use of which is restricted to the treatment of infections caused by penicillinase-producing cocci (mostly staphylococci).

Note: After oral administration serum levels are low and invariably unpredictable, hence the oral route is not recommended.

9.3.7.1.3 Aminopenicillins

A. Amoxicillin

Synonyms Amoxycillin; Amocilline; Amolin; Amopenixin; Amoram; Amoxipen; Anemolin; Aspenil; Betamox; Cabermox; Delacillin; Efpenix; Grinsil; Helvamox; Optium; Ospamox; Pasetocin; Penamox; Penimox; Piramox; Sawacillin; Sumox.

Biological Source It is a **semi-synthetic antibiotic** related to **penicillin** with side-chain containing a basic amino moiety.

Preparation It may be prepared by carrying out the acylation of 6-aminopenicillanic acid with D-(-)-2-(p-hydroxyphenyl) glycine.

Chemical Structure Please refer to Section 9.3.7.1.

It is usually obtained as its trihydrate product.

Characteristic Features

Amoxicillin Trihydrate $[C_{16}H_{19}N_3O_5S.3H_2O]$: [*Synonyms* Alfamox; Almodan; Amoxidin; Amoxypen; Clamoxyl; Cuxacillin; Flemoxin; Ibiamox; Moxaline; Polymox; Robamox; Sigamopen; Silamox; Trimox; Utimox; Zamocillin].

1. It is obtained as fine, white to off-white, crystalline powder, bitter taste.
2. Exposure to high humidity and temperature beyond 37°C adversely affect the stability of amoxicillin.
3. It has specific optical rotation $[\alpha]_D^{20}$ + 246° (C = 0.1).
4. It has uv$_{max}$ (ethanol): 230, 274 nm (ε 10850, 1400); (0.1N HCl) : 229, 272 nm (ε 9500, 1080); (0.1N KOH): 248, 291 (ε 2200, 3000).
5. **Solubility Profile:** In mg . ml^{-1}: water 4.0; methanol 7.5; absolute ethanol 3.4. It is found to be insoluble in hexane, benzene, ethyl acetate and acetonitrile.

Uses

1. Its antibacterial spectrum is very much similar to that of **Ampicillin,** except that its activity is less against *Streptococcus*; *N. meningitidis*; *Clostridium; Salmonella*; and *Shigella*.
2. It is found to be more acid stable than **ampicillin** and absorption is not affected appreciably by food intake.
3. It is the drug of choice for various infections caused by *Enterococcus faecalis (enterococcus) Branhamella catarrhalis* or *Bacteroides fragilis* (mild to moderate infections).
4. It is an alternate drug for infections by penicillinase-producing *Staphylococcus* (combined with clavulanic acid), *N. gonorrhoeae* (with probenecid), *E. coli* (with clavulanic acid) or *Pasteurella multicida* (with clavulanic acid).

Note: **It cannot be given parenterally in conditions with severe infections.**

B. Ampicillin

Synonyms Albipen; Amfipen; Ampipenin; Bonapicillin; Britacil; Doktacillin; Domicillin; Dumopen; Nuvapen; Omnipen; Penicline; Tokiocillin.

Biological Source   It is orally active, semi-synthetic antibiotic which is structurally related to penicilline *i.e.*, penicillin with side-chain having a basic amino function.

Preparation   The outline of the synthesis is that 6-APA is appropriately acylated with D-glycine under specific experimental parameters. Kajfez *et. al.*, in 1976 put forward an alternate method of synthesis.*

Chemical Structure   Please see Section 9.3.7.1. It is mostly obtained as its trihydrate product.

Characteristic Features

1. It is obtained as crystals that get decomposed between 199–202°C.
2. It has specific optical rotation $[\alpha]_D^{23}$ + 287.9° (C = 1 in water).
3. It is found to be sparingly soluble in water.

Uses

1. It is the **first aminopenicillin antibiotic** which exhibits its *in vitro* spectrum against Gram-positive cocci very much similar to but usually somewhat less effective than that of penicillin G, with an exception that it is somewhat effective against *Enterococcus faecalis* (enterococcus).
2. It is $1/20$ as effective against *Streptococcus pyogenes.*
3. It is the drug of choice for treatment of infections due to sensitive strains of Strep Group B, *Enterococcus faecalis* (combined with **gentamycin**); *Listeria monocytogenes* (with or without **gentamycin**); *E. coli* (with or without **gentamycin**); and *Prot mirabilis,* and *Salmonella* (not typhi).
4. It is employed invariably as an alternative drug against *Kl pneumoniae* (with **sulbactam**), indole-positive *Proteus (M. morganii, Pr vulgaris* and *Providencia rettegri*; with **sulbactam**), *Salmonella typhi, Shigella, Gardnerella vaginalis, H. influenzae* (serious infections; initially combined with **chloramphenicol**) or *Nocardia.*

Note: 1.   A good number of these organisms rapidly acquire resistance by elaboration of penicillinase, hence it is invariably administered in combination with sublactam.

2.   It causes allergic reactions typical of other penicillins and is found to be five-times as allergenic as penicillin G.

Ampicillin Sodium [$C_{16}H_{18}Na_3O_4S$]   [*Synonyms* Alpen-N; Amcill-S; Ampicin; Cilleral; Omnipen-N; Penbritin-S; Pentrex; Polycillin-N; Synpenin; Viccillin.]

Preparation   It is prepared by *first* dissolving ampicillin in a suitable organic solvent, and *secondly* by precipitating it as its sodium salt by the addition of sodium accetate.

Characteristic Features

1. It is obtained as white to off-white, crystalline powder, hygroscopic in nature; the L(+) form decomposes at about 205°C.
2. Its dissociation constants are pKa$_1$ 2.66; pKa$_2$ 7.24.
3. L(+) form has specific optical rotation $[\alpha]_D^{20}$ + 209° (C = 0.2 in water).
4. It is found to be very soluble in water, isotonic NaCl or dextrose solutions.

---

* F. Kajfez *et al., J. Heterocycl. Chem.*, **13**, 561, (1976)

5. It has been observed that L(+) form is less active as an antibiotic than the corresponding D(–) isomer.

Uses It is employed for IM or IV administration; and its actions and uses are similar to *Ampicillin.*

C. Bacampicillin

Biological Source It is a **semi-synthetic antibiotic** related to penicillin. It is an acyloxymethyl ester through the **thiazolidine** carboxyl moiety (*i.e.,* a *'prodrug'*), and is duly hydrolyzed to **ampicillin** by esterases in the gut.

Chemical Structure Please refer to Section 9.3.7.1.

Characteristic Features

Bacampicillin Hydrochloride [$C_{21}H_{27}N_3O_7S.HCl$]: [*Synonyms* Ambacamp; Ambaxin; Bacacil; Bacampicine; Spectrabid.]

1. It is obtained as white crystals from a mixture of acetone and petroleum ether having mp 171-176°C. (decomposes).
2. It has specific optical rotation $[\alpha]_D^{20}$ + 161.5°; and also reported as + 173° (Bodin).
3. The pH of a 2% (w/v) aqueous solution ranges between 3 to 4.5.
4. **Solubility Profile:** It is found to be soluble 1g in 15ml. water, 7ml. alcohol and 10 ml. chloroform.

Uses
1. It is an oral prodrug converted to **ampicillin** *in vivo.*
2. It is an improved version of **aminopenicillin** with modified and enhanced Gram-negative activity against *H. influenzae, Enterococcus, Shigella* and *Salmonella.*

9.3.7.1.4 Extended-Spectrum Penicillins The various typical examples of **extended-spectrum (antipseudomonal) penicillins** are **carbenicillin** and **ticarcillin** wherein the penicillins contain an *additional-COOH moiety in the side-chain* and their overall activity is certainly broad-spectrum. Another type of **extended-spectrum penicillins** essentially include the **acylureido penicillins,** namely: **Mezlocillin** and **Piperacillin,** which are found to be much more active against *Pseudomonas aeruginosa* together with other Gram-negative organisms, such as: *Klebsiella pneumoniae* and *Haemophilus influenzae.*

These aforesaid antibiotics shall now be discussed in the sections that follows:

A. Carbenicillin

Biological Source It is a **semi-synthetic antibiotic** related to **penicillin** that essentially has an additional carboxylic function present in the side-chain.

Chemical Structure Please refer to Section 9.3.7.1.

Preparation First of all the starting esters may be prepared by acylating 6-aminopenicillanic acid (*i.e.,* 6-APA) with monoesters of phenylmalonic acid. The resulting esters are subsequently hydrolyzed with the help of an appropriate *esterase,* for instance: **α-chymotrypsin** or **pancreatin,** and extracting the liberated acid with a suitable organic solvent.

Characteristic Features

Carbenicillin Disodium [$C_{17}H_{16}Na_2O_6S$]: [*Synonyms Anabactyl; Carbapen; Carbecin; Geopen; Hyoper; Microcillin; Pyocianil; Pyopen.*]

1. It is obtained as white to off-white, crystalline powder having a bitter taste, odourless; and hygroscopic in nature.
2. The pH of a 1% (w/v) aqueous solution is 8.0.
3. It gives rise to two distinct values for dissociation constant *viz.*, pKa_1 2.76 and pKa_2 3.50.
4. **Solubility Profile:** 1 g in 1.2 ml water; 2.5 ml ethanol; and almost insoluble in chloroform and ether.

Uses

1. It is a **carboxy benzyl penicillin** with enhanced antibacterial profile against non-β-**lactamase** producing Gram-negative bacilli, precisely *Pseudomonas aeruginosa*.
2. It has been observed that the D-and L-isomers actually show very slight differences in their biologic activity, besides they undergo rapid interconversion when in solution; hence, most logically the racemic mixture is employed invariably.
3. It may be safely administered to a maximum extent of 4 g per day so as to obtain serum concentration exceeding 50-60 mcg ml^{-1}, which concentrations normally inhibit most *Pseudomonas aeruginosa* strains.
4. It has been observed that the clinical efficacy may be increased appreciably by the combination therapy of carbenicillin disodium either with *tobramycin* or *gentamycin* in their respective full therapeutic dosages.

   Note: There is an obvious possibility of a chemical interaction between aminoglycosides and β-lactam antibiotics, whereby the amino moieties of the aminoglycoside molecules afford to attack the β-lactam ring, ultimately result into the formation of a covalent adduct and finally the inactivation of the antibiotics. This serious drawback is easily overcome by their administration through different routes.

5. It is particularly effective in UTIs by virtue of its attainment of very high urine levels through IM.

B. Ticarcillin

Biological Source   It is a broad-spectrum, semi-synthetic antibiotic related to penicillin; and it also essentially has an additional carboxylic function at *alpha* position in the side-chain.

Chemical Structure   Please refer to section 9.3.7.1.3.

Preparation   It may be prepared by the conversion of 2-(3-thienyl) malonic acid monobenzyl ester to the corresponding acid chloride which is subsequently condensed with 6-APA, followed by hydrogenation to convert the ester to the free acid.*

---

* Belgian, Pat 646,991.

Characteristic Features

Ticarcillin Disodium [C$_{15}$H$_{14}$N$_2$Na$_2$O$_6$S$_2$] [*Synonyms* Aerugipen, Monapen; Ticar; Ticarpen; Ticillin]

1. It is obtained as creamy-white, hygroscopic non-crystalline powder.
2. It is found to be quite unstable in an acidic medium.
3. It has dissociation constant pKa (acid form) 2.44 and 3.64.
4. The pH of a concentrated solution (> 100 g. mL^{-1}) is approximately 7.0.
5. Its aqueous solutions are relatively stable; and the acidic solutions comparatively unstable.

Uses

1. Its antibacterial profile very much resembles to that of *Carbenicillin* (Section 9.3.7.1.4.A).
2. It is found to be twice as active against *Ps aeruginosa*.
3. Though it has an inherent tendency to develop resistance readily; however, with many infections the resistance is obviated by inclusion of clavulanic acid.
4. For the treatment, control and management of Gram-negative infections, it is invariably combined with either **gentamycin** (Section 9.3.1.2) or **tobramycin** (see section 9.3.1.7) so as to enhance activity and delay resistance to an appreciable extent.

C. Mezlocillin

Biological Source   It is a **semisynthetic, broad-spectrum antibiotic** related to **penicillin** and **azlocillin;** and belong to the class of acylureido penicillins.

Chemical Structure   Please refer to Section 9.3.7.1.

Characteristic Features

Mezlocillin Sodium Monohydrate [C$_{21}$H$_{24}$N$_5$NaO$_5$S$_2$.H$_2$O]   [*Synonyms Baycipen; Baypen; Mezlin*]:

1. It is obtained as either yellowish-white powder or as pale yellow crystalline substance.
2. It has dissociation constant pK$_a$ 2.7.
3. It is found to be soluble in water, methanol and DMF; and insoluble in acetone nd ethanol.

Uses

1. It is one of the most active penicillins against *Ps aeruginosa*, with a potency almost at par with **gentamycin.**
2. It is found to be more potent against *Klebsiella* and a host of other enteric bacilli than is **carbenicillin** and **ticarcellin** (A and B above).
3. It is employed frequently as an **'alternative drug'** against infections caused by *Acinetobacter, Bacteroidis fragilis* (G.I. strains), *Enterobacter, E. coli, Kl pneumoniae, Morganella morganii, Pr vulgaris, Providencia rettegeri, Ps aeruginosa* (UTIs) or *Serratia*.

D. Piperacillin

Biological Source   It is a **broad spectrum semi-synthetic antibiotic** related to **penicillin** bearing essentially an acylureido function.

Chemical Structure   Please refer to Section 9.3.7.1.

Characteristic Features

Piperacillin Sodium [C$_{23}$H$_{26}$N$_5$NaO$_7$S]   [*Synonyms Isipen; Pipril Pentcillin; Pipracil*]: It is obtained as white crystals having mp 183-185°C (decomposes). 1g gets dissolved in approximately 1.5 ml water or methanol, and 5 ml of ethyl alcohol.

Uses
1. It is an **extended-spectrum (antipseudomonal) penicillin.**
2. It is usually administered IV.
3. Its activities are very much similar to **mezlocillin sodium** (sec C above).

9.3.7.1.5 Beta-Lactamase Combinations   β-**Lactamases** are the enzymes that help in opening up the β-lactam rings of penicillins, **cephalosporins** and also the related compounds exclusively at the **β-lactam bond.** Generally, the **β-lactamases** may be classified into *three* major categories, namely:

(*a*) Substrate selectivity and inhibition,
(*b*) Acidity/basicity of the enzyme protein, and
(*c*) Intra-and extracellular location of enzyme.

Penicillinases   are the enzymes which get excreted exclusively from the *bacterium* and the *genes* located on plasmids. These are broadly regarded as **Type II β-lactamases;** and are essentially responsible for the penicillin-resistant Gram-positive organisms, Gram-negative cocci, besides a host of Gram-negative bacilli.

It has been observed that the penicillinase-resistant penicillins usually get bound to the penicillinases; however the actual dissociation of the **'drug'-enzyme complex** is rather quite rapid. In actual practice, they have been successfully supplanted by three substances, namely: **clavulanic acid, sulbactam** and **tazobactam.** All these are regarded as newer breeds of β-lactamase inhibitors that specifically acylate the enzymes by creation of a **'double-bond' (greater electronic bondage)** and consequently afford dissociation very slowly, thereby significantly enhancing the potency of the penicillins against certain organisms and ultimately increase their therapeutic efficacy.

The combination of **β-lactamase inhibitors** with other antibiotics helps to expand the spectrum of the **antibiotic** to a significant extent which may be observed evidently by carrying out the *in vitro* studies.

There are *three* **important β-lactamase inhibitors** duly recognized, namely: **clavulanic acid, sulbactam,** and **tazobactam,** which shall now be discussed individually and also the combinations with antibiotics which are available commercially in the sections that follow:

A. Clavulanic Acid

Synonyms   MM 14151

Biological Source   It is a β-Lactamase inhibitor, and an antibiotic obtained as a fermentation product of *Streptomyces clavuligerus,* structurally related to the penicillins. **Clavulanic acid** enjoys the status of being the first ever reported naturally occurring **fused β-lactam containing oxygen.***

---

* *J. Antibiot.,* **29**, 668, 1976

Chemical Structure Please refer to Section 9.3.7.1.

Characteristic Features

Clavulanate Potassium [$C_8H_8KNO_5$]: It is obtained as a white powder having a bitter taste. 1g is soluble in 2.5 ml of ethanol or in less than 1 ml of water.

Uses

1. The sulphur at position 1 of the β-lactam ring has been strategically replaced by oxygen (less electro negative); and also there is an ethylidene function present at position 2, that significantly increases reactivity with the typical exopenicillinases of *Staphylococcus aureus* and *Epidermatitis* and the Gram-negative β-lactamases of the Richmond Types II and III (*Haemophilus, Niesseria, E. coli, Salmonella* and *Shigella*), IV (*Bacteroides, Klebsiella* and *Legionella*) and V. Interestingly, these are all plasmid-mediated enzymes; and the chromosomally mediated enzymes are not inhibited at all.
2. It is absorbed well orally, but is also suitable for parenteral administration. The half-life is about 1 hour.
   Clavulanate Amoxicillin Trihydrate (*i.e., combination of potassium salt with* **amoxicillin trihydrate**).

Synonyms Augmentin; Amoksiklav; Co-Amoxiclav; Ciblor; Klavocin; NeO-Duplamox.

Uses

1. It is a **β-lactam antibiotic** with a β-lactamase inhibitor.
2. It extends the *in vitro* activity of **amoxicillin** to include **β-lactamase** producing strains of *H. influenzae, E. coli; Pr. Mirabilis*; and *S. aureus*.
   Note:
   (*a*) **It is pertinent to mention here that it may not extend the spectrum to various bacteria not usually killed by amoxicillin (such as: Pseudomonas aeuruginosa) in the absence of β-lactamase resistance.**
   (*b*) **Clavulanate Ticarcillin Disodium** (*i.e.*, **combination of potasium salt with ticarcillin disodium**):

Synonyms Betabactyl; Timentin.

Uses

1. It is employed for parenteral treatment of UTIs, skin and soft tissue, and lower respiratory tract infections, and sepsis caused due to suceptible bacteria.
2. The combination exerts an appreciable increase in activity that takes place against particularly the β-**lactamase**-producing strains of *S. aureus, H. influenzae, gonococcus, E. coli*, and *Klebsiella*.
   Note: It fails to inhibit the β-lactamases generated by majority of strains of pseudomonas, Enterobacter and certain other Gram-negative bacilli; besides, β-lactamase-producing strains of those bacteria which eventually remain resistant to ticarcillin.

B. Sulbactam

Synonyms Penicillanic acid sulfone; Penicillanic acid 1, 1-dioxide; CP-45899.

Biological Source It is also a **semi-synthetic β-lactamase** inhibitor; and is structurally related to the **penicillins.**

Preparation 6-APA is diazotized to result into the formation of the unstable diazo derivative, which is subsequently and rapidly converted to the corresponding 6, 6-dibromo compound by carrying out the reaction in the presence of bromine. Finally, the resulting product is subjected to catalytic hydrogenolysis of the bromine atoms from the product.*

Chemical Structure Please refer to Section 9.3.7.1.

Characteristic Features
1. It is obtained as white crystalline solid having mp 148-151°C.
2. It has specific optical rotation $[\alpha]_D^{20}$ + 251° (C = 0.01 in pH 5.0 buffer).
3. It is found to be soluble in water.

Sulbactam Sodium [$C_8H_{10}NNaO_5S$] [*Synonyms* Betamaze; Unasyn; CP-45899-2.]

Uses
1. It shows greater activity against **Type-I β-lactamases** than clavulanic acid, but fails to penetrate the cell walls of Gram-negative organisms.
2. It also exert its own feeble antibacterial activity.
3. It is absorbed by the oral route but is also suitable for parenteral administration.

Sulbactam Ampicillin [*i.e.*, mixture of sodium salt with ampicillin sodium]: [*Synonyms* Bethacil (inj.); Loricin; Unacid; Unacin (inj.)]

Uses It extends the antibacterial profile of ampicillin to include **β-lactamase**-producing strains of *Acinetobacter, Bacteroides*, besides other anaerobes, such as: *Branhamella, Enterobacter, E. coli, Klebsiella, Neisseria, Proteus,* and *Staphylococcus.*

C. Tazobactam

Synonyms CL-298741; YTR –830H.

Biological Source It is a **β-lactamase inhibitor** and structurally related to the **penicillins.** It also supplants the general approach of expanding the antibacterial spectrum of certain antibiotic(s) (*e.g.,* **piperacillin sodium**) to include some **β-lactamase-producing strains.**

Chemical Structure Please see section 9.3.7.1.

Characteristic Features

Tazobactam Sodium [$C_{10}H_{11}N_4NaO_5S$] [*Synonyms* YTR-830; CL-307579]: It is an amorphous solid having mp > 170°C (decomposes).

Tazobactam Piperacillin [*i.e., mixture of tazobactam sodium with piperacillin sodium*] [*Synonyms* Tazocilline; Tazocin; Zosyn;]: The combination product is administered by IV-infusion over 30 minutes duration. The usual total daily dose is usually 12 grammes of piperacillin and 1.5 grammes of tazobactam gives as 3.375 gramms every 6 hours. It is found to be active *Vs* more Gram-negative bacilli.

---

* *J. Org. Chem.,* **47**, 3344, 1982.

9.3.8 Polypeptide Antibiotics

Interestingly, a plethora of **polypeptides** of bacterial origin that are found to comprise of D- and L-amino acids, do exert a marked and pronounced antibiotic activity. It is, however, pertinent to mention here that these specific antibiotics have two inherent major anomalies, namely: *first*, very poor absorption from the intestinal tract; and *secondly*, possess high degree of nephrotoxicity* when used systemically. Generally, the **polypeptide antibiotics** exert a predominantly Gram-positive spectrum; however, there are a few-exceptions that are solely active against Gram-negative organisms, such as: the strongly basic **polymyxins.**

It has been observed that these **polypeptide antibiotics** have a tendency to occur as mixtures of very close structurally related compounds. Nevertheless, the exact composition of commercial mixtures depend to a great extent upon the skilful usage of selected strains of producing organisms. Besides, a precise and reliable strength of therapeutic response against certain susceptible organisms is exclusively based on the quantitative microbial assay.

The various important members of 'polypeptide antibiotics' are, namely: **cycloserine; polymyxin-B; colistin (polymixin-E), bacitrasin; vanomycin;** and **teichoplanin,** which shall now be treated separately as under:

9.3.8.1 Cycloserine

Synonyms   Closina; Farmiserina; Micoserina; Orientomycin; Oxamycin; Seromycin; PA-94.

Biological Sources   It is a **polypeptide antibiotic** substance produced by *Streptomyces garyphalus* sive *orchidaceus.***

Preparation   It may also be synthesized by the method of Stammer *et al.****

Chemical Structure

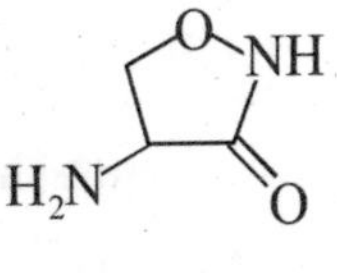

Cycloserine

D-4-Amino-3-isoxazolidinone; $C_3H_6N_2O_2$.

Characteristic Features
1. It is obtained as crystals that decompose at 155-156°C.
2. Its specific optical rotations are: $[\alpha]_D^{23} + 116°$ (C = 1.17); $[\alpha]_{546}^{25} + 137°$ (C = 5 in 2N NaOH).
3. It has uv$_{max}$: 226 nm ($E_{1cm}^{1\%}$ 402).
4. Its aqueous solutions have a pH 6.
5. It is fairly soluble in water; and slightly soluble in methanol and propylene glycol.

---

* A toxic substance that causes damage to kidney tissues.
** Kuehl, Jr. *et al. J. Am. Chem. Soc.,* **77**, 2344, (1955).
*** Stammer *et al. J. Am. Chem. Soc.,* **77**, 2346, (1955).

6. It is found to form salts readily with acids and bases.
7. Its aqueous solutions buffered to pH 10 with Na_2CO_3 may be stored without any loss of activity upto a duration of one week between 0-10°C (*i.e.*, at refrigerated temperatures).

Uses

1. It exhibits a fairly broad spectrum of activity; however, its therapeutic efficacy is exclusively associated with its inherent inhibitory effect on *Mycobacterium tuberculosis*.
2. It precisely inhibits alanine racemase, which action precludes the incorporation of D-alanine strategically into the pentapeptide side-chain of the specific **murein*** component of bacterial cell walls. Perhaps this unique features is solely responsible for its antibiotic activity.
3. It is invariably regarded as an **'antibiotic of second choice'**; and is frequently used in conjunction with **isoniazid** in the control, management and treatment of tuberculosis who usually fail to respond to the **first-line agents.****
4. It is readily absorbed orally and is subsequently exerted quickly through the kidneys (*i.e.*, newly 50% without any metabolic alteration whatsoever).

9.3.8.2 Polymixin B

Polymyxins represent a group of cycle polypeptide antibiotics produced by various species of *Bacillus*. However, **polymyxins A to E** were primarily isolated from *Bacillus polymyxa*. Subsequently, it was shown that both **polymyxin B** and **polymycin E** (or **colistin**) were mixtures of two components each. The structures of **polymyxin B₁** and **polymyxin B₂**; and **polymyxin E₁ (colistin A)** and **polymyxin E₂ (colistin B)** are as given below:

$$X \longrightarrow Dab \longrightarrow Thr \longrightarrow Dab \longrightarrow Dab$$

Dab → Y → Leu → Dab
Thr ← ← Dab ← Dab

Polymyxins	X	Y
Polymyxin B₁	6-methyloctanoic acid	D-Phe
Polymyxin B₂	6-methylheptanoic acid	D-Phe
Polymyxin E₁ (Colistin A)	6-methyloctanoic acid	D-Leu
Polymyxin B₂ (Colistin B)	6-methylheptanoic acid	D-Leu

H_2N—_/—COOH
NH₂
Dab
[L-α, γ-Diaminobutyric acid]

Actually, these molecules essentially contain ten amino acids, of which six happen to be **L-α-, γ-diaminobutyric acid (L-Dab)**, having a fatty acid*** strategically bonded to the N-terminus; besides, a cyclic peptide portion meticulously designed *via* an amide bond located in between the *γ-amino* of one of the **Dab-residues** and the **carboxyl terminus.** Interestingly, the γ-amino functions

---

* Murien: Chloride (Cl⁻).
** Rifampin and Rifabutin.
*** 6-Methyloctanoic acid; or 6-Methylheptanoic acid.

of the remaining Dab residues distinctly attribute a rather strong basic property to the various antibiotics. This particular characteristic feature confers detergent-like properties and perhaps permits them to either get bound or cause damage to bacterial membranes.

Characteristic Features

Polymyxin Hydrochloride

1. It is obtained as nearly colourless powder that gets decomposed at 228-230°.
2. It has specific optical rotation $[\alpha]_D^{23}$-40° (C = 1.05).
3. It is very soluble (> 40%) in water and methanol; the solubility decreases considerably in higher alcohols; and almost insoluble in ethers, esters, ketones, hydrocarbons and the chlorinated solvents.
4. It usually gives rise to water insoluble salts with the help of a host of precipitants, such as: **helianthic acid** ($C_7H_9O_4$) **picric acid; and Reinacke salt.**

$$H_4N\ [Cr\ (NH_3)_2\ (SCN)_4]$$

Picric Acid   Reinecke Salt

Polymyxin B: It is a mixture of **Polymyxins B$_1$ and B$_2$.** The mixture also contains minimal amounts of the more toxic **polymyxins A, C and D.** Both **polymyxins B$_1$ and B$_2$** essentially possess a cyclopeptidic structure and comprise of six residues of α, γ**-diaminodutyric acid (DABs).** However, the latter characteristic feature affords an exceptionally strong basic property to the **polymixin antibiotics.**

It has specific optical rotation $[\alpha]_{5461}$-106.3° (1N. HCl).

Uses

1. It is used topically in ointments (usually 5000 or 10,000 Units/g) and ophthalmic solutions (10,000 Units/ml).
2. It was employed formerly for control, management and treatment of infections of the intestinal tract caused by *Shigella, Pseudomonas aeruginosa,* and *E. coli.*

Polymyxin B Sulphate [*Synonyms* Aerosporin; Mastimyxin;]: It is the sulphate salt of a substance produced by the growth of *Bacillus polymyxa* (Prazmowski) Mignla belonging to the natural order *Bacillaceae.* It has a potency of not less than 600 Units of **polymyxin B.** mg^{-1}, calculated on the anhydrous basis.

Preparation   The filtered broth obtained from the fermentation process (section 9.3.7) is eventually treated with a **'certified dye'**, and the resulting **polymyxin B-dye salt complex** thus precipitated is collected by means of filtration, washed with water and finally treated with an alcoholic solution of a lower aliphatic amine sulphate. The **polymyxin B sulphate** thus produced is filtered off and subsequently purified and lypholized. Polymyxin B is a mixture of **polymyxin B$_1$ ($C_{56}H_{98}N_{16}O_{13}$),**

and **polymyxin B$_2$ (C$_{55}$H$_{96}$N$_{16}$O$_{13}$)** the only vital point of difference is nothing but the composition of the N-acyl moiety (see Section 9.3.8.2).

Characteristic Features

1. It is a white to buff-coloured powder; either odourless or having a very faint odour.
2. It has dissociation constant pKa 8 to 9.
3. Its solutions are either slightly acidic or are neutral to litmus (pH 5 to 7.5).
4. It is found to be freely soluble in water; and slightly soluble in alcohol.

Uses

1. The antimicrobial spectrum of activity of **polymyxin B** sulphate for its *in vitro* and *in vivo* profile is solely restricted to Gram-negative organisms, namely: *Aerobacter, Escherichia, Haemophilus, Klebsiella, Pasteurella, Pseudomonas, Salmonella, Shigella,* most *Vibrio* and *Yesinia;* all strains of *Pr. providencia* and most of *Serratio marceseens* are found to be unaffected by this antibiotic.
2. It is used topically either for the treatment or the prevention and treatment of external ocular infections caused by susceptible microorganisms, especially *Ps aeruginosa*.
3. In topical therapy, it is invariably combined with **neomycin, gramicidin** and **bacitracin.**
4. It also forms an integral component in **glucocorticoid ophthalmological topical preparations.**
   Note: Substances like soap, which is a triglyceride of fatty, acids, and hence specifically antagonize cationic surface-active agents, is found to impair the activity of the antibiotic.

Polymyxin B Sulphate mixture with Trimethoprim [*Synonyms* Polytrim]: The combination of polymyxin B sulphate with trimethoprim enhances the overall antibacterial profile rather than each one used alone.

Polymycin B$_1$ [C$_{56}$H$_{98}$N$_{16}$O$_{13}$]

Polymyxin B$_1$ Pentahydrochloride [C$_{56}$H$_{98}$N$_{16}$O$_{13}$·5HCl]: It is obtained as a white powder. It has specific optical rotation $[\alpha]_D^{25}$-85.11° (C = 2.33 in 75% ethanol).

Polymycin B$_2$ [C$_{55}$H$_{96}$N$_{16}$O$_{13}$]: It has specific optical rotation $[a]_{5461}^{22}$-112.4° (2% acetic acid).

9.3.8.3 Colistin

Synonyms   Polymyxin E; Colimycin; Coly-Mycin; Colisticina; Totazina.

Biological Source   It is a cyclopolypeptide antibiotic produced by *Bacillus colistinus (Aerobacillus colistinus)* first isolated from Japansese soil). It is comprised of **colistins A, B and C.***

---

* Suzuki *et al., J. Biodiem. (Tokyo),* **54,** 25 (1963).

DAB = α, γ -diamobutyric acid

Polymyxin E_1(Colistin A) : R = (+)-6-Methyloctanoyl

Polymyxin E_2 : R = 6-Methylheptanoyl

Uses   This antibiotic has more or less the same spectrum and therapeutic application as that of **polymyxin B.**

Colistin Sodium Methanesulphonate [$C_{58}H_{105}N_{16}Na_5O_{28}S_5$] [*Synonyms* Colistimethate sodium; Alficetin; Methacolimycin]: It is the injectable form of colistin. It is soluble in water and fairly stable in the dry form. It is inactive in itself but releases active polymyxin in the body.

Colistin Sulphate [*Synonyms* Malimyxin; Multimycine]: It is mostly used either orally or topically.

Colistin Formaldehyde-Sodium Bisulphite*: It is obtained as crystals that decompose between 290-295°. It is found to be soluble in water; and slightly soluble in methanol, ethanol, acetone and ether.

Polymyxin E_1 [$C_{53}H_{100}N_{16}O_{13}$] [*Synonym* Colistin A]: It has specific optical rotation $[\alpha]_{5461}^{22}$-93.3° (2% acetic acid).

Polymyxin E_2 [$C_{52}H_{98}N_{16}O_{13}$]: It has specific optical rotation is $[\alpha]_{5461}^{22}$-94.5° (2% acetic acid).

Note: The use of methacolimycin nowadays is rarely justified on account of the availability of less toxic alternative antibiotics.

9.3.8.4 *Bacitracin*

Synonyms   Altracin; Ayfivin; Fortracin; Penitracin; Topitracin; Zutracin.

Biological Source   It is a polypeptide antibiotic complex produced by *Bacillus subtilis* and *licheniformis* (family: *Bacillaceae*).** The commercial **bacitracin** is found to be a mixture of at least nine bacitracins. The purification of **bacitracin** may be affected by '**carrier displacement method**'.

Chemical Structure   The major component of the mixture is '**Bacitracin A**', which is essentially a dodecylpeptide having five of its **amino-acid-residues** arranged strategically in a cyclic structure as shown below:

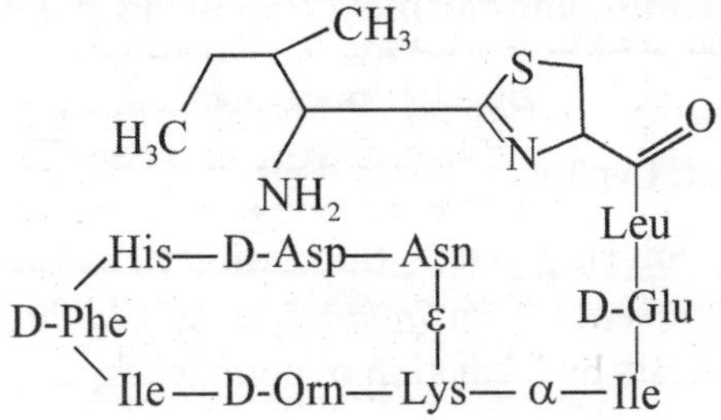

Bacitracin A

---

* Koyama *et al. Japan*. pat. **57**, 4898 (1957).

** Anker *et al. J. Bacteriol.* **55**, 249 (1948).

Characteristic Features

1. It is obtained as a Grayish-white powder having a very bitter taste, odourless and hygroscopic in nature.
2. It is found to be soluble in water and ethanol; and almost insoluble in ether, chloroform, and acetone.
3. It is fairly stable in acid solution and unstable in alkaline solutions.
4. It affords a loss in potency most probably on account of the transformation of **bacitracin A to bacitracin F,** and the latter does not have any antimicrobial activity.
5. Its solutions undergo rapid deterioration at room temperature, and ultimately affords precipitation.
6. Its activity is significantly negated by salts of many of the heavy metals.
7. Its aqueous solutions invariably retain their potency for several weeks when stored in a refrigerator.

Uses

1. It is found to be effective exclusively against Gram-negative organisms.
2. Its applications are more or less limited to such infections only which may be treated either by topical application or by local infiltration.
3. It is significantly effective topically in the control, management and treatment of the following cutaneous bacterial infections where the pathogenic organism is specifically **bacitracin-sensitive,** such as: impetigo-contagiosa; falliculitis; pyoderma; ecthyma; furunculosis; decubitus, ulcer; infectious eczematoid dermatitis; scabies and dermatophytosis.
4. **Bacitracin** also finds its applications in the treatment of various ophthalmological conditions.
5. Its zinc salt invariably is preferred for topical therapy; and is the form most often incorporated into combinations.
6. It is mostly combined with **neomycin** and **polymyxin B sulphate.**

Note: 1. Due to the relatively high incidence of nephrotoxicity (albuminuria, cylindruria, azotemia, accumulation of drug) which essentially follows its parenteral administration precludes systemic usage except in life-endangering staphylococcal infections, such as: pneumonia, empyema, particularly in infants wherein other antibiotics have proved to be either ineffective or in the treatment of antibiotic-associated (pseudomembranous)-enterocolitis caused by Cl difficile.

2. Development of bacterial resistance is much less frequent and slower for bacitracin as compared to penicillin, and for most organisms it is found to be almost nil.

9.3.8.5 *Vancomycin*

Synonyms   Vancocin; Vncoled; Lyphocin (Lyphomed).

Biological Source   It is an **amphoteric glycopeptide antibiotic** substance produced by *Streptomyces orientalis* (Family: *Streptomycetaceae*) from *Indonesian* and *Indian* soil that essentially inhibits bacterial nucleopeptide biosynthesis by formation of complexes.

Chemical Structure   The structure of the primary component of the mixture has been established beyond any reasonable doubt to be a **complex tricyclic aglycone** linked **glycosidically** to *glucose* and **vincosamine** functions. The vancomycin molecule essentially contains one free carboxylic acid moiety, two chloro substituted aromatic residues, and seven amide bonds, one of which is a prominent **primary-amide.**

The apparently novel feature of **vancomycin** is the tricyclic structure exclusively generated by *three* phenolic oxidative coupling reactions.

Vancomycin

Preparation   It is produced by the submerged fermentation process as described earlier under penicillins.

Characteristic Features

Vancomycin Monohydrochloride [$C_{66}H_{75}Cl_2N_9O_{24} \cdot HCl$] [*Synonyms* Lyphocin; Vancor;]:

1. It is obtained as white solid, free-flowing powder, odourless and having a bitter-taste.
2. It has uv_{max} (H_2O): 282 nm ($E_{1cm}^{1\%}$ 40).
3. Its solubility in water is more than 100 mg. ml^{-1}.
4. It is found to be moderately soluble in dilute methanol; and insoluble in the higher alcohols, acetone and ether.
5. Its solubility in neutral aqueous solutions is enhanced by low concentrations of urea.
6. The acidic solutions precipitate out the antibiotic on addition of either NaCl or $(NH_4)_2 SO_4$.

Uses

1. It has a Gram-positive antibacterial spectrum.
2. It specifically acts on bacterial cell walls by inhibiting murein biosynthesis by virtue of its complexation with the D-alanyl-D-alanine precursor and hence is **bactericidal,** which eventually renders it particularly useful in serious infections besides in the immunocompromised patients.
3. It also exerts to a certain extent the **'secondary modes of action'** *i.e.*, enhancing cytoplasmic membrane permeability and impairing RNA synthesis.
4. **Vancomycin hydrochloride** is widely recommended for the control, management and treatment of serious infections, such as: septicemia, endocarditis, wound infections caused by Gram-positive bacteria, specifically in those patients who are allergic to **β-lactam antibiotics.**

5. **Vancomycin HCl** is also found to be effective in *Enterococcus faecalis* strains that are inadequately controlled and managed by **β-lactam antibiotics.**
6. **Vancomycin** is not absorbed orally; however, oral administration is usually recommended for the treatment of staphylococcal-enterocolitis and antibiotic-associated pseudomembranous colitis produced by *Clostridium difficile.*
7. IM administration is rather painful and very often associated with local necrosis; therefore, systemic therapy with **vancomycin** makes use of IV-infusion extended over a span of 20 to 30 minutes.

Note: (*i*) **It is irritating to tissue and hence may cause thrombophlebitis, or pain at the site of injection and neurosis takes place if extravasted; also produces chills, fever, occasional urticaria and maculopapular rashes with hypotension (Red Man's Syndrome), nephrotoxicity and ototoxicity and, rarely, thrombocytopenia and neuropathy.**

(*ii*) **Recently, the plasmid-mediated resistant strains of enterococcus have virtually clamped restriction for the use of vancomycin in hospitals with a view to control the spread of resistance.**

9.3.8.6 *Teicoplanin*

Synonyms   Tiecoplanin A_2; Teichomycin A_2; Targocid; Targosid; MDL-507.

Biological Source   It is a **glycopeptide antibiotic** complex produced by *Actinoplanes teichomyceticus* nov. sp.; structurally related to **vancomycin** and comprised of a mixture of five **teicoplanins,** which essentially differ only in the nature and length of the fatty acid-chain attached to the sugar residue.

Characteristic Features

1. It is obtained as an amorphous powder having mp 260°C (decomposes).
2. It has uv_{max} in 0.1 N HCl 278 ($E_{1cm}^{1\%}$ 53); and in 0.1 N NaOH: 297 ($E_{1cm}^{1\%}$ 74).
3. It is found to be soluble in aqueous solution at pH 7.0; partially soluble in methanol, ethanol; and insoluble in dilute mineral acids, and also in non-polar organic solvents.

The various physical parameters of the five major components of teicoplanin are as follows:

(*i*) **Teicoplanin A_2-1: ($C_{88}H_{95}Cl_2N_9O_{33}$):** It is a white amorphous powder which darkens at 220°C and decomposes at 255°C.

(*ii*) **Teicoplanin A_2-2: ($C_{88}H_{97}Cl_2N_9O_{33}$):** It is a white amorphous powder, darkens at 210°C and gets decomposed at 250°C.

(*iii*) **Teicoplanin A_2-3: ($C_{88}H_{97}Cl_2N_9O_{33}$):** It is a white amorphous powder, darkens at 210°C and decomposed at 250°C.

(*iv*) **Teicoplanin A_2-4: ($C_{88}H_{99}Cl_2N_9O_{33}$):** It is a white amorphous powder, darkens at 210°C and gets decomposed at 250°C.

(*v*) **Teicoplanin A_2-5: ($C_{89}H_{99}Cl_2N_9O_{33}$):** It is a white amorphous powder, darkens at 210°C and gets decomposed at 250°C.

Uses

1. **Teicoplanin** has almost similar antibacterial profile to **vancomycin** (Section 9.3.8.5), but possesses a longer duration of action, and may be administered by IM as well as IV injection.

2. It is also employed against Gram-positive pathogens that are resistant to established antibiotics.
3. The '*Red-Neck Syndrome*' as observed upon rapid administration of **vancomycin** is rarely seen, besides the incidence of autoxicity also seems to be reduced considerably.

9.3.9 Tetracyclines

The **tetracyclines** are a conglomerate of broad spectrum orally active **actinomycete antibiotics** produced by cultures of *Streptomyces* species, and possessing appreciable therapeutic value. **Chlortetracycline** was the first bonafide member of this group isolated from *Streptomyces aureofaciens* and discovered by Duggar in 1948. It was immediately followed by **oxytetracycline** in 1950 from the cultures of *Streptomyces rimosus;* and in 1953 **tetracycline** was eventually discovered in the antibiotic mixture from *S. aureofaciens* as a minor antibiotic.

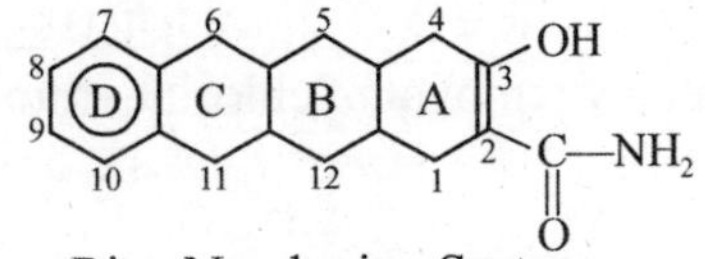

Ring Numbering System
(IUPAC)

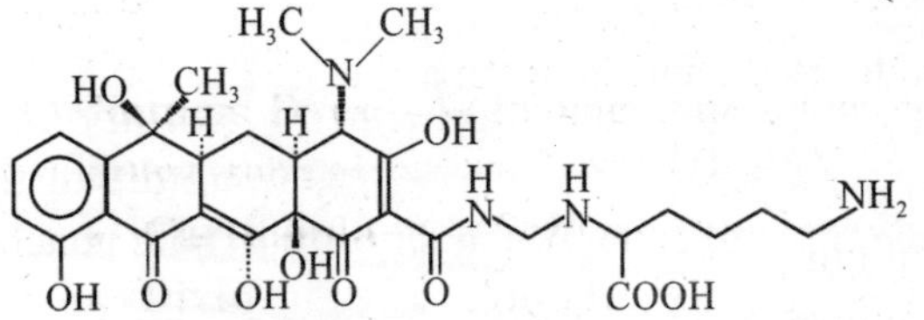

Lymecycline

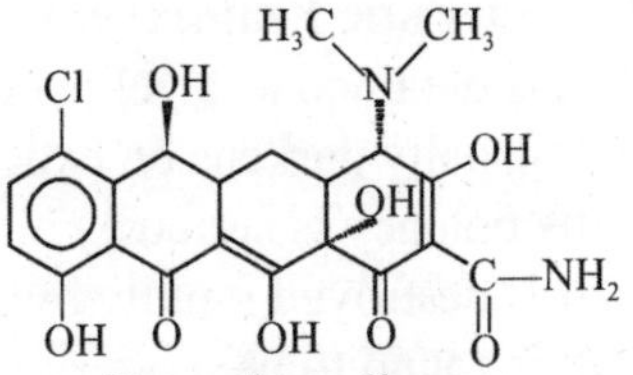

Demeclocycline

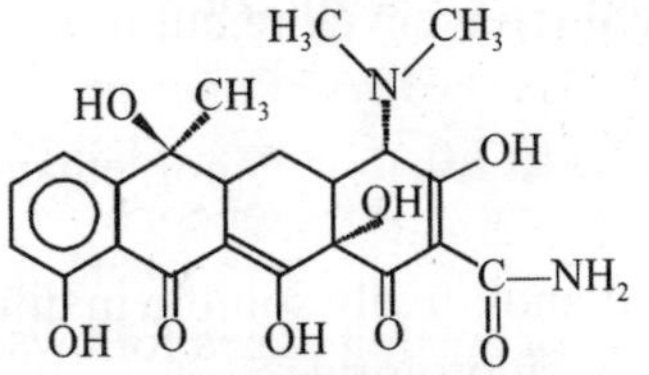

Tetracycline

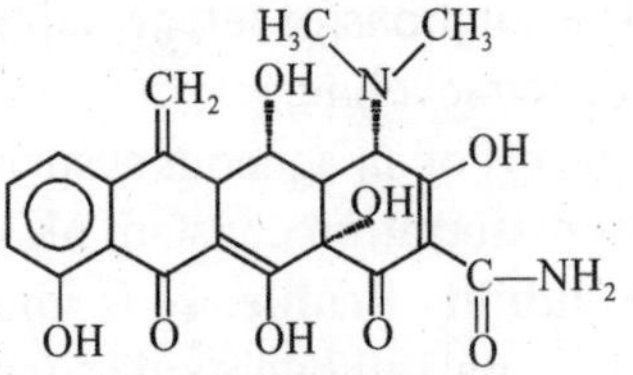

Methacycline

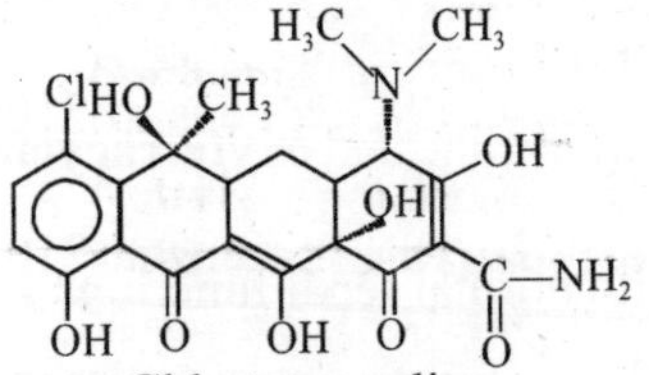

Chlortetracycline

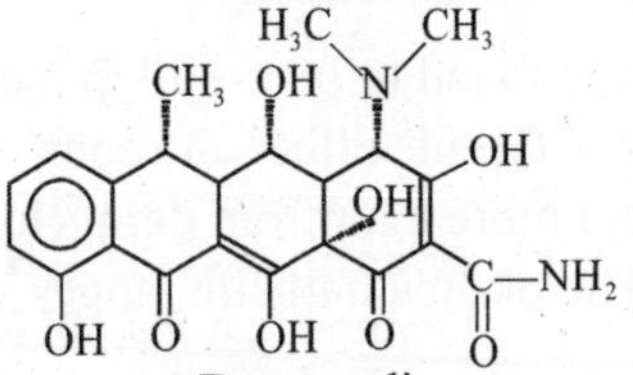

Doxycycline

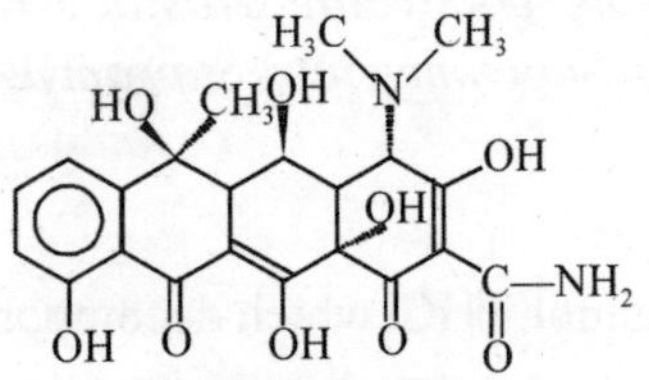

Oxytetracycline

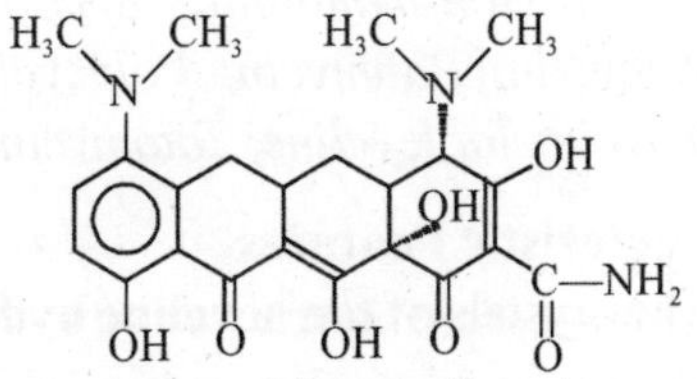

Minocycline

Consequently, the intensive and extensive research and development in the selection of **mutant strains,** and specifically in the manipulations and manifestations to monitor and control both 'methylation' and 'chlorination' procedures have resulted in the fermentative production of a good number of **tetracycline variants,** namely: **demeclocycline, methacycline, doxycycline, minocycline, lymecycline** as given below:

These compounds shall now be discussed individually as under:

9.3.9.1 Tetracycline

Synonyms Deschlorobiomycin; Tsiklomitsin; Abricycline; Ambramycin; Bio-Tetra; Cyclomycin; Dumocyclin; Tetradecin;

Biological Source It is obtained from a *Streptomyces* species cultured in an appropriate nutrient medium.

Preparation It may be prepared by removal of chlorine from chlortetracycline and subjecting it to hydrogenation.

Chemical Structure Please see Section 9.3.9.

Characteristic Features
1. It is obtained as a yellow crystalline powder; odourless, and stable in air.
2. It usually darkens on exposure to strong sunlight.
3. Its potency is seriously affected in solutions of pH < 2.
4. It is destroyed rapidly by alkali hydroxide solutions.
5. It is found to be more soluble than chlortetracycline.
6. It is rather more stable within the physiological and moderately alkaline spectrum of pH.
7. The solutions of **tetracycline** gets darkened more rapidly than **chlortetracycline** but less than oxytetracycline.
8. The pH of an aqueous suspension (1 mg . mL^{-1}) ranges between 3.0 to 7.0.
9. Its dissociation constant pKa are: 3.3; 7.7; 7.9.
10. **Solubility Profile:** 1g is soluble in ~ 2500 mL water; ~ 50 mL ethanol; freely soluble in dilute HCl or alkali hydroxide solutions; and almost insoluble in ether or chloroform.

Uses
1. It is found to be useful in the treatment of toxoplasmosis.
2. The GI side effects are comparatively less than those from chlortetracycline and **oxytetracycline** but more than from **demeclocycline.**
3. The plasma half-life ranges between 6 to 11 hours in patients with normal renal function.

**Tetracycline Hydrochloride [C$_{22}$H$_{24}$N$_2$O$_8$.HCl] [*Synonyms* Achro; Achromycin; Ala Tet; Ambracyn; Ambramicina; Bristaciclina; Cefracycline; Cyclopar; Diocyclin; Hostacyclin; Mephacyclin; Panmycin; Polycycline; Quadracycln; Remicyclin; Sanclomycine; Supramycin; Tetramycin; Topicycline; Totomycin; Unicin.*

Characteristic Features
1. The crystals of **tetracycline hydrochloride** are obtained from butanol + HCl which decomposes at 214°C.

2. Its specific optical rotation $[\alpha]_D^{25}$-257.9° (C = 0.5 in 0.1 N HCl).
3. It is freely soluble in water; soluble in methanol, ethanol; and insoluble in ether and hydrocarbons.
4. The pH of a 2% (w/v) aqueous solution ranges between 2.1-2.3.

9.3.9.2 Chlortetracycline

Synonyms 7-Chlorotetracycline; Acronize; Aureocina; Aureomycin; Biomitsin; Centraureo; Chrysomykine; Orospray.

Biological Source It is obtained from the substrate of *Streptomyces aureofaciens.*

Chemical Structure Please refer to Section 9.3.9.

Characteristic Features

1. It is obtained as golden-yellow crystals having mp 168-169°C.
2. It has specific optical rotation $[\alpha]_D^{23}$-275.0° (methanol).
3. It has uv$_{max}$ (0.1 N HCl): 230, 262.5, 267.5 nm, and (0.1N NaOH): 255, 285, 345 nm.
4. Its solubility in water ranges between 0.5-0.6 mg mL^{-1}, very soluble in aqueous solutions above pH 8.5; freely soluble in the cellosolves, dioxane and carbitol; slightly soluble in methanol, ethanol, butanol, acetone, benzene, ethyl acetate; and almost insoluble in ether and petroleum ether.

Uses

1. It exerts antiamebic activity.
2. It is the first tetracycline antibiotic available for topical application, including ophthalmic purposes.
3. Though its general use has been replaced by other tetracycline antibiotics in human beings, but it is still employed in veterinary medicine.

9.3.9.3 Oxytetracycline

Synonyms Glomycin; Riomistin; Hydroxytetracycline.

Biological Sources It is an antibiotic substance obtained from the elaboration products of the actinomycete, *Streptomyces rimosus,* grown on a suitable medium. **Oxytetracycline** may also be obtained from *Streptomyces xanthophaeus.*

Chemical Structure Refert to Section 9.3.9.

Characteristic Features

1. It is obtained as pale yellow to tan, odourless, crystalline powder.
2. It is fairly stable in air, but an exposure to strong sunlight gets darkened.
3. Like tetracycline it also gets deteriorated in solution of pH less than 2, and is quickly destroyed by alkali hydroxide solutions.
4. Its saturated solution is almost neutral to litmus and shows a pH ~ 6.5.
5. **Solubility Profile:** 1g in 4150 mL water; 100 ml ethanol; > 10,000 ml chloroform; 6250 mL ether; and freely soluble in diluted HCl or alkaline solutions.
6. **Stability:** Its crystals exhibit no loss in potency on heating for a duration of 4 days at 100°C; whereas the hydrochloride crystals show < 5% inactivation after 4 months at 56°C. It has been

observed that the aqueous solutions of the hydrochloride at pH 1.0 to 2.5 are quite stable for at least 30 days at 25°C. It has been observed that the aqueous solutions of the hydrochloride at pH 1.0 to 2.5 are quite stable for at least 30 days at 25°C. However, its solutions at pH 3.0 to 9.0 show no detectable loss in potency on storage at + 5°C for at least 30 days. Half life in hours at aqueous oxytetracycline solutions at 37°C: pH 1.0 = 114; pH 2.5 = 134; pH 4.6 = 45; pH 5.5 = 45; pH 7.0 = 26; pH 8.5 = 33; and pH 10.0 = 14.

Oxytetracycline Hydrochloride [$C_{22}H_{24}N_2O_9$.HCl] [*Synonyms Alamycin, Duphacycline; Engemycin; Geomycin; Oxlopar; Oxybiocycline; Oxycyclin Oxy-Dumocyclin; Oxytetracid; Oxytetrin; Tetran; Vendarcin*]

It is obtained as yellow platelets from water and is found to be extremely soluble in water (1 g/mL). It is also soluble in absolute ethanol: 12,000 g/mL; and in 95% (v/v) ethanol: 33,000 g/mL.

Note: Its concentrated aqueous solutions at neutral pH hydrolyze on standing and consequently deposit crystals of oxytetracycline.

Oxytetracycline Dihydrate [$C_{22}H_{24}N_2O_9$.2H$_2$O] [*Synonyms Abbocin; Clinimycin; Oxymycin; Stevacin; Terramycin; Unimycin*]

It is obtained as needles from water or methanol which decompose at 181-182°C. Its specific optical rotations are: $[\alpha]_D^{25}$-2.1° (0.1N NaOH); and $[\alpha]_D^{25}$-196.6 (0.1N HCl). It has uv$_{max}$ (pH 4.5 phosphate buffer 0.1 M): 249, 276, 353 nm ($E_{1cm}^{1\%}$ 240, 322, 301). It is found to be soluble in water at 23°C at various pH's: pH 1.2 = 31, 400 g/mL; pH 2.0 = 4600 γ/mL; pH 3.0 = 1400 γ/mL; and pH 9.0 = 38,600 γ/mL. It is soluble in absolute ethanol 12,000 γ/mL and in 95% (v/v) ethanol 200 g/mL.

9.3.9.4 *Demeclocycline*

Synonyms   Bioterciclin; Declomycin; Deganol; Ledermycin; Periciclina; Demethylchlortetracycline (obsolete).

Biological Source   Demeclocycline is related to tetracycline and produced by *Streptomyces aureofaciens.*

Preparation   A suitable strain of *S. aureofaciens* is grown in an appropriate liquid nutrient medium under controlled experimental parameters of pH, temperature, and extent of aeration. Subsequently, the duly harvested broth is acidified carefully and filtered. The **demeclocycline** is isolated from the resulting filtrate, either by solvent extraction or by chemical precipitation.

Chemical Structure   Refer to section 9.3.9.

Characteristic Features

Demeclocycline Hydrochloride [$C_{21}H_{21}ClN_2O_8$·HCl] [*Synonyms: Clortetrin; Demetraciclina; Detravis; Meciclin; Mexocine*]

1. It is obtained as yellow, crystalline powder, odourless and having a bitter taste.
2. The pH of 1 in 100 solution is ~ 2.5.
3. It essentially has *three* distinct dissociation constants, namely: pKa$_{1, 2, 3}$: 3.3, 7.2, 9.3 attributed by *three separate zones* in its complex molecule as shown below:

4. **Solubility Profile:** 1g soluble in ~ 60 mL water; 200 mL ethanol or 50 mL methanol; sparingly soluble in alkali hydroxides or carbonates; and almost insoluble in chloroform.

Uses

1. It is an intermediate-acting tetracycline and causes comparatively a greater extent of **phytotoxicity** than other members of its class.
2. Its better absorption and slower exeretion by the body render blood levels that distinctly afford certain minor therapeutic advantages than other members of its class.

Demeclocycline Sesquihydrate It has mp 174-178°C (decomposes); and specific optical rotation $[\alpha]_D^{25}$-258° (C = 0.5 in 0.1 N H_2 SO_4).

9.3.9.5 Methacycline

Synonyms Metacycline, Bialatan; 6-Methylene-5-hydroxytetracycline.

Biological Source It is broad spectrum, semi-synthetic antibiotic related to **tetracycline,** which is obtained from *Streptomyces rimosus.*

Preparation It may be prepared by a chemical dehydration reaction from **oxytetracycline;** besides, it has a methylene function at C-6 position.

Chemical Structure Please refer to Section 9.3.9.

Characteristic Features

Methacycline Hydrochloride [$C_{22}H_{22}N_2O_8$.HCl] [*Synonyms Adriamicina; Ciclobiotic; Germiciclin; Metadomns; Metilenbiotic; Londomycin; Optimycin; Physiomycine; Rindex; Rondomycin*]:

1. It is invariably obtained as crystals containing 0.5 mole water and 0.5 mole methanol; and also from a mixture of methanol + acetone + concentrated HCl + ether. It is a yellow crystalline powder which decompose at ~ 205°C and has a bitter taste.
2. It has uv$_{max}$ (methanol + 0.1 N HCl): 253, 345 nm (log ε 4.37, 4.19).
3. It is found to be soluble in water; sparingly soluble in ethanol; and practically insoluble in chloroform and ether.

Uses

1. The utility of methacycline is particularly associated with good oral absorption.
2. It has a prolonged serum half-life.

9.3.9.6 *Doxycycline*

Synonyms   Jenacylin; Supracyclin; Vibramycin.

Preparation   Methacycline (*i.e.,* 6-deoxy-6-demethyl-6-methylene-5-oxytetracycline) is either dissolved or suspended usually in an inert organic solvent, for instance: *methanol* and subjected to hydrogenation under the influence of catalytic quantities of noble metals, namely: *Rhodium* or *Palladium* to yield a mixture of the 6α-and 6β-methyl epimers. The desired epimer *i.e.,* **α-6-deoxy-5-hydroxytetracycline,** is subsequently isolated by specific chromatographic methods (US Pat 3,200,149).

Chemical Structure   Refer to Section 9.3.9.

Characteristic Features

Doxycycline Hydrochloride Hemiethanolate Hemihydrate [$C_{22}H_{25}Cl\,N_2O_8$.$1/2C_2H_6$0.$1/2H_2O$]
[*Synonyms Doxycycline hyclate; Azudoxat; Diocimex; Doxatet; Doxychel hyclate; Duradoxal; Hydramycin; Paldomycin; Sigadoxin; Tetradox; Unacil; Vibramycin hyclate; Vibra-Tabs; Zadorin*]:

1. It is obtained as light yellow, crystalline powder from ethanol + HCl; and gets charred without melting at ~ 201°C.
2. It has specific optical rotation $[\alpha]_D^{25}$-110°C (C = 1 in 0.01 N methanolic HCl).
3. It has uv$_{max}$ (0.01N methanolic HCl): 267, 351 nm (log ε 4.24, 4.12).
4. It is found to be soluble in water.
5. Both the inherant ethanol and water of crystallization (1/2 mol of each) are usually lost by subject to drying at 100°C under reduced pressure.
6. Its dissociation constant has three values, namely: pKa 3.4, 7.7, and 9.7 (see **demeclocycline**).
7. **Solubility Profile:** It is very slightly soluble in water; freely soluble in dilute acid or alkali hydroxide solution; sparingly soluble in ethanol; and practically insoluble in ether or chloroform.

Uses
1. The 6α-isomer of **doxycycline** is found to be more active biologically than the corresponding 6β-epimer hydrochloride.
2. It is active against Gram-positive organisms wherein it is almost *twice* as potent as **tetracycline;** and having an exception that it is virtually 10 times as potent against *Streptomyces viridans.*
3. Interestingly, strains of *Enterococcus fecalis* that are observed to be more resistant to other **tetracyclines** may prove to be sensitive to this drug.
4. Against Gram-negative organisms it is found to be twice as potent as tetracycline.
5. It is considered to be the drug of first choice for the prophylaxis of *traveler's diarrhea,* commonly caused by enterotoxigenic *E. coli.*
6. It is found to be the best amongst the *'tetracyclines'* against anaerobes.
7. It is absorbed almost completely *i.e.,* 90 to 100% through oral administration than the rest of tetracyclines, and its absorption does not seem to be retarded by intake of foods.
8. Its plasma-protein binding is almost 93%.
9. Its volume of distribution stands at 0.75 mL g^{-1}.
10. It is found to penetrate rapidly body fluids, cavities and cells.
11. It is invariably eliminated upto 65% through hepatic metabolism, and the balance 35% through biliary/renal exertion.

12. The rate of exertion is rather slow and the half-life is the longest among the **'tetracyclines'**, namely, 12 to 22 hr.

Note: 1. Photosensitization usually takes place more frequently as compared to other shorter-acting tetracyclines.

2. Complexation with Ca^{2+} is to a lesser extent than other tetracyclines; besides, it is not affected by either dairy products or foods.

9.3.9.7 *Minocycline*

Synonyms   Minocyn.

Biological Source   It is a semi-synthetic antibiotic obtained from 6-demethyl tetracycline.

Preparation   **6-Demethyl tetracycline** is first dissolved in tetrahydrofuran (solvent) containing aliquot quantity of methanesulphonic acid, and is subsequently reacted with dibenzyl azodicarboxylate to form 7-[1, 2-bis (carbobenzoxy) hydrazino]-6-demethyl-tetracycline. The resulting-product is subjected to Pd-catalyzed hydrogenation in the presence of formaldehyde to yield the desired product minocycline.

Chemical Structure   Refer to section 9.3.9.

Characteristic Features
1. It is obtained as bright yellow-orange amorphous solid.
2. Its specific optical rotation $[\alpha]_D^{25}$-116° (C = 0.524).
3. It has uv$_{max}$ (0.1N HCl): 352, 263nm (log ε 4.16, 4.23); (01 N NaOH) : 380, 243 nm (log ε 4.30; 4.38).

Uses
1. It is readily absorbed from the intestinal tract.
2. It has a slow renal clearance to afford prolonged blood levels; and is normally characterized by relatively lower MICs as compared to other tetracycline antibiotics for certain pathogenic organisms.

Minocycline Hydrochloride [C$_{23}$H$_{27}$N$_2$O$_7$.HCl] [*Synonyms Klinomycin Minomycin; Veetrin*]

Characteristic Features
1. It is obtained as yellow, crystalline powder, odourless, slightly bitter taste and slightly hygroscopic in nature.
2. It is fairly stable in air when protected from light and moisture; however, strong uv-light and/or moist air causes it to darken rather rapidly.
3. Its **potency*** in solution is primarily affected on account of *epimerization*.
4. The pH of 1 in 100 solution ranges between 3.5 to 4.5.
5. It distinctly gives rise to *four* dissociation constant values, namely: pK$_{a1}$ 2.8; pK$_{a2}$ 5; pK$_{a3}$ 7.8; and pK$_{a4}$ 9.3; mainly due to an additional dimethylamino moiety at e-7 position (compare with demeclocycline, Section 3.9.4).

---

* **Potency:** It is equivalent to not less than 785 mcg of minocycline mg^{-1}.

6. **Solubility Profile:** 1 g in nearly 60 mL water and ~ 70 mL alcohol; soluble in solutions of alkali hydroxides or carbonates; and almost insoluble in chloroform and ether.

Uses

1. Generally, it is found to be 2-4 times as potent as tetracycline against majority of **Gram-positive bacteria.**
2. It is found to exhibit an equally low-potency against *Enterococcus fecalis.*
3. It is almost 8 times as potent as **tetracycline** against *Streptococcus viridans.*
4. It is 2 to 4 times as potent as **tetracycline** against Gram-negative organisms.
5. It is now the drug of choice for treating infections caused by *Mycobacterium marinum.*

   Note: It particularly differs from other tetracyclines wherein the bacterial resistance to the drug is not only of low incidence but also of a lower order; which is especially true to staphylococci, in which cross-resistance is observed to be as low as 4%.

6. It is absorbed by the oral route to the extent of 90-100%.
7. Diminution in absorption is caused exclusively by food and milk and substantially by iron preparations and nonsystemic antacids.
8. It is normally protein-bound in plasma between 70-75%.
9. Its **'volume of distribution'*** ranges between 0.14 to 0.7 mLg^{-1}.
10. Its half-life varies between 11 to 17 hours.

9.3.9.8 *Lymecycline*

Synonyms   Armyl; Ciclolysol; Mucomycin; Tetralisal; Tetramyl; Tetralysal; N-Lysinomethyl tetracycline.

Biological Source   It is a **semi-synthetic antibiotic** related to **tetracycline.** It is a classic example of an antibiotic developed by qualified chemical modification of the primary amide function at C-2.

Preparation   It may be prepared by the method suggested by Tubaro and Raffaldoni.**

Chemical Structure   Refer to Section 9.3.9.

Characteristic Features

Lymecycline Sodium [$C_{29}H_{37}N_4NaO_{10}$]: It has uv_{max} (CH_3 OH): 376 nm. It is used as a potent antibacterial agent.

9.3.9.9 *Biosynthesis of Chlortetracycline*

The various steps involved in the **biosynthesis of chlortetracycline** are as stated below:

1. A malonamyl-CoA residue probably caters for as a 'primer'; and eight such malonate entities undergo stepwise condensations with the addition of C_2 units and followed by decarboxylation to yield a linear C_{19} *polyketide.*
2. Subsequently, the carbonyl-methylene condensations give rise to the **tetracyclic pretetramide nucleus.**

---

* **Volume of Distribution**   It is pharmacokinetic parameter representing a proportionality constant that relates drug concentration in a reference fluid, typically plasma, to the amount of drug distributed throughout the body.

** Tubaro and Raffaldoni, *Bull. Chim. Farm.,* **100,** 9 (1961).

3. Importantly, **methylation** at the *C-6 position* of the pretetramide is normally regarded an initial step in the biosynthesis of most tetracyclines; however, this particular step is usually left out in the creation of the naturally occurring dimethyl tetracyclines.

4. Hydroxylation at the C-4 position followed by dearomatization to produce a **4-keto intermediate** appears to precede 7-chlorination.

5. It is necessary that halogenation should precede introduction of the 4-amino group, which is methylated in a stepwise manner.

6. Terminal reactions in the biosynthetic sequence are carried out in *two* stages: *first,* hydroxylation at C-6 position; and *secondly,* reduction of double bond in ring B.

7. It is, however, interesting to absence that the presence of a 7-halogen substituent evidently blocks 5-hydroxylation.

The various steps involved in the **biosynthesis of chlortetracycline** may be summarized as given below:

Biosynthesis of Chlortetracycline

9.3.10 Miscellaneous Antibiotics

In general, the **'antibiotics'** are such a divergent group of medicinal compounds that usually fall into *Four* major categories, namely:

(*a*) Antibiotics based on Mechanism of Action,

(*b*) Synthetic Antimicrobial Agents,

(*c*) Antifungal Agents, and

(*d*) Anticancer Antibiotics.

A few typical and potent antibiotic substances shall be discussed under the so called **'miscellaneous antibiotics'** because of the simple reason that these compounds could not be accommodated under various Sections from 9.3.1 through 9.3.9 discussed earlier in this chapter on **'Antibiotics'**.

9.3.10.1 Antibiotics Based on Mechanism of Action

An intensive and elaborated research findings, with regard to the various established mechanism of action of certain antibiotics, may further sub-divide this group into the following heads, namely:

(*i*) Disruption of DNA-metabolism,

(*ii*) Inhibition of Protein Synthesis,

(*iii*) Inhibition of Cell wall formation, and

(*iv*) Alteration in Cellular Membrane function.

These *four* sub-groups shall now be discussed separately with the help of *one important example* in the sections that follows:

9.3.10.1.1   Disruption of DNA-Metabolism   The antibiotics belong to this specific category help to disrupt the DNA metabolism of the pathogenic organisms thereby inhibiting their growth effectively.

A. Rifampin

Synonyms   Rifampicin; Rifaldazine; Rifamycin; Abrifam; Eremfat; Rifa; Rifadin(e); Rifaldin; Rifabrodin; Rifoldin; Rimactan(e); R/AMP.

Biological Sources   The **rifamycins** are '**ansamycin antibiotics**'* produced by cultures of *Amycolatopsis mediterranei* (previously known as *Nocardia mediterranei* or *Streptomyces mediterranei*). The crude antibiotic mixture was found to consist of *five* closely related substances *i.e.*, **rifamycins A-E.**

The most clinically useful **rifamycin** is **rifampin**, a semi-synthetic derivative produced from **rifamycin SV** *via* a **Maanich reaction** by making use of formaldehyde and N-amino-N′ methylpiperazine.

Preparation   **Rifamycin SV,** which may be prepared by the method of Maggi *et al.*,** is converted to the 8-carboxaldehyde derivative, known also as **3-formylrifamycin SV.** It is finally condensed with 1-amino-4-methylpiperazine to give rise to a Schiff base, which is **Rifampin.**

Chemical Structure

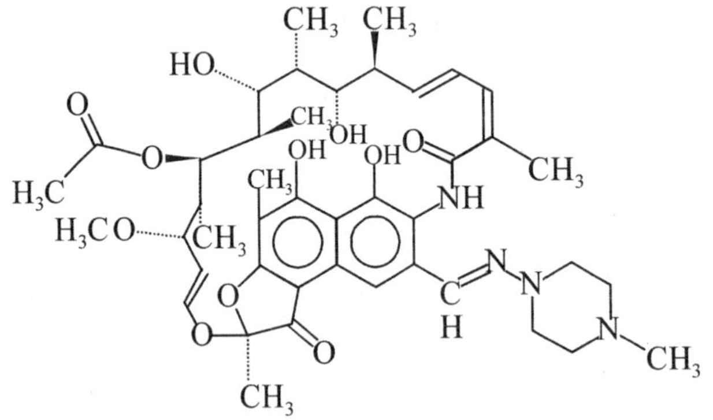

---

   * **Ansamycin Antibiotics (or Ansamycins)** These are a class of macrocyclic compounds wherein the non-adjacent positions on an aromatic ring system are usually spanned by the long aliphatic bridge (**Latin:** ansa = handle). The aromatic portion may comprise of either a *substituted benzene* ring or a *substituted naphthalene* or *naphthaquinone* moiety. The macrocycle present in the **ansamycins** is normally closed by an *amide* rather an ester linkage, *i.e.*, ansamycins are '**Lactams**'.

** Maggi *et al. Chemotherapia*, **11**. 285, (1966).

3-[[(4-Methyl-1-piperazinyl) imino]-methyl]rifamycin; [$C_{43}H_{58}N_4O_{12}$].

Characteristic Features

1. It is obtained as red to orange platelets from acetone that decompose at 183-188°C.
2. It has absorption max. (pH 7.38): 237, 255, 334, 475 nm (ε 33200, 32100, 27000, 15400).
3. **Rifampin** has two values for its dissociation constant, namely:
   (a) pKa_1 1.7 related to the 4-hydroxy function, and
   (b) pKa_2 7.9 related to the 3-piperazine nitrogen.
   Rifampin behaves as a **'zwitterion'** *i.e.*, it behaves both as an acid and as a base.
4. It is odourless; and fairly unstable in light, heat, air and moisture.
5. It is found to be very stable in DMSO; rather stable in water; freely soluble in CH_3Cl, DMSO; soluble in ethyl acetate, methanol, tetrahydrofuran; and slightly soluble in water (pH < 6), acetone and carbon tetrachloride.

Uses

1. It acts as a broad-spectrum antibiotic effective against most **Gram-positive organism,** especially *Staph pyogenes, Strep pyogenes, viridans* and *pneumoniae.*
2. It shows variable activity against **Gram-negative organisms,** particularly *H.influenzae, meningococci,* and *gonococci.*
3. Importantly, both *Mycobacterium tuberculosis* and *Mycobacterium leprae* are *very susceptible to* **rifampin.**
4. Its clinical usage is mainly in the treatment of tuberculosis. However, it is invariably employed in combination with other antitubercular drugs, such as: isoniazid and PAS.
5. It is considered to be an *excellent drug* for prophylaxis of *Meningococcal meningitis* and *pneumonia* caused due to *H.influenzae* Type B; and also in the treatment of *meningococcal* carrier state.
6. It is remarkably absorbed 100% after oval administration; however, the food in the stomach seems to delay absorption of the drug.
7. In plasma it is protein-bound upto 98%.
8. The volume of distribution is 0.9 mL. g^{-1}.
9. Almost 85% of the drug gets eliminated through biotransformation in the liver.
10. One of its **'active metabolite'** gets secreted directly into the bile, where it is therapeutically effective.

   Note: The most serious untoward adverse reactions involve hepatotoxicity, and the apparent enhanced risk of toxicity in persons having incidence of liver-damage e.g., chronic alcoholics suffering from cirrhosis*, may obviously preclude the use of this antibiotic.

9.3.10.1.2 Inhibition of Protein Synthesis There are certain antibiotics that specifically retard the anabolism of proteins *i.e.*, protein synthesis, at the ribosome level. For instance, **chloramphenicol** that binds preferentially to the 50S subunit of microbial 70S ribosomes and disrupts **peptidyl transferase** which catalyzes peptide bond formation exclusively. It is also found to specifically inhibit mitochondrial 70S ribosomes that ultimately results in the dose-related bone marrow suppression.

---

* A chronic disease of the liver marked by formation of dense perilobular connective tissue, degenerative changes in the parenchymal cells, structural alternation of the cords of liver lobules, fatty and cellular infiltration.

A. Chloramphenicol

Synonyms Ak-Chlor; Amphicol; Anacetin; Aquamycetin; Chlovamex; Chloromycetin; Chloramfen; Intramycetin; Leukomycin; Novomycetin; Pantovernil; Ronphenil; Synthomycetin; Tifomycine; Veticol.

Biological Sources It is a broad-spectrum antibiotic originally obtained by Burkholder from a culture of *Streptomyces venezuelae* that was initially isolation in 1947 from soil samples collected in the vicinity of Caracas (Venezuela). As the organism incidentally was not reported previously, Bürkholder thought it proper to baptize it as **venezuelae. Chloramphenicol** was also isolated from the moon snail, *Lunatia heros.*

Chloramphenicol attracted surmountable fame and glory for being the first truly discovered broad-spectrum antibiotic having its span from Gram-negative, Gram-positive organisms, a variety of rickettsial pathogens to a few-specific viruses.

Preparation **Chloramphenicol** enjoys the reputation of being the first even naturally occurring antibiotic known to contain a **nitro function,** besides being a derivative of dehydroacetic acid. Nevertheless, its stereochemical configuration is very much identical to that of **(–)-norpseudoephedrine;** and is the only one of the four related stereoisomers that essentially possess the antibiotic activity stated earlier.

It may be obtained either from the natural source or by the synthetic route as given under:

(*a*) **Natural Source:** It may be obtained from the filtrate of a *Streptomyces venezuelae* culture by extraction with ethyl acetate. In case, the charcoal extract is rich in **chloramphenicol,** the latter may be crystallized from the ethyl acetate by affecting dilution with several volumes of deodourized kerosene oil.

(*b*) **Synthetic Route: Chloramphenicol** may be synthesized by many different routes of preparation, but one of the better known starts with *para*-nitroacetophenone and, and after due conversion it into *para*-nitro-2-amino-acetophenone, proceeds through the following steps, namely:

Step I: Acetylation of the primary –NH$_2$ moiety,

Step II: Interaction with formaldehyde (HCHO) to induct the terminal primary –CH$_2$OH function,

Step III: Reduction with **aluminium isopropoxide Al [OCH (CH$_3$)$_2$]$_3$** to yield a mixture of the racemates of the *threo* and *erythro* forms of *para* –NO$_2$ Ph CH(OH) CH(NH$_2$) CH$_2$OH,

Step IV: Isolation of the *threo* racemate and its resolution using **camphorsulphonic acid,** and

Step V: Condensation of the (–)enantiomorph with methyl dichloroacetate.

Chemical Structure

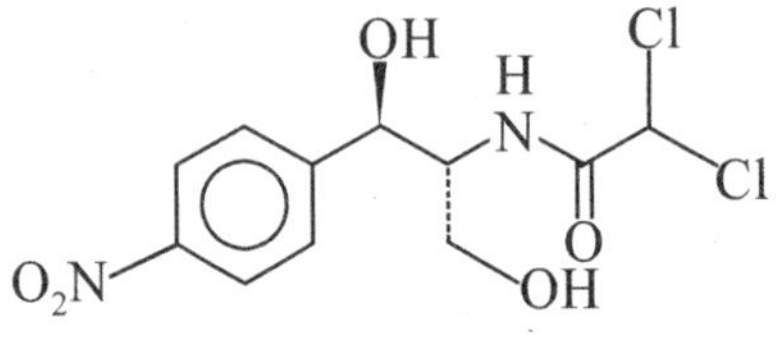

Chloramphenicol

[R-(R*, R*)]-2, 2-Dichloro-N-[2-hydroxy-1-(hydroxymethyl)-2-(4-nitrophenyl) ethyl]acetamide; $[C_1H_{12}Cl_2N_2O_5]$.

Characteristic Features

1. It is obtained either as needles or as elongated plates from water or ethylene dichloride having mp 150.5-151.5°C.
2. It usually sublimes under in the vacuum.
3. It appears as white to grayish white or yellowish white crystals.
4. It is practically odourless and possesses an intense bitter taste.
5. It has specific optical rotation $[\alpha]_D^{27} + 18.6°$ (C = 4.86 in ethanol); $[\alpha]_D^{25}–25.5°$ (ethyl acetate).
6. The pH of a saturated solution ranges between 4.5 and 7.5.
7. It is found to be reasonably stable either in neutral or moderately acidic medium; but rapidly gets destroyed in an alkaline medium.
8. It has dissociation constant pKa 5.5.
9. **Solubility Profile:** It is found to be very soluble in methanol ethanol, butanol, ethyl acetate, acetone; fairly soluble in ether; insoluble in benzene, petroleum ether, vegetable oils; and soluble in 50% (w/v) acetamide solution to an extent of 5%.

Uses

1. The drug is found to be effective in **Rickettsial diseases*** including epidemic, murine and serub typhus, Rocky Mountain spotted fever, rickettsial pox and **Q fever.****
2. It is also effective in chlamydial diseases including the **psittacosis*****-lymphogranuloma**** group.
3. **Chloramphenicol** is useful in a good number of Gram-negative and Gram-positive bacterial infections including the anaerobes (especially *Bacteroides fragilis*).
4. It is extensively used topically for superficial conjunctival **infections***** and **blepharitis****** caused by *E. coli, H. influenzae, Moraxella Lacunata, Staphylococcus aureus, and Streptococcus hemolyticus*.
5. **Chloramphenicol** is very well absorbed through the oral route and crosses rapidly into the cerebrospinal fluid.
6. It is absorbed readily from the GI tract, having a bioavailability of 90%.
7. The drug in blood is bound to serum albumin to the extent of 60%.

---

* **Rickettsial Disease**   A disease caused by an organism of the genus *Rickettsia*. The most common types are: spotted-fever group (Rocky Mountain spotted fever and rickettsial PoX), epidemic typhus, endemic typhus.

** **Q Fever**   It is caused by the rickettsial organism, *Coxiella burnetii* and is contracted by inhaling infected dusts, drinking unpasteurized milk from infected animals.

*** **Psittacosis**   An infections disease caused by *Chlamydia psittacoci* of parrots and other birds that may be transmitted in humans.

**** **Lymphogranuloma**   Infections granuloma of the lymphatics, Hodgkin's disese.

***** **Conjunctival Infections**   Infections in the mucons membrane that lines the eyelids and is reflected into the eyeball.

****** **Blepharitis**   Ulcerative or nonulecrative inflammation of the hair follicles and glands along the edges of the eyelids.

8. Its volume of distribution stands at 0.7 mL g^{-1}.
9. Biotransformation in liver ranges between 85-95%.
10. Its half-life is normally between 1.5 to 5 hours; except over 24 hours in neonates 1 to 2 day old; and 10 hours in infants 10 to 16 days old.

Note: 1. The plasma levels should be monitored very closely due to the significant variability with half-life.

2. Bone-marrow injury is the major toxic effect.

3. It causes serious *hematopoieitic** disturbances, such as: *thrombocytopenia***, *granulocytopenia**** and *aplastic anemia.*****

Chloramphenicol variants are as follows, namely:

(*a*) **Chloramphenicol Palmitate [*Synonyms* Chlorambon; Chloropal; Chlorolifarina]:**

1. It is obtained as crystals from benzene having mp 90°C.
2. It is practically tasteless and hence may be used as suspensions in pediatric formulations.
3. It has specific optical rotation $[\alpha]_D^{26} + 24.6°$ (C = 5 in ethanol).
4. It has uv_{max} (ethanol): 27 nm ($E_{1cm}^{1\%}$ 179).
5. It is very slightly soluble in water (1.05 mg mL^{-1} at 28°C); and petroleum ether (0.225 mg mL^{-1})
6. It is found to be freely soluble in methanol, ethanol, chloroform, ether and benzene.

(*b*) **Chloramphenicol Monosuccinate Sodium Salt [$C_{15}H_{15}Cl_2N_2NaO_8$] [*Synonyms* Protophenicol]:** It is freely soluble in water upto 50% (w/w).

Biosynthesis of Chloramphenicol The various steps involved in the biosynthesis of chloramphenicol are as follows:

1. Experimental studies with radioactive precursors have established a **Shikimic acid-phenylpropanoid pathway.**
2. Pathway evidently branches from normal phenylpropanoid metabolism prior to the formation of phenylalanine or tyrosine.
3. *para*-Aminophenylpyruvic acid (I) seems to be an early metabolite in the biosynthetic pathway.
4. Subsequent steps involved are, namely: transamination, hydroxylation, acylation, reduction of carboxyl moiety and terminal oxidation of the amino function.

   The above steps (1) through (4) are summarized below:

---

* **Hematopoietic** A substance that assists in or stimulates the production of blood cells.

** **Thrombocytopenia** An abnormal disease in number of the blood platelets.

*** **Granulocytopenia** An abnormal reduction of granulocytes in the blood.

**** **Aplastic Anemia** A serious complication of infection with human parvovirus B-19 infection in patients with chronic hemolytic anemia, such as: sickle-cell disease.

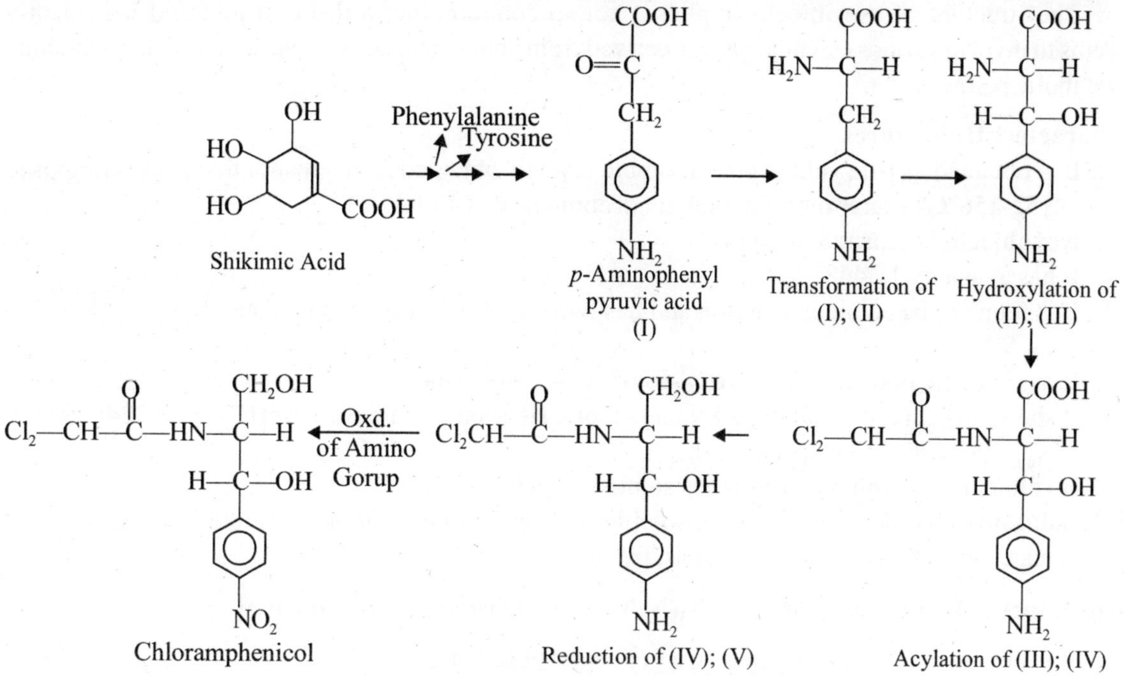

Biosynthesis of Chloramphenicol

9.10.1.3 Inhibition of Cell-Wall Formation

A number of naturally occurring substances have been isolated and characterized that are found to exert their action by inhibiting specifically the cell-wall formation *in vivo*.

Examples

A. Novobiocin

Synonyms Biotexin; Cardelmycin; Cathocin; Cathomycin; Inamycin; Speromycin; Vulcamycin; Vulkamycin; Albamycin; Streptonivicin.

Biological Sources **Novobiocin** is produced by *Streptomyces spheroides* and *Streptomyces niveus*.

Chemical Structure

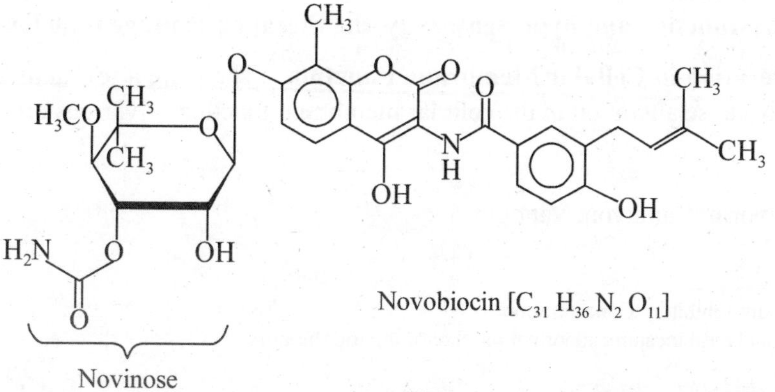

Novobiocin [$C_{31}H_{36}N_2O_{11}$]

Novinose

The structure of **novobiocin** implies a not so common biosynthetic origin; and it evidently seems to involve various essential groups derived from amino acid, acetate and above all carbohydrate metabolic pathways.

Characteristic Features

1. It is obtained as pale yellow orthorhombic crystals obtained from ethanol that get decomposed at 152-156°C (a rarer modification get decomposed at 174-178°C.
2. **Novobiocin** is sensitive to light.
3. It has a density 1.3448.
4. It is found to be acidic in reaction and has two dissociation constant values, namely: pKa_1 4.3; pKa_2 9.1.
5. It has specific optical rotation $[\alpha]_D^{24}$-63.0° (C = 1 in ethanol).
6. It shows uv_{max} (0.1 N NaOH; 0.1N methanolic HCl; Phosphate Buffer pH 7): 307; 324; 390 nm ($E_{1cm}^{1\%}$ 600, 390, 350 respectively).
7. It is found to be soluble in equeous solution > pH 7.5.
8. **Solubility Profile:** It is almost insoluble in more acidic solutions; soluble in acetone, ethyl acetate, amyl acetate, lower alcohols, pyridine.

Novobiocin Monosodium Salt [$C_{31}H_{35}N_2NaO_{11}$]   [*Synonyms:* **Robiocina**]

1. It is obtained as minute crystals that get decomposed at 220°C.
2. Its specific optical rotation $[\alpha]_D^{24}$-38° (C = 2.5 in 95% ethanol); and $[\alpha]_D^{24}$-33° (C = 2.5 in water).
3. The pH of a 100 mg mL^{-1} solution is 7.5.
4. It is found to be freely soluble in water.
5. It has a half-life of approximately 30 days at 25°C and of several months at 4°C.

Uses

1. The activity profile of **novobiocin** is predominantly Gram-positive.
2. It has been observed that it is unusually sensitive to *Staphylococci* (**MIC*** ranges between 0.1 to 2.0 mcg. mL^{-1}); however, resistance gets developed rather readily.
3. It finds its therapeutic application as an '**alternate drug**' for controlling **penicillin-resistant staphylococci.**
4. It also exerts antiviral activity.
5. It exhibits efficacy in canine respiratory infections.

Note: Based on its relatively high incidence of adverse reactions, such as: blood dyscrasia**, hepatic dysfunction and hypersensitivity, the therapeutic usage is no longer justified.

9.3.10.1.4   Alteration in Cellular Membrane Function   There are a few antibiotic substances which essentially cause alteration in the cellular membrane function of various organisms.

A. Candicidin

Synonyms   Levorin; Candivon; Vanobid.

---

* **MIC** = Minimum Inhibitory Concentration;

** **Dyscrasia** An old term meaning abnormal mixture of the four humors.

Biological Source   It is a **heptane macrolide antifungal antibiotic complex** composed of candicidins A, B, C and D (major component). It is produced by a strain of *Streptomyces griseus*.

Chemical Structure

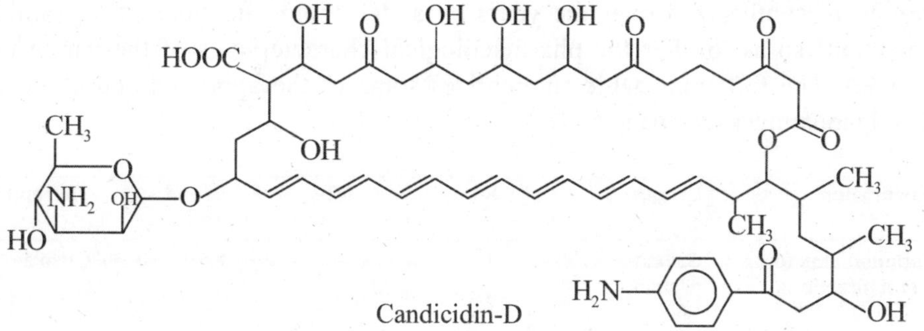

Candicidin-D

Characteristic Features

1. It is obtained as small yellow needles or rosettes from aqueous tetrahydrofuran or a mixture of pyridine/acetic acid/water.
2. It has uv_{max} : 403, 380 ($E_{1cm}^{1\%}$ 1150), 360 nm.
3. **Solubility Profile:** It is almost insoluble in water, alcohols, ketones, esters, ethers, hydrocarbons and other lipophilic solvents; soluble in DMSO, DMF, and lower aliphatic acids (formic acid, acetic acid); very soluble in 80% equeous tetrahydrofuran solution; and addition of 5-25% of water to alcohols greatly enhances its solubility.
4. It readily forms soluble salts in alkaline solutions.

Candicidin D $[C_{59}H_{84}N_2O_{18}]$ **[Levorin A$_2$]:** It is found to be indentical with **levorin A$_2$.** *

Uses

1. It is mostly used as a topical antifungal agent.
2. It is also found to exert antichlolesteremic activity.

9.3.10.1.5   Synthetic Antimicrobial Agents   There are a host of purely synthesized tailor-made medicinal compounds that have been used as antimicrobial agents in the ever increasing therapeutic armamentarium to combat human diseases across the globe. The various synthetic antimicrobial agents may be categorized as stated below:

(*i*)   Sulphonamides and Trimethoprim
(*ii*)   Nitroimidazoles
(*iii*)   Quinolones and Fluoroquinolones
(*iv*)   Agents for systemic UTIs
(*v*)   Agents for *Mycobacterium tuberculosis* Infections.
(*vi*)   Antifungal agents, and
(*vii*)   Anticancer antibiotics.

The aforesaid categories of synthetic antimicrobial agents shall now be treated individually with some typical potent examples in the sections that follows:

---

* Bosshardt, Bickel, *Experientia,* **24**, 422, (1968).

9.3.10.1.5.1 **Sulphonamides and Trimethoprim** **Sulphonamides**—the first and foremost antimicrobial agents, since discovered in 1930s, still hold the glory and fame of the modern antibiotic era. In general, **sulfanilamide** (*i.e.*, *para*-aminobenzene sulphonamide), obtained as a structural analogue of *para*-**aminobenzoic acid (PABA),** is basically the core compound from which hundreds of congeners were synthesized over the years by suitable modifications at N_1 (amide) or N_4 (*p*-amino function) so as to alter the pharmacological characteristics of the parent compound (sulphanilamide). The following table summarizes some of the approved and clinically useful widespread sulphonamides (see page 667).

S. No.	Classification	Drug(s)	R1	R2	Brand Name	Theraputic Uses
I	Sulphonamides for general Infections	1. Sulpha-nilamide	H	H	Rhinamid	Obsolete
		2. Sulpha-pyridine		H	M2B 693	Pneumonia; *Dermatitis herpetiformis.*
		3. Sulpha-Thiazole		H	Cibazol	Bubonic plague staph. infections
		4. Sulpha-Diazine		H	Diazyl	Rheumatic fever; Chancroid due to *Haemophilus ducneyi.*
		5. Sulpha-merazine		H	Solume-dine	General infection
		6. Sulpha-dimidine (sulpha-methazine)		H	Pirmazin	Meningal infections
II	Sulphonamides for Urinary Infections	1. Sulpha cetamide	CH₃—C—H	H	Albucid	UTIs; topical for eye and skin infections.
		2. Sulpha-furazole		H	Sulfalar	UTIs; topically for vaginitis.
		3. Sulfacytine		H	Renoquid	Acute UTIs.
III	Sulphonamides for Intestinal Infections	1. Sulpha-Guanidine		H	Shigatox	Bacillary dysentry;
		2. Phthalyl-sulpha-Thiazole		H	Thalazole	Bacteriostatic effect in GIT.
		3. Succinyl-sulpha thiazole		HO.C.CH₂CH₂.C—	Sulfauxi-dine	Cholera; Bacillary dysentry.
IV	Sulphonamides for *Local Infection*	Mafenide	H	X = CH₂NH₂	Sulfonyl	*Psuedomonas aeruginosa;* severe burns.

[Adapted From: Kar, Ashutosh, **'Medicinal Chemistry'**, 4th ed 2006, New Age International Publishers, New Delhi.]

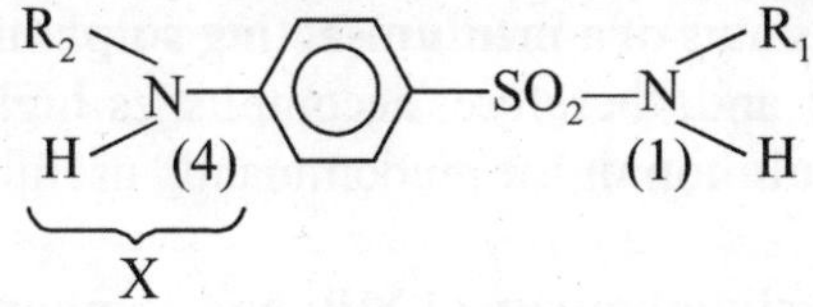

Sulphonamide

Sulphonamides are regarded as **'antimetabolites'** which are found to be the structural analogues of PABA; the latter being a substrate in the biosynthesis of folic acid and also an absolutely necessary metabolite for microorganism which in turn utilizes it as a vital source of *single-carbon-units* required for the biosynthesis of *amino acids, purines* and *pyrimidines*.

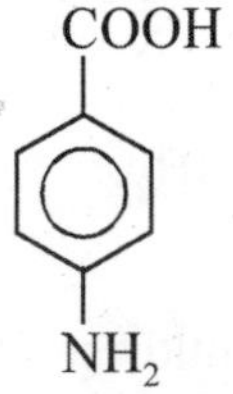

p-Amino
Benzoicacid
(PABA)

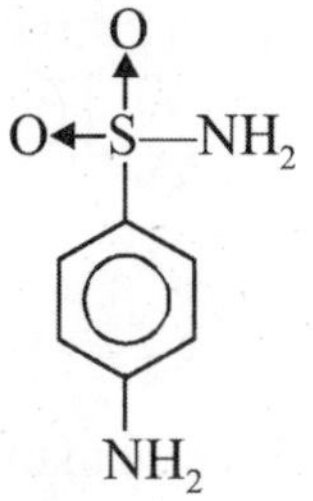

Sulphanilamide

$$\left[\begin{array}{c} \textbf{Sulphonamides Structural} \\ \textbf{Analogues of (PABA)} \end{array} \right]$$

It has been observed that **sulphonamides** inhibit competitively the enzyme **tetrahydroptetroyl synthetase'** that makes use of PABA as a *substrate* ultimately in generating the *'petroyl moiety'* in the **Folic Acid** as given below:

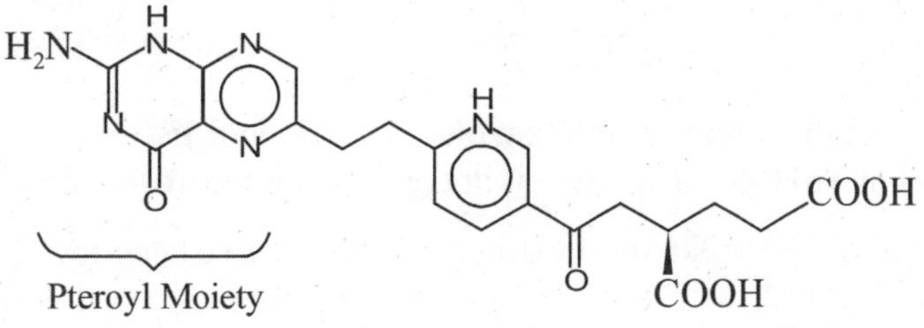

Pteroyl Moiety

Folic Acid

Sulphonamides are of *two* types, namely: *unionized form e.g.,* **sulphamethoxazole;** and ionized form *e.g.,* **sodium sulfisoxazole,** as shown below:

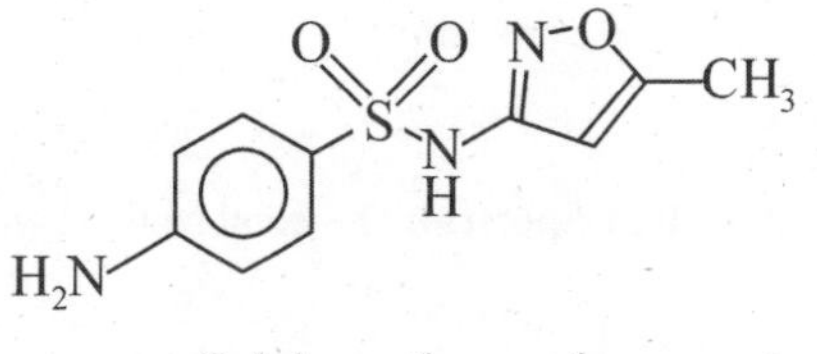

Sulphamethoxazole
[Unionized Form]

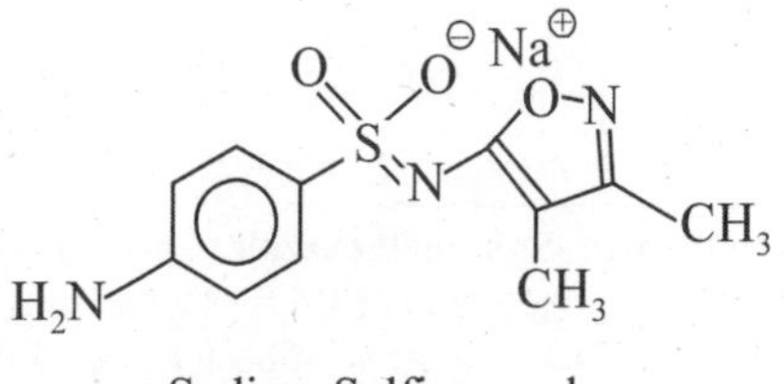

Sodium Sulfisoxazole
[Ionized Form]

Sulphamethoxazole enjoys the status of a **medium-acting sulphonamide** which is comparatively less soluble than **sulfisoxazole;** and, therefore, accomplishes higher blood-levels. Interestingly, **sulfisoxazole** is a **short-acting sulphonamide** predominantly useful for UTIs caused by susceptible pathogenic bacteria.

The unique combination of **trimethoprim (TMP) and sulphamethoxazole (SMZ)*** affords a broad-spectrum *'antibiotic product'* which is found to be active (invariably bactericidal) against a plethora of Gram-positive *cocci* and Gram-negative *rods*. However, certain microorganisms are evidently resistant to this combination, namely: *Mycobacterium tuberculosis* and species of *Pseudomonas, Mycoplasma* and *Bacteroides.*

Trimethoprim

The therapeutic advantages of this combination are as follows:

1. It particularly inhibits the sequential steps in the formation of tetrahydrofolic acid. The resulting inhibition is magnified by the independent actions at two consecutive metabolic steps; and thus the **bacteriostasis**** *phenomenon* gets converted into the **bactericidal***** one. The double blockade broadens appreciably the antibacterial spectrum from that of each drug used alone.
2. The most significant usage of **TMP-SMZ** combination is in the control, management and treatment of UTIs, specifically recurrent, chronic or complicated infections not easily manaeuvrable and controllable by individual drugs; such as: UTIs caused by *E. coli, Klebsiella-Enterobacter* and *Proteus species.*
3. TMP-SMZ combination provides the treatment and serves as *prophylaxis of choice* particularly in immunocompromised patients for *pneumonia* caused by *Pneumocystis carinii* and *enterocolitis* caused by *Isospora.*
4. By virtue of the fact that **sulphamethoxazole,** exhibits poor tissue distribution, and also the pharmacokinetics of **TMP-SMZ** mixture is not optimal for the treatment of systemic infections.

9.3.10.1.5.2 **Nitroimidazoles:** Nitroimidazole, is a 5-membered heterocyclic nucleus having two N-atoms at positions 1 and 2, with the nitro group at position 5. Several structural variants of nitroimidazole have been duly synthesized and sereened for their antibacterial activities.

5-Nitroimidazole

---

* **Trimethoprim-Sulfamethoxazole (Co-trimoxazole, TMP-SMZ, Bactrium, Spectra).** This combination is generally available in a fixed ratio of 1:5 for IV and oral administration.
** **Bacteriostasis:** The arrest of bacterial growth.
*** **Bactericldal:** Destructive to or destroying bacteria.

Two such potent compounds, namely: **Metronidazole** and **Tinidazole,** shall now be discussed as under.

A. Metronidazole

Synonyms   Bayer 5630; RP-8823; Arilin; Clont; Deflamon; Elyzol; Flagyl; Fossypol; Klion; MetroGel; Metrolag; Metrolyl; Orvagil; Rathimed; Trichazol; Tricocet; Vagilen; Zadstat.

Preparation   **Metronidazole** is prepared by the condensation of 2-methyl-5-nitroimidazole with ethylene chlorohydrin by subjecting it to heating in the presence of a large excess of the **chlorohydrin.** The surplus chlorohydrin is removed, the residue is extracted with water and the resulting extract is alkalinized and extracted with chloroform. Chloroform is removed under vacuo to obtain crude **metronidazole** which is finally recrystallized from ethyl acetate.

Chemical Structure

Metronidazole

2-Methyl-5-nitroimidazole-1-ethanol; $(C_6H_9N_3O_3)$.

Characteristic Features

1. It is obtained as cream-coloured crystals having mp 158-160°C, odourless, stable in air and darkens on exponore to light.
2. Its solubility profile at 20°C (g/100 ml): water 1.0; ethanol 0.5; ether < 0.05; chloroform < 0.05; and sparingly soluble in DMF.
3. The pH of a saturated aqueous solution is 5.8.
4. It has dissociation constant pKa 2.62.

Uses

1. It is found to be bactericidal to **anaerobic** and **microaerophilic*** microorganisms, including: *Bacteroides; Clostridium sp.; Endolimax nana; Entameba histolytica; Fusobacterium vincentii; Gardnerella vaginalis; Giardia lamblia; Peptococcus; Peptostreptococcus;* and *Trichomonas vaginalis.*

   Interestingly, all these organisms critically reduce the nitro moiety, and subsequently produce the metabolites that specifically inhibit DNA synthesis.
2. It is the drug of choice since long for the treatment of **trichomoniasis****, and more recently in combination with **iodoquinol** for the treatment of symptomatic amebiasis (except in brain).
3. As it is absorbed so effectively from the oral route, hence its adequate concentrations in the

---

   * **Microaerophilic:** Growing at low amounts of oxygen.
** **Trichomoniasis**   Infestation with a parasite of the genus *Trichomonas i.e.*, Genus of flagellate parasitic protozoa *e.g., T. hominis*—a benign trichomonas found in the large intestine; *T. tenax*—a benign trichomonas that may be present in the mouth; and *T. vaginalis*-a species found in the vagina that produces discharge.

lower bowel invariably are not sufficient enough to cause eradication of amebas, so that it is combined with iodoquinol to render it a first-choice combination.

4. It is also recommended as the drug of first-choice for the treatment of Dracunculus (guinea worm) infestations.

5. It has been employed successfully in the treatment of antibiotic-associated **pseudomembranous colitis*** either through IV or orally.

6. It has been reported to be of value in **Crohn's disease** i.e., inflammatory bowel.

7. Its half life is about 6-12 hour.

   Note: Metronidazole may reasonably be anticipated to be a carcinogen. (Ref: Seventh Annual Report on Carcinogens (PB95-109781, 1994) p 257.

B. Tinidazole

Synonyms Fasigin; Fasigyn; Pletil; Simplotan; Sorquetan; Tricolam; Trimonase.

Chemical Structure

Tinidazole

1-[2-(Ethylsulfonyl) ethyl]-2-methyl-5-nitro-1H-imidazole; ($C_8H_{13}N_3O_4S$).

Characteristic Feature It is obtained as colourless crystals from benzene having mp 127–128°C.

Uses

1. It is used as an effective antiprotozoal agent for Trichomonas and Giardia.

2. It is also employed widely for the treatment of amebic dysentry.

3. It is broadly used as an antibacterial agent.

4. A combination with **norfloxacin [Nortee. –Z$^{(R)}$** (German Remedies Ltd.) containing **norfloxacin** 400 mg + **tinidazole** 600 mg] is invariably employed for the treatment of serious types of dysentry caused due to food poisoning, loose motion etc.

9.3.10.1.5.3 **Quinolones and Fluoroquinolones** **Quinolone antibacterial drugs** have gained entry into the therapeutic armamentarium since 1964 with the evolution of **nalidixic acid**-a purely synthetic molecule, used exclusively for UTIs. Within a very short span (1968-1970) *two* more structurally related analogues, namely: **oxolinic acid** and **cinoxacin** were introduced. However, all these drugs has shown a serious disadvantage by virtue of two major short-comings: (*a*) exhibited limited antibacterial spectra; and (*b*) rapid development of resistance to these bacteria.

   In the usual constant, routine, untiring, sincere efforts towards designing newer and safer drug molecules an attempt was made whereby *two* new chemical entities were introduced into the parent

---

* Inflammation associated with antibiotic therapy. It is caused due to a toxin produced by *Clostridium difficle* and is marked by formation of a pseudomembrane on the mucosa of the colon; symptoms diarrhoea with gross blood and mucus, abdominal cramps, fever and leukocytosis.

structure, namely: (*a*) 6-fluoro; and (*b*) 7-(1-piperazinyl). These structural modifications properly expanded not only the spectrum but also enhanced the potency besides preventing the development of plasmid-mediated resistance. This significantly made the wonderful discovery of the so called **'fluoroquinolones'** that showed **bacteriostatic** action *at low concentrations* and **bactericidal at high concentrations.**

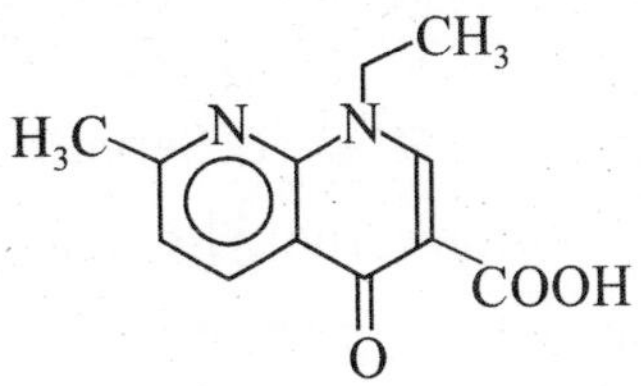

| Nalidixic Acid | Oxolinic Acid | Cinoxcin |

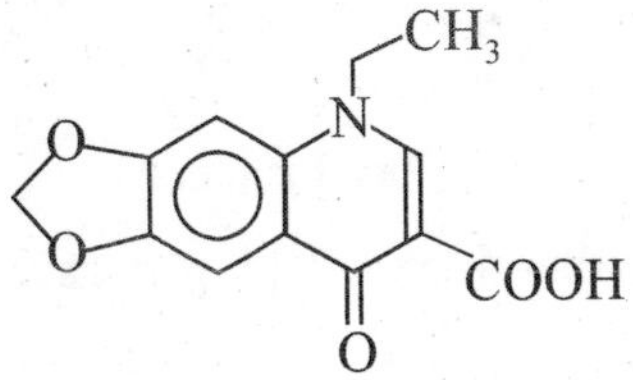

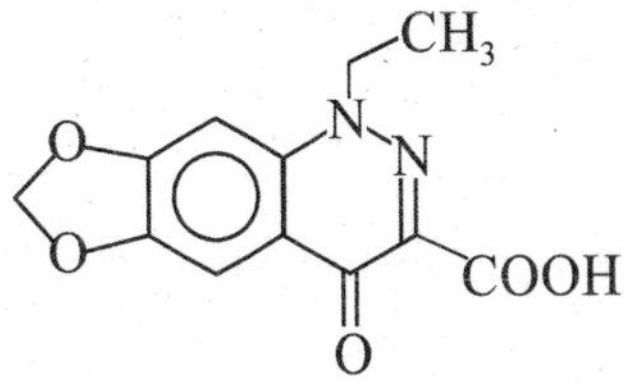

It is, however, pertinent to state here that the mechanism of action of **fluoroquinolones** predominantly involves inhibition of DNA gyrase, a member of the topoisomerase group of enzymes that essentially regulate the superhelicity of DNA within the cells. Evidently, inhibition of DNA gyrase leads to inhibition of DNA replication phenomenon, and ultimately cell death is accomplished. The latest marketed fluoroquinolones exert merely minimal activity against the mammalian topoisomerases. Another important feature with regard to the apparently enhanced activity of the **fluoroquinones** *vis-a-vis* **nalidixic acid** is solely due to the much greater affinity of the former for getting bound to the DNA gyrase. Interestingly, clinical studies have revealed that certain extent of acquired resistance has been observed not so commonly with the newer designed fluoroquinolones and another most vital and important revelation is that till date absolutely not even a single incidence of **plasmid-mediated resistance** has been reported in any clinical isolates.

Thus, **fluoroquinolone** based synthetic compounds occupy a very strategically-useful status in combatting dreadful microbial infections in uman beings. A few potent compounds belonging to this category are, namely: **ciprofloxacin, lomefloxacin, norfloxacin, ofloxacin, spafloxacin** and **trovafloxacin,** which shall now be elaborated squarely in the sections that follows:

A. Ciprofloxacin

Synonyms   Bay q 3939.

Preparation   It is a **fluorinated quinolone antibiotic** prepared by the condensation of 3-chloro-4-fluoroaniline with diethyl ethoxymethylenemalonate to yield the *imine* that is thermally cyclized to form ethyl 7-chloro-6-fluoro-4-hydroxy quinoline-3-carboxylate. Subsequent N-alkylation with cyclopropyl iodide followed by nucleophilic displacement of the 7-chloro function by N-methyl piperazine; and finally the hydrolysis of the ester affords the desired product.*

---

* *J. Med. Chem.*, **19**, 1138, 1976.

Chemical Structure

Ciprofloxacin

1-Cyclopropyl-6-fluoro-1, 4-dihydro-4-oxo-7-(1-piperazinyl)-3-quinolinecarboxylic acid; $(C_{17}H_{18}FN_3O_3)$.

Characteristic Features

1. It is mostly obtained as pale-yellow crystals that get decomposed at 255-257°C.
2. It is found to be amphoteric in nature.
3. Its dissociation constant pKa is 6 and 8.8.
4. 1g of it is soluble in 25 ml of water.

Ciprofloxacin Monohydrochloride Monohydrate [$C_{17}H_{18}FN_3O_3.HCl.H_2O$] [*Synonyms* Baycip; Ciflox; Ciloxan; Ciprinol; Cipro; Ciprobay; Ciproxan; Ciproxin; Flociprin; Septicid; Velmonit]: It is obtained as light-yellow crystalline powder having mp 318-320°C.

Uses

1. It is recommended for use in the treatment of bone and joint infections, infectious diarrhoea caused by *Shigella* or *Compylobacter*), lower respiratory tract infections, skin infections and UTIs.
2. It is found to be the drug of choice for the treatment of infections caused by **Compylobacter jejuni***.
3. Besides, it is an unlabeled but authoritatively alternative drug for the treatment of gonorrhea, salmonella, and **yersinia*** infections.
4. The oral bioavailability is about 70-80%.
5. Its half life is about 4 hour.
6. Ciprofloxacin has improved activity against Gram-positive bacteria, particularly certain *Staphylococci* and *Streptococci* species.

B. Lomefloxacin

Preparations   The active 2-chloro group of 2, 6-dichloro-3-nitropyridine is nucleophillically displaced by 3-methyl-N-carbettoxy-piperazine; then the 6-chloro is displaced with ammonia, and the resulting amine is acylated to the acetamide. The nitro group is reduced, diazotized and subsequently treated with HBF_4 to yield the fluoro derivative. The balance of the synthesis is analogous to that for **ciprofloxacin.**

---

   * **Compylobacter jejuni**   A subspecies of *C. fetus* formerly called *Vibrio fetus.* It can cause an acute enteric disease characterized by diarrhea, abdominal pain, fever, nausea, and vomiting.

 ** **Yersinia**   A genus of **Gram-negative organism.**

Chemical Structure

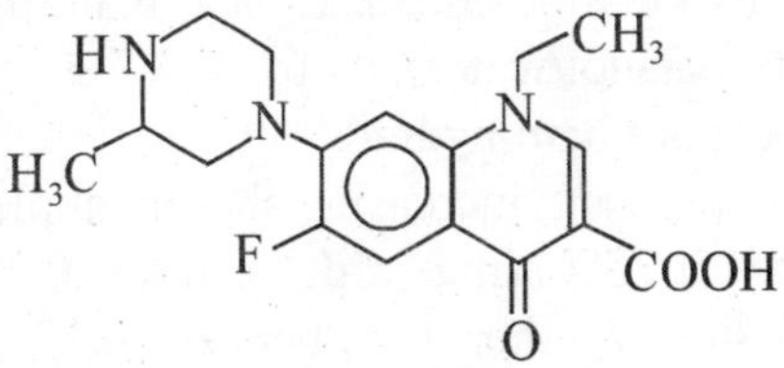

Lomefloxacin

1-Ethyl-6, 8-difluoro-1, 4-dihydro-7-(3-methyl-1-piperazinyl)-4-oxo-3-quinoline carboxylic acid; $(C_{17}H_{19}F_2N_3O_3)$.

Characteristic Features It is obtained as colourless needles from ethanol having mp 239-240.5°C.

Lomefloxacin Monohydrochloride [$C_{17}H_{19}F_2N_3O_3$.HCl] [Synonyms NY-198; Bareon; Chimono; Lomebact; Maxaquin; Uniquin]: It is obtained as colourless needles having mp 295°C with decomposition and is found to be soluble in water.

Uses

1. It is invariably recommended only for treatment of UITs and bronchitis caused by *H. influenzae* or *Branhamella catarrhalis*.
2. It is found to cover Gram-negative bacteria frequently responsible for UTIs but does not necessarily possess the activity to cover the same bacterial infections that respond to either **ciproploxacin** or **ofloxacin.**

C. Norfloxacin

Synonyms Baccidal; Barazan; Chibroxin(e); Chibroxol; Floxacin; Fulgram; Gonorcin; Lexinor; Noflo; Nolicin; Noracin; Noraxin; Norocin; Noroxin(e); Norxacin; Sebercim; Uroxacin; Utinor; Zoroxin;

Preparation Similar to **Ciprofloxacin.***

Chemical Structure

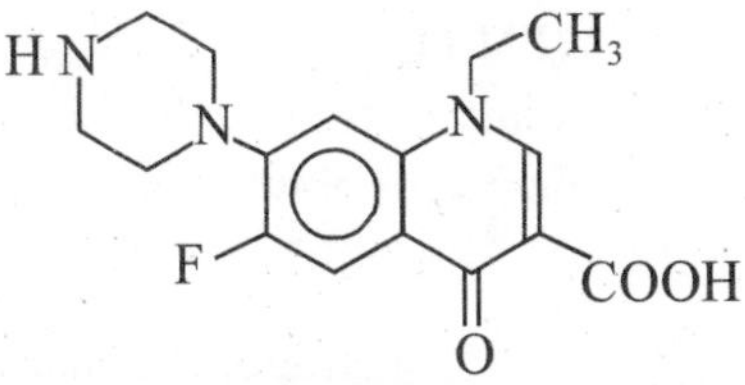

Norfloxacin

1-Ethyl-6-fluoro-1, 4-dihydro-4-oxo-7-(1-piperazinyl)-3-quinoline-carboxylic acid; $(C_{16}H_{18}FN_3O_3)$.

Characteristic Features

1. It is obtained as white to light-yellow crystalline powder having mp 220-221°C.

---

* H. Koga *et al., J. Med. Chem.,* **23**, 1358, (1980).

2. It has uv$_{max}$ (0.1N NaOH): ~ 274, 325, 336 nm (A$^{1\%}_{1cm}$ ~ 1109, 437, 425).
3. It has *two* distinct values of dissociation constant: pKa$_1$ 6.34; pKa$_2$ 8.75.
4. It shows partition coefficient (octanol/water): 0.46.
5. It is hygroscopic in air and forms a hemihydrate.
6. Its solubility in water is pH dependent, increasing sharply at pH < 5 or at pH > 10.
7. **Solubility Profile:** Solubility at 25°C (mg . mL^{-1}): water 0.28; methanol 0.98; ethanol 1.9; acetone 5.1; chloroform 5.5; diethyl ether 0.01; benzene 0.15; ethyl acetate 0.94; octanol 5.1; glacial acetic acid 340.

Uses

1. It is used in the treatment of lower urinary tract infections.
2. It is also employed in penicillin-resistant gonorrhea.
3. It is a limited-spectrum fluoroquinolone.
4. It has incomplete oral absorption.

D. Ofloxacin

Synonyms **Ofloxacine**; DL-8280; HOE-280; Excin; Flobacin; Floxil; Floxin; Oflocet; Oflocin; Oxaldin; Tarivid; Visiren.

Preparation It is a broad-spectrum **fluorinated quinolone antibacterial;** and may be prepared by a method analogous to that for **Ciprofloxacin.***

Chemical Structure

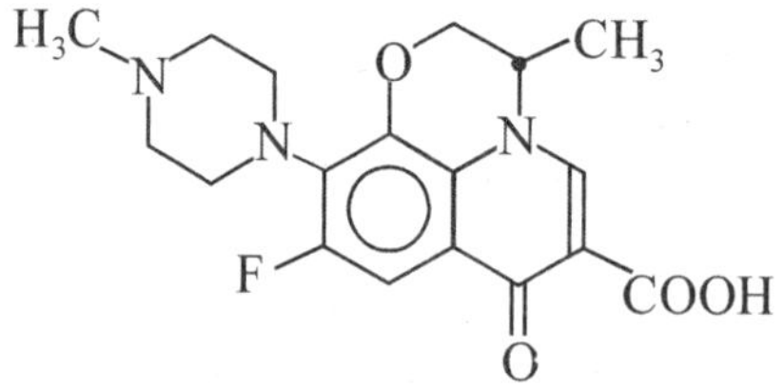

Ofloxacin

(±)-9-Fluoro-2, 3-dihydro-3-methyl-10(4-methyl-1-piperazinyl)-7-oxo-7H-pyrido [1, 2, 3-de], 4-benzoxazine-6-carboxylic acid; (C$_{18}$H$_{20}$FN$_3$O$_4$).

The C-atom to which the —CH$_3$ moiety is attached, in the oxazine ring, is *chiral* and the therapeutically used substance is a racemic mixture; whereas the (+)-form has twice the activity of the (–)-form.

Preparation It may be prepared by a method analogous to that for *Ciprofloxacin.*

Characteristic Features

1. It is obtained as colourless needles having mp 250-257°C, with decomposition.
2. Its dissociation constant pKa is 7.9.
3. It is found to be poorly soluble in water or ethanol.

---

* H. Egawa *et al. Chem. Pharm. Bull.* **34**, 4098 (1986).

Uses　In general, it is found to be an **intermediate-spectrum fluoroquinolone.**

E. Sparfloxacin

Synonyms　Spara; Zagam; AT-4140; CI-978; PD-131501.

Biological Sources　It is a protein-synthesis inhibitor with antibiotic and antineoplastic activity. It is obtained from the fermentation both of *Streptomyces sparsogenes* var *sparsogenes.** It may also be obtained from *Streptomyces cuspidosporus.***

Preparation　US Pat 4,795, 751 (1989); *J. Med. Chem.* **33**, 1645, 1990.

Chemical Structure

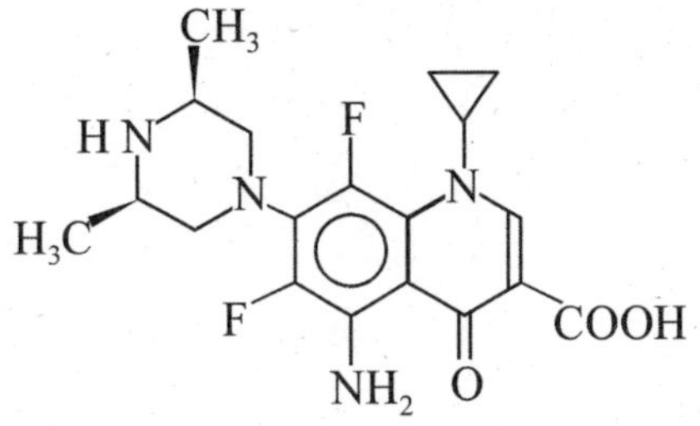

Sparfloxacin

(*cis*)-5-Amino-1-cyclopropyl-7-(3, 5-dimethyl-1-piperazinyl)-6, 8-difluoro-1, 4-dihydro-4-oxo-3-quinolinecarboxylic acid; $(C_{19}H_{22}F_2N_4O_3)$.

Characteristic Features
1. It is obtained as crystals from a mixture of chloroform and ethanol having mp 266–269°C with decomposition.
2. It has two distinct values for dissociation constants. pKa_1 6.25; pKa_2 9.30.
3. **Solubility Profile:** It is sparingly soluble in glacial acetic acid or chloroform; very slightly soluble in ethanol; almost insoluble in water or ether; and soluble in dilute mineral acids or fixed bases (ca 0.1N).

Uses
1. It is a newer **fluoroquinolone** with much improved activity against *Streptococcus pneumoniae,* besides other lower respiratory pathogens covered by **grepafloxacin.**
2. It is found to be more active against *Mycoplasma* than other fluoroquinolones.
3. It exhibits an excellent oral bioavailability profile (92%) and gets metabolized chiefly by **hepatic glucuronidation** rather than **cytochrome P450-mediated pathways.** Evidently, it does not affect the clearance of other drugs (*e.g.*, **cimetidine, cyclosporine, digoxin, theophylline** and **warfarine**) that usually takes place with certain **fluoroquinolones.**
4. Its half-life is 20 hours.

---

* S.P. Owen *et al. Antimicrob Ag. Chemother.* 772 (1962).
** E. Higashide *et al. Takeda Kykusho Nempo.* **25**, 1 (1966).

F. Trovafloxacin

Synonyms Trovan; CP-9921g.

Preparation It is also a **fluorinated quinolone antibacterial** and may be prepared as per US Pat 5,164,402 (1992).

Chemical Structure

Trovafloxacin

$(1\alpha, 5\alpha, 6\alpha)$-7-(6-Amino-3-azabicyclo [3.1.0]hex-3-yl)-1-(2, 4-difluorophenyl)-6-fluoro-1, 4-dihydro-4-oxo-1, 8-naphthyridine-3-carboxylic acid; $(C_{20}H_{15}F_3N_4O_3)$.

Characteristic Features It is usually obtained as white to off white powder.

(*a*) **Trovafloxacin Hydrochloride [$C_{20}H_{15}F_3N_4O_3$.HCl]:** It is mostly obtained as pale-yellow crystals from a mixture of acetonitrile and methanol having mp 246°C (decomposes).

(*b*) **Trovafloxacine Monomethanesulfonate [$C_{20}H_{15}F_3N_4O_3$.CH$_4$O$_3$S] [*Synonyms:* Trovafloxacin Mesylate]**

Uses

1. It is an altogether **newer fluoroquinolone** that exhibits a better activity against certain respiratory pathogens as compared to the **older fluoroquinolones,** for instance: **ciprofloxacin.**
2. It is found to be more active against *Streptococcus pneumonial* (including **penicillin-resistant strains**), *Staphylococcus aureus* (including **methicillin-resistant strains**), *Enterococcus faecalis.*
3. It is observed to be highly active against *chlamydia, Mycoplasma,* and *Ureaplasma;* besides, it also covers important anaerobes, for instance: *Bacterioides frogilis,* and the Gram-negative *Enterobacteriaceae,* including *Ps aeruginosa.*
4. **Trovafloxacin** is recommended for a very broad range of infections including oral and IV treatment of nosocomial and community-acquired pneumonia, acute exacerbations of chronic bronchitis, acute sinusitis, complicated intra-abdominal and pelvic infections, diabetic-foot infection, uncomplicated UTIs, prostatitis, cervicitis, and uncomplicated gonorrhea.
5. It has an excellent oral bioavailability (88%).
6. It has a half-life of 10 hours.
7. It hardly shows any untoward photosensitivity as other **fluoroquinolones.**

9.3.10.1.5.4 **Agents for Systemic UTIs** There are a few purely synthetic drug molecules which are being used exclusively for various systemic urinary tract infections (UTIs). The *two* typical and potent drugs belonging to this category are, namely: **methenamine** and **nitrofurantoin,** which shall now be discussed as under:

A. Methenamine

Synonyms Hexamine; Hexamethylamine; Aminoform; Ammoform; Crystamin, Cystogen; Formin; Uritone; Urotropin.

Preparation **Methenamine** may be prepared by the interaction of a moderate excess of ammonia water to formaldehyde solution, and evaporating the mixture to absolute dryness.

Chemical Structure

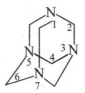

Methenamine

1, 3, 5, 7-Tetraazatricyclo [3.3.1.-1^{3,7}] decane; ($C_6H_{12}N_4$).

Characteristic Features

1. It is obtained as colourless, lustrous crystals or a white crystalline powder, or granules almost odourless which sublimes at about 263°C without melting and with partial decomposition.
2. It is found to be somewhat volatile at low temperature.
3. Its aqueous solution is alkaline to litmus.
4. One subjecting it to ignition it burns with a smokeless flame.
5. **Solubility Profile:** 1g dissolves in 1.5 mL of water; 12.5mL ethanol; 320 mL ether; and 10 mL chloroform.
6. The pH of a 0.2 molar aqueous solution is 8.4.

Uses

1. It is found to be an extremely effective urinary tract anti-infective agent provided it is made to act in an acidic medium.
2. As it is exerted quite rapidly, hence it attains effective antiseptic concentrations in the urine.
   Note: Methenamine depends on its action solely on the liberation of free formaldehyde. Thus, it attains 20% of theoretical value at pH 5.0; 6% at pH 6.0; and nil at pH 7.6.
3. It is of particular value in the treatment of *E. coli* infections of the urinary tract.
4. It is also useful specifically in patients with *renal insufficiency.* By virtue of its low systemic toxicity, failure to excrete the drug produces absolutely very little harmful consequences; of course, unless and until the renal insufficiency is of a severe nature.
   Note: The drug should not be used in patients having hepatic insufficiency.

B. Nitrofurantoin

Synonyms Berkfurin; Chemiofuran; Cyantin; Cystit; FuaMed; Furachel; Furalan; Furadantin; Furadantine MC; Furadoin; Furantoina; Furobactina; Furophen T-Caps; Ituran; Macrodantin; Parfuran; Trantoin; Urantoin; Urizept; Urodin; Urolong; Uro-Tablinen; Welfurin.

Preparation   It is prepared by the interaction of 1-aminohydanoin sulphate and 5-nitro-2-furaldehyde diacetate.*

Chemical Structure

Nitrofurantoin

1-(5-Nitro-2-furfurylideneamino) hydantoin; $(C_8H_6N_4O_5)$.

Characteristic Features

1. It is obtained as orange-yellow needles, crystals or fine powder from dilute acetic acid that get decomposed at 270-272°C. It is found to be odourless and gives a bitter aftertaste.
2. It has dissociation constant pKa 7.2.
3. It shows uv_{max} : 370 nm ($E_{1cm}^{1\%}$ 776).
4. **Solubility Profile:** It has solubility (mg/100 mL): water (neutral pH 7) 19.0; 95% (v/v) ethanol 51.0; acetone 510; DMF 8000; peanut oil 2.1; glycerol 60; and polyethylene glycol 1500.

Nitrofurantoin Monohydrate $[C_8H_6N_4O_5.H_2O]$ [*Synonyms* Macrobid]

Uses

1. It is found to be effective against a majority of urinary tract pathogens, including certain strains of *E. coli; Enterobacter; Klebsiella, Proteus Spp.; Staphylococcus aureus*; and *Streptococcus faecalis.*
2. It is also effective against many *staphylococci, clostridia,* and *Bacillus subtilis.*
3. It is invariably indicated for the treatment of infections of the urinary tract caused by the aforecited organisms: pyclonephritis; cystis and pyelitis.
4. An acidic urine favours activity; and in chronic bacteriuria, it is a second-or third-choice agent.
5. Interestingly, as a prophylactic in the prevention of recurrences it is found to be effective, being slightly superior to methenamine mandelate but inferior to sulfamethiazole.
6. It has a half life for only 0.3 hour.

9.3.10.1.5.5 **Agents for Mycobacterium Tuberculosis Infections**   One of the most dreadful diseases across the world is tuberculosis which is caused by the pathogenic organisms *Mycobacterium tuberculosis.* The **antimycobacterial drugs** existing *generally are usually divided into two main categories. namely: first-line drugs,* which essentially comprise of the natural products, such as: **streptomycin** (see section 9.3.1.6), **rifampin** (Section 9.3.10.1.1.A) and **rifabutin,** plus a good number of purely synthetic compounds including **ethambutol, isoniazid (INH)** and **pyrazinamide;** *second-line drugs,* are invariably employed in *three* specific events, for instance: (*a*) organisms resistant to first line drugs, (*b*) patient idiosyncrasy prohibit use of the first-line agents, and (*c*) serious adverse and untowrd effects, and these mostly include **cycloserine** (Section 9.3.8.1) and

---

* Swirska *et al . Przem. Chem.,* **11**, (34), 306, (1955).

caperomycin belonging to the class of natural products, whereas *para*-**aminosalicylic acid (PAS)** and **ethionamide** belong to the synthetic origin.

It is, however, pertinent to mention here that, in general, *tuberculosis* is always treated with a combination **antimycobacterial agents** to minimise the emergence of resistance organisms and also to broaden its spectrum of activity.

It is thought worthwhile to discuss one synthetic drug each from the **first-line** and **second-line agents** in this section:

A. Pyrazinamide

Synonyms Pyrazineacarboxamide; Prezetamid; Pyrafat; Pirilene; Piraldina; Tebrazid; Unipyranamide; Zinamide.

Preparation **Pyrazinamide** may be prepared by the thermal decarboxylation of 2, 3-pyrazinedicarboxylic acid to form the monocarboxylic acid, which is esterified with methanol and finally subjected to controlled ammonolysis.*

Chemical Structure

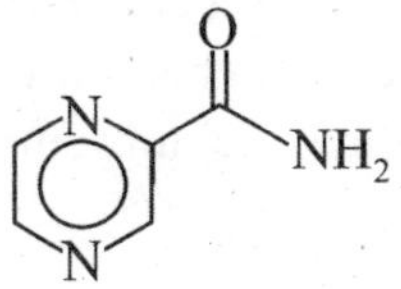

Pyrazinamide

Pyrazine carboxamide; ($C_5H_5N_3O$).

Characteristic Features
1. It is obtained as white to practically white crystals from either ethanol or water having mp 189-191°C. It is found to sublime at 60°C.
2. Its dissociation constant pKa is 0.5.
3. It has uv_{max}: 269 nm ($E_{1cm}^{1\%}$ 660).
4. **Solubility Profile** (mg. mL^{-1}): water 15; methanol 13.8, absolute ethanol 5.7; isopropanol 3.8; ether 1.0; isooctane 0.01; chloroform 7.4.
5. Its aqueous solutions are found to be neutral.

Uses
1. It is used as an antituberculosis drug used for initial treatment in combination with **isoniazid** and **rifampin.**
2. It is invariably administered with **isoniazid,** which it potentiates.

   Note: All patients intended to be treated with the drug must have thorough prior liver-function tests, which tests also should be repeated periodically during therapy.

---

* *J. Am. Chem. Soc.* **74**, 3617 (1952).

B. Ethionamide

Synonyms   Amidazine; Ethioniamide; Bayer 5312; Nisotin; Actina; Trescatyl; Ethimide; Iridocin; Tio-Mid.

Preparation It may be prepared by the method suggested by Libermann *et al.**

Chemical Structure

Ethionamide

2-Ethyl-4-pyridinecarbothioamide; $(C_8H_{10}N_2S)$.

Characteristic Features

1. It is obtained as minute yellow crystals from ethanol that get decomposed at 164-166°C.
2. It is found to be very sparingly soluble in ether and water; sparingly soluble in methanol, ethanol, propylene glycol; soluble in hot acetone, dichloroethane; and freely soluble in pyridine.

Uses

1. It is mostly used as a potent tuberculostatic agent.

9.3.10.1.5.6 **Antifungal Agents: Immunocompromised hosts** are usually pretty gullible and prone to dreadful pathogenic fungi solely responsible for causing a large number of infections. Generally, all fungi are eucaryotic organisms and by virtue of this fact they behave more like human cells than are bacteria. It is, however, pertinent to mention here that the antibacterial compounds may not necessarily either inhibit the growth of fungi or able to kill them completely; and, therefore, it has been virtually a difficult task to identify rather selective and specific targets within the fungal cells. The latest range of systemic antifungal agents invariably and largely target cell membrane synthesis or their integrity. In the recent past, significant emphasis has been attached towards the development of antifungal drugs based on the cardinal fact that the fungal membranes essentially contain a sterol, **ergosterol,** which is not present in any human cell membranes.

Broadly speaking fungi that cause painful human infections are of *four* major categories, namely: (*a*) **yeast**-*i.e.*, *Candida albicans,* usually found in the normal flora that may conveniently overgrow in various vital organs of the body, such as: bladder, intestine, vagina, mouth, skin and even infect the blood stream; besides another organism known as *Cryptococcus neoformans* which specifically causes meningitis or pneumonia; (*b*) **filamentous dermatophytes** *i.e.*, long, interwoven, irregularly placed fungal parasite that grows in or on the skin, which normally cause skin infections, for instance: ringworm (tinea corporis), athelete's foot (tinea pedis) and nail infections (onychomycosis); (*c*) **dimorphic fungi**-*i.e.*, which essenially have both filamentous and yeast-like structures, and are

---

* Libermann *et al. Compt. Rend.* **242**, 2409 (1956).

responsible for causing either exclusively primary pulmonary or secondary disseminated infections by such organisms as: *Blastomyces, Coccidioides, Histoplasma, Paracoccidioides;* and (*d*) **filamentous fungi**-*i.e.*, fungi having long, interwoven and irregularly shaped structures *e.g.*, *Aspergilus* that may duly attack on a variety of sites in the body.

In actual practice, there are *three* well-known **natural products** that are invariably used as the antifungal agents, namely: **griseofulvin, polyenes (amphotericin** B), and **undecylenic acid,** that are employed to treat *dermatophytic infections*. Besides, there are some synthetic antifungal agents that are exclusively used to combat the dermatophytic infections, such as: *allylamines* (**naftifine, terbinafine**); *5-fluorocytosine;* and the *"azoles"* (**fluconazole, miconazole**).

First, of all the antifungal agents derived from the natural products shall be discussed, followed by a brief discussion of the purely synthetic products in the sections that follows:

Natural Products

A. Griseofulvin

Synonyms   Amudane; Curling Factor; Fulcin; Fulvicin; Grifulvin; Grisactin; Grisefuline; Grisovin; Gris-PEG; Grysio, Lamoryl; Likuden; Neo-Fulcin; Polygris; Poncyl-FP; Spirofulvin; Sporostatin.

Biological Sources   **Griseofulvin** is an antibiotic substance produced by *Penicillium griseofulvum* Diercks and also by *Penicillium janezewskii* Zal. [Same as *P. nigricans* (Banier) Thom]. It is produced by *Penicillum patulum.*

Preparation   It is produced commercially by employing the submerged process using *P. patulum.*

Chemical Structure

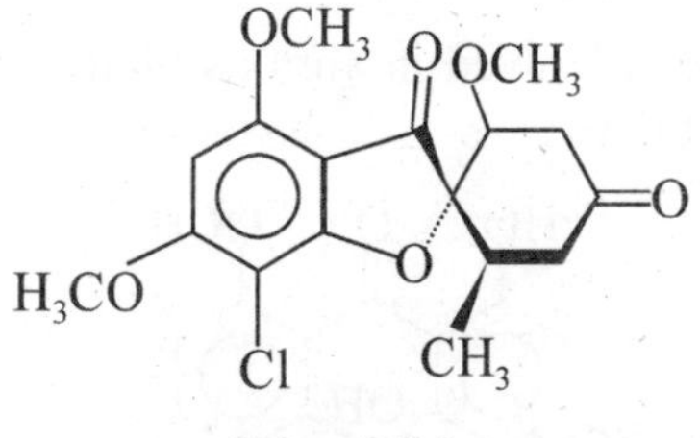

Griseofulvin

(1′S-*trans*)-7-Chloro-2′, 4, 6-trimethoxy-6′-methylspiro[benzofuran 2(3H), 1′-[2] cyclohexene]-3, 4′-dione; ($C_{17}H_{17}ClO_6$).

Characteristic Features

1. It is obtained as white to creamy white, powder, wherein particles of the order of 4 µm in diameter usually predominate. It may also be obtained as octahedra or rhombs from benzene having mp 220°C; and is odourless.
2. It has specific optical rotation $[\alpha]_D^{17} + 370°$ (in saturated chloroform solution).
3. It has uv_{max}: 286, 325 nm.
4. Its solubility in DMF at 25°C is 12-14 g per 100 mL; slightly soluble in ethanol, methanol, acetone, benzene, chloroform, ethyl cetate, acetic acid; almost insoluble in water, petroleum ether.

Uses

1. **Griseofulvin** is **fungistatic** and not **fungicidal,** and serves as an effective agent in the treatment of superficial fungal infections.
2. When administered systemically it is found to be highly effective in the control and management of *tinea captitis, tinea corporis, tinea unquium* (onychomycosis) and the chromic form of *tinea pedis* normally caused by the dermatophytes, namely: *Microsporon, Trychophyton,* and *Epidermophyton.*
3. As it evidently exerts a fungistatic activity thereby only arresting reproduction of the organism, it is absolutely necessary to continue medication long enough so that the entire epidermis undergoes shading and replaced so as to get rid of reinfecting organisms.
   Mechanism of Action: Griseofulvin gets deposited in the **keratin precursor cells** and is carried outwards into the epidermis as normal skin-growth proceeds. It also obviates for a long latency from the time medication is commenced until evidence of improvement takes place.
4. Its half-life is 24-36 hours.
5. It is the drug of choice for mucocutaneous infections.

Biosynthesis of Griseofulvin   The various steps involved in the **biosynthesis of griseofulvin** are as follows:

1. **Griseofulvin** is produced biosynthetically from the head-to-tail condensation of 7-acetate units to yield **polyketide**—as the basic precursor.
2. **Griseophenone C** is obtained as an early intermediate in the biosynthetic pathway.
3. Subsequent methylation and chlorination are assumed to precede the oxidative coupling of the benzophenone to give rise to the formation of **dehydrogreseofulvin-a spiran.**
4. Obviously, the last and ultimate step is the production of **griseofulvin** *via* reduction.

The aforementioned intermediates involved in various biotransformations from step (1) through (4) may be summarized as given below:

Polyketide [Basic Precursor] → Griseophenone C [Early Intermediate] → A Benzophenone [Oxidative Coupling] → Dehyrogriseofulvin [A Spiran] → Griseofulvin

Biosynthesis of Griseofulvin

B. Amphotericin B

Synonyms   Ambisome; Amphozone; Fungizone; Fungilin; Ampho-Moronal.

Biological Sources   It is a polyene antibiotic produced by M 4575 obtained from the soil of the Orinoco river region of Venezuela.*

Preparation   **Amphotericin B** may be prepared by the growth of selected strains of *Steptomyces nodosus* in a suitable culture medium under specific controlled parameters of temperature, pH and aeration. Subsequently, after due extraction from the medium, the crude product is purified by treatment with different solvents at a controlled acidity (pH).

Chemical Structure $(C_{47}H_{73}NO_{17})$

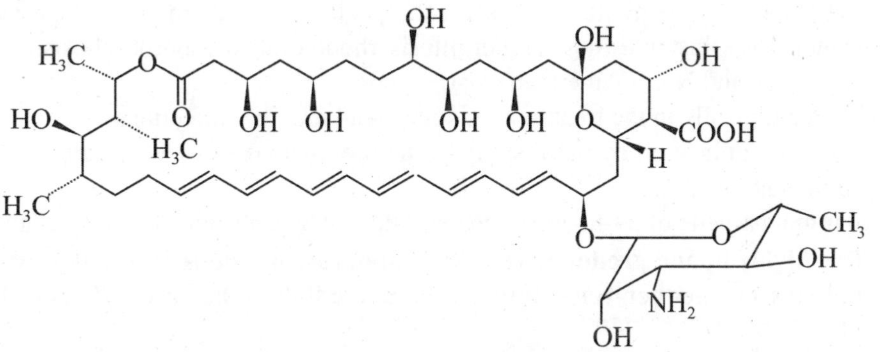

Amphotericin B

Characteristic Features
1. It is obtained as yellow to orange powder or as deep yellow-prisms or needles from DMF that gradually get decomposed above 170°C; and is odourless.
2. It has uv_{max} (methanol): 406, 382, 363, 345 nm.
3. It shows specific optical rotation $[\alpha]_D^{24} + 333°$ (acidic MDF);-33.6° (0.1N methanolic HCl).
4. It has dissociation constant pKa (acid) 5.7, (amine) 10.0.
5. Solids and solutions are fairly stable for long durations between pH 4 and 10 when stored at moderate temperatures out of direct contact with light and air.
6. **Solubility Profile:** It is found to be soluble at pH 2 or pH 11 in water: about 0.1 mg mL^{-1}; soluble in DMF 2-4 mg mL^{-1}; in DMF + HCl: 60–80 mg mL^{-1}; in DMSO: 30-40 mg mL^{-1}. However, its aqueous solubility may be enhanced to nearly 50 mg mL^{-1}, by complexation with **sodium desoxycholate**.

---

* Walters *et al. J. Am. Chem. Soc.*, **79**, 5076, (1957).

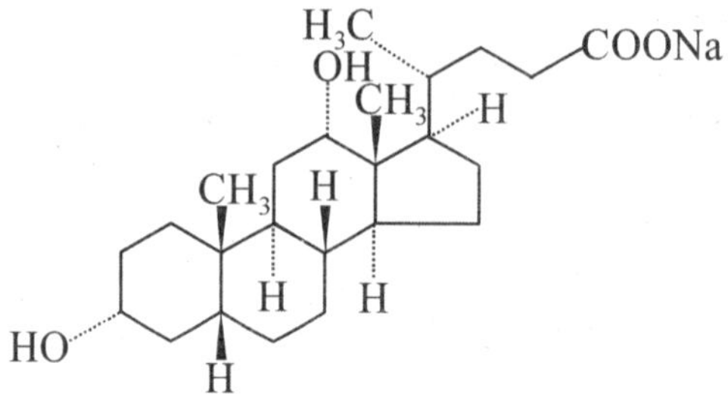

Sodium Desoxycholate

Uses

1. It exhibits the widest spectrum of antifungal activity of any systemic antifungal drug.
2. It is proclaimed to be an extremely useful drug when given by IV route for the management and therapy of a host of systemic fungus diseases, especially coccidioidomycosis, cryptococcosis, systemic moniliasis, histoplasmosis, aspergillosis, rhodotorulosis, sporotrichosis, phycomycosis (mucormycosis), and North American blastomycosis.
3. It also is used topically in the treatment of superficial monilial infections.
4. It also finds its application by nasal spray in the prophylaxis of aspergillosis in immunocompromised patients.
5. It has an initial half-life of 24-hours, which is followed by a terminal half-life of about 15 days.

   Note: It is highly bound predominantly to β-lipoproteins and is exercted gradually by the kidneys but neither renal failure nor hemodialysis has a consistent effect on the plasma levels.

C. Undecylenic Acid

Synonyms   10-Undecenoic acid; Declid; Renselin; Sevinon.

Preparation   It is obtained either by pyrrolysis of ricinoleic acid or by vacuum distillation of castor oil. It is also found to occur in sweat.

Chemical Structure

$$CH_2 = CH (CH_2)_8 COOH$$

Undecylenic Acid

Characteristic Features

1. It is obtained as liquid or crystals having mp 24.5°C.
2. It has a distinct odour suggestive of perspiration.
3. It shows various densities as: d_4^{24}(vac.) 0.9072; d_{25}^{25} 0.9102; d_{45}^{45} 0.8993; $d_4^{79.9}$ (vac.) 0.8653.
4. It has n_D^{25} 1.4486.
5. It shows various bp: bp_{760} 275°C (decomposes); bp_{130} 230-235°C; bp_{90} 198-200°C; and $bp_{1.0}$ 131°C.
6. It has neutralization value 304.5; and iodine value 137.8.
7. It is found to be insoluble in water, but soluble in chloroform, ethanol and ether.

Undecylenic Acid Zinc Salt [$C_{22}H_{38}O_4Zn$] [*Synonyms* Zinc undecylenate]: It is obtained as an amorphous white powder having mp 115–116°C. It resembles zinc stearate in appearance and physical properties. It may be prepared by dissolving zinc oxide in dilute undecylenic acid and concentrating the solution

Synthetic Products: The various important synthetic antifungal products are:

A. Allylamines   Recently, two new allylamines have been synthesized that are found to be potent antifungal agents:

(a) Naftifine

Synonyms   Naftifungin.

Chemical Structure   It is an antimycolytic allylamine.

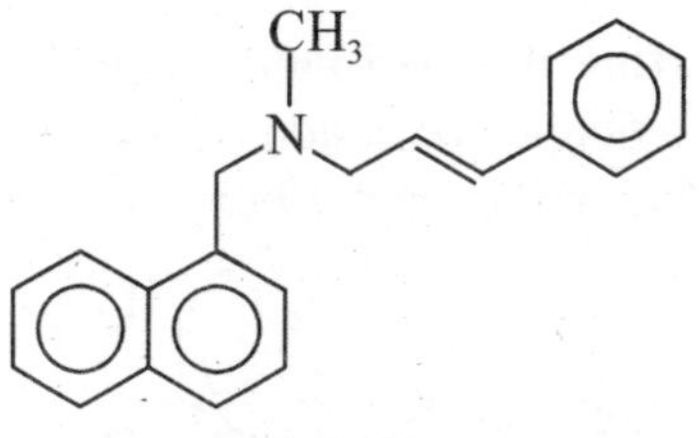

Naftifine

(E)-N-Methyl-N-(3-phenyl-2-propenyl)-1-naphthalene methanamine; ($C_{21}H_{21}N$).

Characteristic Features   It is a colourless viscous oil $bp_{0.015\ torr}$ 162-167°C.

Naftifine Hydrochloride   [$C_{21}H_{21}N.HCl$] [*Synonyms* Exoderil; Naftin; AW-105-843; SN-105-843]: It is obtained as colourless crystals from propanol having mp 177°C.

Uses   It is mostly employed as a topical antifungal agent in the treatment of various skin infections.

(*b*) Terbinafine

Synonyms   Lamisil; SF-86-327.

Preparation   It is an antimycotic allylamine related to naftifine and may be prepared by the method provided by Lednicer *et al.**

Chemical Structure

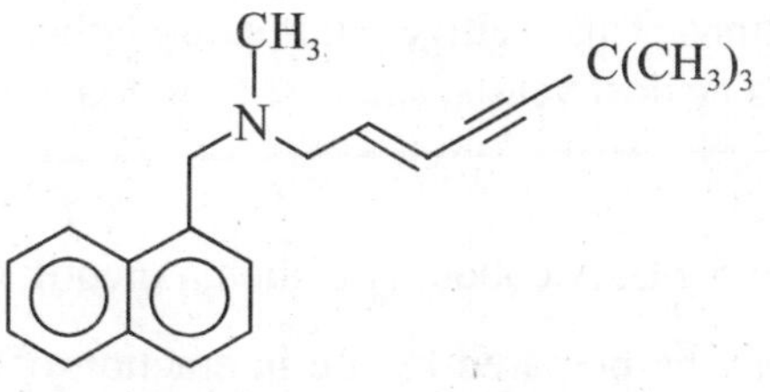

Terbinafine

---

* D. Lednieer *et al., Org. Chem. of Drug Syn.* Vol. 4, Wiley, NY, p-55 (1990).

trans-N-Methyl-N (1-napthylmethyl)-6, 6-dimethylhept-2-en-4-ynyl-1-amine; $(C_{21}H_{25}N)$.

Characteristic Features

Teribnafine Hydrochloride $[H_{21}H_{25}N.HCl]$

1. It is obtained as white to off-white crystalline powder or as crystals from a mixture of 2-propanol + diethyl ether having mp 195-198°C (alteration in crystal structure commences nearly at 150°C).
2. **Solubility Profile:** It is freely soluble in methanol and methylene chloride; soluble in ethanol; and slightly soluble in water.

Uses

1. It is the *first allylamine* known so far as a systemic drug recommended in the treatment of all dermatophytes, namely: *Trichophyton, Epidermophyton,* and *Microspora*.
2. It is also used for topical therapy of dermatophytes including various types of *tinea* infections.

Mechanism of Action   **Terbinafine hydrochloride** selectively inhibits the *fungal squalene epoxidase* responsible for causing a *fungicidal action* by virtue of the intracellular accumulation of the toxic sterol, *squalene*; it is also found to exert a *fungistatic action* by depletion of *ergosterol*.

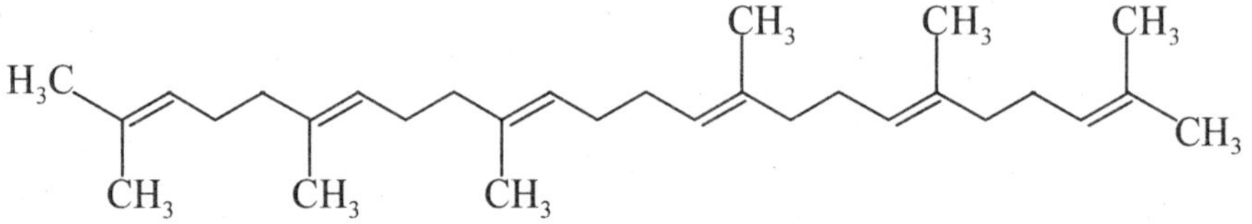

Squalene

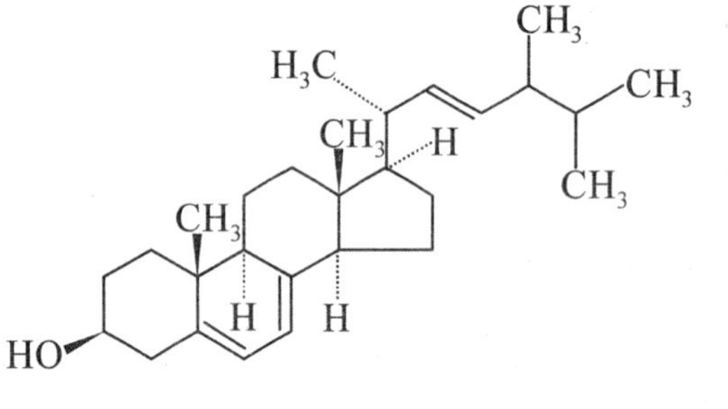

Ergosterol

B. Fluorocytosine   It essentially has basic pyrimidine nucleus that has been duly substituted with fluoro-, amino-, and oxo-functions. This relatively not-so-complicated molecule was introduced in early seventies as a potent drug against yeasts, such as: *Candida* and *Cryptococcus*.

(*a*) Flucytosine

Synonyms   5-Fluorocytosine; 5-FC; Alcobon; Ancobon; Ancotil; Cytosine, 5-fluoro-.

Preparation   **Flucytosine** may be prepared by the interaction of **5-fluorouracil** with $POCl_3$ to yield **2,4-dichloro-5-fluoropyrimidine** which is subsequently reacted with ammonia (NH_3) to give rise to **2-chloro-4-amino-5-fluropyrimidine.** Heating the latter in a medium of concentrated HCl forms the desired product.

Chemical Structure

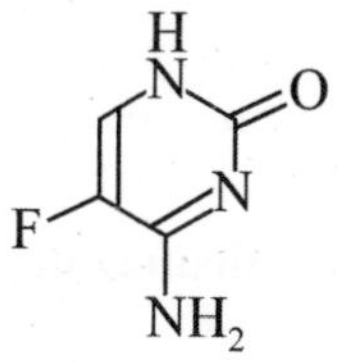

Flucytosine

4-Amino-5-fluoro-2(H)-pyrimidinone; ($C_4H_4FN_3O$).

Characteristic Features

1. It is obtained as a odourless, white off-white crystalline powder with a mp 295-297°C (decompose).
2. It is found to be fairly stable in light, non hygroscopic; stable for at least 3 months at 45°C.
3. It has dissociation constants as pKa 2.9 and 10.7.
4. Its uv_{max} (0.1 N HCl): 285 nm (ε 8900).
5. **Solubility Profile:** Solubility in water: 1.5g/100 ml at 25°C; 1g in 12 mL 0.1N HCl; slightly soluble in ethanol; and almost insoluble in chloroform, ether.

Uses

1. **Flucytosine** gets converted in the fungus to **5-fluorouracil** in the presence of fungal deaminase, which is subsequently incorporated into RNA, that interferes with normal protein synthesis. It has been observed that certain fungal organisms are relatively more sensitive to interference from the drug than are the human cells, and hence it is definitely, useful in the radical treatment of some fungal infections.

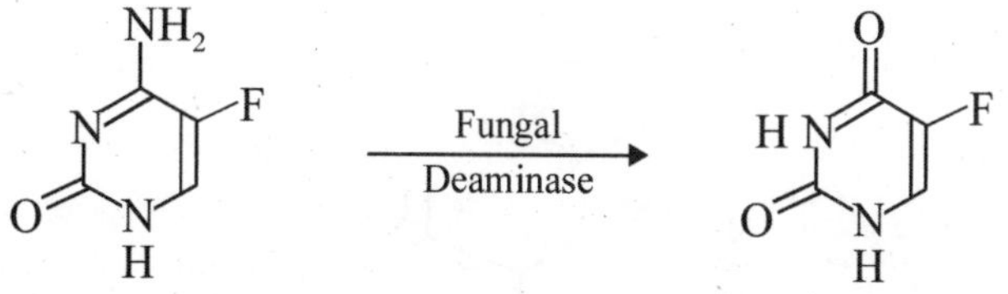

Flucytosine   5-Fluorouracil

2. It has been found that majority of clinical isolates of *Cryptococcus;* and 40-92% of *Candida* are sensitive to the drug.
3. It is the *drug of choice* to treat *chromomycosis;* and of *second choice* to treat systemic *candidiasis.*
4. It may be logically combined with amphotericin B [section 9.3.10.1.5.6.(B)] for the *first-choice treatment* of *aspergillosis* or *cryptococcosis,* especially associated with *meningitis.*
5. It has a normal half-life 0.5-1 hour.

C. Azoles In general, the chemical compounds containing either **'imidazole'** or **'triazole'** moieties are invariably clubbed together and baptized as **"azoles"**.

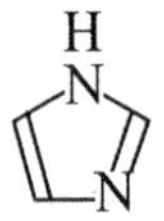

Imidazole 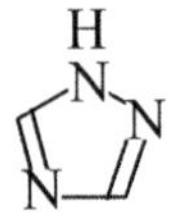   Triazole

The **imidazole** bearing antifungal agents are: **miconazole, clotrimazole, econazole,** and **ketoconazole** as given below:

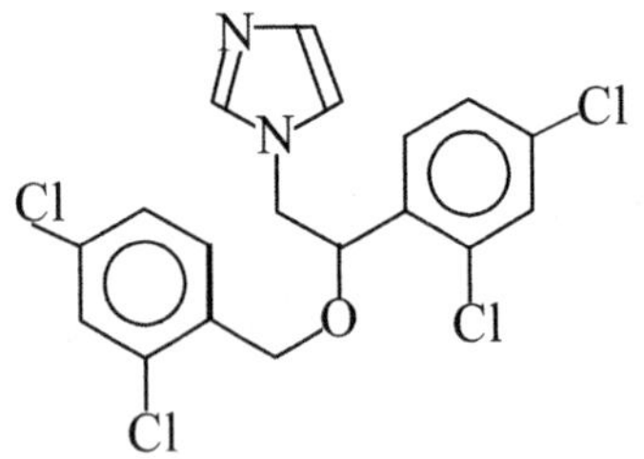

Miconazole 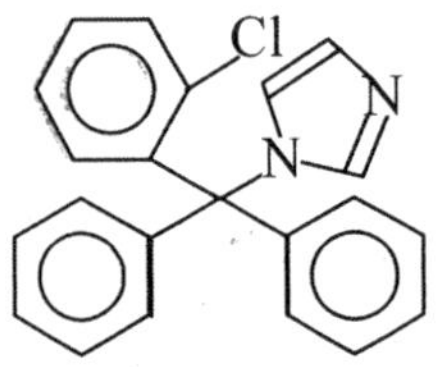   Clotrimazole 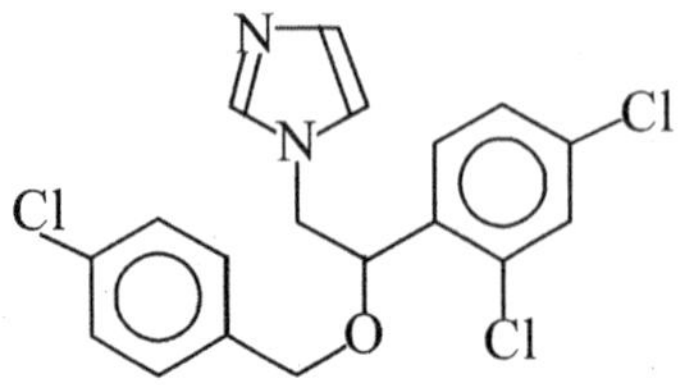   Econazole

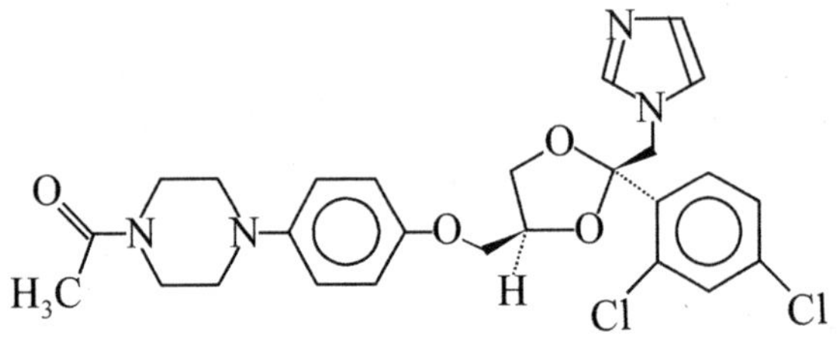

Ketoconazole

The **triazole** containing antifungal agents are, namely: **fluconazole,** and **itraconazole** as shown under:

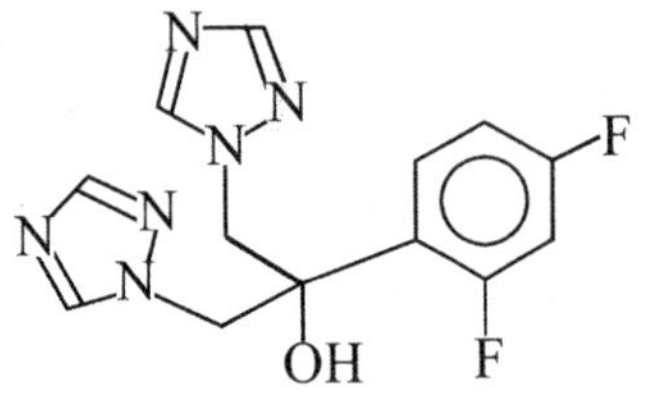

Fluconazole

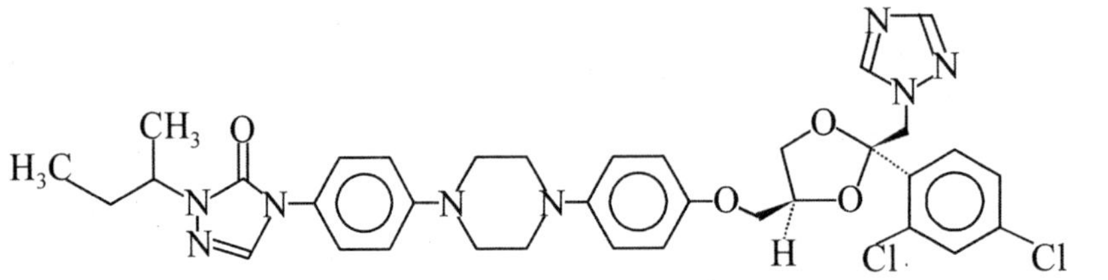

Itraconazole

It is thought worthwhile to discuss at least one representative drug from each of the aforesaid *two* class of compounds:

(*a*) Miconazole

Synonyms   Micatin; Monistat.

Preparation   It is a topical drug for mucocutaneous infections exclusively. **Miconazole** may be prepared* by alkylation of imidazole with 2, 4-dichlorophenacyl bromide followed by reduction of the ketone function to a corresponding secondary alcohol which is subsequently converted to the alkoxide. Finally, the Williamson alkylation with α, *p*,-dichlorotoluene gives rise to the desired product.

Characteristic Features

Miconazole Nitrate [$C_{34}H_{32}N_2O_5$] [*Synonyms* Aflorix; Albistat; Andergin; Brentan; Conoderm; Conofite; Daktarin; Deralbine; Dermonistat; Florid; Fungiderm; Micotef; Prilagin; Vodol]: It is obtained as crystals having mp 170.5°C.

(+)-Form Nitrate   It has mp 135.3°C; and $[\alpha]_D^{20} + 59°$ (methanol).
(–)-Form Nitrate   It has mp 135°C; and $[\alpha]_D^{20}$-58° (methanol).

Uses

1. It exerts significant fungicidal action to various species of *Aspergillus, Blastomyces, Candida, Cladosporium, Epidermophyton, Histoplasma, Microsporon, Paracoccidioides,* and *Trichophyton.*
2. In *tinea pedis* (*i.e.,* **Athlete's Foot**) a mycological cure rate of 96% has been duly accomplished with the nitrate salt, which appreciably exceeds that of any other drugs except **clotrimazole** and **econazole.**
3. It is recommended for topical usage in *vulvovaginal candidiasis,* successful cure rate varies from 80-95% which is significantly superior to that accomplished with **nystatin** (65%), and **amphotericin B** (75%).
4. It has been observed that pruritus is cured even after a single application.
5. It is also found to be very effective against certain vaginal infections caused by *Trichophyton glabratus.*
6. **Miconazole** base is very useful in the topical treatment of various ophthalmic mycoses.
7. **Miconazole** base has been recommended very successfully for the systemic cure and treatment of a number of deep and systemic mycoses, such as: *Candidiasis* and *Cryptococcosis.*

Mechanism of Action   It specifically inhibits ergosterol synthesis, thereby disrupting the fungal cell membranes. Thus, the drug rapidly penetrates deep into the *stratum corneum* where it remains in relatively high concentration upto 96 hours, which situation perhaps contributes its remarkable efficacy against the *dermatophytoses.*

---

* *J. Med. Chem.,* **12**, 784, (1969).

(*b*) Fluconazole

Synonyms   Biozolene; Diflucan; Elazor; Triflucan.

Characteristic Features   It is an orally active **bistriazole antifungal agent** which is obtained as white crystals having mp 139°C. It is also obtained as crystals from a mixture of ethyl acetate and hexane that melts about 138-140°C.

Uses

1. It is found to be a highly selective inhibitor especially of *fungal cytochrome P-450* together with *sterol C-14α-demethylation* that is responsible for the inhibition of ergosterol synthesis.
2. **Fluconazole** is a broad-spectrum bistriazole antifungal substance which is observed to be primarily fungistatic with appreciable activity against *Cryptococcus neoformans* and *Candida spp*.
3. It is duly recommended for *systemic candidiasis, oropharyngeal* and *esophageal candidiasis; and cryptococcal meningitis.*
4. The bioavailability of oral fluconazole is more than 90% compared with IV administration.
5. The volume of distribution is $0.8 gL^{-1}$.
6. The plasma half-life is about 30 hours.

   Note: **Fluconazole may particularly alter cytochrome P-450 pathways of metabolism of a good number of therapeutic agents, such as: cyclosporine, phenytoin, sulphonyl ureas, and warfarin.**

9.3.10.1.5.7 **Anticancer Antibiotics**   A plethora of **anticancer antibiotics** have been derived exclusively from natural origin that are used either independently or in combination with other chemotherapeutic agents. Of course, it may not be within the scope of this text to deal with the entire compounds used in anticancer chemotherapy, but an attempt is made to discuss a few most potent drugs in the sections that follow, namely: **doxorubicin, daunorubicin, dactinomycin** and **mitomycin C.**

A. Doxorubicin   It has already been discussed in this chapter under Section 9.3.2.1.

B. Daunorubicin

Synonyms   Daunomycin; Leukaemomycin C; Rubidomycin; Cerubidin; RP-13057.

Preparation   It is an anthracyclinic antibiotic related to the rhodomycins. It is produced from the fermentation broths of *Streptomyces peucetins* or S. *coeruleorubidus*. **Daunorubicin** is a glycoside formed by a tetracyclic aglycone, **daunomycinone** ($C_{21}H_{18}O_8$) and an aminosugar, **daunosamine** ($C_6H_{13}NO_3$), 3-amino-2, 3,6-trideoxy-L-lyxo-hexose. However, it may also be synthesized by the method of Acton *et al.**

---

* E.M. Acton *et al.*, *J. Med. Chem.* **17**, 659 (1974).

Chemical Structure

Daunorubicin

(8S-*cis*)-8-Acetyl-10-[(3-amino-2, 3, 6-trideoxy-α-L-lyxo-hexopyranosyl) oxy]-7, 8, 9, 10-tetrahydro-6, 8, 11-trihydroxy-1-methoxy-5, 12-naphthacenedione; ($C_{27}H_{29}NO_{10}$).

Characteristic Features   It is obtained as crystals having mp 208–209°C.

Daunorubicin Hydrochloride [$C_{27}H_{29}NO_{10}$.HCl] [*Synonyms* Cerubidine; Daunoblastina; Ondena.]

1. It is obtained as thin red needles that decompose at 188-199°C.
2. The pH of an aqueous solution containing 5 mg mL^{-1} ranges betwen 4.5 to 6.5.
3. The specific optical rotation $[\alpha]_D^{20}$ + 248 ± 5° (C = 0.05-0.1 in CH_3 OH).
4. The colour of aqueous solution changes from pink at acid pH to blue at alkaline pH.
5. It has uv$_{max}$ (methanol): 234, 252, 290, 480, 495, and 532 nm ($E_{1cm}^{1\%}$ 665, 462, 153, 214, 218, and 112).
6. **Solubility Profile:** It is soluble in water, methanol, aqueous alcohols; and almost insoluble in chloroform, ether and benzene.

Uses

1. It is invariably employed for the treatment of severe (acute) lymphocytic and nonlymphocytic leukemias, usually as a component of combination chemotherapeutic regimens. It has been found to undergo very quick reductive metabolism specifically in the liver to give rise to the active **dauno-rubicinol.**
2. It inhibits DNA synthesis by means of a series of bio-chemical reactions, such as: intercalation into DNA, inhibition of topoisomerase II, and production of oxygen radicals. It may prevent cell division in such doses that do not interfere with nucleic acid synthesis.
3. In combination with other drugs it is included in the **first-choice-chemotherpy** of acute *myclocytic leukemia* in adults (for induction of remission) and also in the acute phase of *chromic mycloytic leukemia.*
4. The half-life of distribution is 45 minutes. The half-life of its active metabolite, **daunorubicinol,** is nearly 27 hours.

C. Dactinomycin

Synonyms   Actinomycin D; Meractinomycin; Actinomycin A_{IV}; Actinomycin C_1; Actinomycin I_1; Actinomycin X_1; Cosmegen.

Preparation   It is an antibiotic substance belonging to the **actinomycin** complex, elaborated during the culture of *Streptomyces parvulus*. After extracting from the fermentation broth by suitable solvents, it is subsequently subjected to purification through various chromatographic and crystallization processes (*US Patent: 2, 378, 876*).

Chemical Structure

Dactinomycin [$C_{62} H_{86} N_{12} O_{16}$]

Characteristic Features

1. It is obtained as a bright-red crystalline powder, light sensitive and should be protected appropriately. It melts at 246°C with the decomposition.
2. It should be protected from excessive heat and moisture.
3. It essentially contains in one mg an amount of antibiotic activity of not less than 900 mcg of dactinomycin.
4. **Solubility Profile:** It is found to be soluble 1g in 8 mL ethanol; 25 mL water (at 10°C); 1 L water (at 37°C) and approximately 1666 mL ether.

Uses

1. It is an antineoplastic substance that specifically inhibits DNA-dependent RNA-polymerase, recommended for use in **Wilm's tumour*; rhabdomyosarcoma**,** carcinoma of the testis and the uterus.
2. It is an essential component of the first-choice combinations for the control, management and treatment of **choriocarcinoma,*** embryonal rhabdomyosarcoma,** and **Wilm's tumour.**
3. It is still recommended for use against **Ewing's sarcoma,****** testicular carcinoma, and sarcoma botyroides (*i.e.*, resembling a bunch of grapes).
4. Dactinomycin appreciably potentiates radiotherapy (*i.e., radiation recall*).

---

  *   **Wilm's turmour**   A rapidly developing tumour of the kidney that usually occurs in children.
 **   **Rhabdomyosarcoma**   An extremely malignant neoplasm, originating in skeletal muscle.
***   **Choriocarcinoma**   An extremely rare, very malignant neoplasm, usually of the uterus but sometimes at the site of the ectopic pregnancy.
****   **Ewing's sarcoma**   A diffuse endothelial mycloma forming a fusiform swelling on a long bone.

5. It is found to be a secondary (efferent) immunosuppressive agents.
6. It has half-life approximately upto 36 hours.

Note: It must be handled with exceptional care, to prevent inhaling particles of it and exposing the skin to it.

D. Mitomycin C

Synonyms   MMC; Ametycine; Mitocin-C; Mutamycin.

Preparation   Mitomycin C is one of the three very intimately related entities isolated from the antibiotic complex produced by *Streptomyces caespitosus,* an organism from the Japanese soil.

Chemical Structure

Mitomycin C [$C_{15}H_{18}N_4O_5$]

Characteristic Features

1. It is obtained as blue-violet crystals or crystalline powder, that does not melt below 360°C.
2. It has uv$_{max}$ (methanol): 216, 360, 560 nm ($E_{1cm}^{1\%}$ 742, 742, 0.06).
3. **Solubility Profile:** It is found to be soluble in water, methanol, acetone, butyl acetate and cyelohexanone; slightly soluble in benzene, carbon tetrachloride, ether; and almost insoluble in petroleum ether.

Uses

1. It predominantly inhibits DNA synthesis by virtue of cross-linking double-stranded DNA through guanine and cytosine.
2. It is specifically recommended for the palliative treatment of **disseminated adenocarcinoma*** *of the stomach and the pancreas that have failed other treatment.*
3. It is an integral component of *second--line combinations* for the control, management and treatment of *cervical, gastric, pancreatic carcinomas,* and above all *non-small-cell bronchogenic carcinoma.*
4. It is usually introduced into the bladder in **papilloma.****
5. It is mostly employed as an *alternative drug* in the therapy of *head and neck* **squamous***** *cell carcinoma, bladder carcinoma,* and *osteogenic sarcoma.*

   Note: The active form of nitromycin C is produced metabolically *in situ* and evidently caters as an alkylating agent to suppress DNA synthesis categorically.

---

   * Adenocarcinoma   A malignant adenoma (*i.e.*, a neoplasm of glandular epithelium) arising from a glandular organ.
  ** Papilloma   A benign epithelial tumour.
*** Squamous   Scalelike.

FURTHER READING REFERENCES

1. Bambeke FV *et al.,* **Glycopeptide Antibiotics from Conventional Molecules to New Derivatives,** *Drugs,* **64:** 913-36, 2004.
2. Berdy, J. *et al.* (eds): **Handbook of Antibiotic Compounds,** Vols. 1-8, Boca Taton, FL, USA : CRC-Press, 1982.
3. Brakhage, A: *Biosynthesis of β-Lactam Compounds in Microorganisms.* **Comprehensive Natural Products Chemistry,** Vol. 4, Elsevier, Amsterdam, 1999.
4. Calam, C.T.: **Process Development in Antibiotic Fermentation.** Cambridge, UK: Cambridge University Press, 1987.
5. Cavalleri, B. and Parenti F: Antibiotics [glycopeptides (Dalbaheptides)]. **Kirk-Othmer Encyclopedia of Chemical Technology,** 4th edn., Vol. 2. Wiley, New York, 1992.
6. Coute JE: **Manual of Antibiotics and Infections Diseases,** 8th ed., Williams & Wilkins, Baltimore, 1995.
7. Croom KF and Goa KL: **Levofloxacin—A Review of its use in the Treatment of Bacterial Infections in the United States,** *Drugs,* **63:** 2769-802, 2003.
8. Davies, J.E.: Aminoglycoside-aminocyclitol Antibiotics and Their Modifying Enzymes. In: Loraian, V., ed. **Antibiotics in Laboratory Medicine,** 3rd ed. Baltimore, Williams &-Wilkins, 1991.
9. Fenton C, Keating CM, and Curran MP: **Daptomycin,** *Drugs, 64:* 445-55, 2004.
10. Hughes, M.A.: **Biosynthesis and Degradation of Cyanogenic Glycosides. Comprehensive Natural Products Chemistry,** Vol. 1, Elsevier, Amsterdam, 1999.
11. Jawetz *et al.,* **Medical Microbiology,** 20th ed., Appleton & Lange, Norwalk CT, 1995.
12. Kwon-Chung, KJ and JE Benett: **Medical Mycology,** Lea & Fabiger, Philadelphia, 1992.
13. Kucers A., Bennett, N. McK, and Kemp R.J. Eds.: **The Use of Antibiotics,** J.B. Lippineott, Philadelphia, 1987.
14. Lancini *et al.,* **Antibiotics: an Interdisciplinary Approach,** Plenum Press, New York, 3rd edn., 1995.
15. Luengo JM: Enzymatic Synthesis of Penicillins, **Comprehensive Natural Products Chemistry,** Vol. 4. Elsevier, Amsterdam, 1999.
16. Mandell GL, Bennett JE, and Dolin R, **Mandell, Douglas, and Benett's Principles and Practice of Infectious Diseases,** 4th ed, Churchill Livingstone, Inc., New York, 1995.
17. Page MI (ed.): **The Chemistry of β-Lactams,** Chapman & Hall, New York, 1992.
18. Sutcliffe J and NH Georgopapdakou, Eds.: **Emerging Targets in Antibacterial and Antifungal Chemotherapy,** Chapman and Hall, New York, 1992.
19. Vanden HB, DWR Mackenzie, G. Cauwenbergh, JV Custem, E Drouket, and B Dupont Eds.: **Mycoses in AIDS Patients,** Plenum Press, New York, 1990.
20. Wellington K and Noble S: **Telithromycin,** *Drugs,* **64:** 1683-94, 2004.
21. Wise EM: Antibiotics (Peptides). **Kirk-Othmer Encylopedia of Chemical Technology,** 4th edn. Vol. 3., Wiley, New York, 1992.

10 Drug Molecules of Marine Organisms

- Introduction
- Classification of Drug Molecules
- Marine Natural Products: An Upgradation Profile
- Summary
- Further Reading, References

10.1 INTRODUCTION

The phrase **'drug molecules'** has been appropriately and judiciously employed in line with the classical concept, that is a specific chemical entity which essentially possesses a marked and pronounced phamacological activity emphatically on the mammalian organism. In fact, it is the dedicated and concerted efforts of expert researchers from various specialized scientific fields that a new drug molecule is isolated, characterized and subsequently subjected to a rigorous preclinical and successful clinical studies and ultimately baptized as a therapeutically effective and potent **'drug'**.

Interestingly, innumerable products derived from the marine organisms in several **'crude forms'** have been widely used across the globe by the traditional practitioners for thousands of years. However, scientific as well as logical approach to such marine organisms could materialize only during the last five decades or so. Krebs* and Faulkner** gave the most comprehensive and excellent reviews on the chemistry of thousands of compounds obtained exclusively from the marine organisms during the eighties.

Kaul and Daftari*** presented the latest review on pharmacology of chemically well-defined molecules belonging to marine organisms. In the light of the ever mounting evidences pieced together over the recent past it has more or less strengthened the belief and hypothesis that there exists not only an ample hidden treasure but also a tremendous scope for the emergence of newer drug molecules from the marine environment to combat the human sufferings.

Marine toxins were reported to possess an extremely high potency with regard to their pharmacological actions, and, therefore, sometimes collectively referred to as *'toxins'*. The doctrine and philosophy of *Paracelsus* advocating that 'the clinical efficacy and usefulness of an active principle is nothing but a matter of the right dose administered by the right route' carries a lot of

---

* Krebs, M.C., *Fortschr. Chem. Organ, Naturstoffe,* **48**, 151 (1986).
** Faulkner, D.J., *Nat. Prod. Rep.* I. 251 and 551 (1984): 3.1 (1986): **4**, 539 (1986).
*** Kaul, P.N., and Daftari, P., *Ann. Rev. Pharmacol. Toxicol.* **26**,117 (1986).

value and impact. Nevertheless, the joint efforts by phytochemists and medical scientists may pave the way to assess the plethora of the currently labeled '*marine toxins*' for their usefulness as *drugs* and or as physiological tools that may ultimately decode the mechanisms responsible for various cellular processes solely characteristic of life but unfortunately not revealed as on date.

It is indeed a very critical as well as a crucial turning point when phytochemists, medicinal chemists and pharmacologists will put their knowledge, wisdom, expertise, skill and resources together to unravel the wealth of drugs beneath the sea as they already had accomplished toward the terrestrial plants almost a century ago; and towards soil, samples nearly half-a-century ago for 'antibiotics' when penicillin was discovered by Alexander Fleming.

The present chapter exclusively focuses upon a good complication of certain vital and important 'marine biological' (marine organisms) having established chemical structures and proven pharmacological activities. So far, more than five lakh species of marine organisms have been well-documented both from the ocean and sea across the globe.

Interestingly, quite a sizable number of such marine organisms do possess a wide-spectrum of biological activities, namely: antibiotics, antiviral, antineoplastic, cytotoxic, antimicrobial, antiinflammatory, enzyme inhibitors, prostaglandins, neurophysiological and cardiovascular agents.

10.2   CLASSIFICATION OF DRUG MOLECULES OF MARINE ORGANISMS

The enormous quantum of newer and potent drug molecules derived from the wide spectrum of marine organisms across the world may be judiciously and logically classified based on their specific pharmacologic actions as stated below:

   (*i*) Cytotoxic/Antineoplastic Agents
  (*ii*) Cardiovascular active drugs
 (*iii*) Marine Toxins
 (*iv*) Antimicrobial drugs
   (*v*) Antibiotic substances.
 (*vi*) Antiinflammatory and Antispasmodic Agents
(*vii*) Miscellaneous pharmacologically active substances.

The above mentioned broad classification of marine organisms shall be dealt with at length individually in the sections that follows:

10.2.1 Cytotoxic/Antineoplastic Agents

The two prominent US-based research institutes, namely: US **National Cancer Institute (NCI)** and US **National Sea Grant Office (NSGO)** have discovered thousands of pure and semi-pure compounds derived from the marine origin that distinctly exhibited antineoplastic/cytotoxic activities in a good number of cell lines; besides, *in vivo* actions against both malignant tumours and leukemias in various animal models. In the present context certain duly characterized drug molecules displaying known and potent activities shall be discussed, namely:

(*a*) Cembranes,
(*b*) Macrolides,

(*c*) Depipeptides, and

(*d*) Miscellaneous compounds.

10.2.1.1 Cembranes

Cembranoids, are the 14-membered cyclic diterpenes obtained from a wide variety of soft corals. A good number of cembranoids have been isolated and characterized. It has been observed that most of these compounds do contain an *exocyclic lactone* as their integral part.

A few typical examples of naturally occurring *cembranes* are, namely: sinularin, crassin acetate, cytarabine (Ara-C), fludarabine and aplysistatin. These compounds shall now be discussed individually in the sections that follows:

A. Sinularin

Chemical Structure

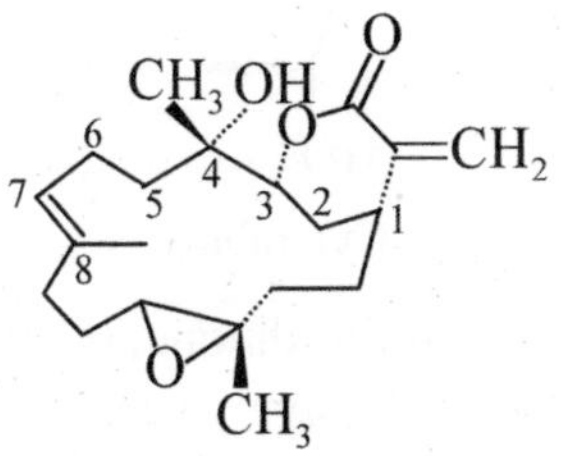

Sinularin

Biological Source   Sinularin and its dihydro congener are obtained from *Sinularia flexibilis.*

Uses   It possesses anticancer activities.

B. Crassin Acetate

Chemical Structure

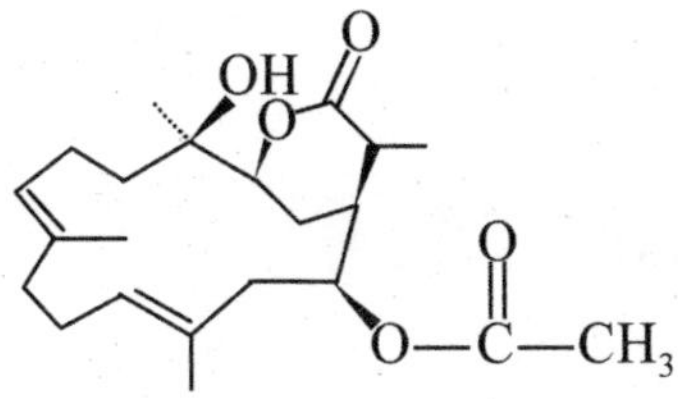

Crassin Acetate

Biological Source   It is obtained from the **Caribbean gorgonian** *Pseudoplexaura porosa.*

Uses   **Crassin acetate** was observed to be comparatively inert to the mammalian systems but on the contrary found to be extremely cytotoxic to human leukemic as well as Hella cells *in vitro* and also to the mouse fibroblasts.

Note: (*a*) The aforesaid activity is almost lost as soon as the exocyclic lactone portion of the compound undergoes cessation (*i.e.*, cleavage) by titration with NaOH.

(*b*) Moreover, the conversion of 'acetate' to 'hydroxyl' via hydrolysis may render this compound more water soluble and useful only if the 'lactone moiety' is kept intact.

C. Cytarabine

Synonyms Ara-C; Alexan; Arabitin; Aracytine; Cytarbel; Cytosar; Erpalfa; Iretin; Udicil; U-19920; CHX-3311; Aracytidine; β-Citosine Arabinoside.

Chemical Structure

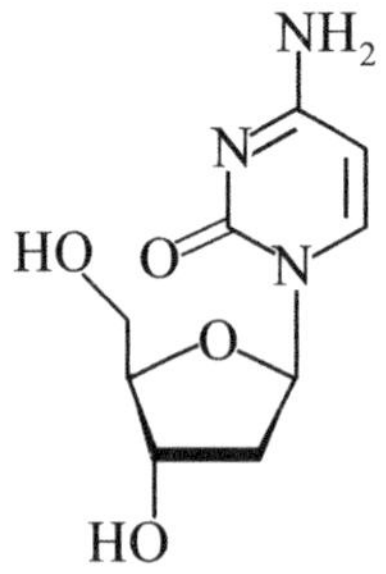

Cytarabine

4-Amino-1-β-D-arabinofuranosyl-2(1H)-pyrimidinone; ($C_9H_{13}N_3O_5$).

Cytarabine is a synthetic compound exclusively based on the knowledge of naturally occurring moieties found to be present in the **'Caribean Sponges'** *e.g.*, **spongosine,** and **spongouridine.**

It may be synthesised* by the acetylation of **uracil arabinoside** followed by treatment with phosphorus pentasulphide (P_2S_5) and subsequent heating with ammonia as given below:

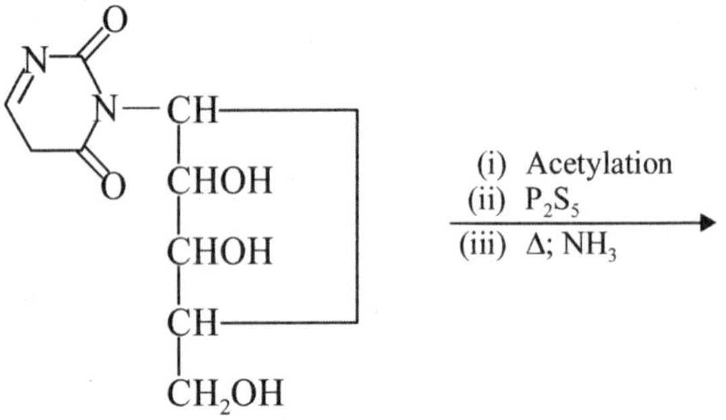

(i)	Acetylation	
(ii)	P_2S_5	→ Cytarabine
(iii)	Δ; NH_3	

Uracil Arabinoside

Characteristic Features

1. It is obtained as prisms from ethanol (50% v/v) having mp 212-213°C.
2. Its specific optical rotation $[\alpha]_D^{23} + 158°$; $[\alpha]_D^{24} + 153°$ (C = 0.5 in water).
3. It has uv$_{max}$ at pH 2 : 281.0, 212.5 nm (ε 13171, 10230); and at pH 12 : 272.5 nm (ε 9259).

Uses

1. It is indicated in both adult and childhood leukemia.

---

* Kar, A.: **Medicinal Chemistry,** New Aage International, New Delhi, 4th, edn., 491, 2006.

2. It is found to be specifically useful in acute granulocytic leukemia, and is more effective when combined with thioguanine and daunorubacine.

3. It is a potent antineoplastic and antiviral agent.

4. It is also employed in the treatment of acute myclogenous leukemia and human acute leukemia.

D. Fludarabine

Synonyms   2-Fluorovidarabine; 2F-Ara A.

Chemical Structure

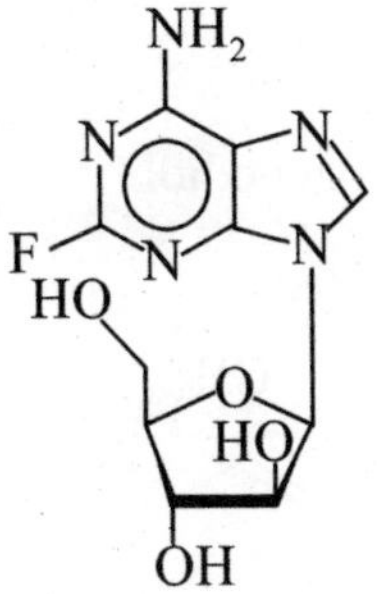

Fludarabine

2-Fluorovidarabine; ($C_{10}H_{12}FN_5O_4$).

Characteristic Features

1. It is obtained as crystals from ethanol and water having mp 260°C.

2. Its specific optical rotation is $[\alpha]_D^{25} + 17 \pm 2.5°$ (C = 0.1 in ethanol).

3. It has uv_{max} (pH1, pH7, pH13): 262, 261, 262 nm ($\varepsilon \times 10^{-3}$ 13.2, 14.8. 15.0).

4. It is sparingly soluble in water and organic solvents.

Uses   It is used as a antineoplastic agent.

E. Aplysistatin

Chemical Structure

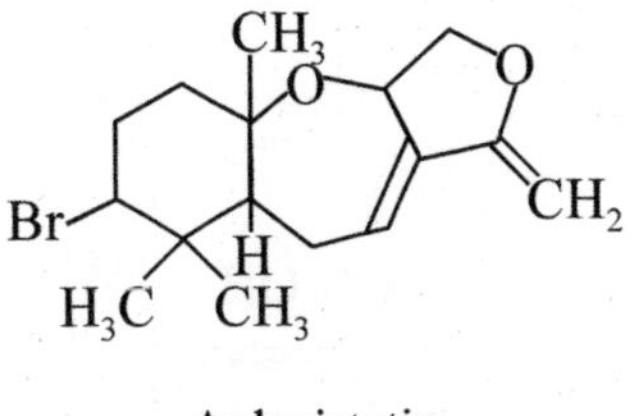

Aplysistatin

Biological Source   **Aplysistatin** is obtained from *Aplysia angasi* (Sea Hare).

Uses   It is used as an antineoplastic agent.

Interestingly, certain **cembranoids** were observed to deciliate protozoa even at a 5 ppm level*

---

* Rerkins, D.L., and Ciereszko, L.S.,: *Hydrobiologia*, **42**, 77 (1973).

thereby implying that perhaps quite a few compounds belonging to this category or their feasible structural analogues might also exhibit either spermicidal and/or parasiticidal properties. It is, however, pertinent to state here that these drug molecules derived from the marine origin obviously require both intensive and extensive preclinical studies by virtue of the fact that most of them are virtually inert to the mammalian systems.*

Non-Lactonic Cembranoid　　There are certain compounds which do not contain a lactone moiety but they do possess cytotoxic actions. A few such examples of **non-lactonic combranoid** are, namely: geranylhydroquinone and asperidol. These *two* drugs are described as under:

A. Geranylhydroquinone

Synonyms　　Geroquinol; Geranyl-1, 4-benzenediol.

Chemical Structure

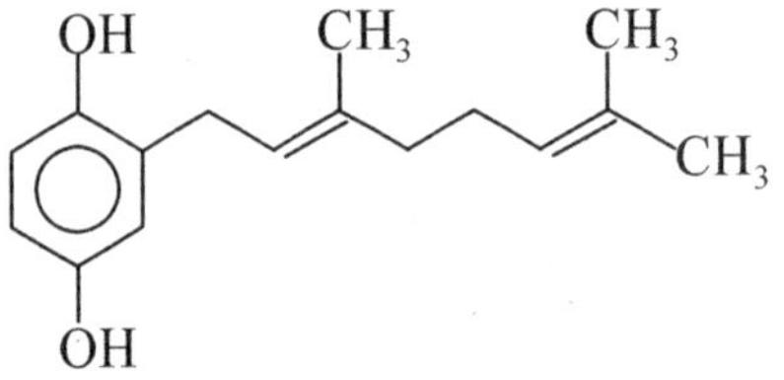

Geranylhydroquinone

trans-(3, 7-Dimethyl-2, 6-octadien-yl)-hydroquinone; ($C_{16}H_{22}O_2$).

Biological Sources　　Geranylhydroquinone is obtained from the chloroform extract of *Aplidium species.*

Characteristic Features　　It is usually obtained as colourless needles from n-hexane/ethyl acetate having mp 61–62°C.

Uses
1. It is found to be cytotoxic to leukemia and mammary carcinoma.
2. It is employed as a radioprotective agent.

B. Asperidol

Chemical Structure

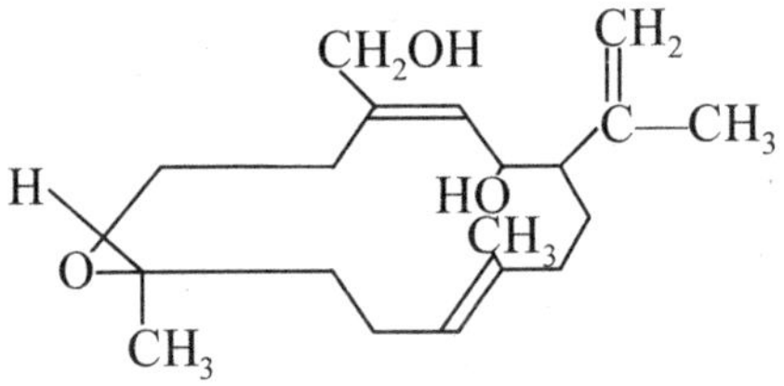

Asperidol

---

* Kobayashi, Y., and Osabe, K.: *Chem. Pham. Bull.* **37**, 631, (1989).

Biological Source   It is obtained from the *gorgonian* coral.

Use   It exhibits cytotoxic activities.

10.2.2 Cardiovascular Active Drugs

During the past three decades a huge number of extracts, fractions and pure isolates from thousands of **marine organisms** were subjected to thorough cardiovascular screening in various research laboratories around the world. Interestingly, most of these compounds did exhibit **cardiovascular activities** perhaps as frequently as observed antibiotic and antineoplastic activities. Unfortunately, as on date hardly any compound could surface out and obtain the FDA approval as a potential drug.

The cardiovascular active drugs may be broadly classified under the following *two* categories, namely:

(*a*) Cardiotonics, and
(*b*) Hypotensive compounds.

These *two* categories shall now be treated separately as under:

10.2.2.1 Cardiotonics

The **cardiotonic compounds** (or **cardiotonics**) showing positive response in either *in vivo* and/or *in vitro* inotropic activities on whole or part of the heart are included in this section.

In general, the **cardiotonics** may be further sub-divided into *two* groups, namely:

(*i*) Marine peptides, and
(*ii*) Marine glycosides

10.2.2.1.1 Marine Peptides   The age-old belief and classical concept that the steroidal nucleus present in the aglycone residues of either **digitalis** or **strophanthus** could only exhibit cardiotonicity was virtually turned down when '**marine peptides**', obtained from *coclenterates*, such as: *Anthopleura xanthogrammica* producing **anthopleurins A, B and C*** (also known as **AP-A, B, C**); and *Anthopleura elegantissima* giving **AP-C.**

Out of these *three* anthopleurins, only **AP-A** has been reported to be showing the most promising cardiotonic activity both on the isolated and *in situ* heart of different species. **AP-A** has a positive edge over the known **cardiac glycosides** because of its unique ability to afford a sustained significant initropic effect under the ischemic conditions. Gross *et al.*** advocated strongly that perhaps AP-A could prove to be extremely beneficial especially in patients having a concomitant β-odrenergic blockade.

Furthermore, the **anemonia toxin II** (also termed as: **Cardiotoxin-II, ATX-II**) isolated from *Anemonia sulcata* (**Sea Anemone**) comprising of at least 47 amino acids demonstrated a very close resemblance to **AP-A.***** Besides, ATX-II was shown to exhibit a significant dose-dependent cardiotonic activities in different mammalian heart experiments.

---

* Norton *et al. J. Pharm. Sci.,* **65,** 1368, (1976).
** Gross *et al. Eur. J. Pharmacol.* **110,** 271 (1985).
*** Kaul, P.N. and Dabtari, P.; *Ann. Rev. Pharmacol. Toxicol.* **26,** 117, (1986).

The cardinal points of difference between **AP-A** and **ATX-II** peptides are as follows:

S. No.	Anthopleurin-A (AP-A)	Anemonia Toxin-II (ATX-II)
1	Alanine is present at the residue 38	Lysine is present at the residue 38.
2	No similar studies as for ATX-II were carried out.	Modification of the acidic-COOH function at the 38 residue leads to absolute inactivation of cardiotonic potency.*
3	If administered systemically gives an immune response; and when given orally loses its activity due to gastric juice (acidic) in stomach.	No such effect has been observed.

Likewise, the two compounds *viz.*, **AP-A** and **ATX-II,** display a number of similarities, namely: (*a*) conformation of the two peptides are almost identical; (*b*) amino-acid sequence similar; (*c*) disulphide bridges are alike; and (*d*) they have the same basicity. Based on these striking points of similarities one may rightly justify the very identical profiles of **cardiotonic activity** of the said two peptides.

A host of other compounds showing **cardiotonic activities** belonging to the class of '**marine peptides**' are, namely: **laminin, octopamine, saxitoxin** and **autonomium chloride.**

These compounds shall now be treated individually in the sections that follow:

A. Laminin

Chemical Structure

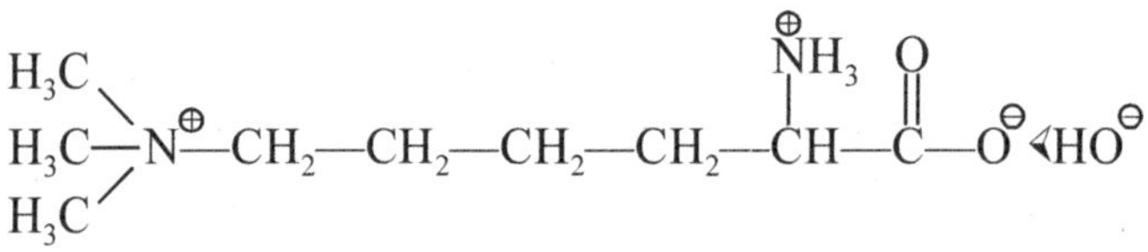

Laminin

Biological Source **Laminin** is obtained from a marine algae *Laminaria angustata.*

Characteristic Features
1. It is the abundant structural component of the basal lamina.
2. It is critical to the stability of the extracellular matrix and to the adhesion of cells to the basement membrane.
3. It belongs to the family of **heterotrimeric glycoproteins** composed of a heavy chain, designated as α (also known as A) and 2 light chains, designated as β (B1) and γ (B2), which are linked by disulphide bonds to form an asymetrical cross-shaped structure.
4. Eight genetically distinct laminin subunits have been identified, namely: $\alpha_1, \alpha_2, \alpha_3, \beta_1, \beta_2, \beta_3, \gamma_1$ and γ_2.

Uses
1. It shows hypotensive effect.
2. It also exhibits diverse biological activities.

---

* Barhanin *et. el. Toxicon.* **20**. 59 (1982).

B. Octopamine

Chemical Structure

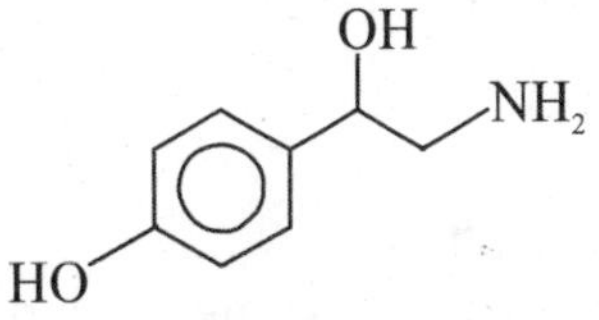

Octopamine

Biological Sources **Octopamine** is found in the salivary glands of *Octopus vulgaris, Octopus macropus* and of *Eledone moschata.*

Characteristic Features D(−)-From:

1. It is obtained as crystals from hot water that gets changed at about 160° to a compound which melts above 250° (decomposes).
2. Its specific optical rotation $[\alpha]_D^{25} - 56.0°$ (0.1 N.HCl); and $- 37.4°$ (water).

DL (±)-Octopamine Hydrochloride ($C_8H_{11}NO_2$.HCl) (Epirenor, Norden, Norfen): It is obtained as crystals which gets decomposed at 170°C. It is freely soluble in water.

Uses
1. The natural D(−) form is almost 3 times more potent than the L(+) from in producing cardiovascular adrenergic responses in anaesthetized dogs and cats.
2. It gives distinct adrenergic responses.
3. In invertebrate nervous systems **octopamine** may function as a neurotransmitter.

C. Saxitoxin

Synonyms Mussel poison; Clam poison; Paralytic shellfish poison; Gonyoulax toxin; STX.

Chemical Structure $[C_{10}H_{17}N_7O_4]^{2+}$

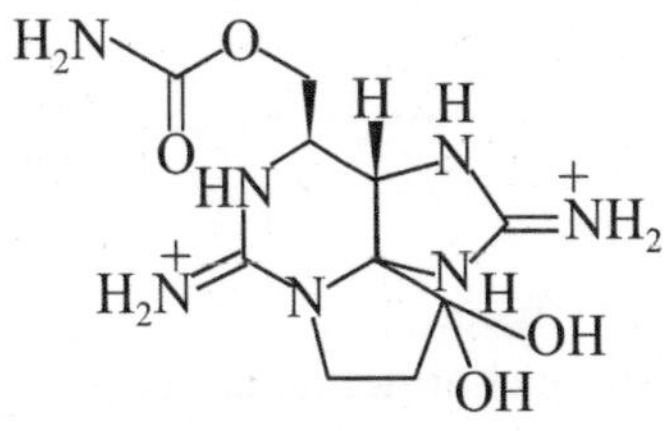

Saxitoxin

Biological Sources **Saxitoxin** is the powerful neurotoxin produced by the dinoflagellates *Gonyaulax catenella* or *G. tamarensis,* the consumption of which causes the California sea mussel *Mytilus californianus,* the Alaskan butterclam *Saxidomus gigantens* and the scallop to become poisonous.*

---

* Ghazarossian *et al. Bichem. Biophys. Res. Commun.,* **59**, 1219 (1974) Sehantz *et al., Can. J. Chem.* **39**, 2117 (1961)

Isolation   **Saxitoxin** may be isolated by the method suggested by Schantz et al.*

Characteristic Features

Saxitoxin Dihydrochloride $[(C_{10}H_{17}N_7O_4)^{2+} . 2HCl]$:

1. It is obtained as a white hygroscopic solid.
2. It has pKa in water: 8:24, 11.60.
3. Its specific optical rotation $[\alpha]_D^{25} + 130°$.
4. It is extremely soluble in water, methanol; sparingly soluble in ethanol, glacial acetic acid; and practically insoluble in lipid solvents.
5. It is found to be fairly stable in acid solutions; and decomposes rapidly in an alkaline media.
6. On boiling for 3 to 4 hours at pH 3 usually causes loss of activity.

Uses

1. It exhibits a hypotensive effect.
2. It is invariably employed as a tool in the neurochemical research.

D. Autonomium Chloride

Chemical Structure

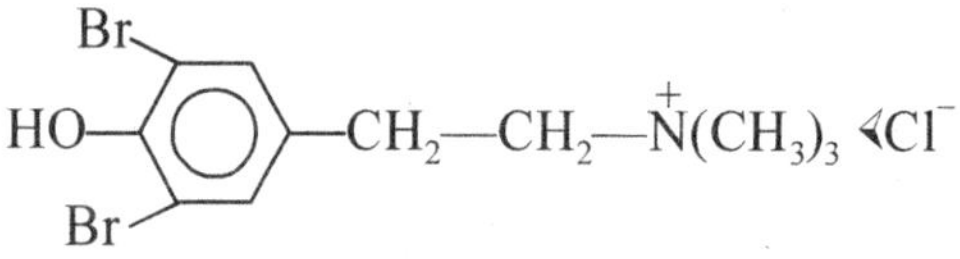

Autonomium Chloride

Biological Source   It is found in *Verongia fistularis.*

Characteristic Features   **Autonomium chloride** possesses an isosteric structure of **adrenaline** and **acetylcholine** as given below:

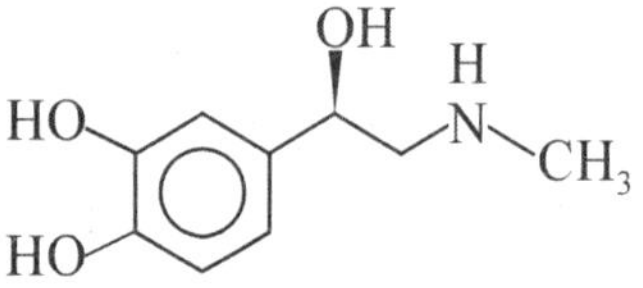

Adrenaline 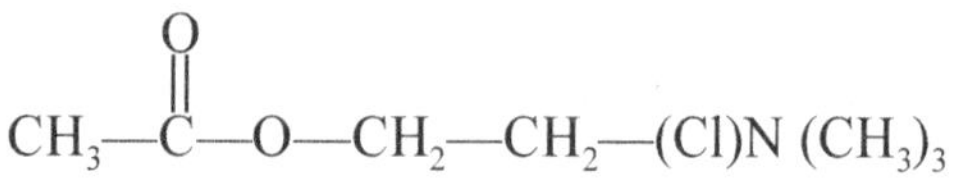   Acetylcholine

Uses

1. It exerts both α- and β-adrenergic effects.
2. **Autonomium chloride** also exhibits cholinergic action.
3. It distinctly shows CNS stimulant activity in *mice* which action is evidently exhibited by an apparent substantial increase in the spontaneous motor activity (SMA).
4. By virtue of the unique dual effects of adrenergic and cholinergic it may prove to be an asset in the control, management and regulation of the behaviour of heart *i.e.*, **cardiotonic effect.**

---

* Schantz *et al. J. Am. Chem. Soc.*, **79**, 5230 (1957).

In addition to the above cited examples of the marine peptides, there are quite a few polypeptides which have been isolated and characterized from a wide spectrum of sea anemones. A few such typical examples are given as under:

S. No.	Biological Source	Compound	Uses
1	Actinia equina	A polypeptide with 147 amino acids	Exhibits bradycardia, rapid hypotension, and respiratory arrest in the rat.
2	Condylactis gigantea	A polypetide with 195 amino acid residue	Exerts a haemolytic action in rabbits.
3	Parasicyonis action stoloides	A poptide with very less number of amino acids	Shows a neurotoxic action.

10.2.2.1.2 Marine Glycosides The **marine glycosides,** in general, are of two types, *viz.*, nonsulphated and sulphated ones. However, **holothurins** and **astrosaponins** are *two* typical examples of **marine glycosides** that generally display cardiotoxic activity having an unusual narrow margin between the effective dose (*i.e.*, ED_{50}) and the lethal dose (*i.e.*, LD_{50}).

Holothurins: These are the aglyconic residues obtained from the family *Holothuroidae* of phylum *Echinodermata* and essentially possess a **steroidal moiety** that very much resemble to the aglycones of the **digitalis glycosides.** In the recent past a large number of the 'hydroxylated steroidal glycosides' have been isolated and characterized from the **holothuroids,** also known as the sea **cucumbers.**

Astrosaponins: These are the **marine glycosides** obtained from the star fishes belonging to the family *Asteroidae.*

In fact, both these **marine glycosides** (*i.e.*, sulphated and non-sulphated) inhibit Na^+, K^+, Mg^{2+} and ATPases, but the holothurins are reported to be far more active on the Na^+, K^+ and ATPase.*

Interestingly, the **astrosaponins** are found to exert an altogether different type of pharmacological actions, such as: antiinflammatory, analgesic, haemolytic, hypotensive; besides having the cytolytic activity on account of its interference in neuromuscular blocking effects and the protein metabolism.

However, the **holothurins** are found to exert both **cardiotonic** and **ichthyotoxic actions.** Besides, they also exhibit haemolytic activity.

Eledoisin: [$C_{54}H_{85}N_{13}O_{15}S$]

Chemical Structure 5-oxoPro-Pro-Ser-Lys-Asp-Ala-Phe-Ile-Gly-Leu-MethNH$_2$.

Biological Source Eldoisin is obtained from the posterior salivary glands of eledone spp. (small octopus spp.) *Eledone moschata.***

Characteristic Features
1. **Eledoisin** is obtained as a sesquihydrate powder that gets decomposed at 230°C.
2. Its specific optical rotation $[\alpha]_D^{22} - 44°$ (C = 1 in 95% acetic acid).
3. It is found to lose its activity gradually when incubated in blood.

Uses
1. Its physiologic action resembles that of the other **tachykinins, substance P** and **physalaemin.**
2. It is found to stimulate extravascular smooth muscle.

   * Gorshkov *et al. Toxicon*, **20**, 655 (1982).
  ** Anastasi, Erspamer, *Brit. J. Pharmacol.*, **19**, 326, (1962); *eidem. Experientia*, **18**, 58, (1962).

3. Eledoisin acts as a potent vasodilator and hypotensive agent.
4. It causes salivation, and enhances capillary permeability in certain specific species.
5. It also stimulates lacrimal secretion.

10.2.2.2 Hypotensive Compounds

There are quite a few potent hypotensive compounds that have been derived from a variety of **marine organisms.** These newer range of medicinally active chemical entities may be categorized into *two* groups, namely:

  (*i*) Marine nucleosides, and
  (*ii*) Hypotensive peptides and other compounds.

  The various **'marine biomedicines'** belonging to each of these *two* categories shall now be discussed as under:

10.2.2.2.1 Marine Nucleosides   **Nucleosides** are formed by the combination of a purine or pyrimidine base in glycosidic linkage with a sugar moiety, such as: adenosine, thymidine etc.; whereas, the *'phosphate ester'* of a nucleoside is known as *nucleotide e.g.,* 5'-guanylic acid; 3'-cytidylic acid.

  In the past two-and-a-half decade a plethora of **marine nucleosides** have been isolated and characterized, and also evaluated for their therapeutic efficacy.

  Cryptotethia crytpa, the well-known **Caribbean sponge** made a spectacular success in the history of marine biomedicine that indeed produced a very rare and unique arabinosylnucleoside which resulted on slightest structural manufestation the wonderful drug of choice used for antileukemic treatment cytarabine or Ara-C (see section 10.2.1.1)*. A good number other nucleosides have been derived from *C. crypta* that showed varying interests. However, *spongosine,* being one such a drug that gained meaningful legitimate recognition because of its highly potential hypotensive activities. *Doridosine,* is another most promising and potent hypotensive nucleoside reported.** These *two* compounds shall now be discussed as under:

A. Spongosine   It is a **nucleoside** and the methoxy derivative of **adenosine.**

Chemical Structure

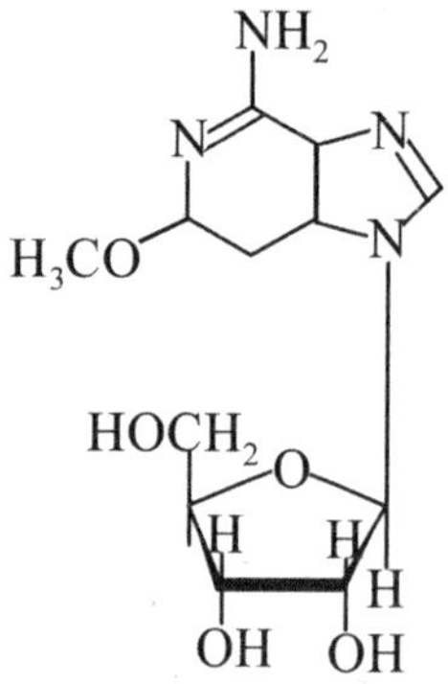

Spongosine

---

  * Cohen, S.S.: *Cancer,* **40,** 509 (1977).
 ** F.A. Fuhrman *et al. Science,* **207,** 193, (1980).

Biological Source   It is obtained from the **Caribbean sponge** *Cryptotethia crypta* and with a minor structural modification of the parent isolated nucleoside known as **arabinosylnucleoside.**

Uses

1. It exhibits various coronary effects resembling to those of **adenosine,** for instance: coronary vasodilation and negative inotropy.
2. It is found to exert more marked and pronounced long-acting effects.
3. It acts as a hypotensive at such as dose level at which **adenosine** is observed to be absolutely inactive.
4. It reduces the rate as well as the force of contraction of heart.

B. Doridosine

Chemical Structure

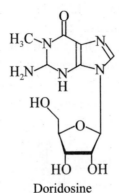

Doridosine

(N′-Methylisoguanosine)

Biological Source   It is obtained from the nudibranch *Anisodoris nobilis*:

Characteristic Features

1. It has been revealed on the basis of the kinetics of the enzymatic degradation of these nucleosides that **doridosine** is not only the most active but also the long-lasting nucleoside.
2. **Doridosine** does not undergo oxidative deamination *in vitro* on being subjected to incubation in the presence of **adenosine deaminase,** while **adenosine** disappears very fast. Perhaps the intensity and the duration of the cardiovascular effects of doridosine is directly related to its half-life *in vivo*.

    Note: The intermediate acting, spongosine happens to disappear in a gradual manner.

Uses

1. It is the most potent hypotensive marine nucleoside known so far.
2. It also exerts hypothermic effect *i.e.*, it lowers the normal temperature of the body.

Hypothermic Effect   Interestingly, both **spongosine** and **doridosine,** when administered *intracerebroventricularly* to guinea pigs, they lower the body temperature by several degrees for a duration ranging between 4-7 hours.* However, this hypothermic effect seems to have no bearing to their prevailing systemic actions.

5′-Deoxy-5-iodobericidin: It is also a **nucleoside** which has been observed to lower the body temperature of mice**. It has been isolated from *Hypnea valentiae* (Red Algae). Perhaps this is the first and foremost compound which possesses the following *two* specific criteria, namely:

(*a*) First iodinated nucleoside discovered, and

(*b*) First 5′-deoxyribosyl nucleoside discovered in nature.

Uses

1. It may prove to be a vital biochemical research tool of immense interest.
2. It is found to be a potent inhibitor of **adenosine kinase.**

10.2.2.2.2 Hypotensive Peptides and Other Compounds A number of peptides have been isolated from the **marine organisms** that exclusively showed distinct and significant hypotensive activities in experimental laboratory animals.

There are certain typical examples, such as: **aaptamine, hymenin** and **uro-tensins I and II,** which shall now be discussed briefly in the sections that follows:

A. Aaptamine

Chemical Structure

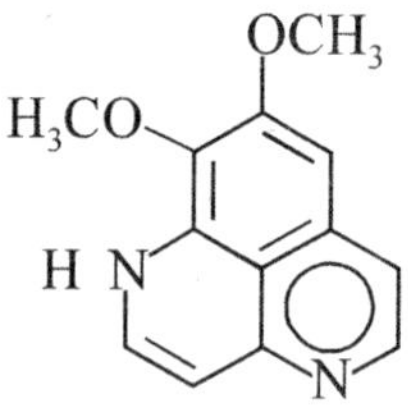

Aaptamine

Biological Source Aaptamine is obtained from *Aaptos aaptos.*

Characteristic Features It has an inherent interesting heterocyclic nucleus besides its structural characteristic and molecular size which may render this molecule a good candidate drug for future intensive as well as extensive pharmacological studies provided it should exhibit a bare minimum level of toxicity.

Uses

1. It has an α-adrenergic blocking effect.
2. In case, it does not undergo a rapid metabolism in mammalian species *in situ,* it may prove to cause a hypotensive effect.

---

* Kaul, P.N.,: *Pure Apl. Chem.,* **54**, 1963 (1982).
** L.P. Davis *et al.: Biochem. Pharmacol.* **33**, 347, (1984).

B. Hymenin

Chemical Structure

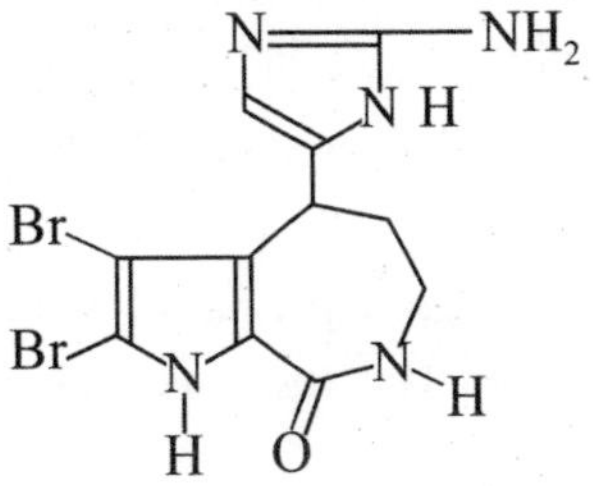

Hymenin

Biological Source **Hymenin** is obtained from *Hymeniacidon aldis*.

Its characteristic features and uses are very much similar to those of aaptamine.

C. Urotensins I and II (U I, U II)

Biological Sources **Urotensins I and II** are obtained from the specific caudal neurosecretory system of *Giltichthys miralilis* (**Telecost**); and also from *Catostomus commersoni*–a fish.

Characteristic Features Both U I and U II are naturally occurring **poly-peptides** which distinctly possess appreciable hypotensive activity as evidently shown in rat, dog, sheep and squirrel monkey.

Uses
1. These **polypeptides** exhibit hypotensive effect that seems to be on account of their vasodilatory action.
2. Nevertheless, the discoverers of these two vasoactive peptides (Laderis and McCannell) proposed that they may possibly prove to be clinically potential drugs, but till date no evidence for their clinical efficacy has yet been reported.

10.2.3 **Marine Toxins**

A host of **marine biotoxins** have been obtained from a wide variety of **marine organisms** in their crude, semipure and other forms between 1960-1970. However, during the eighties a good number of them possessing venomous and toxic properties and having most complex chemical structures have been isolated, characterized with the advent of rather exceedingly sophisticated analytical instruments and a concerted effort of dedicated marine chemists and pharmacologists across the globe.

The **marine toxins** are caused due to either the **external metabolites** (**ectocrine**) or the **endotoxins**.* The endotoxins are found to be the most potent substances.

The **marine toxins** may be classified appropriately under the following categories, namely:

(*a*) Palytoxin,
(*b*) Red-Tide toxins
(*c*) Ciguatera toxins.

---

* **Endotoxin**—A lipopolysaccharide that is part of the cell wall of Gram Negative bacteria.

The aforesaid varieties of toxins shall now be discussed in the sections that follows:

10.2.3.1 Palytoxin

Palytoxin (PTX) was initially reported from the Pacific ocean by Moore and Scheuer* in 1971; and in 1974 by Attaway and Ciereszko** from the Carribean island; incidentally poles apart by two research teams almost at the same-time-span.

Biological Source   It is obtained from **zanathid coral** of the genus *Polythoa* found abundantly both in the Pacific and the Carribean oceans. **It is the most poisonous non-proteinaceous compound known.**

Chemical Structure

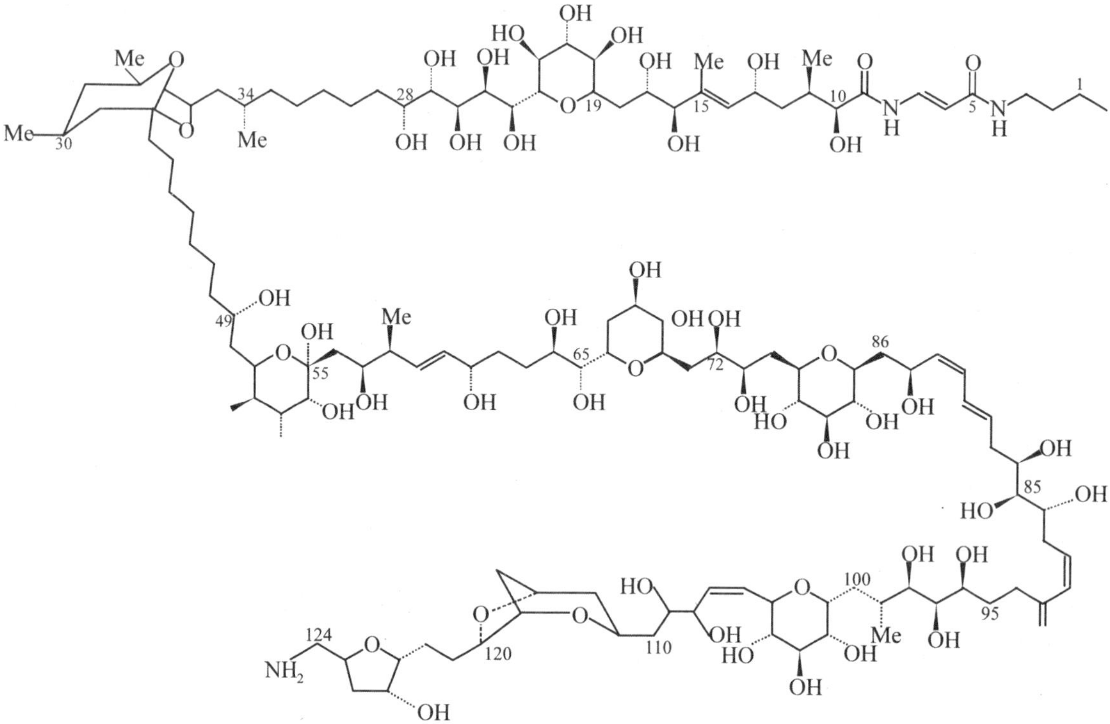

PALYTOXIN
[Polytoxin (C51-55) Hemiacetal]

Polytoxin is regarded as one of the most interesting chemical entity isolated and characterized from a marine organism which is found to be linear, polycyclic, and polyether molecule having molecular formula $C_{129} H_{223} N_3 O_{54}$. Perhaps PTX is the largest **non-peptide marine biotoxin** known till date.

---

* Moore, R.E., and P.J. Schever: *Science,* **172**, 495 (1971).
** Attaway, D.H. and Ciereszko, L.S: *Proc. Soc. Int. Coral Reef Sym.* **7**, 497, (1974).

Characteristic Features

1. **Palytoxin** is a white amorphous hygroscopic solid powder.
2. It does not have any definite mp, but gets charred when heated to 330°C.
3. It has specific optical rotation $[\alpha]_D^{25} + 26°$ (water).
4. It is insoluble in ether, chloroform, acetone; sparingly soluble in methanol, ethanol; and fairly soluble in DMSO, water and pyridine.

Uses

1. It is the most potent coronary vasoconstrictor.
2. It is a versatile physiological tool to evaluate anti-anginal chemotherapeutic agents.
3. Based on the evidence that Na+ – K+ exchange is almost instantaneous and massive in cells following exposure to PTX, it may be inferred beyond any reasonable doubt that it exclusively acts by affecting the Na^+, K^+-AT Pase.*

10.2.3.2 Red Tide Toxins

Starr** (1958) was pioneer in reporting the red tide toxin from the Gulf of Mexico. In fact, the terminology **'red tide'** became known from the very existence of the red coloured *peridinin,* a carotenoid natural pigment, obtained from the periodical blooming of the **dinoflagellates,** thereby imparting to the water a brown to red colouration.

Interestingly, there are only *three* will-known biological species which exclusively produce toxins, namely: (*a*) *Ptychodiscus brevis* [earlier called *Gymnodinium breve*]; (*b*) *Protogonyaulax catenella* [earlier known as *Gaunyaulax catenella*]; and *Protogonyaulax tamarensis*. Because, these organisms possess a mutually beneficial association with the **shell fishes,** the toxins generated by the former get duly accumulated in the latter; and upon subsequent consumption by human beings usually response to a toxic epidemic frequently known as the —**'paralytic shell fish poisoning' (PSP).**

In 1975, Japan (in Owase Bay) first had the incidence of PSP; followed, by Philippines and Thailand in 1983; and in 1986 both at Korea and Taiwan.

The various **red tide organisms** (*i.e.,* **dinoflagellate species**) containing specific *toxins, geographical distributions*, and their *physiological effects* are as stated below:

S. No.	Red Tide Organisms	Toxins Present	Geographical Distribution	Physiological Effects
1	*Protogonyaulax cartenella*	GTXs and STXs	Japan; South America; Pacific USA;	Block membrane Na+ conductance
2	*Alexandrium tamarense (Protogonyaulax tamarensis)*	GTXs and STXs	North Atlantic coastal regions	-do-
3	*Ptychodiscus brevis*	Brevetoxin	Florida; Gulf of Mexico.	Positive intropic and and arrythmogenic.
4	*Protogonyaulax cohorticula*	GTXs	Gulf of Thailand	Paralytic syndrome.
5	*Gymnodinium catenatum*	GTXs and PX	Japan, Tasmania	-do-
6	*Pyrodinium bahamense*	STXs and GTXs	Palau Island	-do-
7	*Prorocentrum lima*	Pectenotoxins	Gulf of Lima	Diarrhetic action.

---

  * Habermann, E.: *Toxicon,* **27,** 1171 (1989).
 ** Starr. T.J.: *Texas Reb. Biol. Med.,* **16,** 813 (1958).

GTX = Gonyautoxins;

STXs = Saxitoxins;

PX = Protogonyautoxin.

The various important red tide toxins, are, namely: **saxitoxin, tetrodotoxin,** and **brevetoxin.** These toxins shall be discussed as under:

10.2.3.2.1 Saxitoxin   It has already been described under Section 10.2.2.1.1.

10.2.3.2.2 Tetrodotoxin

Synonyms   Fugu poison; Maculotoxin; Spheroidine; Tarichatoxin; Tetrodontoxin; TTX.

Chemical Structure

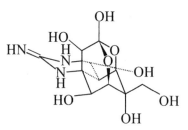

Tetrodotoxin

Octahydro-12-(hydroxymethyl)-2-imino-5, 9:7, 10a-dimethano-10aH-[1, 3] dioxocino [6, 5-d] pyrimidine-4, 7, 10, 11, 12-pentol; ($C_{11}H_{17}N_3O_8$).

Biological Sources   **Tetrodotoxin** is obtained from the ovaries and liver of a large number of species of *Tetraodontidae*, especially the *Spheroides rubripes* **(Globe Fish)**. It is also obtained from the **puffer fish** (*Tetradou* species) which begin a topmost delicacy in Japanese cuisine.

Characteristic Features

1. It usually darkens above 220°C without any decomposition.
2. It has specific optical rotation $[\alpha]_D^{25} - 8.64°$ (C = 8.55 in dilute acetic acid).
3. It is slightly soluble in water, absolute ethanol, ether; and almost insoluble in other organic solvents.
4. It has dissociation constant pKa = 8.76 (water); 9.4 in 50% (v/v) ethanol.
5. The toxin gets destroyed completely both in strong alkali and acid solutions.
6. It is a **marine neurotoxin** *essentially* containing a polar guanidino money.

Uses

1. TTX gets bound particularly to the Na^+ channels on the outside of excitable membranes, thereby inducing Na^+ influx in exchange for K+ influx within a few milliseconds of the accompanying membrane depolarization.
2. It is invariably employed as a valuable pharmacological tool.

Biosynthesis of Tetrodotoxin   **Arginine** is a precursor for **tetrodotoxin.** It has been adequately proved that the remainder of the C-skeleton in it is a C_5 *isoprene unit*, perhaps provided as **isopentenyl diphosphate (IPP)** as given below:

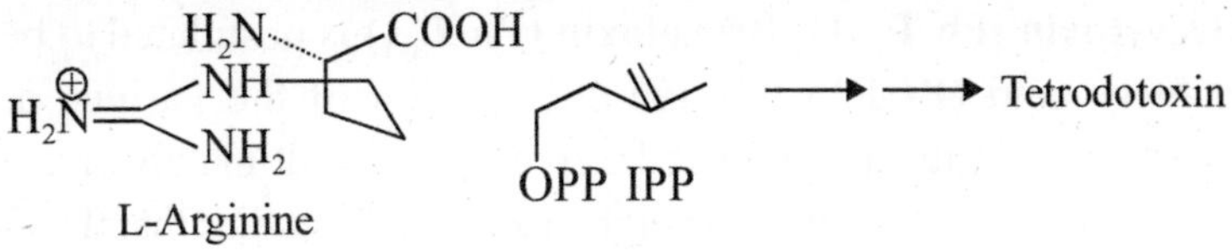

L-Arginine   OPP IPP   → → Tetrodotoxin

10.2.3.2.3   Brevetoxin

Chemical Structure

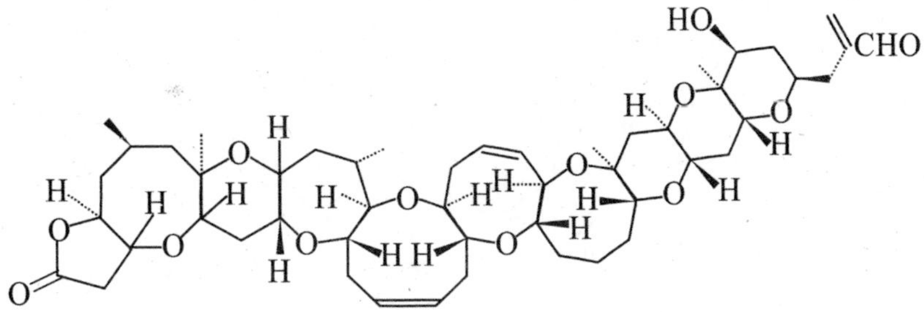

Brvetoxin [Pb Tx-1]

Biological Sources   A plethora of **polycyclic polyether metabolites** have been obtained from the **dinoflagellate** *Ptychodiscus brevis*; and now the **brevetoxins** are commonly known as **PbTx** derived from the generic nomenclature *i.e., P. brevis toxins*.

Characteristic Features

1. These are lipid soluble toxins.
2. The **PbTxs** do not contain any N-atom, which is quite contrary to the STXs and GTXs.
3. The **PbTxs** may be classified into *two* categories, such as: (a) *Hemolytic*, and (b) *Neurotoxic*. However, the latter category are larger in number.
4. The Structure of Pb TX-1, as given above, is the most potent one; and its structure essentially differs from the remaining 9 PbTxs.
5. The toxin Pb Tx-2, is found to be a *cardiotonic* and an *arrythmogenic* in experimental laboratory animal heart studies.

Uses

1. It exerts an excitatory effect on the isolated neuromuscular and other cells. Besides, this effect is further mediated through an increased Na^+ influx subsequent to their strategic binding to *site-5* located upon the voltage-sensitive Na-Channel.
2. Both **Pb Txs** and the **polyether ionophores** (*e.g., norhalichondrins* obtained from *Halichondria okadai* and *okadaic acid*) are found to exhibits marked and pronounced biological actions.
3. It causes both *neurological* and *gastrointestinal* disorders.
4. Pb Txs broadly are splendid activators of voltage-sensitive Na+ channels, with an unique ability to get bounded to very specific receptor sites located on the rat brain synaptosomes. Hence, it may be useful as an important pharmacological tool.

Biosynthesis of Brevetoxin [Pb T$_{x-1}$]   Brevetoxin (Pb T$_{x-1}$) is postulated to be generated from a **polyunsaturated fatty acid (PUFA)** through epoxidation of the various double bonds, and subsequently a concerted sequential opening of the epoxide rings ultimately give rise to the extended polyether structure. It has also been proved through biosynthetic studies that the C-skeleton does not conform to a simple polyketide chain, that fragments from the citric acid cycle together with a 4-carbon starter unit derived from mevalonate are also involved, and that quite a few of the methyls actually obtained from the amino acid *methionine*, as depicted below.

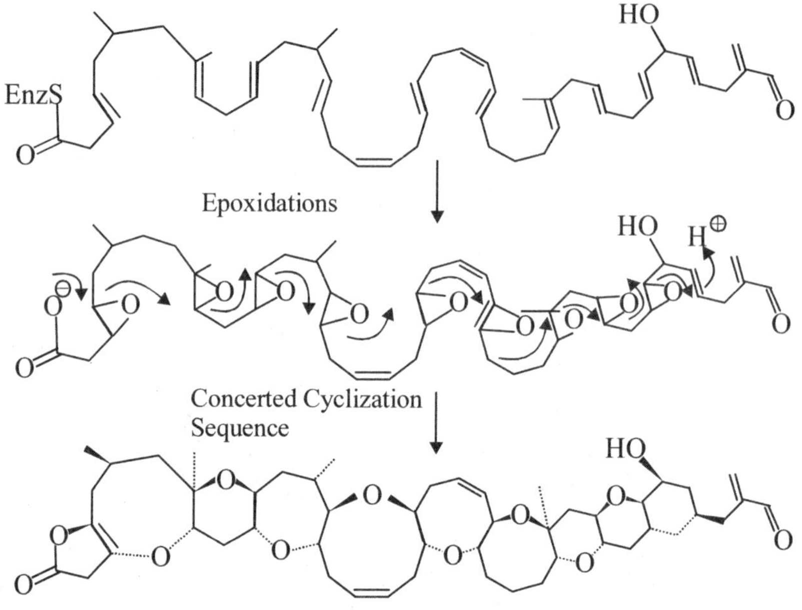

Brevetoxin [Pb T$_{x-1}$]

10.2.3.3   Ciguatera Toxins

It is pertinent to state here that the **ciguatera toxins,** though not directly linked to the '**paralytic shell fish poisoning' (PSP)** of the red tide, are found to be occurring in the toxic *dinoflagellates* that subsequently penetrate the human-food-chain precisely through the *reef fishes* and *not* through the shellfishes.

     In fact, *two* prominent members of this particular category are, namely: **Ciguatoxin (CTX),** and **Maitotoxin (MTX)** which shall now be discussed as under:

10.2.3.3.1   Ciguatoxin   The terminology '**ciguatoxin**' was first and foremost employed to enumerate a disease primarily caused due to the ingestion of *marine snails*. Ciguatera poisoning was thought to be due to the ingestion of blue green algae.

Ciguatoxin [$C_{53}H_{78}NO_{24}$]

Biological Sources **Ciguatoxin (CTX)** is found in *Gymnothorax javanicus* (**Moray Eel**), besides in a variety of coral reef fish, for instance: *Lutjanus bohar* (**Red Snapper**).

Characteristic Features
1. It is one of the most complex examples of a natural polyether structural chemical substance.
2. A **dinoflagellate** *Gambierdiscus toxicus* definitely causes the production of this polyether, thereby synthesizing a comparatively less toxic analogue, that is eventually passed *via* the food chain; and ultimately modified structurally into the extremely toxic **ciguatoxin** within the system of the fish.

Uses
1. It causes neurological, cardiovascular and gastro-intestinal problems.
2. It is found to be exceedingly toxic even at mcg levels, thereby affecting widespread food poisoning (**ciguatera**) both in subtropical and tropical regions that is evidently characterized by diarrhoea, vomiting and sometimes leading to acute neurological problems.
3. **CTX** at low IV doses displays bradycardia and respiratory stimulation in anaesthetized cats and dogs; whereas at higher dose levels there is an apparent depression in both heart rate and respiration followed by hypertension (probably on account of reflex compensation of bradycardia).
4. Interestingly, **CTX** acts as a cardiotonic at a very low concentrations *i.e.*, picogram levels.
5. **CTX**—is found to exert its action at the nerve ends specifically.

10.2.3.3.2 Maitotoxin

Synonym MTX.

Biological Source It is obtained from the toxic **dinoflagellate** *Gambierdiscus toxicus*.

Characteristic Features MTX possesses several characteristic pharmacological features, such as:

1. **MTX** is a Ca^{2+} channel activator.
2. It specifically enhances Ca^{2+} uptake in cultured NG 108-15 neuroblastoma X glioma cells by changing the voltage-dependance of calcium channel activation.
3. **MTX** is found to enhance the rate as well as the force of contraction in rat myocardiac cells immediately followed by arrythmias.

4. **MTX** affords to induce a dose-dependent release of **GABA*** in the reaggregate clusters of striated neurons, that may be blocked by the calcium blocker D-600.

MTX also has a number of characteristic chemical features, namely:

1. Chemical structure of **MTX** not yet known.
2. MTX is a non-peptide having a large molecular weight of 3,425 as estimated by the help of fast atom bombardment mass spectrum.
3. It is found to react with **Dragendorff's Reagent** but fails to give any response with **Ninhydrin Reagent,** suggesting thereby that is basically alkaloidal in nature.
4. The large non-peptide molecule of **MTX** possesses a good number of –OH moieties, ethereal oxygen atoms, and *two* sulphate ester functions.

5. It is found to contain *no* repeatable carbohydrate or amino acid units, no $-\overset{\overset{\displaystyle O}{\|}}{C}-$(carbonyl) moieties, *no* carbocycles, and *no* side chains except either a vinyl or a methyl function.

    Note: Excepting the 'sulphated ester moieties' all other chemical features very closely resemble to those of PTX (*i.e.*; Palytoxin).

Uses   The overall toxicity of **MTX** almost comes at par to that of **PTX;** however, the latter is obviously much more toxic than the former.

10.2.4 Antimicrobial Drugs

A plethora of important **antimicrobial drug** substances have been isolated, characterized and studied extensively over the past three decades particularly from the vast domain of marine organisms. A few typical examples are, namely: **brown algae, red algae** (viz., *three* different species), **gorgonian corals;** and **sponge** (viz., *two* variant species). The chemical substances from these species shall now be discussed briefly as under:

10.2.4.1 *Zonarol*

Chemical Structure

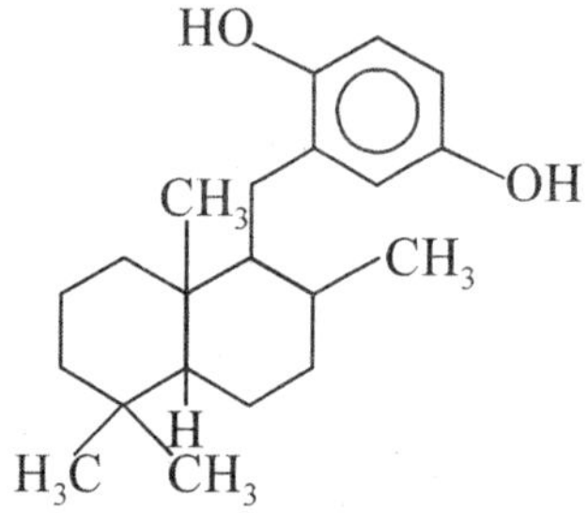

Zonarol

Biological Source   Zonarol and iso-zonarol are both obtained from *Dictyopteris zonaroides* (**Brown Algae**).

---

* **GABA:** γ-Aminobutyric acid.

10.2.4.2 Prepacifenol

Chemical Structure

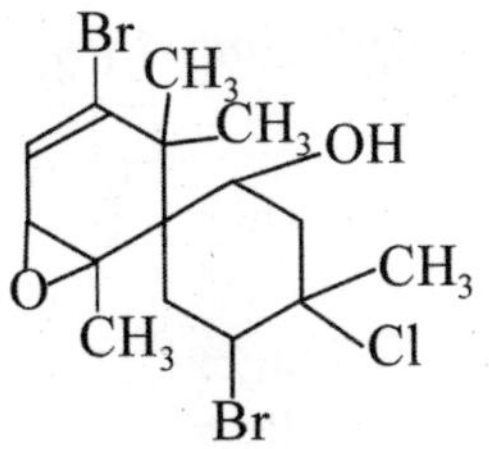

Prepacifenol

Biological Sources   It is obtained from *Laurencia pacifica* and *Laurencia filformis*, the two diffeent species of **Red Algae.**

10.2.4.3 Polyhalo-3-butene-2-one

Chemical Structure

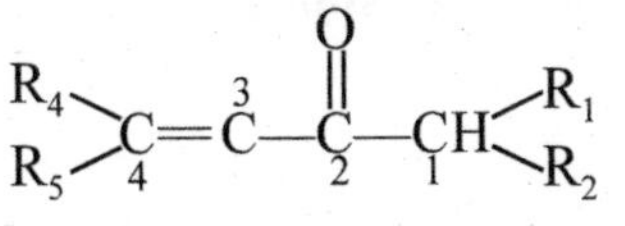

Polyhalo-3-Butene-2-One
[R_1, R_2, R_3, R_4 and R_5 are Haloatoms]

Biological Source   In all four isomers of polyhalo-3-butene-2-one and nearly seven isomer of **polyhalo-acetones** are obtained from *Asparogopsis taxiformis,* another species of **Red Algae.**

10.2.4.4 Tetrabromo-2-Heptanone

Chemical Structure

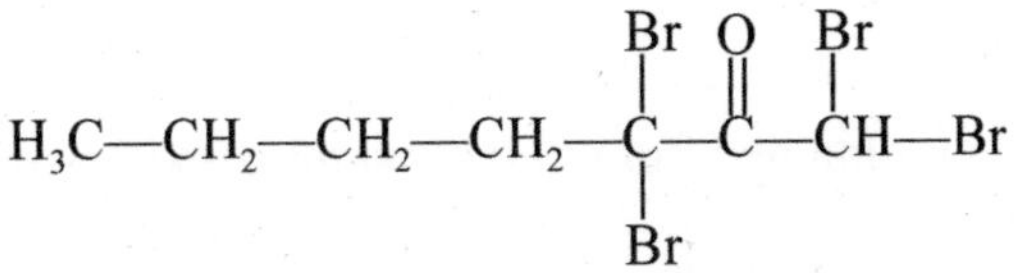

Tetrabromo-2-heptanone

Biological Source   It is obtained from yet another species of **Red Algae** *Bonnemaisonia hemifera.*

10.2.4.5 2-Cyano-4, 5-dibromopyrrole

Chemical Structure

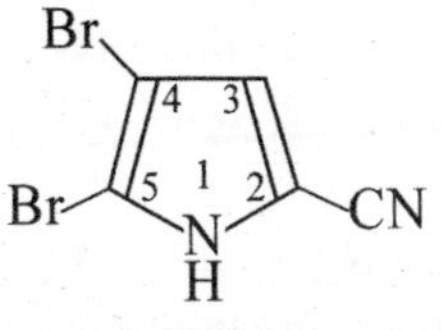

2-Cyano-4, 5-dibromopyrrole

It is perhaps one of the rarest examples of a chemical entity isolated from a **marine organism** which contains a cyano (–CN) function group.

Biological Source   It is obtained from *Agelas oroides,* a specific type of **sponge** found in marine sources.

10.2.4.6   *Aeroplysinin-1 (+) and Aeroplysinin-1 (–)*

Chemical Structures

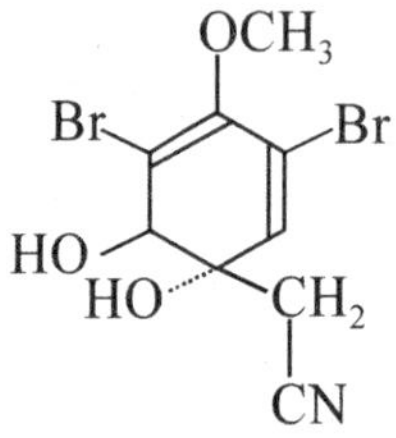

Aeroplysinin-1 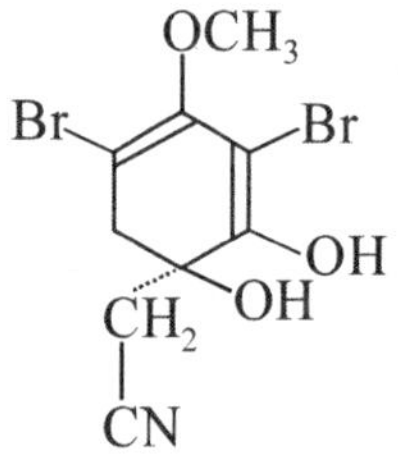 (+)   Aeroplysinin-1 (–)

Biological Sources   The *two* isomers, *viz.*, **aeroplysinin-1(+)** and **aeroplysinin-1(–)** are obtained from *Verongia aerophoba* another species of **sponge.**

10.2.4.7   *Eunicin*

Chemical Structure

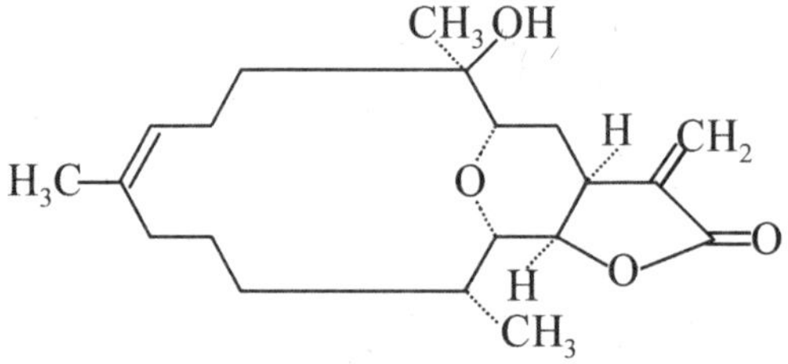

Eunicin

Biological Source   **Eunicin** is obtained from *Eunicia mammosa* the well known **Gorgonian Corals.**

10.2.5   Antibiotic Substances

Interestingly, between a span of almost twenty years (1969-1988) thousands of marine-based extracts, fractions and pure isolates were evaluated for their antibiotic activity. However, the success rate was not only miserable but absolutely nonsignificant. As on date, not even a single **marine-derived antibiotic substance** has been able to either superceded or gained enormous regonition with regard to their broad spectrum of activity and superb quality of the known and available **antibiotics** obtained from the innumerable **terrestrial organisms, semi-synthetic products,** and/for purely synthetic ones.

Nevertheless, the earnest efforts contributed by the **marine-chemists** across the globe have been able to evolve a few antibiotics from the various marine organisms, namely: **okadaic acid, acanthifolicin** and **norhalichondrin** A. These naturally occurring marine antibiotics shall now be discussed in the sections that follows:

10.2.5.1 Okadaic Acid

Synonym   Halochondrine A;

Chemical Structure

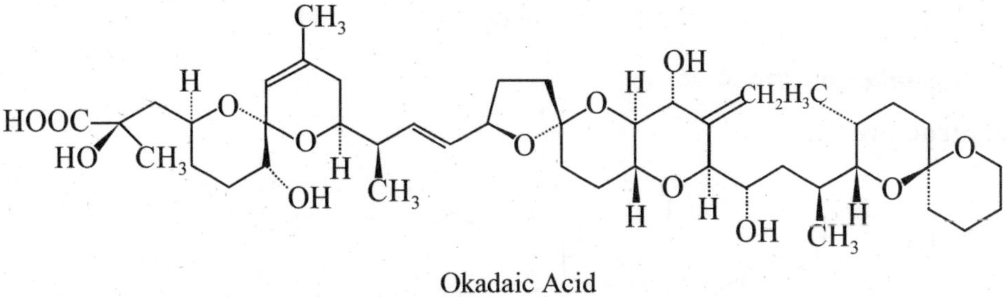

Okadaic Acid

9,10-Deepithio-9, 10-didehydro-acanthifolicin; ($C_{44}H_{68}O_{13}$).

It is the first **ionophoric polyether** identified in marine organisms.

Biological Sources   It is obtained from *Halichondria* (*okadai* or *melanodocia*) (**Marine Black Sponges**).

Characteristic Features   The characteristic features of **okadaic acid** are as follows:

1. It is obtained from dichloromethane/hexane having mp 171-175°C.
2. It has specific optical rotation $[\alpha]_D^{20}$ + 21° (C = 0.33 in chloroform).
3. It is also reported as crystals from benzene-chloroform mixture having mp 164-166°C; and $[\alpha]_D^{25}$ + 25.4° (C = 0.24 in chloroform).

Uses
1. It is an important biochemical tool as tumour promoter and probe of cellular regulation.
2. It was found to be far more cytotoxic to KB-cells and to mice than compared to another **novel ionophoric marine substance acanthifolicin.**
3. It is able to transport divalent cations *e.g.*, Ca^{2+} across the lipoidal membranes conveniently.
4. **Okadaic acid** uniquely causes a prolonged contraction of the human umbilical artery and rabbit aorta without the presence of extracellular Ca^{2+}; and it does not affect the Na^+ and K^+ AT Pase.

10.2.5.2 Acanthifolicin

Chemical Structure

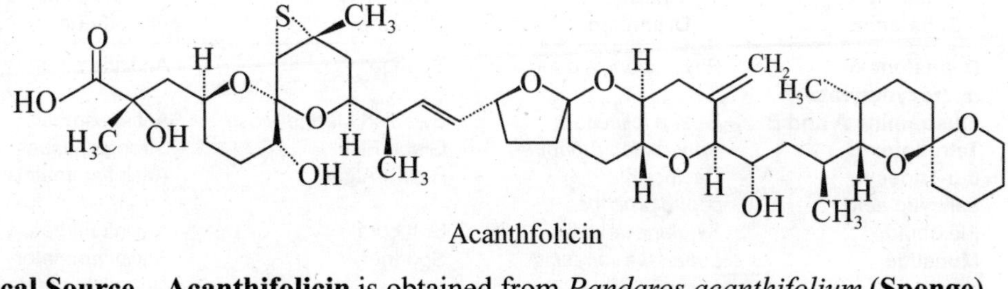

Acanthfolicin

Biological Source   **Acanthifolicin** is obtained from *Pandaros acanthifolium* (**Sponge**).

Characteristic Features

1. It possesses an antibacterial activity.
2. It also exerts cytotoxic actions.
3. It is found to be lethal to mice at low dose level of 0.14 mg kg^{-1} i.v.

Uses   The uses are almost the same as given under **okadaic acid.**

10.2.5.3 Norhalichondrin A

Chemical Structure

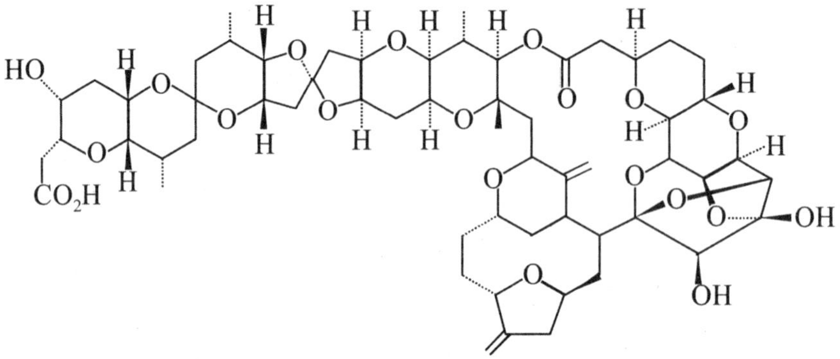

Norhalichondrin A

Biological Source   **Norhalichondrin A** and several other **halichondrin** structural analogues have been obtained from *Halichondria okadai* (**Sponge**).

Characteristic Features

1. It is a **polyether macrolide.**
2. The structure-activity correlational studies with regard to their derivatives; and also their structural fragments are of significant biological interest.

Uses   It is found to exert antitumour activity.

10.2.6 Antiinflammatory and Antispasmodic Agents

A plethora of chemical substances have been isolated from the broad spectrum of **marine organisms** which attribute either **antiinflammatory** or **antispasmodic** activities. A few typical examples are summarized below:

S. No.	Chemical Substance	Marine Organism	Common Name	Biological Activities
1	Dendalone-3-hydroxybutyrate	*Phyllospongia dendyi*	Sponge	Antiinflammatory
2	Flustramine A and B	*Flustra foliaceae*	Swedish Marine Moss	Antispasmodic
3	Tetradotoxin	*Spheroides rubripes*	Globe Fish	Strong antispasmodic.
4	6-n-Tridecyl salicylic acid	*Caulocystis cephalornithos*	Brown Algae	Antiinflammatory
5	Flexibilide	*Sinularia flexibilis*	Soft coral	Antiinflammatory
6	Monalide	*Luffariella variabilis*	Sponge	Antiinflammatory (non-steroidal compound).

10.2.7 Miscellaneous Pharmacologically Active Substances

A good number of **pharmacologically active substances** have been isolated and characterized from marine organisms that invariably exhibit a variety of interesting actions. A few important and typical examples have been grouped together under this section, such as: **Latrunculins; Kainic Acid; Domoic Acid; Vidarabine; Aplysinopsin; 28-Deoxyzoanthenamine; Barettin; Nereistotoxin;** and **Conotoxins.**

The above stated **marine-based chemical substances** shall now be treated individually in the sections that follows:

10.2.7.1 Latrunculins

Latrunculins (LAT) A through D, M and 6, 7-epoxy-LAT A have been isolated and characterized. Interestingly, these are the first and foremost family of natural marine based products essentially having the **2-thiazolidinone moiety.** All, except latrunculin M, are 16- or 14-membered macrocyclic diterpene alkaloids (macrolides) that have been duly isolated and characterized from various corals and sponges, and majority of them do possess certain definite biological activity.

It is, however, pertinent to mention here that out of the *four* toxic **latrunculins A-D,** the first two *i.e.*, **latrunculin A** and **latrunculin B** shall be discussed as under:

Chemical Structures

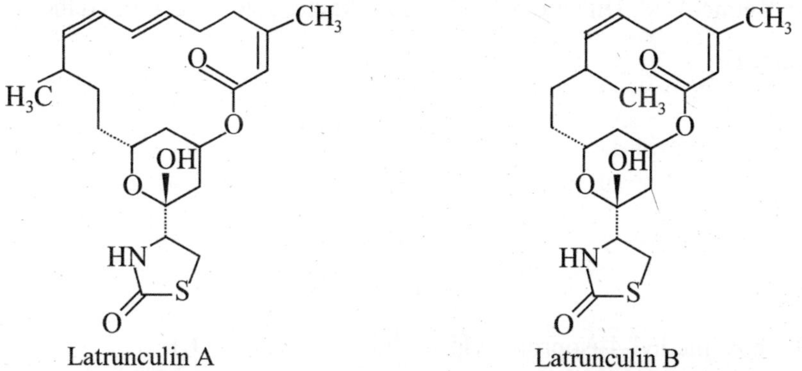

Latrunculin A
$(C_{22}H_{31}NO_5S]$

Latrunculin B
$(C_{20}H_{29}NO_5S]$

Biological Sources Latrunculins are obtained from *Latrunculia magnifica* Keller (**Red Sea Sponge**). They are also found in *Chromodoris elisabethina* (**Pacific Nudibranch**); and the *Spongia mycofijiensis* (**Fijian Sponge**).

Note: When L. magnifica is gently squeezed into an aquarium, the toxins are exuded into it spontaneously. The living fish experience sequentially agitation, hemorrhage, loss of balance and ultimately succumbs to death within a span of 4-6 minute.

Isolation Latrunculins have been isolated from *L. magnifica* by Neeman *et al.**

---

* Neeman *et al.: Marine Biol.* **30**, 293, (1975).

Characteristic Features

Latrunculin A (LAT-A)

1. It is obtained as a foam.
2. It has specific optical rotation $[\alpha]_D^{24} + 152°$ (C = 1.2 in chloroform).
3. It has uv_{max} (methanol): 218 nm (ϵ 23500).

Latrunculin B (LAT-B)

1. It is obtained as crystals.
2. It has specific optical rotation $[\alpha]_D^{24} + 112°$ (C = 0.48 in chloroform).
3. It has uv_{max} (methanol): 212 nm (ϵ 17200).

Uses

1. They are used exclusively in establishing the elucidation of molecular mechanisms of motile processes.
2. At nanomolar concentrations in cultured mouse neuroblastoma and fibroblasts, the **LAT-A** and **LAT-B** distinctly cause significant disruption of microfilament organization without affecting the microtubules, analogous to what the less active **cytochalsins** do.*
3. Unlike cytochalasins, the **LAT-A** and **LAT-B** do not afford any change in the polymerization rate of active filaments.

10.2.7.2 Kainic Acid

Synonyms α-Kainic Acid; Digenic Acid; L_S-*Xylo*-kainic acid; Digenin; Helminal.

Chemical Structure

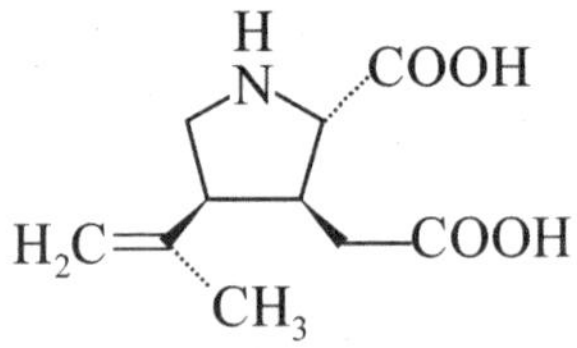

Kainic Acid

2-Carboxy-3-carboxymethyl-4-isopropenylpyrrolidine; ($C_{10}H_{15}NO_4$).

Biological Source   It is obtained from dried *Digenea simplex* (Wulf.) Ag., (**Red Algae**) (*Rhodomelaceae*).

Characteristic Features

1. It is obtained as needles which get decomposed at 251°C.
2. It has specific optical rotation $[\alpha]_D^{24} - 14.8°$ (C=1.01).
3. It shows an intense absorption at 6.05 and 112μ.
4. It is found to be soluble in water; insoluble in ethanol; and fairly stable in boiling aqueous solutions.

---

* Spector *et al.*: *Science*, **219**, 493 (1983).

Uses

1. It is used as a potent convulsant.
2. It is invariably employed as a vital neurobiological tool.
3. It is mostly employed as an **anthelmintic (Nematodes).**

10.2.7.3 Domoic Acid

Chemical Structure   It is a structural analogue of **kainic acid.**

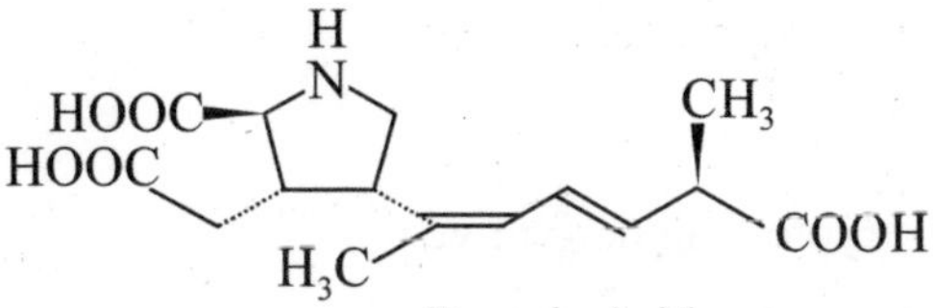

Domoic Acid

[2S-[2α, 3β, 4β (1Z, 3E, 5S*)]]-2-Carboxy-4-(5-Carboxy-1-methyl-1, 3-hexadienyl)-3-pyrrolidineacetic acid; ($C_{15}H_{21}NO_6$).

Biological Source   It is obtained from *Chondria armata* Okamura (*Rhodomelaceae*) (**Red Algae**), also known in Japanese as **'DOMOI';** and hence the name domoic acid.

Characteristic Features

Domoic Acid Dihydrate

1. It has mp 217°C (decomposes).
2. It has specific optical rotation $[\alpha]_D^{12}$ - 109.6° (C = 1.314 in water).
3. It has uv$_{max}$: 242 nm (log ϵ 4.24).
4. Its dissociation constant in water pKa: 2.10; 3.72; 4.93; 9.82.
5. It is found to be soluble in water, acetic acid; and insoluble in methanol ethanol, chloroform, acetone and benzene.

10.2.7.4 Vidarabine

Synonyms   Ara-A; Vira-A; Arasena-A; Adenine arabinoside; Spongoadenosine; CI-673.

Chemical Structure

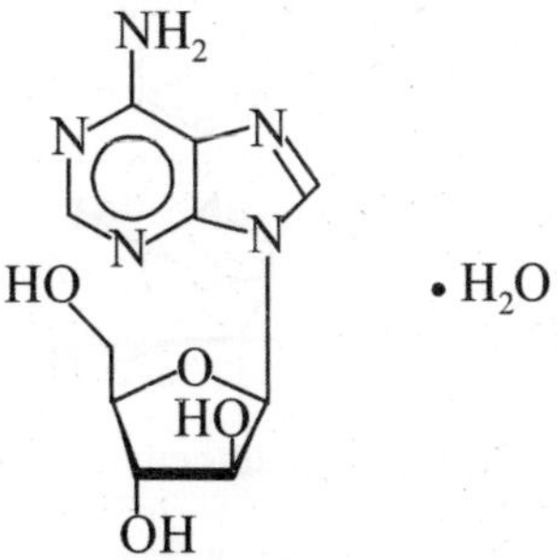

Vidarabine

9-β-D-Arabinofuranosyl-9H-purine-6-amine monohydrate; ($C_{10}H_{13}N_5O_4.H_2O$).

It is a purine nucleoside first ever synthesized as a potential antineoplastic agent.

Biological Source   It is obtained by culturing a strain of *Streptomyces antibioticus*.

Characteristic Features
1. It is obtained as crystals from water having mp 257.0 – 257.5°C (0.4 H_2O).
2. It has specific optical rotation $[\alpha]_D^{27} - 5°$ (C = 0.25).
3. It has uv_{max} (pH1): 257.5 nm (ε 12700); pH 7:259 nm (ε 13400); pH 13 : 259 nm (ε 14000).

Uses   It is mostly used as an antiviral agent.

10.2.7.5 *Aplysinopsin*

Chemical Structure   It is a tryptophan derivative.

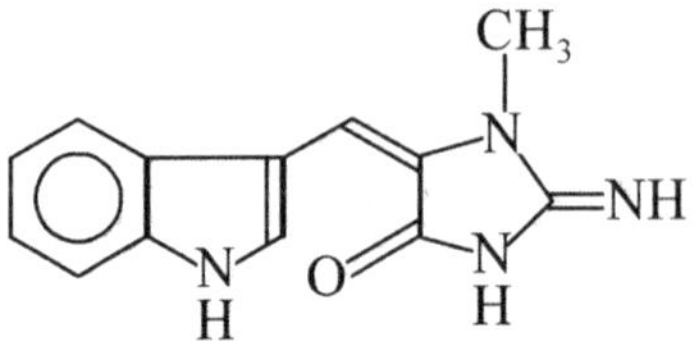

Aplysinopsin

Biological Sources   It is originally obtained from *Verongia spengelii* (**Yellow-Sponge**); and also from *Astroides calicularis* (Anthozoan).

Uses
1. It has cytotoxic activity against **KB.P 388 and L1210 leukemia cell lines.**
2. It has been found to exhibit antidepressant activity very much similar to that of **imipramine.**

10.2.7.6 *28-Deoxyzoanthenamine*

Chemical Structure   It is an **alkaloid** from the **marine organism.**

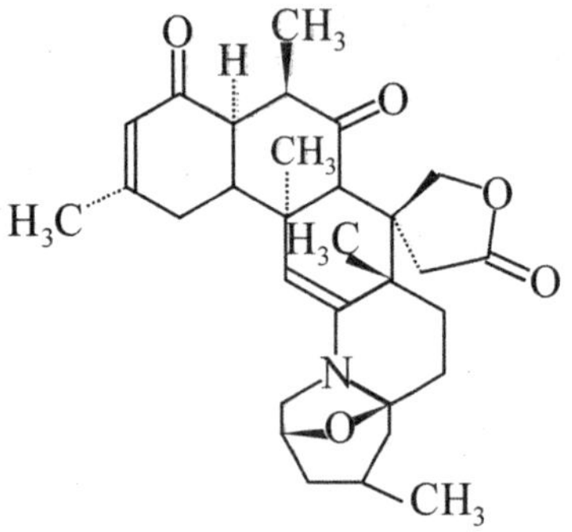

28-Deoxyzoanthenamine

Biological Source   It is obtained from a *Zonathus* sp. from the Bay of Bengal (India).

Uses   It is found to possess strong analgesic as well as antiinflammatory activities.

10.2.7.7 *Barettin*

Chemical Structure   It is structurally an **indole-related alkaloid.**

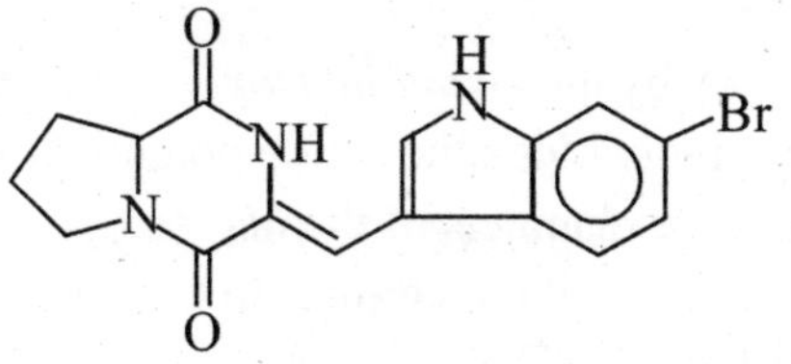

Barettin

Biological Source   It is obtained from *Geodia beretti* (**Cold Water Sponge**).

Uses   It acts as a smooth muscle stimulant.

10.2.7.8 *Nereistotoxin*

Chemical Structure $(C_5H_{11}NS_2)$

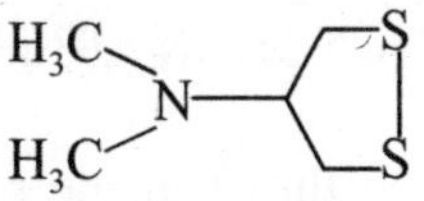

Nereistotoxin

Biological Source   It is obtained from *Lumbriconeris heteropoda*, a marine annelid.

Uses   It is mostly used as an effective *insecticide* by virtue of its inherent ganglion blocking effects.

Note: **Another semisynthetic structural analogue of nereistotoxin, known as cartap is invariably employed as an useful insecticide.**

10.2.7.9 *Conotoxins*

Biological Sources   A plethora of toxins have been obtained and isolated from *Conus geographus*, specifically from the toxic venom of a fish-eating snail. Based on a logical and scientific thought these toxins may be classified into *two* categories, namely:

(*a*) **μ-Conotoxins**   *i.e.*, a congregation of *seven* homologous peptides having 22 residues each*, and

(*b*) **ω-Conotoxins**   *i.e.*, a subgroup in a class of peptides which are exclusively neurotoxic in nature.

Characteristic Features

10.2.7.9.1   μ-Conotoxins   (I) Kobayashi *et al.*** have reported **geographutoxins I and II** that seem to be almost similar to conotoxins **GIIIA** and **BIIIB.*****

10.2.7.9.2   ω-Conotoxins   The inhibition of a depolarization-evoked ATP release from synaptosomes of ray electric organ, evidently by affording the blockade of the Ca^{2+} flux through the

---

   * Cruz *et al.*: *J. Biol. Chem.*, **260**, 9280 (1985).

  ** Kobayashi *et al.*: *Pflugers Arch.*, **407**, 241 (1986).

 *** Sato *et al.*, FEBS *lett* **155**. 177 (1983).

voltage-gated calcium channels were demonstrated by ω-CgTX and the related ω-Cm TX obtained from *Conus magnus.* *

Uses   [m-Conotoxins]

1. Very similar to the actions shown by the *guanidium toxins viz.*, **tetrodotoxin (TTX)** and **saxitoxin (STX),** these toxins also effectively block the action potential of skeletal muscle cells; however, unlike **TTX** they fail to affect the channels of the nerves.
2. It has been proved experimentally that the **conotoxin CIIIA** usually get bound to the same site on the Na+ channel where **STX** and **TTX** are found to bind.

ω-Conotoxins   It has been duly demonstrated that **w-CgTXVIA** shows a very specific high affinity binding to the synaptosomal and membrane preparations from chick brain. Furthermore, it has given a fairly good evidence that this particular toxin acts onto a *new site* on the Ca^{2+} channel, because it has shown an altogether different sites *i.e.*, from both **dihydropyridine** and **verapamil binding sites.** **

10.3   MARINE NATURAL PRODUCTS: AN UPGRADATION PROFILE

In the last two decades an overwhelming thrust in the research towards accomplishment of an upgradation profile of **marine natural products** have taken place across the globe.

However, these wonderful achievements could only be possible either through various microbial transformations or by means of different semisynthetic structural analogues of puupephenone. Interestingly, **marine natural products** were subjected to rigorous bioconversion studies and different specific organic reactions, such as: acetylation, addition of halogen acids (HX), Grignardization, conjugate additions, and other addition reactions.

The important aspects of such modifications of **marine natural products** shall now be discussed briefly with the help of certain typical examples in the sections that follow:

10.3.1   Microbial Transformations

Microbial trransformation may be defined as—'the phenomenon by which certain organism (bacteria) incorporate DNA from related strains into their genetic make-up'.

The two typical examples of microbial transformations *vis-a-vis* the upgradation profile of **marine natural products** are as stated under:

10.3.1.1   *Sarcophine: Bioconversion Studies*

In general, it is almost essential to carry out the **metabolism studies** so as to obtain the legitimate approval of any clinically useful drug. It has already been duly established that **'microorganisms'** may be employed successfully in carrying out the *in vitro* studies so as to predict the drug metabolism

---

* Yeager *et al.*: *J. Neurosci.*, **7**, 2390, (1987).
** L.J. Cruz and B.M. Olivera: *J. Biol. Chem.*, **261**; 6230 (1986).

in the mammalians by virtue of the fact that there exists a very close resemblance of some microbial enzyme systems, particularly fungi, with the **mammalian liver enzyme systems.***

Sarcophine is the **furanochembranoid diterpene** obtained from *Sarcophyton glaucum* having an appreciable yield of 3% dry weight basis. *S. glaucum* is a common soft coral of the Red Sea Pacific, besides other coral reefs. Bernstein *et al.*** advocated that **sarcophine** represents the *major-chemical-defence* entity against the natural predators.

Prepartion   The specimen of *S. glaucum* (Red Sea Soft Coral) was identified and collected from Hurghada (Egypt) in 1994, by snorkelling and SCUBA (-3m). Approximately 1.1kg of frozen coral was subjected to lypholization and subsequently extracted with 95% (v/v) ethanol (3 × 21).

Microbial Metabolism Studies   **Lee's method*** was adopted in carrying out the elaborated microbial metabolism studies. In all, twenty-five authentic **microbial cultures**** were employed for sereening. The method of San-Martin *et al.***** was followed for the exclusive microbial bioconversion studies of sarcophine, which evidently proved that it can be duly metabolized by many fungal species. Further, preparative-scale fermentation was carefully performed by using *Absidia glauca* (**ATCC******-22752**), *Rhizopus arrhizus* (ATCC-11145), and *Rhizophus stolonifer* (ATCC-24795), ultimately gave rise to the isolation of ten (5-14) altogether new metabolities; besides, the known 7β, 8α-dihydroxydeepoxy-sarcophine (4).

It is, however, pertinent to mention here that the structure clucidation of these compounds was entirely based on **2D-NMR spectroscopic studies.** The relative stereochemistry and confirmation of the probable structure of metabolite was ascertained by **X-ray crystallographic studies.**

The various salient features of the **isolated metabolites** are as follows:

1. **Sarcophytols A (2) and B (3)** are simple **cembranoids** isolated from the **Okinawan soft coral** *S. glaucum*. These possess potent inhibitory activities against a wide spectrum of tumour promoters.******* Interestingly, compound (2) helped to mediate dose-dependent diminution of 12-O-tetradecanoyl-phorbol 13-acetate (TPA)-induced transformation of JB6 cells.********
2. The ability and potential to inhibit TPA-induced TB6 cell transformation, it has been duly observed that plethora of the **sarcophine metabolities** (4 to 14) helped to mediate inhibitory responses much higher than exhibited by **sarcophytol A (2)** or **sarcophine (1);** and most prominently 7α-hydroxy-$\Delta^{8(19)}$ **deepoxysarcophine (6),** which was fairly comparable to the 13-*cis*-retinoic acid.

Note: A good number of novel furanocembranoids as antineoplastic agents may be further developed along these lines.

---

   * Clark, A.M. *et. al., Med. Res. Rev.* **5**, 231, (1985).
  ** Bernstein, J., *et al. Tetrahedron*, **30**, 2817, (1974).
  *** Lee, I.S., *et al. Pharm. Res.* **7**. 199, (1990).
  **** University of Mississippi, Dept: of Pharmacognosy Culture Collection Centre.
  ***** San-Martin *et al. J. Phytochem.*, **30**, 2165, (1991).
  ****** **ATTC** = American-Type-Culture-Collection.
  ******* Kobayashi *et al. Chem. Pharm. Bull.*, **27**, 2382, (1979).
 ******** El Sayed *et al. J. Org. Chem.*, **63**, 7449, (1998).

No.	R₁	R₂	R₃	R₄
1	H	CH_3	H	H
7	H	CH_3	$\mathcal{S}$-OH	H
10	H	CH_2OH	H	H
11	H	CH_3	$\mathcal{R}$-OH	H
12	$\mathcal{R}$-OH	CH_3	H	H
13	H	CH_3	H	$\mathcal{R}$-OH
14	H	CH_3	H	$\mathcal{S}$-OH

No.	R
2	H
3	$\mathcal{R}$-OH

No.	R₁	R₂
4	$\mathcal{R}$-OH	$\mathcal{S}$-OH, $\mathcal{R}$-CH₃
5	$\mathcal{S}$-OH	$\mathcal{R}$-OH, $\mathcal{S}$-CH₃

No.	R₁	R₂
4	CH₃	OH
5	OH	CH₃

(6)

10.3.1.2 Manzamine A and ent-8-Hydroxymazamine A: Bioconversion Studies

Higa *et al.** in 1986 first and foremost reported the **manzamines,** a group of **novel polycyclic β-carboline-alkaloids,** from the *Haliclona* (**Okinawan Marine Sponge**). Interestingly, the **manzamines** demonstrated an unique and diverse spectrum of bioactivity, such as: antimicrobial, insecticidal and cytotoxic activities.**

Higa *et al.* isolated **manzamine A (15)** to the extent of ~ 0.85% on anhydrous basis; and elucidated its probable structure with the aid of ^{15}N-NMR spectroscopy exclusively. Further, the same researchers reported the new *ent-8-hydroxymanzamine A (16)* from an unidentified Indo-Pacific, (a sponge belonging to Family *Petrosidae* and Order *Heplosclerida*). Importantly, both the aforesaid compounds exhibited marked and pronounced **cytotoxic activity** against several tumour *cell-lines*; and also displayed appreciable and significant *antimalarial activity* against *Plasmodium falciparum* exclusively (**D6 and W2 clones**).

However, the two compounds (15 and 16) were selected as candidate '**new molecules**' for the intensive microbial bioconversion studies. El Sayed *et al.**** demonstrated that the said two **compounds (15 & 16) may be metabolized by a number of microbial species.**

Preparative-scale fermentation of compounds 15 and 16 under specific experimental parameters have given the following outstanding findings.

---

* Sakai *et al. J. Am. Cham. Soc.*, **108**, 6404, (1986).

** Edrada *et al. J. Nat. Prod.* **59**, 1056, (1996).

*** El Sayed *et al.* Abstract O30, The 39th Annual Meeting of the American Society of Pharmacognosy, Orlando, Fl., July, 1998.

Compounds	Organism (ATCC No.)	Major Metabolite	Remarks
Manzamine-A; (15)	*Fusarium oxysporium* f. *gladioli* (ATCC 11137)	Ircinal A (Compound 17)	—
***ent*-8-Hydroxyman-zamine A; (16)**	*Norcardia sp.* (ATCC 11925) and *Fusarium oxysporium* (ATCC 7601)	12, 34-Oxaman-zamine F (Compound 18)	No cytotoxicity *against different* cell-line (> 10 mcg mL^{-1})

The chemical **structures of compounds 15 to 18** are given below:

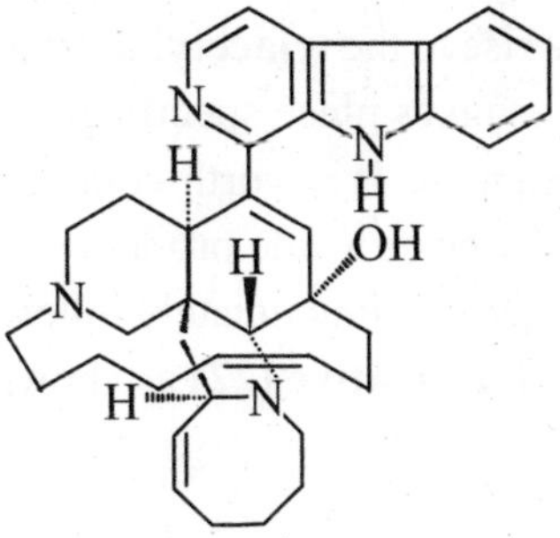

Manzamine A
[15]

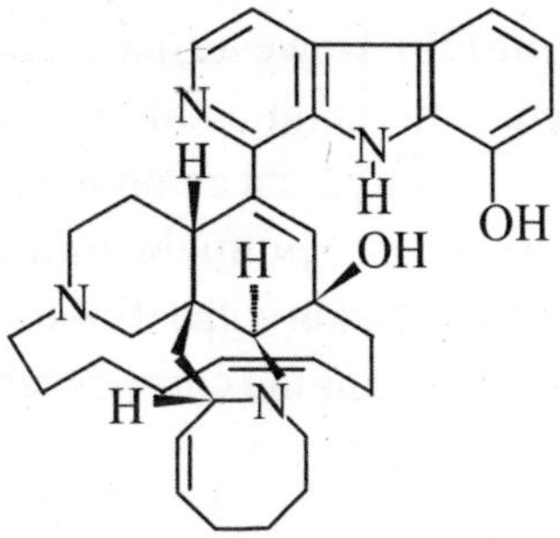

ent-8-Hydroxy-
manzamine A [16]

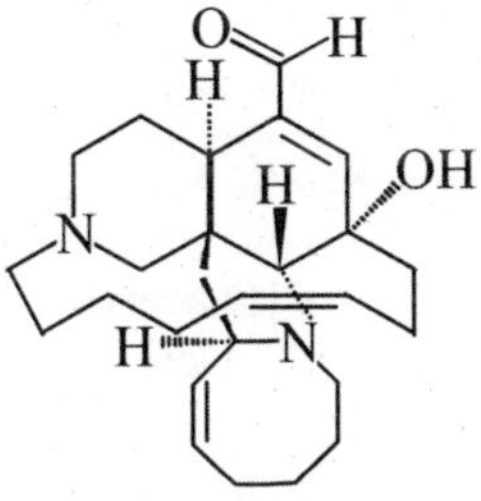

Ircinala
[17]

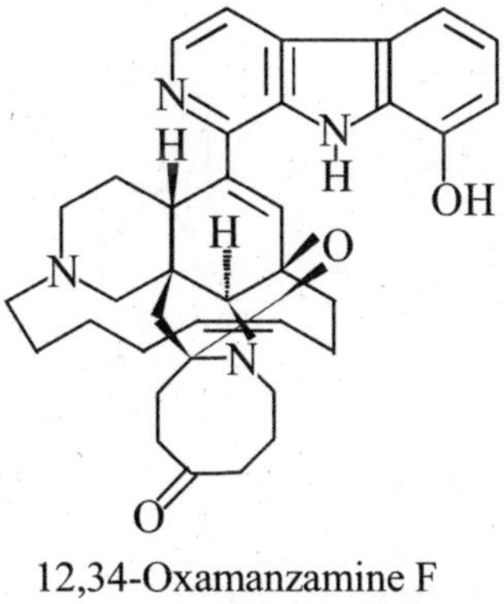

12,34-Oxamanzamine F
[18]

10.3.2 Puupehenone: Semisynthetic Analogues

Puupehenone (19) is a sesquiterpene linked strategically to a C_6-Shikimate function, duly exemplified by the **quinol** (*viz.*, **avarol**)-*quinone* (*viz.*, avarone) pair; and interestingly, belongs to a prominent and distinctive family of **sponge metabolites.** Loya *et al.* (1990)* observed that the diversified biological activities proclaimed for this relatively rare group of compounds is solely due to the characteristic feature of *ilimaquinone* (18A) to prevent categorically and check the replication

---

* Loya, S. *et al., Antimicrob. Agents Chemother.* **34**, 2009, 1990.

phenomenon of the **HIV virus.** It has been established on the basis of the preliminary sereening of puupehenone against the pathogenic organism *Mycobacterium tuberculosis* that it caused inhibition to the extent of 99%. Therefore, it has evidently paved the way towards modifying the chemical structures of **puupehenone** and to evaluate their biological activity.

These structural modifications may be accomplished by the following *four* different ways, which shall be treated separately in the sections that follows:

10.3.2.1 Acetylation and Addition HX

Acetylation of puupehenone (19) should have normally yielded the corresponding **monoacetyl structural analogue (20).** However, it exclusively gives rise to the **triacetyl derivative (21)** through a mechanism whereby the addition of the acetyl moieties takes place specifically at the conjugated double-bond system of the parent compound *i.e.*, puupehenone. It is worthwhile to observe here that the monoacetyl derivative of **puupehenone (20)** is produced as a side product due to the sequence of addition-elimination reaction with HBr/HCl and puupehenone, immediately followed by acetylation which ultimately gave rise to the corresponding **diacetyl derivative (22)** as shown below.

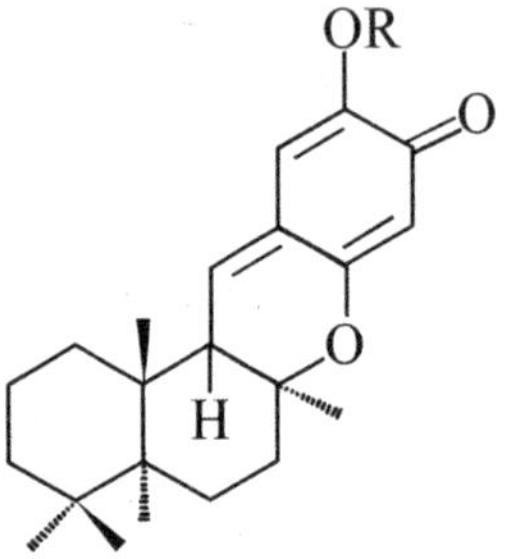

19:R=H; Puupehenone

20:R=O—C—CH$_3$
        (O)
Monoacetyl Puupehenone

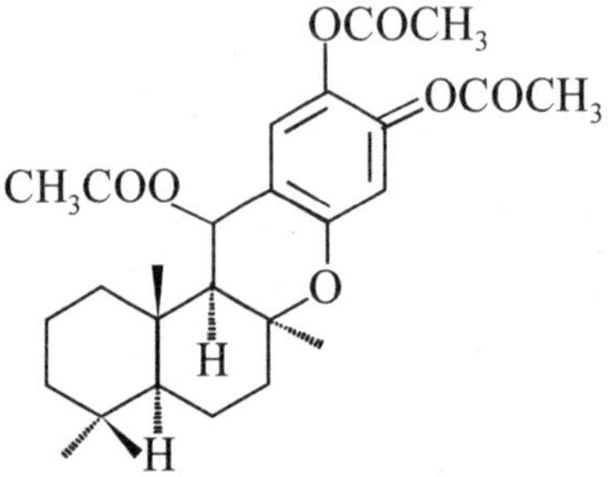

21
[Triacetyl]
Deriv.

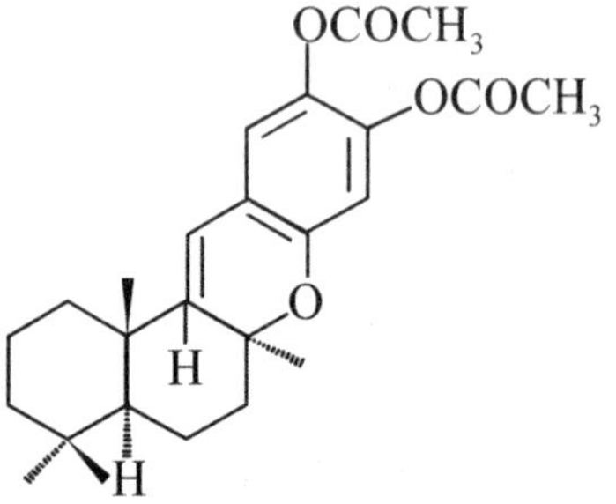

22
[Diacetyl]
Deriv.

10.3.2.2 Grignardization

Grignardization of puupehenone (19) with methyl-magnesium iodide (H$_3$CMgI) in diethyl ether as a reaction medium gave rise to *two* products of addition that solely based upon the stoichiometric proportions of the **Grignard Reagent.**

(*a*) The addition of *three* times molar excess of H$_3$CMgI yielded a product having α-orientation of the CH$_3$ moiety (23). This assignment was, however, based on the extrapolation of NMR features for the 15α-cyanopuupehenol (X) to (23). Exactly in a similar fashion the interaction of puupehenone with ethyl-magnesium bromide produced 15α-ethylpuupehenol (24).

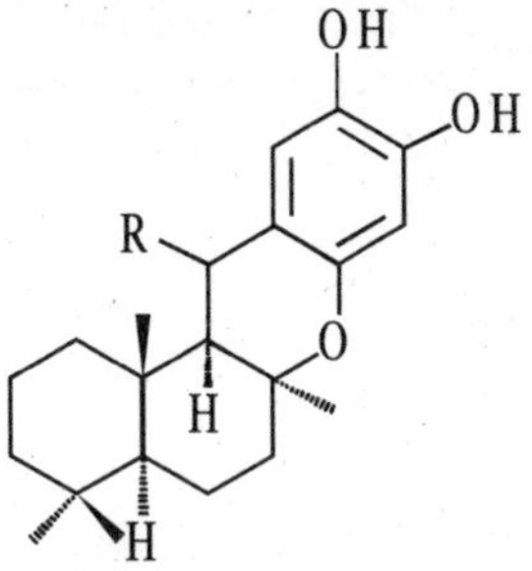

23 : R = α-CH₃;
24 : R = α-C₂H₅;
25 : R = β-CH₃;
26 : R = β-C₂H₅;

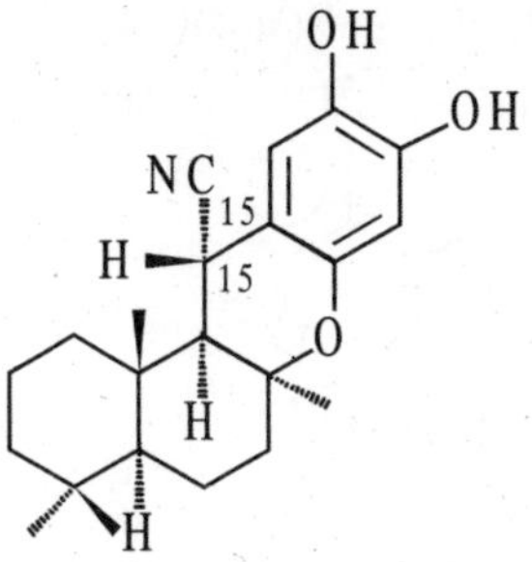

15α-Cyanopuupehenol
X

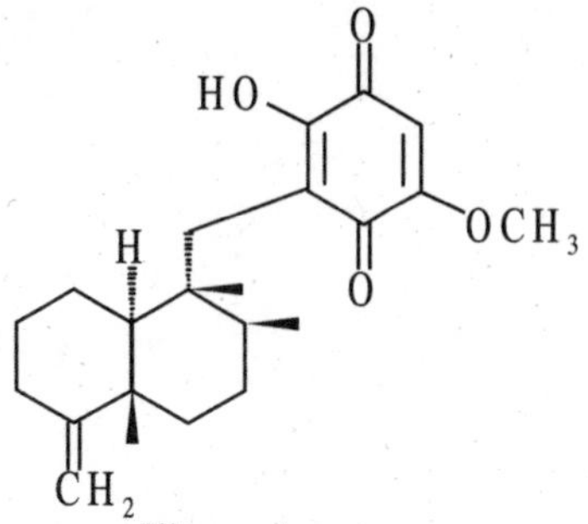

Ilimaquinone
18A

(*b*) **Puupehenone (19)** on being treated with a large excess of H_3C MgI in an ethereal medium, significant decomposition of (19) took place, another **stereochemically different isomer of (23)** was isolated, which has been named as **15β-methyl puupehenol (25).** In an identical treatment with ethyl magnesium iodide ($H_5 C_2$ MgI), gave rise to the corresponding **15β-ethylpuupehenol (26).** However, till date no logical explanation could be forwarded for the formation of the two isomeric species *viz.*, (25) and (26).

Protection of the *two* free -OH moieties present in (23) and (24) by means of acetylation yielded the **stable diacetyl derivatives (27) and (28)** as given below:

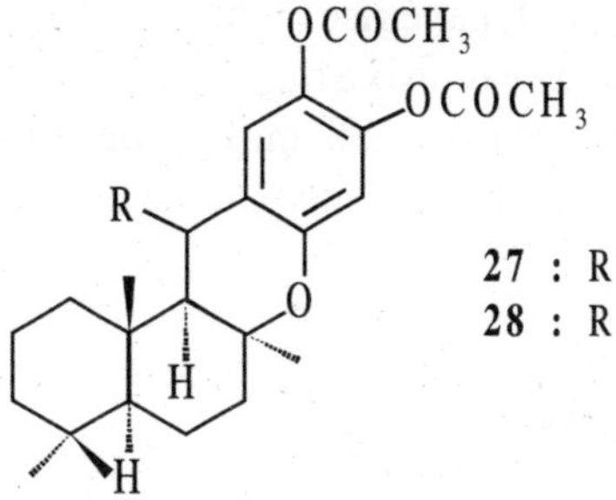

27 : R = α— CH₃;
28 : R = α— C₂H₅;

10.3.2.3 Cyanide and Methoxide Nucleophiles: 1, 6-Conjugate Addition

The probability of the interaction between **puupehenone (19)** with hydrogen cyanide (HCN) in the biological systems formed the basis of an extensive and intensive studies *in vitro* under different aqueous and methanolic experimental parameters. Investigations, revealed that 1, 6-cunjugated nucleophilic addition of HCN was essentially accompanied by oxidation in an environment where there was no restriction with regard to the availability of air/oxygen to the reaction mixture.

Puupehenone (19) in a methanolic solution on being subjected to complete saturation with 100 molar excess of absolutely dried HCN gas produced a quantitative yield of 15α-cyanopuupehenol (X). In order to render the compound (X) significantly stable, it was duly acetylated to give rise to *O*-19, 20-diacetyl-oxy-15α-cyanopuupehenol (29).

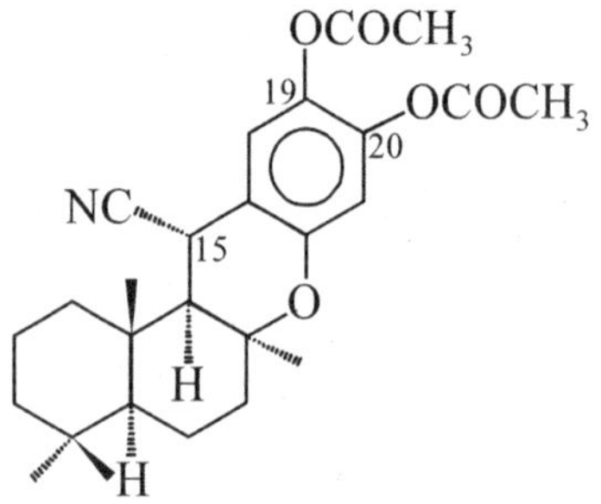

Interestingly, with a view to initiate and simulate the natural living environmental conditions of the sponge, **puupehenone (19)** was strategically combined to a *basic-sorbent,* **Florisil*** pH 8-8.5 in water, duly suspended in distilled-water and completely saturated with pure HCN gas. Thus, it resulted into the formation of **15α-cyanopuupehenol (X)** and **15-cyanopuupehenone (30)** eventually.

It has been observed that **15α-cyanopuupehenone (30)** was a secondary metabolite obtained along with **15α-cyanopuupehenol (X)** in the **Verongid Sponge.** However, it was also synthesized successfully and quantitatively in a direct, spontaneous addition-oxidation of **15α-cyanopuupehenol (X)** in an appropriate admixture of methanol and water at a slightly basic pH environment.

Quite contrarily, the acetylation of **15α-cyanopuupehenone (30)** in the presence of dry pyridine gave rise to the formation of its corresponding **monoacetyl structural analogue (31).**

The interaction of **puupehenone (19)** with **magnesium methoxide [(CH₃O)₂ Mg]** resulted in the conjugate addition of methoxide nucleophile with the production of the corresponding monoacetylated product **15-methoxypuupehenol (32).** Further acetylation of (32) with an appreciable large excess of acetic anhydride [(CH₃CO)₂O] gave rise to the corresponding diacetylated derivative (33), which was subsequently isolated as the exclusive major product. Interestingly, compound (33) may also be obtained by the direct addition of methanol to **puupehenone (19)** at an ambient temperature for a duration of 24 hours, and subsequently subjected to acetylation.

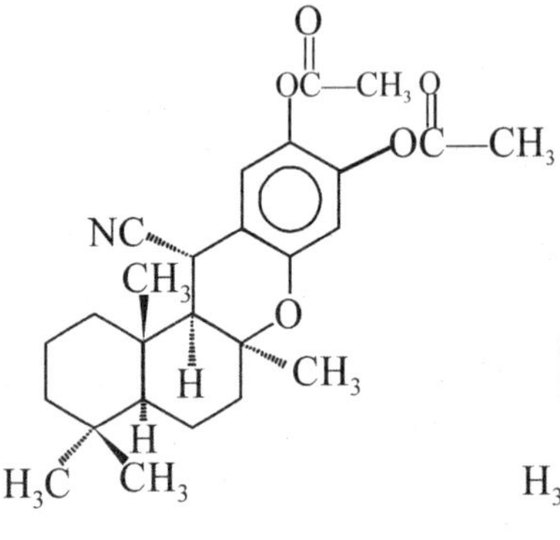

O-19, 20-Diacetyl-oxy-
15α-Cyanopuupehenol
29

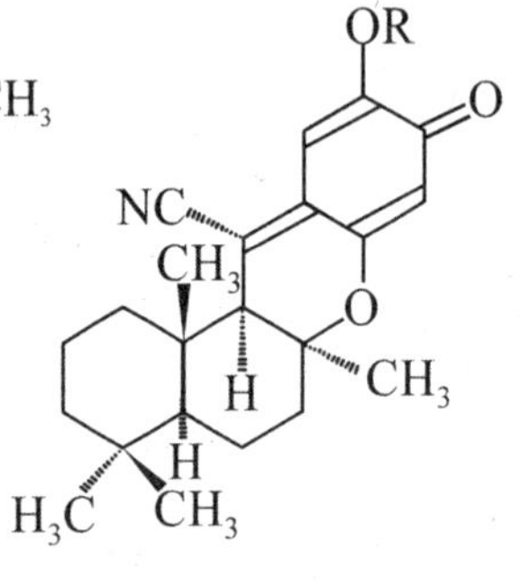

30: R = H (15-Cyanopuupe-
henone)
31: R = OCOCH₃

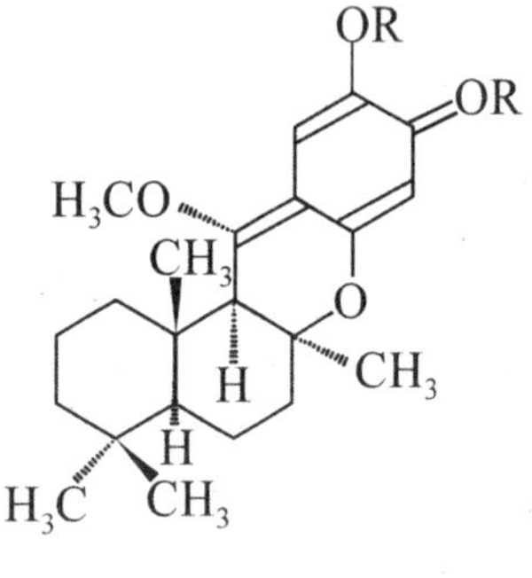

32: R = H (15-Methoxy-
puupehenol)
33: R = OCOCH₃

---

* **Florisil:** A basic-sorbent comprised of activated magnesium silicate-a hard porous granular substance available in variant pH ranges.

10.3.2.4 *Nitroalkane Nucleophiles: Addition Reactions*

Generally, the acidic a-hydrogen bearing compounds were logically employed as **Potential nucleophilic donors** for the addition reactions pertaining to the extension of 1, 6-conjugate system of puupehenone (19). The addition reactions were carried out by making use of **nitromethane [CH$_3$—NO$_2$]** and **nitroethane [C$_2$H$_5$—NO$_2$]** which were reacted with the stoichiometric proportions of **magnesium methoxide [(CH$_3$O)$_2$ Mg]** and the resulting generated ucleophiles were finally added to a solution of **puupehenone (19)** in pure dry benzene. The addition products thus obtained were subsequently subjected to acetylation with actic anhydride [(CH$_3$CO)$_2$O] and finally purified to obtain compounds *O*-19, 20-diacetyl-Oxy-15α-nitromethanepuupehenol (34); and *O*-19, 20-diacetyl-Oxy-15a-nitroethanepuupehenol (35) as given below:

34 : R = H; O-19, 20-Diacetyl-Oxy-15 α-Nitromethanepuupehenol
35 : R = CH$_3$; O-19, 20-Diacetyl-Oxy-15α-Nitroethanepuupehenol

10.4 SUMMARY

In short, the **'marine-world'** evidently and explicitly enjoys the status of holding an enormous and tremendous potential towards the epoch making discovery of a plethora of altogether newer **'lead compounds'** in the development of medicinally potent therapeutic agents that are active against a variety of parasites and infections ailments. The wide range of vat resources tapped from the marine fauna and flora that would certainly help in the evolution of previously known **'chemotypes'** for stemming the influx of crucial drug-resistant microorganisms and insects. In order to explore, tap and above all exploit commercially the relatively virgin biological reserves exclusively depends on the use of rapid technological advancement towards their collection, preservation, identification, and characterization of trace quantum of essential secondary metabolites.

With the advent of recent development and notable advances legitimately accomplished in comparatively safer life-support systems; and amalgamated with most recent technologically advanced computer-aided **sophisticated a nalytical instrumentations***, such as: UPTLC; HPLC; LC-MS;

---

* **HPTLC** = High performance thin-layer chromatography.
  HPLC   = High performance liquid chromatography
  LC-MS = Liquid chromatography-Mass spectroscopy

GC; GC-MS; NMR; 2 D-NMR; FTIR; UV; X-Ray Diffraction; and MS have turned this novel dream-like fiction into a stark reality.

FURTHER READING REFERENCES

1. Baslow, M.H.: **'Marine Pharmaceuticals'**, Williams & Wilkins, Baltimore, 1969.
2. Baker, J., and V. Murphy: **'Handbook of Marine Sciences'**, CRC Press, Cleveland, 1976.
3. Blunt JW and Munro MHG: **Marinlit—A Database of the Literature on Marine Natural Products,** University of Canterbury, 1997.
4. Dewick, P.M.: **'Medicinal Natural Products'**, John Wiley & Sons, Ltd., England, 2nd edn., 2002.
5. D. Chuck Dunbar: **Discovery of Antimalarial Compounds from Marine Inverteprates,** Ph.D. Thesis, University of Mississipi, Oxford, 1996.
6. El Sayed KA *et al., J. Agric. Food Chem.,* **45:** 2735, 1997.
7. Hoppe, H.A. and T. Levring: **'Marine Algae in Pharmaceutical Sciences'**, Vol. 2, de Gruyter, Berlin, 1982.
8. Martin, D., and G. Padilla: **'Marine Pharmacognosy'**, Academic Press, New York, 1973.
9. Nigrelli, R.F.: **'Biochemistry and Pharmacology of Compounds Derived from Marine Organisms'**, Ann. NY Acad. Sc., New York, 1960.
10. Scheuer, P.J.: **'Chemistry of Marine Natural Products'**, Academic Press, New York, 1973.
11. Tursch, B., J.C. : **'Chemistry of Marine Natural Products'**, Vol.2., Academic Press, New York, 1978.
12. Webber, H.H. and G. D. Ruggieri: **'Food Drugs from the Sea Procedings'**, Marine Technol. Soc., Washington, DC, 1976.
13. Worthen, L.R.: **'Food Drugs fom the Sea Proceedings'**, Marine Technol. Soc., Washington, D.C., 1972.
14. Youngken, H.W.: **'Food Drugs from the Sea Proceedings'**, Marine Technol. Soc., Washington, DC, 1969.

GC	=	Gas chromatography
GC-MS	=	Gas chromatography-Mass spectrometry
NMR	=	Nuclear magnetic resonance
2D-NMR	=	Two Dimensional-NMR (or COSY-NMR)
FTIR	=	Fourier transform infrared spectrometry
UV	=	Ultra-violet spectrophotometry
MS	=	Mass spectrometry

11 _____ Nutraceuticals

11.1 INTRODUCTION

Nutraceuticals may be defined as—'*any substance that may belong to a plant, food or an essential component of food providing definitive medicinal usefulness and health promotion as well as physiological benefits, and ultimately minimise the possible risk of the prevailing chronic disease significantly.*'

In the recent past, **nutraceuticals** have legitimately and overwhelmingly acclaimed enormous confidence, acceptance, and recognition amongst the mankind not only as a mere '**health promoting factor**' but also as an excellent '**nutritional contributing factor**'. The ever-increasing comprehensive knowledge with respect to the '**natural inherent nutritive value**' of a relatively large number of *food products*, their chemical constituents *vis-a-vis* biological values has virtually succeeded in combating the human ailments and sufferings to an appreciable extent across the globe.

The wonderful conceptualization of the phrase—'**Mediterranean Cuisine**' by the so called **Western Nutritional Wizards** have implanted ideas or habits by constant urging in their daily food-intakes of such items as: **srpouted beans and lentils, olive-oil-salad with raw vegetables, citrous juices, whole-wheat bread, red/white wines, and extensive usage of garlic, ginger, onion, mustard, and tomato pastes as food-additives.** On the contrary, the **Eastern Nutritional Experts** overwhelmingly advocate the profuse usage of such delicious food items and beverages as: **green-tea, unfermented palm-wine, brined and smoked fish, soyabean milk, soyabean yogurt (curd), fibrous raw fruits and vegetables.**

In a broader perspective one may consider the '**nutraceuticals**' to exert their action synergistically to check deteriorating health conditions, protect cells, and finally to ward off human ailments significantly. In reality, the '**nutraceuticals**' have strategically captured the noticeable professional curiosity of a host of disciplines, namely: health care, food and nutritional scientists, the processed food manufacturers, the pharmaceutical industries, and above all the dietary supplement conglomerates.

Relief from Major Diseases: Nutraceuticals are intimately associated with the **relief, prevention** and/or **treatment** of certain specific and well-known major diseases, such as: coronary diseases, diabetes, cancer, hypertension, nervous debility, impaired digestive problems, and the like. A few other related ailments are: acute arthritis, joint pains, osteoporosis, neural tube problems.

Emergence: **Stephen Defelice*** almost a decade ago vehemently opined that **nutraceutical** is a particular component, for instance: omega oil from salmon (a fish), chenopodium ambrosiodos, pudina oil, tulsi, neem, soy, and orange juice with calcium. It is an universal fact that both **'food'** and **'medicine'** are exclusively based upon *three* vital and important characteristic features, namely:

(*i*) significance to health,
(*ii*) efficacy, and
(*iii*) safety.

Legacy: The history of **'nutraceutical'** dates back to more than 200 years, even though there have been significantly enormous wonderful discoveries accomplished in the field of medicines in the past six decades. The world recognizes the meaningful and excellent progress *vis-a-vis* tremendous achievements in the domain of **science** and **herbal medicines** specifically at a very early stage. The well-known Indian system of **'Ayurveda'** proved to be a main source and provided several techniques whereby many dreadful diseases could be erradicated/cured from a human being. An extensive survey of literature shall reveal that the **'nutraceuticals'** actually came into being around 1500 AD even when people were not really aware about the term **'nutraceutical'**. Several races in the world have generously and profusely contributed towards the phenomenal success, acceptance, and recognition of **'nutraceuticals',** namely: Greeks, Africans, Chinese, Tibetans, Indians, Arabs, Japanese, Thais, Malaysians, Ceylonese, Burmese etc.

Functional Food *Vs* Nutraceutical

Functional Food may be defined as—**"the food usually prepared by the aid of 'scientific intelligence' using definite knowledge about its anticipated merit/usefulness."** In this manner, the **functional food** essentially caters to the body with the necessary quantum of vital carbohydrates, fats, proteins and vitamins, etc, required for its normal as well as healthy survival.

Examples: Vegetables, rice, wheat, fruits, pulses, fish, eggs, poultry products, beef, meat etc.

Nutraceutical may be defined as—**"a food (or a portion of a food) that essentially provides distinct health and medical benefits, even including the prevention and/or treatment of a particular disease."****

Examples: Fortified **'dairy products'** *eg.*, milk powder, baby food, malted milk food; **vitamic C enriched citrus fruits** *eg.*, orange juice, grape juice.

Dietary Supplement***: Based on a number of criteria obtained from the **FDA/CF-SAN Resources,** one may define a **'dietary supplement'** as:

• intended solely to supplement the diet which essentially contains either one or more than one of such dietary requirements as: vitamin, mineral, herb or other botanical product, amino acid,

---

* Stephen Defelice MD., the Founder and Chairman of the private non-profit foundation for **'Innovation in Medicine'** Cranford, NJ, USA, first and foremost coined the term **'pharmaceutical.'**

** Brower V: **Nutraceuticals poised for a healthy slice of the healthcare market.,** *Nat. Biotechnol.,* **16:** 728-31, 1998.

*** FDA/CF SAN-Resources: Food and Drug Administration Web Site. Dietary Supplement Health and Education Act of 1994. [Available at: http://vm.cfsan.fdagm./adms/dietsupp.html.]

dietary ingredient for use by human being to supplement the diet by enhancing the total daily intake, or constituent extract, metabolite concentrate, or various combinations of these ingredients.

- represented for usage as a conventional food or as the exclusive component of a meal or diet.
- intended for ready ingestion in the form of a pill, tablet, capsule, or liquid form.
- labeled explicitly as a **'dietary supplement'**.
- includes essentially such products as: approved **'new drug'**, licensed biological product (*i.e.*, marketed solely as a dietary supplement etc.

11.2 PHYTOCHEMICALS AS NUTRACEUTICALS

In the recent past several newer terminologies have emerged gainfully, noticeably, and widely across the globe to represent strategically the innumerable **nutrients of the future,** namely: **'Phytochemicals'; 'Nutraceuticals'; 'Phytonutrients'; 'Phytofoods',** and **'Functional Foods'.** Importantly, the advent of accumulated knowledge with respect to the **disease-preventing components** present specifically in the natural plant products used as foods are duly recognized as **'nutraceuticals'.**

Nevertheless, **'phytochemicals'** represent a rather more recent evolution of the terminology which categorically emphasizes the inherent plant-source of a relatively larger segment of these important **disease-preventing and protective** chemical entities. In true sense, the potential nutritional role for the **'phytochemicals'** is gaining world-wide recognition and popularity based upon the aggressive on-going research activities specifically highlighting their wonderful and remarkable advantages. The term **'phytonutrient'** expatiates the natural chemical compound's status as **'quasinutrient'.** May be in the near future one would soon encounter the so called **'phytochemicals'** most justifiably as the **'essential nutrients'.**

Researches and other authentic scientific evidences have overwhelmingly revealed that the longivity of our ancestors perhaps could be due to their **correct importance of diet to health** *i.e.* devoid of today's so called 'junk-food', foods laced with chemical additives, preservatives, flavour enhancers, emulsifiers, stabilizers, and the like, which ultimately prevented them succumb to the **'modern diseases'.** A lot of such evidences may be distinctly observed amongst the **'centenarian tribes'** that live in remote **Andean villages** (*i.e.*, Andes Mountains), tribes living in Andaman-Nicobar Islands, tribes living in remote interior villages in African continent etc., who invariably embrace strict and rigid **'traditional dietary practices'.** Obviously, these **'people'** have been duly reported to live extraordinarily **much longer live-spans** which are certainly free of such dreadful human ailments like: heart diseases, cancer, arthritis, respiratory obstructions, impairment in eye-sight etc.

Based on the aforesaid statement of facts together with the stark reality that even as to date a certain small segment of people usually live as **'naturally'** as do the said tribes in the remote Andean villages, researchers have adequately proclaimed **epidemiological*** evidence from **'modern societies'** for definitive clues pertaining to the intricacies of the actual **diet-disease connection.** Importantly, such elaborated and intensive studies helped a long way to the **biochemical researchers** to identify

---

* **Epidemiology:** It is concerned with the traditional study of epidemic diseases caused by infections agents, and with health-related phenomena.

and establish certain **'phytochemicals'** that prominently aid the human body towards **'maintaining a perfect health'**, and also **'combating diseases'**.

Health authorities* recommend an overall guideline for the consumption of such specific diets that are significantly rich in whole grains, fresh fruits, fresh vegetables, reduced fat intake, and animal-protein consumption.

The good number of **phytochemicals** that find their abundant and legitimate use as **Nutraceuticals** may be judiciously classified as enumerated under with typical examples and appropriate plausible explanations wherever necessary.

11.2.1 Terpenoids (or Isoprenoids)

Terpenoids (or **Isoprenoid**) may be defined as—**'any compound either biosynthesized from or containing isoprene** unt** units, including terpenes, carotenoids, fat-soluble vitamins, ubiquinone, rubber and even some steroids.'**

The **Terpenoids** are classified into various categories as described below:

11.2.1.1 Carotenoid Terpenoids

Carotenoids refer to natural compounds that usually render corn yellow, carrots reddish-orange, and tomatos red. Besides, they impart typical distinct natural characteristic colours to gold fish, flamingo, salmon, and also the autumn leaves (*i.e.*, when the nature's green **chlorophyll** get depleted significantly, the carotenoids and phenols remain. They are also found in **Bell-peppers** with different colours that invariably represent a **selection of carotenoids,** namely:

(*a*) **Orange carotenoids** *e.g.*, α-, β-, and γ-carotene.
(*b*) **Red carotenoids** *e.g.*, lycopene and astaxanthin.
(*c*) **Yellow carotenoids** *e.g.*, lutein and zeaxanthin.

As to date approximately **600 carotenoids** have been duly isolated, purified, and characterized in the plant kingdom.

Important Points: The following **important points** need to be considered—

- Nearly half of approximately **fifty carotenoids** that are usually present in the **'normal human diet'** are adequately absorbed into the blood stream.
- Almost 30% of the **actual plasma carotenoids** are duly comprised each of **lycopene** and **β-carotene.**
- Conversion to **Vitamin A** is afforded exclusively by **α-carotene, β-carotene**, and a few **other carotenes** (but **not lycopene** or **lutein**).
- **Hypervitaminosis of Vitamin A** may not be caused due to the excessive intake of **α-carotene** or **β-carotene** by virtue of the fact that the ensuing conversion and absorption rates are exceedingly slow and sluggish.

  Importantly, both **α-carotene** and **β-carotene** deemed to afford reasonable protection against two

---

* Drgsted LO *et al. Pharmacology and Toxicology,* 72 Suppl. **1:** 116-35, 1993.
** **Isoprene:** An unsaturated branched chain, 5C hydrocarbon *i.e.*, the molecular unit of the isoprenoid compounds.

dreadful human diseases *viz.*, **liver cancer** and **lung cancer** as established by extensive and intensive animal and cell culture investigative studies.

- Free liberation of **carotenoids** *viz.*, **lycopene, β-carotene** from vegetables may be accomplished by heating, chopping and/or crushing.
- Significant absorption of **carotenoids** may be observed when they are associated with oils as these are practically insoluble in water.
- **Carotenoids** present in the blood-stream are found to be transported in the most lipid-rich **(LDL*)** cholesterol particles; and, therefore, the tissues having relatively the most abundant **LDL receptors** invariably acquire the most **carotenoid.**
- **α-carotene** possesses essentially 50-54% of the **antioxidant activity** of **β-carotene,** whereas **epsilon carotene** bears 42-50% of the said activity.
- **Carotenes**, in general, also increase appreciably the **immune response** and afford adequate protection to **skin-cells against UV-radiation** (*i.e.*, incorporated in **'Sun-Creams'** profusely).

Following are some of the **typical examples** of **carotenoid terpenoids** together with their **characteristic features,** such as:

1. **Lycopene [Synonyms: ψψ-Carotene; (*all trans*-Lycopene):**

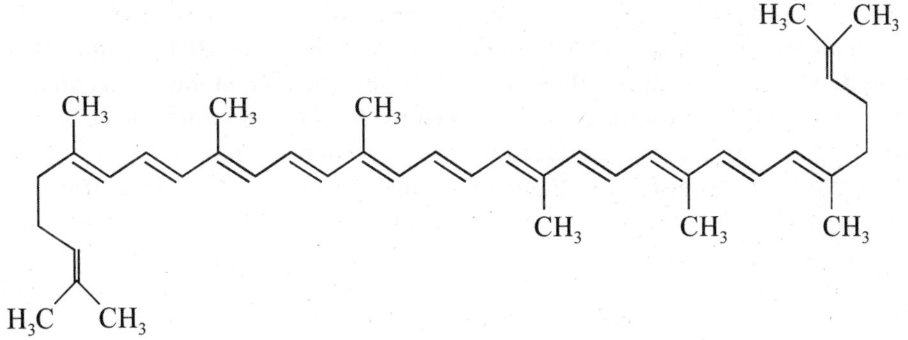

Characteristic Features: These are as given under:

  (*i*) Red colouration of tomatoes, guava, papaya, watermelon, pink grape fruit
 (*ii*) **Lycopene** in the usual and common **'American Diet'** is often derived from **tomato-containing food products.**
(*iii*) Naturally occurring *trans*-Lycopene gets poorly absorbed in the body.
 (*iv*) Conversion of the *trans*-isomer to the *cis*-isomer in the presence of **heat** and **light** actually enhances the latter's bioavailability.
  (*v*) Gets bound to the fibers intimately and tightly—as freed duly by high heat.
 (*vi*) **Lycopene** is found to be more soluble in oil than in an aqueous medium.
(*vii*) **Tomato paste** affords four-fold **'bioavailability'** in comparison to the **fresh tomatoes.**
(*viii*) A **powerful antioxidant** that categorically retards damage caused to DNA and proteins.
 (*ix*) Offers distinctly and appreciably much better **skin protection** against the **UV-light** than β-carotene.

---

* **LDL:** Low-density lipoprotein.

  (*x*) Almost represents **50%** of the total available **carotenoids** found in the **blood serum.**

 (*xi*) **Lycopene** specifically gets accumulated in the various segments of the human-body *viz.*, skin, adrenal glands, prostrate glands, testes etc., thereby rendering adquate protection against **cancer.**

(*xii*) Helps to reduce **LDL-cholesterol levels** considerably.

(*xiii*) **Lycopene** noticeably arrests the **Insulin-like Growth Factor-1 (IGF-1)** stimulation of cancerous (tumour) growth.

   2. **β-Carotene [Synonym: β, β-Carotene; Carotaben; Provatene; Solatene;]:**

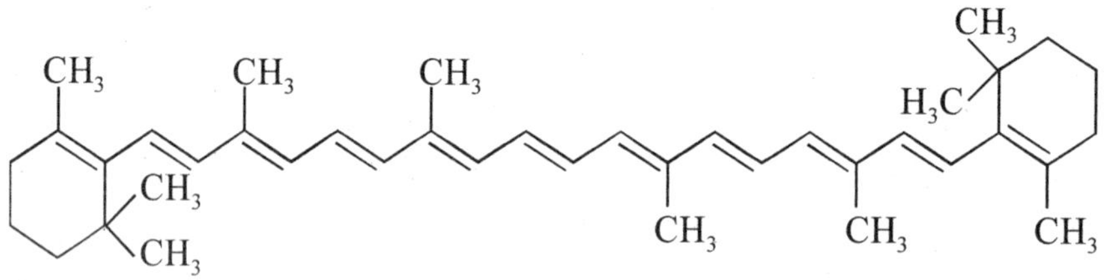

Characteristic Features: The **characteristic features** are as given under:

  (*i*) It is a weak **antioxidant***, but prove to be strong against singlet oxygen.

 (*ii*) The supplements may enrich **LDL-cholesterol-β-carotene content** without affecting other **carotene variants** *e.g.*, **α-carotene; ε, ψ-carotene (or δ-carotene); γ-carotene.**

(*iii*) It may significantly boost the activity of **Natural Killer (NK) immune cells.**

(*iv*) It may appreciably cause **stimulation for the DNA-repair enzymes.**

 (*v*) It definitely provides distinctly better **cornea protection** against the **harmful UV-radiation** (from sun-rays or UV-tubes) in comparison to **lycopene.**

   3. **α-Carotene:**

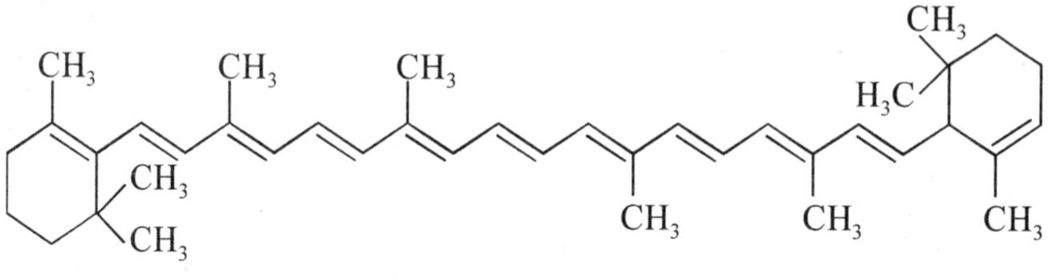

Characteristic Features: The characteristic features are:

  (*i*) It has proved to be almost **ten fold more anti-carcinogenic** in comparison to **β-carotene.**

 (*ii*) It distinctly increases the release of **immunogenic IL-1**** and **TNF-α.*****

---

   * **Antioxidant:** A naturally occurring or synthetic substance that helps protect cells from the damaging effects of oxygen free radicals, and highly reactive compounds formed during normal cell metabolism.

  ** **Immunogenic IL-1:** Immunogenic interleukin-1.

*** **TNF-α:** Tumour necrosis factor-alpha.

4. **Xanthophyll [Synonyms: Lutein; β, ε-Carotene-3, 3′-diol; Vegetable lutein; Vegetable luteol; Bo-Xan;]:**

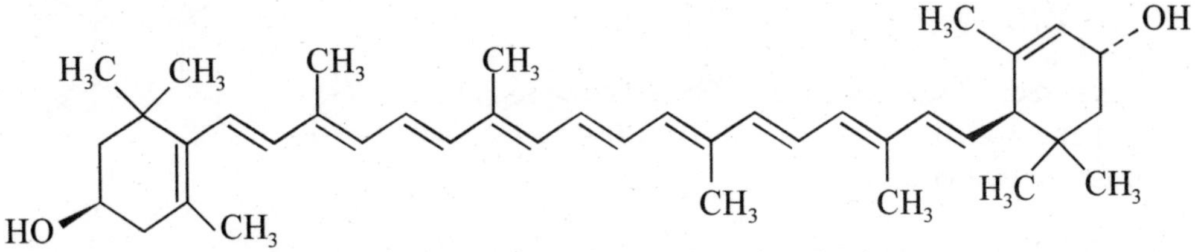

Characteristic Features: The characteristic features of **xanthophyll (lutein)** are as stated under:

(*i*) **Xanthophylls** are important by virtue of the fact that thcy seem to cause protection of **Vitamin A, Vitamin E** and **other carotenoids** from undergoing oxidation *in vivo*.

(*ii*) Substantial evidence is emerging gradually that **xanthophylls** are highly tissue specific.* **Example: Cryptoxanthin,** which appears to be highly protective of cervical, uterine, and vaginal tissues.

(*iii*) **Lutein** and **zeaxanthin** almost comprise of nearly 50% of all **carotenoids** present strategically in the retina.

(*iv*) Likewise, both **leutin** and **zeaxanthin** are the **carotenoids** exclusively present in the **macula**** of the eye.

(*v*) It seems to protect the eye from macular degeneration and cataracts.

(*vi*) It may also render protection against colon cancer.

(*vii*) It imparts **'yellow colour'** to avagado, corn, and yolk of an egg.

(*viii*) Abundantly found in **kale, spinach, watercress,** and **parsley.**

5. **Zeaxanthin [Synonyms: β, β-Carotene -3, 3′-diol;** *all-trans*-β-Carotene -3, 3′-diol; **Zeaxanthol; Anchovyxanthin;]:**

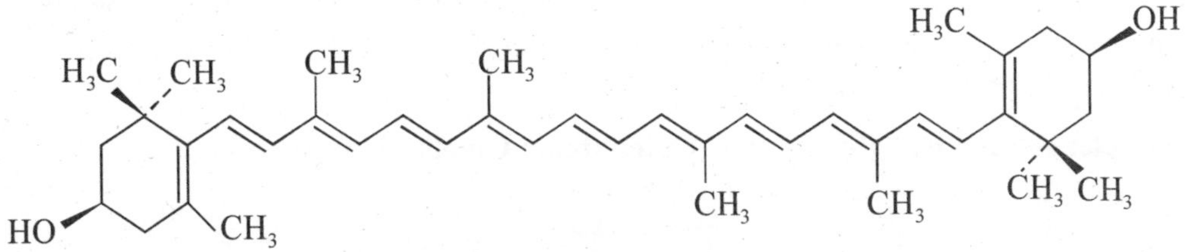

Characteristic Features: These are as given below:

(*i*) **Zeaxanthin** and **lutein** are the only **carotenoids** that are located strategically in the macula of the eye.

(*ii*) Both **zeaxanthin** and **leutin** are almost present in equal quantum in the macula.

(*iii*) It essentially absorbs the damaging **'blue-lighty'.**

(*iv*) It helps to protect the eyes from possible macular degeneration and cataracts.

---

* Parker RS, *J. Nutr.*: **119:** 101-4, Jan.-1989.

** A small spot of coloured area.

6. **Astaxanthin [Synonyms: Ovoester; 3,3′-Dihydroxy-4, 4′-diketo-β-carotene]:**

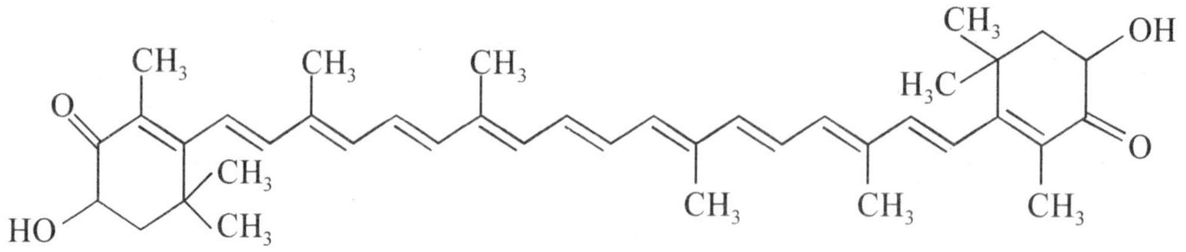

Characteristic Features: The various **characteristic features** of **astaxanthin** are as stated under:

(*i*) It altributes a beautiful pinkish red colour to crab, salmon, and shrimp.

(*ii*) **Astaxanthin** is found to be ten folds more powerful antioxidant in comparison to any other **carotenoid.**

(*iii*) It not only augments the **T-cell production*** but also helps in the release of **cytokine.**

(*iv*) It may also cross the **blood-brain barrier (BBB)** *i.e.*, it serves as a **brain-antioxidant.**

(*v*) It possesses **water-soluble chemical entities** that eventually helps to release the trapped radicals to **Vitamin C.**

11.2.2 Non-Carotenoid Terpenoids

The **non-carotenoid terpenoids** usually do have rather simpler chemical structures. They may be categorized into the following sub-groups, such as:

11.2.2.1 Limonoids [or Terpene Limonoids]

In general, the **limonoids** are particularly found in the peels (*i.e.* outer skins) of several citrus fruits *e.g.*, oranges, mandarins, lemons, grape fruits etc., that specifically directed to the ultimate protection of the lung tissue. the above findings were duly established by means of an elaborated study employing a standardized extract of *d*-**limonene, pinene,** and **eucalyptol** which was fond to be effective in removing grossly the '**congestive** mucous from the lungs of patients having a history of **chronic obstructive pulmonary disease.**

Example: *d*-**Limonene [Synonyms: Cajeputene; Cinene; Kautschin]:**

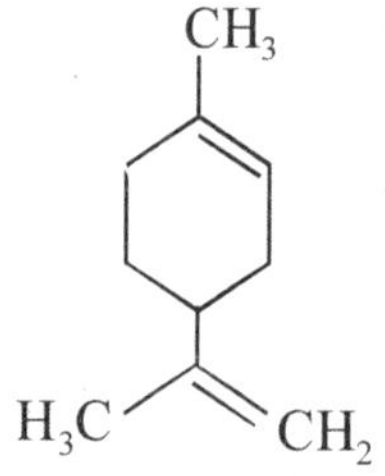

---

* **T-Cells:** T lymphocytes that are differentiated in the thymus and are virtually important in **cell-mediated immunity (CMI),** besides in the regulation of **antibody-mediated immunity (AMI).**

Characteristic Features: These are as stated below:

(*i*) *d*-**Limonene** is found to be 45 times more anticarcinogenic in comparison to **hesperetin.**

(*ii*) It specifically detoxifies the carcinogenic substances, and thereby promotes the ensuing **cancer cell apoptosis*.**

(*iii*) **Limonene** distinctly helps to promote the **'glutathione-S-transferase'** *i.e.*, refers to **detoxification by glutathione addition.**

(*iv*) *d*-**Limonene** has a distinct **orange-like smell;** whereas *l*-**Limonene** possesses a **piney odour** (very much akin to **turpentine**).

11.2.2.2 α-Terpineol

$$CH_3$$

$$H_3C \quad CH_3$$
$$OH$$

Characteristic Features: These are as given below:

(*i*) **α-Terpineol** gives rise to the peculiar carrot flavour to the fresh carrots.

(*ii*) It causes critical arrest of the **'cell-cycle'** in the neoplasmic cells (*i.e.*, cancer cells).

11.2.2.3 Saponins

Saponins represent a group of **amorphous colloidal glycosides** that usually form soapy aqueous solutions.

A number of **'Saponin Glycosides'** have been discussed in details in Chapter 4, and a few typical examples along with their cardinal usages have been given as under:

S.No.	Name	Characteristic Features
(*a*)	**Shatavarin I-IV** [Section: 4.2.8.1.3]	(*i*) Used as galactogogue to promote the flow of milk. (*ii*) Also employed as tonic and diuretic.
(*b*)	**Ginsenoside Rg** [Section: 4.2.8.2.1]	(*i*) In **Chinese System of Medicine** as a general tonic, stimulant and carminative. (*ii*) It possesses **'antistress'** properties. (*iii*) It prolongs the life of elderly persons.
(*c*)	**Glycyrrhizin** [Section: 4.2.8.2.2.]	(*i*) It is used as a flavouring agent in beverages and confectionary. (*ii*) Possesses remarkable expectorant properties.
(*d*)	**Amarogentin** [Section: 4.2.10.2	(*i*) It is used as a bitter tonic in anorexia. (*ii*) It also improves relatively the **'dull appetite'.**

* **Apoptosis:** A pattern of cell death affecting single cells, marked by shrinkage of the cell, condensation of chromatin, and fragmentation of the cell into membrane-bound bodies that are eliminated by phagocytosis (*i.e.*, programmed cell death).

11.2.3 Polyphenolics [or Polyphenol Extracts]

Polyphenolics (or **Polyphenol Extracts)** essentially represent a host of **natural antioxidants,** used as **nutraceuticals,** and found in **apples, green-tea,** and **red-wine** for their enormous ability to combat cancer and are also thought to prevent heart ailments to an appreciable degree.

Polyphenolics may be judiciously classified as given below:

(*a*) Flavonoid polyphenolics,
(*b*) Phenolic acids,
(*c*) Non-Flavonoid polyphenolies.

11.2.3.1 Flavonoid Polyphenolics

Flavonoids are actually **flavone-like** substances which are invariably **antioxidants** and sometimes as **anti-inflammatory agents.**

Mechanism of Action: Flavonoids exert their activity by carefully scavenging the '**free-radicals'** thereby giving rise to a fairly '**stable radical'** which in turn would undergo reaction with another '**flavonoid radical'** to yield **two non-radicals.**

Red wine contains *two* important constituents, namely: **Flavone,** and **Resveratrol** because it is prepared by carrying out the fermentation of the '**pulp'** along with the skin and seeds (though '**ultrafiltration'** is done to minimise both bitterness and astringency); whereas, the **white wine** lacks the said two components because it is usually made by pressing juice away from the solids.

Flavone   Resveratrol

Various **citrus fruits** invariably contain a host of **flavanoids,** such as: **rutin, hesperidin,** and **naringin.**

Rutin   Hesperidin   Naringin

A few typical examples of **flavonoid polyphenolics** are stated below together with their **characteristic features.**

11.2.3.2 Anthocyanins

The term **anthrocyanin** was coined to assign the chemical substance actually responsible for attributing the typical colour of the cornflower (from the **Greek:** *anthos* = flower, and *kuanos* = blue) generally applicable to a group of water-soluble pigments contributing the **red, pink, mauve, purple,** blue, or violet colour of a plethora of fruits and flowers. All these wide-range of pigments invariably come into being as **'glycosides'** (*i.e.*, the **anthocyanins**), and their corresponding **aglycones** (*i.e.*, the **anthocyanidins**); and these are actually derived from the **2-phenylbenzopyrylium cation,** more frequently known as the **flavylium cation.** Interestingly, the nomenclature **'flavylium cation'** categorically emphasis the fact these molecules usually belong to the vast category of the **'flavonoids'** in the broader perspective of the said terminology.

Anthocyanins, whose distinct beautiful explicit colours invariably attract insects and birds; and, therefore, mostly play an important and vital role in the phenomenon of **'pollination** and **'seed-dispersal'.**

Anthocyanins, are water-soluble **glycosides** and **acyl-glycosides of anthocyanidins.** The structure of *six* major **anthocyanidins,** namely: **Cyanidin, Delphinidin, Malvidin, Pelargonidin, Peonidin, Petunidin**—are as given under:

1. **Cyanidin:** R_1 = OH; R_2 = H;
2. **Delphinidin:** R_1 = R_2 = OH;
3. **Malvidin:** R_1 = R_2 = CH_3;
4. **Pelargonidin:** R_1 = R_2 = H;
5. **Peonidin:** R_1 = OCH_3; R_2 = H;
6. **Petunidin:** R_1 = OCH_3; R_2 = OH;

Structures of Major Anthocyanidins

Proanthocyanidins (or **Pycnogenols**) are found to be the short-chained colourless polymers of **anthocyanidins** which usually release the **anthocyanins** either with the **application of heat** or on being subjected to **acidic hydrolysis.**

Characteristic Features: These are as stated under:

(*i*) **Anthocyanins** usually occur in several varieties of **berries** *e.g.*, blackberries, blueberries, black raspberries. In **blueberries** their content actually increases as they get ripened.

(*ii*) White grapes invariably are devoid of any colour due to the fact that they do not have **anthocyanins.**

(*iii*) Abundantly present in **Green Tea** which is consumed profusely by the Chinese and the Japanese.

(*iv*) **Anthocyanins** usually occur in conjunction with the **phenolic acids** in a good number of berries.

(*v*) **Anthocyanins** remarkably protect the **endothelial cells*** from undergoing **oxidative damages** specifically.

---

* **Endothelial Cells:** The layer of epithelial cells that lines the cavities of the heart, the serous cavities, and the lumina of the blood and lymph vessels.

11.2.3.3 Catechin [Synonyms: Catechol; Catechinic Acid; Catechuic Acid; Dexcyanidanol; Cyanidol; Catergen;]

The family of **polyphenolic compounds** usually comprise of *two* types of molecules, namely:

(a) **Monomeric molecules**—which includes: **catechin** and **epicatechin,** and

(b) **Dimeric molecules**—that includes: **procyanidins B1 and B2.**

Characteristic Features: The various **characteristic features** of **catechin** are as enumerated under:

(i) It is an **antioxidant** found in dark, chocolate.

(ii) It is thermo-labile and hence gets lost while drying grapes to obtain raisins.

(iii) **Catechin** particularly affords inhibition of the **catechol-O-methyl transferase norepinephrine degredation.**

(iv) It categorically **enhances the metabolic rate** *i.e.*, helps to '**burn fat**' while substantially increasing the production of free-radical.

(v) **Catechin** can prevent and stop the initiation/progression of neoplasms (cancer).

(vi) It can protect againet the DNA damage; and, therefore, may prove to be of great help for patients undergoing post-operative **radiation therapy** or **chemotherapy.**

(vii) It is an **active constituent** present in **tea** [*Thea sinensis* (Linńe) O. Kuntze] *e.g.*, **green tea solids** range between 15-20%, and **black tea solids** vary between 5-10%.

(viii) It has been duly observed and established that (–) **epigallocatechin 3-O-gallate [EGCG]** is the **most abundant polyphenolic ingredient** found in **green-tea.**

EGCG

- **EGCG** may enhance the basal metabolic rate.
- **EGCG** inhibits the nitration of protein.
- **EGCG** is available in cranberries, and not in black tea.

(*ix*) **Catechins** undergo polymerization to yield **tannins** present in **black tea.**

(*x*) Tea drinking is intimately associated with lowered incidence of cancer in ovary, prostrate gland, stomach, color, and the buccal cavity.

(*xi*) **Catechins** inhibit NF-kB transcription of the ensuing **proinflammatory** and **antiapoptotic** (*i.e.*, **cancer-promoting**) **genes.**

(*xii*) **Theaflavins*** and **Thearubigins**** are the **taninns** obtained from tea, and represent the orange-red/black polymers.

Theaflavine

11.2.3.4 Isoflavones [or 3-Phenylchromone]

Daidzein: $R_1 = R_2 = H$; $R_3 = OH$;

Genistein: $R_1 = R_3 = OH$; $R_2 = H$;

Glycitein: $R_1 = H$; $R_2 = OCH_3$; $R_3 = OH$;

Phytonutrients of this phenol subclass, **isflavones,** usually are derived from **beans** and other **legumes,** which are more or less related to the **flavonoids.** Interestingly, the **isoflavones** invariably function very much similar to the **flavonoids** wherein they predominantly and effectively block the enzymes that essentially promote the tumour growth. The relatively important and well-known isoflavones are **Genistein** and **Daidzein** which are abundantly found in **soy products** and the herb *Pueraria lobata* (Kudzu). People who regularly consume traditiɔnal diets that are rich in soyfoods invariably do not suffer from **breast, uterine,** and **prostrate cancers.**

Pueraria lobata, over the years, have gained immense recognition and popularity as an essential aid for those who consume **'alcohol'** by virtue of the fact that it seems to change the prevailing activity of the specific **alcohol detoxification enzymes** *i.e.*, the speed and momentum at which the **alcohol dehydrogenase** converts **alcohol** into the corresponding aldehydes. The ultimate result is a reduced tolerance for alcohol, and lowering in the **'pleasure response'** to drinking it.***

---

* Obtained from black-tea extracts.

** Weakly acidic class of orange-brown phenolic pigments produced during the fermentation step of tea manufacture.

*** Xie CI *et al. Alcohol Clin Exp. Res.,* **18:** 1443-7, Dec.-1994.

Characteristic Features: These are as given under:

(*i*) **Isoflavones** are found in most concentrated manner in **soy beans** *viz.,* **daidzein, genistein, and glycitein** (upto 2-4 mg/g).

(*ii*) They are commonly found in **legumes** and **pomegranate seeds; besides, parsley and grains.**

(*iii*) The **'genistein'**—an **isoflavanone** inhibits specifically the **tyrosine kinases** involved in **tumorigenesis* (or oncogenesis).**

(*iv*) They help in the elevation of **HDL cholesterol** *i.e.,* **good cholesterol.**

(*v*) They specifically lower the **LDL cholesterol** *i.e.,* **bad cholesterol.**

(*vi*) **Isoflavones** usually serve as **potent antioxidants** against both **hydrogen peroxide** and **superoxide dismutase** (it serves as an anti-inflamatory and radioprotective agent).

(*vii*) **Isoflavone** possesses **estrogenic-like qualities** (*i.e.,* regarded as **phytoestrogen).**

(*viii*) In fact, the **lignans** and **isoflavones** are recognized as the two major groups of **phytoestrogens.**

(*ix*) They also go a big way in reducing and management of **menopausal irregularities.**

(*x*) **Isoflavones** cause prevention of **osteoporosis** (*i.e.,* bone resorption) in **post-menipausal women.**

(*xi*) **Isoflavones** derived from **Soy bean** shown to inhibit the **prostate cancer cells by almost 30%.**

(*xii*) **Genistein** may prevent breast cancer to a certain extent, but promote the existing breast cancer.

11.2.3.5 Hesperetin

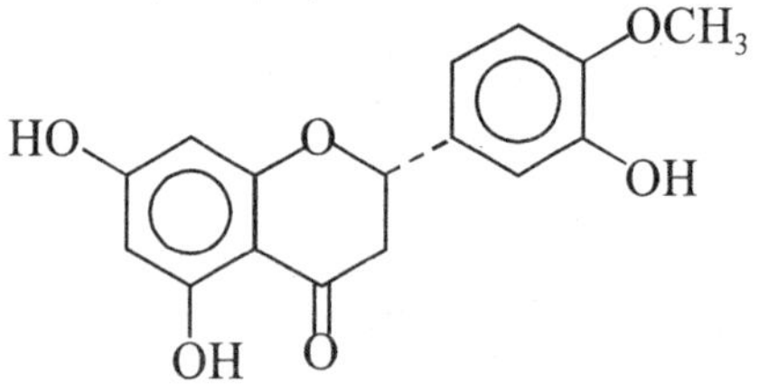

Characteristic Features: These are as given under:

(*i*) **Hesperetin** represents the major flavonoid in oranges and other citrus fruits.

(*ii*) It serves as an **'antioxidant'** which helps to regenerated **Vitamin C** *in vivo.*

(*iii*) It gradually slows down the proliferation of the neoplasm (cancer) cells.

(*iv*) **Hesperetin** also specifically slows down the replication of various **viruses** *e.g.,* **influenza, herpes,** and **polio.**

---

* The production or causation of tumours.

11.2.3.6 Naringin

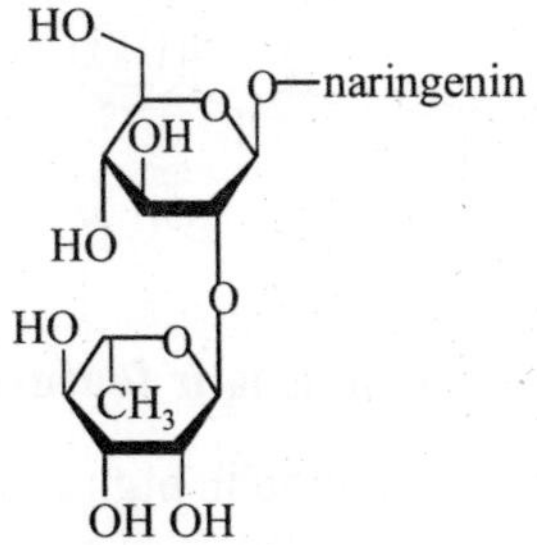

Characteristic Features: The various **characteristic features** are as enumerated under:

  (*i*) **Naringin** provides the **grape fruit** its inherent characteristic bitter taste.
 (*ii*) It may also increase the ability to '**taste**' by direct stimulation of the taste-buds.
(*iii*) **Naringin** particularly reduces **LDL cholesterol** content in blood, but without affecting the **HDL cholesterol.**
 (*iv*) It may, however, interfere with the so called '**intestinal enzymes**', thereby increasing appreciably the **oral-drug absorption.**
  (*v*) **Naringin** is found to increase significantly the **lipid and alcohol metabolism** in the liver while enhancing the **liver antioxidant activity.**
 (*vi*) It helps in a big way to protect against the alcohol-induced stomach ulcers.
(*vii*) **Naringin** protects against the radiation-induced damages in the body to a great extent.
(*viii*) It also possesses **antiapoptotic properties*.**

11.2.3.7 Rutin [Synonyms: Rutoside; Melin; Phytomelin; Eldrin, Ilixathin; Sophorin; Globularicitrin; Paliuroside; Osyritrin; Osyritin; Mytricolorin; Violaquercitrin; Birutan;]

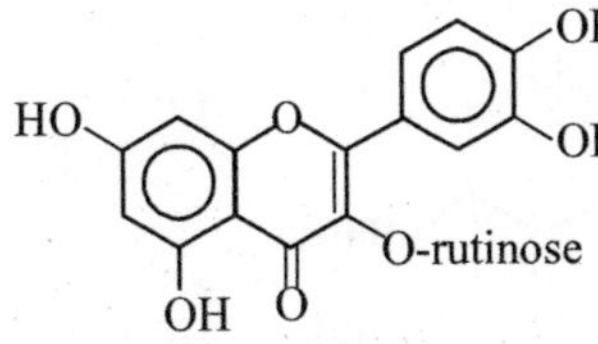

Characteristic Features: These are as follows:

  (*i*) **Rutin** is usally found in buckwheat, asparagus, and a variety of citrus fruits and grapes.
 (*ii*) It has been observed that there is practically very little loss in drying grapes to raisins.
(*iii*) **Rutin** is found to strengthen the capillary walls.

---

* Properties concerned with **programmed cell death.**

11.2.3.8 Quercetin [Synonyms: Meletin; Sophoretin; Cyanidenolon]

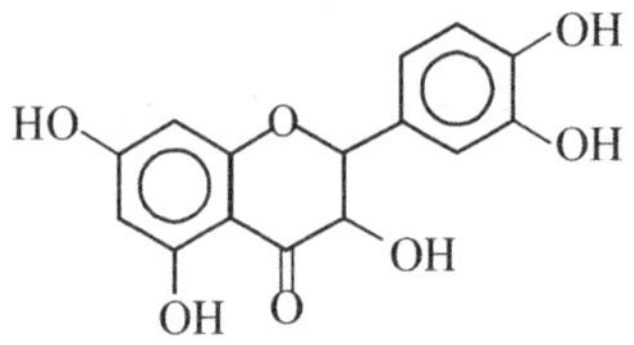

Characteristic Features: The various **characteristic features** of **quercetin** are as follows:

(*i*) **Quercetin** is a **'flavonol'** and usually found in high concentrations in apple skins, red onions, red grapes, green tea, and buckwheat.

(*ii*) It usually does not suffer any **'loss of content'** in drying grapes to raisins.

(*iii*) It is established to serve as a structural backbone to the **citrus flavonoids'**, such as: **rutin** and **hesperetin.**

(*iv*) **Pycnogenols**, a colourless substance, are duly obtained *via* **oligomerization** of **quercetin.**

(*v*) It serves as an efficient and **strong antioxidant,** and also causes reduction of **LDL oxidation** largely.

(*vi*) **Quercetin** is found to act as a **blood thiner,** and as a vasodilator.

(*vii*) It can kill certain **specific viruses** *e.g.*, **herpes.**

(*viii*) **Quercetin** possesses **'antihistaminic activity'** and thereby may relieve **allergic symptoms** caused due to pollen grains, food allergens, dust, dust mite etc.

(*ix*) It is found to specifically inhibit the **COMT* enzyme** thereby causing significant reduction of the ensuing **epinephrine breakdown.****

(*x*) **Quercetin** evidently possesses **sirtunin-like** deacetylase activity.

11.2.3.9 Silymarin [Synonyms: Apihepar; Laragon; Legalon; Pluropon; Silarine; Silepar; Silirex; Silliver; Silmar;]

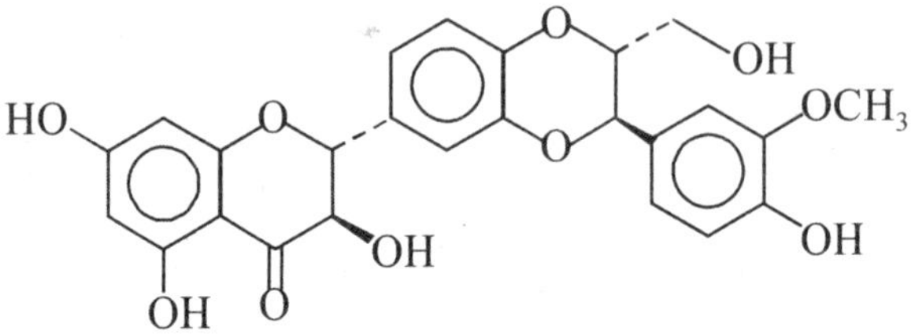

Characteristic Features: These are as stated under:

(*i*) **Silymarin** is an antihepatotoxic principle isolated from the seeds of the **milk thistle** and **antichokes.**

(*ii*) It serves as an excellent **'protective'** against skin-cancer.

(*iii*) **Silymarin** serves as a strong **antioxidant, anti-carcinogenic,** and **anti-inflammatory.**

---

* **COMT:** Catechol-*O*-Methyl Transferase.

** An increased **epinephrine** enhances **fat oxidation** and **energy expenditure** *i.e.*, **"thermogenesis".**

(*iv*) It also serves as an effective **anti-atherosclerotic*** agent.

(*v*) It specifically aids in the mobilization and digestion of fat.

11.2.4 Phenolic Acids

Phenolic acids are present abundantly in **cranberry juice** that essentially help in the reduction of particular adherence of organisms to the cells lining the bladder, and the teeth, which ultimately lowers the incidence of **urinary-tract infections** (UTI) and the usual **dental caries.** It has been duly observed that sweetening slow down the adhesion characteristic properties of the **phenolic acids.** Besides, they categorically reduce the oxidation of the LDL-cholesterol. Importantly, the **phenolic acids** significantly minimize the formation of the specific **cancer-promoting nitrosamines** from the **dietary nitrites and nitrates.** However, the most vital and important **phenolic compounds** that are found in **grapes** (red wine, grape juice, raisins) invariably comprise of **proanthocyanidins, resveratrol,** and **ellagic acid.**

A few typical examples of **'Phenolic Acids'** are briefly described below along with their characteristic features:

11.2.4.1 Ellagic Acid [Synonyms: Benzoaric Acid; Lagistase;]

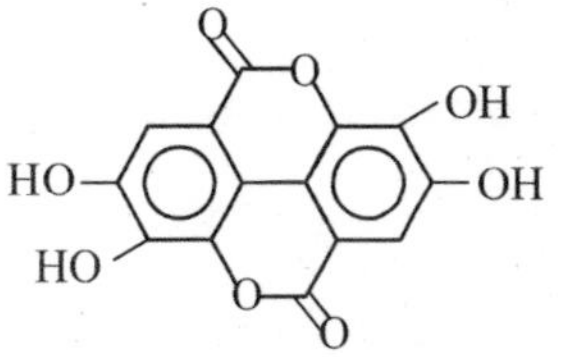

Characteristic Features: The **characteristic features** of **ellagic acid** are as given under:

(*i*) **Ellagic acid** is found to rich in **strawberries,** but 50% more in **raspberries** (chiefly as **ellagitannins**).

(*ii*) It particularly lowers the incidence of oesophagal and colon cancers.

(*iii*) **Ellagic acid** specifically inhibits the formation of **DNA adducts.**

(*iv*) It categorically causes the inhibition of **Phase-I Enzymes,** and potentiates **Phase-II Enzymes.**

11.2.4.2 Chlorogenic Acid

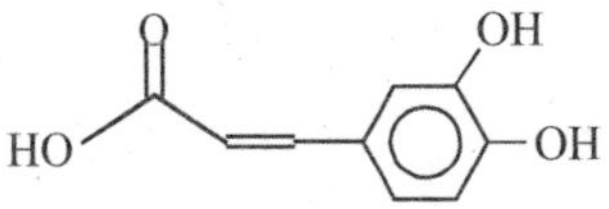

Caffeic Acid

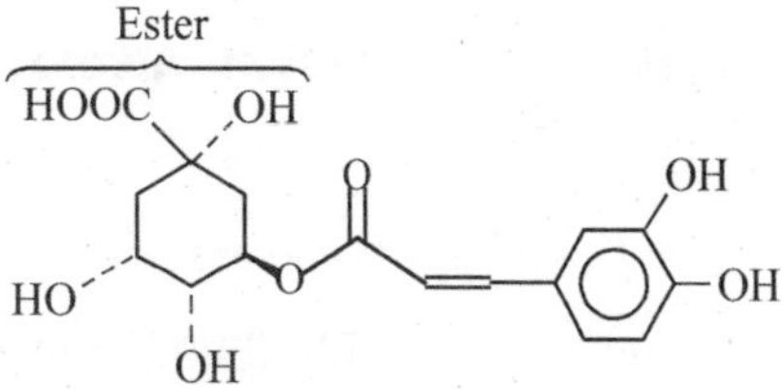

Chlorogenic Acid
(A Caffeic Acid Ester)

Characteristic Features: These are as enumerated below briefly:

---

* Inhibits expression of the adhesion molecules.

(*i*) It is present in relatively higher concentration in **bell peppers, tomatoes,** and **blueberries.**

(*ii*) **Chlorogenic acid** is usually found in the **pulp of grapes** together with **ellagic acid** as given below:

Ellagic Acid

(*iii*) It is most frequently found as an ester of **caffeic acid.**

(*iv*) In fact, **caffeic acid** (*i.e.*, hydroxycinnamic acid) helps to minimize the mutagenicity of polycyclic aromatic hydrocarbons.

(*v*) It serves as a major contributor to the antioxidant activity of coffee.

(*vi*) **Caffeic acid** can regenerate specifically the oxidized Vitamin E.

(*vii*) Chlorogenic acid may prove to be a pro-oxidant in the propagation phase of **LDL-oxidation.**

(*viii*) The **roasting of coffee beans** actually enhances the prevailing **antioxidant activity** to an appreciable extent.

11.2.4.3 para-Coumaric Acid [Synonyms: p–Hydroxy cinnamic acid; β-[4-Hydroxy phe-nyl] acrylic acid;]

Characteristic Features: These are as follows:

(*i*) It is usually present in high concentration in both green and red bell peppers.

(*ii*) *para*-**Coumaric acid** serves as an antioxidant for the color mucosa.

(*iii*) It serves as a flavonoid precursor.

(*iv*) It is found to get bound with nitric acid and its derivatives before they usually get combined with protein amines to result into the formation of '**nitrosamine**'.

11.2.4.4 Phytic Acid [Synonym: Alkalovert]

$$C_6H_6 [OPO(OH)_2]_6$$

Characteristic Features: These are as stated under, namely:

(*i*) **Phytic acid** is invariably found in legumes and whole grains.

(*ii*) It is usually found in high concentration in **flaxseed** and **wheat bran.**

(*iii*) It especially **binds minerals** like: Ca^{2+}, and Fe^{2+}.

(*iv*) Perhaps the **mineral chelation** would reduce the free radicals.

(*v*) It helps to lower the Ca^{2+} **ions absorption** from the gut.

(*vi*) It is observed that the digestion of starch *in vivo* gets reduced appreciably; and, therefore, lower the blood glucose-level considerably.

(*vii*) The **iron-binding phenomenon** (*i.e.*, chelation with Fe^{2+}) helps to slow down the cancerous growth; and hence, minimises the cardiovascular disease significantly.

11.2.4.5 Cinnamic Acid [β-Phenylacrylic Acid]

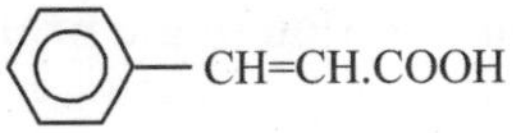

Characteristic Features

(*i*) It is found abundantly in balsam Peru or Tolu, coca leaves, and oil of cinnamon.

(*ii*) It is responsible for attributing the typical cinnamon's characteristic odour and flavour.

(*iii*) **Cinnamic acid** possesses antifungal, antibacterial, and antiparasitic properties.

(*iv*) It has proved to be a **'building block'** for the **lignans.**

(*v*) It is found in higher concentrations in the balsam tree resins, wood, and the inner bark.

(*vi*) Importantly, when combined with **flavonoids** and **benzoic acid** derivatives to result into the formation of **tannins** and **pigments** that specifically impart to the **'vintage wines'** the *colour* and *bouquet*.

11.2.5 Non-Flavonoid Polyphenolics

The **non-flavonoid polyphenolics** do not contain the **benzopyran nucleus.** A few such compounds, such as: **curcumin, resveratrol,** and **lignans** shall now be discussed in the sections that follows:

11.2.5.1 Curcumin [Synonyms: Turmeric Yellow; CI Natural Yellow; CI 75300; Diferuloylmethane;]

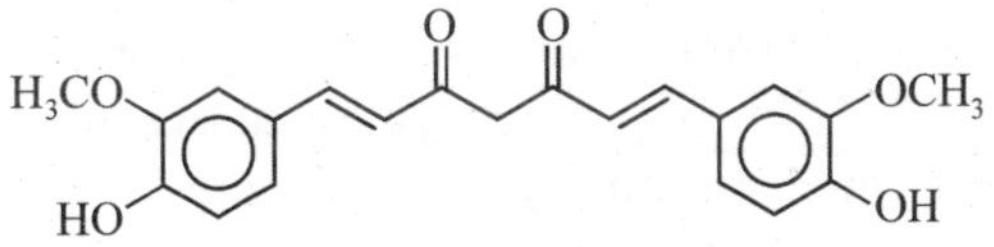

Characteristic Features: The various **characteristic features** of **curcumin** are as stated under:

(*i*) **Curcumin,** a phytochemical, is the major component of the spice **'turmeric'** occur naturally as rhyzomes.

(*ii*) **Curcumin** particularly helps in the inhibition of the **'gene'** that actually gives rise to the formation of the **inflammatory COX-2 enzymes,** and ultimately preventing their production overwhelmingly.*

(*iii*) It is reported to be both strongly anti-inflammatory and strongly antioxidant.

(*iv*) **Curcumin** causes appreciable inhibition for the release of the proinflammatory cytokine **TNF-alpha.****

(*v*) It is highly regarded to be the more effective anti-clotting agent in comparison to acetyl salicylic acid (*i.e.*, **aspirin**) without having any **ulcer-inducing stomach irritation** caused by the latter.

---

* The allopathic drug **'Celebrex'** only inhibits the **COX-2 enzymes.**

** **TNG-alpha:** Tumour Necrosis Factor-Alpha.

(*vi*) It may cause prevention of the color cancer.

(*vii*) It predominantly acts as a scavenger for the **peroxynitrite free-radical.**

(*viii*) **Curcumin** blocks particularly the **amyloid*-β-aggregation** that may eventually help to prevent **Alzheimer's Disease, Hodgkin's disease,** and **carcinoma.**

(*ix*) It distinctly inhibits **NF-kB transcription** of the **proinflammatory** and **antiapoptotic** (*i.e.,* neoplasm-promoting) genes.

11.2.5.2 Resveratrol

Resveratrol depicts the strongest **sirtunin-like deacetylase action** of any known chemical constituent derived from the plant kingdom. In fact, the **sirtuins** have been shown to overwhelmingly extend the ensuing lifespan of **yeast** and **fruit flies.** Contrary to excessive media propaganda and representations, there exist a plethora of other sources of **resveratrol** in addition to the alcoholic beverages (red wine) *e.g.*, **purple grape-juice.**

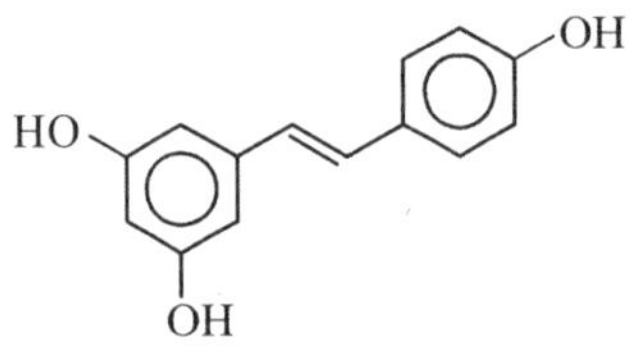

Resveratrol

Importantly, in diverse organisms, calorie restriction invariably slows the **'pace of ageing'** (*i.e.,* helps the rejuvination process) and thereby enhances maximum lifespan significantly. It has been duly established that in the budding yeast **Saccharomyces** *cerevisiae,* the prevailing calorie restriction specifically extends the **'lifespan'** by increasing the activity of **Sir 2,** which being a bonafide member of the conserved **sirtuin family** of **NAD$^+$ dependent protein deacetylases.** Also included in this family are **SIR-2, 1,** a *Caenorhabditis elegans* enzyme that eventually modulates **'lifespan';** and **SIRT 1,** a **human deacetylase** which essentially promotes cell survival by negatively regulating the **p 53 tumour suppressor.**

However, it has been amply demonstrated that the **potent activator resveratrol,** a well-known polyphenol found in red wine, appreciably lowers the **Michaelis constant** of SIRT 1 for the **acetylated substrate** as well as the NAD$^+$, and increases cell survival by stimulating **SIRT 1**-dependent **deacetylation of p 53.** However, in yeast, resveratrol usually mimics the calorie restriction by stimulating **SIR 2,** thereby enhancing both **DNA-stability** and **extension in lifespan upto 70%.**

Characteristic Features: The **characteristic features** of **resveratrol** are given as under:

(*i*) **Resveratrol** is usually found as the **'principle stilkene'** in grapes, in teas (*i.e.,* both green and black), peanuts, and berries.

(*ii*) It is produced by plants within themselves as defense against fungi.

(*iii*) **Resveratrol** serves as an anti-inflammatory agent, and also inhibits **COX-1 enzyme.****

---

* **Amyloid:** A protein-polysaccharide complex having starchilike characteristics produced and deposited in tissues during certain pathological states.

** **COX-1:** It is a constitutive enzyme and plays a role in the production of essential **prostaglandins (PGE).** Inhibition of this enzyme by all the older, **non-selective NSAIDs** is primarily responsible for a number of their side effects.

(*iv*) It aids in the blockade of adhesion of blood cells to vessel walls.

(*v*) It has been duly demonstrated that **resveratrol** distinctly reduces skin as well as breast cancer in mice.

(*vi*) It also inhibits **NF-kB transcription** of proinflammatory and **antiapoptoic*** genes.

11.2.5.3 Lignans

Lignans refer to the plant products of low molecules weight produced primarily by the oxidative coupling of *para*-**hydroxyphenyl propene units,** wherein the two units may be linked together by an oxygen bridge. Nevertheless, the monomeric precursor units are, namely: **cinnamic acid, cinnamyl alcohol, propenyl benzene,** and **allylbenzene.** The terminology **Lignan** or **Haworth Lignan** is applied to such chemical entities that are derived from the coupling propenyl and/or allyl derivatives are termed as **Neolignans.****

Characteristic Features: These are as enumerated under:

(*i*) **Lignans** occur abundantly and have been obtained from the **roots, heartwood, foliage, fruit,** and **resinous exudates of plants.**

(*ii*) They invariably represent the **dimer-stage intermediate** between **monomeric propylphenol units** and **lignin.**

(*iii*) **Lignans** are found to be **optically active.**

(*iv*) The **cinnamic acid dimers** do have the **2-unit composites.**

(*v*) **Lignans** actually strengthens the **plant cell-walls** (*i.e.*, wood).

(*vi*) They are mostly water-soluble, and not-oil soluble.

(*vii*) As to date **flaxseed** is established to be the richest **dietary source for the lignans.**

(*viii*) **Podophylotoxin lignan** *i.e.*, a recognized '**cytotoxic agent**', is mostly used to treat the venereal warts.

(*ix*) It is regarded to be the '**phytoestrogens**'.

(*x*) **Lignans,** in general, may reduce the '**risk of cancer**' in females.

11.2.6 Glucosinolates [or Thioglucosides]

Glucosinolates, formerly known as **thioglucosides,** are the '**anionic glycosides**' solely responsible for the potent and characteristic inherent flavours of numerous *Brassicaceae* (*viz.,* mustard, radish, rutabaga, cabbage); besides, a good number of species related to other botanically close families, such as: *Capparidaceae, Resedaceae,* and *Tropaeolaceae.* The exact content of **glucosinolate** markedly varies with respect to the species, the plant part(s), the cultivation, and the climate conditionalities. It invariably ranges, before cooking: from 0.5 to 1 g.kg^{-1}, and may reach upto 3.9 g.kg^{-1} as could be seen in certain **Brussel Sprouts.**

Basic Structure: The basic structure of the '**glucosinolates**' essentially consists of: (*a*) **glucose residue,** (*b*) **sulphate function,** and (*c*) **variable aglycone,** and the resulting molecule occurring as the respective potassium salt. It has been duly observed that the structural diversity of the '**glucosinolates**' distinctly reflects that of their precursor amino acids. A few typical examples are

---

* **Antiapoptoic:** Neoplasm-promoting.

** Goltleib OR: *Fortschr.Chem.Org.Naturst.,* **35:** 1-72, 1978.

given below that expatiates the formation of **sinigrin, gluconasturtiin, glucobrassicin,** and **sinalbin** from the respective amino acids:

S.No.	Amino Acid	Intermediate	Glucosinolates	Source
1	Homomethionine	Allylglucosinolate	Sinigrin	Black Mustard
2	Homophenylalanine	Phenethrylglucosinolate	Gluconasturtiin	Watercress
3	Tryptophan	3-Indolylmethyl-glucosinolate	Glucobrassicin	Cabbage
4	Tyrosine	p-Hydroxybenzyl-glucosinolate	Sinalbin	White Mustard

General Formula and Postulated Origin of Glucosinolates:

The **biosynthesis of the glucosinolates** are most probably and logically accomplished by the following sequential steps, namely:

(a) Decarboxylation of amino acids to the corresponding aldoximes,

(b) A **'sulphur atom'** (from cysteine) is duly incorporated into the aldoxime,

(c) Resulting product gets **glycosylated** in the presence of **UDP-glucose,** and

(d) The **glycosylated product** is finally **sulphated by phospho-adenosine-phosphosulphate.**

The various sequential steps as explained above in sections (a) through (d) may be summarized as given under:

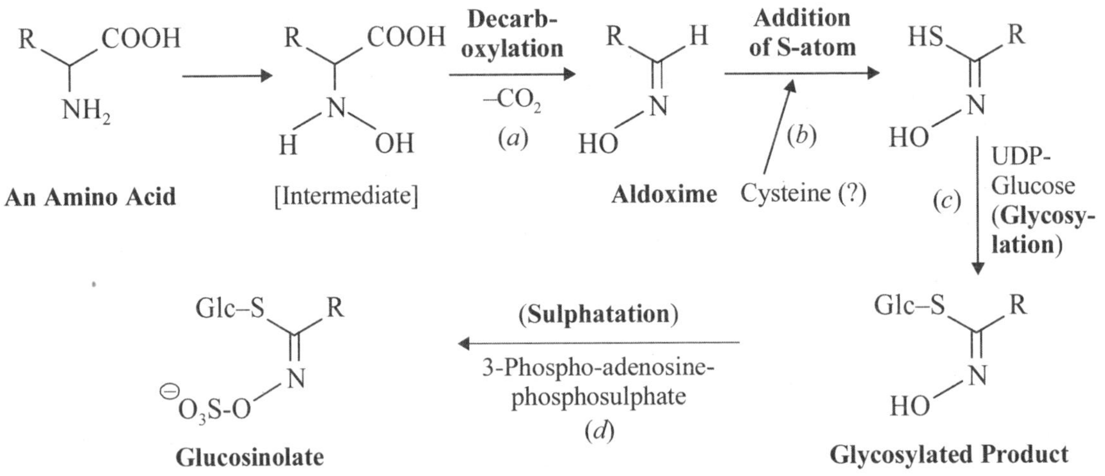

Potentials of Glucosinolate: The various **glucosinolates** described earlier may prove to be of immense beneficiary help to human health. A survey of literatures* have amply revealed that the dietary intake of **glucosinolates** *viz.,* from various vegetable sources as: broccoli, cabbage, cauliflower, and Brussel sprouts might exert a substantial protective support against the **colon cancer.** Importantly, the **isothiocyanates** and the **indole-3-carbinols** do interfere categorically in the **metabolism of carcinogens.**

Mechanism of Action: The **isothiocyanates** and the **indoles** cause inhibition of **procarcinogen activation,** and thereby induce the **'phase-II' enzymes,** namely: **NAD(P)H quinone reductase** or **glutathione S-transferase,** that specifically detoxify the **selected electrophilic metabolites** which are capable of changing the structure of **nucleic acids.**

Example: Regular consumption of **Brussel sprouts** by human subjects (upto 300 g.day^{-1}) miraculously causes a very fast (say within a span of 3 weeks) an appreciable enhancement in the **glutathione-S-transferase,** and a subsequent noticeable reduction in the urinary concentration of a **specific purine meltabolite** that serves as a **marker of DNA-degradation.**

Glucosinolates may be further classified into *two* major groups, namely: (*a*) **Isothiocyanates,** and (*b*) **Indoles,** which shall now be treated individually in the sections that follows:

11.2.6.1 Isothiocyanates

In general, the **isothiocyanates** are solely responsible for causing the hotness of **horseradish, radish,** and **mustard. Isothiocyanates** do have the [–N = C = S] functional moiety present in the chemical constituents. **Mustard oil** essentially comprise of the **allyl thiocyanate.**

A few typical examples of the **isothiocyanates** shall be discussed briefly as under.

11.2.6.1.1 Phenthyl Isothiocyanate

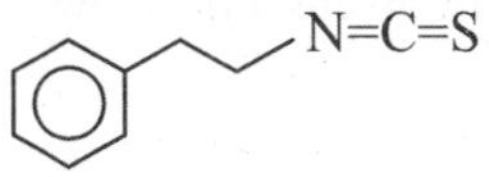

Phenethyl Isothiocyanate

Characteristic Features: These are as given under:

(*i*) **Phenethyl isothiocyanate** offers a '**bitter taste**' to watercress.

(*ii*) It causes effective inhibition of **tumorigenesis** by the aid of polycyclic aromatic hydrocarbons.

(*iii*) It also induces **apoptosis** by **caspase-8 activation,** and **not by p 53.**

(*iv*) It is particularly good against the harmful **nitroamines** in **tobacco smoke.**

(*v*) **Nitrosonicotine,** a major carcinogenic substance, is present in the **tobacco smoke,** and formed by the interaction of **nitric oxide** and **nicotine.**

11.2.6.1.2 Sulforaphane [Synonym: Raphanin;]

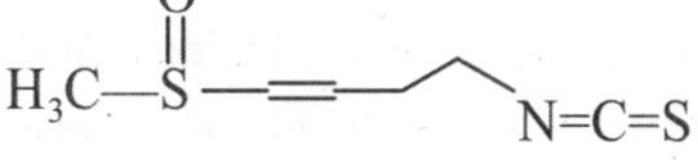

Sulforaphane

Characteristic Features: They are as stated under:

(*i*) It is obtained from the seeds of radish *Ramphanus sativus* L., (*Cruciferae*)

(*ii*) **Sulforaphane** is especially rich in **broccoli.**

(*iii*) It has been proved to be an extremely potent **phase-2 enzyme inducer.**

(*iv*) It predominantly cause specific **cell-cycle arrest** and also the apoptosis of the neoplasm (cancer) cells.

(*v*) **Sulforaphane** categorically produces **δ-D-gluconolactone** which has been established to be a significant inhibitor of the **breast cancer.**

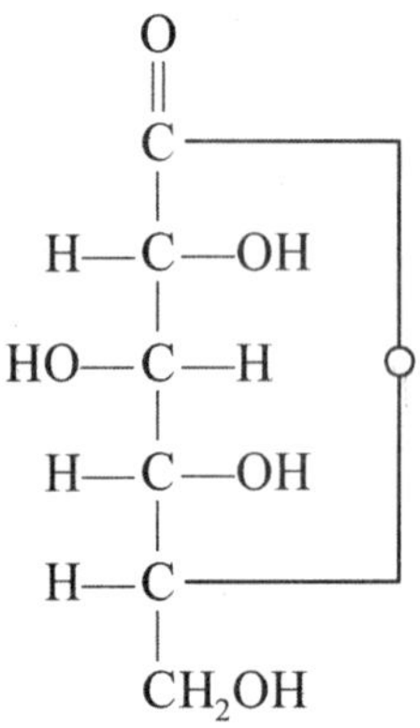

δ-D-Gluconolactone

11.2.6.2 Indoles

The typical example of **indoles** is briefly discussed below:

11.2.6.2.1 Indole-3-Carbinol

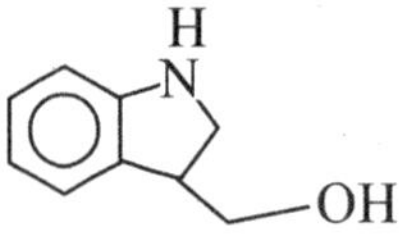

Indole-3-carbinol

Characteristic Features   The various **characteristic features** of **indole-3-carbinol** are as follows:

(*i*) It is found to be the most vital and important indole present in **broccoli.**

(*ii*) **Indole-3-carbinol** specifically inhibits the **Human Papilloma Virus (HPV)** that may cause **uterine cancer.**

(*iii*) It blocks the **estrogen receptors** specifically present in the breast cancer cells.

(*iv*) Interestingly **indole-3-carbinol** downregulates **CDK6,** and upregulates **p21** and **p27** in prostate cancer cells.

(*v*) It affords G_1 **cell-cycle arrest** and **apoptosis of breast** and **prostate cancer cells** significantly.

(*vi*) It enhances the **p 53 expression** in cells treated with **benzo [*a*]pyrene*.**

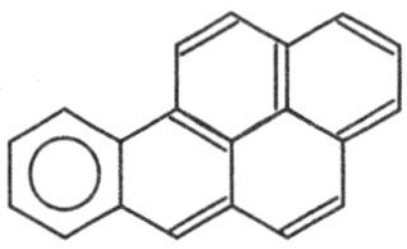

Benzo [*a*] pyrene

(*vii*) It also depresses **Akt, NF-kappaB, MAPK,** and **Bel-2** signalling pathways to a reasonably good extent.

---

* It is reasonably anticipated to be a human carcinogen: **Ninth Report on Carcinogens** (PB 2000-107509, 2000) p III-187.

11.2.7 Thiosulphinates [or Cysteine Sulphoxides]

The major flavour component of **garlic** (*Allium sativum*; Liliaceae/Alliaceae) is a **thiosulphinate** called **allicin. Allicin** is duly formed when the garlic tissue is damaged due to the hydrolysis product of **S-allyl cysteine sulphoxide (alliin)** which is specifically produced by the **pyridoxal phosphate-dependent enzyme allinase.**

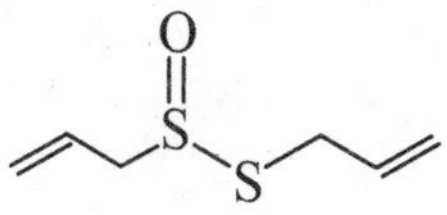

Allicin
[Diallyl Thiosulphinate]

The various garlic preparations used medicinally include steam-distilled oils, garlic macerated in vegetable oils (*e.g.*, soybean oil), dried garlic powder, garlic oil in soft gelatine capsules (known as **'garlic pearls'**), and gel-suspensions of garlic powder. However, careful analyses amply indicate a wide variations in the nature as well as quantum of the **'active constituents'** in the variety of available preparations. Therefore, the freshly crushed garlic gloves typically consists of **allicin** (upto 0.4%), and other **thiosulphinates** (upto 0.1%-chiefly **methyl thiosulphinate**).

Characteristic Features: The **characteristic features** of the **thiosulphinates** are as enumerated under:

(*i*) **Thiosulphinates** are designated as **'organosulphur phytochemicals'** that are abundantly present in **garlic*** and **onions.**

(*ii*) It also comprises of **mercapto cysteins** together with **allylic** sulphides.**

(*iii*) Actually the very presence of the **'allylic sulphides'** contribute to the strong typical characteristic odour of garlic.

(*iv*) **Allicin** protects garlic from the pests.

(*v*) **Allicin** is found to be toxic to insects and the microorganisms.

(*vi*) **Allicin** categorically affords protection against the ulcers by causing inhibition of *Helicobacter pylori.*

(*vii*) **Allicin** is found to lose its stability as soon as it gets removed from **garlic.**

(*viii*) **Allicin** particularly inhibits the proliferation of the cells present in the mammary glands, color, and endometrial.

(*ix*) Garlic may reduce blood pressure in human beings.

(*x*) Garlic can augment the induction of the **nitric-oxide synthetase activity.**

(*xi*) **Garlic** distinctly causes the inhibition of the **platelet** aggregation by the **arachidonic acid, epinephrine,** and other **platelet agonists.**

(*xii*) The incised onions usually releases a chemical component known as: **Propanethial-S-oxide** which gets converted to sulphuric acid in the eyes itself thereby causing a real **'burning sensation'.**

---

* **Garlic**—has more sulphur content in comparison to onions.

** **Allyl**—refers to a hydrocarbon bonded to a S-atom.

(*xiii*) Any type of heating (*i.e.*, cooking) totally destroys the **enzyme allinase** that certainly prevents the formation of many highly useful sulphur containing **chemical entities.**

11.2.8 Phytosterols

Phytosterols usually referred to as—'**any sterol** *i.e.*, **steroidal alcohol, present in the vegetable oil or fat'.**

In a rather broader perspective **sterols** invariably occur in a large segment of plant species. It has been duly observed that both yellow and green vegetables do contain an appreciable quantum; and, of course, their respective seeds specifically concentrate the sterols. Importantly, an extensive and intensive research on these valuable **phytonutrients** has been adequately carried out upon the seeds of certain selected specimens, such as: **soybean, yams, rice, pumpkins,** and **specific herbs.**

Phytosterols invariably engage in competitive uptake of the **dietary cholesterol** in the **entire intestinal passage.** Besides, **phytosterols** have profusely demonstrated the capability to affect complete blockade in the uptake of cholesterol (to which they are intimately structurally related) and also facilitate its subsequent excretion from the body. In fact, **cholesterol** has been duly implicated ever since as a relatively dangerous risk factor associated with the cardiovascular disease.

However, it has been established beyond any reasonable doubt that the prevailing ratio between the **dietary phytosterols** and **cholesterols** was remarkably lower amongst the '**vegetarians**' *vis-a-vis* the '**non-vegetarians**'. This particular observation overwhelmingly underlies the fact that **cholesterol,** *per se*, is not only the **marker of risk** for the aforesaid cardiovascular disease, but also its ensuing ratio with several other **modifying dietary components** may ultimately prove to be a definite better measure of risk factor*.

Interestingly, **phytosterols** invariably block the development of **tumours (neoplasms)** in **colon, breast,** and **prostate glands.** Although the precise and exact mechanisms whereby the said blockade actually takes place are not yet well understood, yet one may strongly affirm that **phytosterols** seem to change drastically the ensuing **cell-membrane transfer** in the phenomenon of neoplasm growth and thereby reduce the inflammation significantly.

β-Sitosterol seems to be the most befitting and typical example amongst the **phytosterols,** and this shall be dealt within the section that follows:

11.2.8.1 β-Sitosterol [Synonyms: α-Phytosterol; Cinchol; Cupreol; Rhamnol; Quebrachol; Sitosterin; Harzol; Prostasal; Sito Lande]

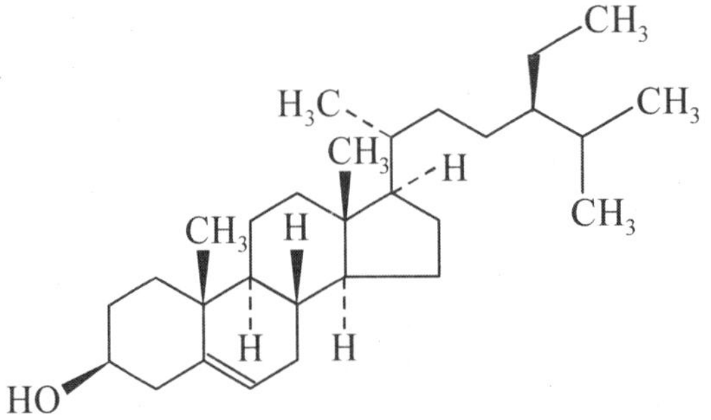

β-Sitosterol

FOOD PHYTOSTEROLS	
FOOD	**β-SITOSTEROL***
Peanut Butter	135
Cashew Nut	130
Almonds	122
Peas	106
Kidney Beans	91
Avocados	76
* milligrams per 100 gramms	

* Nair P *et al. Am. Jr. of Clin. Nitri.*, **40:** (4 Suppl.): 927-30, Oct. 1984.

Characteristic Features: The various characteristic features of **β-Sitosterol** are as given below:

(*i*) **β-Sitosterol** minimises the level of **cholesterol production** by the liver.

(*ii*) It also blocks the **absorption of cholesterol** to a good extent.

(*iii*) It appreciably **lowers the cancerous cell-growth** (as cholesterol is required by the cell membrane).

(*iv*) **β-Sitosterol** causes specific inhibition of the **epithelial cell division** which may in turn drastically **reduce atherosclerosis.**

(*v*) Its structure closely resembles to that of cholesterol.

(*vi*) In fact, **β-stisterol** may be regarded as the **plant equivalent** of the **animal cholesterol.**

11.2.9   Anthraquinones

Anthraquinones are usually characterised by the presence of **phenolic** and **glycosidic** compounds, that are solely derived from **anthracene.** They do possess a variable degree of oxidation *viz.,* **anthrones, anthranols:** and designate the so called **anthraquinone glycosides.** In fact, these molecules *e.g.,* **chrysophanol, aloe-emodin, rhein,** and **emodin** have in common a double hydroxylation at positions C-1 and C-8.

The structures of some **anthraquinone** and **hydroxyanthraquinone** derivatives are as given below:

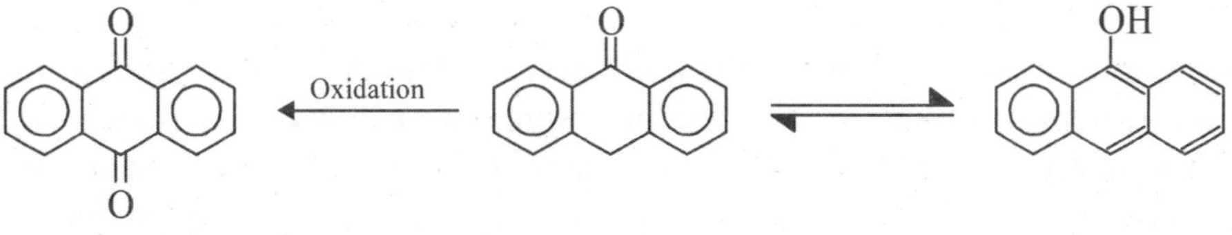

| Anthraquinone | Anthrone | Anthranol |

Structures of Anthraquinone and its Derivatives

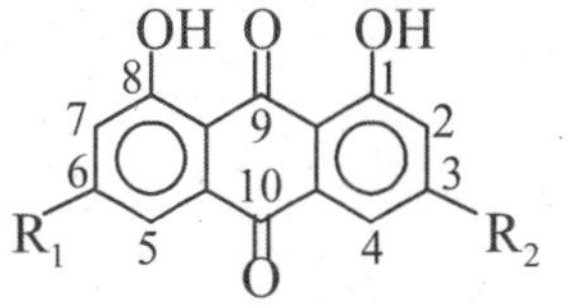

(*a*) **Aloe-emodin**   : $R_1 = H$; $R_2 = CH_2\,OH$;
(*b*) **Chrysophanol** : $R_1 = H$; $R_2 = CH_3$;
(*c*) **Emodin**   : $R_1 = OH$; $R_2 = CH_3$;
(*d*) **Rhein**   : $R_1 = H$; $R_2 = COOH$;

Structures of Some Hydroxyanth raquinone Derivatives

However, the botanical distribution of the various species essentially containing the '1, 8-dihydroxyanthraquinone glycosides' is quite restricted, namely: *Liliaceae* (**aloe**); *Polygonaceae* (**rhubarbs**); *Rhamnaceae* (**cascara, buckthorn**); and *Caesalpinaceae* (**sennas**).

A few typical examples of **anthraquinones** *viz.,* **senna, barbaloin,** and **hypericin** shall now be treated individually in the sections that follows:

11.2.9.1 Senna

Senna the dried leaflets of *Cassia senna* L., essentially contains **Sennosides A and B, glucosides of rhein** and **chrysophanic acid.***

---

* Fairbairne: *Planta Medica,* **12:** 260, 1964.

Following is the structure of **Sennosides** *i.e.*, **anthraquinone glycosides** as observed in **senna** in almost in equal quantum, and also in the rhubarbs where the **Sennoside A predominates.**

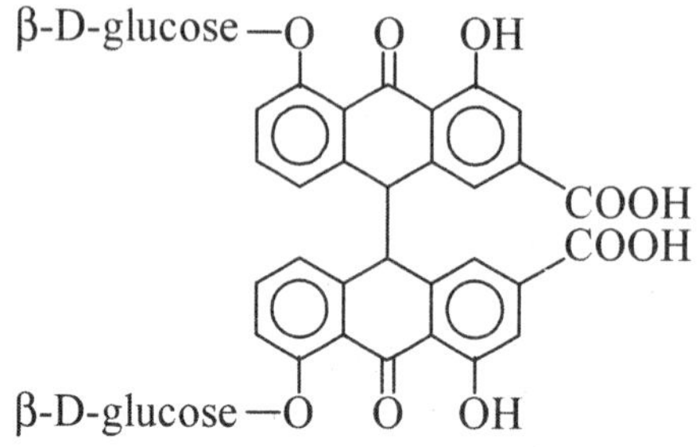

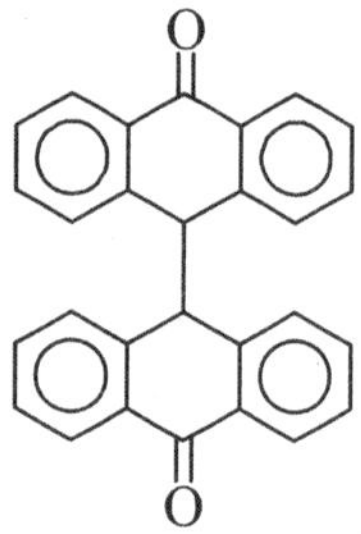

Dianthrone

Characteristic Features: The **characteristic features** of **sennosides** are as stated below:

(*i*) **Sennosides** are **dianthrones.**

(*ii*) The mostly act as purgative for the lower bowel.

(*iii*) **Sennosides** specifically enhances the **peristaltic movement** in the colon (*i.e.*, large intestine).

(*iv*) They possess an inherent nauseating taste.

(*v*) **Sennosides** are distinctly contraindicated for the **hemorrhoids** or **inflammation.**

11.2.9.2 Barbaloin

The major constituents of the **Cascara Bark** are **cascarosides A and B,** that essentially contain both *O*–and *C*–glucoside linkages; and, therefore, represent a pair of optical isomers differing only in the stereochemistry of the C-glucoside bond. The acid hydrolysis does not cleave the C-glucose linkage, and instead gives rise to **barbaloin,** and a mixture of two diastereoisomeric forms, which have been named as **aloin A** and **aloin B.** Hydrolysis of the *O*-glucose linkage generates **chrysaloin,** sometimes also referred to as **deoxybarbaloin.** Both **barbaloin** and **chrysaloin** are also found in the bark, and are believed to be the breakdown products obtained by the enzymatic hydrolysis of the **cascarosides.**

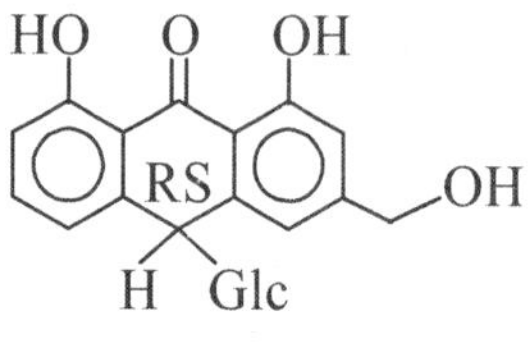

Barbaloin

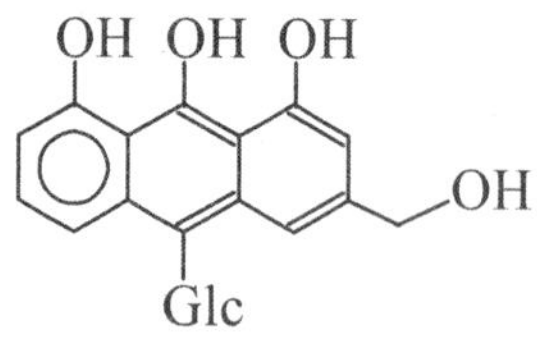

Barbaloin
[Anthranol Tautomer]

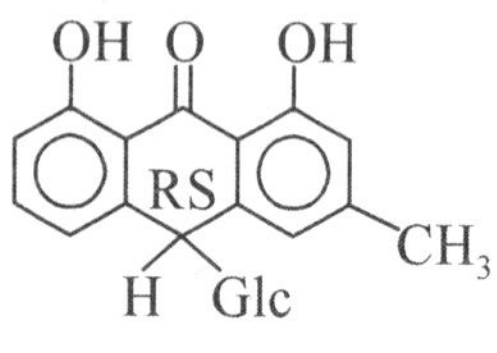

Chrysaloin
[Deoxybarbaloin]

Characteristic Features: These are as given below:

(*i*) It acts as a laxative (lower bowel).

(*ii*) It is largely obtained from the **Aloe Vera plant** which possesses a host of medicinal values, namely:

- Controls diabetes
- Protects Human Immune System
- Prevents AIDS
- Prevents Asthma
- Protects Kidney Function
- Protects Cough and Cold

- Improves Digestive System
- Cures Arthritis
- Manages Cholesterol

- Cleans up Toxins from Intestines
- Cures skin problems and Loss of Hair

11.2.9.3 Hypericin [Synonym: Hypericum Red]

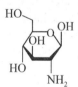

Hypericin

Characteristic Features: The various **characteristic features** of **hypericin** are as enumerated under:

(*i*) It is obtained as a **'Red Pigment'** obtained from *Hypericum perforatum,* otherwise known as **"Saint John's Wort"**.

(*ii*) **Hypericin** finds its usage as **analgesic** or to treat **neuralgic pain.**

(*iii*) It is profusely used as a **'folk remedy'** against **anxiety, depression,** and **insomnia.**

(*iv*) It is found to be free from **purgative properties.**

(*v*) It may sometimes be employed to treat **ulcers** and acute inflammation of the gut.

11.2.10 Glucosamine [Synonym: Chitosamine;]

Glucosamine

Glucosamine is found in **chitin, mucoproteins,** and **micropolysaccharides** *i.e.,* in the naturally occurring plant products. Besides, **glucosamine** is also found naturally in the human body, especially in **cartilage, tendons,** and **ligament tissues.** It forms an integral and essential part towards the production of **glycoaminoglycan (CAG),** that actually constitutes a major segment of the cartilage tissue.* Importantly, it is not available in appreciable quantum in the diet; and, therefore, should be specifically synthesized in the body. As this ability declines progressively with the advancement in age, and hence predisposes the human body to **arthritis.** Several acute and serious types of disease conditions thus come into being, for instance: **osteoarthrhitis (OA), rheumatic arthritis (RA),** and **degeneratic joint diseases** are becoming so common and widespread that they have more or less become a normal part of the **ageing process** and ultimately do affect the hips, knees, hands, and spine.

---

* Briffa J: *Int. J. Act. Comp. Med.,* **15:** 15-16, 1997.

Chondroprotection is the terminology invariably used when the GAGs, namely: **glucosamine,** are duly administered orally so as to proect these joints from undergoing further deterioration with the passage of time.*

Mechanism of Actiion: It has been duly established that **N-acetylglucosamine** causes inhibition of the enzyme elastase in a dose-dependent manner.** However, **elastase** plays a vital and important role in the breakdown of the **articular cartilage, ligaments, tendons,** and **bones** in **rheumatic arthritis (RA).** Besides, **D-glucosamine,** the active principle of **glucosamine sulphate,** happen to be a comparatively small molecule which rapidly undergoes diffusion *via* all the **biological membranes.** It also exhibits a high degree of affinity for the specific cartilaginous tissue and is subsequently introduced right into the **proteoglycan molecules.** Thus, it serves as the most preferred building block for the meticulous synthesis of **GAGs,** and these in turn offer a reasonable and legitimate protection against the ensuing damaging effects of **NSAIDs** as well as steroids. Importantly, the overall manner whereby **glucosamine** acts against **joint degeneration** and **joint protection.**

Hexosamine Pathway gives rise to the formation of the **endogenous glucosamine,** that is intimately associated with the ensuing **insulin responses.** It has been duly established, based on experimental evidences, that **glucosamine** may go a long way to induce **insulin resistance** *via* **hexosamine pathway.** This net effect may be obtained even without the presence of high-glucose concentration, and fat-induced insulin resistance is similar affected by the presence of **glucosamine.*****

From the survey of literature one may safely conclude that **glucosamine** is quite **effective, less toxic, safe,** and a **well-tolerated** alternative drug to **NSAIDs** in the particular treatment of joint degenerative ailments. The actual use of **glucosamine** is apparently widespread in Great Britain, United States, and Europe, and, hence, the pharmacists attached to hospitals and OTC in stores should certainly be informed with respect to its **nutritional supplement** for onward transmission to the 'actual consumers' as its popularity is gaining momentum in geometrical proportion.

11.2.11 Octacosanol [Synonym: Octacosyl Alcohol]

$$H_3C(CH_2)_{26}CH_2.OH$$

Octacosanol is one of the constituents of the **vegetable waxes.** It is an exemplary of a 'nutraceutical'. It is a 28 carbon-chain alcohol which is present in the superficial layers of fruit leaves, and skin of a plethora of plants as well as 'whole grains.**** In fact, a large segment of investigational studies based on **octacosanol** have widely made use of either **wheat germ oil** or **policosanol.** Interestingly, **policosanol** is a natural mixture of '**primary alcohols**' duly purified from the **sugar cane wax** having **octacosanol** as the **major component.**

Characteristic Features: These are as stated under:

(*i*) **Athletes: Octacosanol** supplemented athletes distinctly showed a significant enhancement in the muscle girth measurements thereby ascertaining the formation of lean body mass.

---

* Gottlieb MS: *J Manipulative Physiolog. Ther.*: **20**: 400-14, 1997.
** Kamel M *et al. clin. Exp. Rheum.,* **9**: 17-21, 1991.
*** Hussain MA, *Eur. J. Endocrinol,* **139**: 472-5, 1998.
**** kato S *et al. Br. J. Nut,* **73**: 433-42, 1995.

Studies related to measured grip and chest strength (*i.e.*, an indication of body strength), and reaction time to both auditory and visual stimuli* revealed that exclusively the reaction time to a **visual stimulus** and **grip strength** after ingestion of 1,000 mcg of octacosanol for a duration of 60 days on regular basis.

(*ii*) **Parkinson's Disease (or Motor Neurone Disease):** Clinical studies with Parkinsonian disease subjects, at a dose level of 5 mg of **octacosanol,** for 90 days showed that they improved appreciably.**

(*iii*) **Lipid Metabolism:** Pons *et al.* (1993)*** showed that **hypercholesterolaemic patients** treated with **policosanol** 2 mg per day for 6 months showed extremely promising results, whereby the **'total cholesterol'** was lowered significantly having an apparent safe-profile. Aneiros *et al.***** (1993) carried out the investigations to test the effect successive doses upon the **lipid profile** and **tolerability of treatment** on patient suffering from **primary hypercholesterolaemia** for a duration of 6 weeks initially with 2 tablets of **policosanol** (5g) **once daily,** and followed by 2 tablets **twice daly** for another phase of 6 weeks. They observed that the patients' **blood-lipid profile** were as given below:

Lower-dose level: Significant reduction in **total cholesterol level** and **LDL-cholesterol level;**
Higher-dose level: Further reduction of these *two* levels in patients.

Torres *et al.****** (1995) studied the effect of **policosanol** in patients having a history of **non-insulin-dependent diabetes mellitus (NIDDM),** and enhanced **LDL levels** which may render a major **coronary-artery-disease risk factor.** Patients having **stable gycaemic control** were administered with **policosanol** (5 mg) twice daily for 3 months; and they showed a significantly lowered levels of total **cholesterol** and **LDL-C.** Hence, the above investigative studies evidently shows a prominent, plausible, and possible place of **policosanol** as a **definitive cholesterol lowering nutraceutical** in such patients having **controlled NIDDM.**

(*iv*) **Thromboxane Pathways:** Arruzazabala *et al.******* (1993) investigated the possibility that **policosanol** may substantiate the action of certain **lipid-lowering drugs** causing an effect on the **platelet aggregation.** Furthermore, **policosanol** at a dose level of 200 mg. kg^{-1} also appreciably lowered the mortality with respect to the crebral infarction in **gerbils.********* Conclusively both of these studies would indicate the close involvement of **policosanol** in the **prostaglandin** and the **thromboxane pathways.**

11.2.12 Carnitine [Synonym: γ-Trimethyl-β-hydroxybutyrobetaine;]

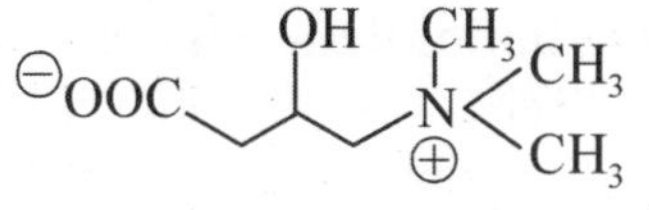

Carnitine

---

*   Saint-John M and Mc Naughton L: *Int. Clin. Nutr. Rev.,* **6:** 81-7, 1986.

**   Snider SR: **Octacosanol in Parkinsonism:** *Ann. Neurol,* **16:** 723, 1984.

***   Pons P *et al. Curr. Ther. Res.,* **53:** 265-9, 1993.

**** Aneiros E *et al. Curr. Ther. Res.,* **54:** 304-12, 1993.

***** Torres O *et al. Diabetes Care,* **18:** 393-7, 1995.

****** Arruzazabala ML *et al. Leukot. Essent. Fatty Acids,* **49:** 695-7, 1993.

******* Arruzazabala ML *et al. Ibid,* **69:** 321-7, 1993.

Carnitine refers to an essential cellular component, which is sometimes referred to as **Vitamin BT,** although it is not generally considered as a Vitamin. In reality, if an amino acid derivative duly synthesized from the amino acids **lysine** and **methionine** present in the liver and kidney, from where it gets adequately released into the **systemic circulation.** Brain also partially synthesizes this chemical entity. Out of the total **carnitine** present in a human body, almost 98% is found in the specific cardiac and skeletal muscle. Importantly, **carnitine** may also be derived from the 'diet' *viz.*, chiefly food of animal origin, and the subsequent quantum ingested therefrom virtually determines the **rate of absorption.***

Stereochemistry: Carnitine is available in *two* **isomeric forms** *viz.*, *d*- and *l*-forms, and the *l*-**isomer** only occurs in the nature. However, the racemic mixture *i.e.*, a mixture of *d*- and *l*-**forms** are invariably marketed as a **nutritional supplement,** which is claimed to be less safer in comparison to the *l*-**form.****

Mechanism of Action: The **mechanism of action** of **carnitine** is solely governed by the falty acid metabolism. The **biochemical reactions** of this **nutraceutical** are predominently based on the reaction taking place between **carnitine** and the **acyl moieties** as given under:

Carnitine + Acyl-co A → Acyl-carnitine + Coenzyme A

Perhaps the above cited reaction would strougly support the analogy that **carnitine** is intimately associated with a plethora of **Coenzyme A-dependent pathways.*****

The first and foremost recognized action of **carnitine** was its direct and articulated involvement in the long-chain faty acid oxidation at the very **mitochondrial level** thereby providing energy. Importantly, **carnitine** serves as a carrier of the **acyl and acetyl** moieties just across the mitochondrial membrane before the β-oxidation can effectively materialize so as to provide 'energy'.**** It is, however, pertinent to state at this point in time that the **emergence of this energy** represents the main pivotal source of energy in the **cardiac** as well as the **skeletal muscle,** thereby legitimately ascertaining the most important role of **carnitine.***** Besides, **carnitine** is strategically responsible for possessing *two* other **cardinal metabolic functions,** namely:

(*a*) Branched chain α-ketoacid oxidation, and

(*b*) Specific detoxification of potentially toxic **Acyl-coA metabolites** from other pathways.

Carnitine is observed to be excreted as 'free carnitine' or as 'acyl carnitine' by the kidneys, whereby more than 90% being reabsorbed by the **proximal renal tubules** genuinely.******

Advantage of Carnitine Supplementation in Haemodialysis Patients:

It has been duly established that **carnitine deficiency** in haemodialysis patients may also lead to serious cardiac problems, that can be even severe. Sakurabyashi *et al.******** (1999) meticulously carried out a clinical study thereby comparing the oral **carnitine** administration in **haemodialysis**

---

*   Kletzmayr J *et al. Kidney Int.,* **55** (Suppl. 69): S 93-S 106, 1999.
**   Li Wan Po A: *Pharm. J.,* 245: 388-89, 1990.
***   Brass EP and Hiatt WR, *J. Am. Coll. Nutr.,* **3:** 207-15, 1998.
****   Grandi M *et al. Int J Clin Pharm Res.,* **17:** 1437, 1997.
*****   Kelly GS, *Alt Med Rev.,* **3:** 345-60, 1998.
******   De Vivo D *et al. Epilepsia,* **39:** 1216-15, 1998.
*******   Sakarabayashi T *et al. Am J Nephrol.,* **19:** 480-4, 1999.

(HD) patients and the **controls** having neither renal nor cardiac diseases. As anticipated, before the actual study was commenced the **observed carnitine levels** in the patients undergoing HD were significantly lower in comparison to the controls. Two months after the regular **carnitine administration** in the said two groups of patients—there was a significant increase in the plasma levels in the patients, and exceeded those of the controls.

Besides, the faulty **myocardial fatty acid metabolism** as observed before the treatment started, that may eventually result in a heart failure in chronic renal patients, was rectified magnificently, thereby putting forward another plausible suggestion with respect to the advantage for the carnitine supplementation in the HD patients particularly.

Other Important Therapeutic Applications of Carnitine: Carnitine finds its abundant vital therapeutically variant applications, and a few important ones shall be enumerated as under:

- **Heart disease:** beneficial usage of **carnitine** for several heart conditions.
- **Angina:** supplementation with **carnitine** may be of great help in patients with **ischaemic heart disease***.
- **Congestive heart failure:** prolonged usage of **carnitine,** at a dose level of 2 g twice daily upto 12 months, showed distinct positive results in terms of improved cardiac events together with greater life-expectancy.
- **Cardiogenic shock: carnitine** acts as a protective means in the **cardiogenic shock****, thereby showing a marked enhancement in the overall survival time.
- **Future applications: carnitine** in the '**glucose metabolism**' and '**insulin deficiency**'; in **Rett Syndrome*****; HIV; muscle weakness in chronic fatigue symptom; beneficial to transfusion-dependent β-thalassemia major subjects, anorexia; diptheria; and male infertility.*****

11.2.13 **Capsaicin [Synonyms: Axsain; Mioton; Zacin; Zostrix;]**

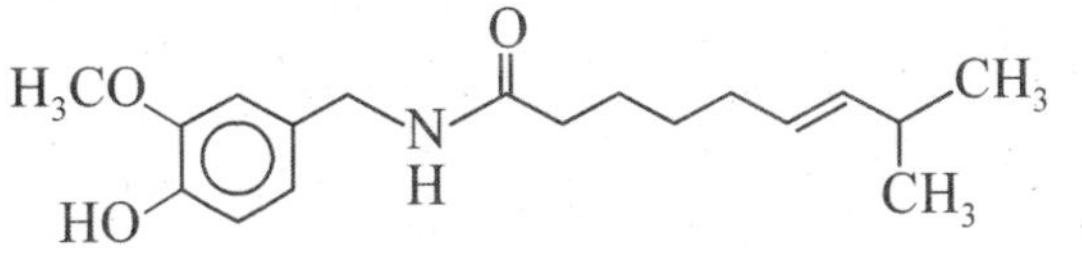

Capsaicin

Capsaicin represents the pungent principle in the fruits of various species of *Capsicum* (*Solanaceae*).

Characteristic Features: These are as follows:

(*i*) **Capsaicin** is obtained from **paparika** and **cayenne.**
(*ii*) It makes chilli peppers '**hot**'.
(*iii*) It finds its usage as a '**pepper spray**' for riot control and self defense.

---

* When blood flow to the heart is reduced, **carnitine levels** in the myocardial muscle may get reduced even upto 40%.
** 'A state of severe tissue hypoperfusion resulting from underlying pump function.
*** 'A neurological disorder, affecting girls, which involves the progressive loss of intellectual and motor skills, resulting in severe mental retardation.
**** Kelly GS, *Alt Med Rev*, **3**: 345-60, 1998.

(*iv*) It causes a '**burning sensation**' for the mammals, but not birds.

(*v*) **Capsaicin** helps to stimulate the **neurons** for burning and abraison sensation.

(*vi*) It is insoluble in water, but soluble in oil and fat.

(*vii*) It can impart a '**cool sensation in mouth**' when mixed with cold milk, alcohol, or ice-cream.

(*viii*) The strength/potency of **capsaicin** never gets lowered either by cooking or freezing.

(*ix*) **Capsaicin** specifically promotes apoptosis in the **pancreatic neoplasm cells.**

(*x*) It exerts practically little effect on the normal pancreatic cells.

(*xi*) **Capsaicin** may critically **relieve chemotherapy-induced neuropathy.**

(*xii*) **Capsaicin** predominently inhibits **NF-kB transcription** of the proinflammatory and antiapoptotic (*i.e.*, neoplasm-promoting) genes.

11.2.14 Piperine

Piperine

Piperine is obtained from **black pepper** (*Piper nigrum L*), and also in *P. longum* L, *P. retrofractum* Vahl. (*P. officinarum* C.D.C.);

Characteristic Features: The **characteristic features** of **piperine** are as stated below:

(*i*) **Piperine** is abundantly found in **hot jalapeno peppers, peppercorns (black pepper).**

(*ii*) It distinctly enhances the intestinal absorption of foods *i.e.*, better digestion.

(*iii*) It is also employed traditionally to mask the taste of the spoiling (putrifying) meat.

11.2.15 Chlorophyll

Chlorophyll a   Chlorophyll b

Chlorophyll is the nature's green pigment specifically found in the plant kingdom. However, the **higher plants** and **green algae** contain **Chlorophyll a** and **Chlorophyll b** in the approximate ratio of 3 : 1. In fact, **Chlorophyll C** is found together with **Chlorophyll a** in a variety of **marine algae.**

Characteristic Features: These are as follows:

(*i*) It is regarded to be the most abundant naturally occurring green pigment in plants.

(*ii*) **Chlorophyll** represents the principal light-abgorbing pigment used profusely in the **photosynthesis.**

(*iii*) **Chlorphyll** seeks its name from the **Greek: chloros = 'yellowish-green'.**

(*iv*) **Chlorophyll** essentially contains the porphyrine ring which is very similar to the **'heme'** (*i.e.*, **haemoglobin**) but contains **Mg** as the central element instead of **Fe.**

(*v*) It forms certain definitive **compact molecular complexes** with some **carcinogenic substances,** such as: **aflatoxin-B1, polyaromatic hydrocarbons** (tobacco smoke), and the **heterocyclic amines** (smoked meat).

(*vi*) It absorbs the red and the violet light more strongly.

(*vii*) **Chlorophyll** present in the leaves undergoes the decaying process in autumn thereby leaving behind the **carotenoid** colours (*e.g.*, yellowish red, yellow).

(*viii*) Chemically, **Chlorophyll a** beans a methyl ($-CH_3$) side chain, whereas **Chlorophyll b** has an aldehydic (–CHO) side chain.

(*ix*) Plants generally comprise of both **Chlorophyll a** and **Chlorophyll b.**

(*x*) The **cyanobacteria*** particularly is devoid of **Chlorophyll b.**

(*xi*) In the UV-region the **chlorophyll a** absorbs **red light** more strongly, whereas **chlorophyll b** absorbs the **violet light** more predominently as given below:

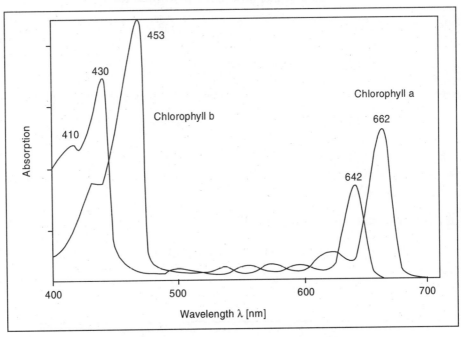

Chlorophyll Light Absorption Spectrum

* **Cyanobacteria:** These are the toxin-producing pond-seum organisms termed as **'blue-green algae'.**

11.2.16 Pectin

Pectin refers to a **polysaccharide** substance usually located in the cell walls of all plant tissues that esseitnally functions as an **intercellular cementing material**. One of the richest sources of **pectin** is **lemon rind** or **orange rind** that comprises of nearly 30% of this particular polysaccharide.

Characteristic Features: These are as stated under:

(*i*) It is available as the soluble fiber in **apples** which perhaps gives the feeling of fullness when eaten.

(*ii*) **Pectin** invariably serves as an antidiarrheal agent.

(*iii*) It possesses an unique property of getting bound to the sugars, and subsequently releasing them gradually as and when required thereby maintaing the blood sugar levels steady almost.

(*iv*) It is found to lower cholesterol in the body.

11.2.17 Dominant Phytochemical Pigments

There are quite a few **dominant phytochemical pigments** or **phytochemical class** that critically provides the most exclusive source of the colouring matter attributed solely to the host of natural **fruits** and **vegetables** which directly or indirectly contribute a lot more as **nutraceuticals**. A good number of such well-known and **dominant phytochemical pigments** are as listed below:

Dominant Phytochemical Pigments

S.No.	Colour	Pigment	Fruit or Vegetable
1	Black	Thearubigens	Black Tea
		Anthocyanins	Black berries
2	Blue/Purple	Anthocyanins	Blueberries, Concord grapes, Eggplant, and Plums
3	Green	Chlorophyll	Asparagus, Broccoli, Cabbage, Green Tea, Kale, and Spinach
4	Orange	β-Carotene	Apricots, Carrots, Cantelope, Mangoes, Sweet Potatoes and Pumpkin
		β-Cryptoxanthin	Oranges, Tangerines
5	Red	Anthocyanins	Apples, Cherries, Crauberries, Pomegranates, Raspberries, Red grapes, and Strawberries
		Lycopene	Pink Grape fruit, Tomatoes, and Watermelon
		β-Cyanins	Beets
6	Yellow	Lutein, Zeaxanthin,	Avocado, Corn,
		Curcumin	Turmeric (Rhizome)

11.2.18 Tocotrienols and Tocopherols

Tocotrienols usually occur in nature *viz.*, in **grains, palm oil** together with their related cousins–the **tocopherols**.

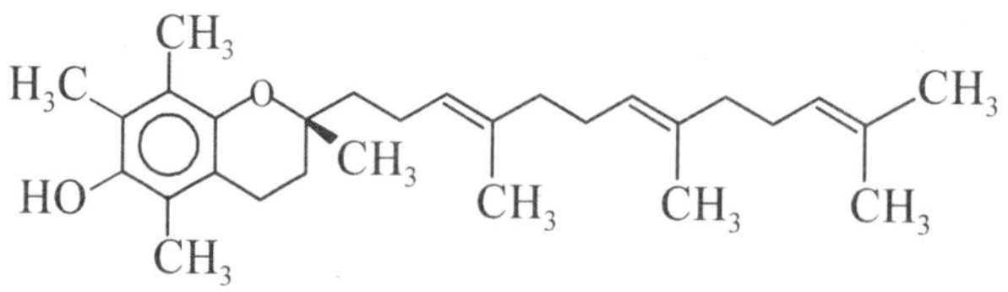

α-Tocotrienol
[From Wheat Bran]

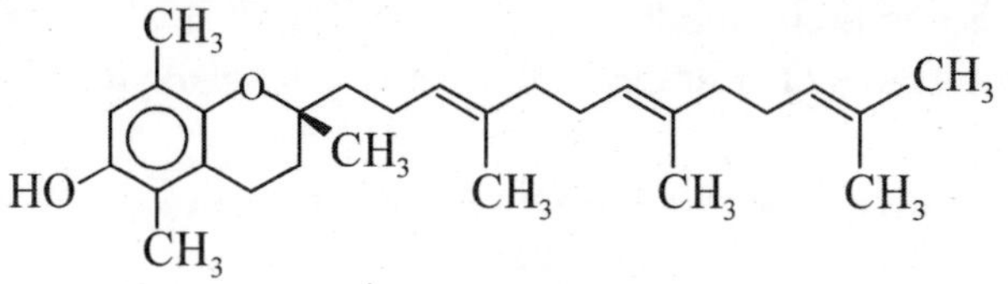

β-Tocotrienol
[From Bran and Wheat Germ Dil]

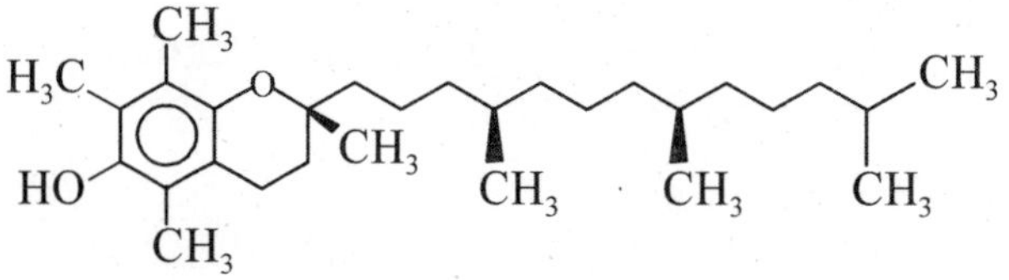

α-Tocopherol
[From Green Vegetables, Grains, Palm oil]

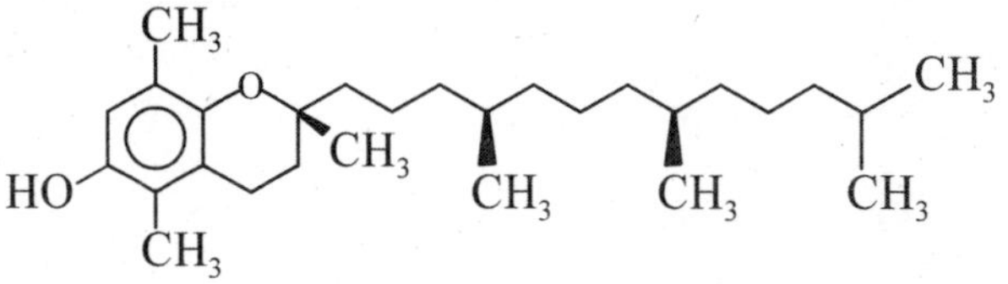

β-Tocopherol
[Naturally occurring form of Vitamin E]

Characteristic Features: These are as enumerated under:

(*i*) **Tocotrienols** seem to cause inhibition of the growth of breast cancerous cells, whereas the **tocopherols** fail to do so.

(*ii*) The biological functionalities of **tocotrienols** and **tocopherols** are quite different.

(*iii*) Biological activity of **tocopherols** resembles to that of **Vitamin E.**

(*iv*) **Tocotrienols** have explicitly shown their distinct **cholesterol-lowering effect.**

11.2.19 α-Lipoic Acid and Ubiquinones

A. **α-Lipoic acid (Thioctic Acid) and Ubiquinones (Coenzymes Q)** have gained ample cognizance as most vital and important **antioxidants** which in turn exhibit their wonderful overall effect to extend the ensuing effects of other **antioxidants** as well.

α-Lipoic Acid [Synonyms: Thioctic Acid; Protogen A; Acetate Replacing Factor; Pyruvate Oxidation Factor; Biletan; Thioctacid; Thioctan; Tioctan;]:

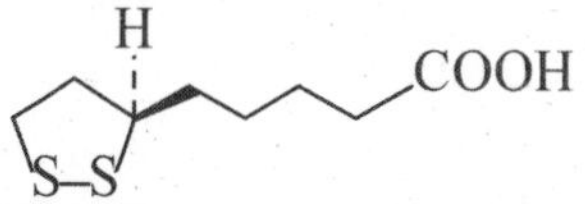

α-Lipoic Acid (*d*-Form)

Characteristic Features: The characteristic features of **α-Lipoic acid** are as follows:

(*i*) In terms of research, **α-lipoic acid,** is regarded to be the **'new kid on the block'** *i.e.,* **nutraceuticals.**

(*ii*) It efficiently serves as a **'hydroxy moiety quencher'** (because of its ability to form **'esters'** rapidly).

(*iii*) The sulphur-sulphur bond in the pentagonal ring system caters as the most reactive segment of the molecule.

(*iv*) It is found to be active on both lipids and tissue fluids.

(*v*) Besides, the available **hydroxyl moieties,** it also strategically scavenges **peroxyl, ascorbyl,** and **chromanoxyl moieties.**

(*vi*) **Thioetic acid** serves as a **'protective agent'** of both **Vitamin E** and **Vitamin C** by virtue of the fact that it critically functions in both **lipid** and **water phases.**

(*vii*) **α-Lipoic acid** articulately affords protection to **catalase, superoxide dismutase (SOD),** and **glutathione,** which play a vital and important role in the **liver-detoxification activities.***

(*viii*) It essentially plays an important role in energy production.

B. Ubiquinones [Synonyms: coenzymes Q; Q-275; Sa;]:

Ubiquinones refer to a group of lipid-soluble benzoquinones directly involved in electron-transport in mitochondria *i.e.*, in the **oxidation of succinate** or **reduced nicotine adenine dinucleotide** (NADH) *via* the **specific cytochrome system.** It predominently occurs in the majority of aerobic microorganisms, from bacteria to higher plants and animals.

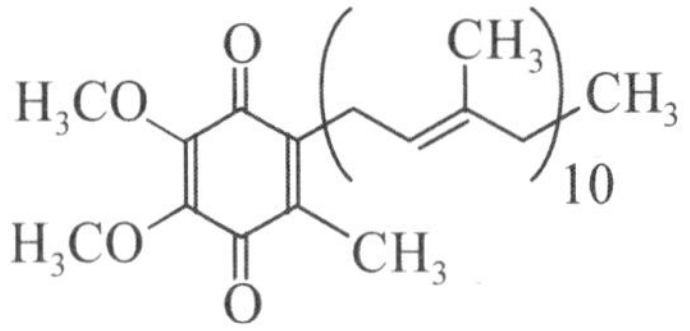

Ubiquinone

Characteristic Features: These are as given under:

(*i*) Coenzyme Q is recognised as a recently discovered antioxidant.

(*ii*) It serves as an important means of energy production.

(*iii*) The clinical aspects of Coenzyme Q reveals that it may be an useful cardiotonic.

11.3   CONTEMPORARY NUTRACEUTICALS

The modern state-of-the-art **nutraceuticals** *i.e.*, **contemporary nutraceuticals** are penetrating the world market based entirely on their legitimate merit(s), safer usages, high degree of efficiency, and above all the superb and excellent means of their therapeutic efficacy across the globe. One may observe the goodness of **'black raspberries'** which are found to be extremely rich in **'antioxidants'**; and therefore, may serve as a powerful tool in the fight against the most dreadful human ailment **'cancer'.** In the same vein one may also consider the so called **'green leafy vegetables'** that are used extensively in the **modern research** essentially comprising of fibre with an exceedingly high content of **galactose**—a carbohydrate that is earnestly believed to help categorically prevent the proteins known as **'lectins'** from getting bound to the inner lining of the colon (large intestine) and thereby causing serious and permanent damage.

In this specific context, a few important **'contemporary nutraceuticals'** shall be discussed briefly as stated under:

---

* Sumathi R *et al. Pharmacol Res,* **27:** 309-318, May-June-1993.

11.3.1 Spiruline

Spiruline (*Spirulina platensis*)—a cyanobacterium having a beneficiary action upon the alimentary biochemical processes for the undernourished and convalescent subjects—is profusely employed in the form of its dry powder capsulated in hard-gelatin capsules as a nutritional supplement. The reasonably significant effect of the **spiruline supplement** is on account of it **relatively higher iron content.***

The mechanism of action of **spiruline** may be attributed by virtue of the high amount in the lipid fraction of **ω** derivative *e.g.,* **γ-linolenic acid.**** However, the singular exclusive presence of **ω-6** vividly records a distinct metabolic gain, because **disaturase enzyme** may not be available in sufficient quantum in the undernourished subjects.***

Spirulina, a commercialized seaweed, should pass the stringent toxicological criteria *viz,* Maximum levels of iodine [≤ 5 g. kg^{-1}], toxic minerals [As: ≤ 3 mg. kg^{-1}; cd: ≤ 0.5 mg. kg^{-1}; Sn and Pb: ≤ 5 mg. kg^{-1}; Hg : ≤ 0.1 mg. kg^{-1}], and the dried seaweeds should pass the following microbiological criteria (per g): faecal *E. coli* ≤ 10, anaerobic microorganisms ≤ 100, aerobic microorganisms $\leq 10^4$, and *Clostridium* ≤ 1.****

11.3.2 Broccoli

Broccoli [*Brassica oleraceae italica;* **Cruciferae/Bracicaceae**] essentially contains **glucarophanin,** the glucosinolate precursor of **sulphoraphane,** as given below, has been amply demonstrated to possess very useful medicinal characteristic features.

Glucoraphanin   Sulphoraphane

It has been observed that **glucoraphanin** helps to induct the specific **carcinogen-detoxifying enzyme systems,** and thereby accelerates the removal of the **xenobiotics.******* Nevertheless, the young sprouted seedlings do comprise of approximately 10-100 folds as much **glucoraphanin** as the fully grown plant; and, therefore, **broccoli** may be regarded as the most valuable dietary vegetable supplement.

Glucoraphanin could prevent **breast cancer** and may also sabotage the uncontrolled cell division of **colon cancer cells.** However, the purely **synthetic compound** exerts its action very much akin to its **natural counterpart** usually known as **oxomate, sulphoraphane,** duly identified and recognized as a cancer preventive agent in **broccoli.**

---

    * Kapoor R and Mehta U: *Indian J Explt. Biol.,* **30**: 904-7, 1992.

  ** Decsi T and Koletzko B: *Nutrition.,* **16**: 447-53, 2000.

 *** Koletzko B *et al. Eur J Pediatr.,* **145**: 109-15, 1986.

**** **Bulletin du Ministere des Affaires Sociales:** Text No: 1705, Nov. 28-1990.

***** **Xenobiotic:** A drug or other substance not normally found in the body.

Mechanism of Action: The body's production of **Phase II enzymes*** is substantially increased by the two aforesaid compounds whereby the enzyme has a tendency to cause detoxification of cancer-causing chemicals, and thus minimise the risk of **cancer.** Oxomate could be administered together with othr **'antineoplastic agents'** like **tamoxifen** *i.e.,* a combination of **phytonutrients** and **drugs,** in an obvious attempt to **muster maximise protection.** Interestingly, **tamoxifen** is at present the only US-FDA approved drug recommended for **breast cancer prevention** particularly in the high-risk women. It actually exerts its therapeutic action by an altogether different mechanism than that of **oxomate.** It has been observed that **tamoxifen** aids a female subject essentially having an **oestrogen-dependent tumours.** However, it may further be expatiated that a drug exclusively based upon the **oxomate** would certainly help prevent cancer formation irrespective of the fact whether the particular tumour is either an **oestrogen-dependent** one or a **non-oestrogen dependent** one.

Stomach Cancer and Ulcers: Sulphoraphane, an active principle found in **broccoli** and **broccoli sprouts** has been observed to cause a bactericidal effect on the specific bacterium responsible for the plethora of **stomach cancers.** In fact, the causative organism, *Helicobacter pyroli,* for specifically debilitating **stomach ulcers** as well as **stomach cancers** could be cured with antibiotics. Jed Fahey** has rightly advocated that—

"If future extended clinical studies reveal that a nutraceutical can either relieve or at least prevent diseases intimately associated with *H. pyroli* in people, it could have significant public health implications not coufined to the United States only but also around the world."

Sulphoraphane showed its proven ability to protect cells against cancer by augmenting their production of **phase 2 enzymes,** *i.e.,* a family of proteins that are responsible for carrying out the detoxification of cancer-causing substances and also damaging the ensuing free-radicals. Nevertheless, its **antibiotic profiles** are not quite explicitly understood as to date, and are likely to take place *via* certain other mechanism.

Brassica Protection Products (BPP) a joint venture by **Fahey and Johns Hopkins University** developed and marketed specialized **chemoprotective food products** and also the **broccoli sprouts.**

11.3.3   Aloe Vera Gel and Aloe Juice

Thre are *two* botanical sources of **'Aloe',** namely:

    (*a*) **Cape Aloe** [*Aloeferox.* Miller].
    (*b*) **Curacao Aloe** [*A. vera* (L.) Burm. *f*: **Asphodelaceae**].

In the usual traditional manner, the juice which is made to flow almost spontaneously right from the incised leaves gets duly collected and carefully concentrated by simple boiling. Thus, the concentrated and thickened juice comprises of the **dark brown masses (Curacao Aloe)** and with distinct **greenish reflections (Cape Aloe).** However, one may obtain the **Aloe Gel** after duly elininating the outermost tissues of the leaf meticulously.

---

   * A family of proteins which detoxify certain cancer-causing agents and damaging free radicals.
   ** **Jed Fahey:** A plant physiologist in the Department of Pharmacology and Molecular Sciences at the Johns Hopkins School of Medicine, USA.

Composition: The **Aloe Vera Gel** composition consists of a rich content of water, besides certain not-so-specific compounds as: **amino acids, enzymes, lipids, sterols,** and most of all, **polysaccharides** (*e.g.,* **pectins, hemicelluloses**).

Characteristic Features: The **characteristic features** of **Aloe Vera Gel** are as stated under:

(*i*) It* contains upto $20 \pm 1\%$ **hydroxy anthraquinone derivatives** *viz.,* Aloin A; α-L-Rha Aloinoside A; Aloin B; and α-L-Rha-Aloinoside B, as given under:

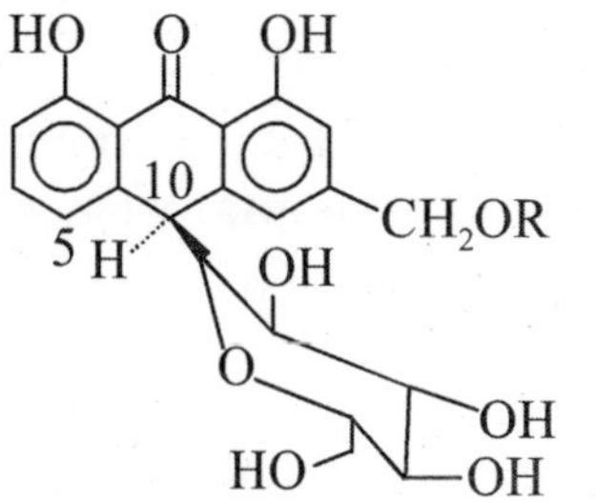

Aloin A: R = H;
Aloinoside A: R = α-L-RHa;

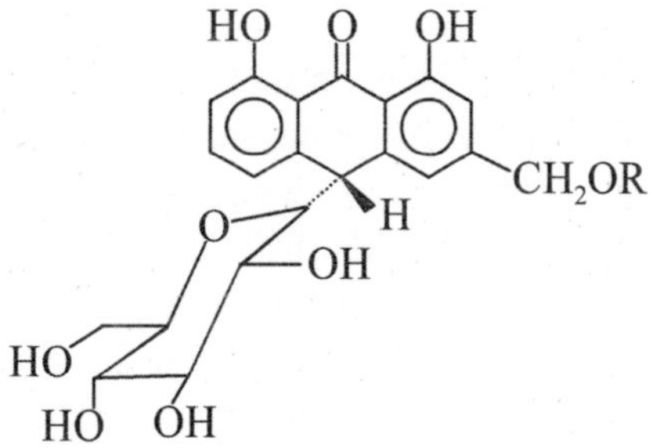

Aloin B: R = H;
Aloinoside B: R = α-L-RHa;

(*ii*) **Aloe Vera Gel** appears to contain various antibacterial and antifungal chemical entities which may potentially delay or inhibit the growth of suh microorganisms which are solely responsible for **food borne illness in humans** and **food spoilage** generally.

(*iii*) It helps to preserve several fresh highly perishable fruits and vegetables *viz.,* table grapes, bananas, strawberrys, apricot, peaches, plums, oranges and the like.

(*iv*) The **Aloe Vera Gel** adequately affords **potential environmental benefits.** Alternatively, it could provide a greener perspective to sulphur dioxide (SO_2) and several other synthetic food preservatives which are invariably used on the agricultural produce thereby increasingly causing serious health hazards.

(*v*) Manufacturers of this **naturaceutical** as health product make a wide spectrum of therapeutic advantages in humans ranging from: diabetes, human immune system, AIDS, digestive system, arthritis, cholesterol management/control, asthma, kidney protection, cough and cold, cleansing of toxins from intestines, skin manifestations, and hair loss.

(*vi*) It is employed extensively in **cosmetic products** to serve as an extremely hydrating ingredient in liquid or creams, sun-lotions, shaving creams, lip-guards, face packs, healing ointments, and various protective creams.

(*vii*) It may also be employed skillfully in the composition of **phytomedicines** traditionally utilized as an adjunct in the **emolient** and **antipruriginous** treatment of various skin disorders, as a trophic protective agent for cracks, abrasions, chaps, frost bite, insect-bites, superficial and limited burns, sunburn, and also for draper rash (in babies).

Mechanisms: Several mechanisms have been duly invoked so as to explain the aforesaid activities, such as:

- stimulation of the complement linked to polysaccharides
- high water content imparting various sequential phenomena *viz.*, **hydrating, insulating,** and **protective properties to the gel.**

11.3.4 Soyfoods

Soyfoods are processed or semi-processed products prepared from **soya bean** or **soja bean** or **Lincoln bean** or **Manchurian bean** or **Chinese pea.** Soya bean is the seed of *Glycine max* (L.) Merrill, and several other species *viz., G. Soja* Sieb & Zucc., *G. hispida* (Moench) Maxim., and *Soja hispida* Moench, belonging to the natural order **Leguminoseae.**

A Chinese investigative study has adequately established the fact that regular consumption of **'Soyfoods'** may drastically reduce the risk of fracture in **postmenopausal women** specifically amongst those who are in the early years following the state of menopause.

It has also been proved beyond any reasonable doubt that there exists a definite linkage between the **'soyfood intake'** and **bone-mineral density.**

In the recent past, **soyboods** are distinctly enjoying an overall strong appeal as an integral component by virtue of the fact they are relatively **free** of the **artery-clogging trans fats,** that are duly formed when these fats are suitably hydrogenated to render them more solid and also extend their shelf-life significantly. Besides, the oil also continues to benefit from an ever-increasing awareness of the innumerable health properties of the antioxidant-rich oil.

11.3.5 Omega-3 Fatty Acids

The **omega-3 fatty acids** represent a class of fatty acids invariably found in **'fish-oils'.** It is especially and abundantly obtained from **Salmon** and some other **cold-water fish.** It has been amply proved and established that the **omega-3 fatty acids** duly help to lower the levels of **cholesterol** and **LDL** (*i.e.,* low-density lipoproteins) in the blood. **LDL** usually represent the so called **'bad-cholesterol'** present in the blood. It serves as a nutritional supplement as well as a natural source of the marine product. The **Omega-3 fish oil** is regarded to be a **nutraceutical,** which is a food providing health supplement. They provide an antiinflammatory action very much within the body that may prove to be extremely beneficial for the particular relief of **inflammatory disorders,** namely: **rheumatoid arthritis.** Generally, eating fish has been reported to cause protection against the age-related **macular degeneration** *i.e.,* a common eye ailment.

Commercial Product
Blackmores Anti-inflammatory Fish Oil-1000
[Manufactured By: Blackmores LTD., 23-Rosebery Street, Balgowlah, Auckland, New Zealand]

Active Ingredients Per Capsule:

Fish Oil (Natural)	1 g (1000 mg)
Containing Omega-3 marine triglycerides 300 mg as:	
Eicosapentaenoic Acid [EPA]	180 mg
Docosahexaenoic Acid [DHA]	120 mg

11.3.6 Pomegranate Juice

The **pomegranate juice** is remarkably quite rich in **antioxidants,** for instance: **anthocyanins,** tannins, and soluble **polyphenols,** that articulately scavenge the **'free radicals'** and thereby help to prevent specifically DNA damage which may ultimately lead to a number of serious health conditions.

It also possesses **antiatherosclerotic activities** *i.e.,* preventing the thickening of the arteries, and thereby slowed down the **oxidation of cholesterol** to almost 50%*.

Pomegranate Juice helps to prevent the ischemic **Coronary heart disease (CHD)****, thereby showing improved flow of blood to the heart by almost 17%. However, no apparent negative effects on lipids, blood-glucose level, haemoglobin A 1c, blood pressure, and above all the body weight of the subject.

11.3.7 Walnuts

In the recent past, the health-conferring benefits of the **walnuts** have shown that are a prominent source of the natural **antioxidant hormone melatonin;** and, therefore, its consumption would certainly help to boost up the blood levels of **melatonin** significantly.

Melatonin

Russel Reiter's findings adequately demonstrated that the **Walnuts** substantically contain **melatonin,** which is duly absorbed when it is eaten. It also improves in patients the ability to **resist oxidative stress** caused on account of certain toxic molecules usually termed as **'free radicals'.**

Melatonin content in **walnuts** ranges between 2.5 to 4.5 ng per g.

The **melatonin supplements** are widely employed by the consumers (*i.e.,* patients) whose sleep patterns are found to be **irregular, engaged in shift work** or **suffering from jet lag.**

11.3.8 Certified Organic Mushroom Nutrace

In a broader sense, **Mushrooms** are quite valuable health food products, which are low in calories, high in vegetable proteins, iron, zinc, chitin, and profusely used in the **Traditional Chinese Medicine (TCM).** In fact, their **legendary** effects on the promotion of good and sound health rightly suggest that the **Mushrooms** are **probiotic** in nature *i.e.,* they help in restoring **bodies health, balance,** and **natural resistance to disease.** The active principles present in them exert to boost the **immune system** *i.e.,* they do possess immune system enhancement properties.

A few typical examples of the **certified organic mushroom nutrace** are as stated under:

---

* *Clin. Nutr.:* **23**(3): 423-33, June-2004.

** Researches carried out at: (*a*) California Pacific Medical Centre, and (*b*) University of California's Non-profit Preventive Medicine Research Institute. **CHD** is the biggest cause of death in several Western countries.

11.3.8.1 Trimyo-Gen™ [Composed of: 33% Cordyceps sinensis (Winter Worm: Summer Grass), 33% Gandoderma lucidum (Reishi), and 33% Schizophyllum commune]

Importantly, the strain of *Cordyceps* was found high in the **Himalayan Mountains** for a short duration in summer, and growing on its natural host—a caterpillar. However, it is now scientifically cultured on organic whole grain substrates, and produced under stringent sterile quality control environment.

11.3.8.2 MycoPlex-7™

It is essentially a **Seven Mushroom Formulation** with a base of the most established **nutraceutical mushrooms.** These mushrooms are of immense use in both **Oriental and Chinese Traditional Medicine (TCM).** It has been shown they exhibit **legendary** effects both as an **adaptogen** and **vitality enhancer.**

FURTHER READING REFERENCES

1. Arruzazabala ML *et al.*: *Leukot. Essent. Fatty Acids,* **49:** 695-7, 1993.
2. Brower V: **Nutraceuticals Poised for a Healthy Slice of the Healthcare Market,** *Nat. Biotechnol.,* **16:** 728-31, 1998.
3. **Bulletin du Ministere des Affaires Sociales:** Text No: 1705, p. 103, Nov. 28-1990.
4. *Clin. Nutr.:* **23**(3): 423-33, June-2004.
5. Hussain MA: *Eur. J. Endocrinol.* **139:** 472-5, 1998.
6. Kato S *et al.*: *Br. J. Nutr.*, **73:** 433-42, 1995.
7. Kelly GS: *Alternative Med. Rev.,* **3:** 345-60, 1998.
8. Parker RS: *J. Nutr.,* **119:** 101-4, Jan-1989.
9. Snider SR: **Octaciosanol in Parkinsonism,** *Ann. Neurol.,* **16:** 723, 1984.
10. Sumathi R *et al.*: *Pharmacol. Research,* **27:** 309-318, May/June-1993.
11. Torres O *et al.*: *Diabetes Care,* **18:** 393-7, 1995.
12. Xie CI *et al.*: *Alcohol. Clin. Exp. Res.,* **18:** 1443-7, 1994.

12 Enzyme and Protein Drug Substances

A. ENZYME AS DRUG SUBSTANCES

12.1 INTRODUCTION

An **enzyme** is usually defined as—'**an organic catalyst produced by the living cells but capable of acting outside cells or even *in-vitro*.** In a broader sense, the **enzymes** may be regarded as **proteins** which categorically alter the rate of **chemical reactions** without requiring the aid of an **external energy source** or being **charged themselves.** Importantly, an enzyme may be able to catalyze a particular reaction several times effectively.

Specific Characteristic Features: The various **specific characteristic features** of **enzyme** are as enumerated under:

(1) Generally, **enzymes** are reaction specific in that they act exclusively on certain substances (known as **'substrates'**).

(2) **Enzyme** and its corresponding substrate or substrates invariably give rise to an **enzyme-substrate complex,** which involves not only **physical shape** but also **chemical bonding.**

(3) **Enzyme** helps in promoting the **'creation of bonds'** either between altogether separate substrates, or induces the cleavage of bonds in a single substrate to result into the formation of the product or products of reaction.

(4) **Metabolism:** Numerous **enzymes** present in human body, whereby each catalyzing one of the several reactions which essentially occur as part of **metabolism.**

(5) **Functionality:** It has been duly observed that each **enzyme** acts at an **optimum temperature** and a **pH,** at which it does function most efficaciously. For most **human enzymes,** these shall be particularly confined to such factors as: **pH of cells, body temperature, tissue fluid, and blood.**

(6) **Impaired Activity: Impaired activity of enzymes** may be caused due to extremes of **pH, temperature, dehydration, UV-radiation,** and the presence of **heavy metals** *viz.*, Pb or Hg.

(7) **Specific Requirements:** Certain enzymes specifically require the dire presence of **coenzymes** (*i.e.*, non protein molecules *e.g.*, **Vitamins**) to enable them function properly; whereas, still others require some **critical minerals,** such as: Fe, Cu, Zn).

(8) **Proenzyme:** It has been observed that certain **enzymes** are obtained as **proenzyme** *i.e.*, in an inactive form; and, therefore, must be duly activated by appropriate means *viz.*, **inactive pepsinogen** is suitably converted to **active pepsin** by the help of hydrochloric acid (HCl) present in the **gastric juice.**

(9) **Activity: Enzymes** do possess a variety of vital and important **activities,** a few of them shall now be discussed briefly as under:

(*a*) **Digestive Enzymes:** These are usually most common and familiar. They are basically the **'hydrolytic enzymes'** which specifically catalyze the addition of water molecules to relatively bigger food-molecules to help them split into rather simpler chemical entities. Quite often the very name of the enzyme explicitly indicates the **'substrate'** with addition of the suffix-**ase.**

Examples: (*i*) **Lipase**—It splits **fat** (triglycerides) into the corresponding fatty acids and glycerol respectively.

(*ii*) **Peptidase**—It splits **peptides** to the corresponding amino acids.

Exceptions: Certain **enzymes** *e.g.*, **pepsin** and **trypsin** do not usually end in –**ase,** because they were duly baptized much before this method of **nomenclature** was actually instituted.

(*b*) **Enzymes for Synthesis Reactions:** The **enzymes for synthesis reactions** help to synthesize a host of **biological products,** such as: **glycogen, hormones, nucleic acids (DNA and RNA), phospholipids for cell membranes, and proteins,** most of them need one if not several enzymes.

Examples: DNA Polymerase—is essentially required for DNA-replication, that actually precedes **mitosis.**

(*c*) **Energy Production:** It also specifically requires a plethora of enzymes.

Examples: Each and every step related to cell respiration needs essentially a particular **enzyme,** for instance: **cytochrome transport system, glycolysis,** and **Krebs cycle.**

(*d*) **Deamination Reactions:** The **deamination reactions** are usually carried out by **deaminases** which critically remove the **amino moieties** from the available pool of excessive **amino acids** so that they may exclusively utilized for **energy.**

10. **Miscellaneous Activities of Enzymes:** These categorically include certain highly specific **enzymes** to perform a definite purpose *in vivo*, A few such typical examples are as given under, namely:

(*a*) **Cessation of Long-chain Fatty Acids:** Specific **enzymes** aid in the splitting of long-chain fatty acids into relatively smaller compounds which in turn used up in the **cell respiration** mostly.

(*b*) **Maintenance of Blood Pressure:** Specific enzymes are usually required for **'blood clotting',** and also for the formation of **angiotensin II** solely required to **maintain and raise the blood pressure.**

Another school of thought describes the **'enzyme'** as—**'a biocatalyst that essentially accelerates specific biological reactions.'** Nevertheless, the recognized concept of biocatalysts is rather broad-spectrum, and generously embraces a variety of **pure substance(s), cell product(s),** and **cell extract(s),** namely:

- pure enzymes,
- plant cells,
- animal cells,
- crude cell extract,
- microbial cells,
- intact non-viable microbial cells.

The sources of **enzymes** that are viable commercially range from **animals, higher-plants,** and **microorganisms.**

Following are certain prevalent and important **enzymes** exploited commercially that belong to the aforesaid categories are as stated under:

(*a*) **Animal Enzymes** *e.g.*, **lipases, rennets, tripsin** etc.
(*b*) **Higher-plant Enzymes** *e.g.*, **amylases, papain, proteases,** and **soybean lipoxygenase.**
(*c*) **Microorganisms** *e.g.*, *Acetobacter lacti, Clostridium aceticum.*

Sasson* (1984) critically advocated that certain **enzymes** are employed overwhelmingly in the **Food and Beverage Industries,** such as:

Papain : obtained from **papaya fruit** used mostly as **meat tenderizer,** and in making **'wort'** from malt (to solubilize residual protein) in breweries to prepare **Beer.**
Protease : used profusely in the manufacture of **detergents,** and in **softening of leather** in **tanning industry.**

In the recent past, the **microbial enzymes** have legitimately acclaimed a wide popularity and overwhelming recognition. In fact, the spectacular production of both **primary and secondary metabolites** by the microorganisms could only be feasible by virtue of the involvement of a host of specific **enzymes.** Thus, one may classify the **enzymes** based upon their **site of action** as given below:

(*a*) **Endoenzymes [or Intracellular Enzymes]:** The **enzymes** that are solely secreted very much within the cell are termed as **endoenzymes.** They essentially are involved in the apt synthesis of different **cellular components, food reserves,** and also serve as **bioenergetic materials.*** * Importantly, as these various processes do occur in the intracellular zones, the **enzymes** involved are also strategically located in the **intracellular region.**
Examples: Isomerases, Phosphorylases, Synthetases etc.
(*b*) **Exoenzymes [or Extracellular Enzymes]:** The **enzymes** that are exclusively secreted outsides the cell are invariably known as **exoenzymes** or **extracellular enzymes.** They usually exert a digestive feature in their overall activity and function. Interestingly, they help in the hydrolysis of relatively complex molecules into much simpler compounds.

* Sasson A: **Biotechnology: Challenges and Promises,** UNESCO, Paris, 1984.
** **Bioenergetic Materials:** Such substances that liberate energy from food stuffs.

Examples: Amylases—hydrolyse **starch** components;
  Lypases—hydrolyse **lipids** (*i.e.,* triglycerides); and
  Proteoses—hydrolyse **proteins** into **amino acids.**

There is a plethora of **endoenzymes** that are specifically generated by **pathogenic** as well as **saprophytic* microorganisms.**

Examples: Cellulase—converts **cellulose** to **cellobiose;**
  Polygalacturonase—
  Pectinmethylesterase—
  Polymethylgalacturonase—

Riviere (1977)** observed that the **endoenzymes,** namely: **asparaginase, invertase,** and **uric oxidase** are noticeably of much higher economic value, and also are quite difficult to undergo extraction because they are critically produced very much inside the cell.

12.2   ENZYME VARIANTS

Over the years a good number of **enzyme variants** have been duly identified and recognized for their specific usages as summarized in the following Table 12.1.

Table 12.1   Enzyme Variants and their Applications

S.No.	Type of Enzyme (Abbreviation)	Applications
1	**Activating Enzyme**	Catalyzes the attachment of an amino acid to the suitable **transfer ribonucleic acid** [t RNA].
2	**Allosteric Enzyme**	Alteration in activity caused due to certain types of **effectors,** known as allosteirc effectors, bind to a nonactive site on the enzyme.
3	**Amylolytic Enzyme**	Catalyzes the conversion of starch to sugar.
4	**Angiotensin-converting Enzyme [ACE]**	Converts **angiotensin I** (a segment of the **renin-angiotensin-aldosterone mechanism** of the kidney) to **angiotensin II** *i.e.,* the ultimate and final step in the **renin-angiotensin mechanism.** The latter helps to stimulate **aldosterone secretion,** and hence Na retention.
5	Autolytic Enzyme	Produces autolysis or cell digestion.
6	**Branching Enzyme**	Transfers a carbohydrate unit from one molecule to another *e.g.,* **glycosyl transferase.**
7	**Brush Border Enzyme**	Serves as the lining of the small intestine and produced by the cells of the **villi** and **microvilli (brush border).**
8	**Coagulating Enzyme**	Catalyses the conversion of **soluble proteins** into **insoluble ones** (*Synonym:* **Coagulase**).
9	**Debranching Enzyme**	Removes a **carbohydrate unit** from molecules which essentially contain **short carbohydrate** units usually attached as side-chains *e.g.,* **dextrin-1, 6-glucosidase.**
10	**Deamidizing Enzyme**	Splits amine off amino acid chemical compounds.
11	**Decarboxylating Enzyme**	Separates specifically carbon dioxide [CO_2] from organic acids *e.g.,* **carboxylase.**
12	**Digestive Enzyme**	Controls digestive processes in the alimentary canal.

(Contd.)

---

* **Saprophytic:** Any organism living on decaying or dead organic matter *e.g.,* **higher fungi.**
** Rivere J: **Industrial Application of Microbiology,** Survey Univ. Press, London, 1977.

13	**Fermenting Enzyme**	Brings about fermentation especially of the **carbohydrates** and produced by **organisms** or **yeasts.**
14	**Glycolytic Enzyme**	Catalyses the oxidation of **glucose.**
15	**Hydrolytic Enzyme**	Catalyses the phenomenon of hydrolysis.
16	**Inhibitory Enzyme**	Blocks or inhibits a chemical reaction.
17	**Inverting Enzyme**	Catalyzes the hydrolysis of sucrose.
18	**Lipolytic Enzyme**	Catalyses the hydrolysis of **fats** (triglycerides) *e.g.*, **lipase.**
19	**Mucolytic Enzyme**	Depolymerizes mucous by splitting **mucoproteins**, *e.g.*, **lysozyme, mucinase** (or **hyaluronidase**).
20	**Oxidising Enzyme**	Catalyses oxidative reactions [*Synonym:* **Oxidase**].
21	**Proteolytic Enzyme**	Catalyses the conversion of proteins into peptides.
22	**Redox Enzyme**	Catalyzes oxidation-reduction reactions.
23	**Reducing Enzyme**	Removes oxygen [O_2] [*Synonym:* **Reductase**].
24	**Respiratory Enzyme**	Acts within tissue cells to catalyze oxidative reactions by releasing energy.
25	**Splitting Enzyme**	Facilitates removal of a portion of a molecule.
26	**Transferring Enzyme**	Facilitates the moving of one molecule to another chemical entity. [*Synonym:* **Transferase**].
27	**Uricolytic Enzyme**	Catalyses the conversion of uric acid to urea.
28	**Yellow Enzyme**	Involves particularly in the cellular oxidations *viz.*, a group of **flavoproteins.**

12.3 ENZYMES OF PHARMACEUTICAL RELEVANCE AND UTILITY

A survey of literature would reveal that there exist quite many enzymes that specifically possess well recognized pharmaceutical relevance and utility. Interestingly, most of them find their highly critical and pivotol role in the therapeutic armamentarium to serve as useful means to provide enormous help in curing human diseases. The following Table 12.2 includes a number of such enzymes that are invariably employed as **'drugs'** along with their particular type, source(s), and applications.

Table 12.2 Drugs (Enzymes) with Pharmaceutical Relevance

S.No.	Drugs (Enzymes)	Enzyme Type(s)	Source(s)	Applications
1	**Bromelain**	Proteolytic	Stem of pineapple plant, *Ananas comosus,*, [*Family:* **Bromiliaceae**].	Soft tissue anti-inflammatory agent.
2	**Chymotrypsin**	—do—	Pancreas of Ox, *Bos taurus*(*Family:* **Bovidae**).	In ophthalmology; and also as anti-inflammatory agent.
3	**Collagenase**	—do—	Fermentation of *Clostridium histolyticum.*	Debredement of skin burns and derma ulcers.
4	**Deoxyribonuclease**	Nucleolytic	Pancreas of Ox, Cow, Buffalo	Lowering the viscosity of bronchopulmonary secretions.
5	**Fibrinolysin**	Proteolytic	Human plasminogen;	Cure of thrombotic disorders.
6	**Hyaluronidase**	Amylolytic	Mammalian (Bovine) testes.	Enhancing of IM injections.
7	**Muramidase**	Mucolytic	Serum, tears, lungs of animals.	Antibacterial and antiviral agent.
8	**Papain**	Proteolytic	Latex of unripe fruits of tropical melon tree (Papaya) [*Carica papaya* (**Caricaceae**)].	Clarification of fruit juices, beer, and as meat tenderizer.
9	**Pancreatin**	Proteolytic, Lipolytic, and Carbolytic	Pancreas of Hog [*Sus serofa* (Suidae)].	Digestive agent for fat, protein and polysaccharides.
10	Pancrealipase	—do—	—do—	Chronic pancreatitis, and cystic fibrosis.

(Contd.)

11	**Pepsin**	Proteolytic	Glandular layer of fresh stomach of hog [*sus scrofa* (**Suidae**)].	Conversion of protein into peptone as well as proteose
12	**Rennin (Chymosin)**	—do—	Glandular layer of fresh stomach of calf [*Bos taurus* (**Bovidae**)].	Commercial manufacture of different types of processed cheese.
13	**Seratiopeptidase**	Proteolytic	Organism belonging to genus *Serratia*.	To increase the effects **antibiotic** due to its inherent anti-inflammatory activity.
14	**Streptokinase**	Plasminogen activator	Culture filtrates obtained from β-hemolytic *Streptococci-* **Group C.**	In thromboembolic disorders.
15	**Urokinase**	Fibronolysis	Kidney-tissue or human urine cultures.	Lysis of blood clots or fibrin in pulmonary embolism.
16	**L-Asparaginase**	Hydrolytic	Obtained from *Escherichia coli*, plant, animal tissues, fungi and yeast.	Interferes with growth of malignant cells.

12.4   BRIEF DESCRIPTION OF ENZYMES USED AS DRUGS

In the following sections a brief description of certain **enzymes** that are specifically used as **drugs** shall be dealt with relevant therapeutic applications;

12.4.1 Bromelain

Bromelain is a proteolytic enzyme particularly present in the pineapple plant. It is usually available as a buff coloured, odourless amorphous powder having poor solubility in aqueous and organic solvents. It is mostly indicated in the cure and treatment of oedema caused due to injury or surgery, and in acute soft-tissue inflammation.

12.4.2 Chymotrypsin

Chymotrypsin refers to the digestive enzyme produced duly by the pancreas and functioning in the small intestine that, with **trypsin,** hydrolyzes proteins to peptones or further. [**Trade names: Avazyme$^{(R)}$; amd Enzeon$^{(R)}$**]. Each mg of **chymotrypsin** contains not less than 1000 USP units. **Chymotrypsin** is largely employed in **ophthalmology** for the critical dissection of zonule of eye-lens for the specific **intracapsular cataract extraction.** It is also indicated for the topical usage to reduce soft-tissue inflammation from abscesses, ulcers, fistulas, as well as necrotic injuries.

12.4.3 Collagenase

Collagenase represents an enzyme that induces certain specific changes in **collagen** to cause its respective degradation. It is invariably obtained from ***Clostridium histolyticum*** by its fermentation; and also bears the capability for the necessary digestion of both **denatured and native collagen.**

The actual potency of **collagenase** is usually given by its capability to digest **normal bovine collagen** *in vitro*, and displays its optimum activity between pH 7 and 8.

Collagenase is mostly used in the form of its **'ointment'** for the specific dedebriment of burns, dermal ulcers, and necrotic ulcers.

12.4.4   Deoxyribonuclease [DNase]

Deoxyribonuclease refers to an enzyme that hydrolyzes and thus depolymerizes **deoxyribonucleic acid (DNA).**

DNase usually loses its activity in an aqueous medium. The optimum activity is exhibited between pH 6 to 7. It has been duly observed that Mg^{2+} ions are an absolute must for its activation.

DNase finds its abundant applications in:

- cure of haematomas and localized abscess formation,
- minimise the specific viscosity of the pulmonary secretions as its **'aerosol preparations'** in **Inhalers,** and
- increase the flow of the expectoration of sputum in typical bronchopulmonary infections.

12.4.5   Fibrinolysin

Fibrinolysin designates a **proteolytic enzyme** duly obtained from the activation of **human plasminogen** by the presence of **streptokinase.** It essentially aids a complicated system of biochemical reactions for the lysis of clots in the vascular system. The principal physiological activator of the **fibrinolytic system is tissue plasminogen activator.** It particularly converts plasminogen in a fibrin-containing clot to plasmin. The fibrin polymer is duly degraded by plasmin into fragments which are subsequently scavenged by **monocytes** and **macrophages.**

Fibrinolysin finds its use in the critical treatment of **thrombotic disorders** essentially caused due to its fibrinolytic inherent nature.

12.4.6   Hyaluronidase

Hyaluronidase is observed duly in the testes and semen. It specifically depolymerizes **hyaluronic acid,** thereby enhancing the ensuing permeability of the connective tissues by dissolving the various substances that hold body cells together. It also acts to disperse the cells of the **corona radiata** about the newly ovulated ovum, thus largely facilitating entry of the sperm.

A few other typical **applications** are as follows:

- reduces the viscosity of tissue cement thereby rendering the tissues easily permeable to tissue fluids; and this characteristic feature has been duly exploited to increase the rate of absorption of both IM and subcutaneous injectables in humans.
- employed in hypodermolysis as an essential aid to the specific subcutaneous administration of relatively large and excessive volume of parentrals in patients.

12.4.7   Muramidase

Muramidase is normally found in blood cells of the **graunulocytic** and **monocytic** series. Its serum and urine level is enhanced in patients having acute or chronic leukemia. It is also mostly present in tears, sweat, and saliva.

Muramidase is observed to hydrolyze **mucopolysaccharides,** and is invariably found to be active in the transformation of **insoluble polysaccharides** of the cell wall to the corresponding **soluble mucopeptides,** particularly in the **Gram-positive organisms.**

By virtue of this unique inherent activity **muramidase** is usually administered IV for the treatment of bacterial or viral infections in human beings.

12.4.8 Papain

Papain refers to a **proteolytic enzyme** derived from the fruit of the **papaya,** *Carica papaya* (**Family:** *Carcicaceae*). It is soluble in water and glycerine and possesses optimum activity ranging between pH 5 to 6. It is usually available as an admixture with **chymopapain.**

Papain finds its use in **medicine** as enumerated under:

- anti-inflammatory agent
- relieve symptoms of **episiotomy***

Papain finds its enormous usage in **industry,** such as:

- clarification of beverages *e.g.*, beer, fruit juices etc.,
- meat tenderizer,
- cheese processing as a substitute of **renin,**
- degumming of silk fibres in textile industry, and
- dehairing of animal skins and hides in leather industry.

1 NF unit of Papain ≡ Activity released by 1 mcg of Tyrosine derived from a Standard Casein Substuate.

12.4.9 Pancreatin

Pancreatin represents one of the active ferments of the pancreas essentially containing a mixture of **enzymes,** namely: **amylase, lipase,** and **protease.** It exhibits its maximum activity in an **alkaline medium.**

Pancreatin finds its abundant uses as stated under:

- used chiefly as a digestant,
- as it becomes **inactive** in an acidic medium, it should be administered orally in combination with a mild alkaline substance *e.g.*, $NaHCO_3$ (sodium bicarbonate),
- for the preparation of predigested or peptonized food, products, and
- conversions of **starch** into **dextrin; proteins** into **amino acids;** and **fats** into **fatty acids** and **glycerols.**

Potency of Pancreatin   Its has been established that:

1 g of **Pancreatin** ≡ 12,000 Units of **Amylase Activity;**
≡ 15,000 Units of **Lipase Activity;** and
≡ 10,000 Units of **Protease Activity.**

---

* **Episiotomy:** Incision of the perineum at the end of the second stage of labour to avoid spontaneous laceration of the prenium and to facilitate delivery.

12.4.10 Pancrealipase

Pancrealipase represents a rather more concentrated version of **pancreatin** whereby the specific **lipase activity** is enhanced significantly. It is derived from the pancreas of the hog, *Sus scrofa* var. **domesticus** belonging to the natural order **Suidae.**

Potency of Pancrealipase: Pancrealipase has the following potencies:

1 g of **Pancrealipase** $\equiv$ 100 Units of **Amylase Activity,**
$\equiv$ 24 Units of **Lipase Activity,** and
$\equiv$ 100 Units of **Protease Activity.**

Pancealipase finds its various applications in therapy, such as:

- cystic fibrosis,
- chronic pancreatitis, and
- pancreatectomy (*i.e.*, surgical removal of pancreas).

12.4.11 Pepsin [*Greek:* Pepsis = digestion]

Pepsin refers to the chief enzyme of gastric juice, that essentially converts proteins into **proteoses** as well as **peptones.** It is usually formed by the major cells of gastric glands, and produces its **optimum activity** at a pH of 1.5 to 2. It is mostly obtainable in the granular form. It has been observed that in the presence of HCl, it helps to digest proteins *in vitro*. **Pepsin** on being heated with either **pancreatic enzymes** or **mild alkali** aptly **loses its biological activity.** It exerts an optimum activity at pH 1.8.

Potency of Pepsin: The potency of **pepsin** is as given under:

Pepsin: capacity to digest **2500 times** its weight of coagulated egg protein;

Modified Pepsin: capacity to digest **10,000 folds** its weight of coagulated-egg protein (**albumin**).

12.4.12 Rennin [or Chymosin]

Rennin (Chymosin) designates the **enzyme** that specifically curdles milk, and usually present in the gastric juice of yound ruminants. In fact, **chymosin** is the most preferred terminology used for **rennin** due to the possible confusion with **renin.**

Renin is obtained either from the glandular layer of the digesting stomach of the **calf,** *Bos taurus* (**Family:** *Bovidae*) or by microbiologically monitored fermentation of *Bacillus cereus, Endothia parasitica*, and *Mucor pusillus*.

Renin is employed for making cheese and junket*. It is also recommended for patients under convalescence and weak in physical status in order to digest milk rather easily.

12.4.13 Seratiopeptidase

Seratiopeptidase is obtained from the microorganism belonging to the **genus** *Serratia* (**E$_{15}$-Species**) which is exclusively present in the gut of silk-worm, but now-a-days solely generated by biotechnology

---

* **Junket:** A dish of sweetened curds of milk.

based fermentation. It is regarded to be a better, more effective, and lesser toxic **microbial enzyme** that certainly has an edge over other enzymes *viz.*, **trypsin** and **chymotrypsin.**

Seratiopeptidase has the following applications, namely:

- possesses **bradykinin** and **histamine** proteolytic and hydrolyzing characteristic activity,
- accelerates and supports the **'wound-healing phenomenon'** which specifically lowers the capillary permeability and cleavage of exudates and proteins,
- retards inflammation,
- liquefaction of thick sputum (*i.e.*, lowering viscosity) on account of proteolytic effect, and
- enhancement of **'antibiotic effects'** by virtue of the effective removal of inflammatory barrier thereby substantially increasing the **actual antibiotic transfer** to the strategically located infected areas.

12.4.14 Streptokinase

Streptokinase refers to an **enzyme** produced by certain specific strains of **Streptococci*** which is capable of converting **plasminogen** to **plasmin** exclusively.

It is found to be water-soluble and exhibits optimum activity at pH 7.

The various **applications** of **streptokinase** are as stated under:

- used as a **fibrinolytic agent** to help in the removal of **bifrin thrombi** from the arteries (*i.e.*, **reperfusion**).
- employed profusely in the treatment of **thromboembolic disorders** pertaining to the lysis of **arterial thrombus, acute coronary artery thrombosis, deep vein thrombosis,** and **pulmonary emboli.**

Mechanism of Action: Streptokinase exerts its activity on account of the particular activation of **plasminogen** into a **proteolytic enzyme** *e.g.*, **plasmin,** that critically carries out the degradation of the **fibrin clots, fibrinogen,** and **certain specific plasma proteins.**

12.4.15 Urokinase

Urokinase is an enzyme obtained solely from human urine, which is used expermentally for dissolving **venous thrombi** and **pulmonary emboli.** It is usually administered IV.

Urokinase** also exerts its action as an activator of the specific **endogenous fibrinolytic system** that eventually help in the conversion of **plasminogen to plasmin;** and also causes degradation of **fibrin clots, fibrinogen,** and **plasma proteins.** It is invariably employed to carry out the dissolution of **fibrin** or **blood clots** present strategically in the **anterior chamber of an eye,** and in **acute massive pulmonary emboli.**

---

* Culture filtrates of β-hemolytic **Streptococci Group C.**

** **Urokinase:** It is found to be less **antigenic** than **enszymes** due to the fact that this is derived solely from the human source.

12.4.16 L-Asparaginase

L-Asparaginase refers to an **enzyme** that serves as an **antineoplastic agent** derived from the organism *Escherichia coli*. It helps to catalyze the hydrolysis of **L-aspargine** to the corresponding **L-aspartic acid** and **NH₃**.

Potency   Each 1 mg of L-Asparaginase ≡ 250 Units

The *two* chief uses of **L-asparaginase** are as given below:

- interferes directly with the growth of **cancerous (malignant) cells** that are incapable of synthesizing **L-asparagine** for their necessary metabolism; and, therefore, it is mostly employed in the usual **chemotherapy of very serious lymphocytic leukemia** in preferred sequential combination with other **antineoplastic drugs,**
- beneficial for induction of required remission in children having relapse of **acute lymphocytic lymphoma,** and
- exhibits **immunosuppressive** therapeutic profile.

B. PROTEIN AS DRUG SUBSTANCES

12.5 INTRODUCTION

Protein [*Greek:* **protos** = first] refers to a class of rather complex nitrogenous compounds that are synthesized by all living organisms, and yield respective array of amino acids when hydrolyzed. Importantly, **proteins** essentially provide the amino acids required for the growth and subsequent repair of impaired animal tissue.

Composition of Proteins: Proteins, are composed of a host of vital elements, such as: C, H, O, N, P, S, and Fe, which ultimately make up the greater segment of the animal and plant tissue. In fact, the **amino acids** do represent the basic structure of **proteins.** Generally, foods invariably contain protein with varying numbers and types of amino acids. However, one may recognize a '**complete protein'** as one that predominantly contains **all the essential amino acids** *viz.,* **arginine, histidine, isoleucine, lysine, leucine, meltionine, phenylalanine, threonine, tryptophan,** and **valine.** In human beings, they are indeed an absolute must for the maintenance of body weight and required growth. **Sources:** Interestingly, the various known and important sources of proteins are, namely: cheese, milk, eggs, meat, fish, and certain vegetables *viz.,* soybeans are recognized as the best sources. Nevertheless, the proteins are invariably found in both animal and vegetable sources of food. It has been duly observed that there are many '**incomplete proteins'** which are found in vegetables; and they do contain some of the so-called **essential amino acids.** Thus, a '**vegetarian diet'** may judiciously make up for this by combining various vegetable groups which complement each other in their basic amino acid groups. This ultimately provides the body with '**complete protein'.**

The **major animal proteins** are as enumerated under in Table-12.3:

Table 12.3   Major Animal Proteins and Their Respective Sources

S.No.	Name of Protein(s)	Source(s)
1	Lactalbumin; Lactoglobulin;	Milk; Milk products;
2	Ovalbumin; Ovaglobulin;	Eggs; Egg powder;
3	Serum albumin;	Blood serum;
4	Myosin; Actin;	Striated muscle fibers/tissues;
5	Fibrinogen;	Blood;
6	Serum globulin;	Serum;
7	Thyroglobulin;	Thyroid gland;
8	Globin;	Blood;
9	Thymus histones;	Thynus gland;
10	Collagen; Gelatin;	Connective tissues;
11	Keratin;	Epidermis; Hairs; Nails; Horny Tissue;
12	Chondoprotein;	Tendons; Cartilage;
13	Mucin; Mucoids;	Secreting glands and animal mucilaginous substances;
14	Caseinogen;	Milk; Milk products;
15	Vitallin;	Egg-yolk;
16	Hemoglobulin;	Red blood cells [RBCs];
17	Lecithoprotein;	Blood; Brain; Bile secretions;

Functionality of Proteins   The ingested **proteins** serve as an important source of **amino acids** essentially required to synthesize the **body's own proteins,** that are quite essential not only for the growth of **new tissue** but also the **repair of damaged tissue.** Importantly, **proteins** constitute an important segment of all the cell membranes. It is proved beyond any reasonable doubt that the excess of amino acids derived from the diet may be conveniently converted to rather **simpler carbohydrates,** and ultimately get oxidized to produce **adenosine triphosphate (ATP)** as well as heat. Thus, 1 g of protein gives rise to 4 kcal of heat.

12.6   PROTEIN VARIANTS

Interestingly, a wide spectrum of **protein variants** have been duly recognized and summarized in Tahle-12.4 together with their applications:

Table 12.4   Protein Variants and Their Applications

S.No.	Type of Protein	Applications
1	**Acute Phase Protein**	Specific role in fighting pathogens is not so clear, but they are believed to influence the **erythrocyte sedimentation rate** (ESR) significantly. **Examples: Complement factor C_3 and C-reactive protein.**
2	**Blood Protein**	Integral component of blood, including hemoglobin in RBCs and serum proteins.
3	**Carrier Protein**	It elicits an immune-response when coupled with a hapten.
4	**Complete Protein**	They contain all the essential amino acids.
5	**Conjugated Protein**	They usually contain the protein molecule along with certain other molecules. **Examples: Chromoproteins** [*e.g.,* hemoglobin]; **glycoproteins** [*e.g.,* mucin]; **lecithoproteins, nucleoproteins, and phosphoproteins** [*e.g.,* casein]
6	**C-Reactive Protein**	It designates an '**abnormal protein**' detectable specifically and exclusively in blood during the active phase of some human diseases *viz.,* rheumatic fever.
7	**Denatured Protein**	Deformation of the amino acid composition and stereochemical structure of amino acid(s) caused due to chemical or physical means.

(Contd.)

8	Derived Protein	Protein derivative duly achieved either by the action of chemical alteration or a purely physical process *e.g.*, heat.
9	G-Protein	Protein which determines the activation of a specific physiologic event. It invariably acts at the cell surface to couple receptors for the **neurotransmitters,** namely: **hormones, epinephrine, odorants,** and **light photons.**
10	Immune Protein	An **immunoglobulin** or an **antibody** produced by the plasma cells that essentially label foreign antigens and initiate the process for their ultimate destruction (death).
11	Incomplete Protein	Protein that essentially lacks one or more of the essential amino acids.
12	Native Protein	Protein which occurs in its natural state *i.e.*, it relates to such a protein that has not yet been denatured.
13	Plasma Protein	Protein which is essentially present in the blood plasma *viz.*, **albumin,** or **globulin.**
14	Serum Protein	Protein that forms an integral component present specifically in the serum portion of the blood.
15	Simple Protein	Refers to such proteins which gives rise to the genesis of only α-amino acids upon hydrolysis *e.g.*, **albumins, albuminoids, globulines, gluteline, histones, prolamines,** and **protamines.**
16	Protein C	Represents plasma protein which specifically inhibits coagulation Factor V and Factor XIII, thereby preventing excessive clotting. Its deficiency may cause thrombosis.
17	Protein Kinase	**Enzyme** that constitute an integral part of the immune reaction; and usually after activation by **cytokines** strategically mediates cellular processes *viz.*, motility and secretion.

12.7 BRIEF DESCRIPTION OF PROTEINS USED AS DRUGS

There are quite a few unique and remarkable proteins that are essentially present in the humans which attribute highly efficacious and critical functions *in vivo*. Some proteins that belong to this category, used normally as therapeutic agents (drugs), have been described briefly in the sections that follows:

12.7.1 Complement Protein (Complement Factor C-3) [Latin; *Complere* = to Complete]

Complement protein refers to a **group of proteins** in the blood which play a vital role in the **body's immune defense mechanisms** *via* a **cascade of interactions.** However, the components of complements are labeled C1 through C9. Nevertheless, C3 and C5 are the most important of these. Complement invariably acts by killing directly the organisms; by opsonizing an antigen, thereby stimulating phagocytosis; and by stimulating inflammation and the B-cell mediated immune response. Importantly, all **complement proteins** usually lie **inactive** in the blood unless and until activated by either the classic or the recognized alternative pathways.

An observed abnormality or deficiency in complement protein strategically refers to an **autosomal recessive trait.** The lack of factor C3 enhances susceptibility to common microbial infections, whereas deficits in C5 through C9 are invariably associated with enhanced incidence of **autoimmune ailments,** such as:

- glomerulonephritis, and
- systemic lupus erythematosus.

It has been duly observed that the lack of any of the more than 25 proteins intimately involved in the complement system may affect the body's defense mechanism adversely.

12.7.2 Gelatin [*Latin:* Gelatina = Gelatin]

Gelatin refers to a derived protein duly obtained by the hydrolysis of **collagen** strategically located in the connective tissues of the skin, bones, and joints of animals. It is used profusely in food products *e.g.*, fruit jellys; in the preparations of pharmaceutical dosage forms *e.g.*, **soft-gelatine capsules** for Vitamin E, garlic pearls etc., and **hard-gelatine capsules** for chloramphenicol, tetracycline, acetamenophen (paracetamol) **Tylenol (R)** in US; and also as a medium for the culture of certain microorganisms.

Gelatin is also employed as a vehicle for some highly specific pharmaceutical injections *e.g.*, **Pitkin's menstrum**—which comprises of **heparin, gelatin, dextrose, acetic acid** and **water.**

Gelatin is also used for the treatment of **'brittle finger nails',** and **'non-mycotic defects'** of the nails in humans.

Types of Gelatin: Gelatin is normally available in *two* distinct forms, namely:

(*a*) **Absorbable Gelatin Sponge:** It is a sterile, white, tough, and finely porous spongy, water-insoluble, and absorbable substance. Even though it is water-insoluble but it is adequately absorbed in body fluids. Nevertheless, it usually takes upto not less than 30 folds its equivalent weight of water.

It has been observed that 9 g of **absorbable gelatin sponge** takes upto 405 g (*i.e.*, 45 times) of **well-agitated oxalated whole blood.**

The various uses of **absorbable gelatin sponge** are as follows:

- as an effective haemostatic,
- as a **localized anticoagulant,** and
- when placed upon a surgical incision after being duly moistened with sterile NaCl solution, it gets slowly absorbed within a span of 4-6 weeks.

(*b*) **Absorbable Gelatin Film: Absorbable gelatin film** refers to a light amber coloured, sterile, non-antigenic thin film invariably produced from a especially prepared **gelatin-formaldehyde solution** by careful drying followed by subsequent sterilization.

Absorbable gelatin film is largely employed in the form of saline-soaked rubber-like thin sheets chiefly in surgical repair of such observed defects in membranes, such as: **dura and pleura matter,** where it grossly serves as a **mechanical means of protection, replacement matrix,** and **temporary supportive structural wall.**

12.7.3 Collagen [Synonym: Ossien]: (Greek: *kolla* = glue, + gennan = to produce)

Collagen refers to a strong, fibrous insoluble protein found in the connective tissue, including the dermis, tendous, ligaments, deep fascia, bone, and cartilage. **Collagen** is the protein typical of dental tissues (except the enamel of teeth), thereby forming the matrix of **dentin, cementum,** and alveolar bone proper. **Collagen fibers** also form the **periodontal ligament,** that eventually attaches the teeth to their respective bony sockets of the lower and upper jaws.

It has been duly observed that there are two important amino acids, namely: **glycine** and **proline** that are strategically located in the central core of the triple helical molecule of the **collagen.** However, **collagen** may be easily differentiated from other accompanying fibrous proteins *e.g.,* **elastin,* reticulin** etc. Interestingly, **collagen** is duly characterized by the presence of a host of **vital amino acids,** such as: **glycine, hydroxyproline, hydroxylysine, proline,** and **tyrosine;** whereas, **elastin** essentially comprises of absolutely **non-polar amino acids,** for instance: **isoleucine, leucine,** and **valine.** Nevertheless, one may come across a plethora of **collagen variants** which solely depends upon the presence of the **'amino-acid sequence'.** When **collagen** is carefully boiled with water it gets duly converted into gelatin.

Collagen finds its typical applications in the preparation of **photographic emulsions, sutures,** and also as a **'gel'** in **food casings.**

12.7.4 Casein [Latin: *caseus* = cheese]

Casein designates the principal protein in milk. It is present in **milk curds.** It essentially provides all the amino acids that are necessary for the growth and development in humans. When milk is subjected to coagulation by **rennin** or **acid, casein** becomes one of the principle ingredients of **cheese.**

Casein actually represents the **phosphoprotein** with a composition of **0.85% P** and **0.75% S.**

Characteristic Features—are as follows:

(*i*) % N = 15 to 16
(*ii*) Sulphated Ash (%) = NMT** 1.5
(*iii*) Loss on Drying (%) = NMT 6
(*iv*) Isoclectric Point = 4.7
(*v*) Specific Gravity = 1.25 to 1.31
(*vi*) Molecular Weight = 75 K*** to 370 K

Casein Variants: Casein has several known variants, such as:

(*a*) **Lactalbumin: Lactalbumin** refers to the albumin of milk and cheese; and it is a **soluble simple protein.** It is present in relatively higher concentration in **human milk** in comparison to the **cow's milk.** When milk is heated, the **latalbumin** aptly coagulates and appears as a film on the surface of the milk.

(*b*) **Lactoglobulin: Lactoglobulin** refers to a protein found most abundantly in milk. Both **casein** and **lactoglobulin** are the most common proteins invariably seen in the cow's milk.

(*c*) **Acid Casein:** The warm skimmed milk when acidified with a diluted mineral acid, the whey usually gets separated. The solid curd is duly separated by any suitable means, residual solid mass is now washed thoroughly, dried and pulverized to obtain acid **casein powder.**

(*d*) **Rennet Casein:** The skimmed milk is adequately treated with an enzyme, **rennet extract,** whereby the product is first separated carefully, and subsequently purified to obtain the **Rennet Casein.**

---

* **Elastin:** It represents a highly cross-linked protein with a distinct hydrophobic character.
** **NMT** = Not More Than;
*** **K** = Thousand;

- **Casein** (or **soluble casein**) is usually recommended as a dietary supplement for protein in both **pre** and **post-operative** care of the patients.
- **Casein** is also employed as a '**base**' in the **proper standardization of the proteolytic enzymes.**
- **Casein** is also exploited as an **emulsifying agent.**
- **Casein** is used in **sizing** of *paper* and *textile.*
- **Casein** is employed as an **unique adhesive agent** for the preparation of large-scale casein paints and casein plastics.

12.7.5 Lectins [Synonyms: Agglutinins; Affinitins; Phasins; Protectins;]

Lectin refers to one of the several plant proteins that specifically stimulate the **lymphocytes** to undergo **proleferation.**

Examples: Phytohemagglutinin; Concanavalin.

Alternatively, **lectins** are **proteins** or **glucoproteins** without having an **immune origin. Lectins** may be isolated from various natural sources, such as: bark, fungi, fresh-eggs, roots, microorganisms, body fluids of lower-vertebrates, invertebrates, sea-weed and sponges, and the mammalian cell membranes.

Importantly, the **lectins** are not used directly as a medicine, but they do have the following usages elsewhere, namely:

- For determining **blood-groups;** and for carrying out **erythrocytic polyagglutination investigative studies.**
- For performing **histochemical studies** related to either **normal and pathological status.**
- For establishing **structural elucidation studies of** the **carbohydrate bearing molecules.**
- For carrying out the **mitogenic stimulation of lymphocytes.**

As tools for studying **cell-surface properties** in **cancer research.**

Natural Sources of Lectins: a few typical **natural sources of lectins** are as given under:

- **abrin:** *Abrus precaturius;*
- **concanavalin A:** *Conovalia ensioformis;*
- **green marine algae:** *Codium fragile;*
- **red kidney bean:** *Phaseolus vulgaris;* and
- **horse gram:** *Dolichos biflorus.*

12.7.6 Yeast

Yeast invariably refers to any of several **unicellular fungi** of the genus **Saccharomyces,** that particularly reproduce by budding. They are capable of **fermenting carbohydrates. Yeasts,** especially *candida albicans,* may cause **systemic infections** as well as *vaginitis.* It has been generally observed that '**yeast infections**' are frequently present in patients with **malignant lymphomas, AIDS, severe diabetes mellitus,** and several other conditions causing **immunocompromise.**

Types of Yeast: There are in fact *two* types of **yeast,** namely:

(*a*) **Brewer's Yeast: Brewer's Yeast** refers to the specific yeast obtained duly during the **brewing of beer'.** However, it may also be used in its **'dried form'** as a good source of **Vitamin B.**

(*b*) **Dried Yeast: Dried Yeast** designates the particular **'dried yeast cells'** obtained from the strains of *Saccharomyces cerevisiae.* It is mostly used as a viable source of **proteins** and **Vitamins** (especially **Vitamin B Complex**).

Interestingly, as to date approximately **350 yeast variants** have been duly isolated, purified, characterized for their specific uses. In a rather broader sense, the **yeasts** have been duly classified according to their actual usages to which they are based upon their **typical morphological characteristic features,** such as:

- **For making Wines** : Winer's Yeast;
- **For making Bakery Products** : Baker's Yeast;
- **For making Lager Beers** : Brewer's Yeast;
- **For making Alcohol** : Distiller's Yeast;
  from Malt Wort, Molasses
- **For making Drugs** : Brewer's Yeast; Baker's Yeast;

Sources of Yeast: The natural habitats of this specific type of microorganism (*i.e.*, **yeast**) are namely: **fruit juice, bread, fermented media,** and **fermenting media.** On a commercial scale the **yeast** is usually produced by making use of **citrus fruits, molasses, grain wort, malt wort, molasses wort** etc.

Chemical Composition of Yeast: Yeast usually contains a wide range of vital and important chemical constituents, namely: nitrogenous ingredients (*i.e.*, **proteins**); vitamins (*e.g.*, **thiamine, riboflavine, folic acid, pantothenic acid, biotine** etc.); enzymes (*e.g.*, **diastase, maltase, zymase** etc.); and **glycogens** and **minerals (ash).**

Applications of Yeast: Following are some of the vital applications of **yeast** in various **food, beverage,** and **pharmaceutical** industries:

(1) **Beverage Industries** *viz.,* Bears, Wines, Alcoholic Beverages such as: Gins, Whiskies, Rums, Vodkas etc.,

(2) **Food Industries** *viz.,* Bakery Products, Biscuit Industries;

(3) **Pharma. Industries** *viz.,* antibiotis, papain etc.

12.7.7 Thaumatin [Synonym: Talin;]

Thaumatin is the sweet-tasting basic protein duly extracted from the fruits of the tropical plant, *Thaumatococcus danielli* Benth., *Marantaceae,* found extensively in West Africa from Sierre Leone to Zaire, in Sudan and Uganda. It is mostly composed of *five* distinct forms *viz.,* thaumatins I, II, III, b, and c. However, **thaumatins I and II** predominate invariably. Importantly, all of them are almost 100,000 times sweeter than sucrose, and do have molecular weights around 22,000.

Characteristic Features: The **various characteristic features** of **thaumatin** are as enumerated under:

(*i*) It has increasingly sweet taste with a licorice-like distinct after taste.

(*ii*) It is strongly cationic having isoelectric point greater than or equivalent to 11.7.

(*iii*) It exhibits UVmax: 278 nm at pH 5.6; and 283,290 nm at pH 13.0.

(*iv*) It is about 750-1600 times sweeter than sucrose on a weight basis; and 30,000 to 100,000 times on a mole basis.

(*v*) Its threshold values are very close to 10^{-4}%.

(*vi*) The **proteins** usually lose sweetness upon heating, whereby the disulphide-bridges undergo strategical cleavages in their basic structures.

(*vii*) **Thaumatin** also loses its sweetness at pHs <2.5, which evidently points to the importance of the very presence of the **tertiary structure** for its inherent sweetness properties.

    Thaumatin finds its enormous usage as a potential low-calorie sweetner. It is also used largely in such products as: **chewing gums, breath freshners. Talin** is its branded product being marketed largely in Japan, United States, and the European countries as well.

FURTHER READING REFERENCES

1. **British Herbal Pharmacopoeia:** British Herbal Medicine Association, London (UK), 1983.
2. Cervoni P *et al.*: **Cardiovascular Agents—Thrombolytic Agents,** In: *Kirk Othmer Encyclopedia of Chemical Technology,* 4th edn., Vol. 5, Wiley, Nw York, pp. 289-293, 1993.
3. **Database on Medicinal Plants Used in Ayurveda:** Vol. 1 (2000), Vol. 2 (2001), Vol. 3 (2001), Central Council for Research in Ayurveda and Siddha, Department of ISM and H, Ministry of Health and Family Welfare (Govt. of India), New Delhi.
4. **Japanese Pharmacopoeia**—XIII, Ministry of Health and Welfare, Tokyo (Japan), 1996.
5. Kaufman PB *et al.:* **Natural Products from Plants,** CRC Press, New York, 1999.
6. **Report on the Task Force on Conservation and Sustainable Use of Medicinal Plants:** Planning Commission, Govt. of India, 2000.
7. **The Ayurvedic Pharmacopoeia of India,** Vol. 1. Pt. 1. Rep. 2001, Vol. 2 (1999), Vol. 3 (2001): Govt. of India, Minisry of Health and Family Welfare, Department of Indian Systems of Medicine and Homeopathy, New Delhi.
8. Wiseman A: **Better by Design: Biocatalysts for the Future,** *Chem. Brit,* 571-573, 1994.
9. Wong S: **Immunotherapeutic Agents,** In: *Kirk-Othmer Encyclopedia of Chemical Technology,* 4th edn, Vol 14, Wiley, New York, pp: 662-676, 1995.
10. Yokotsuka T: **The Quality of Food and Beverages,** Academic Press, New York, Vol. 2, pp. 171-196, 1981.

13 Biomedicinals From Plant-Tissue Cultures

- Introduction
- Profile of Plant-Tissue Cultures
- Biomedicinals in Plant-Tissue Cultures
- Bioproduction of Commendable Secondary Metabolites
- Further Reading References

13.1 INTRODUCTION

In the recent past, the enormous utility and qualified success of the **plant-tissue cultures** in the skilful and meticulous **bioproduction** of a host of **natural biomedicinals** under stringent aseptic laboratory/pilot-scale conditions has virtually opened up several altogether new approaches in the ever-expanding new era of **biotechnology.** Bearing in mind the aforesaid factual statements one may legitimately exploit the application of the interesting **tissue-culture technique** exclusively for carrying out the biosynthesis of **'secondary metabolites'** prevailing particularly in the plants of pharmaceutical importance and significance, musters an excellent promise for the generation of need-based **plant constituents.**

Importance of Biomedicinals from Plant-Tissue Cultures: The importance of biomedicinals from plant-tissue cultures are enumerated under:

(1) To obtain a constant and ample supply of good quality **'biomedicinals'** in comparison to the *conventional older methods.*

(2) To avoid unpredictable factors, such as: absolute neglect of the conservation of environment, careless exploitation of plant species, ever-enhancing labour costs, and unavoidable technical as well as economical constraints associated with the cultivation of the desired medicinal plant species.

(3) To circumvent such critical problems [as in (2) above] the application of plant-tissue cultures may prove to be a great asset and boon.

(4) To obtain **'biomedicinals'** from the **higher plants** are still regarded to be a vital source, inspite of the excellent developments in the field of **pure synthetic chemistry.**

At this material time it has become an absolute necessity to understand the *two* terminologies and their functionalities to a certain extent, namely: (*a*) plant-tissue culture; and (*b*) biomedicinals.

Plant-Tissue Culture

Plant-tissue culture refers to the specific growth of plant tissue *in vitro* on artificial culture media for the experimental research exclusively.

The qunatum leap in **'biotechnology'** has virtually opened up the flood-gate related to the latest available techniques with respect to the various cardinal utilities of **plant-tissue cultures** in the specific bioproduction of several natural plant constituents under stringent aseptic parameters using such techniques that are found to be very much akin to the ones employed for the systematic culture of microbes.

Plant tissue cultures (cell suspension cultures) are theoretically regarded to be the most ideal medium for carrying out an exhaustive studies with regard to **metabolism** and also the underlying **biosynthetic pathways** yielding specifically the **secondary metabolites.** In actual practice, such **cultures** are invariably grown from the **callus tissue** in a duly sterile liquid medium containing the necessary nutrients. At the initial stage the growth is **exponential,** but eventually attains a **stationary phase;** and at this point the batches of cells may be transferred conveniently into a new medium. Interestingly, this particular process helps the number of cells increased continually, which may prove to be of great and distinct advantage, provided the **plant tissue cultures** are employed on a **commercial scale** for various **biomedicinals** judiciously.

As to date commercial application of a plethora of **plant tissue culture technologies** have been duly demonstrated and recognized; however, several teething problems and constraints with regard to high labour costs, and other relevant expenses pertaining to composition of nutrient medium, hardening, and precise delivery of tissue cultured plants still remains to be overcome.

Nevertheless, the **plant-tissue culture technique (PTCT)** has a good number of chief advantages *vis-a-vis* the large-scale **cultivation technique (CT)** which may be summarized briefly as under:

(*i*) **PTCT** affords the advantage of absolutely uniform biomass achievable at every occasion under strictly modulated as well as reproducible parameters, that may be obtained with remote possibility while dealing with the living potential materials.

(*ii*) Importantly, one may conveniently make use of the **plant-cell culture technique (PCCT)** to accomplish the much desired synthesis of such **therapeutically viable agents** (*i.e.*, **medicinal compounds**) that are found to be rather difficult or quite cumbersome to synthesize chemically.

(*iii*) Possible to obtain required useful compounds invariably under rigid and controlled environmental parameters that are certainly quite independent of the unavoidable variants, such as: alterations in climatic profile, and soil conditions.

(*iv*) **Biotransformation reactions** are feasible using **plant-cell cultures.** One may carry out particular desired alterations/modifications in the **'chemical structures'** of certain plant constituents by this specialized technique in comparison to either pure **chemical synthesis** or **microbiologically** (as in **antibiotics**).

(*v*) Plant cells derived from both temperate or tropical environments may be attenuated (multiplied) suitably in order to cause the production of particular metabolites generated by them duly.

(*vi*) **PTCT** may be exclusively used to undertake an elaborative study of the **biosynthesis of secondary metabolites.** However, it may be absolutely feasible to induct labelled precursors strategically to the cell cultures, and subsequently deduce logical and plausible interpretations (or explanations) with respect to the various metabolic pathways of the pre-determined chemical entity.

(*vii*) Possible to preserve and maintain the **'cultured-cells'** quite free from any attack by insects or contamination by various microorganisms.

(*viii*) **PTCT** specifically helps to the ensuing **immbolization of cells*** that may be utilized effectively for carrying out various **biochemical reactions** *i.e.*, biotransformations.

Historic Genesis of Plant-Tissue Culture Technique (PTCT): The genesis of actual **plant-tissue culture technique (PTCT)** dates back to almost 100 years *i.e.*, the very beginning of the twentieth century, whereas its enormous benevolent applications were noticed and recognized across the globe in the past three decades; and its **pharmaceutical potential** duly hailed and appreciated for the benefit of mankind.

One may get a glimpse of the **historic genesis of PTCT** commencing from early 1900 in a sequential manner as eneumerated under:

Haberblandt (1902) : It has been hypothesized that the **isolated plant cells** must be able to undergo propogation (*i.e.*, cultivation) on an **artificial culture medium.** Such investigative studies revealed that one may have an actual assessment of their ensuing capacity as well as typical specific properties as pure **elementary organisms** that are found to be absolutely free from **multicellular system of plant.**

Robbins (1922) and Kotte (1922) : These *two* researchers have independently and **successfully cultured the excised plant roots** for the first time, and hence supported the earlier hypothesis of **Haberblandt** put forward two decades ago.

White (1934) : Further substantiated the researches carried out by both **Robbins** (USA) and **Kotte** (Germany) by successfully performing the culture of **excised tomato root tips.**

White (1939) : Meticulously and successfully reported the **uninterrupted (*i.e.*, continuous) culture of the excised-tomato-root-tips.**

Gautheret (1939) : Demonstrated the classical research carried out upon the **cambial tissue cultures.**
Observed the critical behaviour of the **carrot explants** on a medium essentially comprised of **dextrose** (with cystein hydrochloride + aneurine hydrochloride), inorganic salt mixture, and 3-indole-acetic acid** (in low concentration).

Muir, Hilderbrandt, and Ricker (1954) : Made an epoch making discovery in the growth of **liquid cultures** distinctly comprising of single cells together with small clusters of cells of two plant species, namely: *Nicotiana tabacum* and *Tagetes erecta.*

Reinert (1956) : Demonstrated the occurrence of distinct and highly specific cell divisions in an almost identical preparations having either suspension of single cells or group of cells duly obtained from *Picea glauca*.

---

* **Immobilization of Cells:** It refers to a specific strain of cells duly obtained from suspension cultures which in turn mobilized by suspending in a solution of sodium alginate thereby causing precipitation of the **alginate'** together with the entrapped cells by the aid of $CaCl_2$ solution, followed by **pelleting,** and allowing the product to get hardened in due course.

** A plant-growth hormone.

| Jones, Hilderbrandt, Ricker, and Wu (1960) | : | Critically observed the spectacular growth of plant tissues exclusively in a hanging-drop culture of separated cells duly accomplished from the **callus*** of certain hybrid species of tobacco *viz., Nicotiana tabaccum,* and *Nicotina glutinosa*; |
| Rao *et al.* (1999) | : | Ascertained that the **'synthetic seed technology'** would find its application in both **plant propagation,** and **delivery of tissue cultured plants.**** |

Biomedicinals:

Biomedicine usually refers to the clinical medicine based upon the principles of the so-called **natural sciences** *viz.*, biology, biochemistry, biotechnology etc.

Nevertheless, the present scenaria across the globe entails not only the stability, but also the ensuing viability and potential of newer range of pharmacobiotechnologically developed products. This **new millenium** may eventually see quite a few of them duly approved and okayed by the US-FDA. A few typical examples of **'biotechnology-based products',** otherwise referred to as **biomedicinals,** have already gained world-wide cognizance, namely:

- **Leupine$^{(R)}$**   : For autologus bone marrow transplantation.
- **Proleukin$^{(R)}$** : For renal cell carcinoma.

13.2   PROFILE OF PLANT-TISSUE CULTURES

The profile of **plant-tissue culture** may be adequately expatiated and elaborated in terms of the following different aspects, for instance:

- (*a*) Types of Cultures,
- (*b*) Composition of Culture Medium,
- (*c*) Surface Sterilization of Explants, and
- (*d*) Preparation of Tissue Cultures.

Each of the aforementioned aspects shall now be treated individually in the sections that follows:

13.2.1   Type of Cultures

In a broader perspective, one may rightly observe that the **plant tissue cultures** which initially took off as an intellectual curiosity has recently attained quite a respectable status by virtue of its significant contributions to basic knowledge and biotechnology. Its judicious usage has ultimately led to several practical gainful advantages to pharmaceutical industry and agriculture.

As to date there are *three* major cardinal categories of highly specific and articulated development areas associated with the **plant-tissue culture,** such as:

- (*a*) Culture of specific **isolated plant organs,*****

---

* **Callus:** A mass of unorganized cells.

** Rao PS *et al. 'Synthetic Seed Technology as a Method for Plant Propogation and Delivery of Tissue Cultured Plants,* **In: Trends in Plant Tissue Culture and Biotechnology,** Agro Botanical Publishers (India), 47, 1999.

*** **Isolated Plant Organs:** Roots, leaf primordia, immature embryos, flower structures, and stem-tips.

(*b*) Growth of **callus masses** upon **solidified media,** and

(*c*) Growth of **mixed suspensions of separated cells/small cell clusters** in **liquified media.**

Technique Variants: The **plant-tissue culture** may be duly accomplished using different techniques, namely:

(1) Tissue may be conveniently cultured upon either **liquid nutrient medium** or **solid agar medium.**

    (*a*) **Liquid suspension cultures:** These usually comprise of an admixture fo **cell aggregates, cell clusters (groups),** and **even single cells.** It has been duly observed that the actual growth rate of the **'liquid-suspension cultures'** are mostly **much higher** in comparison to the **solid-agar medium.** Besides, the said technique essentially gives rise to much elegantly **superior control over the growth of biomass** due to the fact the cells are surrounded by the nutrient medium completely.

    (*b*) **Solid-agar Medium:** In this particular instance, the plant-tissue when grown on **solid-agar medium** always gives rise to a **callus.** It is, however, pertinent to state here that the wonderful technique of **callus culture** seems to be much more easier as well as convenient for not only initially and maintaining of cell-lines, but also for carrying out the investigational studies related to **organogenesis** and **meristem culture.**

Importantly, both these aforesaid techniques *viz.*, **liquid suspension culture**, and **callus culture** may be adequately obtained from tissues of several species; however, the ease of initiating the said culture exclusively depends and varies along with the specific type of plant, and the tissue organ employed. Interestingly, one may make use of **any portion of a plant** for the **initial induction** to produce either a **suspension culture** or a **callus.** The required necessary tissue may be duly obtained from various segments of a plant *viz.*, leaf, root, stem, pollen, and seedling, which eventually is made to grow distinctly as a mass of **undifferentiated cells** upon previously enriched solidified in an aseptic environment.

13.2.2 Composition of Culture Medium

Since 1939 various researchers have put forward specific well-defined **culture medium** for the growth of cell cultures that essentially comprise of a host of ingredients, such as:

Carbon source	:	From carbohydrates, starch, steep liquors.
Vitamins	:	To augment the growth of **callus,** and **liquid-suspension cultures;** besides, **meristem culture.**
Plant growth hormones	:	To serve as growth regulators.
Organic supplements	:	To aid the overall growth of certain specific cultures.

Murashige and Skoog* (1962) found an altogether revised medium for rapid growth and bioassay with tobacco tissue cultures; Grambow *et al.*** (1972) studied the cell-division and plant development from protoplasts of carrot cell suspension cultures; Chang and Hsing*** (1980) carried out studies

---

    * Murashige T and Skoog F: *Plant Physiol.*, **15**: 437-497, 1962.

  ** Grambow HJ *et al. Planta*, **103**: 348-355, 1972.

*** Chang WC and Hsing WI, *Nature;* **284**: 341-342, 1980.

of *in vitro* flowering of embryoids derived from mature root callus of **ginseng** (*Panax ginseng*; Shillito *et al.** (1983) investigated agarose plating and a **bead-type culture technique** and stimulate development of protoplast-derived colonies in a number of plant species; Wang (1990)** reported callus induction and plant regeneration of **American ginseng** Hort.; and Arya *et al.**** (1993) described the rapid multiplication of adventitious somatic embryos of *Panax ginseng* (CA Meyer).

Following are the *five* cardinal categories of important ingredients that are absolutely essential as an **ideal nutrient medium** required for **propogation of plant-tissue cultures,** namely:

(1) **Source of Carbon:** Two commonly and abundantly employed source of carbon are **glucose** and **sucrose** invariably used at a concentration ranging between 2-4% (w/v).

(2) **Inorganic Salts:** Importantly, the concentration of K^+ ion (cation) and NO_3^- ion (anion) must be strategicaly adjusted within a range of 20-25 mM (*i.e.*, **millimole**) for each of the said ions; and the concentrations of certain other ions *viz.*, Mg^{2+}, PO_4^{3-}, SO_4^{2-} should vary between 1-3 mM. However, there are some vital and **important micronutrients** that are usually recommended for the **culture medium,** such as: boric acid (H_3BO_3), I^-, besides certain bivalent salts of Zn, Mn, Cu, Co, and Fe which are duly inducted in their chelated form [*e.g.*, sequestered chelates obtained with **ethylene-diamine tetra-acetic acid (EDTA)**].

(3) **Vitamins:** The most essential vitamin required for the **culture medium** is **thiamine hydrochloride** (or **Vitamin B$_1$**); whereas, **pyridoxine hydrochloride** (or **Vitamin B$_6$**), **inositol** (*i.e.*, a part of the **Vitamin B complex,** and **niacin** (or **nicotinic acid**) are invariably employed in **culture medium** to improve significantly the desired **cell growth.**

(4) **Organic Additives:** It has been duly established that the particular incorporation of such **organic additives** as: fresh/pasteurized **coconut milk** (containing **liquid endosperm**), **malt extract, protein hydrolyzates** (*e.g.*, **soy-protein hydrolyzates**), and **yeast extract** are used predominantly to cause an appreciable increase in the actual growth rate of the cells present in the **biomass.******

(5) **Growth Regulators (or Modulators):** **Growth regulators** are essentially required to cause the induction of the desired **cell division** in an affective manner. The various chemical compounds which are mostly used as **growth regulators** together with their optimum operative concentrations are given in the following Table 13.1.

Table 13.1   Chemical Compounds Used as Growth Regulators

S.No.	Chemical Compound (Abbreviation)	Concentration Used (mM)	Remarks
1	2,4-Dichlorophenoxyacetic acid [2, 4-D]	$3 \times 10^{-5} - 5 \times 10^{-5}$	Degraded gradually in plant cells; and are quite stable to autoclaving.
2	Naphthalene acetic acid [NAA]	$3 \times 10^{-5} - 5 \times 10^{-5}$	— do —
3	Cytokines***** *viz.* Kinetin, Benzyladenine	$10^{-7} - 10^{-5}$	Gives **good callus production** when used in conjuction with either **2, 4-D** or **NAA.**

*   Shillito RD, Paszkowski J, and Potrykus I, *Plant Cell Rep.*, **7:** 418-420, 1983.

**   Wang AS: *Science*, **25** (5): 571-572, 1990.

*** Arya S, Arya ID, and Eriksson T: *Plant Cell Tissue and Organ Culture,* **34:** 157-162, 1993.

**** **Biomass:** All of the **living organisms** located in a specified area.

***** **Cytokines:** One of more than 100 distinct proteins produced primarily by WBCs. They provide signals to regulate immunological aspects of **cell growth** and function during both inflammation and specific immune response.

13.2.3   **Surface Sterilization of Explants***

Sterilization essentially refers to the process of completely removing or destroying all microorganisms on a substance by exposure to chemical or physical agents, exposure to ionizing radiation or by filtering gas or liquids *via* porous materials which essentialy remove microorganisms.

    For carrying out extensive and intensive research on **tissue culture propagation** it is almost important and necessary to afford **surface sterilization** of the organ from which the **specific tissue** is required to be excised aseptically or the particular seed material the germination of which shall yield ultimately the **tissue explant.** In actual practice there are quite a few tried and tested frequently employed compounds that find their abundant application as surface-sterilizing agents, namely:

S.No.	Name of Compound	Effective Strength (%)
1	Bromine water	1 to 2
2	Hydrogen peroxide	10 to 12
3	Mercuric chloride	0.1 to 1
4	Silver nitrate	1
5	Sodium hypochlorite	1 to 2

    Procedure: The various steps adopted for the **surface sterilization of explants** are as enumerated under:

(1) Seeds are adequately treated with ethanol (70% v/v) for a short span of 2 minutes; and subsequently washed thoroughly with distilled water.

(2) The resulting seeds are duly subjected to '**sterilization**' by **surface sterilizing agents** for a known prescribed duration.

(3) Seeds thus treated are rinsed once again with enough sterile distilled water, and kept for germination under rigid aseptic environment for a stipulated period.

(4) **Germination** of seeds may be accomplished in several tried and tested methods, namely:

- by placing them on double layers of pre-sterilized filter paper in petri-dishes, duly moistened with sterile DW (distilled water),
- in petri-dishes adequately soaked with sterile cotton plugs, and
- in pre-sterilized culture tubes.

(5) Seeds are duly germinated in complete darkness preferentially at a temperature ranging between 26 to 28 °C.

(6) Finally a small segment of the resulting seedlings are duly utilized for the actual starting of the **callus culture.** Importantly, this step needs to be carried out under perfect sterile conditions so as to avoid any possible risk of contamination inadvertently.

(7) **Aerial Segments of Plant Materials**** are invariably sterilized by subjecting them to sterilization by submerging the specific segments in ethanol (70%, v/v) for a duration of 2-3 minutes in sterile distilled water.

---

* **Explant:** To remove a piece of living tissue from the body and transfer it to an **artificial culture medium** for growth, as in **tissue-culture.**

** **Aerial Segments of Plant Materials:** These are buds, leaves, and stem portions.

13.2.4 Preparation of Tissue Cultures

The actual preparation of **tissue cultures** is accomplished by adopting well-defined methodologies in a sequential manner. The said **tissue cultures** may be prepared either from **suspension cultures** or from **solid cultures,** which shall now be treated separately in the sections that follows:

13.2.4.1 From Suspension Cultures

The various steps adopted generally for the preparation of **'Suspension Cultures'** are as given under:

(1) **Suspension cultures** are first and foremost initiated by careful transference of a previously established **callus tissue** into a sterile agitated liquid nutrient medium* held in an Erlenmeyer Flask (size: 500 mL, or 250 mL) usually termed as **'culture vessels'.**

(2) Composition of the medium for the **suspension cultures** must be exactly the same as meant for the corresponding **callus cultures,** except the addition of agar (for solidification).

(3) **Soft callus** thus generated gives rise to a desired **suspension culture** quite readily without any hazles at all.

(4) The subsequent release of **tissue cells** as well as **tissue fragments** from not so easily crumbling **callus masses.** Thus, one may afford the critical maintenance of a significant extent of **cell separation** *via* sustaining a relatively high level of **auxin**** concentration in the prevailing **liquid medium.**

It is, however, pertinent to mention here that it is absolutely necessary to maintain a suitable and feasible balance between **auxin and yeast extract** or **auxin and kinetin.**

(5) **Incubation** of the **suspension cultures** are carried out invariably at 25±1 °C either in **total darkness** or in **dim and diffused fluorescent light.**

(6) Constant and continuous agitation of the flask cultures is generally accomplished by the help of a **motorized-speed-controllable horizontal shaker** that rotates betwen 100 to 200 RPM.

(7) The labeled and sterile culture flasks are adequately sealed either with **solid-paraffin wax** or with **thick aluminium foil** so as to check the evaporation to a bare minimum level. It takes almost 4 to 6 weeks to obtain a reasonably appropriate and good **cell suspension.**

(8) Cells grown in **suspension cultures** are found to be **meristematic** in nature. These are usually undifferentiable; besides there exists no vivid and apparent evidence that the ensuing cells belonging to either root or shoot tend to be altogether different metabolically.

(9) Finally, the resulting **suspension cultures** are duly subjected to further subculturing by the actual transfer at regular gap of time of both the duly **fractionated known amounts of the suspension culture** and the **untreated suspension culture** into the **fresh sterilized medium.**

13.2.4.2 From Solid Cultures

The various steps involved in the preparation of **tissue cultures** from the **solid cultures** are as enumerated under:

---

* Usually 30 to 50 mL for each 250 mL **Erlenmayer flask.**

** A substance that promotes growth in plant cells and tissues.

(1) Surface sterilized plant material is adequately transferred onto the solidified nutrient medium taken in Erlenmayer flasks, culture tubes, and glass jars aseptically.

(2) These inoculated glass containers (*viz.*, flasks, jars, tubes) are duly incubated between 26 to 28 °C for a period ranging between 3-4 weeks in complete darkness aseptically.

(3) At the end of the incubation period (*i.e.*, 3-4 weeks) the size and shape of the **callus** must be at least 5 to 6 times bigger than the corresponding size of the **explant.**

(4) Importantly, certain **tissue explants** specifically exhibit **some extent of polarity** which evidently gives rise to the formation of **callus** most rapidly at one surface particularly.

(5) **Stem portions** do exhibit the formation of **callus** wherein the specific surface *in vitro* is pointed towards the **root.**

(6) Invariably, the **callus** gets developed rather swiftly originated either from the tissue not immersed in the solidified culture medium or from the tissue that are found to be not in contact with the said medium.

(7) Regular **maintenance of growth in the callus tissue** may be duly accomplished by the aid of 'subculturing' which essentially requires the effective transfer on each occasion of a **specific piece of healthy viable tissue** after each 30 days into the flask having freshly prepared, sterilized, and solidified nutrient medium.

(8) One may evidently observe that even when the usual standard incubation temperature is brought down between 5 to 10°C from 26°C, several cultures would remain healthy and extend their growth usually at a much lower pace but for longer durations without the necesity of 'subculturing'.

(9) Finally, one would distinctly notice that the normal growth of a plethora of tissue cultures, and specifically of those wherein **chlorophyll gets formed** is overwhelmingly stimulated by a certain **low-intensity illumination.***

13.3 BIOMEDICINALS IN PLANT-TISSUE CULTURES

The intensive and extensive investigative studies related to the inherent biosynthetic capabilities of **plant-tissue cultures** meticulously derived and articulately accomplished from a variety of **higher plants** has been carried out in a systematic and methodical fashion stretched over the past three decades across the globe It has been duly observed that in several instances the much desired specific chemical entities could not be generated for one reason or the other; whereas, in others extremely low quantum of such compounds of interest could be achieved precisely.

The observed significantly **poor yields** of the **secondary metabolites*** seem to be caused on account of the prevailing cardinal factors, such as:

(1) Due to apparent differences between duly dipersed, young, and quickly dividing **culture cells *vis-a-vis*** the relatively mature and slow-growing cells pertaining to the variants in product generation based upon a plethora of such vital factors as: regression (or dormancy) in

---

* **Light source** having a 12 hr cycle or continuous exposure is invariably provided in most of the **Incubation Chambers** by the usual fluorescent tubes.

** A molecule derived from a primary metabolite, many serve protective functions.

biosynthetic pathways, non-excretion of viable products from the **culture cells,** and the significant function of time in culture.

(2) These above mentioned drawbacks (in. 1.) may be circumvented by adopting one of the following effective procedures, namely:

- development of immobilized cell systems,
- development of highly specific hairy-root cultures, and
- evolution of such methodologies which may evidently encourage the process of excretion of the desired viable product right into the **culture medium.**

It is indeed worthwhile to mention at this point in time that there are several proven and glaring examples which obviously show that the **callus** as well as the **suspension cultures** are magnificently capable of carrying out the synthesis of several desired **secondary metabolites** having **overwhelming and satisfactory yields** that are found to be fairly comparable to the **intact plant** itself.

A survey of literature would reveal that during the past two decades there have been an excellent progress with regard to the promising discoveries in the field of **biomedicinals** (*i.e.,* medicinally potent substances), a few of them may have the potential to be scaled upto the **commercially viable extent.***

13.3.1   Secondary Metabolites

In the context of the present day knowledge there exists no clear cut, distinct, and sharp line of division between **primary** and **secondary metabolites.** The **secondary metabolites** are now regarded to be an absolute must to the **plant life;** and, therefore, several of them do provide an effective **defence mechanism** against **bacterial, viral,** and **fungal** attack very much analogous to the **immune system of animals.** Importantly, the actual presence of a chemical entity derived from the **secondary metabolism** exclusively rests upon the sensitivity of the analytical procedure detecting its presence precisely.

Example: Azetidine-2-carboxylic acid (I), an amino acid, present in the sugar beet [*Beta vulgaris*; **Family:** *Chenopodiaceae*], was first and foremost detected and analysed and found to be a minor constituent of the plant. Interestingly, there exists a copious evidence indicating that **(I),** which was once regarded restricted to the natural order **Liliaceae,** is perhaps a ubiquitous (*i.e.,* found everwhere) plant constituent.

$$\text{⬦} \!\!-\!\! \text{COOH}$$
$$\underset{\underset{\text{(I)}}{\overset{|}{\text{H}}}}{\text{N}}$$

Function of Secondary Metabolites: Nevertheless, it would be quite unfair to consider the **plant secondary metabolites** as the **'waste products',** as was once even concluded, but now it has been proved beyond any reasonable doubt that they do possess **several most useful functions.** A few such vital functions shall be enumerated as under:

---

* **Commercially viable extent** refers to the productivity for economic considerations, and may be defined in terms of **gram product/culture volume (L)/day.**

(*a*) **Plant Hormones:** In fact, there are *two* types of **plant hormones,** namely:

(*i*) **Plant growth hormone**—responsible for the growth of plant(s) *e.g.,* **Auxin** [indolylacetic acid] **(II); cytokinins** [zeatin] **(III); ethylene** [abscisic acid] **(IV);** and **gibberellins** [gibberellic acid] **(V).**

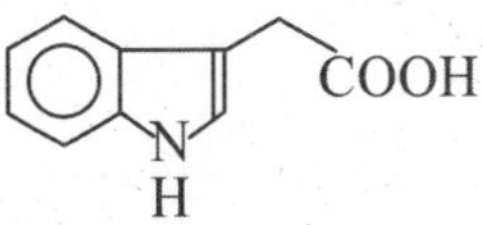

Auxin (II)

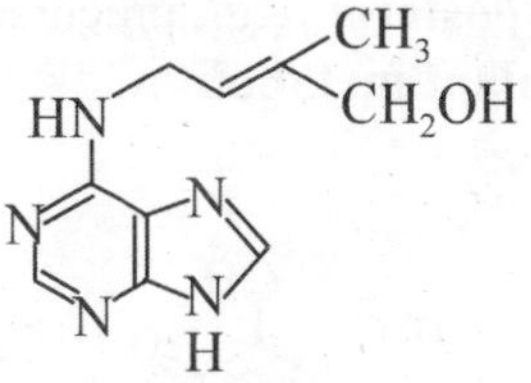

Zeatin (III)

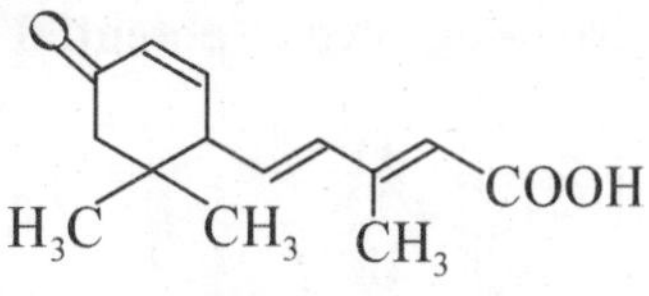

Abscisic Acid (IV)

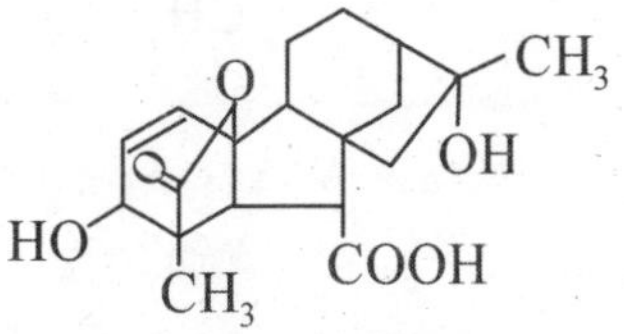

Gibberellic Acid (V)

(*ii*) **Wound hormone**—responsible for the healing of damaged tissue *e.g.,* **traumatic acid (VI):**

$$HOOCCH = CH (CH_2)_8 COOH$$

Traumatic Acid (VI)

(*b*) **Flavonoids and Carotenoids:** A good number of coloured **flavonoids** and **carotenoids** invariably serve to attract specifically **insect and bird pollination** of even the **seed dispersal agents.** However, a few other **secondary metabolites** *e.g.,* the **volatile terpenoids,** repel predominant invaders. It is worthwhile to state here that a relatively large segment of the **secondary metabolites** do exert their marked and pronounced action as **vital fungicides** or **potential antibiotics,** which in turn cause protection of various plants from **fungal or bacterial attacks.**

Examples: Some typical examples belonging to this particular class are, namely: **pterocarpan** [*e.g.,* **pisatin (VII)**], and **sesquiterpenoid** [*e.g.,* **ipomeamarone (VIII)**] which are nothing but **phytolexins** usually generated in response to **specific fungal attack**.

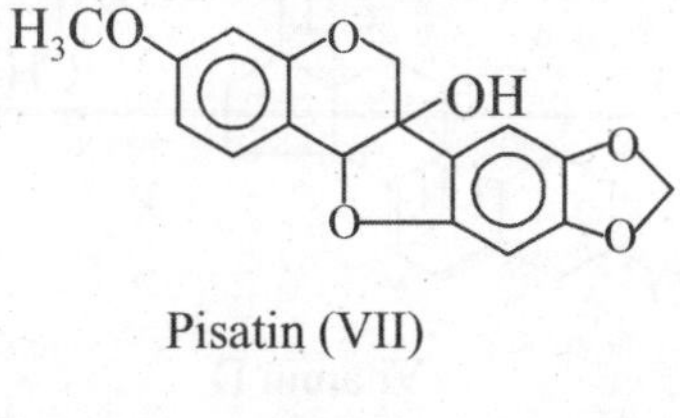

Pisatin (VII)

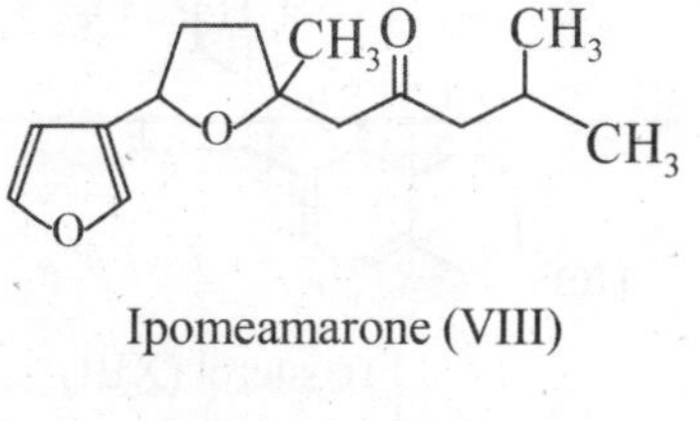

Ipomeamarone (VIII)

13.3.2   Usefulness of Secondary Metabolites

The **usefulness of the secondary metabolites** play an important role either as such to the diet of human beings, such as: **Vitamin C** [*e.g.*, **ascorbic acid (IX), Vitamin E**] *e.g.*, α-tocophenol (X), Vitamin K [*e.g.*, **phylloquinone (XI)**] that are remarkably biosynthesized by plants; or β-carotene [*e.g.*, **precursor of Vitamin A (XII)**], **ergosterol** [*e.g.*, precursor of Vitamin D (XIII)] which are also designated as **potential secondary plant metabolites.**

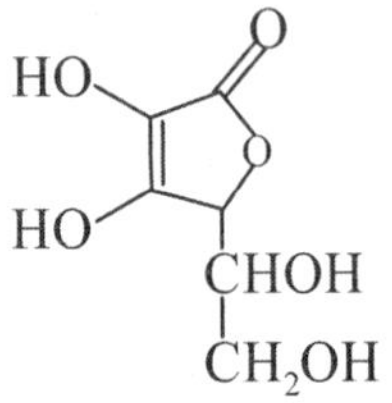

Vitamin C (IX)

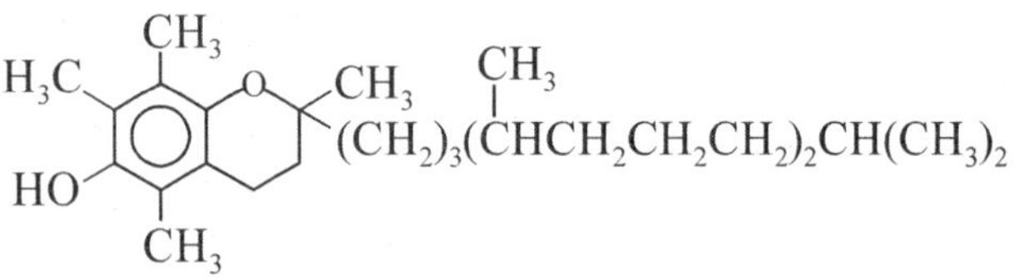

Vitamin E (X)

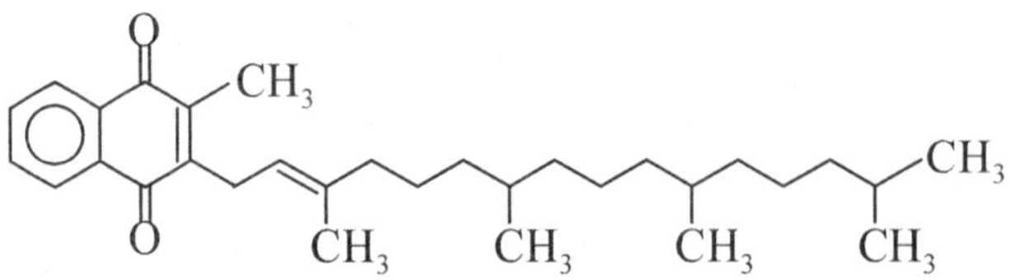

Vitamin K (XI)

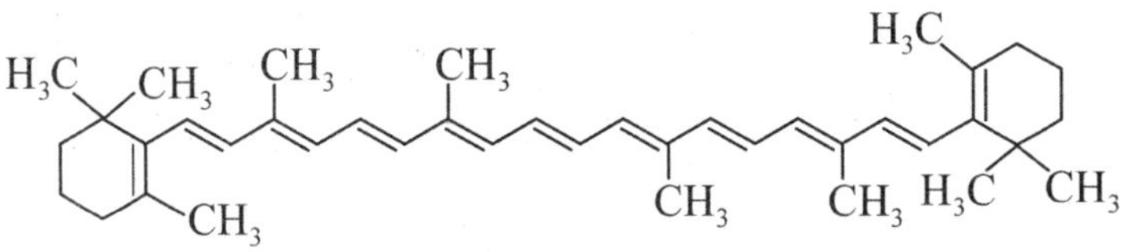

β-Carotene (XII)

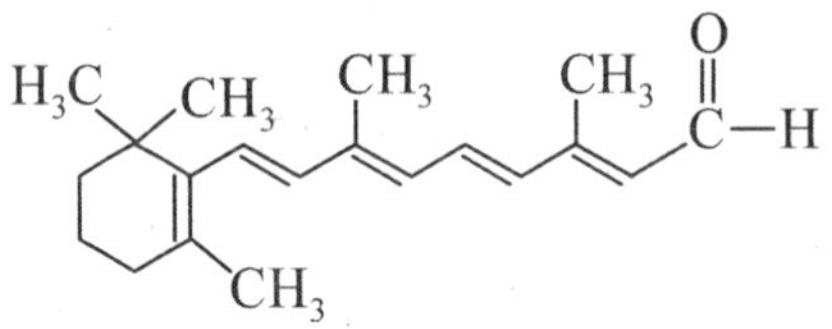

Vitamin A

1 mole of β-carotene yields 2 moles of Vitamin A

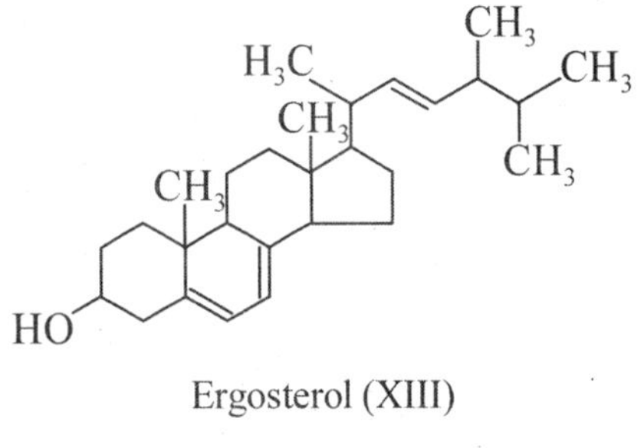

Ergosterol (XIII)

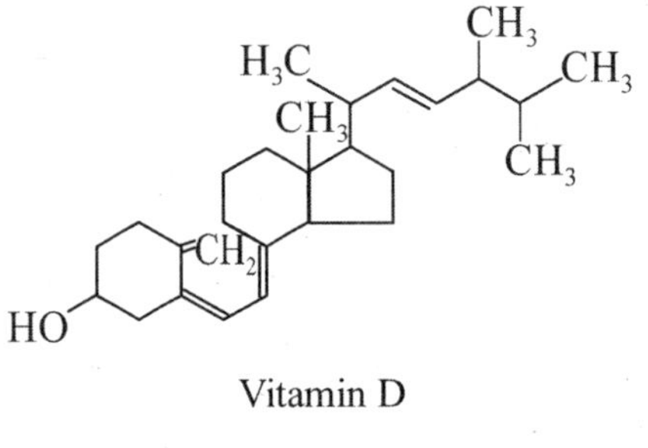

Vitamin D

In addition to the above interesting applications of the **secondary plant metabolites (SPMs)** there are quite a few other noticeable usefulness as enumerated below:

(*a*) **Precursors for Drug Synthesis**—SPMs are also vital and important as precursors for the synthesis of certain drugs *e.g.*, **steroids** and **hormones.**

(*b*) **Plant Poisons (Insecticidal agents)**—Several plants do contain poisonous materials used as insecticidal agents; however, only a few have been duly exploited on a commercial scale, such as: **Nicotine** [*Nicotiana* species: *Family:* **Solanaceae**]; **rotenone** [*Derris* and *Lonchocarpus* species: *Family:* **Leguminosae**]; and **Pyrethrins** [*Chrysanthemum cinerariafolium: Family:* **Compositae**].

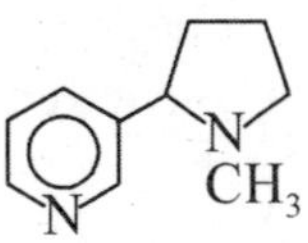

Nicotine 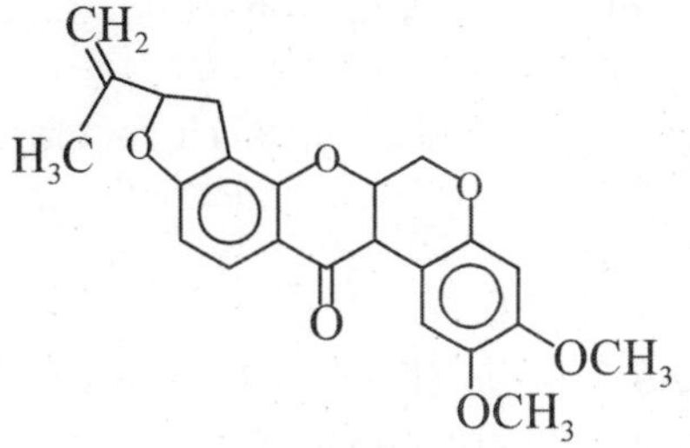   Rotenone 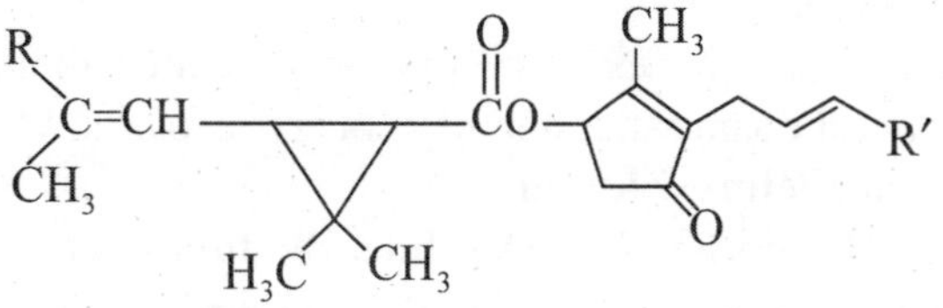   Pyrethrins

(*c*) **Natural Dyes**—As to date quite a few **natural dyes** do find their usefulness in foods and drugs, such as:

- **Carthamin** : *Carthamus tinctorius* (**Compositae**);
- **Bixin** : **Annatto** [*Bixa orellana* (**Bixaceae**)];
- **Crocetin** : **Saffron** [*Corcus sativa* (**Iridaceae**)];
- **Curcumin** : **Turmeric** [*Curcuma longa* (**Zingiberaceae**)].

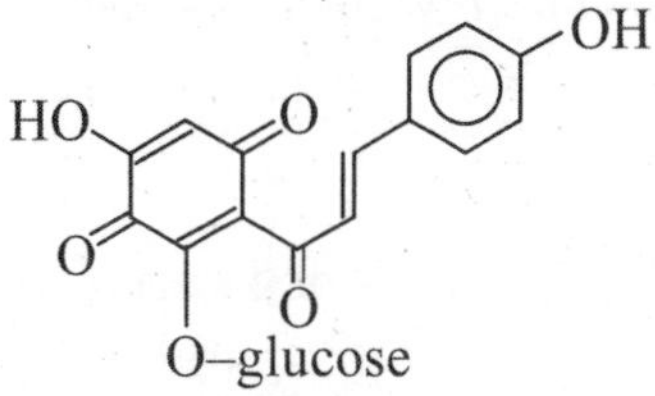

Carthamin 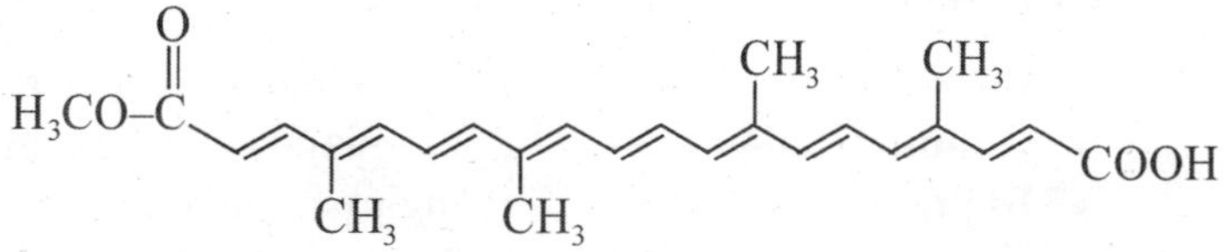   Bixin

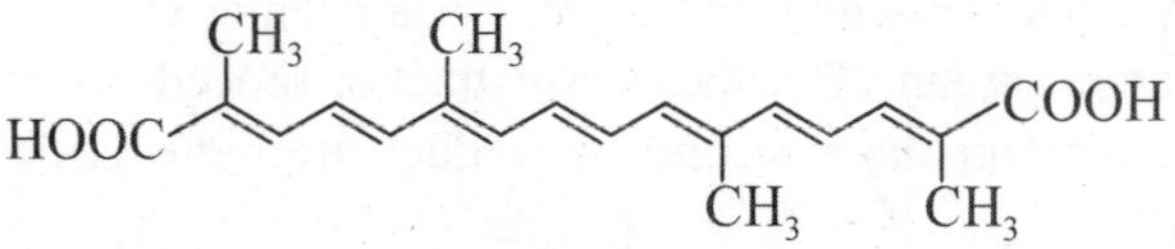

Crocetin 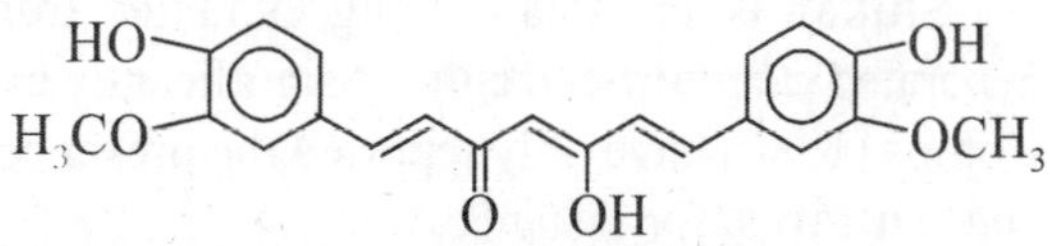   Curcumin

13.3.3 Secondary Metabolites in Chemosystematics

It has been amply demonstrated that the **secondary plant metabolites (SPMs)** may contribute profusely and overwhelmingly to **plant taxonomy, systematics,** and **the study of evolution.** One may observe that the evolution of **chemical** and **morphological characteristic features** are interrelated to an enormous extent; and, therefore, a large segment of these studies related to the **secondary metabolites** invariably serve to confirm the **'morphological classifications'.** Nevertheless, in such specific instances wherein the available morphological relationships seem to be unclear, one may heavily depend upon the so called **'chemotaxonomic markers'** which usually give rise to valuable and critical information(s).

Interestingly, the **biosynthetic pathway** plays an important role while taking into consideration the **chemosystematics** and **plant revolution,** due to the fact that the same kind of **secondary metabolite** may be the **product of two altogether different pathways.** However, the specific enzymes catalyzing the metabolic reactions are of immense importance *vis-a-vis* the products of the reactions, by virtue of the fact that **evolution** solely depends upon the alterations in the **enzyme profiles.**

Plants that essentially possess identical morphological and chemical characteristic profile should have the same ancestor may not prove to be always true perhaps on account of the ensuing **convergent (parallel) revolution.**

Example: Pyrrolizidine alkaloids—are produced by *two* altogether different plant species, namely: *Crotolaria* (Family: **Leguminosae**); and *Senecio* (Family: **Compositae**) by the help of similar pathways; however, these *two* **genera** are absolutely unrelated morphologically. In the light of the above statement of facts it is significantly important to take into consideration all relevant **secondary metabolites** (and not just one particular class) while **classifying the plants** based upon the **biochemical data.**

13.3.4 Newer Products Developed

It has been ascertained that the **secondary metabolites** duly produced from the **plant-tissue cultures** give a yield which is either equal to or greater than that of the **parent plants.** * In fact, almost **thirty natural products** have so far been produced *via* the **plant-cell culture;** and a few such well-known drugs are as follows:

- **Diosgenin** : steroid hormone precursor.
- **Opium Alkaloids** : morphine and its natural congeners
- **Digitalis Glycosides** : digitoxin, digoxin,
- **Essential Oils** : pippermint oil, lemon oil, and
- **Catherenthus Alkaloids** : vincristine, vinblastine.

Shikon is, an Asiatic Drug, obtained from *Lithospermum erythrorhizon* has been adequately generated *via* **plant-cell culture** significantly in larger amounts than the usual extraction procedures.** Robins (1987) have duly reported the presence of certain major secondary products from the **hairy-root cultures,** for instance:***

- **Atropine** : from *Atropa belladona* L,

---

* Staba JE: *J. Nat. Prod.,* **48** (2): 203, 1985.
** Evans WC: **Pharmacognosy,** WB Sannders, London, 15th edn., 2004.
*** Robbins R: *Planta Medica:* **53:** 474, 1987.

- **Hyoscyamine**   : from *Datura stramonium* L.,
- **Nicotine**   : from *Nicotiana tabacum,*
- **Cantharanthene**   : from *C. roses,* and
- **Quinoline Alkaloids**   : from *Cinchona lederiana.*

Based on the scientific evidences one may observe that each **undifferentiated cell** essentially comprises of the necessary genetic information responsible for the production of **secondary metabolites.** It is quite possible to produce commercially **specific plant cells** by integrating their genetic information; and also to increase the production of **secondary metabolites appreciably.** It has been duly observed that the **cell cultures** of several **vital medicinal plants** may effectively produce their **secondary metabolites** in **cultures;** however, the actual yield is comparatively lower to the conventional plant. Last three decades have witnessed the successful achievement of increased yield of desired **secondary metabolities in culture.** Thus, extremely promising results have been achieved for the production of **alkaloids, anthraquinones,** and **cardioactive glycosides.***

13.4   BIOPRODUCTION OF COMMENDABLE SECONDARY METABOLITES

Plant tissue culture has proved to be a viable, feasible and productive alternative method to carry out the production of a plethora of commendable **secondary metabolites** used as **drugs.** In the past *two* decades a copious volume of research has been done in this direction, of which a few typical and important **drugs** shall now be treated in the sections that follows:

(*a*) **Taxol and Related Compounds:** Christen *et al.* (1991)** patented the production of **taxol** from cell cultures. The very next year Fetto-Netto *et al.* (1992)*** reported the cell cultures of *Taxus* species *Taxus cuspidata* and *Taxus canadensis.* It has been observed that the **callus cultures** of *T. cuspidata* could generate **taxol** in quantities almost equivalent to the **stem of the intact plant** (0.02% DW) after 60 days of culture. However, the **immobilized cell cultures** of *T.* cuspidata produced **taxol** very much equivalent to those found in the **bark of the tree** (0.012% DW) after 180 days of culture. All these findings obviously indicated the possibility of making use of **tissue cultures** towards the genuine production of **taxanes.**

(*b*) **Camptothecin:** Wall *et al.* (1966)**** duly reported the presence of **camptothecin,** a *quinoline alkaloid,* from the chinese tree *Camptotheca acuminata;* and subsequently Govindachari *et al.* (1972)***** discovered the same in the indigenous tree *Nothapodytes foetida.* It is an **antitumour alkaloid.**

(*c*) **Medicinal Plants with Anticancer Compounds:** Misawa and Nakanishi (1988)****** reported the presence of certain anticancer compounds in a few well known medicinal plants, such as:

---

* Verpoorte R: **Metabolic Engineering of Plant Secondary Metabolism,** Academic Press, Netherlands, 1999.
** Christen *et al.* United States Patent No.: 5: 019, 504 (1991).
*** Fetto-Neto AG *et al. Bio. Technol.,* **10:** 1572, 1992.
**** Wall *et al.: J. Am. Chem. Soc.,* **88:** 3889, 1966.
***** Govindachari TR and Vishwanathan N., *Phytochemistry,* **11:** 3529, 1972.
****** Misawa M and Nakanishi TM: *Antitumour Compounds Production by Plant Tissue Cultures.* IN: **Biotechnology in Agriculture, Forestry, Medicinal and Aromatic Plants II,** Springer Verlag, Berlin, pp. 192-207, 1988.

- *Cephalotaxus harringtonia,*
- *Podophyllum peltatum,*
- *Tryptergium wilfordii,* and
- *Putterlickia.*

The **tissue cultures** of these medicinal plants have been duly established, and the **cultures** essentially comprised of the desired compounds of the parent plant. Generally, apparent differences were adequately noticed with respect to the yield of the compounds. Kupechan (1972)* observed that in certain specific instances *e.g., T. wilfordii* the **cultures** were able to synthesize appreciably much higher amounts of **tripdiolides** when compared with the intact plant. Kadkade (1982)** carefully observed the **podophyllotoxins** from *P. pelatum* were significantly higher [7.1×10^{-1} % DW] in comparison to the actual plant obtained from the field (*i.e.,* **natural environment**) which stands at [6.4×10^{-1} % DW]. Likewise, the **cephalotoxine** content present in the **cultures** of *C. harringtonia* (in **differentiated tissues**) were found to be much higher in concentrations than the **suspension cultures.**

Conclusively, one may observe that the **potential antineoplastic compounds** may be produced substantially by **tissue cultures** provided the large-scale production could be made feasible if the process can be scaled up in relatively **large bioreactors** followed by critical optimization of experimental parameters required essentially for the **active production.**

(*d*) **Antimalarials:** Fulzele *et al.* (1991)*** reported 0.012% DW of **artemisinin** present in the **shoot cultures** of **Artemisia annua,** whereas He *et al.* (1983)**** reported only 0.008% DW of the same.

Woerdenberg *et al.* (1983)***** duly reported an yield of 0.16% DW of **Artemisinin** in the shoot cultures of *A. annua* growing on MS 1/2 + BA (0.2) + NAA (0.05) medium containing 1% sucrose. However, the respective **Artemisinin** content enhanced with **0.5% sucrose.** Meanwhile, supplementing the **culture medium** with GA (10 mg. L^{-1}), CH (0.5 mg. L^{-1}) and 10 or 20 mg. L^{-1} of **naftifine** remarkably increased the production of **Artemisinin** in the shoot cultures of *A. annua.* Importantly, these wonderful observations do suggest that the duly prepared **shoot cultures** may ultimately prove to be a logical, feasible and viable alternative method for the production of **Artemisinin.**

(*e*) **Adenylate Cyclase Activity Stimulator: Forskolin** is a potent **diterpenoid** isolated from the roots of *Coleus Forskohlii* (an Indian Medicinal Plant) which distinctly possesses **adenylate cyclase activity stimulating profile.** Sen *et al.* (1993)****** duly reported the presence of **forskolin** in the untransformed root cultures of *C. forskohlii.* The roots were carefully grown in various **basal media** and altogether variable **culture conditions.** In actual practice, the **culture media** employed duly for the growth of **root cultures** essentially consisted of MS 25%, sucrose 1%, and either IAA, IBA, or 2-chlorinated derivatives of IAA *viz.,* 4-Cl-IAA

---

   * Kupechan SM *et al. J. Am. Chem. Soc.,* **94,** 7194, 1972.
   ** Kadkade PG: *Plant Sci. Lelt.,* **25:** 107, 1982.
   *** Fulzele DP *et al. Phytotherapy Research,* **5:** 149, 1991.
   **** He XC *et al. Acta. Bot. Sin.,* **25:** 87, 1983.
   ***** Woerdenbag HJ *et al.: Plant Cell Tissue and Organ Culture,* **32:** 247, 1993.
****** Sen J *et al.: Phytochemistry,* **34:** 1309, 1993.

and 5, 6-C 12-IAA. The **tissue cultures** grew very satisfactorily in all the dosages of the chlorinated IAAs. Besides, it also generated more quantum of **forskolin** in comparison to the **cultures** grown in IAA or IBA singly. It has been observed that in a medium comprising 50 mcg. L^{-1} of Cl-IAA the **forskolin** content stood at 0.09% DW, that was evidently comparable to **forkolin** content present in the **wild plant** (0.1% DW). However, at a concentration level of 500 mcg. L^{-1} of IAA or IBA exclusively small amounts of **forskolin** was obtained.

To sum up one may add that the **plant-tissue cultures** continue to remain as a distinct major source for several novel **biomedicinals (phytochemicals),** and the subsequent strategic development in the **Medicinal Plant Biotechnology** together with **Plant Tissue Culture and Technology** have virtually opened up newer avenues both for the propagation of **elite medicinal plants** and **mass cultivation of cells** in **sophisticated PC-based automated Bioreactors** for superb and novel products.

FURTHER READING REFERENCES

1. Brar DS and Khush GS: **Cell and Tissue Culture for Plant Improvement.** In: Basra AS (ed.): *Mechanisms of Plant Growth and Improved Productivity: Modern Approaches,* Mercel Dekker Inc., New York, pp. 229-278, 1994.
2. Brown DCW and Thorpe TA: **Plant Regeneration by Organogenesis.** In: Vasil IK (ed): *Cell Culture and Somatic Cell Genetics*, Academic Press, New York, Vol. 3, 1986.
3. Congress, Office of Technology Assessment: New Developments in Biotechnology: US Investments in Biotechnology—Special Report. OTA-BA-360. Supdt. Documents, Washington DC, 20402-9325, 1988.
4. Debergh P and Zimmerman R (eds.): **Micropropogation,** Kluwer Academic Publication, New York, 1991.
5. Eliet U: **Cell Culture and Somatic Cell Genetic Implants,** Academic Press, San Diego, 1987.
6. Imrie BC and Hacker JB (eds): **Focused Plant Improvement: Towards Responsible and Sustainable Agriculture,** Pergamon Press, London, 1993.
7. Ingram DS and Helgeson JP (eds.): **Tissue Culture Methods for Plant Pathologists,** Blackwell, Oxford, UK, 1980.
8. Marmorosch K and Sato GH (eds.): **Advances in Cell Culture,** Academic Press, California, Vol. 7. 1989.
9. Mohan Ram HY and Kapoor A: ***In vitro* Growth and Development of Hornwort.** In: *3rd International Conference: Plant Tissue and Cell Culture,* Leicester, UK, 1974.
10. Rao AN (ed.): **Tissue Culture of Economically Important Plants,** Asian Network for Biological Sciences, Singapore, 1981.
11. Reinert J and Bajaj YPS (eds.) **Applied and Fundamental Aspects of Plant Cell, Tissue, and Organ Culture,** Springer, Berlin, 1977.
12. Staba EJ: **Plant Tissue Culture as a Source of Biochemicals,** CRC-Press, Boca Raton, 1987.
13. Verporate R: **Metabolic Engineering of Plant Secondary Metabolism,** Academic Publishers, Netherlands, 1999.
14. White PR: **A Handbook of Plant Tissue Culture,** Jaques, Catell, England, 1943.

14 Hi-Tech Products from Plant Sources

- Introduction
- High Throughput Screening (HST)
- Success of HTS of Plant Source Materials for New Lead Chemical Entities
- Hi-Tech Products
- Further Reading References

14.1 INTRODUCTION

Since more than three centuries the World has witnessed the enormous and highly specific therapeutic applications of both **traditional and orthodox medicaments.** Invariably, the use of **'crude natural plant extracts'** comprising of multi-component products duly exerted either **extremely potent/ active entities,** such as: **Digitalis leaf** or **extremely weak/active** components, for instance: **Cinnamon bark.** Interestingly, the **orthodox medicaments** exclusively depend upon mainly single (*i.e.*, a very small quantum of) well defined, duly characterized active-chemical entities predominantly showing highly specific activities at, in a plethora of instances, well-established and known **'biological targets'.**

It is, however, pertinent to state here that these **hi-tech products** (or **medicines**) are invariably fount to be extremely potent; therefore, most of them usually **display pretty narrow gap** prevailing between an **effective dose (ED$_{50}$)** and a **lethal (toxic) dose (LD$_{50}$).** Importantly, one may duly observe that the so called **orthodox medicaments** are meticulously formulated and designed into a good number of dosage forms which may be judiciously **'standardized'** for their ultimate bioavailability *in vivo*.

Following are some of the most **invaluable orthodox drugs,** that are exclusively obtained from chemical compounds frequently occurring in higher plants, are basically **'analgesic'** in character, such as: **morphine** and **codeine; antineoplastic agents** *viz.*, **taxol** and **vincrystine; antimalarials,** for instance: **quinine** and **artimisinine;** and **anti-asthmatics** *e.g.*, **cromoglycate.**

As to date, certain naturally occurring materials from the plant sources (or plant kingdom) still continue to enjoy the most viable and vital commercial source of the **'active principle'. Examples:** The *two* prominent and exclusive examples are as stated below:

(*a*) **Poppy capsule:** Glaxo Wellcome still harvests up to 10,000 MT dry weight of **'poppy capsule'** every year (under license) to provide an authentic genuine source of the **'opiate alkaloids'**, and

(b) ***Digitalis lanata* leaf:** Contractors hired by Glaxo Wellcome also produce 170 MT per annum dry weight of ***Digitalis lanata*** leaf to serve as the prime source of **'digoxin'**—a potent **cardiotonic.**

14.2 HIGH THROUGHPUT SCREENING (HTS)

In an attempt to explore and discover **'new medicines'** that essentially give rise to an altogether distinct and remarkably significant advantages upon the **prevailing practised therapies,** the primary crucial and key starting point is to identify, recognize, and exploit the **'novel biological targets',** which do possess a critical role in the control and management of a plethora of **disease processes.** Interestingly, the immediate text protocol would be to evolve and involve discovery intimately associated with the **'biological assays',** that are quite capable of detecting such substances which may eventually cause articulated modification of the ensuing activity of the **'target'.** It is, however, pertinent to mention at this point in time that the evolved **'lead chemicals'** are predominantly such compounds that are absolutely amenable to a broad-spectrum of **'chemical manipulations'** to achieve the following *two* major objectives, namely:

(a) To substantially optimize their existing **bioactivity** and **bioavailability** profile, and

(b) To look for and develop such rare compounds that may serve as **'potential candidates in their own right'.**

High Throughput Screening (HTS) process is presently the most important and highly procreative power for the useful and ultimate discovery of a variety of **newer lead chemical entities in the pharmaceutical industry.**

Miniaturized Assay: HTS indeed makes use of extremely specific **miniaturized assay formats** having the following salient features:

- Invariably uses **microtitre plates** capable of handling **384 sample variants** that may be assayed most conveniently at $< 50 \mu L$ total assay volume per run effectively,
- Based upon 100% fully automated sophisticated device one may carry out the assay of hundreds of thousands of samples **against each biological target of interest,** and
- Final numbers of samples actually being assayed exclusively depend upon the overall cost involved per assay, that may usually range between INR1 per well to INR 100 per well approximately.

HTS being a complex phenomenon that exclusively demands the following cardinal aspects, such as:

(a) In-depth knowledge with respect to the critical role of **specific biological targets** in the domain of disease progression,

(b) The systematic development of **well-defined bioassays** that are solely capable of discovering desired regulators of the target,

(c) Soft targets with automation-friendly techniques with regard to the respective design, miniaturization, and ultimate **'automation of bioassays',**

(d) Adequate thorough understanding of the **micro-** as well as **macro-structure** of the ensuing 'biological target' in such a manner that the prevailing 'sample-selection strategy' is optimized appropriately,

(e) Engineering excellence and master-piece of meticulously designed **custom-built robots** that may exploited judiciously for desired **storage, retrieval,** and **bioassay** of exceptionally large excess of samples within a span of 1 year, and

(f) Aggressive development of 'numerous software systems' that may go a long way in helping the scientists intimately engaged and associated with the handling of the copious volume of 'data' that emerges eventually.

The **five** vital and important aspects of **HTS** enumerated as under:

(a) **HTS** and Bioassays,
(b) Access to Plants *vis-a-vis* Natural Source Materials,
(c) **HTS** and Selection for Plant Materials,
(d) Identification Process of Plants for Targeted Sets, and
(e) Dereplication and Isolation of Active Compounds.

The aforesaid aspects of **HTS** shall now be discussed briefly in the sections that follows:

14.2.1   HTS and Bioassays

It has been duly observed that the 'ideal bioassays' for **HTS** are those which critically enable **identification of chemical compounds** in *six* different manners, namely:

(a) exerting action upon **specific biological targets,**
(b) engage a minimum number of 'reagent addition steps',
(c) act **predictably and reliably,**
(d) conveniently **amenable** to both **automation and miniaturization**
(e) essentially involve **low-cost ingredients,** and
(f) make use of **effective detection technology.**

Importantly, the 'biochemical targets of interest' in the context of the most enterprising **pharmaceutical lead discovery** which invariably range from **enzymes** to **receptors*** to **ion channels;** however, in the specific instance of infectious disease to the entire microbial cells.

A few typical examples of **HTS and bioassays** are described as under:

Example: (a) **Bradykinin (BK):** A tissue hormone belonging to a group of hypotensive peptides invariably termed as **plasma kinins.** It was first ever obtained by incubation with the venom of *Bothrops jararaca* or with crystalline trypsin. It is used as a vasodilator.

In fact, **bradykinin (BK),** an endogenous neuropeptide gets duly involved in the control and management of different kinds of pain asociated with mammalian central nervous system (CNS). Therefore, systematic approach in inducting adequate antagonism of **BK** to its corresponding receptors is indeed a potential target towards the unique development of altogether new breeds of **analgesic agents.**

---

* **Receptor:** Both nuclear and transmembrane.

(b) ***Candida albicans*** cell-free translation system based upon **Polyurethane** as a **synthetic template** has been adequately proved and established to look for such chemical entities (*i.e.*, compounds) that essentially causes the inhibition of **critical fungal protein synthesis.***

14.2.2 Access to Plants *vis-a-vis* Natural Source Materials

Ten Kate and Laired (1999)** reported duly that the **United Nations Convention on Biodiversity (CBD)** has been ratified in 1992 by almost 175 countries of the world. The most vital and important objectives of **CBD** are as stated under:

(1) To ensure the conservation of biological diversity.
(2) To implement sustainably its various cardinal components, and
(3) To affect equitable and fair sharing of usefulness emerging from its application and usage.

In order to fully respect the **'letter and spirit'** of the said **Convention (CBD)** within the framework are several essential issues, such as:

(a) Sovereignty of countries over their genetic resources, and
(b) Country's reciprocal obligation to facilitate an easy access.

In fact, the *two* mutual contracting parties must establish appropriate means and ways for legitimately honouring the **'benefit sharing'** in the instance of **commercial utilization** of the genetic resources. The concerted efforts of the so-called **three agencies,** namely: (a) **collector,** (b) **source country,** and (c) **industrial collaborator** must prevail in all respects.

Glaxo Wellcome (UK) has come up with a **documented legal policy** to acquire **'natural source materials'** evidently lays down the various cardinal issues, essentially come across by a Pharmaceutical Company, to address such vital aspects as enumerated below briefly:

- that a Pharmaceutical Company shall solely collaborate with such firms or organizations who may amply demonstrate the qualified expertise together with genuine capability to provide **natural source materials** according to the schedule agreed upon in the **'mutual agreement',**
- that only comparatively small quantum of **plant materials** are duly collected from the **sustainable** natural sources,
- that **'endangered species'** *i.e.*, such species which are on the verge of extinction must not be accessed intentionally
- that a well defined 'materials transfer agreement is suitably drawn up which clearly ascertains that **collectors** are duly reimbursed towards the actual cost of collection together with their expertise,
- that the terms and conditions of the agreement should also specify expatiately **all financial benefits** in the event of **commercialization,**
- that the **'agreement'** must clearly state that a significant component of the ensuing **'royalty payment'** should be duly paid back to the source country so as to continue and sustain the **education** and **training** programme at the basic community level, and
- that major portion of **payments** must be affected duly during different successful stages of the ongoing **'drug-development process'** (by Glaxo Wellcome).

---

* Kinsman OS *et al. J. of Antibiotics,* **51**(1): 41-49, 1998.
** Ten Kaite K and Laird SA: **The Commercial Use of Biodiversity,** Earth Scan Publications, London (UK), 1999.

14.2.3 HTS and Selection for Plant Materials

The actual impact of **HTS** and the suitable selection for plant materials always prevails predominantly in the event when a **'target'** belongs exclusively to a **'specific class'** that is rather difficult to find **small molecule hits,** such as:

(*a*) protein-protein interactions,

(*b*) occurrence of a strong precedent, and

(*c*) rationale for natural product-derived activities.

Importantly, the complete compliance of the above three aspects legitimately command the desired **natural product input.**

Examples: The following typical examples would be further useful in the adequate clarifications of the above statement of facts:

(*a*) **Antimicrobial Activity** *i.e.*, the track-record of various drug discoveries from a wide spectrum of **microbial sources, and**

(*b*) **Analgesic Medicaments** *i.e.*, the same rationale shall hold good for the adequate track record of plant species in the production of analgesic medicaments.

Salient Features: The various **salient features** with regard to **HTS and selection for plant materials** are as stated under:

(1) An easy and convenient access to diversified and huge collections of **natural plant materials.**

    Examples:

(*a*) Samples that are collected skilfully in order to add varying diversity to the important collection,

(*b*) Collections may include such samples that are specifically selected based upon various logical reasons *viz.*, microbial producer of a certain chemical entity, or a plant prominently employed **ethnomedically** for a certain prescribed parameter.

(2) A diversity-based point of view certainly requires adequate gaining possession of pre-selected **taxonomic* groups.** Thus, one may make use of a variety of time-tested techniques to critically analyze the **natural taxonomic spread of a plant collection** which may subsequently be extended to minimise the existing gaps so that the ultimate collection distinctly reflects the **'available diversity'** more exhaustively.

(3) **'Chemical Targeting'** and **'Biological Targeting':** Recently, a much more critically focused approach exclusively based upon the **'prior available knowledge pertaining to some selected samples'** amply suggests that they invariably comprise of a good number of:

(*a*) highly specific **chemical classes of interest, and**

(*b*) essentially possess **desirable biological characteristic features.**

Interestingly, the aforesaid **'approach'** may be justifiably considered under *two* categories, namely:

---

* **Taxonomic:** Concerning the laws and principles of classification of living organisms.

(*i*) **Chemical Targeting:** It accomplishes its cardinal objectives in *two* different manners, namely:

- makes use of **natural plant materials** as the prime sources of particular chemical compounds of great interest to a specific disease regimen, and
- provides genuine and authentic sources of chemical class of compounds predicted to possess appropriate **'pharmacophore moieties'**.

In this manner, it would be quite feasible to identify the ensuing **chemical species** that are actively under due consideration in a **prevailing sample collection.**

(*ii*) **Biological Targeting:** It may be regarded as to persue a disease driven process. In actual practice, one may even select **plant samples** that may be utilized for the **'biological evaluation'** thereby providing some sort of relevant information associated with them which in turn could throw ample light with respect to their precise relevance for evaluation *vis-a-vis* a **given therapeutic target.**

Examples:

(*a*) The **ethnobotanical** reports of **traditional medicinal applications** of plant materials, and
(*b*) Commercially available **orthodox medicinals** duly discovered by **definite leads** given by indigenous knowledge.*

14.2.4 Identification Process of Plants for Targeted Sets

As to date a good number approaches have been duly persued, worked out, and adopted in the process of adequate assimilation of the relevant information required necessarily so as to specifically select **plant materials** of particular relevance for a **given disease target.**

Table: 14.1. summarizes the various strategies adopted for the actual identification process of plants for the targeted sets:

Table 14.1 Strategies Adopted for Identification Process of Plants for Targeted Sets

S.No.	Research Group	Adopted Methodology	Comments
1	Ethnobotanical Network	Worked intimately with indigenous colleagues and traditional doctors in different countries.	Low output of actual plant samples for evaluation in laboraory. High output of valuable information(s) of their usage.
2	Pharmaceutical Companies	Make use of information(s) reported in Books, Journals etc.	Chinese Traditional Medicines; Indian Traditional Medicines.
3	Natural Products Alert [NAPRALERT] Database**	The system is maintained at the University of Illinois at Chicago (USA).	Contains huge number of references related to: • Ethnobotanical reports, • Reports of biological activity in scientific literature, and • Phytochemical data.
4	Chemical Information Databases	Dictionary of Natural Products [Chapman and Hall, New York]	Database contains informations on more than 100,000 natural plant products, including the plant species from where the chemical compound actually originates.
5	Literature Survey	To generate semi-purified plant extracts or chemical group of specific interest, or extracts that are enriched in the chemical entities.	Plants having an **ethnomedical application** the extracts may be prepared using recommended **traditional medicine.**

---

* Cox P.: **Ethnobotany and the Search for New Drugs,** Wiley, Chichester, pp. 25-41, 1994.
** Loub WD *et al.: J. Chem. Inform. and Comput. Scs.*, **25**: 99-103, 1985.

In short it may be added that these typical **'targeted'** approaches invariably give rise to the actual involvement of rather smaller quantum of **natural plant samples** *vis-a-vis* a **high throughput random screening programme** [HTRSP].

14.2.5 Dereplication and Isolation of Active Compounds

From actual hands-on experience one may observe critically that before starting a complete **bioassay monitored fractionaion of the active samples** it is absolutely important and necessary to carry out the review with respect to the **tolerance of a given bioassay** of either a **semi-purified** or a **crude** extract of **natural plant materials.** However, the cardinal objective of evaluating such samples in a **planned bioassay** is to identify **chemical entities** that eventually interact with a **specific biological target,** such as: a **receptor** or an **enzyme.**

However, from actual practice it has been duly observed that there are several unwanted, problematic, and trouble-shooter components that directly interfere with the **bioassay** *viz.,*

* **Polyphenolics**—forming complexes with a wide range of proteins, antioxidants, and UV quenchers,
* **Detergent-like Compounds**—causing disruption of cell membranes.

Van Middlesworth and Cannell (1998)* strongly advocated that it is very important and necessary to detect and subsequently get rid of all such **active chemical compounds** as early and swiftly as possible.

Importantly, the physico-chemical characteristic features of a pure isolated compound may provide extremely vital and useful clues with regard to its identity. In fact, the *two* most abundantly used properties, namely: (*a*) **HPLC**-retention time,** and (*b*) **UV-spectral data,** are invariably accomplished *via* well-known **standard analytical procedures.** However, one may easily compare these data *vis-a-vis* the known **reference compounds;** and, therefore, possibly characterize the various components present in a **mixture** without even going through the cumbersome process of **complete isolation** of each individual component.

Preparative HPLC, based on solvent partitioning, perhaps is the most common and widely used method for the isolation of pure chemical entities from various plant source materials.

Meticulous exhaustive studies towards the elucidation of the chemical structure of the pure isolated compound from various plant source materials shall render enormous valuable information(s) together with certain definitive indication of the superb and classical **'drug-like'** qualities present in the molecule.

14.3 SUCCESS OF HTS OF PLANT SOURCE MATERIALS FOR NEW LEAD CHEMICAL ENTITIES

In the recent past, the discovery of a plethora of extremely potent and elegantly novel **euphane tri-terpenes** amply proves and demonstrates the actual enormous ability and potential of several plant

---

* Van Middlesworth F and Cannell RJP: *Dereplication and Partial Identification of Natural Products:* In: Cannell RJP (ed.): **Natural Products Identification,** Humana Press, Totowa, NJ, pp: 343-363, 1998.
** **HPLC:** High performance liquid chromatography [Kar, A: **Pharmaceutical Drug Analysis,** New Age International, New Delhi, **2nd** edn., 2005].

extracts to produce highly beneficial **'chemical leads'** in a defined **HTS-programme.**

The above factual observations may be duly substantiated with the help of the following important investigative experimental results, namely:

(*a*) **Inhibitors of Human Thrombin:** In the usual course of a **'random'** screening exercise to look for certain **'novel inhibitors of human thrombin'** that essentially help in the critical blockade of the actual formation of **blood clots;** and, therefore, may be duly exploited in the treatment, control, and prevention of the **deep-vein thrombosis.** For this meticulous and herculian task, a sizable (approx. 1,50,000) samples adequately derived from both natural sources *viz.*, **plant extracts, microbial extracts, fungal extracts,** and purely **synthetic chemical compounds** were subjected to **vigorous investigative evaluations.** The interesting outcome of this big-job revealed that the **methanolic extracts of *Lantana camara*** leaves, belonging to the natural order **Verbenaceae,** showed **remarkable potent activity.**

Sharma and Sharma (1989)* attributed the inherent toxic effects of the leaves of *Lantana camara* due to the presence of **lantadenes** *i.e.,* a series of **pentacyclic triterpenes.** Later on, Uppal *et al.* (1982)** reported the specific haematological manifestations occurring in sheep with **'lantana poisoning'** associated with the following vital biological effects, such as:

- Enhancement in **blood-coagulation time** and **prothrombin time,**
- Reduction in **blood-sedimentation rate,**
- Total **plasma-protein content,** and
- Total **fibrinogen content.**

The aforesaid observation ascertains the corresponding **thrombin-inhibitory translactone** having the **euphane triterpenes.**

(*b*) **Biological Activity** of the **euphane triterpenes** has been studied both extensived and intensively by Weir *et al.* (1998)***. This investigative study amply revealed their actual **'mechanism of action** as specific inhibitors for **blood clothing** through the strategic acylation of the available **active site(s)** *i.e.,* **Ser 195** residual segment of **thrombin.** It is pertinent to state here that the observed **'acylating activity'** as the very root cause for being genetic against several other particular **serine protease enzymes.** Interestingly, this critical and vital observation forms the basis for both exhaustive exploration and extended exploitation in the ever-expanding domain of **'drug discovery.'**

14.3.1 Use of MS**** for Identification of Potent Biologically Active and Important Drug Molecules

After having isolated the pure chemical constituents from the **natural plant source** it becomes absolutely necessary to analyze such **compound(s)** or **protein(s)** of general interest, to elucidate and identity unambiguously their **exact positions** or **precise retention times (RTS)** by subjecting

---

* Sharma OMP and Sharma PD, *J. Scientific Industrial Research,* **48:** 471-478, 1989.

** Uppal RP and Paul Bs, *Ind. Veterinary J.*, pp 18-24, 1982.

*** Weir MP *et al. Biochemistry,* **37:** 6645-6657, 1998.

**** Mass Spectrometry.

them *via* the **selected adsorption phase** invariably employed in any known sophisticated type of **chromatography.**

Example: HPLC-Chromatograms: Each individual 'sample run' shall give rise to a cluster of several sharp peaks, designating separate chemical compounds present, which may be systematically identified by the help of 'known standards' under identical experimental parameters. Ultimately, it will certainly determine the **Rt*** of the pure **chemical entity** or the **protein of interest.** However, the presence of 'unknown compounds', whose **RTs** are fairly comparable to those of the **standards (reference compounds)** may be identified by the aid of 'multiple forms of chromatography' quite tentatively.

It is pertinent to mention here that either **Mass Spectrometry (MS)** or **Nuclear Magnetic Resonance (NMR) spectroscopy** analysis of the 'unknown peak' should be carried out very carefully and panistakingly so as to identify the 'actual compound of interest' unambiguously.

Identification of Taxol: Taxol, a natural product, obtained from *Taxol brevifolia* Nutt (*Fam.* **Taxaceae**), abundantly used for breast cancer (see Chapter 1) enjoyed the cogent application for its adequate and explicit characterization meticulously by **MS** by McClure *et al.* (1992)** and by **NMR** by Falzone *et al.* (1992)***.

A survey of literature would certainly reveal a good number of chemical compounds, derived from the natural plant sources and invariably used as 'drugs', that have been duly characterized by the said spectral analyses *viz.*, MS, NMR.

14.4   HI-TECH PRODUCTS

Since 1990s a plethora of **hi-tech products** duly obtained from plant source materials have gained qualified success and well-deserved recognition across the globe for the therapeutic usages in humans. It will be worthwhile to discuss a few such **hi-tech products** at this point in time hereunder.

14.4.1   Genistein [*Syn.* Genisteol; Prunetol;]

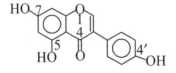

4′,5,7-Trihydroxy isoflavone;

Genistein is the phytoestrogen normally found in **soy products.** It represents the **aglucon of genistin** and of **sophoricoside****.** It serves as a **specific protein kinase inhibitor.**

---

   * **Rt:** It is the time (minutes) recorded duly on the **HPLC-chromatogram** where a given peak of interest occurs.
  ** McClure TD *et al. J. Am. Soc. Mass Spect.,* **3**: 672-679, 1992.
 *** Falzone CJ *et al.: Tetrahed. Lett.,* **33**: 1169-1172, 1992.
**** **Sophoricoside:** It is genistein-4′-glucoside.

Characteristic Features: The various characteristic features of **genistein** are as enumerated under:

(1) It lowers the incidence of breast, prostrate, and several other carcinomas.
(2) It minimises the incidence and number of cancerous tumours; and also to enhance the latency in the animal models of cancer.
(3) In cell-culture models it particularly inibits proliferation of certain types of cancer cells.
(4) Various sophisticated well-defined techniques have been adopted *viz.*, *in vitro* **techniques, cell-culture techniques,** so as to decepher (unfold) the mechanism whereby **genistein** might change the ensuing **cancer-cell kinetics.**
(5) **Genistein** causes the inhibition of **angiogenesis,*** steroid hormone receptors, inhibition of tyrosine kinase, inhibition of radical O_2-species formation, and above all interaction with **topoisomerase.****

14.4.2   Camptothecin

Camptothecin is an **antitumour alkaloid,** which essentially serves a **prototype DNA topoisomerase I*** inhibitor.**

In fact, quite a few products are now the focus of attention, and have virtually undergone extensive preclinical and intensive clinical investigations, or even both of them together, namely:

• 9-amino-20S-camptothecine;
• 9-dimethylaminomethyl-10-hydroxy-20(S)-camptothecine [Topotecan®];
• 7-ethyl-10-[4-(1-piperidino) carbonyloxy-camptothecine [Irinotecan®]; and
• 9-nitro-20(S)-camptothecine.

14.4.3   Rhein [*Syn:* Monorhein; Rheic Acid; Cassic Acid; Parietic Acid; Rhubarb Yellow]

---

* Fotis T *et al. J. Nutr.,* **125:** 790S-79S, 1995.
** Barnes S. and Peterson TG: *Proc. Exp. Biol. Med.,* **208:** 109-115, 1995.
*** **Topoisomerase I:** An enzyme intimately involved in the uncoding of DNA, a prerequisite for **replication** and **transcription.**

Rhein is usually found in the **'free state'** and as **'glucoside'** in *Rheum* species (*Fam. Polygonaceae*) (**rhubarb**) and in **Senna leaves**; besides, in several species of **Cassia** (*Fam. Leguminosae*). The **diacetate salt of rhein** [Diacerein®] is mostly used as **antirheumatic.**

Characteristic Features: The various characteristic features are as follows:

(1) **Rhein** exerts its action as an antineoplastic agent.
(2) Electron microscopic examination of **rhein** reveals that it both disrupts and distorts the membranes pertaining to cells and mitochondria, which expatiates its antitumour effects.
(3) Castiglioni *et al.* (1993)* duly hypothesized that **rhein** strategically changes the **fluidity of membranes** that eventually leads to the ultimate **uptake of glucose.**
(4) The resulting net observed effect of (3) above is substantial reduced available energy for cardinal cellular functions, and hence eventual **cellular necrosis.**

14.4.4 Taxanes

Based on evidences scanned through the literatures one may observe that virtually all parts of *Taxus brevifolia* essentially comprise of a broad spectrum of **diterpenoid structural analogues** invariably known as **taxanes.** Actually these compounds do have a close resemblance to the various **toxic constituents** that are usually found in other *Taxus* species, such as: the **common yew** (*Taxus baccata*).

In the recent past, a successful attempt was made to afford the uninterrupted, constant, and sizable supply of **taxol** and its **corresponding derivatives** for subsequent **drug usage.** Hence, an alternative semi-synthetic route was adopted starting from **closely resembling** and **more accessible structurally related substances.**

Examples: Baccatin III (1) and **10-Deacetylbaccatin III(2):** Interestingly, both these compounds *i.e.*, **(1)** and **(2)** have been effectively transformed into **taxol.** Compound **(2)** may be readily extracted from the twigs and leaves of *T. baccata*.

Baccatin III (1): R = Ac;
10-Deacetylbaccantin III (2): R =H;

14.4.5 Homoharringtonine (HHT)

Homoharringtonine is found to be the most active of the **alkaloids** derived from the bark of the famous Chinese evergreen tree *Cephalotaxus harringtonia*.

---

* Castiglioni S *et al.*: *Anti-Cancer,* **4:** 407-414, 1993.

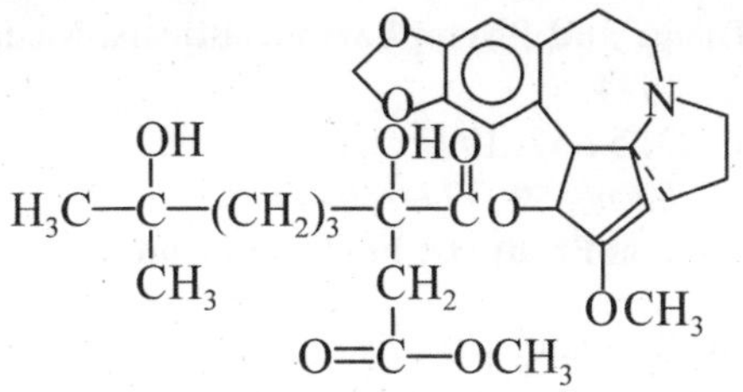

Homoharringtonine

It is extensively employed in the treatment and control of malignancy.* Zhou *et al.* (1995)** reported promising results of **HHT** for the control treatment, and management of **acute nonlymphoblastic leukemias** and **chronic myclogenous leukemia.**

Mechanism of Action: Dwyer *et al.* (1986)*** duly observed that the **HHT** exerts its specific **cytotoxic effects** in the G_1 and G_2 phases of the prevailing cell cycle, which eventually synchronizes with the actual times of **intense protein synthesis.**

The protein synthesis really takes place in *two* distinct major stages, namely:

Stage-I: Initiation: In the course of 'initiation' *mRNA* which essentially possess the code for the '**new protein**', gets hooked on to the **ribosome.** In doing so the *first tRNA* subsequently gets attached to the *mRNA* thereby **commencing the initial amino acid building block process for the protein.**

Stage-II: Elongation: Elongation refers to the particular phenomenon whereby the ensuing *tRNA* securely get attached to the *mRNA.* Thus, the resulting bonds are duly formed amongst the amino acids to give rise to the production of the desired **polypeptide protein.** Here, the **HHT** plays a vital role in causing inhibition of the '**elongation step**'. This unique phenomenon perhaps comes into being by actually competitively inhibiting the particular enzyme, **peptidyl transferase,** that rightly catalyzes the formation of the polypeptide bond, and rather remotely from inhibiting the bonding of *tRNA* to *mRNA* [Zhou *et al.* (1995)]

The aforesaid hypothesis expatiating the probable mechanism of action amply ascertains that **HHT** may cause induction of both **apoptosis** and adequate differentiation of the neoplasm cells, thereby rendering it to be a **potent newer antineoplastic drug.**

FURTHER READING REFERENCES

1. Bajaj YPS (Ed.): **Biotechnology in Medicinal and Aromatic Plants,** Springer Verlag, New York, 1988.
2. Bensky D and Foster S: **Chinese Herbal Medicine, Materia Medica,** Eastland Press, Seattle WA, 1986.

---

* Ohnuma T and Holland JF: *J. Clin. Oncol.,* **73:** 604-606, 1985.
** Zhou DC *et al. Bull. Canc.,* **82:** 987-995, 1995.
*** Dwyer PJ *et al. J. Clin. On col.,* **4:** 1563-1568, 1986.

3. Bisset NG (Ed.): **Herbal Drugs and Phytopharmaceuticals,** Medpharm, Stuttgart (Germany), and CRC-Press, Boea Raton, FL., 1994.

4. Combs SP: *Res. Staff. Phys.,* **43:** 54-57, 1997.

5. Markovits J *et. al. Biochem. Pharm.*, **50:** 177-186, 1995.

6. Olin BR (Ed.): **Review of Natural Products: Facts and Comparisons,** Wolters Kluwer Co., St. Louis MO, 1995.

7. Peterson G,: *J. Nutr.,* **125:** 784 S-789 S, 1995.

15 Indian Traditional Herbal Drugs

- Introduction
- Indian Traditional Herbal Drugs
- Further Reading References

15.1 INTRODUCTION

A large number of natural plant species, specifically those used extensively in various **Indian Traditional Herbal Drugs,** have been, and are still being investigated for ascertaining their specific inherent vital pharmacological and microbiological activities. However, quite a few notable overviews intimately associated with certain specific areas of intensive and extensive research are adequately dealt with practically in most of the chapters in the present compilation.

In the recent past, stretched over to almost two decades the spectacular thrust generated enough interest, inquisitiveness, and incredible latest scientific approach to the search for **'new drugs'** of tremendous potential value and worth in comparison to the modern allopathic system of medicine.

Based upon the high quality, proper standardization procedures, ultra-modern packaging concepts and ideas, exhaustively informative drug-usage literatures, and above all the broad-spectrum methodical promotions both in India and abroad, the **Indian Traditional Herbal Drugs** have undoubtedly made their presence felt amongst the valued consumers. An overwhelmingly plausible and sound confidence amongst the consumers to make use of such available drugs as : OTC products, prescribed medications, long-term usage in chronic ailments, have really turned them into a widely accepted alternative saga of safer and effective medications not only in India but also across the entire globe.

The importance of **'medicinal plants'** right from the very dawn of civilization up to the last couple of decades have witnessed a tremendous cumulative, informative, and educative volume of researches carried out in the ever-expanding field of pharmaceutically significant naturally occurring plant products. Interestingly, the better understanding of the plants as a whole *vis-a-vis* their important chemical constituents have undoubtedly broadend and strengthened one's acceptability and overall confidence in their usages amongst the consumers. Hence, the prevailing biodynamism of the **'active principles'** strategically located in the plant kingdom would certainly provide the mankind with an eternal store-house of clinically beneficial **herbal drugs.**

15.2 INDIAN TRADITIONAL HERBAL DRUGS

The **Indian Traditional Herbal Drugs** have grown in length and breadth with the advent of most sophisticated means of separation *viz.*, **preparative HPLC, preparative HPTLC, GLC,** and the like, ultimately gave birth to a host of **'phytopharmaceuticals'**.

A few very important and highly promising **phytopharmaceuticals** have been duly described in the following sections, wherein each individual class of drugs essentially deals with their name, chemical structure, natural souce(s), and pharmacological activity.

15.2.1 Cardiovascular Drugs

The following **'herbal drugs'**, *viz.*, **escin, curcumin, digoxin,** and **forskolin,** shall now be treated individually in the sections that follows:

15.2.1.1 Escin [Syn: Aescin; Aescusan; Reparil;]

Escin usually obtained as a mixture of **saponins** occurring in the seeds of the **horse chestnut tree,** *Aesculus hippocastanum* L. (*Fam. Hippocastanaceae*)

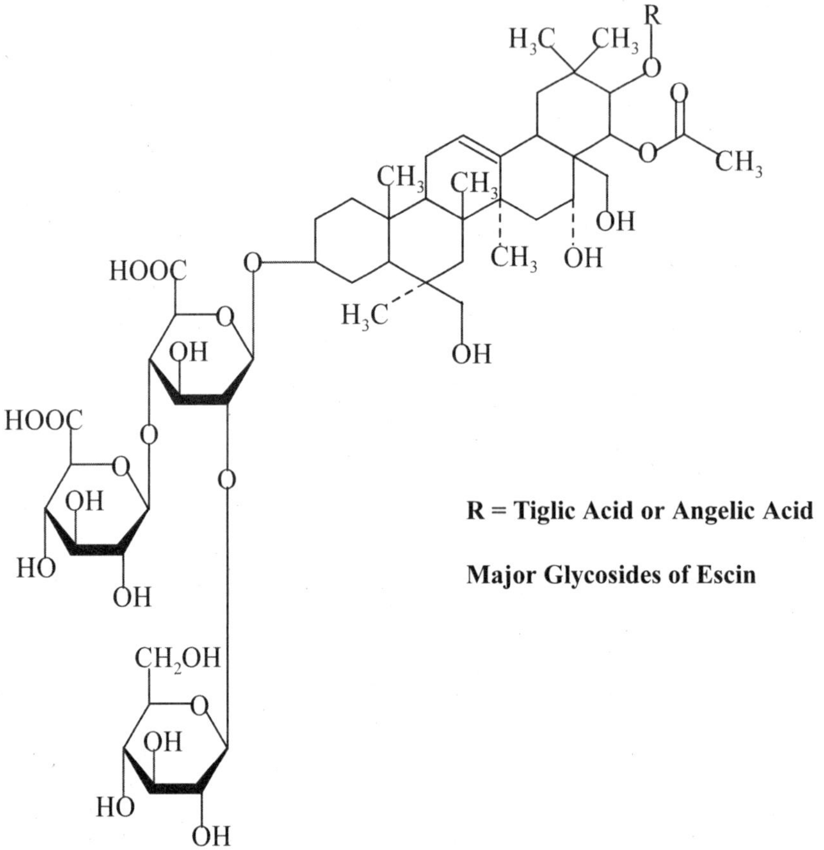

R = Tiglic Acid or Angelic Acid

Major Glycosides of Escin

Escin

Escin is commonly used in the treatment vascular disorders, anti-inflammatory agent.

15.2.1.2 Curcumin[Syn: Turmeric Yellow;]

Curcumin is the natural dye stuff obtained from the root of *Curcuma longa* L. [*Fam:* **Zingiberaceae**]

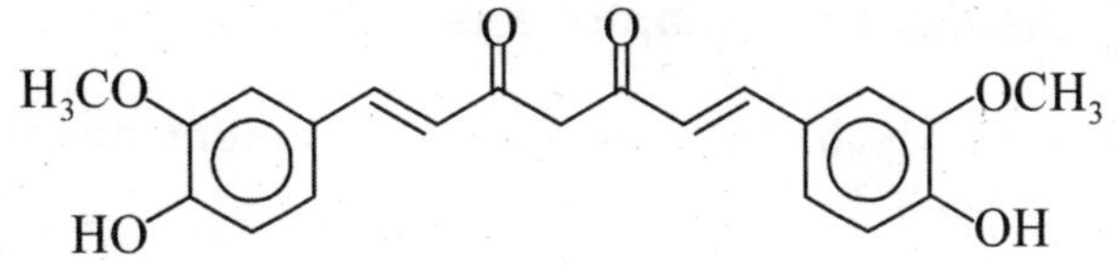

Curcumin

It exerts anti-inflammatory activity.

15.2.1.3 Digoxin [Syn: Digacin; Dilanctin; Endigox; Lanacordin; Lanicor; Lanoxin; Lanoxicaps; Lenoxin; Neo-Dioxanin; Rougoxin;]

Digoxin is the **secondary glycoside** obtained from *Digitalis landa* Ehrh., or *D. orientalis* Lam., (*Fam.* **Scrophulariaceae**). **Digoxin** serves as a potent cardiotonic.

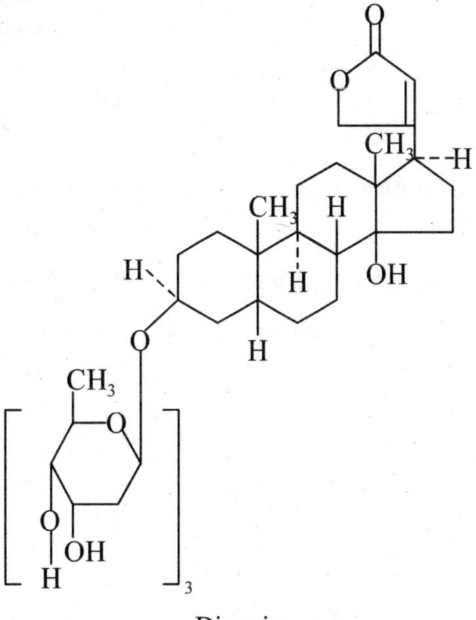

Digoxin

15.2.1.4 Forskolin [Syn: Colforsin; Boforsin;]

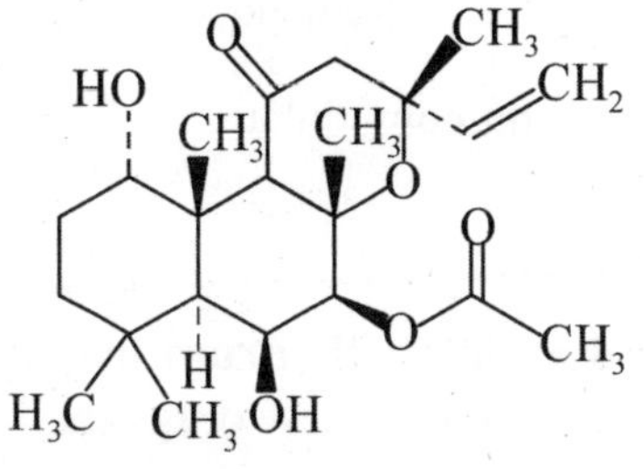

Forskolin [or Colforsin]

Colforsin is a diterpene isolated from *Coleus forskohlii,* Briq. (*Fam:* **Labiatae**).
Forskolin possesses both vasodilating and cardiostimulatory properties.

15.2.2 Immunomodulators and Adaptogens

Indian traditional herbal drugs which specifically serve as **immunomodulators and adaptogens**
are discussed as under:

15.2.2.1 Sitoindoside VII and VIII

The two **acylstearoyl glucosides,** namely (*a*) **Sitoindoside VII,** and (*b*) **Sitoindoside VIII** have
been duly isolated from the roots of *Withania somnifera* L., Dual., [*Syn: Physalis flexuosa*] belonging
to the natural order **Solanaceae.**

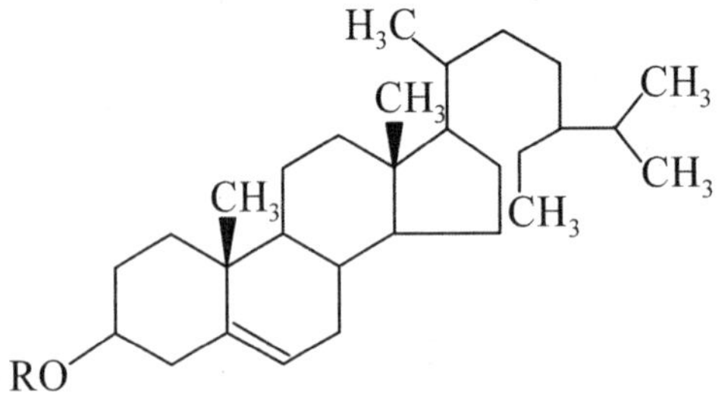

Sitoindoside VII:
R = Glu (6′-*O*-acyl stearoyl)
Sitoindoside VIII:
R = Glu (4′-*O*-acyl stearoyl)

These two naturally occurring **glucosides** are invariably used to relieve the **'stress'** in humans
i.e., they act as an **antistress drug.**

15.2.2.2 Syringin [Syn: Syringoside; Ligustrin; Lilacin; Methoxyconiferine;]

Syringin is obtained from the bark of *Syringa vulgaris* L., **(Lilac Bark),** and also from the **cambial
sap** of **spruce.**

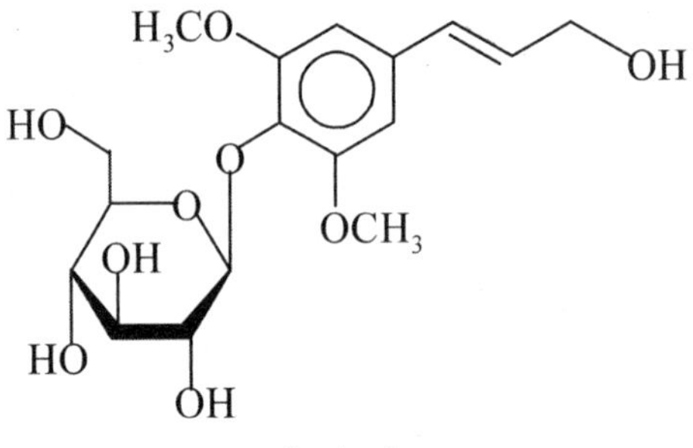

Syringin

Syringin exerts its action as an immunomodulator.

15.2.3 Antidiabetic Drugs

There are quite a few largely used **antidiabetic drugs** that are used in the **Indian Traditional
Herbal Medicines;** however, only a couple of these drugs shall be discussed briefly as under, such
as: **charantin.**

15.2.3.1 Charantin

Charantin is obtained from the fresh green fruits of the plant *Momordica charantia* L., (*Fam.* **Cucurbitaceae**).

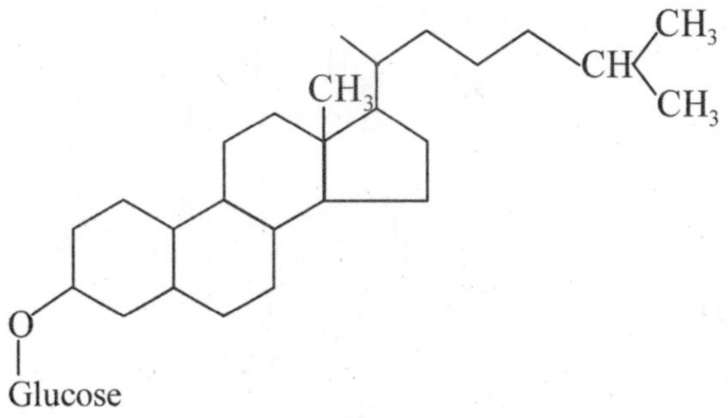

Charantin

It is used for lowering the level of **'blood sugar'** significantly; and, therefore, used profusely for the control and treatment of diabetes mellitus.

Importantly, there exists an appreciable scope for the interaction with various reported **oral hypoglycalmic drugs.*** A survey of literature reveals that there are quite many allied herbal drugs related to *M. Charantia* **(Karela)** that are employed profusely both by the **Vaids**** and **Hakims***** for the effective, control, and management of **diabetes melitus** very much within the **Asian community** in particular, and quite recently in the **European community** in general.

15.2.4 Antineoplastic Drugs

The **Indian Traditional Herbal Drugs** that are exclusively employed as **'antineoplastic drugs'** are:

15.2.4.1 Bryostatins

In fact, the **Bryostatins** belong to a family of seventeen **biologically active macrolides** *viz.*, Bryostatins 1 through 15, A and B. Thse **macrolides** are duly isolated from the **marine bryozoans,** *Bugula neritina* L., and other related organisms.

Bryostatins are usually employed as antineoplastic drugs, which specifically exert a partial agonist effect upon the protein **kinase C.**

---

* Aslam *et al. Lancet.,* **1:** 607, 1979.

** **Vaids:** The professional practitioners of Ayurvedic System of Medicine.

*** **Hakims:** The professional practitioners of Unani System of Medicine.

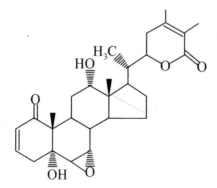

Bryostatin 1

Bryostatins are invariably used as immunomodulators.

15.2.4.2 Nicandrin B

Nicandrin B is obtained from the roots and seeds obtained from *Nicandra physaloides* L. Gaertn. (*Fam:* **Solanaceae**)*.

Nicandrin B

It is primarily responsible for showing *in vitro* cytotoxic activity.**

15.2.5 Antiviral Drugs

It is pertinent to mention here that the phenomenal success accomplished in the management of bacterial infection by the cautious usage of natural antibiotics (see Chapter 9) solely derived from microorganisms was not adequately matched to the same extent in the serious search for **'antiviral**

---

* Rastogi *et al.* **Indian Medicinal Plants,** Vol. 2., PID, New Delhi, 1991.
** *Planta Medica:* **43:** 389, 1981.

drugs'. Evidently, the various viral ailments still remain an important segment of medicine for which critical particular therapeutic treatments are lacking.

In the recent past, there are quite a few vital **'antiviral drugs'** have been identified, tested, and tried safely on humans which essentially belonged to the **Indian Traditional Herbal Medicine.**

Following are some of these **'drugs'** discussed briefly, such as:

15.2.5.1 (+)-Calanolide A

One may observe a very significant discovery in this field to date being the development of a series of **coumarins**—the **Calanolide A** and **Calonolide B** took place in a rather relatively smaller yield from the leaves and twigs of the forest tree *Colophyllum langigerum* (*Fam:* **Guttiferae**).

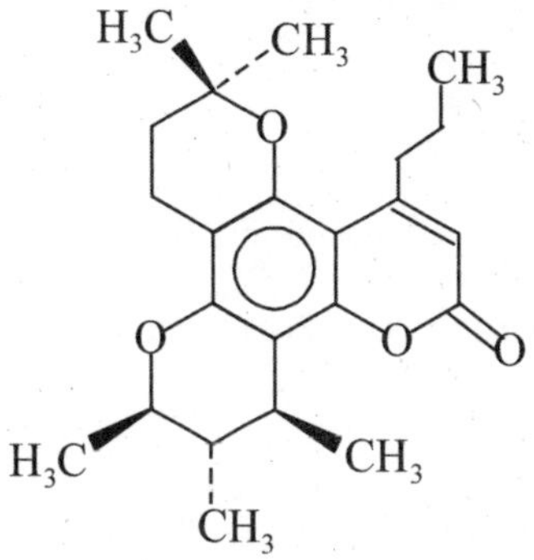

(+)-Calanolide A

(+)-**Calonolide A** possesses anti-HIV activity.

15.2.5.2 6-epi-Castanospermine

Bell and co-workers conducting research, at the London University, London, on certain specific and probable pesticidal non-protein amino acids, observed in the seeds of *Castanos permum austracle* (*Fam:* **Leguminoseae**) an altogether new **alkaloid** known as **6-*epi*-castanospermine,** which essentially has the **tetrahydroxyindolizidine moiety.**

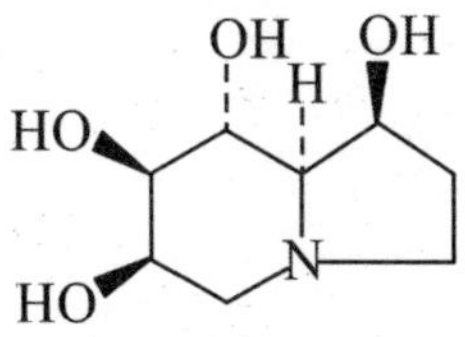

6-*epi*-Castanospermine

It exerts its action as a potent inhibitor of **HIV.** The probable mechanism of action of **6-*epi*-castanospermine** against **HIV** is due to its ability to inhibit **glucosidase I** and **II,** that eventually monitor the formation of **glycoproteins** in the **viral coat,** and thereby without the presence of the essential enveloped structure of the ensuing virus to be able to infect the healthy **WBCs.**

15.2.5.3 Salaspermic Acid

Salaspermic acid is a **pentacyclic terpenoid** obtained from the roots of *Tripterigium wilfordii* (*Fam:* **Celastraceae**).

Salaspermic Acid

It shows inhibition of **HIV reverse transcriptase** and **HIV replication** in the HG lymphocyte cells.

FURTHER READING REFERENCES

1. Evans WC: **Trease and Evans Pharmacognosy,** 15th edn., Saunders, New York, 2004.
2. Mathee G *et al. Planta Medica,* **65**(6): 493-506, 1999.
3. McKee TC *et al. J. Nat. Prod.,* **60**(5): 431-438, 1997.
4. Rastogi RP [Ed.]: **Compendium of Indian Medicinal Plants,** Vol. 1 to 3, CDRI-Lucknow & PID, New Delhi, 1993.
5. Vlientinck AJ *et al. Planta Medica,* **64**(2): 97-109, 1998.

Index

J

K

T